# Handbook of Motivation Science

# Handbook of
# Motivation Science

edited by
James Y. Shah
Wendi L. Gardner

THE GUILFORD PRESS
New York London

A Division of Guilford Publications, Inc.
72 Spring Street, New York, NY 10012
www.guilford.com



Printed in the United States of America

This book is printed on acid-free paper.

Last digit is print number: 9 8 7 6 5 4 3 2 1

**Library of Congress Cataloging-in-Publication Data**

Handbook of motivation science / edited by James Y. Shah, Wendi L. Gardner.
p. cm.
Includes bibliographical references and index.
ISBN-10: 1-59385-568-0 ISBN-13: 978-1-59385-568-0 (hardcover)
1. Motivation (Psychology) I. Shah, James Y. II. Gardner, Wendi L.
BF503.H363 2008
153.8—dc22

2007010671

# About the Editors

**James Y. Shah, PhD**, is Associate Professor of Psychology and Marketing at Duke University. He received his PhD from Columbia University. Dr. Shah's current research focuses on how goals affect people's perceptions, behavior, and subjective experiences, with a particular interest in exploring the different regulatory functions of goals, how personal goals are cognitively structured, and how the regulatory and structural nature of goals affect how one feels and how one acts. He is the author of several journal articles on these topics.

**Wendi L. Gardner, PhD**, is Associate Professor in the Department of Psychology at Northwestern University. She received her PhD from Ohio State University. Dr. Gardner's research involves two broad areas: the social aspects of the self and the unconscious, and rudimentary levels of evaluation and emotion. She has published many journal articles in these areas.

# Contributors

**Henk Aarts, PhD**, Department of Psychology, Utrecht University, Utrecht, The Netherlands

**Nadia Ahmad, PhD**, Department of Psychology, University of Kansas, Lawrence, Kansas

**Jamie Arndt, PhD**, Department of Psychological Sciences, University of Missouri, Columbia, Missouri

**Austin S. Baldwin, PhD**, Department of Psychology, University of Minnesota, Minneapolis, Minnesota

**John A. Bargh, PhD**, Department of Psychology, Yale University, New Haven, Connecticut

**Roger D. Bartels, BA**, Department of Psychology, University of Minnesota, Minneapolis, Minnesota

**C. Daniel Batson, PhD**, Department of Psychology, University of Kansas, Lawrence, Kansas

**Roy F. Baumeister, PhD**, Department of Psychology, Florida State University, Tallahassee, Florida

**Gary G. Berntson, PhD**, Departments of Psychology, Psychiatry, and Pediatrics, Ohio State University, Columbus, Ohio

**Jim Blascovich, PhD**, Department of Psychology, University of California, Santa Barbara, California

**John T. Cacioppo, PhD**, Department of Psychology, University of Chicago, Chicago, Illinois

**Charles S. Carver, PhD**, Department of Psychology, University of Miami, Coral Gables, Florida

**Tanya L. Chartrand, PhD,** Fuqua School of Business and Department of Psychology and Neuroscience, Duke University, Durham, North Carolina

**Clara Michelle Cheng, PhD,** Department of Psychology, American University, Washington, DC

**Woo Young Chun, PhD,** Department of Psychology, Hallym University, Chuncheon, Gangwon-do, Korea

**Cody B. Cox, MA,** Department of Psychology, Rice University, Houston, Texas

**Amy N. Dalton, HBSc,** Fuqua School of Business, Duke University, Durham, North Carolina

**Amanda B. Diekman, PhD,** Department of Psychology, Miami University, Oxford, Ohio

**Ap Dijksterhuis, PhD,** Department of Psychology, Radboud University, Nijmegen, The Netherlands

**Giel Dik, MS,** Department of Psychology, Utrecht University, Utrecht, The Netherlands

**Amanda M. Durik, PhD,** Department of Psychology, Northern Illinois University, DeKalb, Illinois

**Carol S. Dweck, PhD,** Department of Psychology, Stanford University, Stanford, California

**Alice H. Eagly, PhD,** Department of Psychology, Northwestern University, Evanston, Illinois

**Andrew J. Elliot, PhD,** Department of Clinical and Social Psychology, University of Rochester, Rochester, New York

**Melissa J. Ferguson, PhD,** Department of Psychology, Cornell University, Ithaca, New York

**Eli J. Finkel, PhD,** Department of Psychology, Northwestern University, Evanston, Illinois

**Ayelet Fishbach, PhD,** Graduate School of Business, University of Chicago, Chicago, Illinois

**Susan T. Fiske, PhD,** Department of Psychology, Princeton University, Princeton, New Jersey

**Jennifer A. Fredricks, PhD,** Department of Human Development, Connecticut College, New London, Connecticut

**James W. Fryer, MA,** Department of Clinical and Social Psychology, University of Rochester, Rochester, New York

**Shelly L. Gable, PhD,** Department of Psychology, University of California, Santa Barbara, California

**Peter M. Gollwitzer, PhD,** Department of Psychology, New York University, New York, New York, and Department of Psychology, University of Konstanz, Konstanz, Germany

**Heidi Grant, PhD,** Department of Psychology, Lehigh University, Bethlehem, Pennsylvania

**Jeff Greenberg, PhD,** Department of Psychology, University of Arizona, Tucson, Arizona

**Judith M. Harackiewicz, PhD,** Department of Psychology, University of Wisconsin, Madison, Wisconsin

**Cindy Harmon-Jones, BS,** Department of Psychology, Texas A&M University, College Station, Texas

**Eddie Harmon-Jones, PhD,** Department of Psychology, Texas A&M University, College Station, Texas

**Ran Hassin, PhD,** Department of Psychology, Hebrew University of Jerusalem, Jerusalem, Israel

**Andrew W. Hertel, BA,** Department of Psychology, University of Minnesota, Minneapolis, Minnesota

**E. Tory Higgins, PhD,** Department of Psychology, Columbia University, New York, New York

**Alexander Jaudas, DplPsych,** Department of Social Psychology, University of Konstanz, Konstanz, Germany

**John T. Jost, PhD,** Department of Psychology, New York University, New York, New York

**Laura A. King, PhD,** Department of Psychological Sciences, University of Missouri, Columbia, Missouri

**Shinobu Kitayama, PhD,** Department of Psychology, University of Michigan, Ann Arbor, Michigan

**Sander L. Koole, PhD,** Department of Social Psychology, Vrije Universiteit, Amsterdam, The Netherlands

**Arie W. Kruglanski, PhD,** Department of Psychology, University of Maryland, College Park, Maryland

**Julius Kuhl, DrPhil,** Department of Psychology, University of Osnabrück, Osnabrück, Germany

**Mark R. Leary, PhD,** Department of Psychology and Neuroscience, Duke University, Durham, North Carolina

**Angela Y. Lee, PhD,** Department of Marketing, Kellogg School of Management, Northwestern University, Evanston, Illinois

**Lisa Linnenbrink-Garcia, PhD,** Department of Psychology and Neuroscience, Duke University, Durham, North Carolina

**Ido Liviatan, MA,** Department of Psychology, New York University, New York, New York

**Penelope Lockwood, PhD,** Department of Psychology, University of Toronto, Toronto, Ontario, Canada

**Anesu N. Mandisodza, MA,** Department of Psychology, New York University, New York, New York

**Mario Mikulincer, PhD,** School of Psychology, Interdisciplinary Center, Herzlyia, Israel

**Daniel C. Molden, PhD,** Department of Psychology, Northwestern University, Evanston, Illinois

**Beth Morling, PhD,** Department of Psychology, University of Delaware, Newark, Delaware

**Sandra L. Murray, PhD,** Department of Psychology, University at Buffalo, State University of New York, Buffalo, New York

**Jaime L. Napier, MA,** Department of Psychology, New York University, New York, New York

**Elizabeth J. Parks-Stamm, MA,** Department of Psychology, New York University, New York, New York

**Janina Pietrzak, PhD,** Department of Psychology, Warsaw University, Warsaw, Poland

**Rebecca T. Pinkus, MA,** Department of Psychology, University of Toronto, Toronto, Ontario, Canada

**Eva M. Pomerantz, PhD,** Department of Psychology, University of Illinois at Urbana–Champaign, Champaign, Illinois

**Adam A. Powell, PhD,** Center for Chronic Disease Outcomes Research, Minneapolis Veterans Affairs Medical Center, Minneapolis, Minnesota

**Alexander J. Rothman, PhD,** Department of Psychology, University of Minnesota, Minneapolis, Minnesota

**Caryl E. Rusbult, PhD**, Department of Social Psychology, Vrije Universiteit, Amsterdam, The Netherlands

**Michael F. Scheier, PhD**, Department of Psychology, Carnegie Mellon University, Pittsburgh, Pennsylvania

**Michèle M. Schlehofer, PhD**, Department of Psychology, Claremont Graduate University, Claremont, California

**Abigail A. Scholer, MA**, Department of Psychology, Columbia University, New York, New York

**Corwin Senko, PhD**, Department of Applied Psychology, University of Zurich, Zurich, Switzerland

**James Y. Shah, PhD**, Department of Psychology and Neuroscience, Duke University, Durham, North Carolina

**Phillip R. Shaver, PhD**, Department of Psychology, University of California, Davis, California

**Paschal Sheeran, PhD**, Department of Psychology, University of Sheffield, Sheffield, United Kingdom

**Kennon M. Sheldon, PhD**, Department of Psychology, University of Missouri, Columbia, Missouri

**David K. Sherman, PhD**, Department of Psychology, University of California, Santa Barbara, California

**Serena Shim, PhD**, Department of Educational Psychology, Northern Arizona University, Flagstaff, Arizona

**Sheldon Solomon, PhD**, Department of Psychology, Skidmore College, Saratoga Springs, New York

**E. L. Stocks, PhD**, Department of Psychology, University of Texas, Tyler, Texas

**Amy Strachman, PhD**, Department of Psychology, University of California, Los Angeles, California

**Steven J. Stroessner, PhD**, Department of Psychology, Barnard College, New York, New York

**Shelley E. Taylor, PhD**, Department of Psychology, University of California, Los Angeles, California

**Suzanne C. Thompson, PhD**, Department of Psychology, Pomona College, Claremont, California, and Department of Psychology, Claremont Graduate University, Claremont, California

**Yaacov Trope, PhD**, Department of Psychology, New York University, New York, New York

**Jean M. Twenge, PhD**, Department of Psychology, San Diego State University, San Diego, California

**Kathleen D. Vohs, PhD**, Department of Marketing, Carlson School of Management, University of Minnesota, Minneapolis, Minnesota

# Preface

The informed reader of this volume may wonder how motivation science differs from the traditional focus on motivation that has long been central to social psychology. Although the popularity of motivational approaches waned with the start of the cognitive revolution, it has reemerged in earnest over the last two decades as advances in understanding how we construe ourselves and our social world have led the field to reexamine why we do so.

But this reemergence is far more than a simple revisiting of old ideas. Indeed, in the two decades since the *Handbook of Motivation and Cognition* (Sorrentino & Higgins, 1986) so effectively highlighted the intricate and socially significant interrelation of motivation and cognition, the field has not only embraced this integrative approach to motivation but extended it toward other formerly disparate areas of psychology. This has allowed the field to more thoroughly consider the often complex manner in which motivation may interact with social, developmental, and emotional processes, as well as with personality more generally, and explore how these links may be represented and constrained neurologically, physiologically, and even culturally. Such compelling and innovative directions are well represented in this volume.

## THREE R's OF MOTIVATION SCIENCE: RELATIVITY, REGULATION, AND REACTION

In addition to its outward expansion toward other areas of psychology and different levels of analysis, motivational approaches within social psychology have increasingly influenced and inspired each other. This mutual influence has begun to encourage inward consolidation around the common assumptions, themes, and questions that may ultimately come to define this emerging science. Many of these fundamental issues are on vivid display in this volume, but three particularly central themes collectively could be referred to as the three R's of motivation science: motivational relativity, motivational regulation, and motivational reactivity.

## MOTIVATIONAL RELATIVITY

Reminiscent of Einstein, motivation science is focused on the relativity of motivation in both its temporal and structural sense. How do our various needs, for instance, compare and contrast with each other? Moving away from early motivational hierarchies (e.g., Maslow, 1955) that emphasized the "objective" or normative priority and organization of needs, many current motivational approaches assume a subjective relativism in both the priority and mental organization of needs and motives. What needs are most central, then, and how they relate to each other, are thought to be products not only of the inherent qualities of the needs themselves but also of the individuals' distinct history of pursuing them, as well as the constraints and affordances they encounter in the moment and over their lifetime.

An emphasis on motivational relativity also extends to considering how different needs and motives differ with respect to their behavioral and social implications. As compellingly demonstrated in many of the current chapters, qualitative differences in the motives or needs underlying achievement behavior, social interaction, or close relationships can significantly impact the cognitions, behaviors, and emotions involved. Beyond comparing and contrasting needs and motives, an emphasis on relativity has also led motivation scientists to consider how the priority and structure of needs goals and means change over time. A consideration of temporal relativity allows researchers and theorists to begin to understand both the recursive and evolving nature of needs and motives. Although needs may come with some consistency, our pursuit of them may evolve over time. Given such dynamics, how can they be maintained and when should they be abandoned? The present chapters not only offer important insights into these fundamental questions but begin to suggest how both senses of motivational relativity are themselves intertwined. How we compare and contrast our needs in the moment, for instance, surely depends on how we have done so in the past and on the success or failure we have recently encountered.

Starting with Susan T. Fiske's historical overview of the field and its emphasis on core motivations in Part I, Part II of this handbook is devoted to addressing the fundamental issues and questions of relativity. The chapters in the first section of Part II focus on specific, and fundamental, psychological motives core to our definition of self, such as the need for esteem, security, consistency, and achievement. This grouping should familiarize the reader with existing research and theory surrounding a classic set of psychological motives consistently portrayed as central to human functioning and highlight how these motives and needs compare and contrast. The second section of Part II outlines motivational systems that may be applied generally across the varied forms of motivations and provide the structure that arises from, and directs, motivational relativity. These chapters describe, in one form or another, systems that arise to address our fundamental needs and fundamentally alter and constrain the process and experience of motivational states as well as some cognitive and biological "hardware" within which these systems are embodied.

## MOTIVATIONAL REGULATION

An equally important emphasis in motivation science is on the dynamic and often complex process by which our general needs and desires are translated into concrete goals, plans, behaviors, and experiences, with obvious and significant implications for how we see ourselves and others and how we interact with the world around us. Many of the chapters in the present volume lend new insights into traditional regulatory mechanisms or identify new ones. Moreover, the regulation of motivation provides another basis for understanding how individuals, groups, and cultures may differ in comparison to each other and how they may evolve over time.

## THE RECURSIVITY, RESOURCES, AND RESOLUTIONS OF REGULATION

The focus on regulation within motivation science has recently expanded to such a degree as to warrant its own handbook and set of guiding principles. Indeed, in the spirit of the present analysis, motivation regulation may warrant its own three R's, each well represented in this volume. For one, motivation regulation is recursive: It involves a dynamic process of feedback and adjustment as one progresses toward fulfilling a need through goal attainment. How individuals differ in seeking and reacting to feedback has long been a central theme in theories of achievement behavior and optimism and may play an important role in how goals are maintained over time and how effectively they are managed collectively.

There has also been considerable recent emphasis on the personal, situational, and social resources required for effective motivation regulation. Such an emphasis has led researchers to consider not only the nature and potential limits of these resources (as reflected, for instance, in our capacity for self-control, our experience and abilities, the helpfulness or hindrances of others, or the affordances in our environment) but also our ability to perceive and effectively regulate these motivational assets, especially when they are limited and potentially exhausted. And like relativity, a focus on motivational resources has led to a consideration not only of how they may constrain or modify the individual and sometimes social fulfillment of needs in the moment, but also of how such influence may vary over time as resources wax and wane. Finally, there has been a long-standing, if at times implicitly defined, focus on the resolutions required for effective motivation regulation. Such resolutions are required not only between the often disparate needs we have for ourselves but also between the conflicts that may arise between our own needs and the needs of others. Moreover, even after resolving conflicts regarding *what* need or motive to address, individuals still must resolve potential conflicts in *how* best to address the need. To what degree, for instance, should needs be addressed optimally versus efficiently? To what degree should the experience be pleasant or painful? To what degree should we be persistent in pursuing a need versus being pragmatic in our pursuit? The present contributions emphasize or assume many such conflicts and thus provide a compelling basis for defining optimal motivation regulation.

The first section in Part III defines the process and consequences of goal pursuit. The chapters within this section cover the range of systems and strategies used to initiate, sustain, and accomplish goals, such as implicit instigators and the "fit" between motive and environment. The manner in which goal pursuits are maintained over time and defended from temptations, and ultimately abandoned, if necessary, are also explored. Of course, the process and progress of goal pursuit is not invariant across individuals and situations. The second section of Part III introduces some of the important individual, cultural, and developmental moderators of motivational processes and points to important future directions. In combination, the chapters constituting this section offer the reader a fuller picture of the goal pursuit process from initial activation to ultimate satiation, while highlighting how this process may vary as a function of the individual and situation.

## MOTIVATIONAL REACTIVITY

The final part of the handbook addresses a third central theme of this emerging science: the personal and interpersonal reactions to our needs and pursuits. To what extent can motivational approaches help explain our varied and complex emotional experiences and our specific psychological vulnerabilities? How might these approaches lend insight into our complex social reactions, as seen, for instance, in the range of our emotional, cognitive, and behavioral responses to other groups, and their often prejudicial behavior? How might motivational distinctions and motivational systems help explain the dynamics of interpersonal relationships and general social conflict? In organizing these varied reactions, the first section of Part IV looks "inward" in focusing on the implications of motivational processes for well-being and optimal functioning, whereas the second section looks "outward" in focusing on the broader social and societal consequences. The chapters in Part IV address not only the psychological implications of motivational process but also the physical; not only the interpersonal implications but also the even broader societal consequences.

The breadth and organization of this volume is designed in the hope of providing the reader with both a systematic overview of the field and a sense of the emerging themes that promise not only to provide a consolidation of knowledge, but also to suggest compelling new directions and perhaps a broader potential for linking social psychology with traditionally disparate areas of research and levels of analysis. This, of course, is only a beginning, and many important details and directions still need to be established. But as is evident in the present chapters, if the framework for this emerging field is not yet complete, the craftsmanship, creativity, and cooperation of its builders are already on display.

I conclude by acknowledging the effort and dedication of all the contributors, whose hard work is readily on display here. Let me also offer a specific note of gratitude and acknowledgment to Seymour Weingarten and Carolyn Graham of The Guilford Press for their truly extraordinary work in bringing this ambitious collection together. Their efforts, guidance, and administration in all facets of bringing this lengthy process to press cannot be overstated. Their invaluable contributions to this project certainly went well beyond even the typically important contributions of expert and supportive publishers. This volume would not have come together without them, and for this I will always be grateful.

James Y. Shah, PhD

## REFERENCES

Maslow, A. (1955). Deficiency motivation and growth motivation. In M. R. Jones (Ed.), *Nebraska Symposium on Motivation* (pp. 1–30). Lincoln: University of Nebraska Press.

Sorrentino, R. M., & Higgins, E. T. (Eds.). (1986). *Handbook of motivation and cognition: Vol. 1. Foundations of social behavior.* New York: Guilford Press.

# Contents

PART I

# A Historical Perspective

Chapter 1

# Core Social Motivations

## VIEWS FROM THE COUCH, CONSCIOUSNESS, CLASSROOM, COMPUTERS, AND COLLECTIVES

**Susan T. Fiske**

Motivation has a storied past in psychological science. Not only does motivation science inherit many legends (both great figures and great myths), but the field has told many narratives about motivation over time (for reviews, see, e.g., Higgins & Pittman, in press; Pittman, 1998; Weiner, 1985). The current story combines clinical, personality, experimental, and social psychology landmarks to illustrate the background of this handbook. Ancestors to the current volume have each been informed by their own preferred data on the person, providing views from the couch, consciousness, classroom, computer, and collectives. Each view—perhaps reflecting its source—has tended to emphasize certain forms of motives and certain methods of analysis, in keeping with its own perspective.

Contemporary motivation scientists have learned some lessons from their forebears, both following some of their leads and avoiding some of their traps. This chapter is organized around the most fruitful leads, arguing that each approach has characteristically emphasized certain core social motives. Personality and social psychologists have emphasized similar motives over the last 100 years, leading to a consensual list of five (plus or minus) that serves as a heuristic to organize our theories and a framework to understand social surviving and thriving (Fiske, 2003, 2004; Stevens & Fiske, 1995). But this consensus on core motives has emerged gradually over the last century, so the end of the chapter revisits them not only as a framework, but as a culmination of the field's enterprise.

Just as contemporary motivation scientists have followed the leads of our forebears, so also have we avoided many of the old traps. Ironically, chief among them is the listing of motives. The field began by listing instincts (McDougall, 1908), drives (Freud, 1920/

1955), needs (Maslow, 1943), and fundamental activities (F. H. Allport, 1924), to name a few. But it was fruitless to enumerate a motivation unique to each behavior, because that level of detail was both too specific (e.g., can we really speak of a motive to read?) and inaccurate (the same behavior can serve different motives). Besides, it was never clear what the nature of proof should be for any given list. Most of the chapters in this volume avoid listing motives. In organizing this historical chapter around five core motives, I am well aware that others would carve the motives differently, but some backing for the current approach comes from the regularity with which these five emerge. This also makes them a useful organizing tool. And they also cohere theoretically, as the final section argues.

Another trap avoided by current motivation science is the term *instinct*, denoting an innate, unlearned propensity. Instincts take insufficient account of socialization processes. Contemporary motivation scientists also avoid *trait* as a primary explanatory concept (though personality psychology per se seems to have settled on the Big Five; e.g., D. W. Fiske, 1949; Ozer & Benet-Martínez, 2006; Wiggins & Trapnell, 1997). Traits, as Gordon Allport noted (according to Pervin, 1993), are insufficiently dynamic and overly general. Traits predict behavior, but only in complex interplay with situations (Caspi, Roberts, & Shiner, 2005; Lewin, 1936; Mischel, 1968; Mischel & Shoda, 1998). Motivation combines both to operate at a manageable level of analysis, and its agents—goals—are even more specific. For our purposes, a *motive* is a *predisposition to behave in a directed fashion*. Motives act as the motor for action, energizing purposive behavior that serves a function for the individual. Motives operate via specific goals in specific situations.

Related concepts abound in psychology. Boring's (1950, pp. 714–715) *A History of Experimental Psychology* lists 17 terms for the "dynamic principle" that determines a psychological event, in chronological order of appearance in the field: *attention, expectation, preparation, predisposition, Einstellung* (set), *Aufgabe* (instruction), *predetermin[ation], determining tendency, Anlage* (attitude), *instinct, drive, incentive, purpose*, and *need*. Even with all those terms, he never arrived at *motives*. Modern cognates include *tasks, goals, concerns, projects*, and *strivings* (Emmons, 1997). Each new term strives to shed the theoretical baggage of the preceding terms, but all get at the same idea of a mental construct energizing action. That has been the business of psychological science since its inception, with differing delineations of *mental*, as we shall see.

The following sections focus in turn on views ultimately derived from the favored source of data: the psychoanalytic couch (emphasizing narcissistic self-enhancement), accessible consciousness (emphasizing functional trust), the classroom (emphasizing competent control), cognition in human computers (emphasizing informed understanding), and contemporary collectives (emphasizing social belonging). Each section works chronologically through exemplars of its perspective, from early forebears to illustrative chapters in the current collection. The sequence of motives itself bears some relation to their sequence of priority in psychology, but the fit is imprecise, because intellectual history is not tidy.

## ENHANCING SELF: VIEWS FROM THE COUCH

"The great motivational theory of the eighteenth century was hedonism, and it lasted well over into the nineteenth" (Boring, 1950, p. 703; cf. G. W. Allport, 1954b). Hedonism centers around the utilitarian motive to gain pleasure and happiness for the self (Bentham, 1779/1948). The socialized adult version of hedonism associates pleasure, furthermore, with the communal good and with delayed gratification. Ultimately, hedonism gives rise to learning theory's principles of association and law of effect (pleasure leads to repetition of actions that preceded it). Hedonism has had many heirs in scientific psychology—notably Freud, McDougall, Maslow, Murray, and to-be-mentioned contemporary authors.

### Sigmund Freud

Initially, Freud picked up hedonism as the pleasure principle—as in the wish fulfillment functions of dreams (Freud, 1900/1953) and as in the psychopathology of everyday life (e.g., slips of the tongue; Freud, 1901/1951). His mid-career idea of self-preservation, with energy directed inward (the primitive and abnormal form being narcissism), placed the self's own enhancement (enjoying pleasant experiences) at the dynamic center of force and energy. At this point in his career, Freud united normal and abnormal behavior under narcissism (self-love or autoeroticism; Freud, 1914/1953) and mutually opposing motivations, the life and death *instincts* (Freud, 1920/1955). The life instinct strives for pleasure and happiness, creating tension if any needs are unfilled, and resting content when fulfilled. The ultimate state of homeostatic peace is the death instinct, so it too is traceable ultimately to the pleasure principle, oddly enough.

Freud's opus is complex, and it evolved considerably over his lifetime; for present purposes, what matters is his legacy as interpreted by subsequent generations of social and personality psychologists. Freud saw psychic energy as a closed hydraulic system, comparable to the then-modern steam engine as a metaphor: Suppression of psychic energy in one location causes it to emerge elsewhere. This essentially laid the groundwork for drive reduction theories, in which a need remains active, creating pressure to meet it, until it is fulfilled. The reduction in the drive itself is rewarding: hence the class of drive reduction theories.

### William McDougall

The influence of Freud on social psychology was anticipated by one of the field's first two textbooks, McDougall (1908)'s *Introduction to Social Psychology.* He believed that all human behavior (including social interaction) results from inherited *instincts*, as modified by experience. Both Freud and McDougall were influenced by Darwin, but McDougall took the instinct idea to extremes. He listed every instinct imaginable: flight, repulsion, curiosity, pugnacity, parenting, self-abasement, self-assertion, reproduction, construction, gregariousness, acquisition, and more. The problems were that anyone can list instincts, and that the criteria for favoring one list over another have always appeared arbitrary.

Most relevant here, McDougall paired each instinct with a *sentiment* (emotion, value); like Freud, he also claimed that the master sentiment is self-regard. However, for him, self-regard serves the function of unifying the self, creating "character" (McAdams, 1997; McDougall, 1908). Unlike Freud, McDougall believed mainly in conscious effort, volition, and freedom, so he did not advocate the idea of unconscious motives.

However, McDougall, also possibly as influenced by Freud (Boring, 1950, p. 718), did believe in brain energy that is waiting to be discharged. This fits the Freudian drive reduction idea. McDougall believed that organisms always strive toward a goal, a tenet of purposive psychology. Purposive activity, as apart from reflexive activity, he argued, is marked by seven criteria (McDougall, 1923; see also Boring, 1950, pp. 466–467): spontaneity, persistence, variation in direction, ending upon effecting a changed situation, preparation for new situations, improved effectiveness over trials, and totality of the reaction. Purposive activity (i.e., motivated actions) expresses instincts and sentiments, the primary one being self-enhancement.

Admittedly, unlike other theorists in this section, McDougall was not gathering data "from the couch," but he acknowledged the then-current convergence between the complexes of neurotic patients and mental structures of the normal mind (McDougall, 1919, preface to 14th ed. of *Introduction to Social Psychology*). In addition to instincts, his analysis revolved around emotions and sentiments, especially salient in the clinical perspective.

### Abraham Maslow

The influence of Freud on personality psychology is exemplified by Maslow (1943, 1967), though he was also influenced by Gestalt approaches (Weiner, 1985; see "Gestalt Approaches," below) and by functional approaches (see "Trusting Positive Functions," below). He fits the Freudian heritage because he is most famous for his hierarchy of *needs.* Maslow ranked (1) physiological needs (e.g., hunger, sex, shelter) as most fundamental; next came a progression of psychological needs—(2) safety (e.g., security, balance, calm), (3) love (e.g., togetherness, growth together), and (4) esteem (e.g., confidence, mastery, self-regard); and the list culminated in (5) self-actualization (e.g., curiosity, creativity, avocation). All needs are innate, like instincts, and the higher needs cannot be pursued until the lower ones have been met. The higher ones appear later in evolutionary and individual development, are more complex and contingent, but also contribute to surviving and thriving. Maslow viewed the lower ones as deficit-oriented, like Freud, but he viewed the higher ones as "being-oriented," psychological, and associated with positive tensions (Maslow, 1967).

Maslow's privileging of self-actualization as the ultimate need, uniquely human, fits other views from the couch. First, self-actualization echoes Freud's emphasis on the fully functioning human as sublimating primitive narcissism into love and work. Second, self-actualization parallels McDougall's focus on self-regard as building a fully developed, unified character. All three approaches share a sense of primitive, selfish motives giving way to more sophisticated, self-developing motives. All levels relate to the self (as opposed to the collective) and relate to enhancing or improving one's internal experience (as opposed to, say, controlling environmental contingencies or understanding social norms).

### Henry Murray

Murray's (1938) eclectic view of motivation leaps out from his long list of *needs*, roughly clustering into those related to physiology, objects, obtaining power, exerting power, aggression, affiliation, and cognition. Too numerous to mention here, they mostly revolve around self-enhancement. Forced to economize, he concluded that various "considerations commit us to one variety of the now almost abandoned theory of psychological hedonism" (p. 166): pursuit of pleasure, happiness, or well-being. Murray's mentor was Freud's disciple Carl Jung, and he dedicated his book to Freud and McDougall. Certainly his need-listing propensity fits their hedonistic approaches.

But Murray also admitted debts to Lewin (see below), with whom he shared an expectancy–value theory, composed of personal needs interacting with environmental *press*. In this sense, his approach is less biologically driven. He anticipated control-oriented achievement theories (to be described), but his own focus began with self-enhancement.

### Modern Self-Enhancement Theories

Although modern motivation science rarely cites Freud, McDougall, Maslow, or Murray, the idea that people are basically self-serving surfaces in a number of contemporary views (Fiske, 2004; Robins & John, 1997). This operates at all levels, from within individuals to between them to group phenomena.

Within the individual, positive illusions about the superiority of the self (Taylor & Brown, 1988; Taylor & Sherman, Chapter 4, this volume) entail unreasonable optimism and positivity about the self. Motivated reasoning protects self-esteem (Kunda, 1990). Self-affirmation protects self-worth from threats by bolstering another area of self-regard (Steele, 1988). Terror management protects people against thoughts of their own mortality by making salient the enduring values that will outlive them (Greenberg, Solomon, & Arndt, Chapter 8, this volume; Pyszczynski, Greenberg, & Solomon, 1997). Self-discrepancy threatens positive self-feelings, and this threat launches self-regulation (Higgins, 1987; Higgins, Chapter 23, this volume; Molden, Lee, & Higgins, Chapter 11, this volume). The totalitarian ego maintains self-esteem at the cost of accuracy (Greenwald, 1980).

Between individuals, people compare themselves to others partly in the service of enhancing self-regard (Lockwood & Pinkus, Chapter 16, this volume). People are attracted to those who are physically attractive and to those who are similar to self partly because they enhance self-esteem (Fiske, 2004). People hope to be positively evaluated by others (Goodwin, Fiske, Rosen, & Rosenthal, 2002; Stevens & Fiske, 2000). Within a relationship, self-evaluation maintenance requires balancing relationship closeness, own identity, and relative achievement (Tesser, 1988).

Within groups, optimal distinctiveness balances the need to be an individual with the need for group identity, all in the service of positive self-esteem (Brewer, 1991). Social identity operates to maintain a positive view of one's group and oneself as a member of it (Tajfel, 1981). People sometimes stereotype other groups to maintain self-esteem (Fein & Spencer, 1997), and sometimes control prejudice to maintain an unprejudiced self-view (Devine & Monteith, 1999).

### Self-Enhancement: Summary

Starting with analyses of neurotic people and everyday abnormalities, motivational scientists informed by the psychoanalytic couch have emphasized self-enhancement as a prime motivator. Modern advocates of self-enhancement's motivational centrality find that it usefully explains a range of normal personal and social behavior.

## TRUSTING POSITIVE FUNCTIONS: VIEWS FROM CONSCIOUSNESS

Humanists believe in the positive potential of all humans, the basic functionality of the motivational system, and the utility of conscious reports. Most people behave like lay humanists much of the time. People's baseline assumption in the good of at least ingroup others is well established (Fiske, 2004). In motivation scientists, this optimistic functional perspective emerged partly in sympathy with a Jamesian pragmatic view of consciousness, and partly in reaction against the Freudian unconscious with its lurking selfish, aggressive, sexual, and unclean impulses. Early proponents included not only William James but also Gordon Allport, both of whom were oriented toward scientific psychology. Erik Erikson and Carl Rogers were oriented toward clinical settings, but all four emphasized optimism about the functionality of human consciousness, laying the groundwork for trust as a core motive. Modern motivation scientists have eschewed the humanist label because of its vague and unempirical orientation, but the endorsement of functional, conscious motives—communicating an optimistic trust in human nature—remains alive and well.

### William James

The conscious thinker formed the center for James's *The Principles of Psychology* (1890). James, the founding philosopher of psychology, contributed profoundly to the psychology of consciousness, based substantially on his "remarkable introspective talent" (Miller, 1983, p. xxi). Although James believed in each person's self-regard, he emphasized far more the self as having a variety of conscious aspects, each self-aspect "superficial, transient, taken up or dropped at will" (1890, p. 307). James's pragmatism found that the essence of things—even the self—lies in their properties relevant to the perceiver's current interests in the moment. His faith in consciousness focused famously on the will and people's ability to enact their intentions by conscious choice and focused attention. While James admitted that "the mind is active even when the person afterwards ignores the fact," as in sleep (p. 199), he also viewed the apparently slumbering mind as making judgments. Even though he admitted the possibility of delusion, he saw introspection as a source of empirical observation. Thoughts take personal form, in constant flux but sensibly continuous, cognizing the external world by choosing a constantly evolving focus. This then is subjective life, ultimately serving pragmatic functions.

James's *motivations* depend almost entirely on the conscious will, which operates by choice and attentional focus (Fiske, 1989). His ideomotor processes describe the *idea* of the action as implementing the action, as in his apt example of getting out of bed on a chilly morning by imaging the self doing it. In this and in his whole psychology, James believed in human rationality and consciousness as its distinguishing feature. Although himself depressive and sickly, James believed that free will could overcome his difficulties (Boring, 1950; Miller, 1983). Ironically for one of the fathers of scientific psychology (the other being Wundt), James claimed, "I naturally hate experimental work . . . the duty that gets postponed" (quoted in Boring, 1950, p. 511). Nevertheless, James's pragmatism (functionalism) laid the groundwork for much of American can-do empirical psychology. His aphorism captures it well: "My thinking is first and last and always for my doing" (James, 1890, p. 960; see Fiske, 1992, 1993b).

### Gordon Allport

A later occupant of Harvard's Emerson Hall, which originally housed both philosophy and the emerging field of psychology, Gordon Allport supplied the personality side to functional consciousness that James lacked. Allport viewed the personality as consisting of *intentions* and *values* (as transcribed by Smith, 1993). Allport viewed motives as learned, unlike McDougall's innate instincts, and as largely conscious, unlike Freud's primitive motives (Allport, as transcribed by Smith, 1993; Elms, 1993; McAdams, 1997; Smith, 1993). The motives need not be conscious or voluntary, but his writing emphasized consciousness: He reacted strongly against Freud and argued with his colleague Henry Murray (Smith, 1993). He did not assume that the personality would be fixed by biology or early events. Instead, he promoted the *functional autonomy* of motives, meaning that they outlast the context in which they are acquired; motivation often operates independently of its historical origins in a life. His motivation consisted of the heavily cognitive ego, characterized with varied functions: knower, known, egoist, dominator, organizer, center of purpose, system, and personal interpreter of cultural norms. He believed in phenomenology (the conscious interpretation of the situation), along with individual, situational, cultural, and historical approaches.

Allport's idiographic orientation to unique personalities rejected narrow notions of motives as instincts and drives, because they did not account for individuality. He inevitably came across traits, but he found traits overly rigid and insufficiently dynamic, as noted (Pervin, 1993). In his own view, some traits have *motivational*, directive functions; other traits have *expressive*, stylistic functions. Motivational traits are the deeper wellsprings of conduct; expressive traits are variable expressions. But he believed in each individual personality as an integrated whole.

He was a humanist, in the sense of providing (1) an alternative to the prevailing, mechanistic stimulus–response psychology (to be noted); (2) an antidote to Freudian determinism; and (3) an alternative to Freud's emphases on human pathology (Pervin, 1993). More importantly, he was a functionalist: Allport believed that a fully functioning adult will show self-extension (incorporation of self into others, interests, ideas, work), self-objectification (self-insight, sense of humor), and a unifying philosophy of life (one's place in the scheme of things). He wanted to see human potential for democratic and humane behavior. Moreover, his view of human motives was optimistic: "Human nature seems, on the whole, to prefer the sight of kindness and friendliness to the sight of cruelty. . . . [Normal people] like to live in peace and friendship with their neighbors; they prefer to love and be loved" (Allport, 1954a, pp. ix–x). He was egalitarian (McAdams, 1997), as his classic work on *The Nature of Prejudice* (Allport, 1954a) shows. And he was eclectic, listing five motivational strands in his own history chapter in the first edition of the Lindzey *Handbook of Social Psychology* (Allport, 1954b); they overlap considerably with the current set (see the conclusion to this chapter), but for present purposes, the point is that he adhered strictly to none and saw all of them as functional in different ways.

### Related Precursors

The work of several theorists in clinical settings might fit the trusting, consciousness-oriented, functional views, but these theorists are excluded from detailed treatment here because they are only indirect clinical forebears of modern motivation science. For example, Erik Erikson (1950, 1959) directed attention toward developmental progression through stages of *life tasks* and their resolution, the first being trust in a caregiver. He shared humanist notions of positive ego qualities: trust, autonomy, initiative, industry, identity, intimacy, generativity, and integrity. But his legacy lies mostly outside social and personality psychology. Also related to functional trust, the Carl Rogers (1961, 1963) idea of unconditional positive regard emphasized humanistic concerns with people's resilient potential and their conscious assessments, though he focused most closely on clinical clients. Abraham Maslow could have been included here instead of earlier, but as Elms (1993) notes, his form of humanistic psychology never proceeded on solid scientific ground partly because he never took Allport's editorial advice. Also, his form of self-actualization concerned mostly personal benefits, not societal ones; and, like Freud, he focused on dysfunction, not functional approaches.

### Modern Trust Theories

Modern motivation science has avoided clinical associations, probably due to the menacing Freudian monolith. Because motivation science's focus is appropriately empirical, it avoids clinical evidence oriented toward case studies, such as that coming from Erikson, Rogers, and Maslow. And it certainly avoids Gordon Allport's idiographic approach, again because of the empirical requirement of large numbers.

Many readers may view basic trust as a doomed motive, gullible and naive—but in fact, considerable research, at levels from individual to group, indicates the adaptive value of a baseline trusting motive in social beings (Fiske, 2004).

At the individual level, the robust positivity bias in person perception shows that laypeople are basically trusting, and the researchers studying positivity understand that trust (with vigilance for aberrant negativity) is adaptive. Examples include my own (Fiske, 1980) concepts of relative weight in person perception, Kahneman and Tversky's (1979) prospect theory weighting gains and losses, Matlin and

Stang's (1978) Pollyanna hypothesis, Peeters and Czapinski's (1990) motivated vigilance, Sears's (1983) person positivity, Skowronski and Carlston's (1989) valence-based diagnosticity, and Taylor's (1991) mobilization–minimization hypothesis. Trust also appears in work by personality psychologists, as a basis for human relations (Jones, Couch, & Scott, 1997). All of these recognize people's essential trust in others and in life outcomes.

Between individuals, relationships depend on trust (Holmes, 1991), and in experimental game theory, watchful trust outperforms other strategies (Orbell & Dawes, 1993). In groups, communication (Deutsch, 1949), shared goals (Sherif & Sherif, 1953), constructive contact (Dovidio & Gaertner, 1999), and smaller sizes (Yamagishi, 1998) all enable trust.

The best example of the optimistic functional approach in modern motivation science is Mark Snyder and Nancy Cantor's (1998) analysis of functional motives. They argue for the *situational strategy* in personality and social psychology—that is, studying the dynamic interaction between (1) situational regularities that make behavior systematic and (2) people choosing and shaping situations. They argue that these processes share a focus on motivation, defined as movement of and by individuals. They cite Freud's libidinal drives, Erikson's progressive life stages, and Murray's press (already noted), as well as Lewin's locomotion and Floyd Allport's what a person "is trying to do" in life (to be described). Snyder and Cantor argue that social psychology concerns how social situations shape individuals. And personality psychology concerns how dispositional forces move people to actions—that is, regularities in the individual's dynamic systems of adjustment to the environment (borrowing Floyd Allport's admittedly social definition of personality; see below).

Snyder and Cantor's (1998) functionalist strategy concerns reasons and purposes, needs and goals, plans and motives that underlie and generate psychological phenomena. They use the term action *agenda*, referring to outcomes pursued individually, interpersonally, collectively, and societally. Their focus on agendas reflects James's and Gordon Allport's pragmatic, functionalist views, with a focus on processes accessible to conscious analysis. The terms all focus on ends, the outcomes of people's motivated efforts. As they note, purposive psychology describes what movement "is for," as opposed to structural psychology (such as the Big Five work), which describes what "is." As examples, they address agendas in the pursuit of self-understanding, social connection, and societal participation. Each agenda serves goals of furthering individual and social well-being and trusting in human functionality in doing so.

In the current volume, examples of the pragmatic approach, trusting human functionality, appear in Laura King's chapter (see Chapter 34) on positive psychology and more generally its movement to emphasize human resilience and adaptive functioning, as well as Finkel and Rusbult's chapter (see Chapter 36) on accommodation, Batson and colleagues' chapter (see Chapter 9) on prosocial motivation, and Koole and Kuhl's chapter (see Chapter 19) on a functional analysis of volitional affect regulation.

### Trusting Positive Functions: Summary

Some modern descendants of William James and Gordon Allport express the trusting functionality of human motives. The belief in people's resilient, functional motives follows from relying on consciousness as a source of data—a method certainly prominent in James, and to a lesser degree in Allport. That is, if one does not emphasize what is hidden from full view (the inaccessible and the unacceptable), then one can emphasize what is amenable to conscious control (James especially), functional for self (Allport, James), and functional for society (Allport).

## CONTROLLING INCENTIVES: VIEWS FROM THE CLASSROOM

People generally are more motivated (1) the more they value an outcome and (2) the more they expect to achieve it. Such expectancy–value approaches differ from both the psychodynamic view and the functional view of motivation. These approaches tend to come from research settings in which organisms (rodents or people) are presented with clear-cut incentives and learn to control their outcomes by understanding the contingencies of probabilities and values (Boring, 1950; Weiner, 1985).

### Clark Hull and Edward Tolman

Hull (1943) accepted the idea of drives in the rat's classroom (the maze), but he denied purposive psychology and its cognitive trappings, including both the Freudian unconscious and Jamesian consciousness. Hull's drives built on Pavlov's conditioned associations and Thorndike's instrumental law of effect (rewarded stimulus–response pairings encourage repetition); the latter was formulated, ironically, in William James's basement (Weiner, 1985). Hull's resulting mechanistic formula was as follows: behavior = drive × habit, where the *drive* is a need that energizes behavior, and the *habit* is past learning that directs behavior. Drives are nonspecific energizers of behavior, pooling across sources. Habit results from learning (whether associations or stimulus–response linkages).

Tolman (1932) developed a purposive behaviorism, conceiving of *incentives* as the quantity and quality of a reward. Like Freud and Hull, he followed a drive reduction model, and he picked up McDougall's purposive psychology. Hull's (1951) altered model was this: motivation = drive × habit × incentive. Although drive and incentive both energize behavior, the drive is a push from the organism, and the incentive is a pull from the environment. Incentives are learned, whereas drive results from duration of deprivation. Spence (1956) took these ideas to anticipatory goal responses, and Miller (1948) took them to anxiety (an aversive reaction to a dangerous situation). This work bridged to personality psychology (Janet Taylor [Spence]'s [1953] Manifest Anxiety Scale) and social psychology (Zajonc's [1965] drive reduction model of social facilitation). Tolman's intervening variables (the link between the stimulus and response) paved the way to expectancy–value models more tolerant of cognition than those of the early behaviorists.

## Kurt Lewin

Lewin resembled Freud and Murray in hedonism, as well as James and Allport in tapping functional consciousness, but mainly his intellectual origins were Gestalt (below). Nevertheless, "if a Gestaltist, he was a 'hot' Gestaltist" (Jones, 1985, p. 67). On his motivational side, he fits best among the apologists for control motives, with a portrait of individuals responding to environmental incentives. His major motivational theory was organized around the individual's *life space* (Deutsch, 1954; Lewin, 1936, 1951). As Gordon Allport put it, pithily:

> For Murray, personality is the life history. . . . What are [the person's] fantasies? *For Lewin, the person is the life space*. . . . What is the situation? For me, personality is the individual's intentions. . . . What are [the person's] intentions and values? (as transcribed by Smith, 1993, p. 62; emphasis added)

Allport was not entirely fair, for Lewin's life space theory emphasized the *person in the situation*, although admittedly his empirical work and its legacy have emphasized the situation.

Lewin's contribution was more a "way of thinking" (Deutsch, 1954, p. 182; Festinger, 1980) than a precise theory that guided research (Jones, 1985). Essentially, his field theory framework combined person and situation to develop an expectancy–value theory of motivation. In Hull's expectancy–value terms, as noted, drive is the value, and habit is the expectancy, which for rats is the distance to the goal. For Lewin, the comparable terms were *valence* (for value) and *distance* (for expectancy). Distance directly parallels that for the maze rat: As psychological distance in the life space decreases, motivational force increases. People mostly work harder as goals become accessible. Valence also increases motivational force; however, it differs from Hull's habits in being more than mere associations, but actively goal-directed. Valence is a function of the person's tension (need or intention) and perceived properties of the object (Tolman's incentives). However, the parallel with behaviorist approaches should not obscure the fundamental difference in Lewin's orientation: Quite simply, he focused on internal states of the person—both motivations and cognitions—in the context as perceived by the person.

## Achievement Motivation

Lewin's theoretical legacy flows to expectancy–value theories of achievement motivation, combined with Murray's concept of the need for achievement (Weiner, 1985). In John Atkinson's (1964) theory of achievement motivation, the tendency to approach an achievement-related goal is a joint function of need for achievement, probability of success, and incentive value of success. Atkinson, David McClelland (1951), and others further developed Murray's Thematic Apperception Test (TAT) as a reliably scored research tool. McClelland also emphasized other needs striving for accomplishment: achievement, power, and affiliation (with less attention than Freud, for example, to sexual and aggressive drives). The Julian Rotter (1966) expectancy–value theory of social learning addresses perceived freedom—most specifically *locus of control*, either external (controlled by luck, fate, powerful others) or internal (controlled by own actions or dispositions). Beyond locus, Bernard Weiner (1985) contributed *stability* and *control* as perceived causes of people's outcomes—attributions that result in patterns of emotions (e.g., pity vs. anger) and behavior (e.g., help vs. rejection). The achievement motivation work bridges personality and social psychology.

### Social Comparison and Cognitive Dissonance

As noted, Lewin's empirical legacy is mainly the situational part of the person–situation interaction, and as such it lands squarely in social psychology. Leon Festinger most potently transmitted Lewin's influence to subsequent generations of social psychologists, being a dominant figure in the field for two decades (1950–1970; Jones, 1985). Festinger (1954) argued that people have a drive to evaluate their perceptions against social reality, particularly when they perceive a discrepancy. *Social comparison* theory posits a motivation to compare oneself to others, to assess one's relative standing. *Cognitive dissonance* theory posits a motivation to reduce relevant and important cognitive inconsistencies. The most theoretically interesting and empirically tractable inconsistencies are between relevant cognitions (which can be reinterpreted) and a behavior (which is hard to undo). In that sense, it is a drive reduction theory related to people's need to control contingencies between what they do and its effects.

### Effectance Theory

In developmental psychology, Robert White (1959) posited a motive to be competent. He argued that efforts to interact effectively in the environment exhibit all the hallmarks of a motive: direction, selectivity, and persistence. The *effectance motive* aims toward the feeling of interacting effectively in the environment. He argued that it is not a drive reduction motive, and he explicitly argued against both animal learning and psychoanalytic approaches as subsuming this additional intrinsic motive, which operates when other needs are met. His case study is the play of a contented child.

With apologies for nevertheless placing White in drive reduction company, what he shares with other theorists in this section is the emphasis on mastering the contingencies between what one does and what one gets in return from the environment.

### Interdependence Theory

In social psychology, Harold Kelley (1967) also argued for people's motive to gain cognitive mastery of the causal structure of the environment, in the service of predicting and controlling. He noted people's motivation to seek information when it is lacking. His contributions to attribution theory stress the importance of informational regularities in people's behavior: consistency over time, distinctiveness regarding entities, and consensus regarding other actors.

His more directly motivational work, though, concerns his contributions to interpersonal behavior as governed by incentives regarding valued outcomes and their contingencies (Kelley, 1979; Thibaut & Kelley, 1959). People in relationships have joint control over outcomes that matter: reflexive control over some of their own outcomes, fate control over some of their partner's outcomes, and mutual control over outcomes that depend on joint behavior. Interpersonal relationships, in this view, are motivated by *control over outcome dependency.* This control-based approach has influenced a variety of approaches to close relationships (Kelley et al., 1983), ranging from the role of emotion to commitment to gender roles.

### Modern Control Theories

The personality stream in modern control motivation theories focuses on goals: *personal strivings* (Emmons, 1986), *current concerns* (Klinger, 1975), and *personal projects* (Little, 1989). These concepts resemble the broad functional approaches such as Snyder and Cantor's life tasks or Murray's general needs (already noted), but they tend to be narrower and more situation-specific; also, they may not be conscious, but they are intentional (Emmons, 1997). Although Emmons identifies this approach as idiographic (cf. Gordon Allport), some regularities do occur across persons in the types of goals they mention. Not coincidentally, the recurring strivings resemble some of the Big Five traits, as well as the five core social motives that organize the present review—especially self-esteem, self-assertion (control), and affiliation (belonging).

For social psychologists, motives for control appear at all levels. At the within-individual level, laypeople focus on dispositional explanations for others (Jones & Nisbett, 1972). Their own sense of agency appears in Brehm's (1966) reactance theory and Bandura's (1997) self-efficacy theory. Between individuals, people's concern with control can devolve into aggression, under various theories (Anderson & Bushman, 2002). Social exchange approaches indicate people's motivation to control incentives in social relationships (Walster, Berscheid, & Walster, 1973). Interdependence motivations undercut people's spontaneous prejudices (Fiske, 2000). And outcome interdependence defines group life (Campbell, 1958; Deutsch, 1949; Sherif & Sherif, 1953; Thibaut & Kelley, 1959). Between groups, competition over scarce resources explains many theories of group conflict (Campbell, 1965; Sidanius & Pratto, 1999).

In this volume, Thompson and Schlehofer (Chapter 3) directly address control motivations, and Senko, Durik, and Harackiewicz (Chapter 7) focus particularly on achievement motivation. More specifically, Elliot and Fryer (Chapter 15) address the goal construct, Shah and Kruglanski (Chapter 14) emphasize goal management, and Gollwitzer and colleagues (Chapter 21) focus on tenacity in goal pursuit. Individual differences in goal investment (Pomerantz & Shim, Chapter 25) and in theories of self as malleable or fixed (Dweck & Grant, Chapter 26) further illustrate this type of motivational approach. The motive to control is currently in vogue, including in my own work (Fiske, 1993a, 2000).

### Controlling Incentives: Summary

Beginning with incentives in the rat's maze and moving through the human classroom to all tasks of life, many motivational approaches highlight control over incentives, mastery of contingencies, or efforts toward competence. Many are explicitly expectancy–value models coming out of the Hull–Tolman tradition and extending into achievement motivation. But in the legacy of Kurt Lewin, many are less explicitly mathematical and simply emphasize the motive to control one's contingencies and accomplish one's goals, in areas ranging from explanations to relationships.

## UNDERSTANDING SELF AND OTHERS: VIEWS FROM THE HUMAN COMPUTER

People seek prediction as well as control. Not every situation is controllable, but people nevertheless seek to understand their social surroundings in ways that match the understandings of others in their social reference group. The motive for a coherent, socially shared understanding can be traced back to Gestalt psychology; from there, it has moved forward through information-processing theories to motivated social cognition theories.

### Gestalt Approaches

Founded by Max Wertheimer, Kurt Koffka, and Wolfgang Köhler, Gestalt psychology protested the analysis of consciousness into elements, instead emphasizing harmonious fit among elements to form a coherent whole (Boring, 1950; Scheerer, 1954). Its premise—that people perceive meaningful wholes, not sensory parts—began with the perception of patterns and continuity; people perceive the proximal stimulus, filtered through their own interpretive lens from the distal stimulus (Brunswik, 1936). Although this might seem like a solely perceptual phenomenon, not all Gestaltists would agree: "Behavior can be conceptualized as being embedded in a cognitive–emotional–motivational matrix in which no true separation is possible" (Scheerer, 1954, p. 125). The link to motivation lies in people's active construction of their own goals, as opposed, say, to being merely driven by low-level perceptual phenomena or physiological needs. The Lewinian life space, as noted, fits both this Gestalt motivational analysis and the control motives highlighted in the previous section.

In the current context, the Gestalt approach, with its active construction of perception, gave rise in social psychology most directly to the work of Asch and Heider. Basic Gestalt principles include laws of form (imputing organization to the perceptual field), relativity (encoding comparative to standards), object constancy (maintaining identity regardless of sensory input), and dynamics (interacting forces) (Boring, 1950). The perceptual principles translate fairly directly to the social domain.

## Fritz Heider

Heider's rich and dense *The Psychology of Interpersonal Relations* (1958) made two lasting contributions, both cognitive but with implications for motivation science. First, Heider convinced subsequent generations of attribution and social cognition researchers that people's key social observation strategy is the search for invariance, most often resulting in dispositional attributions (Gilbert, 1998). Heider posited that dispositions stand out as figures against a situational ground, so people's preference for subsuming varied behaviors into a single dispositional principle fits Gestalt ideas. The dispositional principle emphasizes inferring another's intent (what the person is *trying* to do) and ability (what the person *can* do). Motivation is relevant both in the perceiver's effort to find coherence in an impression of an individual (e.g., managing inconsistencies) and in the perceiver's imputation of motives to others (also creating coherence).

Heider's other lasting contribution is balance theory—likewise a search for invariance, but here a perceived harmony in relationships. People tend to perceive friends as agreeing and sometimes to perceive enemies as disagreeing. The bias toward inferring harmony between people's relationships to each other and shared attitude objects ("Love me, love my beliefs") appears again to be a motivated urge for consistency and coherence. This fits the understanding motive, but note that it says nothing about achieving accuracy, only a sense of coherence.

## Solomon Asch

Asch's contributions to motivation science appear in the understanding motive's emphasis on both coherent and socially shared understanding. Coherence appears primary in his concept of person perception—namely, that the configuration of traits creates meaning beyond the algebraic combination of elements (Asch, 1946). His elegant experiments demonstrated, for example, *primacy*, or first impressions shaping the meaning of subsequent cues. The studies also emphasized central traits (e.g., warmth) as providing coherence. Apparent were both the adroitness of the human mind in making sense of apparent contradiction (Asch & Zukier, 1984) and the difficulty of undoing a coherent impression, once formed (Asch, 1946). Asch explicitly contrasted Gestalt, holistic impressions with piecemeal, elemental, algebraic formulations, foreshadowing modern dual-process models of impressions (e.g., Brewer, 1988; Fiske & Neuberg, 1990).

His conformity research (Asch, 1956) also foreshadowed the social motivational moderators of perceptual understanding. People's willingness at least sometimes to seek social harmony (agreeing with peers), in contradiction to perceptual evidence, demonstrated a search for social coherence. Socially shared understanding was primary in the conformity research, reflecting a group-level cognitive unity.

Asch framed his Gestalt-inspired contributions as an argument against an oversimplified ego psychology of self-interest (Asch, 1952). Instead, he argued in support of needs for, first, *interested engagement* with one's surroundings, here characterized as the understanding motive; and, second, for *constructing and creating*, here characterized as control (effectance, competence). Third, he emphasized *social interest*, beyond self-interest, which can be characterized as a recognition of social belonging (to be described as the last motive). Asch described social interest as a direct interest in humans and in their character, as a function of surviving (to understand, act, and care) and thriving (to understand, grow, and feel).

## George Kelly

Kelly (1955; see also Robins & John, 1997; Weiner, 1985) originated the notion of humans as naive scientists, motivated to make sense of the observed world. Meaning results from active construction, so his perspective fits with the Gestalt focus on organisms organizing their experience. Kelly postulated that people (and other organisms) channel their reactions by their expectations about events. That is, their understandings (construals) guide their conduct, with a focus on making sense of the world, over other motives such as rewards and punishments or drive reduction. People's main goals, in this view, are prediction and control.

From this follow individual differences in people's *personal constructs*—their everyday theories about themselves and the world. Personal constructs operate as bipolar contrasts (e.g., warm–cold) relevant to particular respondents and the people that they report have played important roles in their lives. Although not a major research focus, this theory contributed to the naive scientist context that informed a generation of work on social cognitive approaches.

### Information-Processing Approaches

The cognitive revolution in psychology laid aside behaviorist dominance in favor of unabashed mentalism. That is, cognitive phenomena—particularly attention, memory, and decision making—were no longer taboo, but on the contrary, the centerpieces of research and theory. The human computer was the metaphor of the day. At first social and personality psychologists focused on pure information-processing explanations for phenomena previously explained in motivational terms. For example, in social psychology, the 1960s had emphasized cognitive dissonance theory (treated earlier under drive reduction control motives), but attitude change theories of the 1970s and 1980s emphasized cognitive heuristics, cognitive responses, and attribution processes. In the same time period, intergroup bias research turned from self-enhancing prejudices to schematic stereotypes.

Granted, some older theories did emphasize rapid, thoughtless types of understanding processes, including *mere exposure* and *propinquity* as increasing liking (respectively, Zajonc, 1968; Festinger, Schachter, & Back, 1950/1963). More recent theories, inspired by the cognitive revolution, have also emphasized rapid processes, in a similar vein, but have emphasized cognitive expectancies in the interpersonal domain: *social prototypes* (Cantor & Mischel, 1977), *significant-other schemas* (Andersen & Chen, 2002), *self-fulfilling prophecies* (Merton, 1948), *expectancy effects* (Rosenthal, 1994), and *behavioral confirmation* (Snyder, 1984). Other modern cognitive theories have emphasized rapid, coherent understanding of the self—as in *self-schemas* (Markus, 1977), or, in a more elaborate but still rapid cognitive process, *self-verification* (Swann, Hixon, Stein-Seroussi, & Gilbert, 1990).

All these theories essentially ignore motivation, except to imply that people seek to understand themselves and others as quickly and easily as possible, in line with a *cognitive miser* framework (Fiske & Taylor, 1984).

Personality research likewise went from focusing on tension reduction constructs such as authoritarianism, achievement motivation, and anxiety, to focusing on cognitive approaches that emphasized learned helplessness, achievement attributions, depressive schemas, and life scripts. But purely cognitive approaches were found lacking, and motivation returned in the dual-process theories as a moderator variable: Social perceivers have been characterized as *motivated tacticians* (Fiske & Taylor, 1991), as in the dual-process models that follow.

### Dual-Process Theories

Motivated social cognition emerged as a more viable explanatory framework than merely cold cognition. A series of dual-process models all contrast faster, relatively automatic, relatively superficial processes with slower, relatively controlled, more elaborate processes (Chaiken & Trope, 1999).

Within individuals, for example, the *continuum model* (Fiske, Lin, & Neuberg, 1999; Fiske & Neuberg, 1990) proposes that people seek rapid initial understandings of others, often based on immediate categorization by demographic or other visual cues. When motivated to be accurate (a stronger understanding motive), people examine additional information, allowing them possibly to go beyond their superficial first impressions. Perceiver values, relationship with the target, or accountability to third parties can increase this accuracy motive. A related theory focuses on different forms of mental representations (Brewer & Feinstein, 1999), but both contrast stereotyping and individuating processes, moderated by motivation—often an understanding motive (Bodenhausen, Macrae, & Sherman, 1999). Attributional processes also can be more *spontaneous* or *intentional* (Uleman, 1999) and can be focused on *identification* or *inference* (Trope & Gaunt, 1999).

Among attitude models, the *elaboration likelihood model* contrasts peripheral cues to persuasion with central cues that elicit more detailed cognitive responses to a persuasive communication (Petty & Cacioppo, 1981; Petty & Wegener, 1999). Likewise, the *heuristic–systematic model* contrasts simplistic short cuts to persuasion with more careful processing of messages (Chaiken, 1980). All these theories presume variations in understanding motives as important moderators of which social cognitive route is taken.

In this volume, contributors in the tradition of understanding motives include *consistency motives* (Harmon-Jones & Harmon-Jones, Chapter 5), *motivated closed-mindedness* (Kruglanski & Chun, Chapter 6), *self-concordance* (Sheldon, Chapter 30), *goal contagion* (Aarts, Dijksterhuis, & Dik, Chapter 17), and *counteractional processes* (Fishbach & Trope, Chapter 18).

### Understanding Self and Others: Summary

Starting from Gestalt approaches emphasizing coherent, holistic understanding, social and personality psychologists transported the understanding motive to people's push for a socially viable understanding, mostly emphasizing a socially shared understanding. Thus Asch's conformity studies illustrate this motive. But Asch's impression formation studies, Heider's balance theory, and Kelly's personal constructs also emphasize the social nature of understanding, in considering social engagement (Asch), interpersonal relationships (Heider), and roles (Kelly). Social cognition research in its initial information-processing guise was social mainly in the sense of using social stimuli instead of nonsocial stimuli, but as interpersonal goals and motives began to emerge, dual-process models began to incorporate more thoroughly the social context of understanding.

## BELONGING WITH OTHERS: VIEWS FROM CONTEMPORARY COLLECTIVES

The motivation to belong is now having its heyday, as this section illustrates. Few psychologists until recently built their theoretical frameworks around social attachment, but now we can't seem to get enough of belonging motives. It's a useful framework, given what we know now, as the concluding section argues.

### Floyd Allport

One of the first social psychology texts (F. H. Allport, 1924), in the spirit of the age, dutifully listed 42 *habits*. These were expressly not McDougall's instincts—a concept Allport labeled "an impediment to the scientific observation of behavior" (1924, p. 81). As the reader harkening back to the opening section of this chapter might expect, habits included every imaginable broad class of behavior from flight to eating to chivalry to reading to learning a trade; Allport selected them as having "early and universal occurrence" (p. 80), as well as importance. However, the list was not intended as an endorsement.

Allport's preferred theoretical standpoint was to start with only the simplest of innate bodily reflexes and immediately move on to "inalienable qualities and tendencies of a social nature" (1924, p. 81). He viewed individuals as profoundly shaped by *social influences*, which he saw as the fundamentally human activities. Social drives for contact and approval were viewed as so fundamental as to be almost innate (p. 427), furthering the development of the individual toward increased success in living. He explicitly focused on the individual in a group—how individuals influence and are influenced by others, including consciousness, to the extent that it concerns other people. Even "thought itself . . . is largely a part of the general social influence" (p. 82). His book came in the context of research that had already demonstrated the motivating fact of others.

Some of social psychology's earliest research demonstrated *social facilitation*, or motivation in the mere presence of other people (Triplett, 1898). Subsequent research showed that all conspecifics—even among cockroaches, baby chicks, and other animals—facilitate the individual's dominant response (Zajonc, 1965). This is perhaps the simplest and most elegant indicator of social influences.

### John Bowlby

Bowlby's (1969, 1973, 1980) approach, though years later than Floyd Allport's, combined the instinct approach with the fundamental role for social contact and responsiveness. His legacy in personality and social psychology fits squarely into issues of *attachment* and belonging in close relationships. Focused on the infant–caregiver bond, his work has much to say about belonging (also understanding and trust), because attachment theory describes a secure relationship as the base that allows exploration of the world. Bowlby's *internal working models* are assumed by social psychologists to be accessible to consciousness (e.g., Hazan & Shaver, 1987, 1994). But his work focused less on belonging per se than on explaining dysfunction as a result of failed attachment. However, his evolutionary theoretical base owes much to the adaptive value of belonging—a theme that has returned in modern theories of belonging.

## Sociological Social Psychology

Independently of Floyd Allport's emphasis on going beyond biological instincts to social influence, and Bowlby's emphasis on biological bases of social bonds, a more macro level of analysis focused on people's core motive to participate in group life. Social group theories emphasized people conforming to *roles* (expectations based on their position) and *norms* (expectations based on group membership). Erving Goffman's (1967) dramaturgical theory, Jacob Moreno's (1953) sociometry, and R. Freed Bales's (1950, 1999) interaction systems exemplify the psychological impact of group membership, structure, and face-to-face interaction. Descendants of these theories appear in *social impact* theories (Latané, 1981; Tanford & Penrod, 1984), which describe how the number, strength, and immediacy of other people influence the individual. *Social influence processes* identified by Cialdini include compliance motivated by liking, approval, and reciprocity—all rules of motivated belonging (Cialdini & Trost, 1998). In all these cases, people are motivated by their place in the group.

## Modern Belonging Theories: Contemporary Collectives

In Europe, group-based, collective theories multiplied to reflect the growing mix of national identity and pan-European identity, as well as the impact of non-European immigration. Social psychologists focused on intergroup relations concentrated on *social identity*—the creation of self-concept centered on a positive, distinctive understanding of one's salient group membership. Social identity contrasts with personal identity, and social identities depend on context. In the original theory (Tajfel, 1981), people are motivated by understanding between-group differences and within-group similarities, as well as by maintaining a positive ingroup identity. In the self-categorization extension, the self-esteem aspect has departed, and people mainly maximize their understanding of between- and within-group variance (Turner, Hogg, Oakes, Reicher, & Wetherell, 1987). These theories defined mainstream European social psychology in the last two decades of the 20th century.

## Modern Belonging Theories: The Individual in the Group

All the previous work indicates that the desire for relationships with other people is arguably crucial to surviving and thriving. First, the need to belong is pervasive, easily established, and reluctantly relinquished (Baumeister & Leary, 1995). Relationships consistently predict well-being. People in every culture and circumstance bond with similar others. People are devastated by rejection: Their self-esteem depends on social acceptance, according to *sociometer theory* (Leary & Baumeister, 2000); they experience a variety of immediate ill effects from ostracism (Williams, Cheung, & Choi, 2000); and ostracism activates pain centers in the brain (Eisenberger, Lieberman, & Williams, 2003).

Second, socially isolated individuals and people with relationship problems suffer a variety of cardiovascular and immunological ill effects, showing higher mortality (House, Landis, & Umberson, 1988; Kiecolt-Glaser, McGuire, Robles, & Glaser, 2002; Stansfeld, Bosma, Hemingway, & Marmot, 1998).

Finally, one can make a social evolutionary argument for the importance of people's motivation to get along with at least some other people. Humans as animals cannot easily get through gestation, infancy, childrearing, and even adult survival as social isolates. Not only are people more likely to reproduce, but their young are also more likely to thrive (and reproduce), when they operate in clusters. For all these reasons, it makes sense that people would be motivated to belong to their group (Fiske, 2004). If the group is the adaptational niche, several roles emerge to help the group function well, so not everyone strives to be the dominant male. Instead, the main tasks are coordination with and acceptance among other group members in a variety of necessary roles (Brewer, 1997; Caporael, 1997).

In this volume, belonging as a motivation appears in Chapter 2 by Leary and Cox (*belonging needs*), Chapter 27 by Morling and Kitayama (*cultural differences in interdependence*), Chapter 28 by Diekman and Eagly (*gender differences in communality*), Chapter 33 by Twenge (*reactions to social exclusion*), Chapter 35 by Murray (*security motivations*), and Chapter 37 by Gable and Strachman (*approach and avoidance social motivation*).

### Belonging with Others: Summary

Floyd Allport rescued early social psychology from the litany of instincts and habits, emphasizing people's irreducibly social aspect; Bowlby posited evolved needs for attachment; and early sociological social psychology founded its analysis on adherence to group roles and norms. Recently, an explosion of work on the need to belong demonstrates the utility of this core social motive. It goes farther, to generate the other core motives, as I suggest below.

## CONCLUSION

Social and personality psychologists over the past century have invented and reinvented recognizable clusters of motivations. The consensus is heartening, though the neglect of prior work is discouraging. What's more, the criteria for prioritizing one set of motives over another are daunting. The effort here is merely to organize the history of motivation science in a heuristic fashion. The foundation for this effort has both methodological and theoretical bases.

The methodological point is a variant on the adage "Where you stand depends on where you sit." In this case, it is "What you posit depends on what you observe." The scientist's observational methods influence the motives that seem most relevant to explaining human nature. This chapter's (perhaps frivolously) alliterative title emphasizes that the important motives differ, depending on whether observers are listening to patients on a couch, examining their own consciousness, watching students in a classroom, modeling cognition on computers, or investigating group members in a collective. If one is listening to patients, then a rather narcissistic, self-serving set of motives comes to the fore. If one examines one's own consciousness, then one almost has to be optimistic about the presumed benevolence, trust, and positivity of human nature. If one bets on students, then one sees striving and controlling of incentives everywhere. If one focuses on information processing, then understanding is key. And if one focuses on the collective level of analysis, then group belonging seems primary. This argues for the nature of the evidence guiding the nature of the analysis. Of course, the reverse causality operates also: Researchers who think that the interesting variance is under the lamppost will look for the key in that location and not see many other perspectives. In either case, the methods both determine and reflect the motives likely to be identified.

The theoretical foundation for listing these particular motives is a social evolutionary base. Using the belonging motive as a theoretical starting point derives from both from its life-or-death effects and from the logic of human adaptation to surviving in groups, as just described. Even better, the belonging motive—wanting to create and maintain relationships—generates the other four motives highlighted here (Fiske, 2004). To function effectively in a group, individuals must be motivated to understand in a socially shared fashion and to have a sense of effective interpersonal control. Individuals must also have enough self-regard to act on their own behalf in the group and must trust others in the group to have fundamentally benign intentions. All of this follows from the group as the relevant adaptational niche.

Could one identify other core motives? Of course. Gordon Allport, to name one hero, identified hedonism (pleasure–pain), egoism (power), sympathy (affiliation), imitation (conforming behavior), and suggestion (socially shared cognition). Although I encountered these five principles only in rereading Allport's history chapter (Allport, 1954a) for this project and had generated the five core motives as described earlier, the systems are roughly and reassuringly parallel: The current chapter's motive of enhancing self is clearly hedonism; the controlling motive is egoism in the power sense; but the remaining three all are variants on belonging, with Allport's sympathy perhaps being closest to my trust, but his imitation and his suggestion closest to my socially shared understanding. May the rest of this volume support a useful consensus and spur further inquiry.

## REFERENCES

Allport, F. H. (1924). *Social psychology.* Boston: Houghton Mifflin.

Allport, G. W. (1954a). The historical background of modern social psychology. In G. Lindzey (Ed.), *Handbook of social psychology* (Vol. 1, pp. 5–56). Reading, MA: Addison-Wesley.

Allport, G. W. (1954b). *The nature of prejudice*. Reading, MA: Addison-Wesley.

Andersen, S. M., & Chen, S. (2002). The relational self: An interpersonal social-cognitive theory. *Psychological Review, 109*, 619–645.

Anderson, C. A., & Bushman, B. J. (2002). Human aggression. *Annual Review of Psychology, 53*, 27–51.

Asch, S. E. (1946). Forming impressions of personality. *Journal of Abnormal and Social Psychology, 41*, 1230–1240.

Asch, S. E. (1952). *Social psychology*. Englewood Cliffs, NJ: Prentice Hall.

Asch, S. E. (1956). Studies of independence and conformity: A minority of one against a unanimous majority. *Psychological Monographs: General and Applied, 70*, 1–70.

Asch, S. E., & Zukier, H. (1984). Thinking about persons. *Journal of Personality and Social Psychology, 46*, 1230–1240.

Atkinson, J. W. (1964). *An introduction to motivation*. Princeton, NJ: Van Nostrand.

Bales, R. F. (1950). A set of categories for the analysis of small group interaction. *American Sociological Review, 15*, 257–263.

Bales, R. F. (1999). *Social interaction systems: Theory and measurement*. New Brunswick, NJ: Transaction.

Bandura, A. (1997). *Self-efficacy: The exercise of control*. New York: Freeman.

Baumeister, R. F., & Leary, M. R. (1995). The need to belong: Desire for interpersonal attachments as a fundamental human motivation. *Psychological Bulletin, 117*, 497–529.

Bentham, J. (1948). *An introduction to the principles of morals and legislation*. Oxford, UK: Blackwell. (Original work published 1779)

Bodenhausen, G. V., Macrae, C. N., & Sherman, J. W. (1999). On the dialectics of discrimination. In S. Chaiken & Y. Trope (Eds.), *Dual-process theories in social psychology* (pp. 271–290). New York: Guilford Press.

Boring, E. G. (1950). *A history of experimental psychology*. Englewood Cliffs, NJ: Prentice Hall.

Bowlby, J. (1969). *Attachment and loss: Vol. 1. Attachment*. New York: Basic Books.

Bowlby, J. (1973). *Attachment and loss: Vol. 2. Separation: Anxiety and anger*. New York: Basic Books.

Bowlby, J. (1980). *Attachment and loss: Vol. 3. Loss: Sadness and depression*. New York: Basic Books.

Brehm, J. W. (1966). *A theory of psychological reactance*. New York: Academic Press.

Brewer, M. B. (1988). A dual process model of impression formation. In T. K. Srull & R. S. Wyer, Jr. (Eds.), *Advances in social cognition* (Vol. 1, pp. 1–36). Hillsdale, NJ: Erlbaum.

Brewer, M. B. (1991). The social self: On being the same and different at the same time. *Personality and Social Psychology Bulletin, 17*, 475–482.

Brewer, M. B. (1997). On the social origins of human nature. In C. McGarty & S. A. Haslam (Eds.), *The message of social psychology* (pp. 54–62). Cambridge, MA: Blackwell.

Brewer, M. B., & Feinstein, A. S. H. (1999). Dual processes in the cognitive representation of personal and social categories. In S. Chaiken & Y. Trope (Eds.), *Dual-process theories in social psychology* (pp. 255–270). New York: Guilford Press.

Brunswik, E. (1936). Psychology in terms of objects. In H. W. Hill (Ed.), *Proceedings of the 25th Annual Celebration of Inauguration of Graduate Studies, University of California* (pp. 122–126). Reading, PA: Addison-Wesley.

Bushman, B. J., & Anderson, C. A. (2001a). Is it time to pull the plug on the hostile versus instrumental aggression dichotomy? *Psychological Review, 108*, 273–279.

Bushman, B. J., & Anderson, C. A. (2001b). Media violence and the American public. *American Psychologist, 56*, 477–489.

Campbell, D. T. (1958). Common fate, similarity, and other indices of the status of aggregates of persons as social entities. *Behavioral Science, 3*, 14–25.

Campbell, D. T. (1965). Ethnocentric and other altruistic motives. In D. Levine (Ed.), *Nebraska Symposium on Motivation* (Vol. 13, pp. 283–311). Lincoln: University of Nebraska Press.

Cantor, N., & Mischel, W. (1977). Traits as prototypes: Effects on recognition memory. *Journal of Personality and Social Psychology, 35*, 38–48.

Caporael, L. R. (1997). The evolution of truly social cognition: The core configurations model. *Review of Personality and Social Psychology, 1*, 276–298.

Caspi, A., Roberts, B. W., & Shiner, R. L. (2005). Personality development: Stability and change. *Annual Review of Psychology, 56*, 453–484.

Chaiken, S. (1980). Heuristic versus systematic information processing and the use of source versus message cues in persuasion. *Journal of Personality and Social Psychology, 39*, 752–766.

Chaiken, S., & Trope, Y. (Eds.). (1999). *Dual-process theories in social psychology*. New York: Guilford Press.

Cialdini, R. B., & Trost, M. R. (1998). Social influence: Social norms, conformity, and compliance. In D. T. Gilbert, S. T. Fiske, & G. Lindzey (Eds.), *The handbook of social psychology* (4th ed., Vol. 2, pp. 151–192). New York: McGraw-Hill.

Deutsch, M. (1949). A theory of cooperation and competition. *Human Relations, 2*, 199–231.

Deutsch, M. (1954). Field theory in social psychology. In G. Lindzey (Ed.), *Handbook of social psychology* (Vol. 1, pp. 182–222). Reading, MA: Addison-Wesley.

Devine, P. G., & Monteith, M. J. (1999). Automaticity and control in stereotyping. In S. Chaiken & Y. Trope (Eds.), *Dual-process theories in social psychology* (pp. 339–360). New York: Guilford Press.

Dovidio, J. F., & Gaertner, S. L. (1999). Reducing prejudice: Combating intergroup biases. *Current Directions in Psychological Science, 8*, 101–105.

Eisenberger, N. I., Lieberman, M. D., & Williams, K. D. (2003). Does rejection hurt?: An fMRI study of social exclusion. *Science, 302*, 290–292.

Elms, A. C. (1993). Allport's *Personality* and Allport's personality. In K. H. Craik, R. Hogan, & R. N. Wolfe (Eds.), *Fifty years of personality and psychology* (pp. 39–54). New York: Plenum Press.

Emmons, R. A. (1986). Personal strivings: An approach to personality and subjective well-being. *Journal of Personality and Social Psychology, 51*, 1058–1068.

Emmons, R. A. (1997). Motives and goals. In R. Hogan, J. Johnson, & S. Briggs (Eds.), *Handbook of personality psychology* (pp. 486–506). San Diego, CA: Academic Press.

Erikson, E. (1950). *Childhood and society.* New York: Norton

Erikson, E. (1959). Identity and the life cycle: Selected papers. *Psychological Issues, 1*, 5–165.

Fein, S., & Spencer, S. J. (1997). Prejudice as self-image maintenance: Affirming the self through derogating others. *Journal of Personality and Social Psychology, 73*, 31–44.

Festinger, L. (1954). A theory of social comparison processes. *Human Relations, 7*, 117–140.

Festinger, L. (1980). Looking backward. In L. Festinger (Ed.), *Retrospections on social psychology* (pp. 236–288). New York: Oxford University Press.

Festinger, L., Schachter, S., & Back, K. (1963). *Social pressures in informal groups: A study of a housing community.* Stanford, CA: Stanford University Press. (Original work published 1950)

Fiske, D. W. (1949). Consistency of the factorial structures of personality ratings from different sources. *Journal of Abnormal and Social Psychology, 44*, 329–344.

Fiske, S. T. (1980). Attention and weight in person perception: The impact of negative and extreme behavior. *Journal of Personality and Social Psychology, 38*, 889–906.

Fiske, S. T. (1989). Examining the role of intent: Toward understanding its role in stereotyping and prejudice. In J. Uleman & J. Bargh (Eds.), *Unintended thought: The limits of awareness, intention, and control* (pp. 253–283). New York: Guilford Press.

Fiske, S. T. (1992). Thinking is for doing: Portraits of social cognition from daguerreotype to laserphoto. *Journal of Personality and Social Psychology, 63*, 877–889.

Fiske, S. T. (1993a). Controlling other people: The impact of power on stereotyping. *American Psychologist, 48*, 621–628.

Fiske, S. T. (1993b). Social cognition and social perception. *Annual Review of Psychology, 44*, 155–194.

Fiske, S. T. (2000). Interdependence and the reduction of prejudice. In S. Oskamp (Ed.), *Reducing prejudice and discrimination* (pp. 115–135). Mahwah, NJ: Erlbaum.

Fiske, S. T. (2003). Five core social motives, plus or minus five. In S. J. Spencer, S. Fein, M. P. Zanna, & J. Olson (Eds.), *The Ontario Symposium: Motivated social perception, Vol. 9* (pp. 233–246). Mahwah, NJ: Erlbaum.

Fiske, S. T. (2004). *Social beings: A core motives approach to social psychology.* New York: Wiley.

Fiske, S. T., Lin, M. H., & Neuberg, S. L. (1999). The Continuum Model: Ten years later. In S. Chaiken & Y. Trope (Eds.), *Dual-process theories in social psychology* (pp. 231–254). New York: Guilford Press.

Fiske, S. T., & Neuberg, S. L. (1990). A continuum of impression formation, from category-based to individuating processes: Influences of information and motivation on attention and interpretation. In M. P. Zanna (Ed.), *Advances in experimental social psychology* (Vol. 23, pp. 1–74). San Diego, CA: Academic Press.

Fiske, S. T., & Taylor, S. E. (1984). *Social cognition.* New York: Random House.

Fiske, S. T., & Taylor, S. E. (1991). *Social cognition* (2nd ed.). New York: McGraw-Hill.

Freud, S. (1951). *The psychopathology of everyday life.* New York: New American Library. (Original work published 1901)

Freud, S. (1953). The interpretation of dreams. In J. Strachey (Ed. & Trans.), *The standard edition of the complete psychological works of Sigmund Freud* (Vol. 4, pp. 1–338; Vol. 5, pp. 339–627). London: Hogarth Press. (Original work published 1900)

Freud, S. (1953). On narcissism: An introduction. In J. Strachey (Ed. & Trans.), *The standard edition of the complete psychological works of Sigmund Freud* (Vol. 14, pp. 67–102). London: Hogarth Press. (Original work published 1914)

Freud, S. (1955). Beyond the pleasure principle. In J. Strachey (Ed. & Trans.), *The standard edition of the complete psychological works of Sigmund Freud* (Vol. 18, pp. 3–64). London: Hogarth Press. (Original work published 1920)

Gilbert, D. T. (1998). Ordinary personology. In D. T. Gilbert, S. T. Fiske, & G. Lindzey (Eds.), *The handbook of social psychology* (4th ed., Vol. 2, pp. 89–150). New York: McGraw-Hill.

Goffman, E. (1967). *Interaction ritual: Essays on face-to-face behavior.* Garden City, NY: Doubleday.

Goodwin, S. A., Fiske, S. T., Rosen, L. D., & Rosenthal, A. M. (2002). The eye of the beholder: Romantic goals and impression biases. *Journal of Experimental Social Psychology, 38*, 232–241.

Greenwald, A. G. (1980). The totalitarian ego: Fabrication and revision of personal history. *American Psychologist, 35*, 603–618.

Hazan, C., & Shaver, P. (1987). Romantic love conceptualized as an attachment process. *Journal of Personality and Social Psychology, 52*, 511–524.

Hazan, C., & Shaver, P. (1994). Attachment as an organizational framework for research on close relationships. *Psychological Inquiry, 5*, 1–22.

Heider, F. (1958). *The psychology of interpersonal relations*. New York: Wiley.

Higgins, E. T. (1987). Self-discrepancy: A theory relating self and affect. *Psychological Review, 94*, 319–340.

Higgins, E. T., & Pittman, T. S. (in press). Motives of the human animal: Comprehending, managing, and sharing inner states. *Annual Review of Psychology, 59*.

Holmes, J. G. (1991). Trust and the appraisal process in close relationships. In W. H. Jones & D. Perlman (Eds.), *Advances in personal relationships* (Vol. 3, pp. 57–104). London: Kingsley.

House, J. S., Landis, K. R., & Umberson, D. (1988). Social relationships and health. *Science, 241*, 540–545.

Hull, C. L. (1943). *Principles of behavior.* New York: Appleton-Century-Crofts.

Hull, C. L. (1951). *Essentials of behavior.* New Haven, CT: Yale University Press.

James, W. (1890). *The principles of psychology* (2 vols.). New York: Holt.

Jones, E. E. (1985). Major developments in social psychology during the past five decades. In G. Lindzey & E. Aronson (Eds.), *Handbook of social psychology* (3rd ed., Vol. 1, pp. 47–107). New York: Random House.

Jones, E. E., & Nisbett, R. E. (1972). The actor and the observer: Divergent perceptions of the causes of behavior. In E. E. Jones, D. E. Kanouse, H. H. Kelley, R. E. Nisbett, S. Valins, & B. Weiner (Eds.), *Attribution: Perceiving the causes of behavior* (pp. 79–94). Morristown, NJ: General Learning Press.

Jones, W. H., Couch, L., & Scott. S. (1997). Trust and betrayal: The psychology of getting along and getting ahead. In R. Hogan, J. Johnson, & S. Briggs (Eds.), *Handbook of personality psychology* (pp. 466–481). San Diego, CA: Academic Press.

Kahneman, D., & Tversky, A. (1979). Prospect theory: An analysis of decisions under risk. *Econometrica, 47*, 313–327.

Kelley, H. H. (1967). Attribution theory in social psychology. In D. Levine (Ed.), *Nebraska Symposium on Motivation* (Vol. 15, pp. 192–240). Lincoln: University of Nebraska Press.

Kelley, H. H. (1979). *Personal relationships.* Hillsdale, NJ: Erlbaum.

Kelley, H. H., Berscheid, E., Christensen, A., Harvey, J. H., Huston, T. L., Levinger, G., et al. (1983). *Close relationships.* New York: Freeman.

Kelly, G. A. (1955). *The psychology of personal constructs.* New York: Norton.

Kiecolt-Glaser, J. K., McGuire, L., Robles, T. F., & Glaser, R. (2002). Emotions, morbidity, and mortality: New perspectives from psychoneuroimmunology. *Annual Review of Psychology, 53*, 83–107.

Klinger, E. (1975). Consequences of commitment to and disengagement from incentives. *Psychological Review, 82*, 223–231.

Kunda, Z. (1990). The case for motivated reasoning. *Psychological Bulletin, 108*, 480–498.

Latané, B. (1981). The psychology of social impact. *American Psychologist, 36*, 343–356.

Leary, M. R., & Baumeister, R. F. (2000). The nature and function of self-esteem: Sociometer theory. In M. P. Zanna (Ed.), *Advances in experimental social psychology* (Vol. 32, pp. 1–62). San Diego, CA: Academic Press.

Levin, K. (1936). *Principles of topological psychology.* New York: McGraw-Hill.

Lewin, K. (1951). *Field theory in social science.* New York: Harper.

Little, B. R. (1989). Personal projects analysis: Trivial pursuits, magnificent obsessions, and the search for coherence. In D. M. Buss & N. Cantor (Eds.), *Personality psychology: Recent trends and emerging issues* (pp. 15–31). New York: Springer-Verlag.

Markus, H. R. (1977). Self-schemata and processing information about the self. *Journal of Personality and Social Psychology, 35*, 63–78.

Maslow, A. H. (1943). A theory of human motivation. *Psychological Review, 50*, 370–396.

Maslow, A. H. (1967). A theory of metamotivation: The biological rooting of the value-life. *Journal of Humanistic Psychology, 7*, 93–127.

Matlin, M. W., & Stang, D. J. (1978). *The Pollyanna principle.* Cambridge, MA: Schenkman.

McAdams, D. P. (1997). A conceptual history of personality psychology. In R. Hogan, J. Johnson, & S. Briggs (Eds.), *Handbook of personality psychology* (pp. 3–39). San Diego, CA: Academic Press.

McClelland, D. C. (1951). *Personality.* New York: Sloane.

McDougall, W. (1908). *Introduction to social psychology.* London: Methuen. (14th ed., 1919)

McDougall, W. (1923). *Outline of psychology.* New York: Scribner.

Merton, R. K. (1948). The self-fulfilling prophecy. *Antioch Review, 8*, 193–210.

Miller, G. A. (1983). Introduction to W. James (1890/1983), *The principles of psychology.* Cambridge, MA: Harvard University Press.

Miller, N. E. (1948). Studies of fear as an acquirable drive: I. Fear as motivation and fear-reduction as reinforcement in the learning of new responses. *Journal of Experimental Psychology, 38*, 89–101.

Mischel, W. (1968). *Personality and assessment.* New York: Wiley.

Moreno, J. L. (1953). *Who shall survive?: Foundations of sociometry, group psychotherapy and sociodrama.* Beacon, NY: Beacon House.

Mischel, W., & Shoda, Y. (1998). Reconciling processing dynamics and personality dispositions. *Annual Review of Psychology, 49*, 229–258.

Murray, H. A. (1938). *Explorations in personality: A clinical and experimental study of fifty men of collage age.* New York: Oxford University Press.

Orbell, J., & Dawes, R. M. (1993). Social welfare, cooperators' advantage, and the option of not playing the game. *American Sociological Review, 58*, 787–800.

Ozer, D. J., & Benet-Martínez, V. (2006). Personality and the prediction of consequential outcomes. *Annual Review of Psychology, 57*, 401–421.

Peeters, G., & Czapinski, J. (1990). Positive–negative asymmetry in evaluations: The distinction between affective and informational negativity effects. In W. Stroebe & M. Hewstone (Eds.), *European review of social psychology* (Vol. 1, 33–60). Chichester, UK: Wiley.

Pervin, L. A. (1993). Pattern and organization: Current trends and prospects for the future. In K. H. Craik, R. Hogan, & R. N. Wolfe (Eds.), *Fifty years of personality and psychology* (pp. 69–83). New York: Plenum Press.

Petty, R. E., & Cacioppo, J. T. (1981). *Attitudes and persuasion: Classic and contemporary approaches.* Dubuque, IA: Brown.

Petty, R. E., & Wegener, D. W. (1999). The elaboration likelihood model: Current status and controversies. In S. Chaiken & Y. Trope (Eds.), *Dual-process theories in social psychology* (pp. 41–72). New York: Guilford Press.

Pittman, T. S. (1998). Motivation. In D. T. Gilbert, S. T. Fiske, & G. Lindzey (Eds.), *The handbook of social psychology* (4th ed., Vol. 1, pp. 549–590). New York: McGraw-Hill.

Pyszczynski, T., Greenberg, J., & Solomon, S. (1997). Why do we need what we need?: A terror management perspective on the roots of human social motivation. *Psychological Inquiry, 8*, 1–20.

Robins, R. W., & John, O. P. (1997). The quest for self-insight: Theory and research on accuracy and bias in self-perception. In R. Hogan, J. Johnson, & S. Briggs (Eds.), *Handbook of personality psychology* (pp. 649–674). San Diego, CA: Academic Press.

Rogers, C. R. (1961). *On becoming a person.* Boston: Houghton Mifflin.

Rogers, C. R. (1963). Actualizing tendency in relation to "motives" and to consciousness. In M. R. Jones (Ed.), *Nebraska Symposium on Motivation* (Vol. 11, pp. 1–24). Lincoln: University of Nebraska Press.

Rosenthal, R. (1994). Interpersonal expectancy effects: A 30-year perspective. *Current Directions in Psychological Science, 3*, 176–179.

Rotter, J. B. (1966). Generalized expectancies for internal versus external control of reinforcement. *Psychological Monographs, 80*(1, Whole No. 609).

Scheerer, M. (1954). Cognitive theory. In G. Lindzey (Ed.), *Handbook of social psychology* (Vol. 1, pp. 91–142). Reading, MA: Addison-Wesley.

Sears, D. O. (1983). The person-positivity bias. *Journal of Personality and Social Psychology, 44*, 233–250.

Sherif, M., & Sherif, C. W. (1953). *Groups in harmony and tension: An integration of studies on intergroup relations.* New York: Harper.

Sidanius, J., & Pratto, F. (1999). *Social dominance: An intergroup theory of social hierarchy and oppression.* New York: Cambridge University Press.

Skowronski, J. J., & Carlston, D. E. (1989). Negativity and extremity biases in impression formation: A review of explanations. *Psychological Bulletin, 105*, 131–142.

Smith, M. B. (1993). Allport and Murray on Allport's *Personality*: A confrontation in 1946–1947. In K. H. Craik, R. Hogan, & R. N. Wolfe (Eds.), *Fifty years of personality and psychology* (pp. 57–64). New York: Plenum Press.

Snyder, M. (1984). When belief creates reality. In L. Berkowitz (Ed.), *Advances in experimental social psychology* (Vol. 18, pp. 248–306). New York: Academic Press.

Snyder, M., & Cantor, N. (1998). Understanding personality and social behavior: A functionalist strategy. In D. T. Gilbert, S. T. Fiske, & G. Lindzey (Eds.), *The handbook of social psychology* (4th ed., Vol. 2, pp. 635–679). New York: McGraw-Hill.

Spence, K. W. (1956). *Behavior theory and conditioning.* New Haven, CT: Yale University Press.

Stansfeld, S. A., Bosma, H., Hemingway, H., & Marmot, M. G. (1998). Psychosocial work characteristics and social support as predictors of SF-36 health functioning: The Whitehall II study. *Psychosomatic Medicine, 60*, 247–255.

Steele, C. (1988). The psychology of self-affirmation: Sustaining the integrity of the self. In L. Berkowitz (Ed.), *Advances in experimental social psychology* (Vol. 21, pp. 261–302). San Diego, CA: Academic Press.

Stevens, L. E., & Fiske, S. T. (1995). Motivation and cognition in social life: A social survival perspective. *Social Cognition, 13*, 189–214.

Stevens, L. E., & Fiske, S. T. (2000). Motivated impressions of a powerholder: Accuracy under task dependency and misperception under evaluative dependency. *Personality and Social Psychology Bulletin, 26*, 907–922.

Swann, W. B., Jr., Hixon, J. G., Stein-Seroussi, A., & Gilbert, D. T. (1990). The fleeting gleam of praise: Cognitive processes underlying behavioral reactions to self-relevant feedback. *Journal of Personality and Social Psychology, 59*, 17–26.

Tajfel, H. (1981). *Human groups and social categories.* New York: Cambridge University Press.

Tanford, S., & Penrod, S. (1984). Social influence model: A formal integration of research on majority and minority influence processes. *Psychological Bulletin, 95*, 189–225.

Taylor, J. A. (1953). A personality scale of manifest anxiety. *Journal of Abnormal and Social Psychology, 48*, 285–290.

Taylor, S. E. (1991). Asymmetrical effects of positive and negative events: The mobilization-minimization hypothesis. *Psychological Bulletin, 110*, 67–85.

Taylor, S. E., & Brown, J. D. (1988). Illusion and well-being: A social psychological perspective on mental health. *Psychological Bulletin, 103*, 193–210.

Tesser, A. (1988). Toward a self-evaluation maintenance model of social behavior. In L. Berkowitz (Ed.), *Ad-*

*vances in experimental social psychology* (Vol. 21, pp. 181–227). San Diego, CA: Academic Press.

Thibaut, J. W., & Kelley, H. H. (1959). *The social psychology of groups.* New Brunswick, NJ: Transaction.

Tolman, E. C. (1932). *Purposive behavior in animals and men.* Oxford, UK: Appleton-Century.

Triplett, N. (1898). The dynamogenic factors in pacemaking and competition. *American Journal of Psychology, 9*, 507–533.

Trope, Y., & Gaunt, R. (1999). A dual-process model of overconfident attributional inferences. In S. Chaiken & Y. Trope (Eds.), *Dual-process theories in social psychology* (pp. 161–178). New York: Guilford Press.

Turner, J. C., Hogg, M. A., Oakes, P. J., Reicher, S. D., & Wetherell, M. S. (1987). *Rediscovering the social group: A self-categorization theory.* Cambridge, MA: Blackwell.

Uleman, J. S. (1999). Spontaneous versus intentional inferences in impression formation. In S. Chaiken & Y. Trope (Eds.), *Dual-process theories in social psychology* (pp. 141–160). New York: Guilford Press.

Walster, E. M., Berscheid, E., & Walster, G.W. (1973). New directions in equity research. *Journal of Personality and Social Psychology, 25*, 151–176.

Weiner, B. (1985). *Human motivation.* New York: Springer-Verlag.

White, R. W. (1959). Motivation reconsidered: The concepts of competence. *Psychological Review, 66*, 297–333.

Wiggins, J. S., & Trapnell, P. D. (1997). Personality structure: The return of the Big Five. In R. Hogan, J. Johnson, & S. Briggs (Eds.), *Handbook of personality psychology* (pp. 737–765). San Diego, CA: Academic Press.

Williams, K. D., Cheung, C. K. T., & Choi, W. (2000). Cyberostracism: Effects of being ignored over the Internet. *Journal of Personality and Social Psychology, 79*, 748–762.

Yamagishi, T. (1998). *The structure of trust: An evolutionary game of mind and society.* Tokyo: Tokyo University Press.

Zajonc, R. B. (1965). Social facilitation. *Science, 149*, 269–274.

Zajonc, R. B. (1968). Attitudinal effects of mere exposure. *Journal of Personality and Social Psychology, 9*, 1–27.

# PART II

# Forms and Systems of Motivation

# DIFFERENT FORMS OF MOTIVATION

Chapter 2

# Belongingness Motivation

## A MAINSPRING OF SOCIAL ACTION

**Mark R. Leary**
**Cody B. Cox**

In the first edition of Lindzey's *Handbook of Social Psychology*, published in 1954, Gardner Murphy proposed that a full understanding of human behavior must begin with an examination of the "raw material" of human nature—the "primitive mainsprings of social action" that underlie social and cultural behavior (p. 601). Murphy pointed out that theories of social motivation tend to fall into three general types: one-drive theories (such as psychoanalytic theory) that trace most if not all behavior to a single motivational process; drive catalogs that identify large numbers of basic motives or needs (such as McDougall's system of instincts); and middle-range theories that identify a limited number of basic, flexible tendencies upon which other, more complex motives are built. Murphy himself offered such a middle-range model of motivation, in which complex social motives—such as motives for conformity, communication, leadership, love, and prestige—are derived from more basic categories of visceral, activity, sensory, and emergency drives.

Midway through his chapter, Murphy (1954) mentioned, almost in passing, that people are motivated to be accepted and supported by others. He noted that "in every society . . . there appears to be a considerable amount of satisfaction from sheer functioning as a member of a group," and that studies of group dynamics reveal "the very strong positive satisfactions of discovering closeness with others" (p. 602). However, he did not seem to place any special emphasis on the motive to be accepted, relative to the other motives he discussed.

In the years since Murphy's (1954) chapter was published, many other psychologists have also noted that people desire to be accepted by others. And, like Murphy, most of them have not placed any special importance on belongingness, viewing it as just another motive alongside motives for affiliation, achievement, power, self-esteem, differentiation, cognition, meaning, and so on. The primary theme of the present chapter is that the human motive for social acceptance and belonging should not be viewed as simply one among many equally important and potent social motives. Rather, we argue that the need for acceptance and belonging (or *belongingness motivation*) is a fundamental social motive that underlies and helps to explain a great deal of human behavior. In fact, this motive is so basic to human behavior that the first premise of virtually every theory of social or cultural behavior could be that people "have a pervasive drive to form and maintain at least a minimum quantity of lasting, positive, and significant interpersonal relationships" (Baumeister & Leary, 1995, p. 497). We are not claiming that other social motives do not exist, or that all social behavior may be traced to the need to belong. However, as we hope to show, the belongingness motive provides a fundamental psychic "engine" or "energy source" (to use Murphy's [1954] metaphor) for a great deal of human social behavior.

This chapter is organized as follows. We first review evidence, previously described in much greater detail by Baumeister and Leary (1995), that belongingness motivation should be considered a fundamental motive that is not reducible to other motives, and we grapple with the question of whether belongingness should be considered a single motive or a set of motives. We then examine an array of social psychological phenomena that appear to stem from people's need for acceptance and belongingness, showing the generality and the applicability of belongingness for understanding aspects of attraction, conformity, group behavior, attitudes, self-presentation, culture, and other behavior. Operating from the assumption that a fundamental motive will be mediated by neural and neurochemical systems, we then explore possible physiological mechanisms that underlie people's quest for belonging.

## EVIDENCE FOR THE NEED TO BELONG

Many theorists have acknowledged that people seek to develop and maintain social bonds with other people (e.g., Bowlby, 1969; Horney, 1945; James, 1890; Maslow, 1968), but none has accorded belongingness motivation the prominence that we believe it deserves. The fullest exposition of the centrality of belongingness to human behavior was offered by Baumeister and Leary (1995), who reviewed an extensive body of evidence to support the notion that the need to belong is a fundamental human motive. Without revisiting all of the evidence they offered for this claim, we begin by briefly summarizing just a few major points.

Baumeister and Leary (1995) pointed out that people form social bonds very easily, without special eliciting circumstances (and even in adverse situations when the presence of other people is associated with negative experiences). People in every culture belong to small primary groups (Mann, 1980) and form a variety of relationships with family members, friends, mates, and others. Cultures differ in the type, number, and permanence of the relationships that people form, but there are no societies in which people do not form social connections with one another. Furthermore, psychological research has repeatedly demonstrated that people quickly and easily develop group identifications (e.g., Billig & Tajfel, 1973; Sherif, Harvey, White, Hood, & Sherif, 1961), attachments with caregivers (Bowlby, 1969), and relationships with strangers (Wilder & Thompson, 1980). Thus the need to belong appears to be universal and innate, occurring in all normal individuals in all cultures, without any special circumstances needed for it to emerge.

Once social bonds form, people are very reluctant to allow them to dissolve, even when relationships have no functional value and may even cause distress or harm. For example, people who are part of time-limited relationships (e.g., participants in weekend retreats or encounter groups, fellow cruise passengers, and members of seasonal teams) may find the end of their time together upsetting and vow to maintain contact afterwards. In the case of established relationships, events that undermine connections—as when people move away—are distressing and accompanied by going-away rituals and promises to maintain the relationship. And, as Baumeister and Leary (1995) observed, "These patterns seem to occur even if the dissolving relationship (e.g., with neighbors) had no important or instrumental function and there is no realistic likelihood of further contact" (p. 502). Reunions also signify people's interest in maintaining at least occasional contact with those with whom they once had ongoing relationships. Perhaps most interesting are instances in which people maintain unsatisfying, unhappy relationships, as when people seem unwilling to leave bad relationships and abusive spouses. Clearly, people are strongly motivated both to establish and to maintain social connections with other people.

Another piece of evidence to support the importance of belongingness motivation is that a great many of people's thoughts, emotions, and conversations involve the state of their interpersonal relationships, indicating that relationships are personally important. People think a great deal about other people, drawing inferences about their characteristics, making attributions for their behavior, and trying to discern how others perceive them. Similarly, changes in social connections are a primary source of emotions. Given that negative emotions arise from events that people perceive as threats to their well-being (Frijda, 1986), the strong aversive emotions that accompany real, potential, and imagined threats to social connections—such as hurt feelings, loneliness, anger, sadness, and jealousy—suggest that damage to social bonds constitute a perceived threat (Leary, Koch, & Hechenbleikner, 2001). Conversely, the formation and strengthening of interpersonal bonds are typically accompanied by positive emotions, such as happiness and joy, suggesting that these events are highly desired.

Of course, people may be happy when their desires are met and unhappy when they are not, but such reactions do not necessarily indicate that those desires should be regarded as "needs" or fundamental motives. Rather, the concept of a need implies that failure to satisfy the need results not only in distress but in dysfunctional outcomes. Indeed, deprivation effects may be the defining features that distinguish needs from mere wants or wishes. People who do not satisfy important needs typically demonstrate evidence of deprivation by experiencing adverse effects and being particularly motivated to satisfy the needs. Along these lines, people who do not experience adequate belongingness show an array of adverse effects, including stress, depression, poor psychological adjustment, a lowered ability to self-regulate, and compromised physical health (for a review, see Baumeister & Leary, 1995). Furthermore, they tend to dwell on their weak social connections and seek ways to strengthen them. Moreover, like other basic motives, the need to belong shows evidence that it can be satiated. People who have adequate social bonds are less interested in seeking additional relationships than those whose need to belong is unfulfilled.

A final consideration in assessing whether belongingness ought to be regarded as a fundamental need involves its evolutionary significance. Many theorists have noted that interpersonal relationships and group memberships were an absolute necessity for the survival and reproductive success of *Homo sapiens* and their hominid ancestors (Barash, 1977; Baumeister & Leary, 1995; Hogan, Jones, & Cheek, 1985). Lacking speed, ferocity, and evasive behaviors (such as winged flight, tree clambering, or burrowing), our ancestors survived throughout evolutionary history primarily because they lived in cooperative social groups that provided mutual protection and support. Natural selection would have favored those individuals who established and maintained supportive relationships with others, and those who had no urge to associate with and be accepted by others would have fared quite poorly in the struggle to survive and reproduce. The fact that human beings (as well as other social mammals) appear to have physiological systems designed to mediate relationships with conspecifics further supports the notion that people are biologically prepared to seek and maintain social relationships. We will return later to the physiology of belongingness.

## ONE MOTIVE OR MANY?

Baumeister and Leary (1995) implicitly conceptualized the need to belong as a single motive that involves fostering and maintaining a wide array of relationships with other people. In their review of the literature, they presented evidence regarding people's relationships with friends, romantic partners, family members, group members, and even strangers. In a broad sense, there seems to be little doubt that people are motivated to establish and maintain lasting, positive, and significant interpersonal relationships of all kinds. Yet one may raise the question of whether belongingness motivation reflects a single broad motive that can be directed toward establishing relationships with an array of targets (e.g., friends, family members, mates, group members), or whether it actually consists of several discrete motives that direct efforts to establish relationships with various categories of individuals.

The possibility that people possess several distinct belongingness motives is raised by evolutionary psychology's assumption that the mind is composed of many domain-specific mechanisms or modules that evolved to handle particular adaptive challenges. Given that different adaptive problems require different solutions, a separate mechanism is needed for each qualitatively different problem (see Symons, 1992). In the interpersonal arena, different kinds of relationships are characterized by different behavioral and emotional features; pose different problems that require different solutions; and, at least in the ancestral environment, would have involved different implications for survival, reproduction, and inclusive fitness.

Along these lines, Kirkpatrick and Ellis (2001) identified four fundamental types of social collectives to which people seek to belong, to which we add a fifth. First, people form into macro-level groups, such as tribes, villages, communities, or nations. The members of these groups may or may not have direct contact with all other members, but they nonetheless identify as members of these collectives because the groups offer various benefits, such as access to resources and defense against members of other groups. Second, people form instrumental coalitions—groups of people who work directly together to achieve mutually desired goals. Hunting parties were perhaps the earliest instrumental coalitions. Today, people join committees, teams, gangs, work groups, army units, civic organizations, unions, neighborhood associations, and other task-oriented groups.

Third, people form relationships for the purpose of mating. Indeed, they may form different sorts of mating relationships, ranging from one-time liaisons to long-term monogamous pairings. Fourth, people in every culture have an array of kin relationships that are maintained primarily on the basis of genetic relatedness rather than (or in addition to) social exchange, because each person has a biological interest in the well-being of genetic relatives.

To these, we add a fifth category—namely, supportive friendships. Friendships develop on the basis of a mutual communal orientation in which each individual can rely on the support of his or her friends. Friendships provide ongoing companionship and support that span time, roles, and tasks, and provide an interpersonal insurance policy for occasions when one is in dire need. People seem to have a limited number of friendship niches that they desire to keep filled (Tooby & Cosmides, 1996).

Presumably, most people are motivated to form and maintain all five kinds of relationships, at least sooner or later. Furthermore, belongingness in each kind may be monitored and regulated by a different system (Kirkpatrick & Ellis, 2001). However, we believe that a strong qualification is in order. Specifically, two facts raise the possibility that people may be motivated to be accepted generically, as well as motivated to form certain kinds of relationships.

First, as Baumeister and Leary (1995) noted, one relationship may, to an extent, substitute for another. This is most obvious when relationships are of the same type: A new friendship or romantic relationship may quickly replace a former one, and people may wish to belong to one or more instrumental coalitions but may not care very much precisely what the group does or who else is in it. However, some substitution also occurs across relationships. For example, people in new romantic relationships often withdraw from their same-sex friends, seeming to need them less than before. Similarly, a person without close friends may derive a great deal of social satisfaction from working in instrumental groups or spending more time with family members. To be sure, the substitution is rarely total; family members do not fully replace friends or lovers, for example. But the fact that substitution occurs at all suggests that all relationships may satisfy some generic need to belong, in addition to whatever special features each type of relationship may have.

Second, as Kirkpartick and Ellis (2001) noted, the criteria for acceptance into and rejection from these various kinds of relationships differ greatly. Community memberships are typically based on shared heritage or attitudes; instrumental coalitions on competence and ability to contribute to the group; mating relationships on mate value; kin relationships on genetic relatedness and willingness to sacrifice for family members; and friendships on the basis of being a reliable source of companionship and support. In light of this, it seems unlikely that a single mechanism could have evolved to monitor one's inclusion in all five types of groups. Even so, many criteria for acceptance and rejection apply across all kinds of relationships. A person who behaves in an untrustworthy, selfish, duplicitous, or cruel fashion toward other individuals is not valued as a relational partner, no matter what type of relationship we might imagine. Just as people can be said to be generally motivated to eat, yet also to be motivated to eat certain kinds of foods (as when a deficiency causes cravings for foods containing a particular nutrient), people may be said to have a general need to belong, even though they are also motivated to establish and maintain certain kinds of relationships that provide specific benefits.

## IMPLICATIONS OF THE NEED TO BELONG FOR UNDERSTANDING HUMAN BEHAVIOR

As noted earlier, the assumption that people have a pervasive drive to form and maintain a minimum number of lasting, positive, and significant interpersonal relationships can be viewed as the first and most fundamental principle in social psychology. Little else in social psychology makes sense without reference to the fact that people desire to be accepted and to avoid rejection. A species that was otherwise identical to *Homo sapiens* but that lacked this basic motive would behave quite differently than modern human beings do. We are not in any way suggesting that all interpersonal behavior emerges from the need to belong; clearly, behavior is determined by a wide array of factors, many of which have nothing whatsoever to do with belongingness. Even so, we maintain not only that a great deal of interpersonal behavior directly reflects concerns with belongingness, but also that, whatever other goals people may pursue, they typically do so in ways that do not jeopardize their acceptance by other people. Thus concerns with social acceptance not only determine certain behaviors directly, but also constrain most other behaviors in which people engage.

Space does not permit us to discuss all of the areas of psychology that may be illuminated by considering the need to belong. Thus, to provide a sense of how important belongingness is in human behavior, we overview only seven relevant topics: conformity and compliance; interpersonal attraction; enhancing personal acceptability; intergroup processes; attitudes and social influence; aggression; and cultural institutions.

### Conformity and Compliance

A great deal of behavior has been explained with reference to the fact that people regularly conform to social norms, bringing their opinions and behaviors into line with those of other people. Traditionally, theorists have distinguished two general reasons why people conform: because others' behavior provides useful information regarding the most effective or accurate response (*informational influence*), or because others' beliefs and actions provide information regarding socially appropriate ways to respond, and deviations from these norms are criticized and punished (*normative influence*) (Kelley, 1952). Although informational influence is largely unrelated to belonging, normative influence emerges directly from people's concerns with rejection. Given that people who violate social norms and deviate too extensively from the behaviors of the majority tend to be devalued, marginalized, and ostracized (Marques, Abrams, Pàez, & Hogg, 2001; Schachter, 1951), it is not surprising that people routinely conform, even when doing so requires them to disregard their own sensory perceptions and personal values (Asch, 1955). People are sometimes willing to sacrifice their well-being, violate their standards, and hurt others in the pursuit of acceptance and belonging.

Of course, people conform more to the standards of certain individuals and groups than to others. Merton and Kitt (1950) adopted the concept of *reference group* to describe the groups to which people most strongly tailor their attitudes and behavior. In our view, reference groups may be conceptualized as consisting of those individuals whose acceptance a person most strongly desires; this explains why people conform so strongly to reference groups.

Conformity is often regarded as a superficial, and typically undesired, acquiescence to others' judgments. However, the belongingness perspective suggests that the inclination to conform is both natural and adaptive. Because satisfaction of most personal and social needs typically requires people to be at least minimally accepted by others, an individual who never accommodated his or her behaviors to social norms or the actions of other people would be unable to satisfy even the most basic needs. The problem, then, is not that people conform, but rather that some of the norms that guide people's behavior lead to actions that are harmful to themselves or others.

## Interpersonal Attraction

Although people are highly motivated to establish and maintain an array of relationships, they are nonetheless selective in their choices of those with whom they interact and establish interpersonal connections. Research has identified many factors that affect the degree to which people like and desire to relate to others, but one prevailing finding is that people are most inclined to like and pursue relationships with those they believe are likely to like and accept them (Aron, Dutton, Aron, & Iverson, 1989; Gold, Ryckman, & Mosley, 1984). This pattern is also reflected in people's preference for those similar to them on almost any dimension—racial and ethnic background, attitudes, level of physical attractiveness, educational level, social status, and so on. Many explanations have been offered for the link between similarity and attraction, but one may be the fact that people believe they are most likely to be accepted by those to whom they are similar. Put differently, people are not inclined to waste their time trying to establish relationships with those who—by virtue of differences in personality, attitudes, background, or lifestyle—are not likely to become or remain a source of belongingness.

Recently, Leder (2004) showed that people report greater feelings of love toward individuals they believe have the potential to provide them with closeness, support, validation, acceptance, and other evidence of psychological intimacy. Again, it seems that people naturally gravitate toward those they believe are likely to accept them. Furthermore, once in a close relationship, people regulate their closeness with their partners depending on how accepted they feel. According to Murray, Holmes, and Griffin's (2000) dependency regulation model, people are willing to extend themselves to relationship partners only to the degree that they feel secure about the relationships. Furthermore, people usually abandon relationships in which they feel insufficiently valued and accepted. The recognition that one is no longer accepted typically results, sometimes after efforts at reconciliation, in the dissolution of a relationship.

## Enhancing Personal Acceptability

Not only do people tend to seek out and like those who may accept them, but they also devote a great deal of effort to making themselves acceptable to others as well. Most obviously, people use a wide array of self-presentational tactics to convey particular impressions of themselves to others (Leary, 1995). Of course, the impressions that people try to convey depend on their goals in a particular situation, and often those goals have little to do with belonging. For example, people may wish to appear intimidating to influence others to do as they wish, or to seem helpless to gain others' assistance. Yet it seems likely that people devote more self-presentational effort to trying to be accepted by other people than to any other interpersonal goal.

Jones and Pittman (1982) identified ingratiation, self-promotion, and exemplification as three fundamental self-presentational strategies that are designed to convey images of being likeable, competent, and exemplary, respectively. These three self-presentational strategies are fundamentally important, in part, because they are the most important determinants of interpersonal acceptance. People who are viewed as likeable, competent, and exemplary are more valued as social interactants and relational partners than those who are not. Thus people desire to foster these kinds of impressions (and try not to behave in ways that negate them), and are quite attuned to evidence that others see them as unlikeable, incompetent, or deviant. Much of self-presentation is directed toward fostering and maintaining social acceptance (Leary, 1995).

People promote their acceptance in other ways as well. For example, research shows that people distance themselves from those who outperform them on tasks that are important to their own identity. According to *self-evaluation maintenance* theory (Tesser, 1988), people do this to maintain a favorable self-evaluation, but concerns with belongingness may also be involved. Being outperformed by another person has implications for one's social acceptance, particularly if the other person is a member of one's social network, because those who are superior on some personally relevant dimension render one's own social value lower. Thus people may either distance themselves from the other person or belittle the other's accomplishments (Tesser, 1988), thereby taking steps to make sure that their unique position is not superseded by others who may be more capable.

A similar effect may be seen in Brewer's (1991) work on *optimal distinctiveness*. According to optimal distinctiveness theory, the maintenance of a person's social identity is driven by two basic needs—a need for group inclusion and belonging (assimilation), and a need for distinctiveness from other group members (differentiation). Because people seek to maintain an optimal level of assimilation and differentiation, perceiving that one is either too similar to or too dissimilar from other group members leads to behaviors that rectify the imbalance. Viewing optimal distinctiveness from the standpoint of belongingness sheds a somewhat different light on the process, however. In our view, only a single motive underlies optimal distinctiveness phenomena. Although people undoubtedly possess a genuine need for belongingness and inclusion, we doubt that they also possess a "need" for differentiation. People strive for differentiation not because they need to be different, but rather to maximize their value to the group, and thus to enhance their belongingness. A fully assimilated individual who is just like everyone else is essentially redundant and dispensable. Maximizing one's social acceptance requires people to be sufficiently assimilated to share fundamental attributes with the group, but sufficiently differentiated to be uniquely valued.

## Intergroup Processes

People are highly motivated to be accepted, but they do not indiscriminately or promiscuously seek acceptance from everyone they meet. This fact can perhaps be seen most clearly in intergroup phenomena through which people create boundaries between themselves and others, such as ingroup favoritism, outgroup derogation, and prejudice. The process of establishing belongingness with one group seems to be accompanied by the process of forgoing, if not discouraging, belongingness with other groups. The *minimal group* paradigm has repeatedly shown how little is required for members of one group to erect boundaries between themselves and others, devaluing, disadvantaging, and rejecting members of other groups (Diehl, 1990). People regularly treat members of other groups in ways that undermine the connections between them, often for no apparent reason.

Although the ease with which people distance themselves from and discriminate against others may seem inconsistent with a pervasive and powerful need to belong, such behaviors may in fact promote social acceptance. For starters, people do not need to be accepted by everyone. Once they are accepted by a minimum number of supportive individuals with whom they can establish cooperative, mutually beneficial relationships of various kinds, further relationships are of relatively little value. (As the number of one's relationships grows, the marginal utility of additional relationships decreases.) Not only are additional relationships less valuable, but, given constraints on one's time and energy, attempting to pursue and maintain additional relationships may undermine the relationships that one already has. The costs of unbridled sociality are very high (Kurzban & Leary, 2002), so people conserve time and energy by actively discouraging further relationships. Perhaps this is why people seem to have a relatively small number of friendship niches (Tooby & Cosmides, 1996) and usually do not pursue new friendships unless one of those niches becomes vacant.

In making choices among groups and relationships, people presumably assess the potential value of those relationships. Because such decisions must often be made quickly in the absence of concrete information about others' characteristics, people may rely on heuristics to assess the degree to which a potential relationship is likely to provide desired outcomes, including social acceptance and support. As noted earlier, acceptance is generally facilitated by similarity, so proxies for psychological similarity (e.g., skin color, ethnicity, language, and indicators of social status) may be used, resulting in the dismissal of members of superficially dissimilar groups.

Derogating and rejecting members of other groups may foster acceptance in yet another way. External threats increase ingroup cohesion and enhance members' attraction for one another (Dion, 1979). Thus, when group members implicitly collude to identify members of another group as the "enemy," the connections among ingroup members may be strengthened.

## Attitudes and Social Influence

Traditionally, attitudes have been conceptualized as intrapsychic structures, and attitude change has been viewed primarily as a cognitive process (albeit one that may be influenced by social factors). Yet there is no question that attitude acquisition and change are strongly affected by people's interpersonal concerns, including their concerns with social acceptance.

People tend to adopt attitudes that are likely to result in social acceptance from people whose acceptance they value—a point emphasized by Smith, Bruner, and White's (1956) discussion of the *social adjustment* function of attitudes. This is not to say that people do not sometimes hold attitudes that others disapprove of, but the general pattern is to have attitudes that facilitate rather than impede acceptance. And when people's private attitudes differ from those of significant others whose acceptance is important to them, they often express attitudes that are more similar to those of the others than is actually the case (see Schlenker, 1980, for a review).

Consistency processes, such as those assumed to underlie cognitive dissonance, also have a strong interpersonal component. Without denying that people prefer intrapsychic consistency over dissonance, it is also clear that people are at least as concerned with *appearing* consistent to others as with actually being consistent. The effects of performing counterattitudinal actions on attitudes are particularly pronounced when people's counterattitudinal behaviors are public and people are concerned with their image in other people's eyes (Schlenker, Forsyth, Leary, & Miller, 1980). In such cases, apparent attitude change is motivated by self-presentation concerns arising from the desire to appear consistent, presumably because inconsistency and hypocrisy undermine social acceptance and disqualify people as relational partners in good standing.

Similarly, many of the strategies by which people influence one another play upon the target's desire to be accepted. For example, the process of *reciprocal concessions*, in which people meet others' concessions with concessions of their own, seems to rely on people's desire to be seen as fair and conciliatory. Because obstinate, uncompromising individuals are not viewed as good friends or coalition partners, people feel compelled to reciprocate when others concede.

## Aggression

A wide variety of factors promote aggressive behavior, including frustration, aversive stimuli (e.g., heat, pain), and aggressive role models. One important set of precipitating events that has not received adequate attention involves those that connote interpersonal rejection. People who feel rejected often become angry and lash out at those who have rejected them (Buckley, Winkel, & Leary, 2004; Downey, Feldman, & Ayduk, 2000; Twenge, Baumeister, Tice, & Stucke, 2001).

The link between rejection and aggression is noteworthy not only because it demonstrates another important consequence of unfulfilled belongingness, but also because of what it implies about the nature of the belongingness motive. If, as emotion theorists suggest, anger and aggression are typically reactions to perceived threats (Frijda, 1986), the fact that rejection reliably makes people angry and inclined to aggress suggests that rejection is appraised as a serious threat to well-being.

The irony, of course, is that behaving aggressively is rarely a successful strategy for enhancing acceptance. Occasionally, aggression (or even threats of aggression) may deter rejection or abandonment (as in the case of an abusive spouse whose threats deter the partner from leaving), but almost always at the cost of liking and goodwill. Why, then, do people want to hurt those who reject them? In a review of the literature on the link between rejection and aggression, Leary, Twenge, and Quinlivan (2006) have recently examined several processes that might account for the effect. Although they conclude that the current literature is not adequate to resolve the issue of which explanation is most plausible, they discuss two possibilities that point specifically to the role of belongingness. First, Leary and colleagues suggest that feeling accepted may inhibit aggression in the face of stimuli that might otherwise make people respond aggressively. Because aggression nearly always damages interpersonal relationships, people generally avoid acting aggressively toward those who accept them. However, once acceptance from others is no longer forthcoming, those restraints are loosened, increasing the likelihood of aggression. Put differently, rejection greatly lowers the social costs of behaving aggressively. Thus, aside from whatever effects rejection may have on aggression directly, it may also loosen the constraints on aggressive behavior.

Second, aggression may function to drive away those who do not accept us. People who do not accept us are unlikely to provide valued outcomes (such as support and companionship); may exact costs that are not reciprocated; or, even worse, may try to do us harm. Thus, in a strictly pragmatic sense, there is not only nothing to gain by relating to them, but possibly good reasons to dissuade them from interacting with us at all.

## Cultural Institutions

If belongingness is a fundamental human motive, we would expect to see widespread evidence of cultural institutions that offer opportunities for belonging. Perhaps the most obvious examples are the innumerable social groups to which people belong. Many groups have explicit purposes that can be achieved only through working with other people (e.g., political action groups, sports teams, neighborhood associations, and professional groups), and people may join these groups for reasons other than belongingness per se. Even so, one gets the impression that the appeal of joining these groups comes as much from the satisfaction of belongingness as from accomplishing the group's stated goals.

Even churches, temples, and synagogues—groups that, on the surface, exist for personal religious study and worship—provide important opportunities for interaction and belonging, and a climate of welcoming acceptance is viewed as essential for attracting and retaining members. Indeed, many people would hesitate to attend a church that did not sponsor occasional social events (dinners, picnics, interest groups) or that discouraged its members from interacting with one another. It is informative that people can more easily articulate the differences between the sorts of people who attend their own versus other churches than can describe how their own church's doctrine differs from that of other churches (Stark & Bainbridge, 1985); this suggests that people's choice of which church to attend is heavily influenced by interpersonal factors.

In addition to groups that have a purported nonsocial purpose, many other groups exist primarily, if not exclusively, to promote the belongingness of their members. Social fraternities and sororities, for example, may engage in various service activities, but their primary purpose is to foster the social lives of their members. (The fact that their members call one another "brothers" and "sisters" highlights the emphasis placed on forming close relationships.) Furthermore, in the case of certain leisure and recreation groups, a group's ostensible purpose—to play cards, bowl, ski, practice yoga, or discuss popular books, for example—is often secondary to the opportunity to interact with and form relationships with other people.

On the dyadic level, the most obvious example of a cultural institution that promotes belonging is marriage. Marriage exists in almost every society to recognize the special social status of married individuals and to provide means of protecting the marital relationship from outsiders. But marriage may also reflect an institutional means of satisfying the desire for acceptance by offering a sanctioned way to promote long-term belongingness. The traditional marriage vow that promises unfaltering commitment "till death do us part" may reflect an institutionalized mechanism for helping to maintain belongingness.

Modern technological advances also reflect people's need for social connection. In the United States, the Internet is most commonly used as a means of communication via e-mail, and of the more than 200 million people who use the Internet worldwide, approximately 25% report visiting Internet chatrooms or online discussions (Madden, 2003). Online games also promote a sense of community, even though the players are not in one another's presence and may not even know one another's identities. Software developers develop multiplayer options for their games because they realize that providing an interpersonal feature will enhance the game's success.

## Summary

These and other patterns of social behavior make sense only with reference to the fact that people are pervasively and powerfully motivated to be accepted and to avoid rejection. People's social behaviors would be quite different had human beings evolved under conditions that did not put such a premium on social acceptance. To repeat a point made earlier, we are not claiming that all behavior, or even all social behavior, stems from the belongingness motive. Most notably, patterns of behavior involving dominance, status, and power typically involve efforts to influence other people without regard to social acceptance. Even so, however, people sometimes seek power and status to promote their social acceptance (Leary, Cottrell, & Phillips, 2001), and influence must often be exercised in ways that do not sacrifice one's own belonging.

## THE PHYSIOLOGICAL UNDERPINNINGS OF BELONGINGNESS

Given the adaptive significance of social acceptance, one would expect to find neurological substrates that facilitate the development and maintenance of social bonds. Over the last 30 years, researchers have become increasingly interested in the physiological aspects of social relationships (Levine, Caspi, & Laufer, 1997), focusing on the physiological underpinnings of parent–child bonding, mating/romantic relationships, and everyday social interactions.

Researchers have identified areas of the central nervous system that are involved in social relationships, as well as neuropeptides and endogenous neurochemicals that facilitate social interactions and bonding. Unfortunately, two factors have impeded progress in this area. First, some promising candidate neuropeptides are difficult to study in human beings because they do not cross the blood–brain barrier. As a result, their effects cannot be studied experimentally with peripheral administrations of the chemicals (Insel, 2000). Additionally, only a small number of laboratory animals demonstrate the kinds of selective affiliation and relationship development that are characteristic of human beings (Insel, 1997), which limits the ability to use animals as models. For example, only 3% of mammals display biological monogamy that resembles pair bonding in human beings (Insel, 2003).

One unlikely animal popular in this research area is the prairie vole found in midwestern North America. Prairie voles are useful both because they display a variety of selective social behaviors and because they are very similar to the nonsocial montane vole, which allows for comparisons between two closely related animals that demonstrate great differences in social behavior (Insel, 1997). Research with the prairie vole has identified several neurochemicals that appear to affect bonding, and the evidence for two of these appears particularly compelling. Specifically, oxytocin and vasopressin consistently play important roles in social affiliation and possibly bonding. Oxytocin and vasopressin are very similar compounds, differing in only two amino acids (Insel, 1997), and the gene for both of these neuropeptides occupies the same chromosome (Carter, 1998).

In prairie voles, the effects of oxytocin and vasopressin appear to be sexually dimorphic. Male prairie voles that receive a vasopressin antagonist do not form pair bonds after mating, whereas female voles that receive an oxytocin antagonist do not form bonds after mating (Insel, 1997). However, strong doses of either oxytocin or vasopressin can induce pair bonding, which may indicate sex differences in sensitivity to these neuropeptides (Curtis & Wang, 2003). Likewise, newborn voles treated with oxytocin antagonists do not develop a normal preference for their mothers (Nelson & Panksepp, 1998).

Similarly, oxytocin plays a role in social recognition among rats. Rats given infusions of oxytocin show an increased recognition for other rats to which they have been previously exposed. In contrast, rats whose receptors for oxytocin are "knocked out" lose the ability to recognize familiar rats. This debility is specific to social memory, and other forms of memory function normally (Ferguson, Aldag, Insel, & Young, 2001). Vasopressin may play a similar role in facial recognition in human beings. Intranasal administration of vasopressin raises the electromyogram response to an emotionally neutral face to the level of the response of control groups to an angry face, which may indicate that vasopressin affects the overall response to social stimuli (Thompson, Gupta, Miller, Mills, & Orr, 2002).

Experimental research on the effects of oxytocin in human beings is difficult because oxytocin does not cross the blood–brain barrier (Curtis & Wang, 2003), though this may not be true of vasopressin (Thompson et al., 2002). Even so, research on oxytocin and vasopressin suggests that both are involved in human bonding. For example, breast stimulation releases oxytocin into the circulatory system in women during lactation. Given that oxytocin release may be a subjectively pleasant experience, the affective experience of the release may be then conditioned to the infant, thereby promoting maternal bonding (Carter, 1998). Additionally, evidence indicates that oxytocin is released during orgasm in both men and women (Riley, 1988).

In understanding how oxytocin and vasopressin facilitate social bonding, researchers have examined the locations of oxytocin and vasopressin receptors in the brain. The distribution of oxytocin and vasopressin receptors is species-specific (Carter, 1992). Insel (2003) has noted that the oxytocin receptors in prairie voles (the highly social species) are concentrated in the reward centers of the brain, such as the nucleus accumbens, whereas the oxytocin receptors in the montane vole (the less social species) are located in regions of the brain associated with nonsocial behavior. The specific locations of these receptors may explain the different behavioral effects of oxytocin in these two species, particularly given that they do not differ in the distribution of receptors for other hormones. Indeed, after inserting a prairie vole vasopressin receptor gene into a mouse genome, researchers produced unique affiliative behaviors in the genetically altered mice by exposing them to vasopressin (Young, Nilsen, Waymire, MacGregor, & Insel, 1999).

Oxytocin and vasopressin receptors in the human brain have also been found in dopaminergic systems often associated with reward centers (Insel, 2000). Dopamine plays an important role in the reward system and may also facilitate the rewarding affective quality of social bonds (Carter, 1998). Noting that this pathway seems similar to pathways implicated in drug use, Insel (2003) has suggested that the pathways that evolved for social interaction may be utilized by addictive drugs, extending MacLean's (1990) speculation that substance abuse is an attempt to generate neurochemicals that are produced naturally during positive social interactions.

Brain areas involving social bonding are also implicated in research involving opioids and attachment. According to the brain opioid theory of social attachment, social contact causes the release of endogenous opioids, whereas social isolation lowers basal opioid levels, which motivates individuals to seek social contact (Nelson & Panksepp, 1998). One example of this pattern can be seen in rat pups. The ultrasonic vocalizations that rat pups emit when isolated are eliminated if pups either are placed with an anesthetized littermate (which provides the presence of a conspecific, albeit a nonresponsive one) or receive low doses of an opioid such as morphine. However, if an opioid antagonist, such as naltrexone, is administered, then the presence of a littermate does not affect ultrasonic vocalizations (Carden, Hernandez, & Hofer, 1996; see also Nelson & Panksepp, 1998). Also, administering morphine (an opioid) reduces the pursuit of social interaction in several species, including nonhuman primates (Martel, Nevison, Simpson, & Keverne, 1995).

Activity in the hypothalamic–pituitary–adrenal (HPA) axis is also associated with social bonding. In her review of the literature on the neuroendocrinology of attachment, Carter (1998) observed that social interactions decrease HPA axis activity and that negative interactions reduce it. For example, HPA hormones increase after an animal is separated from others and decrease during reunion (Carter, 1998). Oxytocin and vasopressin may also reduce HPA activity. As a result, peptidergic systems utilizing oxytocin and vasopressin may inhibit innate defensive behaviors (such as automatic defensive or aggressive responses to unfamiliar stimuli) and allow social bonds to develop (Carter, 1998).

As noted, rejection typically results in negative emotions, if not acute feelings of being hurt (Leary & Springer, 2000; MacDonald & Leary, 2005), so we should expect to find that rejection experiences involve neurophysiological systems that are associated with negative affect and pain. Panksepp, MacDonald, and others have proposed that during the course of mammalian evolution, the system that promotes and maintains social connections was built on top of more primitive systems that mediate physical pain (MacDonald, Kingsbury, & Shaw, 2005; Panksepp, 1998). Specifically, MacDonald and Leary (2005) argue that the "hurt feelings" that result from interpersonal rejection utilize the same system as *pain affect*—the emotionally aversive component of physical pain that can be distinguished from its physically aversive sensations. In support of this idea, Eisenberger, Lieberman, and Williams (2003) found in a functional magnetic resonance imaging study that social exclusion activates the anterior cingulate cortex (ACC), which has been implicated in the negative affect associated with physical pain. (However, if the social exclusion is inadvertent, the right ventral prefrontal cortex is also activated.) These findings suggest that the negative affect following social exclusion may utilize some of the same neurological mechanisms as physical pain.

In brief, researchers have begun to develop models of neurophysiological mechanisms that may underlie social affiliation and bonding. Oxytocin and vasopressin clearly play an important role in bonding, and research seems to indicate that these neuropeptides also suppress defensive behaviors toward individuals with whom the bond is shared. Neurochemicals in the reward system may also make bonding a phenomenologically rewarding experience, while activation of the ACC makes social exclusion phenomenologically painful.

Much of this research raises the provocative idea that people (and nonhuman animals that show similar patterns of affiliation and bonding) are motivated to seek social connections because such connections affect neurophysiological systems that involve reward centers, and thus are inherently pleasurable. At its root, then, belongingness motivation may be fed by a desire for the pleasurable experience of being connected to another person. This research is in its infancy, and questions may be raised regarding the degree to which the systems identified in nonhuman animals are responsible for either the human need to belong or the rewarding features of interpersonal acceptance. Even so, given that social connections have been important throughout human evolution, specific neurological mechanisms seem to have evolved to support the pursuit and development of social bonds.

## CONCLUSIONS

We once heard of a social scientist who had contracted to write a scholarly book about hermits, setting out to locate and interview people who not only lived alone but avoided human contact and eschewed relationships of all kinds. He tracked down dozens of individuals whom other people identified as recluses, but he was eventually forced to abandon the project because he was unable to find even one bona fide well-adjusted hermit. Many of the so-called hermits lived alone, sometimes in very isolated places, yet had ongoing contact with friends or family members. (One fellow lived by himself in a tin-covered hole in the desert, but he regularly walked to town to have dinner with his mother.) Others were homeless people who often roamed the streets by themselves during the day but joined other homeless people at night. A good number were simply people, most of them elderly, who lived alone not out of choice, and who would have preferred greater social contact and more close relationships. The researcher did locate some true hermits, but they were uniformly seriously psychologically disturbed, unable to hold jobs or form meaningful personal relationships.

Perhaps there are a few well-adjusted people somewhere who happily and easily live for extended periods of time with no social relationships whatsoever and with no desire to develop such relationships—but we doubt it. The drive to form some minimum number of lasting, positive, and significant interpersonal relationships is such a critical aspect of human nature that we consider it inconceivable that otherwise normal individuals would have no desire to connect with other people through friendships, romantic or mating relationships, instrumental coalitions, or kinship. Human beings are fundamentally not only social animals (as are many other group-living species) but also, for lack of a better term, "relationship animals." No other species forms such a broad array of distinct relationships with conspecifies as human beings do, nor have lives that are so markedly affected by the development, maintenance, and dissolution of relationships. The need for acceptance and belonging is indeed a "mainspring of social action" (Murphy, 1954) that is connected, in one way or another, to most of the machinery of human life.

## REFERENCES


Aron, A., Dutton, D. G., Aron, E. N., & Iverson, A. (1989). Experiences of falling in love. *Journal of Social and Personal Relationships, 6*, 243–257.

Asch, S. E. (1955, November). Opinions and social pressure. *Scientific American*, pp. 31–35.

Barash, D. P. (1977). *Sociobiology and behavior.* New York: Elsevier.

Baumeister, R. F., & Leary, M. R. (1995). The need to belong: Desire for interpersonal attachments as a fundamental human motivation. *Psychological Bulletin, 117*, 497–529.

Billig, M., & Tajfel, H. (1973). Social categorization and similarity in intergroup behavior. *European Journal of Social Psychology, 3*, 27–52.

Bowlby, J. (1969). *Attachment and loss: Vol. 1. Attachment.* New York: Basic Books.

Brewer, M. (1991). The social self: On being the same and different at the same time. *Personality and Social Psychology Bulletin, 17*, 475–482.

Buckley, K. E., Winkel, R. E., & Leary, M. R. (2004). Reactions to acceptance and rejection: Effects of level and sequence of relational evaluation. *Journal of Experimental Social Psychology, 40*, 14–28.

Carden, S. E., Hernandez, N., & Hofer, M. A. (1996). The isolation and companion comfort responses of 7- and 3-day-old rat pups are modulated by drugs active at the opioid receptor. *Behavioral Neuroscience, 110*, 324–330.

Carter, S. C. (1992). Oxytocin and sexual behavior. *Neuroscience and Biobehavioral Reviews, 16*, 131–144.

Carter, S. C. (1998). Neuroendocrine perspectives on

social attachment and love. *Psychoneuroendocrinology, 23*, 779–818.

Curtis, T., & Wang, Z. (2003). The neurochemistry of pair bonding. *Current Directions in Psychological Science, 12*, 49–53.

Diehl, M. (1990). The minimal group paradigm: Theoretical explanation and empirical findings. In W. Stroebe & M. Hewstone (Eds.), *European review of social psychology* (Vol. 1, pp. 263–392). Chichester, UK: Wiley.

Dion, K. L. (1979). Intergroup conflict and intergroup cohesiveness. In W. G. Austin & S. Worchel (Eds.), *The social psychology of intergroup relations* (pp. 211–224). Monterey, CA: Brooks/Cole.

Downey, G., Feldman, S., & Ayduk, O. (2000). Rejection sensitivity and male violence in romantic relationships. *Personal Relationships, 7*, 45–61.

Eisenberger, N. I., Lieberman, M. D., & Williams, K. D. (2003). Does social rejection hurt?: An fMRI study of social exclusion. *Science, 302*, 290–292.

Ferguson, J. F., Aldag, J. M., Insel, T. R., & Young, L. J. (2001). Oxytocin in the medial amygdala is essential for social recognition in the mouse. *Journal of Neuroscience, 21*, 8278–8285.

Frijda, N. (1986). *The emotions*. Cambridge, UK: Cambridge University Press.

Gold, J. A., Ryckman, R. M., & Mosley, N. R. (1984). Romantic mood induction and attraction to a dissimilar other: Is love blind? *Personality and Social Psychology Bulletin, 10*, 358–368.

Hogan, R., Jones, W. H., & Cheek, J. M. (1985). Socioanalytic theory: An alternative to armadillo psychology. In B. R. Schlenker (Ed.), *The self and social life* (pp. 175–198). New York: McGraw-Hill.

Horney, K. (1945). *Our inner conflicts: A constructive theory of neurosis*. New York: Norton.

Insel, T. R. (1997). A neurobiological basis of social attachment. *American Journal of Psychiatry, 154*, 726–735.

Insel, T. R. (2000). Toward a neurobiology of attachment. *Review of General Psychology, 4*, 176–185.

Insel, T. R. (2003). Is social attachment an addictive disorder? *Physiology and Behavior, 79*, 351–357.

James, W. (1890). *The principles of psychology*. New York: Holt.

Jones, E. E., & Pittman, T. S. (1982). Toward a general theory of strategic self-presentation. In J. Suls (Ed.), *Psychological perspectives on the self* (pp. 231–263). Hillsdale, NJ: Erlbaum.

Kelley, H. H. (1952). Two functions of reference groups. In G. Swanson, T. Newcomb, & E. Hartley (Eds.), *Society for the Psychological Study of Social Issues: Readings in social psychology* (pp. 410–414). New York: Holt.

Kirkpatrick, L. A., & Ellis, B. J. (2001). An evolutionary approach to self-esteem: Multiple domains and multiple functions. In M. Clark & G. Fletcher (Eds.), *The Blackwell handbook of social psychology: Vol. 2. Interpersonal processes* (pp. 411–436). Oxford, UK: Blackwell.

Kurzban, R., & Leary, M. R. (2001). Evolutionary origins or stigmatization: The functions of social exclusion. *Psychological Bulletin, 127*, 187–208.

Leary, M. R. (1995). *Self-presentation: Impression management and interpersonal behavior.* Boulder, CO: Westview Press.

Leary, M. R., Cottrell, C. A., & Phillips, M. (2001). Deconfounding the effects of dominance and social acceptance on self-esteem. *Journal of Personality and Social Psychology, 81*, 898–909.

Leary, M. R., Koch, E. J., & Hechenbleikner, N. R. (2001). Emotional responses to interpersonal rejection. In M. R. Leary (Ed.), *Interpersonal rejection* (pp. 145–166). New York: Oxford University Press.

Leary, M. R., & Springer, C. (2000). Hurt feelings: The neglected emotion. In R. M. Kowalski (Ed.), *Behaving badly: Aversive behaviors in interpersonal relationships* (pp. 151–175). Washington, DC: American Psychological Association.

Leary, M. R., Twenge, J., & Quinlivan, E. (2006). Interpersonal rejection as a determinant of anger and aggression. *Personality and Social Psychology Review, 10*, 111–132.

Leder, S. (2004). *Intimacy motivation: Testing a theory of romantic love*. Unpublished master's thesis, Wake Forest University, Winston-Salem, NC.

Levine, J., Caspi, N., & Laufer, N. (1997). Immediate effects of chlorpromazine and perphenazine following neuroleptic washout on word association of schizophrenic patients. *Schizophrenia Research, 26*, 55–63.

MacDonald, G., Kingsbury, R., & Shaw, S. (2005). Adding insult to injury: Social pain theory and response to social exclusion. In K. Williams, J. Forgas, & W. Von Hipple (Eds.), *The social outcast: Ostracism, social exclusion, rejection, and bullying* (pp. 77–90). New York: Psychology Press.

MacDonald, G., & Leary, M. R. (2005). Why does social exclusion hurt?: The relationship between social and physical pain. *Psychological Bulletin, 131*, 202–223.

MacLean, P. (1990). *The triune brain in evolution: Role in paleocerebral functions*. New York: Plenum Press.

Madden, M. (2003). *America's online pursuits*. Washington, DC: Pew Internet and American Life Project.

Mann, L. (1980). Cross-cultural studies of small groups. In H. Triandis & R. Brislin (Eds.), *Handbook of cross-cultural psychology: Vol. 5. Social psychology* (pp. 155–209). Boston: Allyn & Bacon.

Marques, J. M., Abrams, D., Pàez, D., & Hogg, M. A. (2001). Social categorization, social identification, and rejection of deviant group members. In M. A. Hogg & R. S. Tindale (Eds.), *Blackwell handbook of social psychology: Vol. 3. Group processes* (pp. 400–424). Oxford, UK: Blackwell.

Martel, F. L., Nevison, C. M., Simpson, M. J. A., & Keverne, E. B. (1995). Effects of opioid receptor blockade on the social behavior of rhesus monkeys living in large family groups. *Developmental Psychobiology, 28*, 71–84.

Maslow, A. H. (1968). *Toward a psychology of being* (2nd ed.). Princeton, NJ: Van Nostrand.

Merton, R. K., & Kitt, A. (1950). *Contributions to the theory of reference group behavior.* Glencoe, IL: Free Press.

Murphy, G. (1954). Social motivation. In G. Lindzey (Ed.), *Handbook of social psychology* (pp. 601–633). Cambridge, MA: Addison-Wesley.

Murray, S. L., Holmes, J. G., & Griffin, D. W. (2000). Self-esteem and the quest for felt security: How perceived regard regulates attachment processes. *Journal of Personality and Social Psychology, 78*, 478–498.

Nelson, E. E., & Panksepp, J. (1998). Brain substrates of infant–mother attachment: Contributions of opioids, oxytocin, and norepinephrine. *Neuroscience and Biobehavioral Review, 22*, 437–452.

Panksepp, J. (1998). *Affective neuroscience: The foundations of human and animal emotions.* London: Oxford University Press.

Riley, A. J. (1988). Oxytocin and coitus. *Sexual and Marital Therapy, 3*, 29–36.

Schachter, S. (1951). Deviation, rejection and communication. *Journal of Abnormal and Social Psychology, 46*, 190–207.

Schlenker, B. R. (1980). *Impression management: The self-concept, social identity, and interpersonal relations.* Monterey, CA: Brooks/Cole.

Schlenker, B. R., Forsyth, D. R., Leary, M. R., & Miller, R. S. (1980). A self-presentational analysis of the effects of incentives on attitude change following counterattitudinal behavior. *Journal of Personality and Social Psychology, 39*, 553–577.

Sherif, M., Harvey, O. J., White, B. J., Hood, W. R., & Sherif, C. W. (1961). *Intergroup conflict and cooperation: The Robber's Cave experiment.* Norman: University of Oklahoma Press.

Smith, M. B., Bruner, J. S., & White, R. W. (1956). *Opinions and personality.* New York: Wiley.

Stark, R., & Bainbridge, W. S. (1985). *The future of religion: Secularization, revival, and cult formation.* Berkeley: University of California Press.

Symons, D. (1992). On the use and misuse of Darwinism. In J. H. Barkow, L. Cosmides, & J. Tooby (Eds.), *The adapted mind: Evolutionary psychology and the generation of culture* (pp. 137–159). New York: Oxford University Press.

Tesser, A. (1988). Toward a self-evaluation maintenance model of social behavior. In L. Berkowitz (Ed.), *Advances in experimental social psychology* (Vol. 21, pp. 181–227). San Diego, CA: Academic Press.

Thompson, R., Gupta, S., Miller, K., Mills, S., & Orr, S. (2002). The effects of vasopressin on human facial responses related to social communication. *Psychoneuroendocrinology, 29*, 35–48.

Tooby, J., & Cosmides, L. (1996). Friendship and the banker's paradox: Other pathways to the evolution of adaptations for altruism. *Proceedings of the British Academy, 88*, 119–143.

Twenge, J. M., Baumeister, R. F., Tice, D. M., & Stucke, T. S. (2001). If you can join them, beat them: Effects of social exclusion on aggressive behavior. *Journal of Personality and Social Psychology, 81*, 1058–1069.

Wilder, D. A., & Thompson, J. E. (1980). Intergroup contact with independent manipulations of in-group and out-group interaction. *Journal of Personality and Social Psychology, 38*, 589–603.

Young, L., Nilsen, R., Waymire, K. G., MacGregor, G. R., & Insel, T. R. (1999). Increased affiliative response to vasopressin in mice expressing the V-sub(1a) receptor from a monogamous vole. *Nature, 400*, 766–768.

Chapter 3

# The Many Sides of Control Motivation

## MOTIVES FOR HIGH, LOW, AND ILLUSORY CONTROL

**Suzanne C. Thompson**
**Michèle M. Schlehofer**

Personal control has been one of the most pervasive and enduring ideas in psychological research and theory. Numerous theories posit a important role in human behavior for control constructs such as *self-efficacy* (Bandura, 1977), *personal causation* (deCharms, 1968), *effectance motivation* (White, 1959), *perceived control* (Thompson, 1981), *helplessness* (Seligman, 1975), *self-control* (Baumeister & Heatherton, 1996), *perceived behavioral control* (Ajzen, 1985), *control in aging* (Baltes & Baltes, 1986; Lachman, 2006), *primary and secondary control* (Rothbaum, Weisz, & Snyder, 1982), *compensatory control* (Schulz & Heckhausen, 1996), *controllability* (Heider, 1958), and *agency* (Deci & Ryan, 1987).

Along with the central role that control perceptions are presumed to play in many aspects of human life, having a sense of control has consistently been found to have adaptive effects. Perceived control is associated with emotional well-being, reduced physiological impact of stressors, enhanced ability to cope with stress, improved performance, less pain, and a greater likelihood of making difficult behavior changes (Thompson & Spacapan, 1991). Across a variety of environments from the classroom to the workplace to the medical center, and in diverse populations from children to older adults, it is generally adaptive to have a sense of control.

### WHY IS CONTROL ADAPTIVE?

Several perspectives on why perceived control has these positive effects have been offered. One idea is that personal control gives assurance about future outcomes. For example, according to Miller's (1979) *minimax* hypothesis, having a sense of control assures people that they will be able to act to avoid the worst future outcomes, and this assurance reduces anxiety and stress. Outcomes may also be enhanced because having control gives people information about the future environment that reduces their uncertainty and leads to more adaptive behavior (Kofta, 1993). Another reason why a sense of control improves performance and helps people to make difficult changes is that people are unlikely to exert effort unless they have some indication that their behavior will result in desired outcomes. Thus people are more likely to take action if they have a sense of control that their actions can lead to better outcomes. The benefit of control may also relate to the deficits associated with a lack of control. Helplessness—the perception of no control over important outcomes—can lead to depression, apathy, and negative physiological outcomes associated with stress (Seligman, 1975). Having perceived control helps people avoid the aversiveness of perceived uncontrollability.

Yet another view is that control is adaptive because of an innate desire to feel efficacious and able to change one's environment. According to White (1959), humans have an intrinsic need to feel that they can act effectively on the environment and to discover the ways in which they can effect change. Having a sense of control satisfies this need to feel like an effective agent. The evidence for this motive can be found in the actions of small infants and throughout the lifespan (White, 1959). For example, children have a strong drive to explore and manipulate their environment. Along the same lines, in his evolutionary account, Geary (1998) argues that humans possess an innate desire to achieve control over their environment, especially the resources that support survival and reproduction. An innate desire for control has evolutionary advantage, because those who possess it are more likely to act to acquire control over resources that are necessary for individual survival and the continuation of their genes. Thus, in addition to the many specific benefits of a sense of control—such as assurance about future outcomes, the increased likelihood of acting to obtain better outcomes, and the avoidance of helplessness effects—perceived control may be beneficial because it satisfies an innate need to feel efficacious and to control resources.

*Personal control*, as defined by psychological researchers, is a cognition—a judgment that one has the ability, resources, or opportunities to take action to increase the likelihood of obtaining positive outcomes or avoiding negative ones. In this chapter, we explore the motivational properties of the personal control cognition. One set of questions focuses on various aspects of the motive for control: Are people in fact motivated to have control? Is it control per se that is desired? For what types of people and under what circumstances is there a motive to have personal control? Are people also motivated to avoid having control, or to seek out illusory rather than realistic control? A second set of questions addresses the effects of control motivations on cognition, behavior, and non-control-related motivations.

## ASPECTS OF THE MOTIVE FOR CONTROL

### Are People Motivated to Acquire Control?

Given the positive effects associated with having a sense of control, it would not be surprising to find that people are motivated to have control. There are several lines of evidence to support this idea. The way people respond to protect or restore control when it has been undermined by a stressful or low-control experience shows a push to retain perceptions of control. For example, Friedland, Keinan, and Regev (1992) proposed that stress undermines a sense of control and leads to behavior to restore perceived control. In support of this, they found that participants who were in a high-stress condition (e.g., expecting to be shocked for one task) were more likely to choose an option that gave them illusory control on a different task, even if the illusory control came at the expense of a lower likelihood of success on the second task. Thus participants who were stressed were willing to accept the probability of poorer immediate outcomes in order to feel a sense of control. Along the same lines, work on compensatory control has found that if people's control perceptions are undermined in one area, they will act to exert control in other areas. Evidently, the desire to have control motivates individuals to find another source of control when one source has been lost (Schulz & Heckhausen, 1996; S. C. Thompson, Sobolew-Shubin, Galbraith, Schwankovsky, & Cruzen, 1993).

Another situation in which people are likely to be motivated to have control is when there is a desirable outcome. When an outcome is more desirable, personal control is likely to be more impactful in reducing anxiety and directing behavior toward the goal. Thus personal control should be more highly desired in situations of high need or desire for the outcome. The earliest research on this topic demonstrated a desirability effect on the perception of getting an outcome. Marks (1951) conducted an experiment in which school-age children were asked to choose a particular type of card from a deck in a random draw. Participants were awarded "points" for some cards and lost points for the selection of other cards. Children had higher expectations that the desired card would be selected in any given draw. Two years later, Irwin (1953) replicated this study with a college student sample, and again found support for the hypothesis that the perceived probability of desirable outcomes was higher than that of less desired outcomes.

In a series of studies tying the desirability effect more closely to personal control, Biner and his colleagues found that people with a need for an outcome seemed to overestimate their control over getting the outcome. Biner, Angle, Park, Mellinger, and Barber (1995) found that participants who were motivated to get a food incentive because they were hungry had higher beliefs that they would obtain the outcome through their actions. Similarly, they found that state lottery players with lower incomes (and presumably more in need of the outcome) had higher confidence that they would win the lottery than those with higher incomes. In a subsequent study, participants who were food-deprived and therefore had a stronger need for the outcome of a food incentive were more likely to want to be personally involved in playing the game that could win them the incentive (Biner, Huffman, Curran, & Long, 1998). Personal involvement enhances a sense of control, and thus the preference for self-involvement is evidence for wanting to have personal control. Although this study found that a motive to have control led to actions that would enhance perceived control, control perceptions were not directly assessed.

In a study that directly examined how the desire for the outcome enhanced control estimations, Thompson and colleagues (2004) found that if participants received a monetary reward each time a green screen appeared on the computer, they had higher ratings of their control over getting the green screen to appear than if they did not receive a monetary reward for the green screen. Thus, when the outcome was more desirable because it led to a monetary reward, people were especially prone to thinking they had control over it. When these results are taken together with those of the Marks (1951), Irwin (1953), and Biner and colleagues (1998) research, it appears that people are prone to overestimate the likelihood of getting good outcomes (the desirability effect); that this effect is stronger when the need for the outcome is higher; and that the effect, at least in part, is based on the propensity to have higher perceptions of personal control when motivated to have control. Thus the research on reactions to losses in control and on situations where people have a strong desire for an outcome supports the contention that people are motivated to have control.

### Control Per Se or Good Outcomes?

Although there is a fair amount of evidence that control is desirable, and that people in general are motivated to have control, is it control per se that is wanted or the presumably better outcomes that people receive when in control of a situation? A few studies have investigated this question, but the findings are not consistent. Rodin, Rennert, and Solomon (1980) concluded that people would not work to obtain control per se if they did not have sufficient information to exercise the control (make an informed choice between options). Thus they did not find that control is valued for its own sake. On the other hand, Schorr and Rodin (1984) set up a situation in which some participants could get personal control in a second task if they put more effort into a first task. Participants in that situation worked harder on the first task. This result held even when differences in the ability to get good outcomes for oneself on the second task were controlled for. Thus people were motivated to get control per se, not just to get better outcomes. One difference between these two studies is that with inadequate information, the participants in the studies described by Rodin and colleagues may not have felt a sense of control over outcomes. Choices without the information to make them effective are not likely to feel like control. Because having personal control is almost always associated with the belief that one can get better outcomes, it is difficult to tease the two concepts apart. Still, the Schorr and Rodin study seems to indicate that control is desirable for itself. It is possible that White (1959) and Geary (1998) are correct in asserting an innate desire to feel effective and to gain control over the environment. However, in some circumstances, this motivation may be overridden by other motives, such as obtaining the best possible outcomes. Even if an innate desire for control exists, it is not likely that it is dominant in every situation.

### Individual Differences in Desire for Control

Not everyone is strongly motivated to have personal control. A program of study by Burger (1991a) has shown that there are reliable personality differences in how much control is wanted, as measured by the Desirability of Control Scale (Burger & Cooper, 1979). To satisfy their desire for mastery and control, those who score higher on this scale set higher and more challenging aspiration levels, are more persistent, and do better on more difficult and challenging tasks. Others, who score low on the scale, seem less motivated to pursue personal control.

Another factor that affects desires for control is locus of control. Those with an external locus of control believe that the source of important reinforcements in their lives resides outside themselves (Rotter, 1966). Given this orientation, it is likely that the desire to have personal control will be low. For example, Reich, Zautra, and Manne (1993) found that for patients with rheumatoid arthritis, age and locus of control interacted in the effects of spousal encouragement to take control. Older patients with an external locus of control experienced more distress if their spouses urged them to take control. The combination of two factors that reduce the desire for control (age and external locus of control) led to little motivation to strengthen one's own personal control. Similarly, Reich and Zautra (1991) showed that older adults with an external locus of control gained more from an intervention that emphasized dependency and reliance on others than from one that enhanced personal control.

Not surprisingly, age also affects the motive to have control. Although adults may maintain fairly high levels of personal control throughout much of the age span (Mirowsky, 1995), the desire for control may not remain as high. Older adults may have less desire for control in specific areas; for example, there is a tendency for older people to prefer less control over health-related decisions than younger adults do (Thompson, Pitts, & Schwankovsky, 1994; Woodward & Wallston, 1987). The lower desire for control over health outcomes appears to be due to diminished self-efficacy in this area as people age. A diminished capacity to make decisions and a lower confidence in one's ability to negotiate situations successfully both seem to play a part (Woodward & Wallston, 1987).

Thus there is individual variation in how strongly personal control is desired or useful. Those with low scores on the Desirability of Control Scale, those with an external locus of control, and older individuals are less likely to prefer to have control.

### Is There a Motive to Have No Control?

Although most of the research on perceived control has focused on the adaptiveness of personal control and the human motivation to possess control, having personal control may not always be purely positive. Several features of personal control can make it undesirable. First, the control that people are able to enact is probabilistic. Those with personal control are able to increase their chances of success or of avoiding a misfortune, but even with control, failure is possible. Second, other agents may also have control to achieve the outcome that is desired, and their control may have a higher probability of getting the desired outcome. Third, exercising control and attempting to get a particular outcome can be costly, requiring the expenditure of personal resources such as time, money, or attention. Finally, those who have control may be seen as responsible for negative consequences arising from the situation.

These features of personal control make it likely that under some circumstances people would prefer not to have control. One condition that affects the desirability of control is the relative effectiveness of the self versus other people in obtaining the desired result (Burger, 1991a). Burger, McWard, and LaTorre (1989) found in three experiments that undergraduate participants did not choose self-administration of stressors such as drawing a blood sample on oneself if they believed that another agent was more skilled than they were at this task. By forgoing one source of control (self-administration), participants were able to maintain an overall perception of control over their general well-being. This suggests that people may be selective in choosing areas to control that further their greater interests, and relinquishing control in areas where it does not lead to better outcomes.

A second condition in which people may be motivated not to have control is when the situation has the potential for regret or blame (Burger, 1991a; Thompson, Cheek, & Graham, 1988). The attribution of blame is closely linked to control perceptions (Alicke, 2000). People who are judged to have control over an outcome are likely to be held responsible for that result by themselves and by others. Even in relatively minor situations—for example, selecting a movie or restaurant for a group to attend—individuals may be motivated to avoid having control so that they cannot be held responsible for a poor choice. In more important situations, where personal, moral, or legal responsibility is at stake, individuals are likely to be even more strongly motivated to forgo control to avoid regret or blame.

A third circumstance that may engender the motivation to avoid having control occurs because exercising control and attempting to get a particular outcome can be costly, requiring the expenditure of personal resources such as time, money, or attention. Although in the actor's current assessment, the outcome may not be worth the control effort, not attempting to get the outcome could be regretted later or judged negatively by others. For example, some people who smoke may prefer to believe that they do not have control over their smoking behavior, because it absolves them of trying to quit smoking—an action they would prefer not to take. Having control may imply an imperative to use it. So with personal control, people may feel compelled to act or may be held to account for not acting in a situation where they would prefer not to exercise the control. Thus a lack of personal control may be desired when actors prefer not to exercise control and want to avoid personal regret and blame from others for *not* taking action.

Finally, Thompson and colleagues (1988) suggest that personal control can have negative effects if control efforts result in failure. Perceived control that is not effective and results in failure can have several maladaptive effects, including a wasted investment of resources, enhanced disappointment, and a lack of preparation to cope when the desired outcome is not achieved. On the other hand, those with a low sense of their own ability to get a desired outcome are more likely to be prepared for failure, and to adjust their expectations and effort accordingly. This suggests that personal control may not be desired when the outcome is important, but the chances of success are low. For many people, being prepared for failing to obtain a desired situation may be preferable to having some chance to work to obtain it.

In summary, although the motive to have personal control may be pervasive, it is clear that in many common situations, people may be motivated not to have control. These situations include ones where another agent is more effective, where there is a potential for blame or regret (either for acting or for not acting to achieve the outcome), and where the effort expended to exercise control results in a lack of preparation for failure.

## Illusory versus Actual Control

In addition to preferring not to have control at times, some research suggests that people will prefer illusory control to real control in some situations. Having *illusory control* refers to overestimating one's personal control by judging that one has control in a purely chance situation or overestimating the effectiveness of one's strategies to get a desired outcome or avoid a misfortune. In general, people overestimate their control, especially when they act with the intention of getting the desired outcome and when there is a clear connection between their action and the outcome (Thompson, Armstrong, & Thomas, 1998). The propensity to overestimate one's control is assumed to be driven by the motivation to have control—which, in fact, it may often be. However, Thompson, Kent, Thomas, and Vrungos (1999) have suggested that in some circumstances, people are motivated to have illusory instead of real control. This will occur when individuals feel anxious about a threat, but do not want to make difficult behavior changes that would protect them from the threat. In that case, illusory control in the form of easy, but largely ineffective, strategies can reassure people that they are protecting themselves without requiring the difficult changes. Thompson and colleagues examined this idea in the context of young adults protecting themselves against HIV. Using samples of sexually active heterosexual students and gay men from the community, the researchers measured the propensity to use illusory control, perceived vulnerability to HIV, and the use of illusory protective strategies (e.g., screening partners or taking a sexual history). As predicted, it was found that in both samples, those with a propensity to illusory control in general were more likely to use illusory protection strategies and to feel that these provided a sense of control over avoiding HIV. Illusory control strategies have the advantage of providing a sense of safety and reducing anxiety without the necessity for taking inconvenient or difficult action to provide real protection. Thus people may be motivated to have illusory rather than real control if they wish to avoid the more difficult course of action.

To return to the question of whether people are motivated to have control, the simple answer is "yes." Personal control is desired for a variety of reasons, and there is evidence that people will work to establish or restore a sense of control. Although far less research has been directed toward understanding the motive not to have control, it is also clear that personal control is not an unmixed blessing and not always desirable. At times, the disadvantages of personal control, such as being held responsible for a bad outcome or not taking action, will motive people to abrogate control. In addition, when personal control implies engaging in difficult behaviors, illusory control that reduces anxiety without necessitating behavior change may be more desirable than actual control.

Additional research is needed for a better understanding of when people are motivated to have control and when they are not. In addition, the desirability of personal control versus the belief that better outcomes will be obtained needs more examination. Research has proceeded to address the ways that a motive for control affects other motives, cognitions, and behaviors, which we cover in the next section.

## THE EFFECTS OF CONTROL MOTIVATION

Having a strong motive to have control has a variety of effects, which can be classified into three categories: effects on cognitions, behaviors, and other motivations.

### Effects on Cognitions

Being motivated to have control over one's environment has multiple implications for cognitions and cognitive processing style, including control overestimation, high aspirations and expectations, vigilant processing style, and increased attributional analysis.

#### *Illusory Control Perceptions*

Although people in general are likely to show illusory control, there is evidence that individuals high in control motivation are especially susceptible to these overestimations. Burger's (1979, Experiment 2; 1986, 1991b) research has demonstrated that individuals high in desire for control are most likely to hold illusions of control over purely chance-based gaming situations. This is especially the case if the situation is familiar (e.g., a game that contains typical objects, such as standard playing cards); if the individual has established a previous history of wins in the game (e.g., a "winning streak"); or when the situation has characteristics mimicking situations in which one has control over the outcome (e.g., being able to toss one's own dice in a die-toss game). For example, individuals playing the lottery are more likely to select their own numbers—as opposed to buying machine-picked numbers—if they are high on control motivation, even though selecting their own numbers does not increase the probability of winning (Burger, 1991b, Experiment 1).

What happens when one's personal control is undermined? Will individuals high in control motivation restore their sense of control in such situations via illusory control perceptions? There is initial evidence to suggest individuals with high control motivations engage in behaviors that work to reestablish a sense of personal control when such feelings are undermined—even if the control that is achieved is illusory. Keinan (1994, 2002) has suggested that engaging in magical and superstitious thinking is one method by which individuals with a high need for personal control can restore their sense of control. In a test of this hypothesis, Keinan (2002) conducted a study in which participants differing in control motivations were exposed to a stressful or nonstressful situation (tested on an exam day or not on an exam day) and then provided with an opportunity to elicit the superstitious behavior of "knocking on wood." The results show that those high in control motivation enacted more "knock on wood" behaviors and reported more desires to knock on wood. However, these findings varied by stress. Although being under stress—a situation known to undermine individuals' sense of control (Fisher, 1986; Lazarus & Folkman, 1984)—increased the propensity or desire to knock on wood, these increases were significantly greater for those high in control motivation, suggesting that engaging in superstitious behaviors helps one regain a sense of control over one's situation.

Other research suggests, conversely, that those who are low on desire for control are more likely to believe in superstitious behavior, and to believe that such behavior has an effect on outcomes. Burger (1991b, Experiment 2) found that individuals playing bingo who had low control motivation were significantly more likely to rely on superstitious behaviors during play than those with high control motivation, suggesting that superstitious behaviors are one method by which individuals enhance personal control over the outcomes of a game. Rothbaum and colleagues (1982) suggest that leaving outcomes up to fate, luck, or divine intervention can be a type of secondary control that enhances personal control indirectly. Indirect enhancement of control may generally be more appealing to those low in control motivation. On the other hand, those high in desire for control may use secondary control methods only when other options are not available. At present, it is unclear whether these indirect methods do indeed work to promote personal control; this is one area in which further empirical research is needed.

### *High Aspirations and Expectations*

In addition to producing overestimations and illusions of control, control motivations have implications for one's aspirations and expectations in any given situation. Individuals who have a high desire for control generally have greater aspiration levels than those low in desire for control (Burger, 1985a, 1991a). Those high in desire for control may have a tendency to select harder tasks, which are viewed as opportunities to demonstrate their ability to assert control and mastery over difficult, challenging situations (Burger, 1985a). Those low in control motivation, on the other hand, are not as concerned with proving their mastery, and as such may set more realistic goals (Burger, 1985a).

In an experimental demonstration of this effect, Burger (1985a, Experiment 1) had participants either high or low in desire for control complete anagrams that were perceived as ranging from easy to difficult (in actuality, all anagrams were only mildly difficult). Participants, furthermore, had total choice over which anagrams to complete. As would be expected, although those high and low in control motivation performed equally well on the anagram tasks, those high in desire for control chose more often than those low in desire for control to work on anagrams they perceived as more difficult. Thus it appears that having strong control motivations can lead individuals to have high performance aspirations. However, the assumption that individuals high in control motivation choose more difficult tasks *because* they are perceived to present an opportunity to assert their control and mastery has yet to be empirically tested.

### *Vigilant Processing Style*

There is also evidence to suggest that being motivated to have control can encourage one to employ a more effortful and vigilant information-processing style. In a test of this idea, Pittman and D'Agostino (1989, Experiments 1 and 2) conducted an experiment in which a sense of uncontrollability was instilled in participants completing a concept identification task by providing noncontingent feedback. These individuals presumably would be motivated to reinstate a sense of control. The study found that these participants recalled more sentence pairs from a list (Experiment 1), took longer to read a subsequent unrelated article (Experiment 2), and recalled more information from the article (Experiment 2), suggesting that the motive to restore control can lead individuals to engage in more effortful, vigilant information processing. Pittman and D'Agostino suggest that these effects occurred because a loss of control calls one's understanding of the way things work into question, leading one to scrutinize the environment more carefully in an effort to reassert a sense of understanding and control. The result is an information-processing style that is more thorough and effortful.

The effects of control motivation on information processing are likely to be generalized, not just situation-specific. Swann, Stephenson, and Pittman (1981) temporarily deprived research participants of control on an experimental task, after which they provided them with the opportunity to ask a potential partner for a second task questions about him- or herself. Supporting the notion that control motivations promote a generalized vigilant processing style, participants demonstrated generalized information seeking on this second task: They tended to ask questions of the potential partner that were likely to elicit a great deal of personal information.

Finally, work with depressed individuals also provides support for the notion that those motivated to have control engage in more effortful processing (Weary, Marsh, Gleicher, & Edwards, 1993). Experimental manipulations of control deprivation (Burger & Arkin, 1980; Pittman & Pittman, 1980), correlational research with depressed individuals (Gleicher & Weary, 1991; Marsh & Weary, 1989), and longitudinal studies in which depressive symptomatology is predicted from control constructs (Brown & Siegel, 1988; Lewinsohn, Steinmetz, Larson, & Franklin, 1981; Lewinsohn, Hoberman, & Rosenbaum, 1988) have suggested that depression is characterized by expectations of uncontrollability over life events. Thus depressed individuals should have high control motivation, and therefore should engage in a processing style that is more vigilant, effortful, and detailed. Hildebrand-Saints and Weary (1989) conducted a replication of Swann and colleagues' (1981) research, modified to examine differences between depressed and nondepressed participants. As hypothesized, depressed individuals sought out more diagnostic information than nondepressed participants, even when the information was not relevant to the task at hand. The authors explain these effects by suggesting that depressed individuals, having prior experiences with uncontrollability, have stronger control motivation—motivation that leads to more effortful cognitive processing.

### *Increased Attributional Analyses*

Control motivations also have implications for attributional analyses (Kelley, 1971; Wortman, 1976). It has long been suggested that people often make attributions that work to promote effective control (Heider, 1958; Kelley, 1967, 1971). People with high control motivation, in particular, tend to seek explanations for their behavior that allow them to maintain a strong sense of environmental control, such as attributing successes to effort and ability (Burger, 1987, 1991a; Pittman & Pittman, 1980). Although self-serving attributions for success and failures are widespread phenomena, those high in control motivation have been found to display self-serving attributions to a greater degree (Burger, 1991a). To test this empirically, Burger (1985a, Experiment 5) had participants either high or low in desire for control engage in a number-guessing task. Participants were given instructions suggesting that the presentation of numbers in the task followed a logical pattern, when in fact the presentation was random. The results indicate that participants high in desire for control were more likely to attribute their performance to effort and ability (as compared to luck) than those low in desire for control; additionally, this effect strengthened with better actual task performance.

Empirical demonstrations of this effect also come from the body of research on depressed individuals and attributional processes. Again, depressed individuals have presumably high motives for control, due to previous experiences of uncontrollability. Marsh and Weary (1989) conducted a study examining the relationship between depression and attributional complexity. The findings indicate that those individuals who were mildly or moderately depressed engaged in more complex attributional processing, as measured by the Attributional Complexity Scale (Fletcher, Danilovics, Fernandez, Peterson, & Reeder, 1986). Those who were not depressed (who should presumably experience uncontrollable outcomes less frequently, and therefore should demonstrate lower control motivations) or who were severely depressed (who had presumably become helpless, and thus should succumb to cognitions of uncontrollability) engaged in less attributional complexity.

What types of attributions will individuals with a high level of control motivation make if placed in a low-control situation? Will these individuals make attributions that lead to a reestablishment of control? As might be expected, the research suggests that these individuals, when placed in a low-control situation, will indeed engage in attributional analyses that allow them to regain control. If stress impairs perceptions of control, then it would follow that those high in desire for control would be more likely to form attributions that help them regain control when placed in a high-stress situation. In an initial test of this hypothesis,

Keinan and Sivan (2001) had participants differing in control motivation complete measures of their current subjective stress level and their tendency to make causal attributions. They found that among participants under less stress at the time of measurement, desire for control did not influence the number of causal attributions made. However, when under greater stress, those high in desire for control made more causal attributions than did those lower in desire for control. This implies that those individuals with high control motivation engage in attributional analyses when control is undermined (such as when under stress) in order to reassert control. Although these findings have yet to be replicated in an experimental setting, they are promising in supporting the notion that those high in control motivation actively seek out attributions that allow them to restore a sense of control in low-control situations.

It has been suggested that control motivation, in addition to influencing attributions for individuals' own successes and failures, influences the attributions the individuals make concerning others' successes and failures (Miller & Norman, 1975). Due to high control motivation, individuals will selectively process or distort information received in order to increase the confidence of their attributions during the course of an interpersonal interaction. Thus, in general, individuals with strong control motivation are more likely to provide exaggerated dispositional attributions for others' behavior, as doing so leads to increased effective control. For instance, Miller, Norman, and Wright (1978, Experiment 1) conducted a study in which, after observing two individuals (one of whom was a target) participate in a staged prisoner's dilemma game, participants overexaggerated the amount of dispositional information that could be inferred from a target's behavior when envisioning interacting with the target in a conflict situation. In a subsequent experiment, Miller and colleagues (Experiment 2) found that this was especially true of those individuals holding high personal control needs, as measured with the Cialdini and Mirels (1976) Personal Control Scale. These individuals were most likely to believe that they knew the target player's personality, and that they could describe the target's personality to another individual.

Indeed, those with high control motivation whose control is undermined may make any control-enhancing attribution available to them, regardless of whether it is connected to the original event responsible for instilling perceptions of control deprivation. These attributions may be enough to satisfy motives for control, despite the fact that they do not directly reinstate the situation-specific control that was lost. In one of the initial studies on this topic, Pittman and Pittman (1980) found that participants were more likely to make use of any available information in the forming of attributions in a subsequent, unrelated setting if they first completed a task in which their control over task outcomes was undermined than were those not given this initial experience.

In a test of a person-by-situation interactive model on interpersonal attribution processes, Smith and Brehm (1981) explored whether people exhibiting the Type A coronary-prone behavior pattern—a pattern marked by competitiveness and strivings for achievement—would be motivated to enhance perceptions of control via attributions for competitors' successes and failures. Smith and Brehm replicated Miller and colleagues' (1978) study, in which participants watched two individuals (one of whom was a target) participate in a staged prisoner's dilemma game, after which they were asked to rate the extent to which the target's personality could be inferred from the interaction and to which they could describe the target's personality. Smith and Brehm, however, modified this study to include the individual difference variable of Type A or B personality characteristics. Type A individuals, in comparison to Type B individuals, were more motivated to succeed at the game. This motivation, in turn, led to dispositional attributions of their opponent's behavior: The Type A participants were more likely to believe that they knew and could describe to another individual the other player's personality. The researchers suggest that such attributions are made because they work to increase participants' perceptions of control over the outcome. Thus those individuals with a highly competitive personality (such as the Type A pattern) might be particularly motivated to engage in attributional processes that foster a sense of control, especially in situations that challenge a sense of control. In support of this, Keinan and Tal (2005) found that under high-stress conditions, Type A individuals were more likely than Type B individuals to make causal attributions for events.

When all these findings are taken together, it appears that having high control motivation can have multiple effects on cognitions, including influences on susceptibility to illusions of control, aspirations and expectations for success, processing style, and attributional analyses. Those with high control motivation are more susceptible than those with lower control motivation to illusions of control. In addition, being motivated to have control can lead people to have greater aspirations and expectations for success, although the underlying mechanisms for this effect have not been empirically validated. Finally, having greater control motivation can lead individuals to process information in a more vigilant and effortful manner, and to make control-instilling attributions in order to maintain or increase their sense of control. However, some important questions remain unanswered.

One important question that is in need of clarification is an understanding of the types of cognitions that work to increase control perceptions. Although researchers have suggested that cognitions such as superstitious and magical thinking (Keinan, 1994, 2002), effortful processing (Pittman & D'Agostino, 1989), and attributions that provide internal explanations for successes (Miller et al., 1978) work to increase individuals' perceptions of control, these assumptions have not been, for the most part, empirically validated. Future research should explore the extent to which these and other cognitions work to increase control perceptions, and the extent to which certain types of control-enhancing cognitions are preferred over others.

Second, questions remain as to whether certain changes in cognitions are global in nature among those with high control motivation, or whether they primarily occur when control is undermined. The majority of existing research has examined attributional analyses and information processing in an experimental setting in which individuals first experienced a loss of control. Thus it is unclear whether people with high control motivation engage in effortful information processing and control-instilling attributional analyses globally, or only when their sense of control is undermined. Future research should explore the generalizability of these effects for individuals differing in dispositional control motivation, in situations varying in controllability.

## Effects on Behaviors

In addition to affecting cognitions, a high motivation to have control over one's environment has behavioral implications. Empirical research suggests that individuals with high control motivations tend generally to perform better on laboratory tasks (Burger, 1985b, 1987) and to act as though they have greater control over the environment (Hammond & Horswill, 2002). In an experimental test of how motivation for control can affect driving behavior, participants who were either high or low on desire for control completed a driving simulation task in which their speed and gap acceptance (the amount of space between two vehicles that they were willing to pull into) were measured (Hammond & Horswill, 2002). Those high in desire for control drove faster and pulled out into smaller gaps in traffic during the simulation than those low in desire for control. These findings provide clear preliminary evidence of the role that control motivation plays in influencing behavior: A strong motivation to have control over their environment may lead individuals to act as though they have more control over their environment.

The aforementioned example provides evidence of the effect of having control motivation on behaviors in relatively controllable situations. What about a situation in which desire for control is high, but control over the environment is not perceived as available? Would such a situation still translate into behavioral changes? There is evidence to suggest that the effects of control motivation on behaviors are indeed moderated by perceptions that control is possible. Sprott, Brumbaugh, and Miyasaki (2001) examined the behavior of playing in a state-sponsored lottery among individuals either high or low in the general dispositional trait of desire for control and high or low in perceived ability to influence lottery outcomes (illusory control beliefs that the outcome of the lottery was within or outside of their control). Neither desire for control nor perceived ability to influence lottery outcomes independently predicted lottery-playing behavior. However, an interaction between these two variables was found, such that individuals who both were high in control motivation and perceived themselves as having the ability to influence their lottery outcomes (e.g., by engaging in behaviors such as choosing their own lottery numbers) were most likely to play the lottery. A similar interaction indicating that both control motivation and perceived control are necessary to engage behavior was found regarding dental treatment anxiety. Patients who had a high desire for control in that setting, but did not have a high level of personal control, were more likely to avoid treatment (Sartory, Heinen, Pundt, & Johren, 2006). As such, control motivation may not be sufficient for evoking changes in behavior; it is only when control motivation is high and individuals perceive a direct connection between their actions and a particular outcome that the effects of control motivation on behavior become apparent.

This last point has been demonstrated in an academic setting. Shell and Husman (2001) examined how perceptions of control were related to students' self-reports of their study time and effort. Furthermore, they examined two distinct aspects of control: *competency* cognitions (believing that one is academically capable—i.e., smart) and cognitions pertaining to *contingency* (believing that one's effort has an influence on academic outcomes—i.e., hard work results in higher grades). The findings indicate that these two different control cognitions have different implications. While competency beliefs (believing, for instance, that one is a good student or is smart) were associated with high grades, contingency beliefs (believing, for instance, that one's hard academic work will lead to higher grades) were related to the amount of time spent studying. Thus, supporting the findings from the study by Sprott and colleagues, perceiving one's actions as having a direct influence over one's outcomes is necessary for behavioral change, regardless of whether one perceives oneself as self-efficacious.

In conclusion, although the body of literature on the behavioral effects of control motivation is still growing, there is consistent evidence demonstrating that being motivated to have control can lead to behavioral changes. First, it seems that having high control motivation can lead individuals to behave as though they have a great amount of actual control. There is also evidence to suggest that high control motivation leads participants to perform well on experimental tasks. Finally, what is clear from the Shell and Husman (2001) and Sprott and colleagues (2001) studies is that high control motivation may not be in and of itself enough to lead to behavioral changes; it must also be accompanied by perceptions that one's actions can lead to desired outcomes.

It should be noted that the effects of control motivation on behaviors may not necessarily be direct. That is, control motivation may have behavioral implications via influencing non-control-related motivations, such as motivation to perform well on a task. We now turn to this relationship—the relationship between control motivations and other motivation.

### Effects on Other Motivations

As alluded to earlier, there is yet another way in which control and motivation may be linked: A high sense of personal control may affect motivational states, such as motivations to perform well on tasks. McCombs and Whisler (1989) propose a theory of *adaptive motivation*, by which they suggest that having a sense of control helps us accomplish our life goals. This type of motivation starts with the premise that we all have an innate desire to achieve and maintain a sense of self-worth and self-esteem. Personal life goals, and expectations for reaching them, are developed in such a way as to maintain this sense of self-worth (e.g., personal goals may be set to be obtainable, thus ensuring the probability that we will reach them and, as a result, feel good about doing so). Our perceptions of control influence our expectations for success and failure at reaching our personal goals. The notion of adaptive motivation asserts that we tend to pursue obtainable activities or personal goals that allow us to maintain a sense of control and self-worth. These control perceptions, in turn, motivate us to reach additional personal goals.

Indeed, there is a growing body of empirical evidence to support the notion that control judgments influence individuals' performance motivations. For instance, research has consistently demonstrated that students are more motivated to perform well when they perceive a high degree of control over their academic choices and decisions (Bar-Tal & Bar-Zohar, 1977; DiCintio & Gee, 1999). In a review of 36 studies relevant to the topic of control and children's academic performance, Bar-Tal and Bar-Zohar (1977) concluded that children who believe they have control over their academic environment have increased motivations to perform well on academic tasks. Among at-risk students, it has been found that increased perceptions of control lead to decreases in students' boredom, confusion, and desire to do something other than academics (DiCintio & Gee, 1999).

There is evidence outside the academic arena to support the contention that high perceptions of control increase motivations to perform well on various tasks. Harrison and Liska (1994) conducted a workplace-based study of employees who had an opportunity to join a company-sponsored exercise program. They found that perceptions of self-efficacy were motivating; having efficacy over goal attainment led to increased commitment to keep an exercise goal. Those with lower self-efficacy perceptions, on the other hand, saw more barriers to exercising and had more health concerns, including obesity, aches and pains, smoking habits, and more use of sick time. In a similar vein, Wong and Bridges (1995) found that male adolescent soccer players who held a high level of perceived control over sport-specific outcomes perceived themselves as more competent players and were more motivated to perform well on the field. Although this study was correlational in nature, it does suggest that having perceptions of control may increase performance motivations.

In a series of experiments, Lawrence Perlmuter and his colleagues have consistently demonstrated that a high degree of control over one's environment leads to increased motivation to perform well, and subsequently to better task performance. In their studies, participants were placed in a condition in which they either did or did not have the ability to make a decision over their task. It should be noted that Perlmuter and colleagues have found that the mere act of giving participants a choice over their task is enough to invoke a sense of control in participants, regardless of whether participants actually *make* a choice that is relevant to the experimental task at hand (Bailey, Perlmuter, Karsh, & Monty, 1978; Chan, Karbowski, Monty, & Perlmuter, 1986). Once evoked, these motivations led to greater performance on not only the experimental task, but unrelated tasks as well (Perlmuter, Scharff, Karsh, & Monty, 1980), suggesting that perceptions of control can "spill over" to produce a general state of high performance motivation. In addition, Perlmuter and colleagues' research has found that choosing outcomes for others is not enough to lead to an increase in perceptions of control (Bailey et al., 1978), suggesting that choice increases task performance by increasing motivations to perform well on subsequent tasks.

Control motivation can also work to protect intrinsic motivation from the negative effects of extrinsic rewards on task performance. Feehan and Enzle (1991) had college student participants complete a task in which they were to construct a truck from Legos. Although participants were rewarded for taking part in the study, a sense of illusory control over the payment schedule was instilled for some of the participants by providing them with a "choice" over the payment schedule, in which one schedule was clearly preferable over the others. At the end of the task, the participants were given additional free time during which they could continue to work with the Legos. Their results indicate that those who perceived control over the payment schedule displayed increased intrinsic motivation over the task, as evidenced by playing with the Legos for a longer length of time in comparison to those rewarded on a forced payment schedule or those not rewarded. It is important to note that this intrinsic motivation remained high, despite the fact that the participants were extrinsically motivated (via financial compensation) for their time and effort. Thus it appears that perceptions of control can help mitigate the effects of extrinsic reward on intrinsic motivation.

These findings, however, may only hold for those individuals who do not already have high control motivation. E. P. Thompson, Chaiken, and Hazelwood (1993) examined the moderating role of desire for control on intrinsic motivation, utilizing methodology similar to the study conducted by Feehan and Enzle (1991). Participants in the Thompson and colleagues study were either given a small monetary reward or received no reward for their work on a brainstorming task, and were then given the option of spending additional time on a similar task. The results showed that among those rewarded, people high in desire for control spent less time on the secondary task, while those low in desire for control spent more time on the secondary task. Thus, for those individuals highly motivated to have control, receiving extrinsic motivation for engaging in the task resulted in a decrease in intrinsic motivation, while for those not highly motivated to have control, receiving extrinsic motivation resulted in increased intrinsic motivation. These findings suggest that control motivation plays a key role in the operation of undermining effects.

Taken together, the above-mentioned studies suggest a strong link between control motivation and motivation to perform well on a variety of tasks—including not only those tasks that are presented in the context of an experiment, but also those that are academic in nature or related to health behaviors. It would seem, therefore, that there is at least preliminary support for McCombs and Whisler's (1989) notion of adaptive motivation, although clearly more work needs to be done to fully test this theory. Although there appears to be a causal link between control motivation and performance motivation, it remains to be seen whether goal attainment (or failure) leads to changes in control motivation, as is suggested by McCombs and Whisler's model. Future research should longitudinally examine all stages of McCombs and Whisler's model in order to fully understand the role control motivation plays in the continuous adjustments of goals and motivations.

Second, the research covered in this section has tended to focus on how perceptions of control or actual control—not control motivation per se—influence other motivations. Thus questions remain as to whether dispositional differences in a general motive for control evoke differences in other motivations, or whether perceptions of control (and the extent to which these perceptions match actual control) are really key.

In conclusion, the research covered in the sections above provides support for the contention that control motivation can and does influence individuals in a myriad of ways, including cognitively, behaviorally, and motivationally. Having a strong motivation to control their surroundings can affect not only people's performance motivation, but also how they process information, the types of attributions they make for their own and others' behavior, their susceptibility to illusions of control, and their behavior. As the majority of studies have experimentally instilled a loss of control in participants to test these effects, the challenge for future research is to explore whether a dispositional motive for control per se or a more situationally based motive for control (spurred by a sudden loss of control) is responsible for these effects.

## CONCLUSIONS

Evidence for our human desire to control our environment is ubiquitous. We observe ourselves and others strive to make a difference, to experience our ability to change our environment, to set goals and accomplish them, to be effective, and to know that we have ways to avoid harm. All these are manifestations of the desire to have personal control—the perception that we can act to get what we want or to avoid undesired consequences. In this chapter we have addressed general questions regarding the motive to have control, and have covered the various ways that the desire for control can affect cognitive processing, subsequent behaviors, and the strength of other motivations. In doing so, we have identified several avenues for further research to advance understanding of how the motive for control affects human thinking and behavior.

Control motivation may not be limited to wanting more control. Going beyond a focus just on motives for more control, we suggest that, at times, control motivation includes avoiding personal control and relying on illusory rather than actual control. Although there is research to suggest that "personal control avoidance" motivation exists, and may even be fairly common, only a few studies have examined its effects. A comprehensive understanding of control motivation will include the interplay of the motive to have personal control when that best suits one's needs and the motive to relinquish it when other concerns take precedent. Research on the cognitive, behavioral, and motivational aspects of control avoidance motivation is needed to complete the picture.

## REFERENCES

Ajzen, I. (1985). From intentions to actions: A theory of planned behavior. In J. Kuhl & J. Beckman (Eds.), *Action-control: From cognition to behavior* (pp. 11–39). Berlin: Springer-Verlag.

Alicke, M. D. (2000). Culpable control and the psychology of blame. *Psychological Bulletin, 126*, 556–574.

Bailey, S. E., Perlmuter, L. C., Karsh, R., & Monty, R. A. (1978). Choice for others and the perception of control. *Motivation and Emotion, 2*, 191–200.

Baltes, M. M., & Baltes, P. B. (1986). *The psychology of control and aging*. Hillsdale, NJ: Erlbaum.

Bandura, A. (1977). Self-efficacy: Toward a unifying theory of behavioral change. *Psychological Review, 84*, 191–215.

Bar-Tal, D., & Bar-Zohar, Y. (1977). The relationship between perception of locus of control and academic achievement. *Contemporary Educational Psychology, 2*, 181–199.

Baumeister, R. F., & Heatherton, T. F. (1996). Self-regulation failure: An overview. *Psychological Inquiry, 7*, 1–15.

Biner, P. M., Angle, S. T., Park, J. H., Mellinger, A. E., & Barber, B. (1995). Need state and the illusion of control. *Personality and Social Psychology Bulletin, 21*, 899–907.

Biner, P. M., Huffman, M. L., Curran, M. A., & Long, K. R. (1998). Illusory control as a function of motivation for a specific outcome in a chance-based situation. *Motivation and Emotion, 22*, 277–291.

Brown, J. D., & Siegel, J. M. (1988). Attributions for negative life events and depression: The role of perceived control. *Journal of Personality and Social Psychology, 54*, 316–322.

Burger, J. M. (1979). The desirability of control. *Motivation and Emotion, 3*, 381–393.

Burger, J. M. (1985a). Desire for control and achievement-related behaviors. *Journal of Personality and Social Psychology, 48*, 1520–1533.

Burger, J. M. (1985b). Desire for control, locus of control, and proneness to depression. *Journal of Personality, 52*, 71–89.

Burger, J. M. (1986). Desire for control and the illusion of control: The effects of familiarity and sequence of outcomes. *Journal of Research in Personality, 20*, 66–76.

Burger, J. M. (1987). Effects of desire for control on attributions and task performance. *Basic and Applied Social Psychology, 8*, 309–320.

Burger, J. M. (1991a). Control. In V. J. Derlega, B. A. Winstead, & W. H. Jones (Eds.), *Personality: Contemporary theory and research* (pp. 286–312). Chicago: Nelson-Hall.

Burger, J. M. (1991b). The effects of desire for control in situations with chance-determined outcomes: Gambling behavior in lotto and bingo players. *Journal of Research in Personality, 25*, 196–204.

Burger, J. M., & Arkin, R. (1980). Desire for control and the use of attributional processes. *Journal of Personality, 56*, 531–546.

Burger, J. M., & Cooper, H. M. (1979). The desirability of control. *Motivation and Emotion, 3*, 381–393.

Burger, J. M., McWard, J., & LaTorre, D. (1989). Boundaries of self-control: Relinquishing control over aversive events. *Journal of Social and Clinical Psychology, 8*, 209–221.

Chan, F., Karbowski, J., Monty, R. A., & Perlmuter, L. C. (1986). Performance as a source of perceived control. *Motivation and Emotion, 10*, 59–70.

Cialdini, R. B., & Mirels, H. L. (1976). Sense of personal control and attributions about yielding and resisting persuasion targets. *Journal of Personality and Social Psychology, 33*, 395–402.

deCharms, R. (1968). *Personal causation: The internal affective determinants of behavior.* New York: Academic Press.

Deci, E. L., & Ryan, R. M. (1987). The support of autonomy and the control of behavior. *Journal of Personality and Social Psychology, 53*, 1024–1037.

DiCintio, M. J., & Gee, S. (1999). Control is the key: Unlocking the motivation of at-risk students. *Psychology in the Schools, 36*, 231–237.

Feehan, G. G., & Enzle, M. E. (1991). Subjective control over rewards: Effects of perceived choice of reward schedule on intrinsic motivation and behavior maintenance. *Perceptual and Motor Skills, 72*, 995–1006.

Fisher, S. (1986). *Stress and strategy.* Hillsdale, NJ: Erlbaum.

Fletcher, G. J. D., Danilovics, P., Fernandez, G., Peterson, D., & Reeder, G. D. (1986). Attributional complexity: An individual differences measure. *Journal of Personality and Social Psychology, 51*, 875–884.

Friedland, N., Keinan, G., & Regev, Y. (1992). Controlling the uncontrollable: Effects of stress on illusory perceptions of controllability. *Journal of Personality and Social Psychology, 63*, 923–931.

Geary, D. C. (1998). *Male, female: The evolution of human sex differences.* Washington, DC: American Psychological Association.

Gleicher, F., & Weary, G. (1991). The effect of depression on the quantity and quality of social inferences. *Journal of Personality and Social Psychology, 61*, 105–114.

Hammond, T. B., & Horswill, M. S. (2002). The influence of desire for control on drivers' risk-taking behaviour. *Transportation Research, 4*, 271–277.

Harrison, D. A., & Liska, L. Z. (1994). Promoting regular exercise in organizational fitness programs: Health-related differences in motivational building blocks. *Personnel Psychology, 47*, 47–71.

Heider, F. (1958). *The psychology of interpersonal relations.* New York: Wiley.

Hildebrand-Saints, L., & Weary, G. (1989). Depression and social information gathering. *Personality and Social Psychology Bulletin, 15*, 150–160.

Irwin, F. W. (1953). Stated expectations as functions of probability and desirability of outcomes. *Journal of Personality, 21*, 329–335.

Keinan, G. (1994). Effects of stress and tolerance of ambiguity on magical thinking. *Journal of Personality and Social Psychology, 67*, 48–55.

Keinan, G. (2002). The effects of stress and desire for control on superstitious behavior. *Personality and Social Psychology Bulletin, 28*, 102–108.

Keinan, G., & Sivan, D. (2001). The effects of stress and desire for control on the formation of causal attributions. *Journal of Research in Personality, 35*, 127–137.

Keinan, G., & Tal, S. (2005). The effects of Type A behavior and stress on the attribution of causality. *Personality and Individual Differences, 38*, 403–412.

Kelley, H. H. (1967). Attribution theory in social psychology. In D. Levine (Ed.), *Nebraska Symposium on Motivation* (Vol. 15, pp. 192–240). Lincoln: University of Nebraska Press.

Kelley, H. H. (1971). *Attribution in social interaction.* Morristown, NJ: General Learning Press.

Kofta, M. (1993). Uncertainty, mental models, and learned helplessness: An anatomy of control loss. In G. Weary, F. Gleicher, & K. L. Marsh (Eds.), *Control motivation and social cognition* (pp. 122–153). New York: Springer-Verlag.

Lachman, M. E. (2006). Perceived control over aging-related declines. *Current Directions in Psychological Science, 15*, 282–286.

Lazarus, R. S., & Folkman, S. (1984). *Stress, appraisal, and coping.* New York: Springer.

Lewinsohn, P. M., Hoberman, H. M., & Rosenbaum, M. A. (1988). Prospective study of risk factors for unipolar depression. *Journal of Abnormal Psychology, 97*, 251–264.

Lewinsohn, P. M., Steinmetz, J. L., Larson, D. W., & Franklin, J. (1981). Depression-related cognitions: Antecedent or consequence? *Journal of Abnormal Psychology, 90*, 213–219.

Marks, R. W. (1951). The effect of probability, desirability, and "privilege" on the stated expectations of children. *Journal of Personality, 19*, 332–351.

Marsh, K. L., & Weary, G. (1989). Depression and attributional complexity. *Personality and Social Psychology Bulletin, 15*, 325–336.

McCombs, B. L., & Whisler, J. S. (1989). The role of affective variables in autonomous learning. *Educational Psychologist, 24*, 277–306.

Miller, D. T., & Norman, S. A. (1975). Actor–observer differences in perceptions of effective control. *Journal of Personality and Social Psychology, 31*, 503–515.

Miller, D. T., Norman, S. A., & Wright, E. (1978). Distortion in person perception as a consequence of the need for effective control. *Journal of Personality and Social Psychology, 36*, 598–607.

Miller, S. M. (1979). Controllability and human stress: Method, evidence, and theory. *Behavior Research and Theory, 17*, 287–306.

Mirowsky, J. (1995). Age and the sense of control. *Social Psychology Quarterly, 58*, 31–43.

Perlmuter, L. C., Scharff, K., Karsh, R., & Monty, R. A. (1980). Perceived control: A generalized state of motivation. *Motivation and Emotion, 4*, 35–45.

Pittman, T. S., & D'Agostino, P. R. (1989). Motivation and cognition: Control deprivation and the nature of subsequent information processing. *Journal of Experimental Social Psychology, 25*, 465–480.

Pittman, T. S., & Pittman, N. L. (1980). Deprivation of control and the attribution process. *Journal of Personality and Social Psychology, 39*, 377–389.

Reich, J. W., & Zautra, A. J. (1991). Experimental and measurement approaches to internal control in at-risk older adults. *Journal of Social Issues, 47*, 143–158.

Reich, J. W., Zautra, A. J., & Manne, S. (1993). How perceived control and congruent spouse support affect rheumatoid arthritis patients. *Journal of Social and Clinical Psychology, 12*, 148–163.

Rodin, J., Rennert, K., & Solomon, S. K. (1980). Intrinsic motivation for control: Fact or fiction. In A. Baum & J. E. Singer (Eds.), *Advances in environmental psychology* (Vol. 2, pp. 131–148). Hillsdale, NJ: Erlbaum.

Rothbaum, F., Weisz, J. R., & Snyder, S. S. (1982). Changing the world and changing the self: A two-process model of perceived control. *Journal of Personality and Social Psychology, 42*, 5–27.

Rotter, J. B. (1966). Generalized expectancies for internal versus external control of reinforcement. *Psychological Monographs, 80*(1, Whole No. 609).

Sartory, G., Heinen, R., Pundt, I., & Johren, P. (2006). Predictors of behavioral avoidance in dental phobia: The role of gender, dysfunctional cognitions, and the need for control. *Anxiety, Stress, and Coping: An International Journal, 19*, 279–291.

Schorr, D., & Rodin, J. (1984). Motivation to control one's environment in individuals with obsessive–compulsive, depressive, and normal personality traits. *Journal of Personality and Social Psychology, 46*, 1148–1161.

Schulz, R., & Heckhausen, J. (1996). A life span model of successful aging. *American Psychologist, 51*, 702–714.

Seligman, M. E. P. (1975). *Helplessness: On depression, development, and death.* San Francisco: Freeman.

Shell, D. F., & Husman, J. (2001). The multivariate dimensionality of personal control and future time perspective beliefs in achievement and self-regulation. *Contemporary Educational Psychology, 26*, 481–506.

Smith, T. W., & Brehm, S. S. (1981). Person perception and the Type A coronary-prone behavior pattern. *Journal of Personality and Social Psychology, 40*, 1137–1149.

Sprott, D. E., Brumbaugh, A. M., & Miyazaki, A. D. (2001). Motivation and ability as predictors of play behavior in state-sponsored lotteries: An empirical assessment of psychological control. *Psychology and Marketing, 18*, 973–983.

Swann, W. B., Jr., Stephenson, B., & Pittman, T. S. (1981). Curiosity and control: On the determinants of the search for social knowledge. *Journal of Personality and Social Psychology, 40*, 635–642.

Thompson, E. P., Chaiken, S., & Hazlewood, J. D. (1993). Need for cognition and desire for control as moderators of extrinsic reward effects: A person × situation approach to the study of intrinsic motivation. *Journal of Personality and Social Psychology, 64*, 987–999.

Thompson, S. C. (1981). A complex answer to a simple question: Will it hurt less if I can control it? *Psychological Bulletin, 90*, 89–101.

Thompson, S. C., Armstrong, W., & Thomas, C.

(1998). Illusions of control, underestimations, and accuracy: A control heuristic explanation. *Psychological Bulletin, 123*, 143–161.

Thompson, S. C., Cheek, P., & Graham, M. (1988). The other side of perceived control: Disadvantages and negative effects. In S. Oskamp & S. Spacapan (Eds.), *The social psychology of health* (pp. 69–93). Beverly Hills, CA: Sage.

Thompson, S. C., Kent, D. R., Thomas, C., & Vrungos, S. M. (1999). Real and illusory control over exposure to HIV in college students and gay men. *Journal of Applied Social Psychology, 29*, 1128–1150.

Thompson, S. C., Kyle, D., Osgood, A., Quist, R. M., Phillips, D. J., & McClure, M. (2004). Illusory control and motives for control: The role of connection and intentionality. *Motivation and Emotion, 28*, 315–330.

Thompson, S. C., Pitts, J., & Schwankovsky, L. (1994). Preferences for involvement in medical decision making: Situational and demographic influences. *Patient Education and Counseling, 22*, 133–140.

Thompson, S. C., Sobolew-Shubin, A., Galbraith, M. E., Schwankovsky, L., & Cruzen, D. (1993). Maintaining perceptions of control: Finding perceived control in low-control circumstances. *Journal of Personality and Social Psychology, 64*, 293–304.

Thompson, S. C., & Spacapan, S. (1991). Perceptions of control in vulnerable populations. *Journal of Social Issues, 47*, 1–21.

Weary, G., Marsh, K. L., Gleicher, F., & Edwards, J. A. (1993). Depression, control motivation, and the processing of information about others. In G. Weary, F. Gleicher, & K. Marsh (Eds.), *Control motivation and social cognition* (pp. 255–287). New York: Springer-Verlag.

White, R. W. (1959). Motivation reconsidered: The concept of competence. *Psychological Review, 66*, 297–330.

Wong, E. H., & Bridges, L. J. (1995). A model of motivational orientation for youth sport: Some preliminary work. *Adolescence, 30*, 437–452.

Woodward, N. J., & Wallston, B. S. (1987). Age and health care beliefs: Self-efficacy as a mediator of low desire for control. *Psychology and Aging, 2*, 3–8.

Wortman, C. B. (1976). Causal attributions and personal control. In J. H. Harvey, W. G. Ickes, & R. F. Kidd (Eds.), *New directions in attribution research* (Vol. 1, pp. 23–52). Hillsdale, NJ: Erlbaum.

Chapter 4

# Self-Enhancement and Self-Affirmation

## THE CONSEQUENCES OF POSITIVE SELF-THOUGHTS FOR MOTIVATION AND HEALTH

**Shelley E. Taylor**
**David K. Sherman**

*Self-enhancement* and *self-affirmation* enable people to manage challenging events. The validity of this statement has been demonstrated repeatedly with respect to challenges as diverse as coping with threatening information, practicing effective health behaviors, maintaining persistence and motivation to achieve difficult goals, coping with daily stress, and managing life-threatening events. Put simply, research on self-enhancement and self-affirmation addresses this important question: How do people restore their balance following a stressful event to the point that they can once again pursue their usual goals and activities? We maintain that processes involving self-enhancement and self-affirmation are key to understanding how psychological health is maintained, and especially how it is restored following challenging events.

### THREAT AND THE SELF

In addressing this question, Taylor's research on cognitive adaptation (Taylor, 1983) and on positive illusions (e.g., Taylor & Brown, 1988) and the research on self-affirmation (e.g., Sherman & Cohen, 2006; Steele, 1988) make very similar points. Both assert that the process of enhancing and/or affirming personal attributes and values musters valuable resources for grappling with challenges. Whereas Taylor has largely studied these processes in populations experiencing naturally occurring threats and in people for whom self-enhancement is a chronic mode of addressing life challenges, research on self-affirmation has more commonly studied these processes experimentally. The findings, however, dovetail well in presenting a picture of how enhancing the self enables people to manage threats to the self.

## Managing Life-Threatening Events

The importance of self-enhancement for managing challenging events was first proposed in a theory of cognitive adaptation (Taylor, 1983). Threatening events can undermine the motivation to pursue and achieve goals, and unexpected setbacks such as the diagnosis of a life-threatening illness, a natural disaster, or an unexpected problem at work or in one's romantic life have the ability to bring purposeful activity to a grinding halt, at least temporarily. In an early study of patients with breast cancer, Taylor (1983) and her colleagues (Taylor, Lichtman, & Wood, 1984) found that self-enhancing beliefs were important for restoring a positive sense of self and for making effective use of psychological resources for coping. Specifically, the women Taylor and colleagues studied experienced positive changes in themselves that they attributed to having grappled with the threat of cancer and defeated it, at least in the short term. Many women said that they considered themselves to be more compassionate, stronger than they had been before, and able to take charge of their lives. They often reported an enhanced sense of purpose in their lives. Many women stated that they believed they now had personal control over their illness and the course of their remaining time.

The women also coped with breast cancer by making social comparisons in a self-enhancing manner (Taylor, 1983). Festinger's (1954) social comparison theory would suggest that people make upward social comparisons in threatening situations in order to learn how to cope more effectively. But Taylor and colleagues (1984) found that rather than comparing themselves to women who were doing better, most of the women compared themselves to those who were doing worse, and used these downward comparisons to bolster the self by inferring how relatively well they were coping with their cancer. (For a discussion of how these social comparisons affect subsequent motivation to perform behaviors, see Lockwood & Pinkus, Chapter 16, this volume.)

When people develop spontaneous self-enhancing perceptions in response to a threatening event, these perceptions are often based on a modest degree of illusion. There is, for example, no evidence that people can personally affect the course of a potentially fatal illness, but such beliefs figure into such accounts nonetheless. Findings like these have been repeatedly replicated in a diverse range of people coping with a wide array of threatening events (Updegraff & Taylor, 2000; Updegraff, Taylor, Kemeny, & Wyatt, 2002). Because that evidence has been extensively reviewed elsewhere (see Updegraff & Taylor, 2000), it will not be reiterated here. However, the fact that self-enhancement so reliably occurs in response to threatening events, with clear beneficial effects on adjustment, raises the intriguing possibility that self-enhancement has more general positive effects—not just those manifested in response to intensely stressful events.

## The Dynamics of Self-Enhancement

Drawing on this idea, Taylor and Brown (1988) put forth a theory of positive illusions, one component of which is self-enhancement. Specifically, because self-aggrandizement had so clearly helped the women with breast cancer adjust to their altered circumstances, they suggested that illusions such as self-enhancement may be adaptive for mental health and well-being more generally. Taylor and Brown reviewed a substantial array of evidence to show that positive illusions (including self-enhancement, the illusion of control, and unrealistic optimism) are highly prevalent in the everyday thinking of normal, well-adjusted people, and that these beliefs contribute actively to the criteria thought to be indicative of the healthy, well-functioning person: the ability to be happy or relatively contented with one's life; the ability to care for and about others; openness to new ideas and people; the capacity for creative and productive work; and the ability to cope with stressful events.

As evidence of the mild but common tendency toward self-enhancement, Taylor and Brown (1988) reviewed literature showing people's disproportionate interest in and recall of information about their positive rather than their negative qualities; their tendency to take credit for good outcomes (Miller & Ross, 1975); their tendency to see themselves more positively than others see them (e.g., Lewinsohn, Mischel, Chaplin, & Barton, 1980); and their tendency to see themselves as more likely than their peers to possess positive attributes and less likely to possess negative attributes (e.g., Alicke, 1985). On the basis that everyone cannot be better than everyone else, Taylor and Brown referred to this finding as evidence of a positive illusion of self-enhancement.

Self-enhancement has not always enjoyed a good reputation. In early work on mental health, positively inflated self-perceptions were regarded as evidence of poor mental health (Jahoda, 1958; Maslow, 1950). Personality psychologists addressing this *defensive neuroticism* view of self-enhancement have maintained that self-enhancing cognitions are reliably associated with adverse outcomes indicative of poor psychological functioning (e.g., John & Robins, 1994; Paulhus, 1998; Shedler, Mayman, & Manis, 1993). In contrast, the *positive illusions* position maintains that self-enhancement is characteristic of most people, and that it ebbs and flows as a function of situational constraints (Taylor & Gollwitzer, 1995). Self-enhancement is most evident in the abstract when it holds the power to inspire and motivate, and less evident when it can be directly disconfirmed by the feedback of specific situations (Armor & Taylor, 1998). In an empirical investigation designed to address these competing accounts, Taylor, Lerner, Sherman, Sage, and McDowell (2003b) comprehensively assessed the relation of self-enhancement to mental health by employing multiple measures of self-enhancement generated by advocates of both theoretical positions, as well as multiple measures of mental health, also reflecting both theoretical positions. As such, the study was able to examine the positive illusions prediction that self-enhancement is positively related to mental health, and the defensive neuroticism position (e.g., Shedler et al., 1993) that self-enhancement is negatively related to indicators of mental health. Across multiple measures, the relation of self-enhancement to mental health was largely linear and positive, as predicted by the positive illusions position. This was true regardless of the theoretical origins of the self-enhancement and mental health measures.

Thus a modest degree of self-enhancement appears to be associated with mental health and resilience in the face of threat. Indeed, recent investigations have found that self-enhancement was associated with reduced posttraumatic stress disorder symptoms after the September 11 terrorist attacks (Bonanno, Rennicke, Dekel, & Rosen, 2005) and with better adjustment among Bosnian civilians in Sarajevo after the civil war (Bonanno, Field, Kovacevic, & Kaltman, 2002). Believing that one has many talents and positive qualities, and more talents and more positive qualities than one's peers, allows one to feel good about the self and to deal with the stressful circumstances of daily life with the resources conferred by a positive sense of self. These self-enhancing beliefs help people thrive in times of stress that might otherwise leave them dispirited and unable to pursue their goals.

## The Dynamics of Self-Affirmation

Self-affirmation theory (Sherman & Cohen, 2006; Steele, 1988) begins with the premise that people are motivated to maintain the perceived worth and integrity of the self. When one experiences a threat to the self—be it a failure experience, information suggesting that one has acted wrongly, or information contradicting one's beliefs—one is motivated to respond to the threat in such a way as to restore self-worth. There are three categories of responses that people can make to such threats to the self. First, people can respond directly to the threat by accepting the failure or threatening information. However, the need to maintain positive self-regard (Taylor & Brown, 1988) often makes this very difficult to do. Second, people can respond directly to the threat by devaluing the threat in some way. We refer to this as a *defensive bias* (Sherman & Cohen, 2002), because the evaluation serves to minimize the threat at the expense of learning from important, though threatening, information. But self-affirmation theory proposes that there is greater flexibility in how people can respond to threats than these two alternatives suggest. People can also respond to threats indirectly, by affirming alternative self-resources. Since the overall goal of the self is to maintain global self-worth and self-integrity, when people affirm the self, this goal is achieved. Consequently, self-affirmation serves a buffering function and helps people deal with the threat.

The original self-affirmation studies suggested that cognitive dissonance stems from a threat to the self-concept. This was demonstrated in studies (e.g., Steele & Liu, 1983) in which people who reflected on important values no longer had the need to reduce their dissonance by engaging in some sort of rationalization. Recent work on self-affirmation has further shown that when people affirm important self-resources, they are less likely to be defensive and to devalue threatening information, and consequently are more open to potentially threatening information (Sherman & Cohen, 2002).

One of the most challenging threats individuals face is health information suggesting the personal potential for ill health. Health information can threaten the self by suggesting that people have acted unwisely—by, for example, smoking, drinking, or practicing unsafe sex. Although it would be optimal if people responded to personal health information by changing their behavior, people can be quite resistant to personally threatening health messages, and subsequently less likely to change their behavior. In her work on motivated inference, Kunda (1987) has shown that people are more likely to scrutinize health information for fault when it is of high personal relevance than when it is not relevant to the self. Thus individuals who have the most to gain from health communications are often the least likely to accept them. For example, one study found that sexually active students who saw an AIDS educational message responded by seeing themselves as being at reduced risk for sexually transmitted diseases—a defensive response (Morris & Swann, 1996).

Sherman, Nelson, and Steele (2000) examined defensive responses to threatening health information in the context of breast cancer prevention. Participants were women who were either coffee drinkers or not, and they reviewed a scientific report linking caffeine consumption to fibrocystic disease, a precursor to breast cancer. The article concluded by suggesting that women can reduce their risk for fibrocystic disease by reducing their caffeine consumption. As in earlier research (Kunda, 1987), coffee drinkers were more critical of the scientific article and thus more resistant to the message than were those who did not drink coffee. Yet coffee drinkers who had completed a values scale for a personally important value prior to reading the threatening messages (and who were thus self-affirmed) were more open to the information contained in the report than were participants who did not drink coffee, and they intended to reduce their coffee drinking accordingly. Because the motivation to maintain self-integrity was achieved by the self-affirmation, people who would otherwise have felt threatened by the health message were less resistant to the threat and more open to the message. A second study (Sherman et al., 2000) found that sexually active students who completed a similar self-affirmation task prior to viewing an AIDS educational video saw themselves as being at increased risk for HIV (relative to no-affirmation controls) and engaged in more positive health behaviors—namely, purchasing condoms and taking educational brochures. Other research has found that the effects of self-affirmation on acceptance of threatening health information related to alcohol intake can persist for at least 1 month (Harris & Napper, 2005), and that self-affirmation can lead high-risk smokers to have greater intentions to quit smoking and self-efficacy to do so after viewing graphic images depicting the negative effects of smoking (Harris, Mayle, Mabbott, & Napper, in press).

Self-affirmations can also affect the type of social comparisons people make in response to threat. Participants in a study by Spencer, Fein, and Lomore (2001) received bogus negative feedback about their intelligence based on a test they had taken. Then some participants completed a self-affirmation task of writing about a personally important value (others wrote about an unimportant value). Participants then had the opportunity to learn more about either a very effective, competent person (which would allow them to make upward social comparisons) or a less effective person (which would allow them to make downward social comparisons). The nonaffirmed people chose to make downward social comparisons, but those who completed the self-affirmation were more likely to make upward social comparisons. This pattern again suggests that self-affirmation can serve as a means to enhance the self, and thus can promote openness to what would be otherwise threatening information.

Thus, in these ways, self-affirmation can serve as a resource for people dealing with challenging events (e.g., potential threats to their health) and enable them to confront challenges more openly and directly.

## SELF-ENHANCEMENT, SELF-AFFIRMATION, GOALS, AND PERFORMANCE

Can self-affirmation and self-enhancement not only restore balance following exposure to threatening events and make people more receptive to useful negative information, but also fuel the ability to set high goals and strive persistently to achieve them? In their original paper, Taylor and Brown (1988) reviewed evidence to suggest that a positive sense of self is associated with working longer and harder on tasks. In particular, such illusions as self-enhancement may help people try harder in situations with objectively somewhat poor probabilities of success; although some failure is inevitable, ultimately these illusions may pay off with more progress than would be the case with lack of persistence (see also Greenwald, 1980).

Armor and Taylor (2003) tested this prediction by manipulating positive illusions. This was accomplished through the introduction of *deliberative* or *implemental* mindsets. Previous research (Taylor & Gollwitzer, 1995) had found that when people are deliberating whether or not to undertake a particular task, their optimism and task- relevant self-assessments are less inflated and more accurate than is the case when they have decided to undertake a task and are preparing to implement it; during implementation, positive illusions are much more evident. In the Armor and Taylor study, participants were either induced to deliberate the merits of participating in a particular task (a scavenger hunt) or told that they would be shortly doing the task (implementation). As in the previous research, deliberation produced reliably pessimistic expectations regarding the task, compared to implementation. Specifically, those who deliberated the pros and cons of participating in a scavenger hunt predicted that they would do more poorly and saw the hunt as inherently more difficult than did those who entertained thoughts of actually doing it. A second investigation replicated these effects and also assessed performance on the scavenger hunt. Those in the implemental mindset condition were not only more motivated to pursue the task, but also did significantly better on the task; that is, they found more objects on the scavenger hunt, albeit not as many as they had predicted they would find. Thus positive illusions, which in this case were induced by an implemental mindset, enhanced task expectations and performance predictions, in turn enhancing performance. The favorable assessment induced by this manipulation ensured that the goal was actively and aggressively pursued. An intriguing question is whether these positive illusions enable people to pursue their goals more flexibly (see Gollwitzer, Parks-Stamm, Jaudas, & Sheeran, Chapter 21, this volume). That is, a heightened awareness of one's positive attributes may facilitate performance not by leading one to focus narrowly on the goal, but by boosting one's general sense of self-worth.

Additional evidence for this perspective comes from an intervention study conducted by Cohen and colleagues at a racially mixed middle school (Cohen, Garcia, Apfel, & Master, 2006). The middle school children completed a 15-minute self-affirmation writing exercise, and wrote about an important value (or a relatively unimportant value, in the control condition) in the context of a normal school assignment. The intervention significantly improved the end-of-semester grades of the African American students and reduced the racial achievement gap by 40%, presumably by reducing the self-threat associated with the possibility of confirming negative stereotypes (Steele, 1997). Thus bolstering self-worth enabled these students to achieve their academic goals.

## THE SELF AND SOCIAL FUNCTIONING

### Do Self-Enhancers Experience Social Costs?

A particular sticking point in the literature on self-enhancement has been whether self-enhancement fosters success with respect to social goals. Are people high in self-enhancement more or less favorably perceived by peers than those low in self-enhancement? Research suggests that self-enhancers can be seen as conceited, hostile, and self-important (Colvin, Block, & Funder, 1995) or as self-centered and narcissistic (Paulhus, 1998). The positive illusions position, however, maintains that self-regard is associated with the capacity for positive and rewarding social relationships. Taylor and colleagues' (2003b) previously described study assessed the social relationships experienced by participants in an effort to compare these two positions. Using several different measures of self-enhancement, they found little evidence that self-enhancers experienced social costs. Those people categorized as high self-enhancers were perceived to be as likeable and as interpersonally capable as those who were characterized as low self-enhancers. In addition, the friendships of high self-enhancers were as long, as close, and as satisfying as those of low self-enhancers. Even when self-enhancing individuals were seen less positively by their friends than they saw themselves, the friendships showed no signs of compromise or lack of closeness. There was accordingly no evidence that self-enhancers experienced social costs.

Recent research (Master & Taylor, 2007) suggests a possible reason why the social costs that would seem to be almost inevitably associated with self-enhancement do not necessarily occur. Master and Taylor (2007) found that highly self-enhancing individuals not only enhance their personal qualities directly through self-affirming statements, but enhance themselves indirectly by affirming the positive qualities of their friends, their families, the institutions with which they are affiliated, and their personal activities. Thus, for example, in their study, students who referred to themselves as performing exceptionally well in their courses were also more likely to report receiving support from their professors, having a great set of friends, and enjoying several rewarding leisure activities. These findings could of course be due to a general positivity effect, rather than to self-enhancement per se. However, analyses that controlled for general positivity revealed that these indirectly self-serving statements made a positive impression on others. Because indirectly self-enhancing statements were approximately 2.5 times more common than directly self-enhancing statements, Master and Taylor suggested that the potential socially adverse effects of blatant self-enhancement may have been muted by the high frequency of indirectly self-enhancing statements expressed by these individuals. That is, instead of coming across as self-centered, these individuals may have come across instead as upbeat people who enjoyed their lives.

## Group-Serving Judgments and Self-Affirmation

The research described above by Master and Taylor (2007) shows how people enhance the groups of which they are members. People often make decisions and evaluate information in ways that favor the interests, reputation, and esteem of their groups. People favor their teams by making negative assessments about other teams (Hastorf & Cantril, 1954) and favor their ingroups by derogating outgroups (Tajfel, 1982). This process helps people maintain motivation when their groups experience challenging or threatening events. For example, after a World Series, baseball players and managers from the winning team made more internal attributions for the outcome of the game ("We won because we played so well"), and players and managers from the losing team made more external attributions ("We ran into a lot of bad luck") (Lau & Russell, 1980). For both groups, such attributions can help them maintain motivation to see themselves as competent and successful.

In a series of studies, Sherman and Kim (2005) examined whether such group-serving judgments serve a self-protective function. They reasoned that people defend their groups, in part, because groups are an important part of how they see themselves (Tajfel & Turner, 1986). When their groups encounter challenging events, people will make biased social judgments to protect the groups, and consequently themselves. However, building on the logic of self-affirmation theory, if people have the opportunity to affirm their global selves in an important but unrelated domain, then they should be less group-serving, and more open to potentially threatening information about their groups.

Sherman and Kim (2005) tested this hypothesis in two studies. Participants were intramural athletes who had just completed a team sports competition and were asked to make attributions for the outcome of the game. Consistent with other research demonstrating group-serving judgments, players who won the game made more internal team attributions for the outcome of the game (i.e., attributions to the team's teamwork) than did team members who lost the game. However, participants who completed a self-affirmation task prior to making their judgments were not group-serving in their attributions; as winners or losers, they were equally likely to attribute the outcome of the game to internal factors. Thus people were more open to the threatening but potentially valuable information that bad teamwork had led to defeat when they were buffered by a self-affirmation. A second study replicated this finding, and found that the effect of self-affirmation was partially mediated by the extent to which the athletes felt that they were worthy team members.

Thus people are less likely to be group-serving in their judgments when their self-worth is affirmed. Other evidence for this point comes from research on outgroup derogation and prejudice. Fein and Spencer (1997) found that people were less likely to evaluate members of stereotyped groups negatively when their self-worth was affirmed. Their argument is a particularly good demonstration of the links between self-enhancement and self-affirmation. They posit that one manner in which people confront the vulnerabilities and frustrations of everyday life is by using stereotypes and prejudices to enhance the self (Wood & Taylor, 1991). But if the self-protective motivation is satisfied by some other means (such as a self-affirmation), then people should be less likely to stereotype others. Fein and Spencer supported this reasoning by demonstrating that after a threat, people made more prejudiced judgments of a member of a stigmatized group, and this process served to increase their state self-esteem (relative to those who did not have the opportunity to stigmatize). However, those who were affirmed by receiving positive feedback did not derogate an outgroup member, because they had less of a motivational need to bolster their self-esteem.

## THE SELF AND BIOLOGICAL FUNCTIONING

### The Biologically Protective Effects of Self-Enhancement

We have suggested that self-enhancement is a resource for fostering goal pursuit and for restoring motivation following a threat. Might self-enhancement accordingly represent a resource with biological implications for managing stress as well, and might self-affirmation reduce stress and illness by buffering the self? Threatening and stressful events take a toll not only on the psyche, but also on biological resources. When engaged by stressful circumstances, the autonomic nervous system and the hypothalamic–pituitary–adrenocortical (HPA) axis become activated and mobilize a person for "fight or flight." Although these responses are protective in the short term, recurrent or chronic activation of these stress-regulating systems can confer damage over the long term with adverse implications for health (e.g., McEwen, 1998).

If self-enhancement helps a person to manage stressful conditions, then biological responses to stress may be lower or less frequent in people who are high in self-enhancement. As a result, self-enhancers may experience a lesser chronic toll on their biological stress-regulating systems then those who lack this resource, by virtue of less wear and tear across the numerous stressful and challenging events to which people are inevitably exposed. Accordingly, one might expect self-enhancement to be associated both with chronically better-regulated stress systems and with lesser acute responses to specific stressful events (see McEwen, 1998).

In contrast to this viewpoint, however, researchers adopting the defensive neuroticism view of self-enhancement have suggested that self-enhancement leads to self-deceptive suppression of negative information about the self (e.g., Eysenck, 1994; Paulhus, 1998; Shedler et al., 1993; Weinberger & Schwartz, 1990). The suppression or repression of negative information is believed to be physiologically taxing, and so if the defensive neuroticism account of self-enhancement is correct, one might expect to see adverse physiological and neuroendocrine profiles associated with self-enhancement, instead of positive ones. Likely manifestations would appear in the form of overly active stress systems, such as higher or poorly regulated autonomic functioning or elevated HPA axis activity, chronically and/or in response to stress.

This hypothesis was explicitly tested by Shedler and colleagues (1993), who examined "the illusion of mental health." They maintained that people who self-enhance on mental health measures, but who are judged by clinicians to be distressed, represent a group at risk for poor mental health and overactive stress-regulating systems. Specifically, they argued and reported evidence that those with "illusory mental health" had higher cardiovascular reactivity during laboratory stressors than those judged to be genuinely mentally healthy (those who rated themselves high in mental health and were perceived by a clinician to be mentally healthy).

In an effort to compare these alternative positions, Taylor, Lerner, Sherman, Sage, and McDowell (2003a) identified individuals who were either high or low in self-enhancement and compared their biological responses to laboratory stress challenges. Consistent with the positive illusions position, and counter to the predications of the defensive neuroticism position, they found that high self-enhancers had significantly lower cardiovascular responses to stress, more rapid cardiovascular recovery, and lower baseline cortisol levels. (Cortisol is an indicator of the functioning of the HPA axis.) Consistent with the viewpoint that self-enhancement represents a psychological resource, the association between self-enhancement and lower baseline cortisol was mediated almost entirely by the psychological resources that people high in self-enhancement demonstrated, such as optimism, a sense of personal mastery, and an extroverted style.

Of particular significance was the fact that self-enhancers not only were protected in the immediate stressful circumstances that demanded their abilities to cope with stress (e.g., lesser cardiovascular reactivity to laboratory challenges), but also demonstrated biological responses to the stressors suggestive of chronically better-functioning stress regulatory systems. Specifically, self-enhancers' baseline heart rate was somewhat lower than that of low self-enhancers; their recovery from stress was significantly faster (the capacity to recover from stressful events is thought to be an important parameter indicative of the chronic functioning of the cardiovascular system); and their baseline cortisol levels were lower. Thus the fact that self-enhancers appear to have biological stress-regulating systems marked by signs of better functioning suggests that self-enhancement may have been a biologically protective resource across previous encounters with stress as well.

The biologically protective effects of self-enhancement are not confined to physiological and neuroendocrine responses to laboratory stressors; they are also manifested in disease course. For example, in a series of studies with people infected with HIV or diagnosed with AIDS, Taylor and colleagues found that those who held unrealistically positive views of their ability to stave off a rapid course of illness actually experienced a less rapid course of illness and a longer time period before death (Reed, Kemeny, Taylor, Wang, & Visscher, 1994; see also Taylor, Kemeny, Reed, Bower, & Gruenewald, 2000, for a review). On the basis of this research, Taylor and colleagues (2000) speculated that positive illusions such as self-enhancement may keep physiological and neuroendocrine responses to stress at low levels, as evidenced in lesser autonomic activation and lower HPA axis responses to stress. Because these systems exert important regulatory effects on the immune system, chronically lower stress responses of people higher in self-enhancing perceptions might account for a less rapid course of HIV infection. The laboratory evidence noted above—namely, that self-enhancement is associated both with fewer signs of chronic wear and tear on biological stress-regulating systems and with lesser cardiovascular responses to laboratory challenges—is consistent with this pathway.

## Reducing Stress and Illness by Affirming the Self

Both field and laboratory studies suggest that self-affirming activities can serve as a buffer against stressful events and result in positive health outcomes. Keough (1998) conducted a naturalistic field study in which college students wrote a series of essays over their winter break. Participants in the self-affirmation condition wrote two pages about the events of the day, and their feelings about those events in the context of their most important value. Compared to those in control conditions, participants in the self-affirmation condition reported the fewest physical symptoms over winter break and had reduced visits to the health center. A second study replicated this basic finding and found that the self-affirmation was more effective among those who were experiencing more constant threats to the self, as assessed by their self-reported daily hassles.

To test the stress-buffering effects of self-affirmation directly, Creswell and colleagues (2005) had participants complete a self-affirmation procedure—a values scale for their most important value (vs. an unimportant value in the control condition)—prior to engaging in the Trier Social Stress Task (Kirschbaum, Pirke, & Hellhammer, 1993). That is, those in the self-affirmation condition indicated their agreement with an important value (e.g., religion) in a domain of their lives unrelated to the stressful task. Participants were instructed to prepare a speech to be given to two speech evaluators concerning why they would be qualified for a job as an administrative assistant in a psychology department. The speech evaluators (i.e., confederates who were trained to act in a sullen manner) directed the 5-minute speech task and then asked each participant to complete a 5-minute mental arithmetic task by counting aloud backward from 2,083 by 13's. Salivary cortisol measurements were assessed at baseline and at 20, 30, and 45 minutes after stress onset.

During baseline, there were no differences in cortisol levels between participants in the self-affirmation and control conditions. Yet at the 20-minute measurement, and persisting through 45 minutes after the stress task, the participants in the control condition had elevated cortisol levels, whereas the self-affirmation participants did not (Creswell et al., 2005). This finding demonstrates that a self-affirmation manipulation can buffer the self not only at a psychological level, but also at a physiological level.

Thus self-affirmation interventions were associated with positive physiological and health outcomes in two relatively healthy college student samples (Creswell et al., 2005; Keough, 1998). An important question centers on whether similar effects would be obtained in a sample of people confronting disease. A study of women with breast cancer by Creswell and colleagues (2007) examined the relation between self-affirming writing and recovery from breast cancer. This research was based on a reanalysis of data from a study by Stanton and colleagues (2002). Essays that were written by the women were coded for self-affirmation (whether the essays evidenced positive reflection on valued self-domains), cognitive processing (whether the essays evidenced active thinking about the positive aspects of the breast cancer experience), and discovery-of-meaning statements (whether the essays evidenced efforts to find a larger lesson or significance to their breast cancer), to test for potential mediating mechanisms for the writing effects on breast cancer recovery. The number of self-affirming statements made in the essays (e.g., "I have always had a good positive attitude about all things, and that has really helped me during this time") fully mediated the writing intervention effects found on physical symptoms at a 3-month follow-up. Additionally, the frequency of self-affirmation statements predicted enhanced coping and reductions in distress at the follow-up session. Thus it appears that self-affirmation is a potential health intervention for people who are dealing with stressors and threats to the self—an exciting direction for future research.

## BENEFITS OF SELF-ENHANCEMENT AND SELF-AFFIRMATION: EXPLORING SOME CHALLENGES

Both enhancing and affirming the self have clear benefits for goal pursuit and for managing stress, but at least two areas of research present challenges to the generality of these benefits. The first is how one reconciles self-enhancement with obvious needs to monitor reality accurately. The second issue concerns whether these processes characterize some cultures more than others.

### Reconciling Self-Enhancement with Accuracy Needs

Does not self-enhancement entail the risk that falsely positive self-perceptions will promote errors and inaccuracies in the selection of goals or courses of action? For example, might not a person high in self-enhancement overshoot his or her abilities, select tasks that are too difficult, promise more than he or she can deliver, or otherwise thwart or undermine the beneficial outcomes that positive illusions are thought to foster?

Two characteristics of self-enhancement may keep these concerns from being problematic. The first is that although people generally inflate their personal qualities, their relative accuracy is very high, as compared, for example, with friends' assessments of them on those same qualities (Taylor et al., 2003b). Thus, although people may consider themselves to be, for example, more athletic or artistic than is actually true, they have a *relatively* accurate sense of how athletic or artistic they are, and are therefore unlikely to pick professional sports or fine arts as occupations if their talents in these arenas are modest.

The second factor that may keep self-enhancement from promoting errors and inaccuracies in life choices is the fact that self-enhancement is situationally responsive and more evident at the general than at the specific level, when it could be disconfirmed (Armor & Taylor, 2003). Specifically, self-enhancement is greater at the beginning of a project, when it has the power to motivate people to carry through their efforts toward their goals, than at the end of a project, when modest achievements and their discrepancies from hoped-for results might be dispiriting (Shepperd, Ouellette, & Fernandez, 1996). Self-enhancement is more in evidence when personal qualities are ambiguous than when they are concrete, with clear behavioral referents generating the potential for disconfirmation (e.g., Dunning, Meyerowitz, & Holzberg, 1989). Self-enhancement is more in evidence when a course of action has been selected than when it is under debate; as noted, when people are debating the pros and cons of a particular course of action, their perceptions both of that undertaking and of their personal abilities to achieve it are more modest and in line with reality than is the case when they are preparing to implement it (Taylor & Gollwitzer, 1995). Thus people are most likely to be self-enhancing at the general level when the chances that they will be proven wrong are negligible, but they are more modest in specific situations when exaggerated self-assessments may be subject to scrutiny or may lead them down risky paths.

Rather than promoting errors in judgment, self-enhancement and self-affirmation seem to promote more unbiased processing of information (Sherman & Cohen, 2002). One set of studies supporting this point has examined the *disconfirmation bias*—the tendency to spend effort and energy disconfirming information that contradicts strongly held beliefs (Lord, Lepper, & Ross, 1979). One of the reasons why people are so resistant to believe disconfirming information is that it threatens how they see themselves. Consequently, self-affirmation should secure the self and make people more open to belief-disconfirming information. Cohen, Aronson, and Steele (2000) examined this issue with opponents and proponents of capital punishment, who were presented with a persuasive scientific report that contradicted their beliefs about the death penalty's effectiveness as a deterrent for crime. As in past research (Lord et al., 1979), participants were very resistant to this type of information, exhibiting a disconfirmation bias. They found flaws in the methodology of the studies reported; they suspected bias on the part of the authors of the report; and they persisted in their attitudes toward capital punishment. In contrast, participants who completed a self-affirmation task were less critical of the reported research; they suspected less bias on the part of the authors; and they even changed their overall attitudes toward capital punishment in the direction of the report they read. Coupled with the self-enhancement research described above, the self-affirmation studies suggest that by reflecting on important self-resources, people can become less biased, rather than more biased, in their judgments and decisions.

## Culture, Self-Enhancement, and Self-Affirmation

Are the benefits of self-affirmation and self-enhancement cross-cultural or specific to Western cultures? Some cultural psychologists maintain that there is not a universal need for positive self-regard, and that there are instead cultural differences between East Asians and North Americans in the extent to which they self-enhance (Heine, Lehman, Markus, & Kitayama, 1999). As Heine (2003) has noted, there are two forms this argument can assume about cultural differences in self-enhancement: a weak form and a strong form. The weak form argues that East Asians enhance less than North Americans. There is much evidence to support the weak form of the argument. Heine and Hamamura (2007) conducted a meta-analysis on published studies making cross-cultural comparisons in self-enhancement, and found that East Asians showed weaker self-enhancement than Westerners in 79 out of 81 studies. The average effect size for the cross-cultural comparison was large ($d = 0.83$). Thus a great many studies support the argument that East Asians enhance less than Westerners.

The strong form of the argument is that East Asians do not self-enhance (Heine, 2003). As Brown and Kobayashi (2003a) put it, this argument is provocative "because it challenges the claim that self-enhancement needs are universal, arguing instead that people from East Asian cultures feel no desire to enhance their feelings of self-worth" (p. 492). Evidence for the strong form of the argument comes from the meta-analysis finding that across all of the studies, East Asians were not self-enhancing (average $d = 0.01$) (Heine, 2005; Heine & Hamamura, 2007).

A number of researchers have challenged this notion. For example, Kurman (2003) argued that cultural differences in modesty mediate cultural differences in self-enhancement, and that when cultural differences in modesty are statistically controlled for, there are no longer cultural differences in enhancement. Brown and Kobayashi (2003b) argued that East Asians do self-enhance on traits that are important to them, and that past studies showing a lack of self-enhancement reflect are based on studies using traits that are more important to Westerners than to East Asians. They found that East Asians are much more self-enhancing when they rate traits that are important to them rather than unimportant traits (see also Sedikides, Gaertner, & Toguchi, 2003). Other studies, however, have found an opposite pattern—namely, that East Asians are less self-enhancing in domains important to them (Heine, 2005; Kitayama, Markus, Matsumoto, & Norasakkunkit, 1997). For a discussion of how self-enhancement varies cross-culturally, see Morling and Kitayama (Chapter 27, this volume).

The debate about culture and self-enhancement highlights some important issues regarding the measurement of self-enhancement. For example, in the meta-analysis by Heine and Hamamura (2007), one methodology that most clearly demonstrated East Asian self-enhancement was the *self–other bias* (also known as the *better-than-average effect*). However, they note that there are some important methodological issues to consider with this measure. It appears that when people compare an individual in their group (a singular person) to the average person in their group (a mean of a hypothetical distribution), they tend to view everybody in the group as better than their group's average (Klar & Giladi, 1999). Thus methodologically, one important suggestion for studying self-enhancement is to utilize a number of different methodologies to converge on the concept. This strategy was adopted in a recent investigation (Taylor et al., 2003b) in which we compared three distinct measures of self-enhancement. Patterns of results did not vary by whether self-enhancement was assessed comparatively or not.

The question of whether self-affirmation can reduce biased social judgments among individuals from collectivist cultures has received some attention. One possibility suggested by Heine and Lehman (1997) is that members of collectivist cultures may be less motivated to affirm the self, because their culture places less emphasis on maintaining a positive self-image. However, it is also possible that members of collectivist cultures are just as motivated as members of individualist cultures to protect the self, but that they are more responsive to collectivist affirmations (e.g., of social relationships) than to individualist affirmations (e.g., of personal values; see Heine & Lehman, 1997).

A recent study by Hoshino-Browne and colleagues (2005) shed light on this question, and supported the second possibility. Within a cognitive dissonance paradigm, participants (who were either Asian Canadian or European Canadian) made choices for either themselves or their friends. As in Heine and Lehman (1997), when the Asian Canadians made choices for themselves, they experienced no cognitive dissonance and did not justify their choice by spreading the alternatives between the chosen and nonchosen objects. In contrast, when the Asian Canadians made choices for their friends, they appeared to exhibit cognitive dissonance and justified their choice by spreading the alternatives between the chosen and nonchosen objects. Most important and central to our concerns, this tendency was reduced among Asian Canadian participants who completed a collectivist affirmation (i.e., those who had written about a value that was important to their families) and not reduced among those who completed an individualist affirmation. Thus it appears that Asians can be affirmed; however, the affirmation needs to be congruent with the collectivist sense of self.

## TOWARD A NEUROBIOLOGY OF SELF-ENHANCEMENT

The fact that self-enhancement can be central to motivational processes involving goal pursuit and restoration of self-worth following threat implies a centrality to motivation that may have biological underpinnings. The idea that self-enhancement is an intrinsic part of the goal-setting–persistence–performance nexus has recently been given some intriguing credibility from research on the neural bases of attribution. In a neuroimaging study, Blackwood and colleagues (2003) had participants make attributions (i.e., "Was it something about the situation, something about you, or something about your friend?") for such hypothetical actions as "A friend brought you a present" or "A friend thinks you are dishonest." One goal of the research was to examine the neural bases of one indication of self-enhancement—namely, the *self-serving attributional bias*. This bias reflects the tendency to take credit for good actions and deny responsibility for bad ones. The results indicated that the self-serving bias was common and significant, and that it was associated with enhanced activation in the bilateral caudate nucleus, a subregion of the striatum.

Primate studies suggest that motor, cognitive, and motivational systems interact with the striatum, fostering adjustment to changing environmental contingencies in the form of goal-directed behavior. That is, the striatum is a central structure involved in the motivational control of behavior, with the ventral striatum particularly involved in the processing of motivational information. In addition, there are connections between the striatum and the dopaminergic system, and both dorsal and ventral striatum neurons have been implicated in the prediction and detection of rewards. The striatum is regarded as critically involved in reinforcement learning. Striatal activation subserving the self-serving bias therefore may conceivably be understood as reflecting the fact that internal attributions for positive events and external attributions for negative events are rewarding. Moreover, recent research suggests that neurons in the caudate nucleus link the anticipation of expected reward with preparation for goal-directed eye movements, thus relating these processes to preparation for action. The self-serving bias, then, is subserved by regions that have been implicated in motivated behavior.

Blackwood and colleagues (2003) have also suggested that the striatal activations implicated in the self-serving bias may indicate that the self-serving bias is a social routine or habit that functions at the intuitive rather than the deliberative level, to simplify understanding of the complex social world. That is, this brain region is an "old" one, and its activation is thought to reflect automatic rather than controlled processing. As such, the bias may be so automatic and so much a part of the pathways linking anticipated rewards to anticipatory action that in order to attribute events in a non-self-serving manner, an individual may need to employ deliberative and controlled processes to counteract it. While not definitive, such intriguing findings clearly suggest that self-enhancement can play an intrinsic and potentially automatic role in the processes that regulate goal-related performance.

## CONCLUSIONS

Integrating research on self-enhancement and self-affirmation reveals that a positive sense of self can be a vital resource for managing stress and for goal pursuit. The benefits of a strong sense of self are biological as well as psychological, and in this respect, self-affirmation and self-enhancement fit well in the burgeoning literature on positive psychology (see King, Chapter 34, this volume; Taylor & Sherman, 2004). Of particular significance is the fact that self-enhancement and self-affirmation actually increase rather than decrease receptivity to personally relevant negative information. Further research should continue to address the boundary conditions around these benefits, especially the cultural limitations. These caveats notwithstanding, evidence is emerging to suggest that a positive sense of self can be an integral part of the neural pathways underlying motivation and performance.

## ACKNOWLEDGMENT

This research was supported by a National Institute of Mental Health grant (No. MH 056880) to Shelley E. Taylor.

## REFERENCES

Alicke, M. D. (1985). Global self-evaluation as determined by the desirability and controllability of trait adjectives. *Journal of Personality and Social Psychology, 49*, 1621–1630.

Armor, D. A., & Taylor, S. E. (1998). Situated optimism: Specific outcome expectancies and self-regulation. In M. P. Zanna (Ed.), *Advances in experimental social psychology* (Vol. 30, pp. 309–379). San Diego, CA: Academic Press.

Armor, D. A., & Taylor, S. E. (2003). The effects of mindset on behavior: Self-regulation in deliberative and implemental frames of mind. *Personality and Social Psychology Bulletin, 29*, 86–95.

Blackwood, N. J., Bentall, R. P., ffytche, D. H., Simmons, A., Murray, R. M., & Howard, R. J. (2003). Self-responsibility and the self-serving bias: An fMRI investigation of casual attributions. *NeuroImage, 20*, 1076–1085.

Bonanno, G. A., Field, N. P., Kovacevic, A., & Kaltman, S. (2002). Self-enhancement as a buffer against extreme adversity: Civil war in Bosnia and traumatic loss in the United States. *Personality and Social Psychology Bulletin, 28*, 184–196.

Bonanno, G. A., Rennicke, C., Dekel, S., & Rosen, J. (2005). Self-enhancement among high-exposure survivors of the September 11th terrorist attack: Resilience or social maladjustment? *Journal of Personality and Social Psychology, 88*, 984–988.

Brown, J. D., & Kobayashi, C. (2003a). Introduction: Culture and the self-enhancementmotive. *Journal of Cross-Cultural Psychology, 34*, 492–495.

Brown, J. D., & Kobayashi, C. (2003b). Motivation and manifestation: Cross-cultural expression of the self-enhancement motive. *Asian Journal of Social Psychology, 6*, 85–88.

Cohen, G. L., Aronson, J., & Steele, C. M. (2000). When beliefs yield to evidence: Reducing biased evaluation by affirming the self. *Personality and Social Psychology Bulletin, 26*, 1151–1164.

Cohen, G. L., Garcia, J., Apfel, N., & Master, A. (2006). Reducing the racial achievement gap: A social-psychological intervention. *Science, 313*, 1307–1310.

Colvin, C. R., Block, J., & Funder, D. C. (1995). Overly positive self-evaluations and personality: Negative implications for mental health. *Journal of Personality and Social Psychology, 68*, 1152–1162.

Creswell, J. D., Lam, S., Stanton, A. L., Taylor, S. E., Bower, J. E., & Sherman, D. K. (2007). Does self-affirmation, cognitive processing, or discovery of meaning explain cancer-related health benefits of expressive writing? *Personality and Social Psychology Bulletin, 33*, 238–250.

Creswell, J. D., Welch, W., Taylor, S. E., Sherman, D. K., Gruenewald, T., & Mann, T. (2005). Affirmation of personal values buffers neuroendocrine and psychological stress responses. *Psychological Science, 16*, 846–851.

Dunning, D., Meyerowitz, J. A., & Holzberg, A. D. (1989). Ambiguity and self-evaluation: The role of idiosyncratic trait definitions in self-serving appraisals of ability. *Journal of Personality and Social Psychology, 57*, 1082–1090.

Eysenck, H. J. (1994). Neuroticism and the illusion of mental health. *American Psychologist, 49*, 971–972.

Fein, S., & Spencer, S. J. (1997). Prejudice as self-image maintenance: Affirming the self through derogating others. *Journal of Personality and Social Psychology, 73*, 31–44.

Festinger, L. (1954). A theory of social comparison processes. *Human Relations, 7*, 117–140.

Greenwald, A. G. (1980). The totalitarian ego: Fabrication and revision of personal history. *American Psychologist, 35*, 603–618.

Harris, P. R., Mayle, K., Mabbott, L., & Napper, L. (in press). Self-affirmation reduces smokers' defensiveness to graphic on pack cigarette warning labels. *Health Psychology.*

Harris, P. R., & Napper, L. (2005). Self-affirmation and the biased processing of threatening health-risk information. *Personality and Social Psychology Bulletin, 31*, 1250–1263.

Hastorf, A. H., & Cantril, H. (1954). They saw a game: A case study. *Journal of Abnormal and Social Psychology, 49*, 129–134.

Heine, S. J. (2003). Self-enhancement in Japan?: A reply to Brown & Kobayashi. *Asian Journal of Social Psychology, 6*, 75–84.

Heine, S. J. (2005). Where is the evidence for pancultural self-enhancement?: A reply to Sedikides, Gaertner, and Toguchi (2003). *Journal of Personality and Social Psychology, 89*, 531–538.

Heine, S. J., & Hamamura, T. (2007). In search of East Asian self-enhancement. *Personality and Social Psychology Review, 11*, 1–24.

Heine, S. J., & Lehman, D. R. (1997). Culture, dissonance, and self-affirmation. *Personality and Social Psychology Bulletin, 23*, 389–400.

Heine, S. J., Lehman, D. R., Markus, H. R., & Kitayama, S. (1999). Is there a universal need for positive self-regard? *Psychological Review, 106*, 766–794.

Hoshino-Browne, E., Zanna, A. S., Spencer, S. J., Zanna, M. P., Kitayama, S., & Lackenbauer, S. (2005). On the cultural guises of cognitive dissonance: The case of Easterners and Westerners. *Journal of Personality and Social Psychology, 89*, 294–310.

Jahoda, M. (1958). *Current concepts of positive mental health.* New York: Basic Books.

John, O. P., & Robins, R. W. (1994). Accuracy and bias in self-perception: Individual differences in self-enhancement and the role of narcissism. *Journal of Personality and Social Psychology, 66*, 206–219.

Keough, K. A. (1998). When the self is at stake: Integrating the self into stress and physical health research (Doctoral dissertation, Stanford University, 1998). *Dissertation Abstracts International, 58*, 3959B.

Kirschbaum, C., Pirke, K., & Hellhammer, D. H. (1993). The "Trier Social Stress Test"—a tool for investigating psychobiological stress responses in a laboratory setting. *Neuropsychobiology, 28*, 76–81.

Kitayama, S., Markus, H. R., Matsumoto, H., & Norasakkunkit, V. (1997). Individual and collective processes in the construction of the self: Self-enhancement in the United States and self-criticism in Japan. *Journal of Personality and Social Psychology, 72*, 1245–1267.

Klar, Y., & Giladi, E. E. (1999). No one in my group can be below the group's average: A robust positivity bias in favor of anonymous peers. *Journal of Personality and Social Psychology, 73*, 885–901.

Kunda, Z. (1987). Motivated inference: Self-serving generation and evaluation of causal theories. *Journal of Personality and Social Psychology, 53*, 636–647.

Kurman, J. (2003). The role of perceived specificity level of failure in self-enhancement and in constructive self-criticism. *Personality and Social Psychology Bulletin, 29*, 285–294.

Lau, R. R., & Russell, D. (1980). Attributions in the sports pages. *Journal of Personality and Social Psychology, 39*, 29–38.

Lewinsohn, P. M., Mischel, W., Chaplin, W., & Barton, R. (1980). Social competence and depression: The role of illusory self-perceptions. *Journal of Abnormal Psychology, 89*, 203–212.

Lord, C. G., Lepper, M. R., & Ross, L. (1979). Biased assimilation and attitude polarization: The effects of prior theories on subsequently considered evidence. *Journal of Personality and Social Psychology, 37*, 2098–2109.

Maslow, A. H. (1950). Self-actualizing people: A study of psychological health. *Personality Symposium, 1*, 11–34.

Master, S., & Taylor, S. E. (2007). *The dynamics of direct and indirect self-enhancement: Impact on social evaluations.* Manuscript under review.

McEwen, B. S. (1998). Protective and damaging effects of stress mediators. *New England Journal of Medicine, 338*, 171–179.

Miller, D. T., & Ross, M. (1975). Self-serving biases in attribution of causality: Fact or fiction? *Psychological Bulletin, 82*, 213–225.

Morris, K. A., & Swann, W. B. (1996). Denial and the

AIDS crisis: On wishing away the threat of AIDS. In S. Oskamp & S. Thompson (Eds.), *Understanding and preventing HIV risk behavior: Safer sex and drug use* (pp. 57–79). Thousand Oaks, CA: Sage.

Paulhus, D. L. (1998). Interpersonal and intrapsychic adaptiveness of trait self-enhancement: A mixed blessing? *Journal of Personality and Social Psychology, 74*, 1197–1208.

Reed, G. M., Kemeny, M. E., Taylor, S. E., Wang, H.-Y. J., & Visscher, B. R. (1994). "Realistic acceptance" as a predictor of decreased survival time in gay men with AIDS. *Health Psychology, 13*, 299–307.

Sedikides, C., Gaertner, L., & Toguchi, Y. (2003). Pancultural self-enhancement. *Journal of Personality and Social Psychology, 84*, 60–79.

Shedler, J., Mayman, M., & Manis, M. (1993). The illusion of mental health. *American Psychologist, 48*, 1117–1131.

Shepperd, J. A., Ouellette, J. A., & Fernandez, J. K. (1996). Abandoning unrealistic optimism: Performance estimates and the temporal proximity of self-relevant feedback. *Journal of Personality and Social Psychology, 70*, 844–855.

Sherman, D. K., & Cohen, G. L. (2002). Accepting threatening information: Self-affirmation and the reduction of defensive biases. *Current Directions in Psychological Science, 11*, 119–123.

Sherman, D. K., & Cohen, G. L. (2006). The psychology of self-defense: Self-affirmation theory. In M. P. Zanna (Ed.), *Advances in experimental social psychology* (Vol. 38, pp. 183–242). San Diego, CA: Academic Press.

Sherman, D. K., & Kim, H. S. (2005). Is there an "I" in "team"?: The role of the self in group-serving judgments. *Journal of Personality and Social Psychology, 88*, 108–120.

Sherman, D. K., Nelson, L. D., & Steele, C. M. (2000). Do messages about health risks threaten the self?: Increasing the acceptance of threatening health messages via self-affirmation. *Personality and Social Psychology Bulletin, 26*, 1046–1058.

Spencer, S. J., Fein, S., & Lomore, C. D. (2001). Maintaining one's self-image vis-à-vis others: The role of self-affirmation in the social evaluation of the self. *Motivation and Emotion, 25*, 41–65.

Stanton, A. L., Danoff-Burg, S., Sworowski, L. A., Collins, C. A., Branstetter, A., Rodriguez-Hanley, A., et al. (2002). Randomized, controlled trial of written emotional expression and benefit finding in breast cancer patients. *Journal of Clinical Oncology, 20*, 4160–4168.

Steele, C. M. (1988). The psychology of self-affirmation: Sustaining the integrity of the self. In L. Berkowitz (Ed.), *Advances in experimental psychology* (Vol. 21, pp. 261–302). San Diego, CA: Academic Press.

Steele, C. M. (1997). A threat in the air: How stereotypes shape intellectual identity and performance. *American Psychologist, 52*, 613–629.

Steele, C. M., & Liu, T.J. (1983). Dissonance processes as self-affirmation. *Journal of Personality and Social Psychology, 45*, 5–19.

Tajfel, H. (1982). Social psychology of intergroup relations. *Annual Review of Psychology, 33*, 1–39.

Tajfel, H., & Turner, J. C. (1986). The social identity theory of intergroup behavior. In S. Worchel & W. G. Austin (Eds.), *Psychology of intergroup relations* (2nd ed., pp. 33–48). Chicago: Nelson-Hall.

Taylor, S. E. (1983). Adjustment to threatening events: A theory of cognitive adaptation. *American Psychologist, 38*, 1161–1173.

Taylor, S. E., & Brown, J. D. (1988). Illusion and well-being: A social psychological perspective on mental health. *Psychological Bulletin, 103*, 193–210.

Taylor, S. E., & Gollwitzer, P. M. (1995). The effects of mindset on positive illusions. *Journal of Personality and Social Psychology, 69*, 213–226.

Taylor, S. E., Kemeny, M. E., Reed, G. M., Bower, J. E., & Gruenewald, T. L. (2000). Psychological resources, positive illusions, and health. *American Psychologist, 55*, 99–109.

Taylor, S. E., Lerner, J. S., Sherman, D. K., Sage, R. M., & McDowell, N. K. (2003a). Are self-enhancing cognitions associated with healthy or unhealthy biological profiles? *Journal of Personality and Social Psychology, 85*, 605–615.

Taylor, S. E., Lerner, J. S., Sherman, D. K., Sage, R. M., & McDowell, N. K. (2003b). Portrait of the self-enhancer: Well-adjusted and well-liked or maladjusted and friendless? *Journal of Personality and Social Psychology, 84*, 165–176.

Taylor, S. E., Lichtman, R. R., & Wood, J. V. (1984). Attributions, beliefs about control, and adjustment to breast cancer. *Journal of Personality and Social Psychology, 46*, 489–502.

Taylor, S. E., & Sherman, D. K. (2004). Positive psychology and health: A fruitful liaison. In A. Linley & S. Joseph (Eds.), *Positive psychology in practice* (pp. 305–319). New York: Wiley.

Updegraff, J. A., & Taylor, S. E. (2000). From vulnerability to growth: The positive and negative effects of stressful life events. In J. Harvey & E. Miller (Eds.), *Loss and trauma* (pp. 3–28). Philadelphia: Taylor & Francis.

Updegraff, J. A., Taylor, S. E., Kemeny, M. E., & Wyatt, G. E. (2002). Positive and negative effects of HIV-infection in women with low socioeconomic resources. *Personality and Social Psychology Bulletin, 28*, 382–394.

Weinberger, D. A., & Schwartz, G. E. (1990). Distress and restraint as superordinate dimensions of self-reported adjustment: A typological perspective. *Journal of Personality, 58*, 381–417.

Wood, J. V., & Taylor, K. L. (1991). Serving self-relevant goals through social comparison. In J. M. Suls & T. A. Wills (Eds.), *Social comparison: Theory and research* (pp. 23–50). Hillsdale, NJ: Erlbaum.

Chapter 5

# Cognitive Dissonance Theory

## AN UPDATE WITH A FOCUS ON THE ACTION-BASED MODEL

**Eddie Harmon-Jones**
**Cindy Harmon-Jones**

Theories of *cognitive consistency* were prevalent in the 1940s and 1950s (Heider, 1946, 1958; for a review, see Abelson et al., 1968). In this heyday of cognitive consistency theories, Festinger (1957) proposed the theory of *cognitive dissonance*, which ultimately became the consistency theory that generated the most research. Dissonance theory differs from other consistency theories in that it posits the need to specify the resistance to change of cognitions (Wicklund & Frey, 1981), with this resistance determining the manner in which cognitive inconsistency will be reduced. In the early research, resistance to change was often manipulated by behavioral commitment. However, Beauvois and Joule (1996, 1999) have suggested that this focus on behavioral commitment in fact made dissonance not a theory of consistency, but a theory about the psychology of commitment.

In addition to the large volume of research on cognitive dissonance theory itself, the theory has had a wide influence on psychological theory and research. Aronson (1992) identified a number of social psychological theories that could be thought of as dissonance in other guises, including self-affirmation theory (Steele, 1988), symbolic self-completion theory (Wicklund & Gollwitzer, 1982), self-evaluation maintenance theory (Tesser, 1988), self-discrepancy theory (Higgins, 1989), and action identification theory (Vallacher & Wegner, 1987).

Festinger formulated the original theory of cognitive dissonance in the mid-1950s. He theorized that when an individual holds two or more elements of knowledge that are relevant to each other but inconsistent with one another, a state of discomfort is created. He called this unpleasant state *dissonance*. Festinger theorized that the degree of dissonance in relation to a cognition can be expressed as $D/D + C$, where $D$ is the sum of cognitions dissonant with a particular cognition and $C$ is the sum of cognitions consonant with that same particular cognition, with each cognition weighted for importance (for precise mathematical models, see Sakai, 1999; Shultz & Lepper, 1999).

Festinger (1957) theorized that persons are motivated by the unpleasant state of dissonance to engage in psychological work so as to reduce the inconsistency between cognitions. To reduce the dissonance, individuals can add consonant cognitions, subtract dissonant cognitions, increase the importance of consonant cognitions, or decrease the importance of dissonant cognitions. Researchers have most often measured dissonance reduction via attitude change. Attitude change in response to a state of dissonance is expected to be in the direction of the cognition that is most resistant to change. In experimental tests of the theory, knowledge about recent behavior is usually assumed to be the cognition most resistant to change. If one has recently performed a behavior, it is usually difficult to convince oneself that the behavior did not occur. Thus attitude change is often consistent with the behavioral commitment and may justify it.

## EXPERIMENTAL PARADIGMS USED TO TEST THE THEORY

### Free Choice

In 1956, Brehm examined dissonance theory's predictions for postdecision processing. According to the theory, after a decision is made, all of the cognitions that favor the chosen alternative are consonant with the decision, while all the cognitions that favor the rejected alternative are dissonant. The greater the number and importance of dissonant cognitions, and the lesser the number and importance of consonant cognitions, the greater the degree of dissonance experienced by the individual. In a decision situation, dissonance typically becomes greater as the alternatives become closer in attractiveness (as long as each alternative has several distinguishing characteristics). Dissonance caused by a decision can be reduced by viewing the chosen alternative as more attractive and/or viewing the rejected alternative as less attractive. Brehm (1956) conducted an experiment in which participants made either an easy or a difficult decision between two alternatives. The difficult decision was one in which the alternatives were close in attractiveness, whereas the easy decision was one in which one alternative was much more attractive than the other. Participants were asked to evaluate the decision options before and after the decision. Brehm found that when persons made a difficult decision, they changed their attitudes to become more negative toward the rejected alternative. After an easy decision, participants did not change their attitudes.

### Induced Compliance

Festinger and Carlsmith (1959) hypothesized that dissonance should be aroused when a person acts in a way that is contrary to his or her attitudes. To test this prediction, they brought participants into the laboratory and asked them to perform a boring task. Then participants were paid either $1 or $20 to tell "another participant" that the task was interesting. According to dissonance theory, lying for a payment of $20 should not arouse much dissonance, because $20 should provide sufficient justification for the counterattitudinal behavior (i.e., it adds 20 cognitions consonant with the behavior). However, being paid $1 for performing the same behavior should arouse much dissonance, because $1 should be just enough justification for the behavior (i.e., it adds only 1 consonant cognition). As expected, participants in the $1 (low-justification) condition changed their attitudes to be more positive toward the task, whereas participants in the $20 (high-justification) condition did not change their attitudes. It is important to note that in this paradigm the preexisting attitude is the dissonant cognition.

## CHALLENGES TO THE RESEARCH AND ORIGINAL THEORY

After these and other dissonance results appeared in the literature, some theorists began to question whether the results were due to motivation. Some theorists hypothesized that the effects were due to nonmotivational cognitive processes (e.g., Bem, 1972) or to impression management concerns (Tedeschi, Schlenker, & Bonoma, 1971). However, subsequent research confirmed that dissonance is a motivated process. As Wicklund and Frey (1981) noted, dissonance theory does not deal with a purely cognitive process, wherein all cognitions are brought into agreement with one another. Rather, a behavioral commitment is needed in order to elicit dissonance reduction. Dissonance processes come into play when persons hold cognitions that disagree with their actions or goals. In fact, Wicklund and Frey (1981) stated that a "person who has no dissonance-creating decision in his immediate background might well be curious about new or incongruous information" (p. 159).

Dissonance involves negative affect, and a motivated, often effortful search for ways of reducing the negative affect. In support of this, experiments have shown selective exposure to information as a means of dissonance reduction. *Selective exposure* is the tendency to seek out information that agrees with one's goals or beliefs and to avoid information that disagrees. In a study by Walster (1964), students were given the opportunity to read information that was favorable or unfavorable about the profession they intended to pursue. If the source of the information was highly credible, participants were more likely to choose to read the supportive information. If the source of the information was not credible, participants were more likely to choose to read the information that was unfavorable (presumably because they expected it would be easy to refute). This pattern of results has been replicated several times (see, e.g., Frey, 1986, for a review). These results support an active, goal-oriented process, with the purpose of justifying behavior, rather than a process of merely seeking consistency between cognitions. Discrepancy between cognitions only needs to be minimized when it relates to an ongoing behavioral commitment.

Beginning in the late 1960s, researchers began to propose motivational explanations for dissonance effects that differed from Festinger's originally proposed theory. Four primary revisions of dissonance theory have been proposed, and their originators have provided evidence to support the new conceptions. These include Aronson's (1968, 1969, 1999) *self-consistency* theory; Steele's (1988) *self-affirmation* theory; Cooper and Fazio's (1984) model of *aversive consequences*; and Harmon-Jones's (1999, 2000b) *action-based* model. The first three of these are discussed below, and a more detailed examination of the fourth follows.

### Self-Consistency

In his self-consistency theory, Aronson (1968) proposed that dissonance is not due merely to an inconsistency between cognitions. Instead, he posited that dissonance occurs when a person acts in a way that violates his or her self-concept—that is, when a person performs a behavior inconsistent with his or her sense of self. Since most persons have a positive self-concept, dissonance is most often experienced when a person behaves negatively, behaving in an incompetent, irrational, or immoral manner. One of the primary predictions derived from this revision is that individuals low and high in self-esteem should respond with less and more dissonance reduction (e.g., attitude change), respectively, because in dissonance experiments individuals high in self-esteem are induced to act in ways that are more discrepant from their positive self-views. Experiments testing this prediction have produced mixed results.

### Self-Affirmation

Steele (1988) proposed a different alternative to Festinger's dissonance theory. He proposed that persons possess a motive to maintain an overall self-image of moral and adaptive adequacy. He stated that dissonance-induced attitude change occurs because dissonance threatens this positive self-image. Whereas Festinger's dissonance theory posits that individuals are motivated to reconcile inconsistent cognitions, Steele proposed instead that individuals are merely motivated to affirm the integrity of the self. Steele conducted experiments where participants were induced to perform a counterattitudinal action. Afterward, participants either were, or were not, presented with an opportunity to affirm an important value. When participants were allowed to affirm an important value, dissonance-related attitude change did not occur.

However, in 1995, Simon, Greenberg and Brehm presented data supporting an alternative explanation for Steele's findings that was in line with the original theory of dissonance. Festinger's original theory proposed that the degree of dissonance experienced depends on the importance of the dissonant and consonant cognitions. Simon and colleagues hypothesized that making an important value salient can reduce dissonance by reducing the individual's perception of the importance of the dissonant act. They conducted an experiment in which participants who opposed a tuition increase were given high choice to write essays in support of a tuition increase (a counterattitudinal statement). After writing the essay, participants either were given an opportunity to affirm an important value (self-affirmation condition), were asked to write about a value (e.g., ending world hunger) that was not important to them personally but was of general importance (value-salient condition), or neither (control condition). Participants were then asked to rate the degree to which they supported a tuition increase. Participants in the control condition changed their attitudes to be more favorable toward a tuition increase, as expected. Participants in both the self-affirmation and value-salient conditions did not change their attitudes: They had trivialized, or reduced the importance of, the tuition increase issue by thinking about other important values, even when these values were not self-affirming. Blanton, Cooper, Skurnik, and Aronson (1997) and others have published experiments questioning some of the assumptions and predictions of the self-affirmation model of dissonance (see reviews by Aronson, Cohen, & Nail, 1999). Finally, both self-based versions have difficulty explaining the research that shows support for dissonance-derived predictions in the behavior of white rats (e.g., Lawrence & Festinger, 1962).

### Aversive Consequences

Following the results of several experiments (Collins, 1969; Collins & Hoyt, 1972; Cooper & Worchel, 1970; Nel, Helmreich, & Aronson, 1969), Cooper and Fazio (1984) proposed that the discomfort experienced in dissonance experiments was not due to an inconsistency between an individual's cognitions, but rather to feeling personally responsible for producing an aversive consequence. In one experiment supportive of this idea, Cooper and Worchel (1970) replicated and extended Festinger and Carlsmith's (1959) classic experiment. In addition to the conditions of the original experiment, Cooper and Worchel added conditions in which, when the participant tells the confederate that the boring task is interesting, the confederate is not convinced by the lie. They found that attitude change occurred only in the low-justification condition where the confederate believed the lie. The researchers interpreted this result as indicating that dissonance-related attitude change only occurred in the condition in which an aversive consequence was produced. This revision of cognitive dissonance theory was widely accepted.

However, concerns regarding the aversive consequences revision persisted among some. According to Eagly and Chaiken (1993), the aversive consequences revision "transformed . . . the quite general theory that Festinger (1957) had envisioned into a mini-theory that delineates a particular set of circumstances that produce a particular type of attitudinal adjustment within the induced compliance paradigm" (p. 520). Berkowitz and Devine (1989) also lamented the rise of this model, saying, "Gone was the theory's broad sweep" (p. 499).

In addition, the results of experiments that used paradigms other than the counterattitudinal action paradigm are not consistent with the aversive consequences model. Dissonance research using a selective exposure paradigm has demonstrated that persons are more willing to examine materials that confirm their beliefs than materials that dispute their beliefs (Brock & Balloun, 1967; Frey, 1986). Research using a belief disconfirmation paradigm has shown that when persons are exposed to information that challenges their beliefs, they often strengthen their original belief (Batson, 1975; Burris, Harmon-Jones, & Tarpley, 1997). In neither of these experimental paradigms are individuals acting to produce aversive consequences.

Research using a hypocrisy paradigm has shown that persons change their behavior to be more in line with their beliefs when they are reminded of times when they did not live up to their beliefs (Aronson, Fried, & Stone, 1991; Stone, Aronson, Crain, Winslow, & Fried, 1994). In a representative study, students were asked to make a videotape encouraging safe sex practices, which would purportedly be shown to high school students. Students who were then asked to remember times they had failed to practice safe sex chose to take more condoms than did subjects who had not been reminded of past failures to practice safe sex (Stone et al., 1994). In the hypocrisy experiments, dissonance is evoked by inducing participants to perform an act that produces beneficial, rather than aversive, consequences. It is difficult to reconcile any of these lines of dissonance research with a conception of dissonance theory in which the production of an aversive consequence is the only motivator of dissonance-related attitude change.

Certainly, according to the original theory of cognitive dissonance, the production of aversive consequences would be expected to increase the amount of dissonance produced (see Harmon-Jones, 1999). In the original theory, an aversive consequence would be considered an important dissonant cognition, or it would be considered to strengthen the commitment to behavior and thus increase the resistance to change of the behavioral cognition. However, the original theory would deny that an aversive consequence is necessary to produce dissonance.

Why did the past research find that in the induced compliance paradigm, attitude change only occurred when the participant caused an aversive consequence? First of all, the lack of attitude change in the no-aversive-consequences conditions is a null effect. Null effects are notoriously difficult to explain and subject to multiple alternatives. Attitude change may have been produced, but may have been too slight to be detected with the small sample sizes of these experiments. Perhaps not enough dissonance was aroused in these experiments to produce attitude change without the additional help of an aversive consequence. It is also possible that in these experiments, dissonance was produced, but it was either not reduced or was reduced by a route other than attitude change. In dissonance research, the presence of attitude change has often been assumed to reflect the fact that dissonance occurred. However, attitude change is not a direct measure of dissonance. Instead, it is a measure of the individual's response to dissonance.

In 1996, Harmon-Jones, Brehm, Greenberg, Simon, and Nelson published experiments demonstrating that dissonance-related attitude change can occur without the production of aversive consequences in induced compliance experiments. Under the guise of an experiment on memory, participants were exposed to an attitudinal object. Participants were assured of privacy and anonymity, and then were given high or low choice to write a counterattitudinal statement about the object (to manipulate justification). They were asked to discard the statement in the trash after writing it, so that there was no chance of the statement causing an aversive consequence. This manipulation was based on Cooper and Fazio's (1984) statement that "making a statement contrary to one's attitude while in solitude does not have the potential for bringing about an aversive event" (p. 232).

In one experiment (Harmon-Jones et al., 1996), participants were asked to read a boring passage. They were then given high or low choice to write that they found the boring passage interesting. In order to provide a more direct measure of evoked dissonance, nonspecific skin conductance responses (NS-SCRs) were assessed during the 3 minutes between the writing of the statement and the assessment of the participants' attitudes toward the passage. Although no aversive consequences were produced, persons in the high-choice condition changed their attitudes to be more favorable toward the passage. In addition, NS-SCRs suggested that participants in this condition experienced more emotional arousal.

In another experiment, participants who liked chocolate were asked to eat a piece of chocolate and were then given high or low choice to write a statement that they disliked the chocolate (Harmon-Jones, 2000a). This experiment was conducted because reviewers of the first set of experiments had suggested that reading the boring passage was aversive in itself, and that participants in the high-choice condition could have believed they had high choice to read the passage as well as to write the statement. Since eating the chocolate was pleasant rather than aversive, that alternative could not apply in this case. Participants in the high-choice condition changed their attitudes to dislike the chocolate. In addition, self-reported negative affect was increased following counterattitudinal behavior and was reduced following the attitude change. The results obtained in these experiments demonstrate that dissonance-related affect and dissonance-related attitude change can occur in situations in which a cognitive inconsistency is present but the production of aversive consequences is not present. They also demonstrate that the experience of cognitive dissonance evokes an unpleasant state that motivates dissonance reduction. These recent experiments have supported the original conception of dissonance theory against the revisions.

## THE ACTION-BASED MODEL OF DISSONANCE

But why does dissonance evoke this negative motivational state? Why is inconsistency aversive? Festinger proposed no answer to the question of why dissonance processes occur, other than to say that inconsistency is motivating. Brehm and Cohen (1962), Wicklund and Frey (1981), Beauvois and Joule (1996), and others pointed out that a behavioral commitment is an important component of the dissonance process, and that cognitive inconsistencies without implications for behavior are unlikely to provoke dissonance motivation. However, like Festinger (1957), Brehm and Cohen (1962), Wicklund and Frey (1981), Beauvois and Joule (1996), and others did not say why cognitions with implications for behavior are the cognitions that persons are motivated to maintain in a consistent relationship.

Harmon-Jones (1999, 2000b) has proposed an action-based model of cognitive dissonance in an attempt to answer this question. The action-based model concurs with other areas of psychological research in proposing that perceptions and cognitions can serve as action tendencies. The action-based model further proposes that dissonance between cognitions evokes an aversive state because it has the potential to interfere with effective and unconflicted action. Dissonance reduction, by bringing cognitions into line with behavioral commitments, serves the function of facilitating the execution of effective and unconflicted action.

Thus the action-based model proposes both a proximal and a distal motivation for the existence of dissonance processes. The proximal motive for reducing dissonance is to reduce or eliminate the negative emotion of dissonance. The distal motivation is the need for effective and unconflicted action.

After a decision is made, psychological processing should assist with the execution of the decision. The tendency of participants in dissonance research to view the chosen alternative more favorably and the rejected alternative more negatively after a decision is made between the two may help the participants to follow through—to act on the decision in a more effective manner.

As an example of how dissonance processes may operate in the real world, imagine Bob, who has been offered jobs with two different companies. The position offered by one company is more intellectually stimulating, but the other company has friendlier coworkers. One company is located in a city with a pleasant climate, but the other is in a city with a more reasonable cost of living. Bob sees both job positions as similarly attractive, although they are quite different from each other, and he must decide between them. Once Bob makes a decision, he will need to perform actions in order to follow through with his decision. He will need to relocate, learn his new duties, and perform well at them. After his decision, if he continues to see the two positions as similar in attractiveness, he may experience excess regret, which could inhibit him from following through with his decision. On the other hand, if he is able to reduce dissonance, so that he views the chosen position more positively and the rejected position more negatively, he will be likely to have better job performance and greater job satisfaction.

### Theoretical Perspectives Consistent with the Action-Based Model

The action-based model is consistent with views that have been presented previously but have not been given due consideration. One reason for the lack of consideration of these conceptual ideas may be the difficulty of understanding how the effects observed in the laboratory experiments can be produced by a concern over effective action. We propose that dissonance processes constitute a mechanism that has survived because of its adaptive value. Such a mechanism may be able to produce effects in conceptually similar situations that do not have obvious adaptive significance. In some situations, dissonance processes may in fact be maladaptive and dysfunctional, as when persons maintain and bolster a commitment to a decision that clearly harms themselves. However, we propose that dissonance processes have survived because they are adaptive in the majority of situations in which they operate.

Other scientists have advanced similar but not identical conceptions (see Harmon-Jones, 2000d). For example, Jones and Gerard (1967) discussed the concept of an *unequivocal behavior orientation*, which was argued to be an adaptive strategy that forces individuals to bring their relevant cognitions into harmony with each other. The unequivocal behavior orientation "represents a commitment to action in the face of uncertainty. Such a commitment involves the risks of acting inappropriately, but such risks are assumed to be less grave on the average than the risks of hesitant or conflicted action" (p. 185). Jones and Gerard further suggested, "When the time comes to act, the great advantage of having a set of coherent internally consistent dispositions is that the individual is not forced to listen to the babble of competing inner forces" (p. 181).

Another view consistent with the action-based model is Kuhl's (1984, 2000; see also Koole & Kuhl, Chapter 19, this volume) theory of *action control*. Kuhl has proposed that to ensure that the intended action rather than a competing action tendency will be executed, the intended action tendency has to be selectively strengthened and protected against interference until the action is executed. The postdecisional spreading of decision alternatives may serve the function of putting the decision into action (Beckmann & Irle, 1985). Kuhl proposed that the efficiency of action control is determined by whether the individual is in an action-oriented or state-oriented frame of mind. An individual in a state orientation focuses excessively on the past, present, or future, without attending to plans that would implement the action. In contrast, an individual in an action orientation seeks to implement a plan of action and focuses simultaneously on the present state, the intended future state, the discrepancy between the present and future state, and the alternative plans that may transform the present state into the future state. Similar ideas have been proposed by Heckhausen (1986) and Gollwitzer (1990; see also Gollwitzer, Parks-Stamm, Jaudas, & Sheeran, Chapter 21, this volume). Considering that dissonance is primarily a theory about postdecisional or postcommitment processing (e.g., Brehm & Cohen, 1962; Festinger, 1964), it is clear that these non-dissonance-related theories fit with the present conception of the function of the dissonance process. In addition, research on counteractive self-control theory is also consistent with the action-based model, in that it has revealed a number of commitment-supporting psychological strategies that individuals use to stick with their long-term goals and commitments (Fishbach & Trope, Chapter 18, this volume).

Past presentations of the theory of cognitive dissonance have referred to two different constructs as *cognitive dissonance*. One is the inconsistency between cognitions. The second is the unpleasant emotional–motivational state that occurs when a person holds two contradictory cognitions. In order to clarify the processes of dissonance, the action-based model distinguishes between the two. We refer to inconsistency between cognitions as *cognitive discrepancy*, while we call the unpleasant emotion *dissonance*. The unpleasant emotion of dissonance provides motivation.

Changing one's cognitions to bring them in alignment with each other (discrepancy reduction) is one way of reducing the negative emotion of dissonance. This is the method of dealing with dissonance most often measured in research. However, according to the action-based model, this is not the only way persons can deal with the emotion of dissonance. It is also possible to deal with dissonance by trivializing the cognitions (as in Simon et al., 1995; see above). Drinking alcohol after performing a counterattitudinal act has been shown to eliminate attitude change, presumably by reducing the negative emotional state and therefore the motivation (Steele, Southwick, & Critchlow, 1981). The action-based model predicts that reducing dissonance by means other than attitude change is more likely when action is not greatly needed or when the action implications of the cognitions are not high. If action is needed, these methods should lead to less effective action than dissonance reduction through attitude change.

It is also possible to experience dissonance and not do anything to reduce it. The negative emotion of dissonance provides motivation, but the fact that an individual is motivated to do something does not necessarily mean that he or she acts on the motivation. He or she may instead continue to experience cognitive discrepancy, in which case the action-based model predicts that negative affect will remain elevated. The action-based model also predicts that if an individual experiences dissonance and does not reduce it, this will interfere with the effectiveness of his or her behavior. These and other possible ways of dealing with cognitive discrepancies, and with the negative emotion of dissonance, need to be considered by researchers.

Furthermore, the action-based model does not make the claim that dissonance reduction in the direction of a decision always occurs. Sometimes a person makes a decision, and the evidence is overwhelming that the wrong decision has been made. This new information will arouse dissonance. Persons make poor decisions and recognize that poor decisions have been made. When a person realizes that he or she has made a mistake, his or her original decision is no longer the cognition most resistant to change. Consider Bob in the example above, who is taking a new job position. Bob may accept a position, but after beginning the job, realize that it is completely unsuitable for him.

He will probably not be able to reduce the dissonance associated with his decision; in fact, the negative emotion of dissonance will increase because of the new information indicating that the job is unsuitable for him. At some point, if his dissonant cognitions continue to increase, he may reverse his decision and look for a different job.

According to the action-based model, certain types of perceptions and cognitions may lead to less of the aversive state of dissonance, because they are less directly connected to behavior. Indeed, they may assist in explaining why not all inconsistencies evoke dissonance. Similarly, the abstractness of the cognitions involved in the discrepant cognitive relationships may also affect the amount of dissonance aroused, because abstract cognitions may be less strongly related to behaviors.

The action-based model assumes that dissonance processes operate because they are functional—that is, most often useful for the organism. However, the action-based model does not claim that dissonance reduction is always functional. (We think of dissonance processes similarly to the way we think of other functional, motivated behaviors such as eating. Eating is necessary for the survival of the organism; however, disordered eating can be harmful.) A person may make a poor decision. If the person reduces the dissonance associated with the decision, he or she will persist in acting on the decision. What if, after Bob begins his new job, he marries an abusive spouse? Every time his spouse mistreats him, this constitutes a dissonant cognition. But Bob's decision to get married is very resistant to change, so he reduces this dissonance (perhaps by reducing the importance of the incidents, "forgetting" the incidents, exaggerating the importance of the benefits of the relationship, etc.). The dissonance process is not serving Bob well in this instance. The action-based model proposes that dissonance reduction, while not always functional, is functional more often than not. In the majority of cases, it is better for persons to reduce dissonance and act effectively on their decisions. The dissonance reduction mechanism prevents the danger of continuing to experience conflict, which interferes with effective action.

The action-based model proposes that the state that occurs following a decision is typically an action-oriented state. When a person is in an action-oriented state, implementation of decisions is enhanced (Gollwitzer, 1990; Gollwitzer et al., Chapter 21, this volume; Heckhausen, 1986; Koole & Kuhl, Chapter 19, this volume; Kuhl, 1984). We (Harmon-Jones & Harmon-Jones, 2002) integrated these ideas with dissonance theory to propose that this action-oriented state that follows decision making is the state in which dissonance motivation operates and dissonance reduction occurs. We hypothesized that experimentally manipulating the degree of action orientation experienced following a decision should affect the degree of dissonance reduction.

In one experimental test of these ideas, participants first were asked to make either an easy decision or a difficult decision (Harmon-Jones & Harmon-Jones, 2002). Participants completed a mindset questionnaire after the decision. The neutral mindset questionnaire asked participants to list seven things they did in a typical day, while the action-oriented mindset questionnaire asked participants to list seven things they could do to perform well on the exercise they had chosen. Participants were then asked to reevaluate the exercises. Results indicated that participants in the difficult-decision/action-oriented condition changed their attitudes to prefer the chosen exercise more than participants in the other conditions. Enhancing the action-oriented state that normally occurs after a decision increased participants' ability to reduce the dissonance associated with the decision.

In a second experiment testing the action-based model, we (Harmon-Jones & Harmon-Jones, 2002) replicated the results of the first experiment, using a different manipulation of action orientation. In this experiment, action orientation was induced by having participants think of an important decision that they had made and to list the steps they intended to use to follow through successfully with their decision. The participants in the action orientation condition engaged in more attitude change following a difficult decision than did participants in the comparison conditions. This study replicated the results of the previous study, but it used an action orientation induction unrelated to the decision at hand.

### Action Orientation, Frontal Brain Activity, and Spreading of Alternatives

The experiments just described cannot be easily interpreted by other revisions of dissonance theory (see Harmon-Jones & Harmon-Jones,

2002). To further explore the motivation underlying in dissonance processes, we have conducted other research, derived from the action-based model, regarding the involvement of the frontal cortices in dissonance reduction. Over the last two decades, research findings obtained from a variety of methodological approaches have converged impressively to suggest that the left and right frontal cortical regions have different motivational and emotional functions, with the left frontal region being involved in approach-related processes, and the right frontal region being involved in withdrawal-related processes (for reviews, see Coan & Allen, 2004; Harmon-Jones, 2004). For instance, Robinson and colleagues (e.g., Robinson & Downhill, 1995) have observed that it is specifically damage to the left frontal lobe that causes depressive symptoms. They have found that for persons with left-hemisphere brain damage, the closer the lesion is to the frontal pole, the greater the depressive symptoms. In contrast, persons with damage to the right frontal hemisphere are more likely to respond with mania.

The left frontal cortical region has been described as an important center for intention, self-regulation, and planning (Kosslyn & Koenig, 1995; Petrides & Milner, 1982). These functions have often been described as properties of the *will*—a hypothetical construct that guides approach-related behavior. Persons with damage to this region are apathetic, experience less interest and pleasure, and have difficulty initiating actions.

Research using measures of electroencephalographic (EEG) activity has found that increased left frontal cortical activation relates to dispositional tendencies toward approach motivation (Harmon-Jones & Allen, 1997, 1998) and repression (Tomarken & Davidson, 1994), and that decreased left frontal activity relates to depression (Henriques & Davidson, 1991). It is interesting to note that repression has been linked to an increased likelihood of reducing dissonance via attitude change (Olson & Zanna, 1979; Zanna & Aziza, 1976), suggesting that increased left frontal activity may be related to dissonance-related attitude change. Other research has found that left frontal activation is increased during approach toward rewarding outcomes, whereas right frontal activation is increased during withdrawal from aversive outcomes (Sobotka, Davidson, & Senulis, 1992). Thus, as approach-related, action-oriented thinking increases, greater left frontal activation may occur. Moreover, individuals who are more action-oriented may be expected to show increased left frontal activity following a dissonance-arousing decision.

In one experiment testing this hypothesis, participants' EEGs were assessed while they were given low or high choice to engage in a counterattitudinal behavior. Results indicated that immediately after individuals in the high-choice condition committed to writing a counterattitudinal essay, they evidenced increased left frontal activity (Harmon-Jones, Gerdjikov, & Harmon-Jones, in press). This experiment has been conceptually replicated in a no-aversive-consequences induced compliance design.

In another experiment, participants made a difficult decision, and their EEGs were recorded following the decision. They then rerated the decision alternatives. Finally, they completed Kuhl's (1993) trait measure of action control, which contains a subscale relevant to decision processes—the prospective and decision-related action orientation versus hesitation. We predicted that trait action orientation would relate to relative left frontal activity and spreading of alternatives. Results supported these predictions (Harmon-Jones, Peterson, Hubbell, & Harmon-Jones, 2005). Another experiment has revealed that the implemental/action-oriented mindset described above increases relative left frontal cortical activation and attitude change immediately following a dissonance-arousing decision (Harmon-Jones, Harmon-Jones, Fearn, Sigelman, & Johnson, in press).

In these studies, the psychological process (action-oriented dissonance reduction) was manipulated, and the proposed physiological substrate was measured (left frontal EEG). These types of studies are limited in the causal inferences that can be drawn. Because the measured physiological activation may be only one of a number of physiological activations that occur in response to the psychological manipulation, it is possible that one of the other unmeasured physiological activations is more responsible for the psychological process. To provide stronger causal inferences regarding the role of a particular neural structure's involvement in a particular psychological process, it is important to reverse the direction—that is, to manipulate the physiology and measure the psychology. To accomplish this, we recently conducted an experiment in which neurofeedback was used to manipulate left frontal cortical activity. After successful neurofeedback training, participants were given a difficult decision, and their attitudinal spreading of alternatives was measured following the decision. In support of predictions, individuals trained to have decreased left frontal activation showed decreased spreading of alternatives (Harmon-Jones et al., in press).

Taken together, these experiments suggest that the process of dissonance reduction involves the activation of the left frontal cortex. These results are consistent with research demonstrating that the left frontal cortex is involved in approach motivation processes, and with the action-based model of dissonance, which predicts that the process of dissonance reduction involves an approach-related action orientation.

### Emotion as Action Tendency Experiment

To explore the action-based model of dissonance still further, we conducted an experiment to test the hypothesis that dissonance should be increased as the salience of the action implications of cognitions that are involved in a dissonant relationship is increased. Several perspectives consider emotions to involve action tendencies (Brehm, 1999; Frijda, 1986). To the extent that an emotion generates an action tendency, as the intensity of one's current emotion is increased and as the emotion is involved in a dissonant relationship with other information, dissonance should be increased.

Research has demonstrated that the emotion of sympathy (or empathy) increases helping behavior because it evokes altruistic motivation—that is, motivation to relieve the distress of the person in need of help (see Batson, 1991, for a review). We conducted an experiment that tested whether an inconsistency between the emotion of sympathy and knowledge about past failures to act in accord with the sympathy would evoke motivation to reduce this inconsistency (Harmon-Jones, Peterson, & Vaughn, 2003).

In the experiment, we tested the hypothesis that after experiencing sympathy for a target person in need of help, individuals will be more motivated to help that person when they are reminded of times that they failed to help similar persons (see Batson et al., 1997, for evidence that feeling sympathy for one target person can transfer to the target person's group and cause attitude change toward the group). Participants were informed that they would be listening to a pilot broadcast for a local radio station, and that the researchers would like students' reactions to the tape. Participants then listened to a tape-recorded message that was purportedly from a person in need of help (an adolescent with cancer). Before listening to the tape, participants were assigned to one of two conditions: one in which they tried to imagine how the person must feel (high-empathy set), or one in which they tried to remain objective as they listened to the tape (low-empathy set). Then they listened to the tape-recorded message. Afterward, they completed questionnaires assessing self-reported emotional responses and evaluations of the tape-recorded message. Participants then either were asked to list times when they failed to help other persons who were in need of help (in order to induce dissonance) or completed a demographic survey (control condition). Finally, participants were given an opportunity to help by volunteering time to assist the person with addressing letters that would request money from possible donors or by donating money to the person's family. The design was a 2 (low vs. high empathy) × 2 (reminded of times that one did not help vs. not reminded) between-subjects factorial. Consistent with predictions derived from the action-based model, results indicated that more helping occurred in the high-empathy/reminder-of-past-failures condition than in other conditions.

## CONCLUSION

Many recent studies have challenged the dissonance revisions and provided support for Festinger's original conception of dissonance. Clearly, dissonance has much to do with cognitive inconsistency, rather than being due to such limiting conditions as a self-threat or the production of an aversive consequence. Festinger did not propose why cognitive inconsistency produces discomfort and motivates cognitive and behavioral change; however, the newly proposed action-based model of dissonance does propose an underlying motivation. Research on the action-based model suggests that dissonance reduction may serve the function of assisting in the successful execution of a commitment, which may facilitate effective and unconflicted action.

## ACKNOWLEDGMENTS

This chapter and portions of the research described herein were supported by funds from the University of Wisconsin Graduate School, the Wisconsin Alumni Research Foundation, a Wisconsin/Hilldale Undergraduate/Faculty Research Fellowship, and the National Science Foundation (Grant No. BCS-9910702).

## REFERENCES

Abelson, R. P., Aronson, E., McGuire, W. J., Newcomb, T. M., Rosenberg, M. J., & Tannenbaum, P. H. (Eds.). (1968). *Theories of cognitive consistency: A sourcebook*. Chicago: Rand McNally.

Aronson, E. (1968). Dissonance theory: Progress and problems. In R. P. Abelson, E. Aronson, W. J. McGuire, T. M. Newcomb, M. J. Rosenberg, & P. H. Tannenbaum (Eds.), *Theories of cognitive consistency: A sourcebook* (pp. 5–27). Chicago: Rand McNally.

Aronson, E. (1969). The theory of cognitive dissonance: A current perspective. In L. Berkowitz (Ed.), *Advances in experimental social psychology* (Vol. 4, pp. 1–34). New York: Academic Press.

Aronson, E. (1992). The return of the repressed: Dissonance theory makes a comeback. *Psychological Inquiry, 3*, 303–311.

Aronson, E. (1999). Dissonance, hypocrisy, and the self concept. In E. Harmon-Jones & J. Mills (Eds.), *Cognitive dissonance: Progress on a pivotal theory in social psychology* (pp. 103–126). Washington, DC: American Psychological Association.

Aronson, J., Cohen, G., & Nail, P. R. (1999). Self-affirmation theory: An update and appraisal. In E. Harmon-Jones & J. Mills (Eds.), *Cognitive dissonance: Progress on a pivotal theory in social psychology* (pp. 127–147). Washington, DC: American Psychological Association.

Aronson, E., Fried, C., & Stone, J. (1991). Overcoming denial and increasing the intention to use condoms through the induction of hypocrisy. *American Journal of Public Health, 81*, 1636–1638.

Batson, C. D. (1975). Rational processing or rationalization?: The effect of disconfirming information on a stated religious belief. *Journal of Personality and Social Psychology, 32*, 176–184.

Batson, C. D. (1991). *The altruism question: Toward a social-psychological answer.* Hillsdale, NJ: Erlbaum.

Batson, C. D., Polycarpou, M. P., Harmon-Jones, E., Imhoff, H. J., Mitchener, E. C., Bednar, L. L., et al. (1997). Empathy and attitudes: Can feeling for a member of a stigmatized outgroup improve attitudes toward the group? *Journal of Personality and Social Psychology, 72*, 105–118.

Beauvois, J. L., & Joule, R. V. (1996). *A radical dissonance theory.* London: Taylor & Francis.

Beauvois, J. L., & Joule, R. V. (1999). A radical point of view on dissonance theory. In E. Harmon-Jones & J. Mills (Eds.), *Cognitive dissonance: Progress on a pivotal theory in social psychology* (pp. 43–70). Washington, DC: American Psychological Association.

Beckmann, J., & Irle, M. (1985). Dissonance and action control. In J. Kuhl & J. Beckmann (Eds.), *Action control: From cognition to behavior* (pp. 129–150). Berlin: Springer-Verlag.

Bem, D. J. (1972). Self-perception theory. In L. Berkowitz (Ed.), *Advances in experimental social psychology* (Vol. 6, pp. 1–62). New York: Academic Press.

Berkowitz, L., & Devine, P. G. (1989). Research traditions, analysis, and synthesis in social psychological theories: The case of dissonance theory. *Personality and Social Psychology Bulletin, 15*, 493–507.

Blanton, H., Cooper, J., Skurnik, I., & Aronson, J. (1997). When bad things happen to good feedback: Exacerbating the need for self-justification with self-affirmations. *Personality and Social Psychology Bulletin, 23*, 684–692.

Brehm, J. W. (1956). Postdecision changes in the desirability of alternatives. *Journal of Abnormal and Social Psychology, 52*, 384–389.

Brehm, J. W. (1999). The intensity of emotion. *Personality and Social Psychology Review, 3*, 2–22.

Brehm, J. W., & Cohen, A. R. (1962). *Explorations in cognitive dissonance.* New York: Wiley.

Brock, T. C., & Balloun, J. C. (1967). Behavioral receptivity to dissonant information. *Journal of Personality and Social Psychology, 6*, 413–428.

Burris, C. T., Harmon-Jones, E., & Tarpley, W. R. (1997). "By faith alone": Religious agitation and cognitive dissonance. *Basic and Applied Social Psychology, 19*, 17–31.

Coan, J. A., & Allen, J. B. (2004). Frontal EEG asymmetry as a moderator and mediator of emotion. *Biological Psychology, 67*, 7–49.

Collins, B. E. (1969). The effect of monetary inducements on the amount of attitude change produced by forced compliance. In A. C. Elms (Ed.), *Role playing, reward, and attitude change* (pp. 209–223). New York: Van Nostrand Reinhold.

Collins, B. E., & Hoyt, M. F. (1972). Personal responsibility-for-consequences: An integration and extension of the "forced compliance" literature. *Journal of Experimental Social Psychology, 8*, 558–593.

Cooper, J., & Fazio, R. H. (1984). A new look at dissonance theory. In L. Berkowitz (Ed.), *Advances in experimental social psychology* (Vol. 17, pp. 229–264). New York: Academic Press.

Cooper, J., & Worchel, S. (1970). Role of undesired

consequences in arousing cognitive dissonance. *Journal of Personality and Social Psychology, 16*, 199–206.

Eagly, A. H., & Chaiken, S. (1993). *The psychology of attitudes*. Fort Worth, TX: Harcourt Brace Jovanovich.

Festinger, L. (1957). *A theory of cognitive dissonance*. Evanston, IL: Row, Peterson.

Festinger, L. (1964). *Conflict, decision, and dissonance*. Stanford, CA: Stanford University Press.

Festinger, L., & Carlsmith, J. M. (1959). Cognitive consequences of forced compliance. *Journal of Abnormal and Social Psychology, 58*, 203–210.

Frey, D. (1986). Recent research on selective exposure to information. In L. Berkowitz (Ed.), *Advances in experimental social psychology* (Vol. 19, pp. 41–80). New York: Academic Press.

Frijda, N. H. (1986). *The emotions*. Cambridge, UK: Cambridge University Press.

Gollwitzer, P. M. (1990). Action phases and mind-sets. In E. T. Higgins & R. M. Sorrentino (Eds.), *Handbook of motivation and cognition: Foundations of social behavior* (Vol. 2, pp. 53–92). New York: Guilford Press.

Harmon-Jones, E. (1999). Toward an understanding of the motivation underlying dissonance effects: Is the production of aversive consequences necessary to cause dissonance? In E. Harmon-Jones & J. Mills (Eds.), *Cognitive dissonance: Progress on a pivotal theory in social psychology* (pp. 71–99). Washington, DC: American Psychological Association.

Harmon-Jones, E. (2000a). Cognitive dissonance and experienced negative affect: Evidence that dissonance increases experienced negative affect even in the absence of aversive consequences. *Personality and Social Psychology Bulletin, 26*, 1490–1501.

Harmon-Jones, E. (2000b). A cognitive dissonance theory perspective on the role of emotion in the maintenance and change of beliefs and attitudes. In N. H. Frijda, A. R. S. Manstead, & S. Bem (Eds.), *Emotions and beliefs* (pp. 185–211). Cambridge, UK: Cambridge University Press.

Harmon-Jones, E. (2004). Contributions from research on anger and cognitive dissonance to understanding the motivational functions of asymmetrical frontal brain activity. *Biological Psychology, 67*, 51–76.

Harmon-Jones, E., & Allen, J. J. B. (1997). Behavioral activation sensitivity and resting frontal EEG asymmetry: Covariation of putative indicators related to risk for mood disorders. *Journal of Abnormal Psychology, 106*, 159–163.

Harmon-Jones, E., & Allen, J. J. B. (1998). Anger and prefrontal brain activity: EEG asymmetry consistent with approach motivation despite negative affective valence. *Journal of Personality and Social Psychology, 74*, 1310–1316.

Harmon-Jones, E., Brehm, J. W., Greenberg, J., Simon, L., & Nelson, D. E. (1996). Evidence that the production of aversive consequences is not necessary to create cognitive dissonance. *Journal of Personality and Social Psychology, 70*, 5–16.

Harmon-Jones, E., Gerdjikov, T., & Harmon-Jones, C. (in press). The effect of induced compliance on relative left frontal cortical activity: A test of the action-based model of dissonance. *European Journal of Social Psychology*.

Harmon-Jones, E., & Harmon-Jones, C. (2002). Testing the action-based model of cognitive dissonance: The effect of action-orientation on post-decisional attitudes. *Personality and Social Psychology Bulletin, 28*, 711–723.

Harmon-Jones, E., Harmon-Jones, C., Fearn, M., Sigelman, J. D., & Johnson, P. (in press). Action orientation, relative left frontal cortical activation, and spreading of alternatives: A test of the action-based model of dissonance. *Journal of Personality and Social Psychology*.

Harmon-Jones, E., Peterson, H., Hubbell, C., & Harmon-Jones, C. (2005). *Trait action-orientation predicts increased left frontal cortical activity and spreading of alternatives following a difficult decision*. Unpublished manuscript.

Harmon-Jones, E., Peterson, H., & Vaughn, K. (2003). The dissonance-inducing effects of an inconsistency between experienced empathy and knowledge of past failures to help: Support for the action-based model of dissonance. *Basic and Applied Social Psychology, 25*, 69–78.

Heckhausen, H. (1986). Why some time out might benefit achievement motivation research. In J. H. L van den Bercken, E. E. J. De Bruyn, & T. C. M. Bergen (Eds.), *Achievement and task motivation* (pp. 7–39). Lisse, The Netherlands: Swets & Zeitlinger.

Heider, F. (1946). Attitudes and cognitive organization. *Journal of Psychology, 21*, 107–112.

Heider, F. (1958). *The psychology of interpersonal relations*. New York: Wiley.

Henriques, J. B., & Davidson, R. J. (1991). Left frontal hypoactivation in depression. *Journal of Abnormal Psychology, 100*, 535–545.

Higgins, E. T. (1989). Self-discrepancy theory: What patterns of self-beliefs cause people to suffer? In L. Berkowitz (Ed.), *Advances in experimental social psychology* (Vol. 22, pp. 93–136). San Diego, CA: Academic Press.

Jones, E. E., & Gerard, H. B. (1967). *Foundations of social psychology*. New York: Wiley.

Kosslyn, S. M., & Koenig, O. (1995). *Wet mind: The new cognitive neuroscience*. New York: Free Press.

Kuhl, J. (1984). Volitional aspects of achievement motivation and learned helplessness: Toward a comprehensive theory of action-control. In B. A. Maher (Ed.), *Progress in experimental personality research* (Vol. 13, pp. 99–171). New York: Academic Press.

Kuhl, J. (1993). Action versus state orientation: Psychometric properties of the Action Control Scale (ACS-90). In J. Kuhl & J. Beckmann (Eds.), *Volition and personality: Action versus state orientation* (pp. 47–59). Seattle, WA: Hogrefe & Huber.

Kuhl, J. (2000). A functional-design approach to motivation and self-regulation: The dynamics of personality systems interactions. In M. Boekaerts, P. R. Pintrich, & M. Zeidner (Eds.), *Handbook of self-regulation* (pp. 111–169). San Diego, CA: Academic Press.

Lawrence, D. H., & Festinger, L. (1962). *Deterrents and reinforcement.* Stanford, CA: Stanford University Press.

Nel, E., Helmreich, R., & Aronson, E. (1969). Opinion change in the advocate as a function of the persuasibility of his audience: A clarification of the meaning of dissonance. *Journal of Personality and Social Psychology, 12,* 117–124.

Olson, J. M., & Zanna, M. P. (1979). A new look at selective exposure. *Journal of Experimental Social Psychology, 15,* 1–15.

Petrides, M., & Milner, B. (1982). Deficits on subject-ordered tasks after frontal- and temporal-lobe lesions in man. *Neuropsychologia, 20,* 249–262.

Robinson, R. G., & Downhill, J. E. (1995). Lateralization of psychopathology in response to focal brain injury. In R. J. Davidson & K. Hugdahl (Eds.), *Brain asymmetry* (pp. 693–711). Cambridge, MA: MIT Press.

Sakai, H. (1999). A multiplicative power function model of cognitive dissonance: Toward an integrated theory of cognition, emotion, and behavior after Leon Festinger. In E. Harmon-Jones & J. Mills (Eds.), *Cognitive dissonance: Progress on a pivotal theory in social psychology* (pp. 267–294). Washington, DC: American Psychological Association.

Shultz, T. R., & Lepper, M. R. (1999). Computer simulation of cognitive dissonance reduction. In E. Harmon-Jones & J. Mills (Eds.), *Cognitive dissonance: Progress on a pivotal theory in social psychology* (pp. 235–265). Washington, DC: American Psychological Association.

Simon, L., Greenberg, J., & Brehm, J. W. (1995). Trivialization: The forgotten mode of dissonance reduction. *Journal of Personality and Social Psychology, 68,* 247–260.

Sobotka, S. S., Davidson, R. J., & Senulis, J. A. (1992). Anterior brain electrical asymmetries in response to reward and punishment. *Electroencephalography and Clinical Neurophysiology, 83,* 236–247.

Steele, C. M. (1988). The psychology of self-affirmation: Sustaining the integrity of the self. In L. Berkowitz (Ed.), *Advances in experimental social psychology* (Vol. 21, pp. 261–302). San Diego, CA: Academic Press.

Steele, C. M., Southwick, L. L., & Critchlow, B. (1981). Dissonance and alcohol: Drinking your troubles away. *Journal of Personality and Social Psychology, 41,* 831–846.

Stone, J., Aronson, E., Crain, A. L., Winslow, M. P., & Fried, C. B. (1994). Inducing hypocrisy as a means for encouraging young adults to use condoms. *Personality and Social Psychology Bulletin, 20,* 116–128.

Tedeschi, J. T., Schlenker, B. R., & Bonoma, T. V. (1971). Cognitive dissonance: Private ratiocination or public spectacle? *American Psychologist, 26,* 685–695.

Tesser, A. (1988). Toward a self-evaluation maintenance model of social behavior. In L. Berkowitz (Ed.), *Advances in experimental social psychology* (Vol. 21, pp. 181–227). San Diego, CA: Academic Press.

Tomarken, A. J., & Davidson, R. J. (1994). Frontal brain activation in repressors and nonrepressors. *Journal of Abnormal Psychology, 103,* 339–349.

Vallacher, R. R., & Wegner, D. M. (1987). What do people think they're doing?: Action identification and human behavior. *Psychological Review, 94,* 3–15.

Walster, E. (1964). The temporal sequence of post-decision processes. In L. Festinger, *Conflict, decision, and dissonance* (pp. 112–128). Stanford, CA: Stanford University Press.

Wicklund, R. A., & Frey, D. (1981). Cognitive consistency: Motivational vs non-motivational perspectives. In J. P. Forgas (Ed.), *Social cognition: Perspectives on everyday understanding* (pp. 141–163). London: Academic Press.

Wicklund, R. A., & Gollwitzer, P. M. (1982). *Symbolic self-completion.* Hillsdale, NJ: Erlbaum.

Zanna, M. P., & Aziza, C. (1976). On the interaction of repression-sensitization and attention in resolving cognitive dissonance. *Journal of Personality, 44,* 577–593.

Chapter 6

# Motivated Closed-Mindedness and Its Social Consequences

**Arie W. Kruglanski**
**Woo Young Chun**

Human judgments and everyday activities require a subjective construction of knowledge that affords individuals at least a minimal degree of confidence. The cognitive activity underlying such a process could be carried on indefinitely. However, the time available for such a deliberation is typically limited, and the search for information relevant to a given judgment must be terminated at some point. Such termination is motivationally driven by the *need for closure* (NFC). In this chapter we describe a research program centered around this particular motivation, its antecedent conditions, and its personal and social consequences.

As a preview of what is to come, we first describe a theory elucidating the nature of the NFC, its situational and individual determinants, and its general effects on information processing (Kruglanski, 1989, 2004; Kruglanski & Webster, 1996). We then review research investigating effects of the NFC on a variety of social psychological phenomena at the intrapersonal, interpersonal, group, and intergroup levels of analysis.

## THE NEED FOR CLOSURE

The NFC has been defined as a desire for a definite answer to a question, as opposed to uncertainty, confusion, or ambiguity (Kruglanski, 1989). It is assumed that the motivation toward closure varies along a continuum anchored at one end with a strong NFC and at the other end with a strong need to avoid closure. According to the theory, the NFC is elevated by the perceived benefits of possessing closure and/or the costs of lacking them (Kruglanski & Webster, 1996; Webster & Kruglanski, 1998). Likewise, the need to avoid closure is elevated by the perceived benefits of lacking and the costs of possessing closure. Those benefits and costs may vary according to situational factors or individual differences.

## Situational Determinants

Many different contextual benefits or costs are assumed to have an impact on the NFC. For example, a potential benefit of closure may be the ability to act or decide in time for meeting an important deadline. Accordingly, the NFC should be heightened under time pressure (see Chiu, Morris, Hong, & Menon, 2000; Kruglanski & Freund, 1983). An alternative benefit of closure is that it obviates the necessity for further information processing. If so, the NFC should be heightened under a diverse set of conditions that render information processing subjectively difficult, laborious, or otherwise unpleasant. Some such conditions are environmental noise (see Kruglanski, Webster, & Klem, 1993) and tedium or dullness of the cognitive task (see Webster, 1993b). Individuals may also find information processing taxing and arduous when they are fatigued or low on energy (see Webster, Richter, & Kruglanski, 1996), or when alcoholic intoxication limits their capacity for systematic thought (see Webster, 1993a). The NFC is also heightened when closure is known to be valued by significant others, because the possession of definite closure may earn their esteem and appreciation (see Mayseless & Kruglanski, 1987). Finally, the NFC is heightened simply when judgment on some issue is required, compared to situations where the individual is at liberty to abstain from forming a definite opinion. In summary, the NFC is heightened by such diverse factors as environmental noise, task dullness, fatigue, alcohol, or a positive value attached to clear-cut opinions.

Similarly, the NFC may be lowered, and the need to avoid closure may be heightened, by conditions that highlight the costs of closure and the benefits of openness. In some circumstances, the costs of closure may be rendered salient by a fear of invalidity (Kruglanski & Freund, 1983), stemming from concern about committing a costly error of judgment. Under these conditions, the person may be prone to suspend or postpone judgment in order to avoid premature closure. This statement may imply that validity concerns are necessarily at odds with those of closure. Obviously, however, no one will consciously adopt a closure that he or she judges to be invalid. To know that one's name is John, or that it happens to be Tuesday now, means to have closures on these topics *and* simultaneously believe these closures to be true. Nonetheless, psychological concerns for closure and validity often arise fairly independently of each other. What is more important, they pull information processing in diametrically opposite directions. For example, where the NFC is elevated for some reason (e.g., because of fatigue, noise, or other situational impediments to information processing), the individual may consider limited information and/or rely on preconceived notions (prejudices, cultural stereotypes, etc.) in reaching social judgments. By contrast, where the NFC is reduced (e.g., by felt accountability for one's decisions, or by fear of the costs of making a false move), the person may consider ample information before making up his or her mind. Note that the person may not be *cognizant* of sacrificing validity or of excessively postponing closure. Rather, in both cases, the individual may feel that he or she is processing just the right amount of information to make a reasonably secure judgment. In other words, the epistemic dynamics prompted by the NFC are not assumed to be consciously accessible to the knower, but rather to exert their effects implicitly and typically outside of awareness.

It is important to realize that validity concerns may not always lower the NFC or foster openness to new ideas or information. If a particular closure appears valid beyond reasonable doubt—for instance, because its source (e.g., one's parents, an adored guru, or the printed page) appears to have impeccable credibility or indubitable "epistemic authority" (Ellis & Kruglanski, 1992; Kruglanski, 1989; Kruglanski et al., 2005)—validity concerns may magnify the tendency to embrace it rather than to avoid or postpone it until ample further information has been considered.

## Individual Differences

Individuals may exhibit stable personal differences in the degree to which they value closure. Some persons may form clear-cut and often extreme opinions regardless of the delicacy of a situation, whereas others may feel uncomfortable about rendering a definite judgment and prefer to suspend it in even the safest of environments. Such differences may derive from various sources, such as cultural norms (Hofstede, 1980) or personal socialization histories that place a premium on confidence, orderliness, and clarity. To tap such individual differences, Webster and Kruglanski (1994) developed the NFC Scale (NFCS) and established its reliability and validity. The scale has been translated into several languages (Cantonese and Mandarin Chinese, Croatian, Dutch, French, German, Hebrew, Italian, Japanese, Korean, and Spanish); hence it facilitates the cross-cultural investigation of issues associated with closed- and open-mindedness.

Numerous structural analyses conducted with the NFCS in its various versions have consistently demonstrated that a solution with five correlated first-order factors fits the data well, that the factors are unidimensional, and that the five-factor structure is consistent across different national and international samples (Cratylus, 1995; Pierro et al., 1995; Webster & Kruglanski, 1994). Further exploration of commonalities among the facets has also yielded consistent results. Thus Webster and Kruglanski (1994) found support in their data for a single second-order factor, also supported in the Dutch data (Cratylus, 1995). Pierro and colleagues (1995) found virtually identical indexes of fit for a single second-order factor and for a two-factor second-order model in which one factor consisted of the Decisionality subscale and the other of the remaining four facets of the NFCS. Similar results were reported by De Grada, Kruglanski, Mannetti, Pierro, and Webster (1996), who compared an Italian sample with a U.S. sample, and found that both the single second-order factor and the two second-order factors yielded nearly identical fit indexes for both samples. Kossowska, Van Hiel, Chun, and Kruglanski (2002) also found the same structural invariance, partial metric invariance, and partial scalar invariance of the NFCS across Polish, Flemish, Korean, and U.S. samples. These findings indicate that the NFCS has the same basic meaning and structure cross-nationally, and that ratings can be meaningfully compared across different countries and cultures.

### The Urgency and Permanence Tendencies

We posit two general tendencies that the NFC may instill: the *urgency* tendency and the *permanence* tendency. The urgency tendency is the inclination to "seize" on closure quickly. People under a heightened NFC desire closure immediately. Any further postponement of closure is experienced as bothersome, and the individuals' overriding sense is that they simply cannot wait. The permanence tendency is the desire to perpetuate closure, giving rise to the dual inclination (1) to preserve, or "freeze" on, past knowledge and (2) to safeguard future knowledge. Individuals under a heightened NFC may thus desire an enduring closure and (in extreme cases) abhor letting go of closure. The urgency and permanence notions both rest on the assumption that people under a heightened NFC experience its absence as aversive. They may wish to terminate this unpleasant state quickly (the urgency tendency) and keep it from recurring (the permanence tendency).

## INTRAPERSONAL EFFECTS OF THE NFC

In forming judgments about people or events, individuals will seek less information before crystallizing an opinion if at the moment they experience a heightened NFC. To test the possibility of restricted predecisional search for information, Webster and colleagues (1996) asked psychology students to carry out an impression formation task in which each student played a personnel manager faced with a hiring decision. Individuals experiencing a relatively high (vs. low) NFC (manipulated via mental fatigue) requested significantly fewer pages of relevant information prior to forming their impression of the job candidate. Furthermore, when some participants were held accountable for their judgments (a manipulation designed to lower their NFC), they requested significantly more pages of information than those who were not held accountable). In another experiment (Mayseless & Kruglanski, 1987, Study 2), participants were asked to identify barely visible digits appearing on a screen of a tachistoscope. The extent of informational search, operationally defined as the number of times participants operated the tachistoscope, was lowest in the NFC condition (manipulated by stressing the value of unambiguous, clear-cut opinions), intermediate in the control condition, and highest in the need-to-avoid-closure conditions (manipulated by accuracy instructions and incentives).

### Hypothesis Generation

In forming a judgment or an opinion, people often generate a number of alternative hypotheses to account for known facts, and proceed to choose among them on the basis of further relevant information. The "seizing" and "freezing" tendencies evoked by the (nonspecific) NFC may restrict the tendency to keep generating such alternative hypotheses. Mayseless and Kruglanski (1987, Study 3) showed participants photos of parts of common objects (e.g., a comb or a toothbrush) taken from unusual angles to disguise their true identity. Participants listed as many hypotheses as possible concerning an object's identity, and finally selected what they deemed as the most likely identity. It was found that participants in the need-to-avoid-closure condition (manipulated by stressing the value of accurate judgments) generated more hypotheses on the average than participants in the neutral control condition, whereas participants in the NFC condition (manipulated by stressing the value of clear-cut opinions) generated fewer hypotheses on the average than did the control group.

## Subjective Confidence

An ironic consequence of reduced hypothesis generation before forming a judgment may be heightened subjective confidence despite limited consideration of alternatives. If individuals under a high NFC are less aware of competing judgmental possibilities, they may be more confident that the possibility they select is correct. Indeed, elevated judgmental confidence under a heightened NFC has been manifested in numerous studies (Kruglanski & Webster, 1991; Kruglanski et al., 1993; Mayseless & Kruglanski, 1987; Webster, 1993a, 1993b). These findings suggest that subjective certainty is possible in the absence of extensive information processing, and in fact may be inversely related to extensive processing.

## Cue Utilization

Under a heightened NFC, individuals are likely to base their final judgments on early cues. The urgency tendency should dispose persons to "seize" quickly upon early cues and utilize them toward the formation of initial judgments. And the permanence tendency should dispose them to "freeze"—that is, to fixate or perseverate on those particular judgments. Substantial research on a variety of seemingly diverse social psychological topics has supported these ideas.

### *Primacy Effects in Impression Formation*

A *primacy effect* is the tendency to base one's social impressions on early information about that person, to the relative neglect of subsequent, equally relevant information. From the present perspective, primacy effects exemplify the "seizing" and "freezing" tendencies assumed to be manifested under a heightened NFC. If our analysis is correct, the magnitude of primacy effects should be augmented under a heightened (nonspecific) NFC. This prediction was supported in various experiments, in which the NFC was manipulated via time pressure (Kruglanski & Freund, 1983, Study 1) or mental fatigue (Webster et al., 1996), or measured via the NFCS (Webster & Kruglanski, 1994). These studies found that the magnitude of the primacy effect varied positively with the NFC and negatively with the need to avoid closure.

### *Anchoring Effects*

A different instance of early-cue utilization may underlie the *anchoring effect* made famous by Tversky and Kahneman (1974). From the present perspective, anchoring may represent the "seizing" and "freezing" on initial knowledge activated, and hence made accessible, by the anchor. Indeed, Kruglanski and Freund (1983, Study 2) found greater anchoring effects under time pressure (vs. no pressure), assumed to heighten the NFC, and reduced anchoring effects under accountability instructions, assumed to lower the NFC.

### *The Correspondence Bias*

The *correspondence bias* (Jones, 1979), or the *fundamental attribution error* (Ross, 1977) refers to an attributor's tendency to overascribe an actor's behavior to his or her unique attitudes or personality, and to underestimate the extent to which the situation is capable of eliciting such behavior from most people. The effect was originally demonstrated in a study by Jones and Harris (1967) that required participants to judge the true attitude of a target person after reading an opinion essay allegedly prepared by this individual under either a free-choice or a no-choice condition. The intriguing finding was that even when participants learned that the target was given no choice in determining the contents of the essay, and was explicitly instructed by the experimenter to espouse a given position, they still estimated that his or her attitude corresponded to some degree to the one expressed in the essay.

It seems plausible, then, that just as with primacy and anchoring effects, the correspondence bias may reflect the "seizing" and "freezing" on early hypotheses effected by the NFC. To test this possibility, Webster (1993b) asked participants to complete a typical attitude attribution task in which they estimated a target's attitude after hearing her deliver a speech criticizing student exchange programs with foreign universities. The speech was allegedly prepared under either a high- or a low-choice condition. The results showed that the correspondence bias was enhanced in the high-NFC condition (manipulated via task attractiveness or measured via the NFCS) relative to the control condition, and reduced in the low-NFC condition. Of particular interest, in a third study the pattern of results was completely reversed when initial cues implied a *situational* rather than an *attitudinal* attribution. Specifically, individuals under a high NFC were less likely to make dispositional attributions, and those under a low NFC were more likely to do so, when both were compared to the control condition. This suggests that NFC effects are essentially content-free, and that the order of the cues (i.e., their appearance early vs. late in the sequence) rather than their particular substance (implying a dispositional vs. a situational attribution) is critical.

### Stereotype Application

Increased application of prevalent social stereotypes and prejudices to various social judgments may represent a particularly striking case of "seizing" and "freezing" under a heightened NFC. General stereotypes prevalent within a culture constitute knowledge structures that may readily come to mind; hence they may be particularly likely to serve as bases for judging such stereotyped targets when the perceiver is under a high (vs. low) NFC. This possibility was supported in several studies and with several different stereotypic contents, such as the stereotypes of Ashkenazi and Sepharadi Israelis (Kruglanski & Freund, 1983), stereotypes of women in management (Jamieson & Zanna, 1989), and stereotypes of soccer hooligans as well as nurses (Dijksterhuis, Van Knippenberg, Kruglanski, & Schaper, 1996).

### Construct Accessibility

The argument that NFC enhances the tendency to base judgments on prevalent stereotypes, or that it often magnifies the tendency to overascribe actors' behaviors to their attitudes or dispositions, critically assumes that such stereotypes or dispositional (attitudinal) hypotheses are highly accessible to an individual—that is, that they tend to pop into the individual's mind immediately upon his or her encounter with the stimulus. To test this assumption, Ford and Kruglanski (1995) used the priming paradigm employed by Higgins, Rholes, and Jones (1977) in which an ambiguous paragraph about an individual named Donald is interpreted in line with the prime. For example, if the description of Donald is ambiguous in regard to the traits *adventurous* and *reckless*, priming the word *adventurous* in a prior (and allegedly unrelated task) should disambiguate the description in a corresponding direction, as should priming the word *reckless*. In the Ford and Kruglanski (1995) study, participants who scored either high or low on the NFCS (Webster & Kruglanski, 1994) received one of two primes during a memory task: either the negatively valenced adjective *reckless* or the positively valenced adjective *adventurous*. They then performed an impression formation task that required them to characterize a target person with a single word after reading behavioral information about the target that was ambiguous with regard to the adventurous–reckless distinction. In one of the experiments (Study 1), the NFC was manipulated via cognitive load, specifically via rehearsal of an eight-digit number while processing information about a target person. In the second experiment (Study 2), the NFC was assessed via the appropriate scale (Webster & Kruglanski, 1994). The findings of both studies indicated that participants high (vs. low) on a dispositional NFC tended to characterize the target more in terms suggesting recklessness in the *reckless* prime condition, and adventurousness in the *adventurous* prime condition. Furthermore, when in Study 1 the NFC was lowered via accuracy instructions, the differences between the two primes (i.e., *reckless* and *adventurous*) disappeared. Thus, consistent with the "seizing" and "freezing" notion, high-NFC participants exhibited stronger effects of priming than did low-NFC participants.

### Recency Effects

If construct accessibility is what truly matters, then under some circumstances the NFC should lead to recency instead of primacy effects. The moderator variable could be the timing of the goal setting for the information-processing task. Specifically, it should matter whether the impression formation goal is set prior to the informational exposure or following it. When the goal of forming an impression exists from the start, a heightened NFC may indeed foster primacy effects prompted by "seizing" and "freezing" on the early information as soon as it becomes accessible. When the impression formation goal is formed only following the informational exposure, however, judgments may be made from memory, based on previously received notions deemed relevant to the present judgment. In such a case, the most *recently* received information is the most accessible (cf. Higgins, 1996). To test this possibility, Richter and Kruglanski (1999) asked participants to judge descriptive sentences for their grammatical structure and coherence. All the sentences depicted a job candidate. As expected, in a situation where the impression formation goal was introduced following exposure to the stimulus information, participants' judgments were based on memory rather than being formed online, in that a significant correlation was obtained between positivity of recall and positivity of participants' impressions. Furthermore, participants under high time pressure manifested more pronounced recency effects than did participants under no time pressure. Finally, this difference was eliminated when an accuracy motivation (assumed to lower the NFC) was introduced.

## INTERPERSONAL CONSEQUENCES OF THE NFC

The processing of information about one's interaction partners, and the formation online of judgments about their feelings, cognitions, and probable actions, are essential aspects of social relations. The "seizing" and "freezing" tendencies fostered by a heightened NFC should, therefore, exert important effects at the interpersonal level of analysis. We consider three such interactional phenomena: (1) perspective taking and empathy, (2) audience design in interpersonal communication, and (3) the language of interpersonal discourse.

### Perspective Taking and Empathy

According to Davis (1983), the term *empathy* actually covers two conceptually separate phenomena. *Perspective taking* is an aspect of empathy that involves an ability to see things from another person's vantage point. *Empathic concern* represents the extent to which one experiences compassion, sympathy, or caring for another person (Davis, 1983). These two aspects of empathy are interrelated. Perspective taking is likely to affect empathic concern, as one is more likely to feel a concern for others if one appreciates their predicament.

The taking of another person's perspective may often require substantial cognitive effort, as the first thing that typically comes to mind is one's own perspective. Thus perspective taking may require correction, adjustment, and careful consideration of just exactly how another person may differ from oneself. This may necessitate appreciable cognitive labor, especially if the person whose perspective one is attempting to divine differs from oneself substantially on various pertinent dimensions. If the NFC reduces an individual's readiness to put mental effort into the processing of information, and if it disposes the individual to "seize" and "freeze" upon early notions, it may substantially reduce perspective taking and empathic concern when it comes to a person with a dissimilar perspective.

These ideas were examined in two studies conducted by Webster-Nelson, Klein, and Irvin (2003). Participants in their first experiment engaged in a social perception task, wherein they read information allegedly provided by another participant from a previous study. The target information depicted a negative social experience. Half the participants read a description in which the target reported suffering from chronic shyness, as well as feelings of disappointment and dejection after a specific failed attempt to socialize at a party. According to Higgins (1987), these feelings are often the consequence of a discrepancy between one's *actual* and *ideal* selves. The remaining participants read the same description, only the target now reported feelings of guilt and agitation after the social failure, associated with an *actual–ought* discrepancy (Higgins, 1987). These two variations were used to manipulate the similarity between the participants and the targets, as participants were preselected on the basis of possessing one or the other kind of discrepancy. Thus participants were exposed to information about a target who either expressed thoughts and feelings similar to those they might have in the same situation, or about a target who expressed thoughts and feelings different from those they might have. After having read the description, participants answered a number of questions. First, they evaluated the appropriateness of the target's response to the incident. This was designed to assess perspective taking. Furthermore, they indicated the extent to which they felt compassionate, sympathetic, tender, warm, and softhearted with respect to the target.

The main analyses indicated that perceived appropriateness of the target's response (reflecting perspective taking) was *reduced* by a heightened NFC (manipulated via fatigue) when the target was dissimilar from the participant. This condition represented a case when perspective taking would require cognitive effort, which fatigued participants (assumed to experience the NFC) apparently did not exert. No significant differences in perspective taking as a function of fatigue occurred when the target and the participant were similar. An identical pattern of findings emerged for the measure of empathic concern. Specifically, *less* empathic concern was reported by fatigued participants when the target was dissimilar to themselves, whereas no significant differences in empathic concern emerged when the target was similar to the participants.

If perspective taking and empathic concern for dissimilar targets was reduced by the NFC, lowering this need should appropriately reverse this effect. A second study tested this possibility. In this experiment, the NFC was expected to be attenuated if individuals expected to be outcome-dependent on the target, since past research demonstrates that outcome dependency motivates people to make accurate judgments (e.g., Erber & Fiske, 1984) and that accuracy concerns seem to lower the NFC (Mayseless & Kruglanski, 1987).

Of greater interest, the non-outcome-dependent participants behaved pretty much as did participants in the first study. Fatigued (but not nonfatigued) participants rated the target's affective response as significantly less appropriate when the target's discrepancy was dissimilar from that of the participants. No differences in rated appropriateness emerged when targets' affect and participants' discrepancies matched each other. The empathic concern data revealed the same general pattern. Fatigued (vs. nonfatigued) participants exhibited significantly less concern and compassion toward the target's response when the targets' and participants' perspectives were dissimilar, yet no differences as a function of fatigue emerged when these perspectives were similar.

A very different data pattern emerged in the outcome-dependent condition, where no fatigue effects emerged on either perspective taking or empathic concern. It appears that despite their fatigue, outcome-dependent participants were quite capable of adopting the target's perspective and consequently experiencing empathic concern even when the target's perspective was quite dissimilar from their own. These findings are consistent with the notion that empathic deficits owing to fatigue are at least in part motivational in nature (i.e., are related to the NFC that fatigue may induce). Further analyses suggested that the effects of NFC on empathic concern were mediated by perspective taking (Baron & Kenny, 1986). These findings support the notion that "seizing" and "freezing" on one's own perspective may play an important role in such a distinctly interpersonal phenomenon as empathy.

## Interpersonal Communication

A fundamental presumption of communication theory is that in conveying messages to others, speakers take the listeners' perspective into account and refer their utterances to the social reality they share. From this perspective, Clark and Murphy (1982) noted that "in ordinary conversation we tailor what we say to the particular people we are talking to" (p. 287). They term this process *audience design*, and state that "an essential part of [such] design . . . is the use of the speaker's and addressee's mutual knowledge, beliefs, and suppositions, or common ground (p. 288).

Krauss and Fussell (1991, p. 4) argued that assumptions about what others know may be thought of as tentative "hypotheses that participants continuously modify and reformulate on the basis of additional evidence," such as verbal and nonverbal feedback (see also Powell & O'Neal, 1976). Horton and Keysar (1996) found that while speakers did incorporate common ground into their communications in the absence of time pressure, common ground was not used when the speakers were under time pressure. They concluded that this finding supported their *monitoring and adjustment* model, whereby a speaker's initial hypothesis in formulating an utterance is based on the speaker's own knowledge and on information that is salient to him or her. Given sufficient time, however, the speaker will modify or adjust that hypothesis to incorporate the common ground shared with the listener. Of course, the presence or absence of subjectively sufficient time—that is, time pressure—has constituted one of the major ways in which the NFC has been operationalized in past research (Kruglanski & Freund, 1983; Shah, Kruglanski, & Thompson, 1998). It is thus possible that a high level of this need may reduce the amount of effort communicators invest in their search for common ground. As a consequence, communications by high-NFC individuals may be excessively biased in the direction of the communicators' own perspective, which might reduce their comprehensibility to the listeners. Richter and Kruglanski (1999) investigated this hypothesis, using Fussell and Krauss's (1989) two-stage referential task paradigm.

In this particular paradigm, participants are provided with a set of abstract figures and are asked to write descriptions of those figures so that that they themselves (the nonsocial condition) or another person (the social condition) could match the descriptions to the figures on a subsequent occasion. Participants were scheduled to appear in the laboratory for two sessions, corresponding to two separate research phases. In the description phase, participants wrote descriptions of each of 30 figures after having received either social or nonsocial encoding instructions. In the identification phase, carried out 3–5 weeks later, participants attempted to match a series of 90 descriptions written by themselves and others to their respective 30 figures presented on a poster board.

The results showed that participants with high (vs. low) NFC (measured via the NFCS) used significantly fewer words in their descriptions, and they produced significantly more figurative (or less literal) descriptions. Furthermore, the average number of words used by participants with low NFC in the social condition was more than double that for such participants in the nonsocial condition. This difference was much less pronounced and nonsignificant for participants with a high NFC. Did these NFC-driven differences affect communicative efficacy? Apparently so: Significantly more descriptions encoded by low-NFC communicators were correctly matched to the appropriate figures than descriptions encoded by high-NFC communicators.

## The Language of Interpersonal Discourse

If the NFC induces the tendency to seek permanent knowledge and avoid the recurrence of ambiguity, it should foster a bias toward general, transsituationally stable knowledge. Accordingly, people under a heightened NFC should prefer abstract descriptions and category labels over concrete, situationally specific depictions. Consistent with these assumptions, Boudreau, Baron, and Oliver (1992) found that participants expecting to communicate their impressions to a nonknowledgeable other, and thus experiencing decreased concerns about judgmental validity and high NFC, increased the preponderance of global trait labels in their descriptions. In contrast, those expecting to communicate to a knowledgeable other, and hence experiencing increased concerns about validity and low NFC, used a lower proportion of global trait labels (see also Mikulincer, Yinon, & Kabili, 1991).

Assuming the existence of such an abstraction bias under a heightened NFC, how might it affect the use of language in interpersonal discourse, and what effects might it have on interpersonal rapport? Work by Semin, Rubini, and Fiedler (1995) indicates that the abstractness level of questions influences the locus of causal origin for answers. Specifically, questions formulated with action verbs, (e.g., *to help, to write*) cue the logical *subject* of a question as the causal origin of answers. Questions formulated with state verbs (e.g., *to love, to like*) cue the logical *object* of a question as the causal origin for answers. Thus, if asked such simple and mundane question as "Why do you *own* a dog?" (using an interpretative action verb), one is prompted to respond by referring to oneself (the subject of the question) as the causal agent in the answer (e.g., by stating, "Because *I* enjoy the companionship that dogs provide"). If one is asked "Why do you *like* dogs?," however, one is prompted to respond by referring to the object itself (e.g., "Because *dogs* are good companions").

One interesting implication of this effect is that individuals may feel that they disclose more about themselves when asked questions formulated with action verbs as opposed to state verbs, or, more generally speaking, questions formulated at a lower (vs. higher) level of abstractness. As a consequence, respondents asked questions at a low level of abstractness may feel closer and friendlier toward the interviewer, which may elicit reciprocal friendliness on the interviewer's part. By contrast, respondents asked questions at a higher level of abstractness may feel more distant and less friendly toward the interviewer, again inviting a response in kind.

In their first experiment designed to investigate these issues, Rubini and Kruglanski (1997) had participants under high (vs. low) NFC (manipulated via ambient noise) rank-order questions on a list in terms of their likelihood of using them in a real interview. It was found that participants under noise (vs. no noise) assigned higher ranks to questions characterized by a higher (vs. lower) level of abstractness. In a follow-up study, questions selected by participants under high (vs. low) NFC were found to elicit more abstract answers from respondents, and ones focused more on the logical object (vs. subject) of the question. Also, respondents reported feeling less friendliness toward the interviewer whose questions were more (vs. less) abstract. Finally, in a third study, the results of the previous two experiments were replicated in a free-interaction context. In that research, interviewers with high (vs. low) NFC asked more abstract questions, which in turn elicited more abstract answers and ones focused more on the logical object (vs. subject) of the question, and elicited less friendliness from the interviewee. These results suggest that the permanence tendency induced by the NFC may affect the level of linguistic abstractness, and in so doing may affect the nascent social relations among conversation partners.

## GROUP PHENOMENA

### Task versus Socioemotional Orientation

Although members of a small group may perform a variety of task-oriented or socioemotional acts (e.g., Bales, 1950; Fiedler, 1967), the task at hand is likely to constitute the single most accessible notion whereby group members may define their situation. If high-NFC individuals are likely to seize and freeze on a highly accessible construct (Ford & Kruglanski, 1995; Thompson, Roman, Moskowitz, & Chaiken, 1994), a heightened NFC should enhance participants' task orientation and reduce their engagement in acts of a socioemotional nature. To test this prediction, De Grada, Kruglanski, Mannetti, and Pierro (1999) asked University of Rome students in groups of four to role-play the managers of four corporate departments at a meeting designed for a negotiation of a monetary reward to a meritorious worker. Consistent with the present analysis, participants under a high NFC (manipulated via time pressure or measured via the NFCS) produced a higher proportion of task-oriented responses and a lower proportion of positive socioemotional acts than did participants under a low NFC.

### Consensus Striving

As Festinger (1950) has noted, social reality requires a homogeneity of opinions within a group. That is, social uniformity is essential for the maintenance of epistemic certainty. It follows, therefore, that the quest for permanence under a heightened NFC should fuel the desire for consensus.

#### *Experienced Pressures for Uniformity*

De Grada and colleagues (1999) asked participants after a negotiation session in a group to answer a modified version of the Conformity Pressure Questionnaire developed by Kroon, van Kreveld, and Rabbie (1992). As predicted, members of the high-NFC groups reported greater perceived pressure for conformity than those of the low-NFC groups. This finding was confirmed when two independent observers who did not know the composition of the various groups viewed the video-recorded group discussions. It appears, then, that groups composed of high-NFC (vs. low-NFC) individuals do exert greater conformity pressures on their members, and that such pressures are both experienced by the members and perceptible to outside observers.

#### *Changing Others and Changing Self*

Kruglanski and colleagues (1993) asked participants (members of alleged two-member juries) to what extent they wished to reach agreement with the other member, and to what extent they wished to do so quickly. It was found that participants high (vs. low) in NFC (manipulated via ambient noise or measured via the NFCS) reported a significantly greater desire for quick agreement with their partners. Of importance, the way participants under high (vs. low) NFC dealt with disagreement from the other "jury member" differed appreciably as a function of whether they did or did not possess a firm prior opinion. Participants who were provided with a (fictitious) legal analysis allowing them to form a relatively firm opinion about the appropriate verdict were relatively refractory to arguments from the other "juror" and refused to change their minds as a consequence of the discussion. If they desired consensus (as they apparently did), they probably hoped to attain it by the *change other* strategy identified by Festinger (1950)—that is, by exerting influence attempts geared at altering their partner's views to coincide more closely with their own. In contrast, participants who lacked a firm prior opinion exhibited considerable opinion shifts in the direction of the other "juror's" arguments. One might say that their strategy of attaining consensus was via Festinger's (1950) *change self* option—that is, by altering their own views to bring them into closer correspondence with those of the other.

### Rejection of Opinion Deviates

Festinger (1950) identified another way of securing consensus within a group if persuasion attempts should fail—namely, rejection of opinion deviates and redefinition of the group's boundaries, so that only the consensual members remain included in the group. If a heightened NFC augments the desire for consensus, then it should result in a greater tendency to reject opinion deviates. To test this prediction, Kruglanski and Webster (1991) asked participants (University of Maryland students) who favored drug testing for athletes to reach consensus on a case involving compulsory drug testing. In other conditions, participants were allowed to form their decision by a majority rule rather than by consensus. Two confederates participated in the group discussions: One confederate enacted the role of a conformist and argued the majority viewpoint in favor of testing; the other enacted the deviate role and argued the minority viewpoint against testing. As predicted, the ratings of the deviate were significantly lower under high (vs. low) NFC (manipulated via ambient noise). Of importance, rejection of the deviate occurred only in the noise/consensus condition, where the deviant frustrated the other group members' desire for collective closure. No comparable rejection occurred in the noise/majority-rule condition, presumably because collective closure was satisfied via the allowable majority rule. This finding is important because it rules out the possibility that the observed rejection of the deviate was caused by the noise-produced irritation, or in the preceding study by the time pressure. Consistent with this interpretation, in an additional study a conformist who vocally endorsed the consensual view (an "active" conformist) was evaluated more positively, in fact, under the noisy versus the quiet conditions. Thus it seems that noise-induced NFC may instill a striving for consensus, manifested in the rejection of opinion deviates as well as in the adulation of conformists.

### Focus on Shared versus Unshared Information

The tendency of group members to predominantly discuss information they all share has been discovered by Stasser in a series of studies (Stasser & Stewart, 1992; Stasser & Titus, 1985, 1987). Webster (1993a) tested the further notion that a heightened NFC may focus individuals on shared information because of their strong desire for consensus, and because shared information provides a common knowledge base on which consensus can be built. Participants in groups of three discussed three candidates for a student political office on campus. Each participant was provided with background materials consisting of statements made by each of the three candidates regarding several campus-relevant issues, such as parking fees, dormitory policies, class sizes, registration policies, and campus security. Overall, 18 items of information were shared by group members, while 18 were unshared (i.e., they were included in only one member's reading materials). The shared versus unshared items were selected to bias prediscussion preferences in favor of Candidate A. Nonetheless, the *total body* of information received by all members of each group favored Candidate C.

Webster (1993a) found that the tendency to bring up unique information varied inversely with the group members' NFC (manipulated via amount of ingested alcohol), but the differences due to alcohol entirely disappeared in the high-need-to-avoid-closure conditions (manipulated via accountability instructions). These results were mimicked in turn by the proportion of groups who reached the correct solution (i.e., who properly selected C as the best qualified candidate): In the no-accountability condition, the tendency to select C varied inversely with the amount of alcohol ingested, whereas no significant differences as a function of alcohol emerged in the accountability condition. It appears then, that the focus on shared information and the exclusion of unshared information during group discussion are least partly determined by members' NFC, presumably due to their strong desire for group consensus.

### *Group Creativity*

The findings that group members under a high NFC strive for consensus (Kruglanski & Webster, 1991; Kruglanski et al., 1993) and exert uniformity pressures on each other (De Grada et al., 1999) suggest that they may not be particularly innovating or creative. To test this possibility, Chirumbolo, Mannetti, Pierro, Areni, and Kruglanski (in press) asked participants in groups of three to engage in a brainstorming task. It was found that groups under a high NFC (manipulated via ambient noise) displayed lesser ideational fluency (i.e., produced a lesser number of ideas) than groups under a low NFC. This relation was mediated by an appropriate NFC manipulation check. In the second study by Chirumbolo and colleagues, participants in groups of four created advertising slogans for a given product. Some groups were composed of individuals with a high dispositional NFC, whereas other groups were composed of low-NFC individuals. Results indicated that ideational fluency, degree of elaboration, and creativity, as rated by independent judges, were lower in high-NFC (vs. low-NFC) groups. Considered collectively, these results suggest that NFC-driven tendencies to restrict the number of hypotheses generated and to produce conventional ideas (reflecting perceived consensus) act to lower the degree of creativity in interacting groups.

### *Inequality of Participation*

Beyond uniformity pressures, NFC may affect group interaction in another intriguing way. Groups consisting of high-NFC (vs. low-NFC) individuals may manifest a less evenly distributed interaction pattern and greater dominance of the discussion by some individuals over others. This prediction too follows from the quest for opinion uniformity that high-NFC members are expected to exhibit. Uniformity may be obtained more readily when one opinion (or only a few opinions) governs the discussion than when a heterogeneity of opinions is offered that impedes consensus. Accordingly, groups composed of high-NFC members may exhibit more autocratic (or less democratic) patterns of participation and decision making than those composed of low-NFC members.

De Grada and colleagues (1999, Study 2) looked at the number of instances in which members seized the discussion floor and maintained it despite interruption attempts by others. Whereas no significant difference emerged in regard to the asymmetry of obtained turns, the asymmetry of maintained turns was higher in the high-NFC groups than in the low-NFC groups. These results were replicated in an additional study (Pierro, Mannetti, De Grada, Livi, & Kruglanski, 2003) using an identical procedure and method of analysis. This time, the asymmetry of both the obtained and the maintained turns was greater in groups composed of high-NFC individuals. In addition, Pierro and colleagues (2003) asked independent observers who viewed the video recordings of the group interactions to rate each of the four participants in each group on the degree to which he or she appeared to be authoritarian, assertive, dogmatic, and egocentric. It was found that the correlation between autocracy and floor control was significantly higher for groups composed of high-NFC members than for groups composed of low-NFC members. Finally, Pierro and colleagues found that the tendency to control the floor was perceived (by the group members themselves as well as by independent observers) as a demonstration of influence and leadership in the group; this finding combines with the others to suggest that high-NFC (vs. low-NFC) groups indeed foster the emergence of more autocratic leaders. In their final study, Pierro and colleagues manipulated the NFC via time pressure and measured the tendency toward centralization in a group via interaction process analysis (Bales, 1950). Groups under time pressure (vs. no pressure) exhibited significantly greater asymmetry between members in their degree of centrality (assessed via the number of acts emitted as well as acts received). Again then, it appears that groups whose members are under a high NFC exhibit a greater degree of centralization and hierarchical differentiation between members in their degree of influence than do groups whose members are under a low NFC.

## Norm Stability

The pressures toward epistemic permanence and "freezing" on extant knowledge structures fostered by a heightened NFC may induce in members the disposition toward conservatism, traditionalism, and the preservation of group norms (Jost, Glazer, Kruglanski, & Sulloway, 2003a, 2003b).

The relation between NFC and the tendency to preserve group norms was also the subject of recent experimental work by Livi (2002). Participants were given information about a (fictitious) new voice-activated computer software program and were asked to answer in a group format a number of questions allegedly posed by a marketing firm, including the age of potential users, the optimal number of TV commercials, and the optimal advertising budget for effective marketing of the product. Livi utilized a generational procedure, modeled after the one devised by Jacobs and Campbell (1961). Each generation was composed of three members. In the first generation, two of these were confederates who agreed on rather low values (as determined by a pretest) with respect to all three issues being discussed (i.e., on relatively low age of potential users, low optimal number of TV commercials, and low optimal advertising budget)—thus influencing the third member, who was a naive participant. This established an initial norm to which subsequent generations of participants could refer.

After having stated their opinions, one of the confederates left the group and was replaced by a naive participant; after the second cycle, the second confederate was replaced; after the third cycle, the original naive participant was replaced; and so forth for a total of eight generational cycles. Half of the groups were placed under a high NFC by means of a great deal of ambient noise (presumably generated by a faulty air conditioner). The remaining half of the groups was not placed under noise. In support of the present theory, Livi (2002) found that over the several generational cycles investigated, norms were considerably more stable in groups under noise versus no noise. These findings were replicated in Livi's second study, wherein dispositional differences in NFC were substituted for ambient noise.

## INTERGROUP PROCESSES

Hogg and Abrams (1993) have specifically stressed the epistemic functions of ingroups, and have proposed that uncertainty reduction may constitute an important motivational basis underlying ingroup favoritism. To the individual member, the ingroup represents a source of unambiguous social knowledge—a highly valued psychological "commodity." If so, it is easy to see why members may considerably appreciate the ingroup, identify with it, and be generally biased in its favor. It should also therefore be the case that where one's desire for epistemic certainty is heightened, appreciation of one's ingroup should rise. In what follows, we review three such intergroup phenomena to which the "seizing" and "freezing" tendencies seem highly relevant: (1) ingroup bias, (2) ingroup homogeneity effects, and (3) linguistic intergroup bias.

### NFC and the Ingroup Bias

Our conceptual analysis suggests that a heightened NFC should augment the ingroup bias by increasing the subjective value of the social reality provided by the ingroup. Shah and colleagues (1998) investigated this possibility in a study where participants were led to believe that, together with a teammate, they would be competing against a rival team of two participants on a reading comprehension task. Participants received two alleged self-descriptions, one written by their own teammate and the other by a member of the competing team. Participants whose NFC was elevated by time pressure expressed greater liking toward their teammate and lesser liking toward the member of the other team than did participants not exposed to pressure. The former (vs. the latter) participants also perceived themselves as more similar to the ingroup member and less similar to the outgroup member. These findings were strongly replicated in a third study, where the NFC was assessed via the Webster and Kruglanski (1994) NFCS rather than being manipulated via the time pressure.

### Homogeneity of Ingroups and Outgroups

If enhanced ingroup bias under a heightened NFC has to do with the ingroup's provision of a "social reality" to its members, the degree of a group's perceived homogeneity should affect its appeal to high-NFC members. A diverse group membership is likely to disagree on various matters. By contrast, a homogeneous group (one composed of largely similar members) may agree on the same basic premises. Accordingly, it may quickly reach consensus on various attitudes and opinions. Where epistemic confidence is at a premium, as under a high NFC, people should find particularly appealing groups whose membership is homogeneous rather than diverse.

There is, however, one boundary condition for these effects. If the greater appeal to high-NFC persons of homogeneous versus heterogeneous groups is due to the homogeneous groups' potential for provision of a stable social reality, then it should profoundly matter whether a group's membership is similar to or dissimilar from oneself. Only a self-similar group would constitute an adequate source of social reality; hence only a self-similar group would gain advantage from its homogeneity as a "reality provider." A self-dissimilar group, on the other hand, might be expected to differ from oneself on important attitudes and opinions. This may fundamentally undermine its "reality provision" potential, leaving little room for additional effects due to its perceived homogeneity.

To test this prediction, Kruglanski, Shah, Pierro, and Mannetti (2002) provided University of Maryland students with two responses to an alleged survey question (about their perception of average U.S. students' attitudes). These responses were said to be provided either by two University of Maryland students (the ingroup) or by two George Washington University students (a local outgroup), who either agreed among themselves (signifying homogeneity of perceptions) or disagreed (signifying heterogeneity). Participants then rated how much they thought they would like these particular George Washington University students, and how much they would like these particular University of Maryland students. They also rated the degree to which the two University of Maryland (or George Washington University) students were similar to each other, and how similar they were to the participant.

The results showed that the higher members' NFC was, the greater was their liking of the homogeneous versus the heterogeneous ingroup, and the lesser was their dislike for the homogeneous versus the heterogeneous outgroup. Of greatest interest, the preference of high-NFC (vs. low-NFC) individuals for the homogeneous (vs. heterogeneous) ingroup held only when the ingroup was perceived as relatively similar to oneself.

These findings support our analysis regarding the epistemic function of the ingroup as a provider of a social reality for its members. High-NFC (vs. low-NFC) individuals are more attracted to groups that fulfill their epistemic function satisfactorily—that is, to groups whose members' characteristics or opinions are sufficiently homogeneous to afford a coherent sense of "social reality"—as long as this reality is similar enough to their own attitudes and beliefs to be of use.

### Linguistic Intergroup Bias

Research referred to earlier (Boudreau et al., 1992; Mikulincer et al., 1991; Rubini & Kruglanski, 1997) has shown that under a heightened NFC, individuals are likely to exhibit an *abstractness bias*—that is, to be drawn to general labels or trait terms in thinking or talking about others. Such allure of the abstract is compatible with the permanence tendency assumed to arise under a heightened NFC, and to reflect the quest for stable knowledge consistent across situations. But as we also know (cf. De Grada et al., 1999; Kruglanski et al., 1993; Webster & Kruglanski, 1998), persons under a heightened NFC are also likely to exhibit a *consensus bias*—that is, to be attracted to consensual knowledge shared by significant others in their community.

An intriguing question is this: How might the abstractness and consensus biases (both born of the NFC!) interact? This question was addressed in research by Webster, Kruglanski, and Pattison (1997) on the relation between NFC and the *linguistic intergroup bias*. This bias is the tendency by group members to describe positive ingroup and negative outgroup behaviors in relatively abstract terms (implying that the behaviors in question represent relatively stable characteristics of the actor), and to describe negative ingroup and positive outgroup behaviors in relatively concrete terms (implying that the behaviors represent relatively transient, situationally specific occurrences that must not be expected to recur with any frequency) (Maass & Arcuri, 1992).

How might the linguistic intergroup bias be affected by the NFC? NFC-based abstraction and consensus tendencies should work in concert in regard to positive ingroup and negative outgroup behaviors. Both tendencies should contribute to enhanced abstraction level of linguistic descriptions under a high NFC. When it comes to *negative ingroup* and *positive outgroup* behaviors, however, the general abstraction tendency should be at odds with the preference for concrete descriptors implied by ingroup favoritism. Thus differences in descriptive abstractness due to the NFC should be reduced or eliminated in the case of these latter behaviors.

To test these ideas, Webster and colleagues (1997) conducted two separate experiments. In the first of these, participants previously classified as high or low in dispositional NFC (Webster & Kruglanski, 1994) took part in an experiment presented as an investigation of impression formation. The ingroup versus outgroup status of a target person was operationally defined in terms of his or her endorsement of the pro-choice versus the pro-life position on abortion. An ingroup status of the target was assumed to exist when the participant and the alleged target held the same position on abortion, and an outgroup status when their positions on abortion differed. The results of this experiment lent support to the hypothesis. Specifically, individuals with a high (vs. low) NFC (measured via the NFCS or manipulated via ambient noise) adopted a significantly higher level of abstraction when describing positive ingroup and negative outgroup behaviors. Such NFC differences were rendered nonsignificant for negative ingroup as well as for positive outgroup behaviors. These findings support the notion that the permanence tendency fostered by the NFC, even though it produces a general tendency toward abstractness, produces also a tendency toward ingroup favoritism that at times may conflict with the tendency toward abstractness. The latter may be the case where ingroup favoritism demands concrete rather than abstract depictions—that is, when one is describing negative behaviors of the ingroup members or positive ones of the outgroup members.

## CONCLUSIONS

In this chapter we have reviewed theory and research about the antecedents and consequences of the NFC (for a more complete discussion, see Kruglanski, 2004). The NFC is defined as a desire for a definite answer to a question, as opposed to uncertainty, confusion, or ambiguity. A growing body of research supports the notion that the desire to attain closure immediately and retain it permanently has an impact on a broad range of basic social psychological phenomena at the intrapersonal, interpersonal, group, and intergroup levels of analysis. These findings illustrate the fundamental psychological significance of the nexus between social and epistemic processes, and its implications for broad domains of human endeavors.

## ACKNOWLEDGMENTS

This work was supported by a National Science Foundation grant (No. 0314291/0313483) and by a Korea Research Foundation grant funded by the Korean Government (MOEHRD) (No. KRF-2006-332-H00019).

## REFERENCES

Bales, R. F. (1950). *Interaction process analysis: A method for the study of small groups*. Cambridge, MA: Addison-Wesley.

Baron, R. M., & Kenny, D. A. (1986). The moderator/mediator variable distinction in social psychological research: Conceptual, strategic, and statistical considerations. *Journal of Personality and Social Psychology, 51*, 1173–1182.

Boudreau, L. A., Baron, R., & Oliver, P. V. (1992). Effects of expected communication target expertise and timing of set on trait use in person description. *Personality and Social Psychology Bulletin, 18*, 447–452.

Chirumbolo, A., Livi, S., Mannetti, L., Pierro, A., & Kruglanski, A. W. (in press). Effects of need for closure on creativity in small group interactions. *European Journal of Personality.*

Chiu, C., Morris, M. W., Hong, Y., & Menon, T. (2000). Motivated cultural cognition: The impact of implicit cultural theories on dispositional attribution varies as a function of need for closure. *Journal of Personality and Social Psychology, 78*, 247–259.

Clark, H. H., & Murphy, G. L. (1982). Audience design in meaning and reference. In J. F. LeNy & W. Kintsch (Eds.), *Language and comprehension* (pp. 287–299). New York: North-Holland.

Cratylus. (1995). De Nederlandse Need for Closure Schaal [The Netherlands Need for Closure Scale]. *Nederlandse Tijdschrift voor de Psychologie, 50*, 231–232.

Davis, M. H. (1983). Measuring individual differences in empathy: Evidence for a multidimensional approach. *Journal of Personality and Social Psychology, 44*, 113–126.

De Grada, E., Kruglanski, A. W., Mannetti, L., & Pierro, A. (1999). Motivated cognition and group interaction: Need for closure affects the contents and processes of collective negotiations. *Journal of Experimental Social Psychology, 35*, 346–365.

De Grada, E., Kruglanski, A. W., Mannetti, L., Pierro, A., & Webster, D. M. (1996). Un'analisi stutturale comparative delle versioni USA e italiana della scala di "Bisogno di chiusura cognitive" di Webster and Kruglanski [A comparative structural analysis of the U.S. and Italian versions of the "Need for Cognitive Closure" Scale of Webster and Kruglanski]. *Testing, Psicometria, Metodologia, 3*, 5–18.

Dijksterhuis, A., Van Knippenberg, A., Kruglanski, A. W., & Schaper, C. (1996). Motivated social cognition: Need for closure effects on memory and judgment. *Journal of Experimental Social Psychology, 32*, 254–270.

Ellis, S., & Kruglanski, A. W. (1992). Self as epistemic authority: Effects on experiential and instructional learning. *Social Cognition, 10*, 357–375.

Erber, R., & Fiske, S. T. (1984). Outcome dependency and attention to inconsistent information. *Journal of Personality and Social Psychology, 47*, 709–726.

Festinger, L. (1950). Informal social communication. *Psychological Review, 57*, 271–282.

Fiedler, F. E. (1967). *A theory of leadership effectiveness*. New York: McGraw-Hill.

Ford, T. E., & Kruglanski, A. W. (1995). Effects of epistemic motivations on the use of accessible constructs in social judgment. *Personality and Social Psychology Bulletin, 21*, 950–962.

Fussell, S. R., & Krauss, R. N. (1989). The effects of intended audience design on message production and comprehension: Reference in a common ground framework. *Journal of Experimental Social Psychology, 25*, 203–219.

Higgins, E. T. (1987). Self-discrepancy: A theory relating self and affect. *Psychological Review, 94*, 319–340.

Higgins, E. T. (1996). Knowledge activation: Accessibility, applicability and salience. In E. T. Higgins & A. W. Kruglanski (Eds.), *Social psychology: A handbook of basic principles* (pp. 133–168). New York: Guilford Press.

Higgins, E. T., Rholes, W. S., & Jones, C. R. (1977). Category accessibility and impression formation. *Journal of Experimental Social Psychology, 13*, 141–154.

Hofstede, G. (1980). *Culture's consequences*. Beverly Hills, CA: Sage.

Hogg, M. A., & Abrams, D. (1993). Towards a single-process uncertainty reduction model of social motivation in groups. In M. A. Hogg & D. Abrams (Eds.), *Group motivation: Social psychological perspectives* (pp. 33–59). London: Harvester Wheatsheaf.

Horton, W. S., & Keysar, B. (1996). When do speakers take into account common ground? *Cognition, 59*, 91–17.

Jacobs, R. C., & Campbell, D. T. (1961). The perpetuation of an arbitrary tradition through several generations of a laboratory microculture. *Journal of Abnormal and Social Psychology, 62*, 649–658.

Jamieson, D. W., & Zanna, M. P. (1989). Need for structure in attitude formation and expression. In A. R. Pratkanis, S. J. Breckler, & A. G. Greenwald (Eds.), *Attitude structure and function* (pp. 383–406). Hillsdale, NJ: Erlbaum.

Jones, E. E. (1979). The rocky road from act to disposition. *American Psychologist, 34*, 107–117.

Jones, E. E., & Harris, V. A. (1967). The attribution of attitudes. *Journal of Experimental Social Psychology, 3*, 1–24.

Jost, J. T. , Glaser, J., Kruglanski, A. W., & Sulloway, F. J. (2003a). Exceptions that prove the rule: Using a theory of motivated social cognition to account for ideological incongruities and political anomalies: A reply to Greenberg and Jonas (2003). *Psychological Bulletin, 129*, 383–393.

Jost, J. T., Glaser, J., Kruglanski, A. W., & Sulloway, F. J. (2003b). Political conservatism as motivated social cognition. *Psychological Bulletin, 129*, 339–375.

Kossowska, M., Hiel, A. V., Chun, W. Y., & Kruglanski, A. W. (2002). The need for closure scale: Structure, cross-cultural invariance, and comparison of mean ratings between European-American and East Asian samples. *Psychologica Belgica, 42*, 267–286.

Krauss, R. M., & Fussell, S. R. (1991). Perspective taking in communication: Representations of others' knowledge in reference. *Social Cognition, 9*, 2–24.

Kroon, M. B. R., van Kreveld, D., & Rabbie, J. M. (1992). Groups versus individual decision making. *Small Group Research, 23*, 427–458.

Kruglanski, A. W. (1989). *Lay epistemics and human knowledge: Cognitive and motivational bases*. New York: Plenum Press.

Kruglanski, A. W. (2004). *The psychology of closed mindedness*. New York: Psychology Press.

Kruglanski, A. W., & Freund, T. (1983). The freezing and unfreezing of lay inferences: Effects on impressional primacy, ethnic stereotyping and numerical anchoring. *Journal of Experimental Social Psychology, 19*, 448–468.

Kruglanski, A. W., Raviv, A., Bar-Tal, D., Raviv, A., Ellis, S., Bar, R., et al. (2005). Says who?: Epistemic authority effects in social judgment. In M. P. Zanna (Ed.), *Advances in experimental social psychology* (Vol. 36, pp. 346–392). San Diego, CA: Academic Press.

Kruglanski, A. W., Shah, J. Y., Pierro, A., & Mannetti, L. (2002). When similarity brings content: Need for closure and the allure of homogeneous and self-resembling groups. *Journal of Personality and Social Psychology, 83*, 648–662.

Kruglanski, A. W., & Webster, D. M. (1991). Group members' reactions to opinion deviates and conformists at varying degrees of proximity to decision deadline and of environmental noise. *Journal of Personality and Social Psychology, 61*, 212–225.

Kruglanski, A. W., & Webster, D. M. (1996). Motivated closing of the mind: "Seizing" and "freezing." *Psychological Review, 103*(2), 263–283.

Kruglanski, A. W., Webster, D. M., & Klem, A. (1993). Motivated resistance and openness to persuasion in the presence or absence of prior information. *Journal of Personality and Social Psychology, 65*, 861–876.

Livi, S. (2002). *Il bisogna di chiuscora cognitiva e la transmissione delle norme nei piccoli gruppi* [*The *need for cognitive closure and norm-transmission in small groups*]. Unpublished doctoral dissertation, University of Rome "La Sapienza."

Maass, A., & Arcuri, L. (1992). The role of language in the persistence of stereotypes. In G. Semin & K. Fiedler (Eds.), *Language, interaction and social cognition* (pp. 129–143). Newbury Park, CA: Sage.

Mayseless, O., & Kruglanski, A. W. (1987). What makes you so sure?: Effects of epistemic motivations on judgmental confidence. *Organizational Behavior and Human Decision Processes, 39*, 162–183.

Mikulincer, M., Yinon, A., & Kabili, D. (1991). Epistemic needs and learned helplessness. *European Journal of Personality, 5*, 249–258.

Pierro, A., Mannetti, L., Converso, D., Garsia, V., Miglietta, A., Ravenna, M., et al. (1995). Caratteristiche strutturali della versione italiana della scale di bisogno di chiusura cognitiva (di Webster and Kruglanski) [Structural characteristics of the Italian version of the Need for Cognitive Closure Scale (of Webster and Kruglanski)]. *Testing, Psicometria, Metodologia, 2*, 125–141.

Pierro, A., Mannetti, L., De Grada, E., Livi, S., & Kruglanski, A. W. (2003). Autocracy bias in informal groups under need for closure. *Personality and Social Psychology Bulletin, 29*, 405–417.

Powell, R. S., & O'Neal, E. C. (1976). Communication feedback and duration as determinants of accuracy, confidence, and differentiation in interpersonal perception. *Journal of Personality and Social Psychology, 34*, 746–756.

Richter, L., & Kruglanski, A. W. (1999). Motivated search for common ground: Need for closure effects on audience design in interpersonal communication. *Personality and Social Psychology Bulletin, 25*(9), 1101–1114.

Ross, L. (1977). The intuitive psychologist and his shortcomings: Distortions in the attribution process. In L. Berkowitz (Ed.), *Advances in experimental social psychology* (Vol. 13, pp. 279–301). New York: Academic Press.

Rubini, M., & Kruglanski, A. W. (1997). Brief encounters ending in estrangement: Motivated language use and interpersonal rapport in the question–answer paradigm. *Journal of Personality and Social Psychology, 72*, 1047–1060.

Semin, G. R., Rubini, M., & Fiedler, K. (1995). The answer is in the question: The effect of verb causality on locus of explanation. *Personality and Social Psychology Bulletin, 21*, 834–841.

Shah, J. Y., Kruglanski, A. W., & Thompson, E. P. (1998). Membership has its (epistemic) rewards: Need for closure effects on ingroup bias. *Journal of Personality and Social Psychology, 75*, 383–393.

Stasser, G., & Stewart, D. (1992). Discovery of hidden profiles by decision-making groups: Solving a problem versus making a judgment. *Journal of Personality and Social Psychology, 63*(2), 426–434.

Stasser, G., & Titus, W. (1985). Pooling of unshared information in group decision making: Biased information sampling during discussion. *Journal of Personality and Social Psychology, 48*(6), 1467–1478.

Stasser, G., & Titus, W. (1987). Effects of information load and percentage of shared information on the dissemination of unshared information during group discussion. *Journal of Personality and Social Psychology, 53*(1), 83–93.

Thompson, E. P., Roman, R. J., Moskowitz, G. B., & Chaiken, S. (1994). Accuracy motivation attenuates covert priming: The systematic reprocessing of social information. *Journal of Personality and Social Psychology, 66*, 447–489.

Tversky, A., & Kahneman, D. (1974). Judgment under uncertainty: Heuristics and biases. *Science, 185*, 1124–1131.

Webster, D. M. (1993a). *Groups under the influence: Need for closure effects on information sharing in decision making groups*. Unpublished doctoral dissertation, University of Maryland.

Webster, D. M. (1993b). Motivated augmentation and reduction of the overattribution bias. *Journal of Personality and Social Psychology, 65*(2), 261–271.

Webster, D. M., & Kruglanski, A. W. (1994). Individual differences in need for cognitive closure. *Journal of Personality and Social Psychology, 67*, 1049–1062.

Webster, D. M., & Kruglanski, A. W. (1998). Cognitive and social consequences of the motivation for closure. *European Review of Social Psychology, 8*, 133–173.

Webster, D. M., Kruglanski, A. W., & Pattison, D. A. (1997). Motivated language use in intergroup contexts: Need for closure effects on the linguistic intergroup bias. *Journal of Personality and Social Psychology, 72*, 1122–1131.

Webster, D. M., Richter, L., & Kruglanski, A. W. (1996). On leaping to conclusions when feeling tired: Mental fatigue effects on impressional primacy. *Journal of Experimental Social Psychology, 32*, 181–195.

Webster-Nelson, D., Klein, C. F., & Irvin, J. E. (2003). Motivational antecedents of empathy: Inhibiting effects of fatigue. *Basic and Applied Social Psychology, 25*, 37–50.

Chapter 7

# Historical Perspectives and New Directions in Achievement Goal Theory

## UNDERSTANDING THE EFFECTS OF MASTERY AND PERFORMANCE–APPROACH GOALS

**Corwin Senko**
**Amanda M. Durik**
**Judith M. Harackiewicz**

Why do some students expend enormous effort on a class project, while others coast or even withdraw effort? Why do some people respond to early career setbacks with dogged persistence, while others respond with helplessness? Why do some people enjoy challenge, while others shy away from it? These are the sorts of questions that have long interested achievement motivation theorists (Atkinson, 1964; Eccles et al., 1983; McClelland, 1961; Weiner, 1972). In the past 20 years, *achievement goal theory* has been one of the most prominent theories of achievement motivation, having received extensive research attention in the education field in particular (e.g., Ames, 1992; Dweck & Leggett, 1988; Nicholls, 1984). In this chapter we review this research, highlighting a provocative pattern of findings that has emerged in the past several years, and then suggest several new directions for research. But first we review the core features of achievement goal theory.

### ACHIEVEMENT GOAL THEORY

Achievement goal theorists focus mainly on two goals: *performance goals* and *mastery goals*. Both goals concern the pursuit of competence and the assessment of one's own skill level, but they do so in different ways. When pursuing performance goals, people try to validate their ability by outperforming peers, and so they define success versus failure with normative standards. When pursuing mastery goals, they instead try to develop their ability, and so they define success versus failure with self-referential standards. Because these two goals represent different ways of defining competence, theorists have posited that they should promote distinct thoughts, feelings, and behaviors in achievement situations (e.g., Ames, 1992; Dweck & Leggett, 1988; Nicholls, 1984).

Classic achievement goal theorists argued that performance goals should produce outcomes similar to or worse than mastery goals, *but never better* (Dweck & Leggett, 1988; Nicholls, 1984). For example, Dweck and Leggett (1988) theorized that mastery goals and performance goals both produce adaptive behaviors for people high in perceived competence. But for people low in perceived competence, especially when they are faced with a stiff challenge or have encountered an initial failure, performance goals should be less adaptive than mastery goals. This is because people with a performance goal tend to believe that ability is a fairly stable attribute. As such, they are apt to consider mistakes as indicators of low ability and, therefore, to assume that they cannot easily overcome setbacks. By contrast, people with a mastery goal tend to believe that ability is a fairly malleable attribute. As such, they are more apt to consider mistakes a normal part of the learning process and, therefore, to assume that they can overcome setbacks with additional effort or a new strategy. In sum, the standard postulate of achievement goal theory, which we refer to as the *mastery goal hypothesis*, has been that mastery goals are optimal for motivation and performance, and many theorists have therefore argued that mastery goals should be promoted over performance goals in the classroom (e.g., Ames, 1992; Maehr & Midgley, 1991).

A large body of research has been conducted to test this mastery goal hypothesis. Much of it compares the effects of mastery and performance goals on achievement in the class (e.g., grades) and interest in the course material, as well as several other processes that may facilitate or hinder these two important educational outcomes, such as anxiety, learning strategies, and help-seeking behaviors (for reviews, see Ames, 1992; Harackiewicz, Barron, & Elliot, 1998; Rawsthorne & Elliot, 1999; Urdan, 1997). Below, we first provide an overview of the typical methodology used in this field and then review the research findings, some of which are unexpected and do not support the mastery goal hypothesis. We then provide and evaluate several potential explanations for these unexpected findings. Throughout the chapter, we focus our attention on the research conducted in educational domains, though we assume that these findings may generalize to other domains, such as athletic and work settings (Duda & Nicholls, 1992; Van Yperen & Janssen, 2002).

## An Overview of Achievement Goal Research Methods

Although some achievement goal research is conducted in controlled laboratory experiments in which goals are randomly assigned to participants (e.g., Elliott & Dweck, 1988; Harackiewicz & Elliot, 1993; Van Yperen, 2003), the majority of this research, especially that done in the education domain, has been conducted in field settings with the use of correlational methods. In these field studies, students' self-reported pursuit of mastery and performance goals for a course are correlated with various measures of their educational experiences, such as the type of study strategies they employ, the effort they put into the course, feelings of self-efficacy, interest in the course material, and grades in the class.

These studies typically show that mastery and performance goals are uncorrelated, indicating that the two are independent instead of opposing (e.g., Ames & Archer, 1988; Miller, Behrens, & Greene, 1993; Nicholls, Cheung, Lauer, & Patashnick, 1989). That is, in a given achievement situation, individuals may adopt both goals, one goal but not the other, or neither achievement goal. It is important, then, to assess the different ways in which pursuing both a mastery goal and a performance goal may affect achievement outcomes: The two goals may produce independent effects on separate outcomes (e.g., grades and interest); the goals may produce an additive effect on the same outcome, such that pursuing both is better than pursuing only one goal; or the goals may interact, such that a particular combination (e.g., strong pursuit of one goal, weak pursuit of the other) is most likely to produce a given outcome (Barron & Harackiewicz, 2001). In short, the effects of adopting both mastery and performance may take several forms. With this in mind, let us turn to the research findings.

## A Review of Achievement Goal Findings

In both the experimental and correlational studies, mastery goals have been linked to a variety of educationally adaptive outcomes. One such outcome that is especially valued in educational settings is interest in the material (Harackiewicz, Barron, Tauer, & Elliot, 2002; Heyman & Dweck, 1992). Interest is an emotional reaction that individuals experience when they work with material from a particular content area. The experience is characterized by heightened attention, involvement, and personal valuation of the material (Hidi & Harackiewicz, 2000; Renninger, 1990; Schiefele, 1991). Interested students are not passive recipients of material, but rather active agents in their own pursuit of knowledge. For instance, when interest in a domain is deep and enduring, individuals generate their own questions about material that piques their curiosity and seek answers to these questions (Renninger, 1990, 2000). As such, interest can prompt a host of strategies geared toward acquiring knowledge (Hidi, 1990; Renninger, Hidi, & Krapp, 1992; Schiefele, 1991).

Not surprisingly, these strategies have also been linked to students' adoption of mastery goals. For example, compared to those who do not value task mastery, students who pursue mastery goals are more apt to use "deep" learning strategies, such as elaborating the material, connecting it to other concepts, making it self-relevant, and questioning its veracity (Elliot, McGregor, & Gable, 1999; Harackiewicz, Barron, Tauer, Carter, & Elliot, 2000; Nolen, 1996; Wolters, 2004). They tend to be more effective self-regulators, able to successfully monitor their own understanding of the course material (Pintrich, 2000; Pintrich & Garcia, 1991; Wolters, Yu, & Pintrich, 1996). They also tend to persist longer and seek help when confused (Ryan & Pintrich, 1997; Wolters, 2004). In fact, few studies show any negative effects of mastery goals whatsoever. Yet, despite all these positives, mastery goals are seldom linked to what is arguably the *most* important educational outcome: actual achievement (e.g., exam scores or overall course grades). That is, students who vigorously pursue a mastery goal do not typically perform better in the class than students who shun the mastery goal (for a review, see Harackiewicz, Barron, Pintrich, Elliot, & Thrash, 2002; for recent exceptions, see Dweck & Grant, Chapter 26, this volume). Later in this chapter, we review and evaluate several possible explanations for this surprising disconnect between mastery goals and course grades.

The findings for performance goals have been much less consistent than the mastery goal findings. Performance goals *sometimes* have been linked to negative educational experiences. For example, some studies indicate that, relative to students who shun performance goals, those students who pursue performance goals are more apt to rely solely on "surface" learning strategies, such as rote memorization of terms and facts while studying (Elliot et al., 1999; Harackiewicz et al., 2000; Meece & Holt, 1993). They are also sometimes more likely to experience anxiety (Elliot & McGregor, 1999); to cheat (Anderman, Griesinger, & Westerfield, 1998); to avoid seeking help when confused (Ryan & Pintrich, 1997); and to intentionally engage in self-handicapping behaviors, such as procrastinating or staying out late the night before an exam, in order to protect themselves from low ability attributions just in case they do poorly on an upcoming exam (Midgley & Urdan, 2001; Urdan & Midgley, 2001). However, many other studies show no link of performance goals with many of these behaviors (e.g., Ames & Archer, 1988; Nolen, 1988), and some others even show a positive link with deep learning strategies, effort, and task achievement (e.g., Bouffard, Vezeau, & Bordeleau, 1998; Harackiewicz et al., 2000; Pintrich & Garcia, 1991; Skaalvik, 1997).

To help clarify these discrepant findings, Elliot (1999) has distinguished between *approach* and *avoidance* forms of performance goals. *Performance–approach* goals focus on the desire to outperform others and the feelings of pride that accompany that success; *performance–avoidance* goals focus more on the desire to avoid doing worse than others and the feelings of shame that accompany such failure. Elliot and colleagues (Elliot & Church, 1997; Elliot & Harackiewicz, 1996; Elliot & McGregor, 2001; Elliot et al., 1999), and other researchers (e.g., Skaalvik, 1997; Wolters, 2004), have shown that performance–avoidance goals produce many of the negative qualities previously tied to performance goals. For example, students who fear doing worse than others tend to have low self-efficacy, experience high anxiety, possess weak self-regulatory skills, engage in self-handicapping, have low task interest, and earn low course grades. Performance–approach goals, by comparison, tend not to produce these negative experiences, with the exception that students pursuing these goals tend to experience anxiety to a small degree (Elliot & McGregor, 1999). Moreover, performance–approach goals also reliably predict *high* achievement in the classroom (for a review, see Harackiewicz, Barron,

Pintrich, et al., 2002). Thus, it appears that the distinction between approach and avoidance can help explain many of the confusing findings previously tied to a singular omnibus performance goal. This distinction has helped clarify findings immensely, and it is now typical practice in research to measure both approach and avoidance tendencies to test their independent effects.[1]

In sum, mastery goals and performance goals, when framed in an approach manner, promote distinct educational benefits. Operating independently, each goal predicts different outcomes: Mastery goals generally predict interest but not actual achievement in a class or activity, whereas performance–approach goals generally predict high achievement but not interest (Harackiewicz, Barron, Pintrich, et al., 2002). This basic pattern of findings has been shown repeatedly with both middle school students (Wolters et al., 1996) and college students (e.g., Harackiewicz, Barron, Tauer, et al., 2002). Of course, mastery goals may sometimes exert *indirect* effects on achievement by way of promoting other processes, such as deep processing or interest, that do predict grades, but those indirect effects are generally weaker and less consistent than the direct effects of performance–approach goals on grades.

These distinct goal benefits are not easily explained by traditional achievement goal theory, which, readers will recall, postulates that performance goals should produce outcomes similar to or worse than those of mastery goals (Dweck & Leggett, 1988; Nicholls, 1984). Thus, the link of performance–approach goals, but not mastery goals, to high grades has been particularly difficult for goal theorists to reconcile.

One possibility raised by some theorists is that these findings are illusory effects caused by underlying confounds (e.g., Brophy, 2005; Van Yperen, 2003). In particular, because much of the achievement goal research within the education field is correlational in nature, it has been argued that the link between students' self-reported performance–approach goals and actual grades, plus the link between self-reported mastery goals and interest, may actually be caused by confounding variables. For example, perhaps the more talented students get better grades in all their classes, and, incidentally, are the ones most willing to pursue a goal that focuses on outperforming peers. Similarly, perhaps the more intellectually curious students are apt to find school interesting and to value learning and mastery. In both cases, the links between goals and outcomes may merely reflect underlying individual differences in academic ability or personality.

However, it is important to note that several field studies have found the basic effects even when controlling statistically for baseline interest (e.g., Harackiewicz, Durik, Barron, Linnenbrink, & Tauer, in press; Senko & Harackiewicz, 2005b) or indicators of students' ability, such as standardized test scores or previous grades (e.g., Elliot et al., 1999; Harackiewicz, Barron, Tauer, et al., 2002). Thus, it is unlikely that third-variable explanations can account fully for the findings observed to date. Moreover, we have recently replicated these basic findings in a pair of experiments, described in full later in this chapter, in which participants were *randomly assigned* to pursue a mastery goal or a performance goal. The performance goal *caused* greater achievement, but lower interest, than the mastery goal (Senko & Harackiewicz, 2005a).

This is not to say that the outcomes may not also influence subsequent goal pursuit. The link between goals and outcomes may in fact work reciprocally. For example, successful achievement, especially within a classroom context that emphasizes normative evaluation, may further reinforce students' pursuit of a performance–approach goal. Likewise, students who work hard to learn the material and eventually find it interesting would then have their mastery goal pursuit reinforced (Harackiewicz et al., in press). Nevertheless, the important point is that goals do seem capable of *causing* effects on interest, achievement, and other key educational measures. Given that these goal effects have been documented, what else can explain them? In the next two sections, we review and evaluate several possible explanations for why performance goals, but not mastery goals, reliably predict achievement in the classroom. We begin with mastery goals.

## WHY DON'T MASTERY GOALS PREDICT ACHIEVEMENT?

### The Achievement Measure Explanation

As noted previously, much of achievement goal research is conducted in classroom field settings. For practical reasons, these are often large introductory-level courses in which grades are based on multiple-choice exams that assess students' broad understanding of the course content. It is conceivable that these multiple-choice exams typically test surface learning more than deep learning; moreover, deep learning strategies may even be harmful in classes that use these exams (Scouller, 1998). Therefore, performance–approach goals, which are often associated with surface learning strategies, may be better suited for success in these contexts than are mastery goals, which instead are often associated with deep learning strategies. In fact, several theorists regard the link of performance–approach goals to grades as de facto evidence that the classes must be assessing only surface learning (e.g., Midgley, Kaplan, & Middleton, 2001). They propose that mastery goals may become a stronger predictor of grades if teachers' evaluation procedures require evidence of deep learning, and that the effect of performance goals on achievement may even disappear in such classes. In other words, the failure to find mastery goal effects on achievement may trace to how achievement is defined, rather than to some "flaw" inherent in mastery goals.

This achievement measure explanation is intuitively appealing. Yet it has seldom been tested directly, and there is only minimal support for it thus far. For example, Elliot and McGregor (1999) found that performance–approach goals, but not mastery goals, predicted grades on multiple-choice exams *and* essay exams. Barron and Harackiewicz (2003) also tested the achievement measure explanation by assessing the relationships of goals with grades in senior-level seminars at a large university. Grades in these courses were based on the strength of papers and class participation—qualities that presumably necessitate "deeper" learning than found in typical introductory-level courses. Yet, as in the introductory-level courses, performance–approach goals again predicted grades but not interest, and mastery goals again predicted course interest but not grades. In contrast to the prior two studies, Church, Elliot, and Gable (2001) found that mastery goals and performance–approach goals *both* predicted grades in an unusual college chemistry course designed to increase student retention in the chemistry major. It is unknown whether the class emphasized deep learning, though we assume it did to some degree, because it relied on small-group discussion and used absolute instead of normative grading criteria.

In sum, the small amount of research done thus far provides only mixed support for the achievement measure explanation, and performance–approach goals appear to be more reliable than mastery goals at predicting grades in classes that appear to emphasize deep learning. Nevertheless, the hypothesis deserves further testing—for example, by directly comparing goal effects across classes or activities that vary in the degree to which evaluation procedures emphasize deep learning of the course material. Taking this idea further, it would be useful to test goal effects on exams that not only assess deep understanding, but also *require* students to elaborate beyond the available information covered in class or textbooks. The achievement measure explanation suggests that mastery goals would predict success on exams that involve generating new uses for and ideas about the material. Students who adopt mastery goals and find the material interesting may be especially capable of integrating the material in novel ways. Their curiosity may help them use the material in creative ways, rather than in ways that already have been covered in class by the instructor or in the textbook. In other words, mastery goals may predict performance on exams that require independent thinking, rather than just deep processing of content that has been fleshed out through direct instruction.

## The Tangential Studying Explanation

If we assume that mastery goals still fail to predict achievement even when the evaluation procedures require "deep learning," what else can explain the surprising disconnect between these goals and grades? One possibility is rooted in the high personal interest that mastery-oriented students often have in their course material. Recall that personal interest prompts students to generate curiosity questions and to pursue answers through further contact with the material (Renninger, 2000). We propose that this interest may, ironically, sometimes undermine performance in the class by allowing students to pursue their own learning agenda instead of the teacher's. That is, due to their heightened course interest, students may delve into a particular subset of the material at great depth, or even explore topics that are tangential to the course material, to the neglect of some less interesting material that the teacher deems important. Consequently, despite having engaged the material deeply, they may find themselves unprepared for some topics covered on an exam and therefore perform less than optimally.

As an example, consider a hypothetical student, Jessica, who finds her history class fascinating. While studying, she becomes so enthralled with a historical figure that she spends much of her study time comparing the person to famous modern politicians—not because she thinks those comparisons will be tested, but simply to satisfy her intellectual curiosity. Unfortunately, due to time constraints, she may have only skimmed over some of other course material that, though just as important for the purposes of the exam, was less interesting to her. She may therefore be underprepared for parts of the exam.

Senko and Miles (2007b) recently provided an initial test of this *tangential studying* hypothesis. They developed a measure of tangential studying that asked students whether they deliberately focus their study efforts on the more interesting material, even if it is tangential to the exam material (e.g., "If certain sections of material are more interesting, I spend most of my time reading those sections" and "I rarely get to the dry material because I spend so much time on the interesting material"). College students in an introductory psychology course completed measures of goal pursuit in the second week of class. Toward the end of the semester, they completed other measures concerning their interest in the course material and their study strategies (i.e., surface strategies, deep strategies), including the degree to which they engaged in tangential studying.

The results supported the hypothesis. First, they replicated the basic finding from previous studies: Mastery goals predicted course interest but not course grade, whereas performance–approach goals predicted course grade but not interest. More importantly, mastery goals also predicted greater tangential studying: Students who pursued mastery goals for the class were also more likely to report neglecting drier topics in favor of personally interesting ones while studying. This link between mastery goals and tangential studying was mediated by those students' interest in the course material, thus hinting at a potential negative consequence of interest in this context (cf. the *seductive details effect*; Harp & Mayer, 1998). Tangential studying in turn predicted lower course grades. Thus, although mastery goals did not directly predict exam performance, they did seem to *indirectly* undermine students' exam performance by virtue of facilitating high interest in the course topic, which in turn seemed to promote undisciplined study efforts. By contrast, the performance–approach goal was negatively related to tangential studying. Students who pursued performance–approach goals were disinclined to pursue their own learning agenda; nor, then, did they inadvertently hamper their own exam performance.

## Summary and Research Directions

We have submitted two possible explanations for why mastery goals do not reliably predict grades in the classroom. The first is that the achievement measures (i.e., exams), perhaps testing superficial learning in many cases, do not adequately match the learning strategies of mastery-oriented students. These measures may instead favor the learning strategies of performance-oriented students. The second explanation is that mastery-oriented students, due to their high interest in the course material, sometimes inadvertently sabotage their own achievement by selectively focusing on the material that most interests them (Senko & Miles, 2007b). Both ideas have received little research attention thus far. Additional studies are therefore needed to test whether, in accord with the achievement measure explanation, mastery goals more strongly predict achievement in classes that evaluate students' depth of learning than in those that test surface understanding. The tangential studying explanation, of course, suggests that mastery goals will continue to have no relationship with grades in classes that emphasize deep learning.

According to the tangential studying argument, mastery goals should instead directly aid achievement only when the students' and teacher's learning agendas are aligned. In such cases, mastery-oriented students' deep learning should pay dividends, because the material that interests them would also be important for the exam; they will not be engaging in tangential studying in these cases. Lacking this alignment, though, any potential benefit of deep learning is likely to be counteracted by the tangential studying detriment. This alignment may be more common in self-directed learning courses in which students help choose the topics of study (Rogers & Freiberg, 1994), or in vocational courses, which, perhaps more than most college courses, directly and clearly bear on students' career paths. In both types of classes, mastery-oriented students may be more apt to share their teacher's learning agenda and to perform well as a result.

## WHY DO PERFORMANCE–APPROACH GOALS PREDICT ACHIEVEMENT?

Tangential studying may help explain why mastery goals fail to predict grades, but it does not explain why mastery goals predict interest in the first place. Nor does it fully explain why performance–approach goals do successfully predict grades. For example, in the study by Senko and Miles (2007b), tangential studying provided a bridge between mastery goals and grades, but it was not strongly related to performance–approach goals. What does explain these relationships between performance–approach goals and grades, and between mastery goals and interest? In this section, we propose that they may be partially explained by differences in the perceived difficulty of the two goals.

Mastery and performance–approach goals rely on different standards for defining success. Success in meeting a performance goal is often defined with a normative, external standard: You succeed after surpassing most, if not all, peers. By contrast, success in meeting a mastery goal is defined with a self-referential and often subjective standard: You succeed when you feel that you have "learned" or "developed" a skill. Therefore, as noted by Dweck and Elliott (1983, p. 656), mastery goals "may be less tyrannical than performance goals in terms of whether and when they are attained." In other words, it may often be easier to attain a mastery goal, because its standard for performance is more easily negotiated than is a performance goal's standard.

We propose that not only is a mastery goal easier to attain, but it also *appears* easier to attain than a performance–approach goal. This difference in the perceived difficulty of mastery and performance–approach goals may activate a series of processes that help account for the unique benefits of these goals for task interest and actual achievement, respectively. We base this hypothesis largely on principles of *goal-setting theory* (Locke & Latham, 1990). Goal-setting theory postulates that people perform tasks better when pursuing specific, difficult goals (e.g., writing seven manuscript pages a day) instead of specific, easy goals (e.g., writing one paragraph a day) or vague goals (e.g., "doing my best"). This effect, demonstrated in numerous studies (see Locke & Latham, 1990), occurs in part because the high expectations conveyed by difficult goals generate greater pressure to excel and, as a result, spur greater effort. On the other hand, specific, difficult goals sometimes also *reduce* task interest, presumably because the performance pressure can be unpleasant and undermine confidence (Mossholder, 1980).

Although goal-setting theory concerns task-specific goals, the same general processes may also operate with more abstract achievement goals. Specifically, the performance–approach goal—the harder goal—may in some cases arouse greater performance pressure and effort, and this in many cases may augment performance. By contrast, the mastery goal—the easier goal—may minimize pressure, thereby facilitating feelings of progress and, as a result, cultivating interest in the activity.

We conducted two experiments to test this goal difficulty hypothesis (Senko & Harackiewicz, 2005a). In each, participants played two sets of Boggle—a popular word game in which players use adjacent letter cubes to form as many words as possible. In Study 1, they were randomly assigned to a goal condition after being shown several word-finding strategies. Those in the performance–approach goal condition were asked to try to do better on the game than our previous participants, whereas those in the mastery goal condition were asked to try to develop a greater mastery of several word-finding strategies that we introduced to them beforehand. Performance on the word game and task interest, measured at the session's end, were the primary outcome measures. Goal difficulty perceptions and other process measures were also collected during the session.

The results of Study 1 were consistent with our hypotheses. The performance–approach and mastery goals yielded unique benefits: Participants pursing a performance–approach goal performed better than those pursuing the mastery goal, yet participants pursuing the mastery goal found the activity more interesting than those pursuing the performance–approach goal. Moreover, participants pursuing a performance goal rated their goal as more difficult to attain than did those pursuing a mastery goal, and this in turn ignited greater feelings of pressure while doing the activity. Mediation analyses suggested that these processes helped explain the benefits of the mastery goal and the performance–approach goal for interest and achievement, respectively. These effects occurred despite participants being equally committed to the mastery and performance goals; thus, the effects do not reflect differences in goal investment, another variable that can exert strong effects on achievement outcomes (Pomerantz & Shim, Chapter 25, this volume).

Study 2 was nearly identical to Study 1, except that we also attempted to demonstrate the role of goal difficulty perceptions by *directly manipulating* the perceived difficulty of the mastery goal. Participants were assigned a performance–approach goal, a "standard" mastery goal, or an allegedly difficult mastery goal. In the third condition, participants were informed by written instructions that the mastery goal would probably be difficult to achieve simply because it would take a good deal of time to master the word-finding strategies they had just been taught. The effects of the performance–approach and the standard mastery goals were identical to those in Study 1. Moreover, as expected, participants pursuing the difficult mastery goal experienced the session just like those pursuing the performance–approach goal did. Not only did they report higher goal difficulty perceptions than those in the standard mastery goal condition, but they also experienced more pressure, performed better, and reported less task interest. In other words, goal difficulty, not goal type, mattered most.

These two goal difficulty experiments provide preliminary support for our hypothesis that mastery and performance–approach goals differ in how difficult they appear to achieve, and that this in turn may help explain why the two goals promote interest and achievement, respectively. It remains for further research to extend these findings from the laboratory back into the classroom setting. These experimental studies also have important implications for how we interpret the pattern of findings from field research in which students' goals are self-reported. As noted earlier, one possible explanation for the relations between mastery goals and interest, and between performance–approach goals and achievement, is that these correlations merely reflect underlying individual difference confounds such as students' ability level. Although several studies have found those correlations even when statistically controlling for baseline interest levels and ability levels, it is still impossible to fully eliminate such third-variable explanations in those studies. By showing the same unique goal benefits with an experimental methodology, however, these two studies further validate that mastery and performance goals can have different *causal* links to grades and interest.

Although we suspect that performance goals are generally viewed as more difficult than mastery goals, there of course are probably exceptions. Situational factors may influence the difficulty of either goal. For instance, perceptions of peers' apparent skill level may influence how difficult a performance goal appears. In fact, elite athletes often claim to perform their best when facing strong competition (akin to a challenging performance–approach goal), but well beneath their potential when facing weaker competition (akin to an easy performance–approach goal). Based on the logic of our goal difficulty hypothesis, competing against a talented opponent should elevate the perceived difficulty of winning and, as a result, should also potentially improve one's own performance. Senko and Miles (2007a) found empirical support for this hypothesis in a recent experiment. Participants practiced two games of Boggle and then were given feedback about how many words they found. Additionally, those in the "superior" condition were informed by the feedback that they had performed above average compared to prior participants; those in the "inferior" condition were informed that they had performed below average; and those in a baseline control group were not told anything about their normative ranking on the practice puzzles. All participants then considered a mastery goal or a performance–approach goal for an additional pair of puzzles, and reported how difficult they thought each would be to achieve. Two key findings emerged. First, participants in the "superior" group perceived the performance–approach goal to be easier than did those in the "inferior" group, thereby demonstrating that a performance goal's apparent difficulty can be affected by information about peers' ability levels. By contrast, the perceived difficulty of the mastery goal was unaffected by the normative midsession feedback. Second, and perhaps more important, participants in the baseline control group rated the difficulty of the performance–approach goal as high as did those in the "inferior" group, thus demonstrating that a performance–approach goal may typically seem rather difficult to achieve.

The perceived difficulty of the mastery goal is more likely to be affected by features of the activity itself. For example, a mastery goal may appear more difficult if the activity seems complex instead of simple to learn and master. This hypothesis was tested in a second experiment (Senko & Miles, 2007a). Participants learned a novel multiplication technique. Intended to help people solve multiplication problems more efficiently, the technique requires doing math operations in one's head rather than writing them out on paper (for more details, see Barron & Harackiewicz, 2001). Before the tutorial, participants in the "simple task" condition were led to believe that the technique is simple to learn and use; those in the "complex task" condition were led to believe that the technique is fairly complex; and those in the baseline control group were told nothing about the task's complexity. Then, in advance of learning the technique and using it on a problem set, they all reported how difficult they expected it would be to achieve a mastery goal or performance–approach goal. Two key findings emerged. First, participants perceived the mastery goal to be harder if told that the task was complex than if told that it was simple, thereby demonstrating that a mastery goal's perceived difficulty can be affected by characteristics of the activity. By contrast, the perceived difficulty of the performance–approach goal was unaffected by the task's description. Second, participants in the baseline condition rated the mastery goal as easy as did those in the "simple task" condition, thus demonstrating that the mastery goal may typically seem rather easy to attain in learning situations.

As a whole, these goal difficulty studies (Senko & Harackiewicz, 2005a; Senko & Miles, 2007a) indicate that performance–approach goals often appear harder than mastery goals, and that this may help account for the common finding that performance–approach goals, but not mastery goals, predict grades in the classroom. These studies also suggest that mastery goals may more strongly predict grades if the class material is exceptionally challenging, as this would make the mastery goal more difficult and, therefore, perhaps activate some of the same motivational processes more commonly activated by the performance–approach goal. Although there is no direct test of this possibility, two studies provide some intriguing support (Church et al., 2001; Grant & Dweck, 2003; see also Dweck & Grant, Chapter 26, this volume). In difficult chemistry courses, both studies found that students pursuing a mastery goal did in fact earn higher grades than those who shunned the mastery goal. Perhaps this was to some degree due to the mastery goal being unusually difficult in this course. Of course, this hypothesis awaits a more direct test in future research.

## Research Directions

There are several possible directions for research into the role played by goal difficulty perceptions. One direction is to study how the type of task may affect whether performance–approach goals benefit task performance. Social facilitation research and test anxiety research both suggest that high arousal facilitates performance on tasks that are well learned or relatively simple, but that it hampers performance on novel tasks that are highly complex or require creativity (e.g., Amabile, 1979; Zajonc, 1965). Insofar as performance–approach goals usually appear harder and arouse more pressure and effort, it may be that the benefits of performance goals for task achievement are restricted to tasks that are well learned or only moderately complex. With exceptionally complex tasks, the benefits of performance–approach goals may disappear or may be even reversed (e.g., Barron & Harackiewicz, 2001; Butler, 1988). Some early studies did test this, and a meta-analysis by Utman (1997) indeed found that performance goals hampered achievement on complex experimental activities. However, because the studies examined in that meta-analysis did not distinguish between performance–approach and performance–avoidance goals, it is difficult to know whether the negative effects on complex tasks were due to high levels of performance pressure or to an avoidance orientation. It would be useful for additional research to examine how goal difficulty perceptions may moderate the effects of mastery and performance–approach goals on simple versus complex (or creativity) tasks.

Research is also needed to further chart the motivational processes that might be triggered by goal difficulty. For example, it is conceivable that performance–approach goals, due to their enhanced difficulty, heighten students' vigilance toward cues in the classroom that may facilitate their goal attainment. We base this proposal largely on the logic of *construal theory* (Freitas, Salovey, & Liberman, 2001; Liberman & Trope, 1998; Trope & Lieberman, 2003). According to this theory, people take either low-level or high-level construals for their activities. People often adopt lower-level construals under duress, as when facing an impending deadline or doing a difficult task. In such circumstances, they focus on the finite details of an activity so that they can develop an effective plan for attaining their goal. When thinking more long term about a goal, however, they tend to adopt higher-level construals that focus on the abstract meaning of the goal and the utility of meeting it. In short, high-level construals focus on *why* a task is worth accomplishing, whereas low-level construals focus on *how* to accomplish it.

Inasmuch as performance–approach goals seem harder, it may be that they trigger lower-level construals for the class. This in turn may prompt students pursuing a performance–approach goal to become extra attentive to the teacher's demands and expectations, allowing them to identify the key course material to study. For example, teachers often remark that it is the performance-oriented students who inquire, "What exactly will be on the exam?" or "How important will this be for the exam?" The tangential studying findings provide tentative support for this, in that performance-oriented students were highly unlikely to engage in tangential studying, the strategy that appears to sabotage mastery-oriental students' achievement (Senko & Miles, 2007b). If students pursuing performance–approach goals are in fact especially attentive to evaluation cues, then perhaps they also excel at preparing *effectively* for exams. Contrast this with mastery goals. By being perceived as easier and therefore encouraging high-level construals for a class, mastery goals may facilitate the development of interest, but, for the same reason, they may also be less likely to promote vigilance toward meeting the demands of the course. In fact, this may help explain why mastery goals promote the type of tangential studying described earlier; high-level construals may focus students more on their own learning agendas than on the teacher's agenda.

If students pursuing performance–approach goals do in fact tend to be highly vigilant, then they may also be particularly adept at *changing* their study strategies to match their teachers' demands. That is, due to their vigilance, perhaps they are strategic in their study efforts, relying on surface learning strategies when sufficient but also quick to use deeper strategies when necessary. There is already tentative support for this hypothesis. Entwistle (1988) noted that many competitive students—who would be apt to pursue performance–approach goals (Harackiewicz, Barron, Carter, Lehto, & Elliot, 1997)—tend to use a "strategic approach" to studying, characterized by cue seeking, careful planning, and using any learning strategy that will produce the best grades.

This possibility is especially intriguing in light of an assumption tacitly endorsed by many achievement goal theorists. Because performance goals often predict shallow learning strategies more consistently and more strongly than they predict deep learning strategies, some theorists have suggested that the association of performance–approach goals with grades must mean that the exams in those courses tested only shallow learning (e.g., Midgley et al., 2001). If the exams instead more rigorously tested students' depth of understanding, so the argument goes, the link to grades would likely disappear. Consequently, rather than interpret the connection between performance–approach goals and grades as a benefit of performance goals, they suggest that this link reflects flawed educational practices. The underlying assumption of that perspective is that performance-oriented students would use only shallow learning strategies even in classes that do rigorously test students' depth of learning. In contrast, we propose that performance-oriented students, being sensitive to class demands and strategic in their approach to studying, would instead adopt deep learning strategies in those classes. Indeed, this would help explain why performance goals have predicted achievement in a variety of classes, ranging from introductory-level courses in which grades are based on "curved" multiple-choice exams that assess broad, surface understanding of the course material to seminar courses in which grades are based on deeper learning of the course material. Clearly, additional research is needed to test these competing perspectives directly.

Finally, we do not wish to imply that perceived goal difficulty alone can account for the full body of research findings concerning mastery and performance–approach goals. For example, goal difficulty perceptions are unlikely to account for why performance goals are more strongly linked than mastery goals to help avoidance. Other factors clearly help explain goal effects, too. For example, as noted earlier, whether a goal is framed in an approach or avoidance manner can determine whether the goal is adaptive or maladaptive (Elliot, 1999). So too can the degree of congruence between a student's goal and broader cultural factors, such as the classroom climate, the school environment, or broader societal mores (Ames, 1992; Harackiewicz et al., 1998; Maehr & Midgley, 1991; Urdan, 2004). In short, we view goal difficulty perceptions as a potential complement, not a substitute, to other factors that can help pinpoint when and why mastery and performance goals exert their distinct influences.

## CONCLUSION

Achievement goal theory has generated a body of research that, as a whole, has enhanced our understanding of the motivational benefits and drawbacks of pursuing different types of goals in the classroom. Much of the research has focused on identifying which goals predict which educational outcomes, such as school achievement or interest. Along the way, the traditional goal hypothesis favoring mastery goals has in many ways been vindicated, with the important exception that mastery goals have seldom been shown to predict actual achievement in the classroom. This disconnect between mastery goals and grades, and the reliable link between performance–approach goals and grades, together present a strong challenge to the traditional mastery goal hypothesis. Therefore, to maintain the viability of achievement goal theory, it is important now to focus research attention on the goal-relevant processes that can help explain these unexpected effects. We have attempted to do so in the current chapter. In a manner consistent with Elliot and Fryer's (Chapter 15, this volume) call for greater integration of achievement goal theory with other theories of motivation, we have drawn from goal-setting theory and construal theory to explore why mastery and performance–approach goals provide distinct educational benefits.

In particular, we have proposed that one reason why mastery goals predict interest but not grades, whereas performance–approach goals predict grades but not interest, is that the two goals differ in how difficult they appear to achieve. This in turn may activate a set of processes that accounts for these distinct goal effects. Mastery goals, by virtue of being easier, may encourage a higher level of construal that focuses students' attention on the broader utility of the course, thus facilitating the development of their interest in the material. However, in so doing, mastery goals may also encourage students to pursue their own learning agendas. This may sometimes hinder students' performance if their own agendas do not overlap well with the instructor's agenda. By contrast, we have speculated that performance–approach goals, by virtue of being harder and elevating performance pressure, encourage a lower-level construal that leads students to become highly attentive to the demands of the activity and to expend efficient effort to meet those demands. Inasmuch as they are able to ascertain the instructor's learning agenda for an exam, this approach may often facilitate their performance in the class.

Of course, this is largely conjecture. To our knowledge, there are not yet any tests of whether mastery and performance–approach goals encourage different levels of construal. Nor are there any tests of whether performance–approach goals heighten students' vigilance to the instructors' expectations. Nevertheless, we hope that these speculations will encourage research in these directions, or, at the very least, will prompt fellow achievement goal theorists to develop and test alternative explanations for effects that have thus far frustrated and confused many of us.

## NOTE

1. Theorists have recently begun to apply the approach–avoidance distinction to mastery goals (Elliot & McGregor, 2001; Linnenbrink & Pintrich, 2000). Mastery–approach goals focus on trying to learn and develop a skill, whereas mastery–avoidance goals focus on trying to avoid failing to learn (Linnenbrink & Pintrich, 2000) or trying to avoid declining in skill level (Elliot & McGregor, 2001). Because the prior research on mastery goals has clearly used an approach form of the goal, and because little research has been done on mastery–avoidance goals, we refer to the approach form of the goal whenever discussing mastery goals in this chapter.

## REFERENCES

Amabile, T. M. (1979). Effects of external evaluation on artistic creativity. *Journal of Personality and Social Psychology, 37*, 221–233.

Ames, C. (1992). Classrooms: Goals, structures, and student motivation. *Journal of Educational Psychology, 84*(3), 261–271.

Ames, C., & Archer, J. (1988). Achievement goals in the classroom: Students' learning strategies and motivation processes. *Journal of Educational Psychology, 80*, 260–267.

Anderman, E. M., Griesinger, T., & Westerfield, G. (1998). Motivation and cheating during early adolescence. *Journal of Educational Psychology, 90*, 84–93.

Atkinson, J. W. (1964). *An introduction to motivation.* Princeton, NJ: Van Nostrand.

Barron, K. E., & Harackiewicz, J. M. (2001). Achievement goals and optimal motivation: Testing multiple goal models. *Journal of Personality and Social Psychology, 80*, 706–722.

Barron, K. E., & Harackiewicz, J. M. (2003). Revisiting the benefits of performance–approach goals in the college classroom: Exploring the role of goals in advanced college courses. *International Journal of Educational Research, 39*, 357–374.

Bouffard, T., Vezeau, C., & Bordeleau, L. (1998). A developmental study of the relation between combined learning and performance goals and students' self-regulated learning. *British Journal of Educational Psychology, 68*, 321–330.

Brophy, J. (2005). Goal theorists should move on from performance goals. *Educational Psychologist, 40*, 167–176.

Butler, R. (1988). Enhancing and undermining intrinsic motivation: The effects of task-involving and ego-involving evaluation on interest and performance. *British Journal of Educational Psychology, 58*, 1–14.

Church, M. A., Elliot, A. J., & Gable, S. L. (2001). Perceptions of classroom environment, achievement goals, and achievement outcomes. *Journal of Educational Psychology, 93*, 43–45.

Duda, J. L., & Nicholls, J. G. (1992). Dimensions of achievement motivation in schoolwork and sport. *Journal of Educational Psychology, 84*, 290–299.

Dweck, C. S., & Elliott, E. S. (1983). Achievement motivation. In P. H. Mussen (Series Ed.) & E. M. Hetherington (Vol. Ed.), *Handbook of child psychology: Vol. 4. Social and personality development* (4th ed., pp. 643–691). New York: Wiley.

Dweck, C. S., & Leggett, E. L. (1988). A social-cognitive approach to motivation and personality. *Psychological Review, 95*, 256–273.

Eccles, J. S., Adler, T. F., Futterman, R., Goff, S. B., Kaczala, C. M., Meece, J., et al. (1983). Expectancies, values and academic behaviors. In J. T. Spence (Ed.), *Achievement and achievement motives* (pp. 75–146). San Francisco: Freeman.

Elliot, A. J. (1999). Approach and avoidance motivation and achievement goals. *Educational Psychologist, 34*, 169–189.

Elliot, A. J., & Church, M. A. (1997). A hierarchical model of approach and avoidance achievement motivation. *Journal of Personality and Social Psychology, 72*, 218–232.

Elliot, A. J., & Harackiewicz, J. M. (1996). Approach and avoidance achievement goals and intrinsic motivation: A mediational analysis. *Journal of Personality and Social Psychology, 70*, 461–475.

Elliot, A. J., & McGregor, H. A. (1999). Test anxiety and the hierarchical model of approach and avoidance achievement motivation. *Journal of Personality and Social Psychology, 76*, 628–644.

Elliot, A. J., & McGregor, H. A. (2001). A 2 × 2 achievement goal framework. *Journal of Personality and Social Psychology, 80*, 501–519.

Elliot, A. J., McGregor, H. A., & Gable, S. (1999). Achievement goals, study strategies, and exam performance: A mediational analysis. *Journal of Educational Psychology, 91*, 549 563.

Elliott, E. S., & Dweck, C. S. (1988). Goals: An approach to motivation and achievement. *Journal of Personality and Social Psychology, 54*, 5–12.

Entwistle, N. (1988). Motivational factors in students' approaches to learning. In R. Schmeck (Ed.), *Learning strategies and learning styles: Perspectives on individual differences* (pp. 21–51). New York: Plenum Press.

Freitas, A. L., Salovey, P., & Liberman, N. (2001). Abstract and concrete self-evaluative goals. *Journal of Personality and Social Psychology, 80*, 410–424.

Grant, H., & Dweck, C. S. (2003). Clarifying achievement goals and their impact. *Journal of Personality and Social Psychology, 85*, 541–553.

Harackiewicz, J. M., Barron, K. E., Carter, S. M., Lehto, A. T., & Elliot, A. J. (1997). Predictors and consequences of achievement goals in the college classroom: Maintaining interest and making the grade. *Journal of Personality and Social Psychology, 73*, 1284–1295.

Harackiewicz, J. M., Barron, K. E., & Elliot, A. J. (1998). Rethinking achievement goals: When are they adaptive for college students and why? *Educational Psychologist, 33*, 1–21.

Harackiewicz, J. M., Barron, K. E., Pintrich, P. R., Elliot, A. J., & Thrash, T. M. (2002). Revision of achievement goal theory: Necessary and illuminating. *Journal of Educational Psychology, 94*, 638–645.

Harackiewicz, J. M., Barron, K. E., Tauer, J. M., Carter, S. M., & Elliot, A. J. (2000). Short-term and long-term consequences of achievement goals: Predicting interest and performance over time. *Journal of Educational Psychology, 92*, 316–330.

Harackiewicz, J. M., Barron, K. E., Tauer, J. M., & Elliot, A. J. (2002). Predicting success in college: A longitudinal study of achievement goals and ability measures as predictors of interest and performance from freshman year through graduation. *Journal of Educational Psychology, 94*, 562–575.

Harackiewicz, J. M., Durik, A. M., Barron, K. E., Linnenbrink, E. A., & Tauer, J. M. (in press). The role of achievement goals in the development of interest: Reciprocal relations between achievement goals, interest and performance. *Journal of Educational Psychology.*

Harackiewicz, J. M., & Elliot, A. J. (1993). Achievement goals and intrinsic motivation. *Journal of Personality and Social Psychology, 65*, 904–915.

Harp, S. F., & Mayer, R. E. (1998). How seductive details do their damage: A theory of cognitive interest in science learning. *Journal of Educational Psychology, 90*, 414–434.

Heyman, G. D., & Dweck, C. S. (1992). Achievement goals and intrinsic motivation: Their relation and their role in adaptive motivation. *Motivation and Emotion, 16*, 231–247.

Hidi, S. (1990). Interest and its contribution as a mental resource for learning. *Review of Educational Research, 60*, 549–571.

Hidi, S., & Harackiewicz, J. M. (2000). Motivating the academically unmotivated: A critical issue for the 21st century. *Review of Educational Research, 70*, 151–179.

Liberman, N., & Trope, Y. (1998). The role of feasibility and desirability considerations in near and distant future decisions: A test of temporal construal theory. *Journal of Personality and Social Psychology, 75*, 5–18.

Linnenbrink, E. A., & Pintrich, P. R. (2000). Multiple pathways to learning and achievement: The role of goal orientation in fostering adaptive motivation, affect, and cognition. In C. Sansone & J. M. Harackiewicz (Eds.), *Intrinsic and extrinsic motivation: The search for optimal motivation and performance* (pp. 196–230). San Diego, CA: Academic Press.

Locke, E. A., & Latham, G. P. (1990). *A theory of goal setting and task performance.* Englewood Cliffs, NJ: Prentice Hall.

Maehr, M. L., & Midgley, C. (1991). Enhancing student motivation: A schoolwide approach. *Educational Psychologist, 26*, 399–427.

McClelland, D. C. (1961). *The achieving society.* Princeton, NJ: Van Nostrand.

Meece, J. L., & Holt, K. (1993). A pattern analysis of students' achievement goals. *Journal of Educational Psychology, 85*, 582–590.

Midgley, C., Kaplan, A., & Middleton, M. (2001). Performance–approach goals: Good for what, for whom, under what circumstances, and at what cost? *Journal of Educational Psychology, 93*, 77–86.

Midgley, C., & Urdan, T. C. (2001). Academic self-handicapping and achievement goals: A further examination. *Contemporary Educational Psychology, 26*, 61–75.

Miller, R. B., Behrens, J. T., & Greene, B. A. (1993). Goals and perceived ability: Impact on student valuing, self-regulation, and persistence. *Contemporary Educational Psychology, 18*, 2–14.

Mossholder, K. W. (1980). Effects of externally mediated goal setting on intrinsic motivation: A laboratory experiment. *Journal of Applied Psychology, 65*, 202–210.

Nicholls, J. G. (1984). Achievement motivation: Conceptions of ability, subjective experience, task choice, and performance. *Psychological Review, 91*, 328–346.

Nicholls, J. G., Cheung, P. C., Lauer, J., & Patashnick, M. (1989). Individual differences in academic motivation: Perceived ability, goals, beliefs, and values. *Learning and Individual Differences, 1*, 63–84.

Nolen, S. B. (1988). Reasons for studying: Motivation orientations and study strategies. *Cognition and Instruction, 5*, 269–287.

Nolen, S. B. (1996). Why study?: How reasons for learning influence strategy selection. *Educational Psychology Review, 8*, 335–355.

Pintrich, P. R. (2000). An achievement goal theory perspective on issues in motivation terminology, theory, and research. *Contemporary Educational Psychology, 25*, 92–104.

Pintrich, P. R., & Garcia, T. (1991). Student goal orientation and self-regulation in the college classroom. In M. L. Maehr & P. R. Pintrich (Eds.), *Advances in motivation and achievement* (Vol. 7, pp. 371–402). Greenwich, CT: JAI Press.

Rawsthorne, L. J., & Elliot, A. J. (1999). Achievement goals and intrinsic motivation: A meta-analytic review. *Personality and Social Psychology Review, 3*, 326–344.

Renninger, K. A. (1990). Children's play interests, representation, and activity. In R. Fivush & J. Hudson (Eds.), *Emory cognition series: Vol. 3. Knowing and remembering in young children* (pp. 127–165). Cambridge, UK: Cambridge University Press.

Renninger, K. A. (2000). Individual interest and its implications for understanding intrinsic motivation. In C. Sansone & J. M. Harackiewicz (Eds.), *Intrinsic and extrinsic motivation: The search for optimal motivation and performance* (pp. 375–404). San Diego, CA: Academic Press.

Renninger, K. A., Hidi, S., & Krapp, A. (1992). *The role of interest in learning and development.* Hillsdale, NJ: Erlbaum.

Rogers, C. R., & Freiberg, J. (1994). *Freedom to learn* (3rd ed.). New York: Merrill/Macmillan.

Ryan, A. M., & Pintrich, P. R. (1997). "Should I ask for help?": The role of motivation and attitudes in adolescents' help seeking in math class. *Journal of Educational Psychology, 89*, 329–341.

Schiefele, U. (1991). Interest, learning and motivation. *Educational Psychologist, 26*, 299–323.

Scouller, K. (1998). The influence of assessment method on students' learning approaches: Multiple choice question examination versus assignment essay. *Higher Education, 35*, 453–472.

Senko, C., & Harackiewicz, J. M. (2005a). Achievement goals, task performance, and interest: Why perceived goal difficulty matters. *Personality and Social Psychology Bulletin, 31*, 1739–1753.

Senko, C., & Harackiewicz, J. M. (2005b). Regulation of achievement goals: The role of competence feedback. *Journal of Educational Psychology, 97*, 320–336.

Senko, C., & Miles, K. M. (2007a). *How task complexity and peers' ability affect the pursuit of achievement goals*. Manuscript in preparation.

Senko, C., & Miles, K. M. (2007b). *Pursuing their own learning agenda: How mastery-oriented students jeopardize their class performance*. Manuscript submitted for publication.

Skaalvik, E. M. (1997). Self-enhancing and self-defeating ego orientation: Relations with task and avoidance orientation, achievement, self-perceptions, and anxiety. *Journal of Educational Psychology, 89*, 71–81.

Trope, Y., & Liberman, N. (2003). Temporal construal. *Psychological Review, 110*, 403–421.

Urdan, T. C. (1997). Achievement goal theory: Past results, future directions. In M. L. Maehr & P. R. Pintrich (Eds.), *Advances in motivation and achievement* (Vol. 10, pp. 99–141). Greenwich, CT: JAI Press.

Urdan, T. (2004). Predictors of academic self-handicapping and achievement: Examining achievement goals, classroom goal structures, and culture. *Journal of Educational Psychology, 96*, 251–264.

Urdan, T., & Midgley, C. (2001). Academic self-handicapping: What we know, what more there is to learn. *Educational Psychology Review, 13*, 115–137.

Utman, C. H. (1997). Performance effects of motivational state: A meta-analysis. *Personality and Social Psychology Review, 1*, 170–182.

Van Yperen, N. W. (2003). Task interest and actual performance: The moderating effects of assigned and adopted purpose goals. *Journal of Personality and Social Psychology, 85*, 1006–1015.

Van Yperen, N. W., & Janssen, O. (2002). Fatigued and dissatisfied or fatigued but dissatisfied? Goal orientations and responses to high job demands. *Academy of Management Journal, 45*, 1181–1171.

Wolters, C. A. (2004). Advancing achievement goal theory: Using goal structures and goal orientations to predict students' motivation, cognition, and achievement. *Journal of Educational Psychology, 96*, 236–250.

Wolters, C. A., Yu, S. L., & Pintrich, P. R. (1996). The relation between goal orientation and students' motivational beliefs and self-regulated learning. *Learning and Individual Differences, 8*, 211–238.

Weiner, B. (1972). *Theories of motivation*. Chicago: Markham.

Zajonc, R. B. (1965). Social facilitation. *Science, 149*, 269–274.

Chapter 8

# A Basic but Uniquely Human Motivation

## TERROR MANAGEMENT

**Jeff Greenberg**
**Sheldon Solomon**
**Jamie Arndt**

The fundamental question for motivation science is this: Why do people behave the way they do? Beginning with the assumption that an organism's behavior facilitates the satisfaction of needs and attainment of goals, motivation science explicates what those needs and goals are; why they exist; and how innate and acquired affective, cognitive, and behavioral propensities, in response to specific environmental factors, affect their fulfillment. Human motivation is multidimensional and multilayered; virtually any human action can serve numerous motives, which vary in terms of their degree of specificity and conscious awareness on the part of the actor. Accordingly, motivational theories and associated research programs range from broad conceptual analyses of human behavior (e.g., Freud's psychoanalytic theory) to concrete micro-level analyses of specific mechanisms that guide behavior (e.g., Hull's drive theory).

Freud saw human actions as typically serving distal unconscious motives very different from the proximal motives to which they are attributed. Research on cognitive dissonance, motivated reasoning, terror management, and goal priming (e.g., Arndt, Greenberg, Solomon, Pyszczynski, & Simon, 1997; Aronson & Carlsmith, 1963; Bargh & Chartrand, 1999; Brehm, 1956; James & Greenberg, 1989; Kunda, 1990; Nisbett & Wilson, 1977) demonstrates that human behavior is indeed often if not always guided by motives operating outside conscious awareness. But what are the most basic motives that direct and energize behavior?

Powers (1973, 1978) developed a hierarchical model of motivation based on levels of abstractness, which we believe best captures the multilayered nature of human motivation and provides insights into what the most basic human motives are. His cybernetic model (e.g., Powers, 1978) influenced Carver and Scheier's (1981) cybernetic theory of self-regulation, Pyszczynski and Greenberg's (1992) self-regulatory perseveration theory of depression, and Vallacher and Wegner's (1987) theory of action identification. The basic idea is that any action serves multiple goals, which range from very specific, concrete goals to very general, abstract ones.

Toward the abstract end, human motivation has to do with the broad purposes of life—the last "why" questions. Imagine a businessman doing something very simple, tying his shoes on a weekday morning. Imagine an interviewer asking him why he is moving his fingers that way. "So I can tie my shoes," he replies. Why is he tying his shoes? "So they will stay on my feet." Why does he need them on his feet? "So I can go to work." Why is he going to work? "So I can meet the expectations of my boss." Why does he want to meet the expectations of his boss? "So I can be successful in my career." Why does he want to be successful? "So I can provide good things for my family." Why does he want to do that? "So I can feel like I'm a good husband and father." Why does he want to feel that way? "So I can feel like a person of worth." But why does he want to feel like a person of worth? This last question is precisely the one that sparked the development of *terror management theory* (TMT).

## TERROR MANAGEMENT THEORY

Our motivational analysis begins with the Darwinian observation that as products of evolution, humans, like all other animals, are equipped with many biological systems designed to keep them alive. Some systems maintain a stable internal biochemical environment by homeostatic regulation of blood flow, respiration, nutrient intake, temperature, and so forth. Other systems are geared toward addressing external threats to survival. Essential in this regard, humans share with reptiles, birds, and other mammals an amygdala, which serves a critical role in fight-or-flight reactions to threat: It regulates neurotransmitters and hormones that cause sympathetic nervous system arousal and, in humans, provoke such emotions as fear and anger.

These commonalities notwithstanding, each species is characterized by particular distinctive structures and processes and by consequent behavioral capabilities. According to evolutionary theory, these distinctive features are the results of natural selection in specific environments that provide advantages in terms of gene perpetuation for some qualities over others. Birds, for example, presumably acquired the adaptation of wings and the capacity for flight because those creatures with the ability to lift themselves off the ground were more successful in avoiding predators and seeking prey. The physical adaptations that distinguish humans include the opposable thumb, bipedalism, and—of vital importance for understanding human motivation—the development of the cerebral cortex (in terms of sheer relative size and distinctly human neural connections between forebrain and mid- and hindbrain structures; see, e.g., Helmuth, 2001).

The brain provides us humans with uniquely complex and useful forms of subjective experience. Most central to the current analysis are the capacities for language and symbolic thought, thinking about the past and the future, and reflecting on the self as an object in the world (Becker, 1971; Deacon, 1997; Donald, 1991). These facilities have proven highly adaptive, because they allow us to shift attention from the ongoing flow of current sensations to (1) think about ourselves; (2) gauge our emotions, thoughts, goals, and preferences in relation to our circumstances; (3) explicitly recall useful information from the past; (4) consider and plan hypothetical possibilities for the future; and (5) communicate these emotions, thoughts, preferences, goals, memories, and possibilities to others.

These marvelous abilities have allowed us humans to, paraphrasing Langer (1975), escape the confines of animal realism, transcend the boundaries of time and space, and thereby proliferate throughout the planet—surviving in all terrestrial environments, and thriving in most of them. Because of our unprecedented cognitive flexibility, we not only adapt well to an incredibly wide variety of novel circumstances (see, e.g., Kanazawa's (2004) recent argument that general intelligence is a "domain-specific" adaptation to novelty), but we also routinely alter our environments to enhance their capacity to serve our preferences and goals. Indeed, the most serious physical threat to the long-term perpetuation of humankind is probably overpopulation; we have had too much success in propagating ourselves for the entire planet to bear.

But a more personal, pressing, and fundamentally psychological problem has also emerged from humans' evolving cognitive capabilities. Here we are, each of us individual organisms, with big brains built in so many ways to enhance our chances (and our genes' chances) for survival. What could be bad about that? Well, a couple of things. First, awareness of ourselves as objects existing in the world, juxtaposed with the capacity to imagine future possibilities, rendered our ancestors aware of a wide variety of potential threats to their continued existence, many of which were fatal and uncontrollable (e.g., floods, famines, earthquakes, hungry predators, hostile neighbors, and physical illnesses). Second, no matter how well we dodge these threats, death—the end of existence, the failure of all systems designed to keep us alive—is inevitable.

Imagine when the recognition of vulnerability and ultimate mortality became explicitly clear to our forebears. It must have been a monumental insight that changed everything:

> And with the rise and gradual conception of the self as the source of personal autonomy comes of course, the knowledge of its limit, the ultimate prospect of death. The effect of this intellectual advance is momentous. . . . It is in a fairly recent phase of that evolutionary course that the realization of death as the inevitable finale of every life has overtaken mankind. As a naked fact, that realization is unacceptable. Nothing perhaps is more comprehensible in that people, savage or civilized would rather reject than accept the idea of death as an inevitable close of their brief earthly careers. (Langer, 1975, pp. 90–91)

How did humans, evolving over billions of years to endure and respond to threats to survival with feelings of terror and defensive action, manage the awareness of perpetual vulnerability to an inevitable fate of nonexistence? Building on the work of Otto Rank, Gregory Zillborg, and Norman Brown, Ernest Becker (1971, 1973) proposed that humans utilized the imaginative capacities that created this existential dilemma to construct *cultural worldviews*—shared conceptions of reality that imbue life with order, stability, meaning, and permanence, and that provide bases for viewing ourselves as enduringly significant contributors to a meaningful reality rather than as mere transient animals groping for survival. In Becker's (1973, p. 5) words,

> It doesn't matter whether the cultural hero system is frankly magical, religious and primitive or secular, scientific and civilized. It is still a mythical hero system in which people serve in order to earn a feeling of primary value, cosmic specialness, of ultimate usefulness to creation of unshakeable meaning. They earn this feeling by carving out a place in nature, by building an edifice that reflects human value, a temple, a cathedral, a totem pole, a skyscraper, a family that spreads three generations. The hope and belief is that the things that man creates in society are of lasting worth and meaning, that they outlive or outshine death and decay, that man and his products count.

The specific contents of shared cultural conceptions of reality have presumably been shaped over the course of human evolution by a variety of historical events, ecological influences, and pragmatic concerns (for cultural materialists [e.g., Marvin Harris, 1979], these are the only factors that determine the nature of cultural constructions). However, we assert that one fundamental determinant of their character is their ability to quell the potential for terror inherent in the human awareness of vulnerability and mortality by imbuing life with meaning, and the individuals who subscribe to them with significance.

If this TMT analysis is correct, a great deal of our human cognition and behavior should be directed toward sustaining faith in the accepted cultural worldview and in our personal significance within the context of that worldview. And social validation should play a particularly large role in this sustenance, because to the extent that the same physical reality (i.e., the universe) can be apprehended in a variety of mutually exclusive ways by different cultural worldviews, our bases of meaning and self-worth are ultimately shared fabricated fictions.

How then do we come to believe in and subscribe to an ultimately fictitious view of reality? We become imbedded in cultural worldviews through the socialization process. Indeed, human children recapitulate the phylogenic process in the sense that with increasing cognitive development, the capacity to grasp their vulnerability and ultimate mortality grows as well. Because children are born helpless and are dependent from the very beginning, their original basis of security is the love and protection of their parents. The parents serve as conveyors of the cultural worldview as they expose the children to roles and values through language and stories. As the children grow, television, peers, and teachers take on an increasing role in conveying and validating the prevailing worldview.

What children learn very early is that as long as they feel valued by living up to the internalized cultural standards of value, they are loved and protected. When they fall short, the protection may be lost. As children mature and individuate from their parents, they come to realize the limits of the parental protection. They must grab onto larger bases of security, such as a deity, science, or one's country. This is accomplished by adopting social roles provided by the culture and adhering to the standards of value associated with them. Through this socialization process, we each live out our lives ensconced within an individualized but largely culturally derived orderly and meaningful construal of reality, in which we are significant beings qualified for transcendence of death through an eternal soul and/or permanent contributions to the world (e.g., offspring, group memberships, and culturally valued achievements).

TMT first appealed to us because, as Becker (1971, 1973, 1975) cogently argued, it seems to fit so much we have learned about humans both from history and from the social sciences. We humans by and large conform to our culture's ways, following its norms and obeying its authorities. We defend our cherished beliefs and rituals vehemently; indeed, many people are (somewhat ironically, as research has recently explored) quite willing to die for them. Religious, governmental, and educational institutions reinforce cultural beliefs and values in a myriad of ways. Cultural belief systems provide explanations of where the world and we humans come from, what we should strive for, and how we will persist in some form after our individual deaths. Until the last century, concepts of deities and souls were part of virtually every known worldview; as Robert J. Lifton (1968) argued, even the clearest recent exceptions, communist cultures, have attempted to sell immortality in the form of being part of an endlessly progressing collective.

In our view, the two most illuminating implications of TMT for understanding social behavior concern self-esteem and prejudice. By explicating how self-esteem comes to serve an anxiety-buffering function, the theory can explain the groping for self-esteem that seems to play such a prevalent role in human behavior—including the facts that those with high self-esteem fare much better in life than those lacking in self-regard, and that threats to self-esteem engender anxiety, anger, and all sorts of defensive reactions (from self-serving attributions to murder). The theory also offers an explanation for what is humankind's most tragic and well-documented flaw: the inability to get along peacefully with those different from ourselves. If culturally derived worldviews serve a deep security-providing psychological need and yet are fragile social constructions, it makes perfect sense that we respond to those espousing alternative worldviews with a combination of disdain, efforts to convert those others to our views, and aggression.

Of course, broad consistency of a theory with general trends in human behavior is necessary, but not sufficient, for accepting the theory's validity. We should be able to use the theory to generate novel, testable hypotheses that are supported by research. Indeed, the remainder of this chapter is devoted to an overview of research generated by TMT, emphasizing recent and current directions. We begin with a concise overview of the existing body of published research, which now exceeds 350 studies. Then we describe work examining the role of mortality concerns in six domains that have recently been given considerable attention: striving for meaning, creativity, health-related behaviors, mental health, legal decision making, and political preferences.

## THE BASIC EVIDENCE SUPPORTING TMT

The primary strategy we have developed for testing hypotheses derived from TMT is to remind people of their own death (*mortality salience*, or MS) and assess whether doing so intensifies bolstering of the psychological structures posited to protect people from their mortality concerns: their worldview and their self-worth. From the perspective of the theory, a core cultural belief that serves a terror management function is that we humans are more than just animals; rather, we are "super-natural" life forms, and hence not fated to absolute annihilation with death like all of nature's other denizens. If so, reminders of mortality should exaggerate our general human disinclination to acknowledge aspects of our corporeality.

### Denying Our Animality

A substantial body of research spearheaded by Jamie Goldenberg supports this idea (for a review, see Goldenberg, Pyszczynski, Greenberg, & Solomon, 2000). This research has shown that MS increases both disgust reactions to reminders of animality and preference for an essay trumpeting the uniqueness of humans over one emphasizing our similarities to other animals. Studies have also shown that MS leads to negative reactions to corporeal aspects of human reproductive behavior, such as breastfeeding (Cox, Goldenberg, Arndt, & Pyszczynski, 2007) and the physical aspects of sex (see Goldenberg, Pyszczynski, et al., 2000); such reactions are particularly strong if neuroticism is high, or if individuals are reminded of their similarity to other animals. In addition, when physical aspects of sex are made salient, the accessibility of death-related thought increases, unless participants are reminded of romantic love prior to the administration of the accessibility measure.

These findings support the idea that cultures provide constructs such as romantic love in part to imbue such corporeal activities as sex with meaning, thereby reducing the threatening connection of these behaviors to other animals. Fine dining; proper concealment of urination and defecation; body adornment (clothing and jewelry); and specific rituals concerning sex, circumcision, and menstruation are other cross-culturally observed examples of our human efforts to distance ourselves from animals.

## Striving for Self-Esteem

Beyond raising us above mere animals, cultures provide a sense that when we display cherished attributes and abilities, we are truly significant contributors to a meaningful world. If this culturally derived sense of self-esteem serves a terror management function, then reminders of death should increase striving to display such culturally valued qualities. A variety of studies have supported this idea. For example, MS increases displays of driving skill in those who base their self-esteem in part on such skill (Taubman-Ben Ari, Florian, & Mikulincer, 1999); increases identification with the body in those high in body self-esteem (Goldenberg, McCoy, Pyszczynski, Greenberg, & Solomon, 2000); increases monetary contributions to valued charities (Jonas, Schimel, Greenberg, & Pyszczynski, 2002); increases following of salient cultural norms (Jonas, Martens, Johns, Greenberg, & Reiss, 2007); increases identification with successful ingroups (Dechesne, Janssen, & van Knippenberg, 2000); and increases displays of physical strength in individuals whose self-esteem is predicated on this attribute (Peters, Greenberg, Williams, & Schneider, 2005). Most recently, we have found that MS increases the desire to be famous (Greenberg, Kosloff, Solomon, & Cohen, 2007).

MS has also been shown to lead to self-esteem protection in the form of increased self-serving attributional bias (Mikulincer & Florian, 2002); increased striving for optimal distinctiveness in response to threats (Simon, Greenberg, Arndt, et al., 1997); reduced body monitoring in those with low body esteem (Goldenberg, McCoy, et al., 2000); and reduced identification with unsuccessful or negatively framed ingroups (e.g., Arndt, Greenberg, Schimel, Pyszczynski, & Solomon, 2002). Complementing this work showing that MS increases self-esteem striving is a body of work showing that high and boosted self-esteem buffers anxiety in response to threat and reduces defensive responses to reminders of death (Arndt & Greenberg, 1999; Greenberg et al., 1992, 1993; Harmon-Jones et al., 1997). Taken together, these findings show that efforts to view ourselves as more than mere animals and to live up to cultural standards of value serve a terror management function: to keep the potential for anxiety engendered by the awareness of mortality at bay.

## Prejudice and Intergroup Conflict

According to TMT, one important reason why people so often can't get along with each other is that when others violate or threaten the validity of a person's worldview, because of the security-providing function of that worldview, the person has to defend it by somehow putting the others in their place—by derogating them, attempting to convert them, or (in extreme but historically all too prevalent cases) annihilating them. In support of this idea, a large body of research has shown that MS leads to harsh punishment of those who violate values of the participant's worldview, and to disdain and aggression against others who criticize that worldview or espouse a very different one (these reactions are often referred to as *worldview defense*; see Greenberg, Solomon, & Pyszczynski, 1997). In a complementary fashion, this research has also shown that MS leads to greater rewards and more positive reactions to others who uphold values of the worldview or otherwise help validate the worldview. This body of work suggests that in addition to real conflict over resources and cultural transmission of stereotypes, the need for terror management plays a substantial role in prejudice and intergroup conflict.

### Close Relationships

Another well-developed line of research spearheaded by Mario Mikulincer and Victor Florian (for a review, see Mikulincer, Florian, & Hirschberger, 2003) has shown that close relationships play a significant role in terror management. For example, MS increases interest in forming close relationships, and it increases valuing of current romantic partners as well as one's parents (Cox, Arndt, Pyszczynski, Greenberg, & Solomon, 2007). Additional studies have shown that secure attachment can mitigate certain responses to MS. Finally, studies have shown that contemplating threats to close relationships like extended separation increase the accessibility of death-related thought. Mikulincer and colleagues (2003) have proposed that this work indicates that close relationships serve as an anxiety buffer, in addition to the worldview and the sense of self-worth. However, we believe that close relationships may be a central component of many people's terror management because they play such a vital role in validating the individual's worldview and sense of self-worth. Further research will be needed to test between these two possibilities definitively.

## THE COGNITIVE ARCHITECTURE OF TERROR MANAGEMENT PROCESSES

Research has also focused on elucidating the cognitive dynamics underlying terror management processes (for reviews, see Arndt, Cook, & Routledge, 2004; Pyszczynski, Greenberg, & Solomon, 1999). The dual-defense model that emerged from this research suggests that because of the developmental process through which people learn to associate the mitigation of existential distress with maintaining a sense of symbolic value, knowledge of mortality becomes a central construct in people's cognitive networks of self-relevant beliefs. The activation of death-related thought then motivates two different systems of defense, depending on whether cognitions pertaining to one's mortality are in focal attention or accessible but outside of conscious awareness. Although these basic processes share certain characteristics with other automatic and self-regulated goal pursuits (cf. Bargh & Chartrand, 1999), there are some notable differences that highlight the unique role of the awareness of death in people's cognitive functioning.

Explicit thoughts of death first provoke *proximal defenses* designed to remove death-related cognitions from conscious awareness. People generally don't like to think about their vulnerability to mortality, and thus will employ a variety of often pseudorational means to avoid doing so—such as suppressing death-related thoughts, or engaging in cognitive and motivational biases to deny or minimize vulnerability (e.g., Arndt, Greenberg, Solomon, et al., 1997; Greenberg, Arndt, Simon, Pyszczynski, & Solomon, 2000). This explains why immediately after thinking about death, death thought accessibility is generally low but then increases following a delay (Greenberg, Pyszczynski, Solomon, Simon, & Breus, 1994). These effects speak to the very active role that the mind can take in managing conscious death-related concerns, and they offer convergent insights regarding the dynamics of intentional mental control of disturbing thoughts. For example, reminding people of their mortality extends Wegner's (e.g., 1992) pioneering work on thought suppression (which instructed participants to avoid thinking about a particular topic) by uncovering a domain of self-initiated and naturally occurring thought suppression. However, such responses only reflect the tip of the defensive iceberg.

Once proximal defenses are relaxed, there is a delayed increase in death thought accessibility outside of focal attention. In laboratory research, the necessity of a delay in using explicit mortality primes to increase death thought accessibility can be circumvented by priming death subliminally (e.g., Arndt, Greenberg, Pyszczynski, & Solomon, 1997) or by having participants contemplate their mortality under conditions of high cognitive load, which reduces the effectiveness of ensuing efforts to suppress death-related thought (Arndt, Greenberg, Solomon, et al., 1997). Increased death thought accessibility outside of focal attention signals a heightened potential for anxiety (Greenberg et al., 2003), which then instigates worldview- and self-esteem-relevant *distal defenses*—the terror management defenses we have been describing. This deep activation (Wegner & Smart, 1997) of death-related thought increases the accessibility of constructs associated with the individuals' culturally prescribed investments in meaning and esteem.

This model is similar to other spreading activation and related models (e.g., McKoon & Ratcliff, 1992): Because knowledge of mortality occupies a prominent and deeply rooted position within a network of knowledge structures that function as self-protective beliefs, when death is activated, accessibility spontaneously spreads to other interconnected constructs that function to provide meaning and value. Thus, for example, subliminal death primes, or explicit mortality primes after a delay, spontaneously increase accessibility of nationalistic cognitions for men and relationship cognitions for women, presumably because these respective domains represent important beliefs for these gender groups (Arndt, Greenberg, & Cook, 2002). Notably, however, Arndt, Greenberg, and Cook (2002) found that this sequence of activation depends on the elements of a person's belief system that are both dispositionally and situationally salient as symbolic investments, and that it is only elicited by the unconscious reverberation of death-related thought. This suggests that the nature of "automatic" goal activation can (at least in certain contexts) depend on the specific motivational dynamics implicated by particular conscious and unconscious thoughts (cf. Cesario, Plaks, & Higgins, 2006).

With the increased accessibility of these worldview-relevant domains, unconscious death thoughts trigger distal or symbolic defenses—experientially based strategies to bolster faith in the cultural worldview and one's self-worth that ultimately provide protection from deeply rooted existential fears. Consistent with this characterization of distal defenses, studies show, for instance, that the increased worldview investment found after MS does not occur when participants are induced to process information in a rational mode, but is quite robust when participants are induced to process information in a more experiential, intuitive manner (Simon, Greenberg, Harmon-Jones, et al., 1997). Beyond the mechanisms through which these different classes of defense manifest themselves, this model also specifies at least one critical function that symbolic defenses serve for the individual: Specifically, the successful engagement of symbolic defenses then restores relative psychological equanimity, in part by reducing the heightened accessibility of death-related thoughts that instigated the response (e.g., Arndt, Greenberg, Solomon, et al., 1997). Moreover, for depressed individuals, worldview defense in response to MS can increase the perceived meaningfulness of life (Simon, Arndt, Greenberg, Solomon, & Pyszczynski, 1998).

## ISSUES FOR THE THEORY AND THE RESEARCH

We believe that this large and continually growing body of work attests to the value of TMT. It seems to be generative and highly supported by the extant research. However, concerns regarding the theory and research have been raised; although extensive discussion of these criticisms can be found elsewhere (e.g., Greenberg et al., 1997, Pyszczynski, Greenberg, & Solomon, 1997; Pyszczynski, Greenberg, Solomon, Arndt, & Schimel, 2004; Pyszczynski, Greenberg, Solomon, & Maxfield, in press), we briefly acknowledge and address the three most common concerns.

### The Conceptual Problem of Suicide

As noted earlier, we think that TMT generally accords very well with the way people behave in the world—and, indeed, that it offers a parsimonious explanation for many large-scale historical events and mundane human activities. However, suicide stands as one glaring exception. If the unconscious fear of death is a driving force in human behavior, why do some people seek out death? This is a challenging question. Suicide is a difficult problem for any theory of human motivation. Whether people desire control, pleasure, self-integrity, belonging, achievement, power, or growth, suicide thwarts all of these. From an evolutionary perspective, why would an organism built for survival and effective perpetuation of its genes take itself out of the gene pool? Some elaborate explanation might be offered for suicide in elderly people. But what about teen suicides, or murder–suicides in which people kill their children and themselves? From virtually any motivational perspective, suicide is an anomaly—a failure of the motivational self-regulatory system.

Nevertheless, we believe that TMT offers some valuable insights into suicide. Suicides that reinforce one's qualification for death transcendence fit the theory particularly well. Middle Eastern suicide bombers typically believe that their actions make them heroes and martyrs, who gain access to eternal joy in a heaven replete with 72 virgins and the like. Mario Mikulincer (personal communication, 2001) informed us of two particularly interesting cases in Israel that illustrate how literal such beliefs can be. One suicidal terrorist had armor protecting his penis; the other had doused himself with cologne. Similarly, notes to the 9/11 terrorists before their murderous actions acknowledged the normality of fearing death, but emphasized that they must overcome this to reach the greater rewards of eternal heaven (see, e.g., Pyszczynski, Solomon, & Greenberg, 2003). Recent studies have supported a terror management view of such acts of martyrdom, finding that MS increases Iranians' interest in joining the cause of suicidal martyrdom against the United States (Pyszczynski et al., 2006). Lest we are tempted to think that such reactions occur only among Islamic extremists, a second study in that research found that MS also increased U.S. students' endorsement of using extreme violence, including nuclear weapons, in the "war on terrorism." Interestingly, Routledge and Arndt (2007) recently found that presenting British participants with an alternative avenue for symbolic immortality eliminated an MS-induced increase in self-reported willingness to sacrifice oneself for the country, suggesting that such self-sacrifice may indeed reflect a way to manage concerns over one's obliteration upon physical death.

Other examples of suicide that can be seen as serving terror management include traditional Japanese hari-kiri, which is often committed to restore the honor of one's ancestral line, and less ritualized suicides by individuals who believe that an afterlife awaits. Suicides are also typically attempted by people having difficulty sustaining the structures that serve terror management: faith in a meaningful view of reality and in one's value within the context of that reality. Stripped of this protection, such people may be unable to bear the terror they feel. As Shakespeare noted in a number of plays (e.g., *Julius Caesar*), dying is ironically the one way to rid ourselves of the fear of death. Dostoevsky made a similar observation in *The Possessed* when a character in the novel explained the reason for his impending suicide: "I wish to deprive myself of life, because the idea has occurred to me, because I don't want to have the fear of death . . . " One can see the reality of these literary insights in people on death row. It is not uncommon for such people to be placed on suicide watch. Faced squarely only with impending death, ending their fear sooner may be preferable to later.

Other suicides seem to be motivated by revenge (e.g., getting back at a loved one who has betrayed the person). Still other suicides seem to be motivated by the need to escape intense physical pain. In these cases, it may be that these other emotion-driven pressing motives simply override the fear of death. And, of course, some suicide attempts are half-hearted efforts designed not to end one's life but to get desired help or attention. In many of these instances, intoxication by alcohol or other drugs helps people attempt suicide. By blocking self-awareness, consideration of future consequences, impulse control, and anxiety, these substances allow people to overcome their imminent fear in order to end their misery. The only type of suicide really difficult for TMT to account for would be a sober atheist's calmly killing him- or herself in a manner that does not serve his or her symbolic immortality, and in the absence of an impending threat of death such as a terminal illness.

## Does the Research Support a Unique Role of Death?

Conceptually, we believe that death is of unique psychological importance. Death is the only certain future event we all will face. It portends the ultimate futility of all the systems and activities we direct toward staying alive, and it undermines all other needs and desires. Specifically, it eliminates self-integrity, growth, control, pleasure, achievement, power, belonging . . . you name it. Of course, death can be viewed as a complex concept (see, e.g., Florian & Mikulincer, 2004). Indeed, the original MS induction—which consists of two open-ended items concerning emotions aroused by thoughts of (1) one's own death, and (2) what happens as one dies and once one is dead—may confound reminding people of mortality with other variables (negative affect, general aversiveness, etc.). However, from the beginning, our research team has been sensitive to this issue and has worked to determine the convergent and discriminant validity of our MS inductions.

The first published paper on MS (Rosenblatt, Greenberg, Solomon, Pyszczynski, & Lyon, 1989) reported six studies that employed interaction predictions, multiple comparison conditions, an alternative operationalization of MS, and measures of affect and physiological arousal. These studies made the original case that thoughts of death are specifically what increase harsh judgments of others who violate the worldview and positive reactions to those who uphold it. Since then, many studies have provided additional support for the unique role of thoughts about death. Terror management predictions have been supported by wide-ranging operationalizations of reminders of death, including the open-ended items described above, death anxiety scales, writing a single sentence about death, proximity to funeral homes and cemeteries, and subliminal death primes. We believe that the variety of instantiations used makes any single alternative explanation unlikely.

Furthermore, the subliminal death primes (e.g., Arndt, Allen, & Greenberg, 2001; Arndt, Greenberg, & Cook, 2002; Arndt, Greenberg, Pyszczynski, et al., 1997; Dechesne et al., 2000; Jonas & Greenberg, 2004), which typically consist of 10 outside-of-awareness exposures to a single word, *dead*, constitute a particularly pure operationalization. This work has shown that these effects are not replicated by parallel exposure to the words *fail* or *pain*. These findings also show that MS effects are not really the result of making mortality salient at all, but rather of increasing the accessibility of death-related thought. Indeed, the specific role of accessible death thought in terror management processes has been supported by extensive research reviewed earlier on the dual-process model of defense, as well as by the research showing increased death thought accessibility in response to threats of creatureliness, relationship disruption, and worldview threat (e.g., Schimel, Hayes, Williams, & Jahrig, 2007).

Additionally, these various death reminders have been compared with making thoughts about a wide variety of alternative topics salient, including meaninglessness, cultural values, the self, failure, uncertainty, giving a speech in public, worries after college, general anxiety, dental pain, general pain, intense unpredictable bouts of pain, social exclusion, and paralysis. In each case, our research has found different effects for reminders of mortality. McGregor, Zanna, Holmes, and Spencer (2001) reported similar effects for a temporal discontinuity induction and an MS induction. However, research suggests that the temporal discontinuity induction actually increases the accessibility of death-related thought (Chaudary, Tison, & Solomon, 2002). In addition, van den Bos and Miedema (2000) found similar effects of MS and an uncertainty salience induction in reactions to people being treated unfairly. But over a dozen published studies have shown that MS and uncertainty salience have quite different effects on other tasks and judgments (e.g., Landau, Johns, Greenberg, et al., 2004; Routledge, Arndt, & Goldenberg, 2004).

Although we believe that examining comparison conditions adds to the strong case for the unique effects of death-related thought, we are not suggesting that threats other than death cannot increase defense and bolstering of the individual's worldview and self-esteem. Indeed, TMT was developed specifically to explain why people respond defensively to threats to their cherished beliefs and to their self-esteem. Thus it is perfectly consistent with the theory that direct threats to psychological structures posited to serve terror management should activate defenses of those structures. We would also suggest that the knowledge of mortality is never really too far from consciousness, and so we view our MS inductions as intensifications of ongoing worldview and self-esteem maintenance processes. Of course, this latter point is particularly difficult to assess empirically.

## Where Is the Terror?

From the very first MS study, research has carefully examined affective reactions to a reminder of mortality. Although the threat of impending death clearly triggers terror, as reactions to fires, airplane turbulence, and terrorist acts (notably the 9/11 attacks on the World Trade Center and the Pentagon) attest, whether our MS induction would arouse even traces of such terror was not at all clear or predictable from TMT. Indeed, the theory is about why and how, given the capacity for the threat of death to arouse terror, people are able to function with equanimity despite the knowledge that death is inevitable and could occur at any time for a host of reasons that cannot be anticipated or controlled.

MS inductions have consistently failed to arouse detectable negative affect, whether measured through self-report or through psychophysiological measures. The one exception is the study by Arndt and colleagues (2001), who found a small and brief increase in corrugator activity during exposure to subliminal death primes. However, this indication of negative affect lasted less than 10 seconds and did not mediate subsequent worldview defense. Although this lack of affective responses to MS has never troubled terror management theorists and researchers (see, e.g., Rosenblatt et al., 1989), others have argued that it challenges the validity of the theory (see Solomon, Greenberg, & Pyszczynski, 1997). From an early stage, TMT articles proposed that terror management defenses avert the experience of anxiety; in fact, they proposed this to be their primary function. Rather than serving to ameliorate anxiety in response to MS, the defenses function to protect from the potential to experience anxiety that is signaled by the heightened accessibility of death-related thought. In support of this view, Greenberg and colleagues (2003) found that giving participants exposed to an MS induction a placebo reported to block the potential to experience anxiety mitigated the typical increase in worldview defense.

## NEW BRANCHES OF TERROR MANAGEMENT RESEARCH

Terror management research is proliferating in diverse directions, thanks to many different researchers around the world; indeed, supportive findings have been reported in a dozen countries in addition to the United States. Even a cursory overview of this work would be beyond the scope of this chapter. Therefore, we limit ourselves to discussing some recent directions we have been pursuing that have already borne substantial fruit. We begin with work focusing on fundamental aspects of the worldview—the imposition of structure and meaning. Then we focus on work examining the role of terror management concerns in particular domains of human affairs: creativity, physical and mental health, the law, and finally politics (with foci on responses to terrorism and the attraction of charismatic leaders).

### Structure and Meaning as Antidotes to Terror

> People die and murder, nurture and protect, go to any extreme, in behalf of their conception of the real. More to the point, perhaps, they live out the details of their daily lives in terms of what they conceive to be real: not just rocks and mountains and storms at sea, but friendship, love, respect, are known as false or real. Indeed, we institute such intersubjective realities, even give them embodiment in the layout of the village, in forms of address, in ritual and myth. This is the domain of meaning making, without which human beings in every culture fall into terror. The product of meaning making is Reality. (Bruner, 1996, p. xv)

TMT proposes that structuring subjective reality and imbuing it with meaning are essential components of how worldviews provide us with psychological equanimity. Living within an orderly, stable, and meaningful reality is a critical prerequisite for believing that we humans are significant beings in a meaningful world, rather than animals fated only to death. If this idea is correct, MS should increase efforts to structure social reality in simple and benign ways. From this perspective, many of the early MS studies could be viewed as showing that MS leads to categorizing people more simply as good or bad, thereby leading to a polarization of preferences.

The first direct evidence that MS encourages reliance on simple structures is a set of studies showing that MS increases stereotypic thinking and preferences for stereotype-consistent outgroup members over counterstereotypic outgroup members (Schimel et al., 1999). Then, in a series of seven studies, Landau, Johns, and colleagues (2004) demonstrated a variety of additional ways in which MS encourages both simple and benign structuring. One aspect of viewing the world as stable and meaningful is perceiving people as consistent. Primacy effects in person perception contribute to this by assimilating subsequent information into initial impressions of an individual. Landau, Johns, and colleagues (Study 1) therefore hypothesized and found that MS would increase primacy effects. Similarly, in Study 2, they hypothesized and found that MS increased the use of the representativeness heuristic, in which people judge a person's group membership based on the extent to which the person seems to fit the stereotype of that group.

Additional studies tested the hypothesis that MS would particularly motivate preference for structuring in people high in *personal need for structure* (PNS). In Studies 3 and 4, Landau, Johns, and colleagues (2004) found that MS increased preference for balanced over imbalanced social relations and for a consistently introverted or extroverted person over an inconsistent person, but only among high-PNS people. In a more recent set of studies, Landau, Greenberg, Pyszczynski, Solomon, and Martens (2007) found that these effects extended to self-perception as well as perception of others. Specifically, MS led high-PNS people to view themselves in less complex and more certain ways.

Another pair of studies from Landau, Johns, and colleagues (2004) tested the idea that MS would increase high-PNS people's desire to believe that the world is a just and benign place. Believing that good things happen to good people and bad things happen to bad people makes the world seem both orderly and meaningful. In Study 5, high- and low-PNS participants read about a college student disfigured in an unprovoked attack. After an MS manipulation, the participants were given the opportunity to read titled bits of information about the victim, with the titles implying either positive or negative information about the person. Negative information would bring the event more in line with belief in a just world. Supporting predictions, Landau, Johns, and colleagues found that for high-PNS people, MS increased preference for negative over positive information about the victim. Interestingly, low-PNS participants actually increased preference for positive information after MS—a result we discuss later.

To provide further support for the role of just-world beliefs in terror management, in Study 6 Landau, Johns, and colleagues (2004) had participants read about the attack and then read either negative or positive information about the victim. Reading positive information about a victim should threaten belief in a just world. Thus Landau and colleagues predicted and found that this scenario would lead to especially high death thought accessibility in high-PNS participants. Hirschberger (2006), using Israeli participants, has recently provided complementary evidence that MS increased blaming of victims, especially when the victims' injuries were severe and they were not responsible for their injuries—precisely the conditions under which the threat to just-world beliefs is greatest. And, as found by Landau, Johns, and colleagues in Study 6, Hirschberger found that it is just such victims who elicit increased death thought accessibility.

In addition to believing in the justice of outcomes, people can believe in an orderly, benign world by thinking that everything happens for a reason and that bad events lead to good outcomes. To assess whether such a believe in benevolent causation contributes to terror management, in Study 7 Landau, Johns, and colleagues (2004) had high- and low-PNS participants exposed to MS or a control condition read two summaries of movie scripts. In one summary, a protagonist witnesses his apartment building burn down, but later through a separate series of events finds love. In the other summary, the apartment fire leads the protagonist to meet the woman with whom he falls in love. In support of predictions, MS increased high-PNS people's preferences for the "bad causes good" scenario over the "bad simply precedes good" scenario. Thus MS encouraged preference in high-PNS people for the story that reinforces the idea of benevolent causation—that bad events will turn out for the best.

A third set of studies examined the implications of this analysis for aesthetic preferences (Landau, Greenberg, Solomon, Pyszczynski, & Martens, 2006). Art serves a number of functions, but one is to reinforce an orderly and meaningful view of reality. Representational, mythic, and religious art all seem to serve this function, whereas more chaotic abstract art does not. Perhaps this is why people so often react to abstract art negatively—because it doesn't provide the expected reinforcement of an orderly, meaningful world, and may even imply the opposite (a random, meaningless, or absurd universe). Thus Landau, Greenberg, Solomon, and colleagues (2006) tested the idea that MS would increase preference for meaningful representational art over abstract art, especially among high-PNS people.

In the first study they did not measure PNS, but simply asked participants in MS and control conditions their impressions of a set of abstract paintings. Consistent with hypothesis, MS reduced liking for the abstract art. In the second study, high- and low-PNS participants after an MS manipulation rated their liking for two representational and two abstract paintings. MS increased high-PNS participants' preference for representational over abstract art. In the third study, they utilized an apparently abstract painting by Jackson Pollock that became meaningful and representational because of its title. They had high and low-PNS participants in MS and control conditions view the painting with either the meaning-imbuing (and actual) title, *Guardians of the Secret*, or a meaningless numeric title, *No. 12*. Without the meaningful title, MS led to reduced liking for the painting in high-PNS participants. In contrast, with the meaningful title, MS had no effect on liking for the painting.

In a final study, Landau, Greenberg, Solomon, and colleagues (2006) imbued abstract art with meaning in a different way. One way to derive meaning from abstract art is to recognize the feeling the art seems to be expressing (hence the term *abstract expressionism*). Providing a personal frame of reference is one way to facilitate recognition of such feeling in abstract art. So in this study, before participants in MS and control conditions were shown and asked how much they liked a Wassily Kandinsky painting of kinetically swirling colors and shapes that seem to convey a sense of chaos and disorder, they were requested to imagine either a chaotic situation (being in a very strange place where nothing seems comprehensible) or an orderly situation (being in a place where everything seems familiar and orderly). As in the prior studies, in the orderly-situation condition, MS led high-PNS participants to dislike the Kandinsky painting. However, if these participants had imagined a chaotic experience, MS did not reduce liking for the painting.

Taken together, these studies suggested that following MS, high-PNS people disliked art that lacks meaning. Interestingly, in the art and social perception studies, MS did not lead to a preference for structure and meaning in low-PNS people. Generally, MS had no effect for such people. However, in Study 5 of Landau, Johns, and colleagues (2004), these people actually responded in a less structuring way, and nonsignificant trends in this direction were found in a number of the other recent studies as well. This suggests that low-PNS people do not rely on simple structures to quell their mortality-related concerns. Perhaps they derive meaning from more complex, idiosyncratic conceptions of the world. Other research shows that low-PNS people value openness and are relatively low in conscientiousness. So perhaps their self-worth is tied to openness rather than conformity to rigid or predictable conceptions of the world.

In a fourth series of studies, Landau, Greenberg, Arndt, and Routledge (2007) recently examined the terror management function of one of the most basic sources of order and meaning: conceptions of time and self-continuity over time. In the first two studies, Landau and colleagues found that MS led to more negative attitudes toward people or arguments that violate cultural conventions for keeping and abiding by clock time. In addition, those who were high in PNS responded to MS and a threat to clock time by using more definitive temporal intervals to structure their own time.

Four additional studies explicated the nature of MS-induced temporal structuring in considering the past, present, and future. Briefly, in a third study, some participants were asked to organize past events in a personally meaningless fashion. When combined with MS, this threat to experiential temporal coherence led to a compensatory boost in the perceived meaningfulness of the past. Furthermore, in another study, high-PNS participants receiving an MS induction perceived more meaningful connections between events in their personal past and their current sense of self, suggesting a heightened concern with establishing continuity between their personal past and present. Continuing to document the influence of MS on current temporal structuring, yet another study in this series found that high-PNS participants responded to MS by using more causal words in spontaneously describing their day, suggesting a greater concern with imposing causal coherence on the separate elements of their recent experience. In the final study of this series, after receiving an MS induction, participants were more interested in an opportunity to transcend time symbolically by immortalizing their name on a star.

## Creativity and Terror Management

The TMT research just reviewed seems to show that MS increases defensive reliance on conventional bases of structure and meaning. Of course, as argued by many theorists and researchers, there clearly seems to be another side to motivation—one that reflects self-expanding and personal-growth-oriented behavior (e.g., Aron & Aron, 1994; Deci & Ryan, 2002; Maslow, 1970; Rank, 1941). Over the last few years, TMT research has begun to examine the interplay between these different motivations (for theoretical considerations, see Greenberg, Pyszczynski, & Solomon, 1995; Pyszczynski, Greenberg, & Goldenberg, 2003), particularly with respect to how death-related concerns influence creative action.

Based on the classic theorizing of Otto Rank (e.g., 1941), Arndt, Greenberg, Solomon, Pyszczynski, and Schimel (1999) suggested that intimations of mortality may render creative action a source of guilt. From this perspective, creative engagement, by virtue of serving to distinguish one from prevailing social norms and from dependency on conventional structure and meaning, threatens the social connection that provides protection from mortality concerns. Consistent with this reasoning, Arndt and colleagues found that participants in such situations experienced increased guilt, and also increased their efforts to embed themselves in a sense of collective validation through enhanced social projection.

Subsequently, Arndt, Routledge, Greenberg, and Sheldon (2005) found that informing participants that they were quite similar to others enabled creative action after MS to transpire guilt-free, and Arndt, Routledge, and Vess (2007) found that participants reminded of death were more creative when the creative action was prompted by a task that enhanced connectedness than when it served individuation. An additional study in Arndt, Routledge, and colleagues took the analysis one step further in finding that after MS and creative writing, attention to social connectedness, relative to individuation, increased positive mood, creative problem solving, and vitality. This is the first research to uncover effects of MS on indices generally regarded as reflecting positive psychological well-being. Finally, Routledge, Arndt, and Sheldon (2004) also found that when creativity can inspire a more open-minded orientation, it can reduce worldview defense after MS. This shows how growth-oriented pursuits can ameliorate propensities for defenses that adversely affect others.

## A TERROR MANAGEMENT LENS ON BEHAVIORAL HEALTH RISK AND PROMOTION

The notion of dual defenses against existential fears has played a pivotal role in the application of TMT to understanding health risk and promotion, as well as the way in which health vulnerabilities can elicit concerns about mortality. For example, recent studies indicate that certain health threats have the potential to instigate conscious death concerns and thus to provoke direct defenses. Arndt, Cook, Goldenberg, and Cox (2007) demonstrated that the salience of cancer can act as such a threat. Whereas in the absence of cognitive load, cancer salience did not increase death thought accessibility (as a simple priming effect might predict), the salience of cancer did heighten death thought accessibility when participants were under high cognitive load.

One implication here is that people will be especially likely to suppress the death-related thoughts instigated by health threats when they feel particularly vulnerable to the threats they are encountering. When perceived vulnerability is low, however, concern with mortality should be minimal, and thus suppression should be less necessary. Consistent with this reasoning, Arndt, Cook, and colleagues (2007) found that female participants led to believe they were more vulnerable to breast cancer showed lower levels of death thought accessibility than participants led to believe they were less vulnerable, suggesting that the former participants were indeed engaging in active suppression—an effect that was mediated by how threatening participants found the vulnerability information to which they were exposed.

The proximal–distal defense distinction is important for understanding how individuals respond in health relevant domains. For example, Greenberg and colleagues (2000) found that participants reacted to conscious thoughts of death by denying vulnerability to those factors (i.e., levels of emotionality) that they were told were associated with a short life expectancy (notably, such effects did not emerge when thoughts of death were allowed to fade from focal attention). Although this may seem to paint a bleak picture of people responding to vulnerability information with an ostrich-like reaction of burying their heads in the sand, people fortunately also possess the fortitude to enact productive health-oriented responses. For example, when consciously reminded of their mortality, people also increase their intentions to exercise more (Arndt, Schimel, & Goldenberg, 2003, Study 1), and to use sunblock with a high sun protection factor to (presumably) reduce the risk of skin cancer (Routledge, Arndt, & Goldenberg, 2004, Study 1). Indeed, individual differences in health optimism and health coping appear to predict when people will respond to conscious thoughts of death with productive or avoidant health-based reactions (Arndt, Routledge, & Goldenberg, 2006).

Consistent with the dual-defense model of terror management, this research suggests that conscious thoughts of death will provoke health-oriented reactions that are at least guided by pseudorational principles; however, several recent lines of research indicate that a very different health-relevant story emerges when people try to manage unconscious intimations of mortality. The defenses employed against unconscious death salience often have little to do with health per se; rather, the operative motivation in these contexts is to maintain a sense of meaning and value, and as such may often override the motivation to take care of one's health. In this way, the TMT analysis affords insights extending beyond the rationally oriented risk perception models that are widespread in health psychology research.

Consider, for example, the findings mentioned above in which immediately following an explicit contemplation of mortality, participants increased their intentions to exercise. It should be noted that this finding was observed regardless of the relevance of physical fitness to participants' self-esteem. In contrast, when a delay intervened between MS and the assessment of fitness intentions, only those individuals for whom fitness was relevant to self-esteem increased their exercise intentions, suggesting the manifestation of a drive to maintain feelings of self-worth (Arndt et al., 2003, Study 2).

Unfortunately, the pathways to self-esteem that are prescribed in our society do not always encourage adaptive health trajectories. Thus, for example, in Routledge, Arndt, and Goldenberg (2004, Study 1), when a delay intervened between the manipulation of MS and assessment of sun lotion endorsement, people for whom tanning was relevant to their self-worth actually lowered their intentions of using safe sun products. Furthermore, evidence indicates that these contingencies of self-worth are quite malleable; for example, they can be swayed by the many advertisements with which we as consumers are bombarded. In support of this notion, Routledge, Arndt, and Goldenberg (Study 2) found that when participants were exposed to an advertisement that propagated the associations among tanned skin, attractiveness, and self-esteem, thoughts of death outside of focal attention increased tanning intentions, and even did so among those who had not previously indicated that tanned skin was important to their sense of self-worth.

Importantly, recent studies also indicate that the effect can be pushed in the other direction; that is, exposing people to information that suggests a link between paler skin and attractiveness leads MS to decrease tanning intentions (Arndt, Cox, Cohen, Goldenberg, & Routledge, 2007). Additional findings consistent with this overall analysis are provided by Taubman Ben-Ari and colleagues (1999) research on risky driving behavior, and by Goldenberg, Arndt, Hart, and Brown (2005) in their studies on women's dieting. In this latter research, MS led to restricted eating behavior among women, and particularly for overweight women in group contexts in which they were made aware of their failure to attain the societal ideal of thinness. Indeed, these specific effects of MS were mediated by an individual's perceived discrepancy from attaining this societal ideal of thinness.

The distal/symbolic effects of mortality concerns on health-relevant behaviors suggest that there can be adaptive and maladaptive outcomes for one's health, depending on both situational and dispositional self-esteem contingencies. Another important factor to consider in how the existential concerns evoked by the awareness of death can affect health behavior is the extent to which the health behavior implicates individuals' concerns with the physicality, or creatureliness, of their bodies. As noted earlier, in accord with the notion that the body can pose an existential threat, a number of experiments have demonstrated that when existential concerns are heightened via an MS prime, individuals respond with more negative attitudes and behavioral avoidance of the physical body (see Goldenberg, Pyszczynski, et al., 2002, for a review).

Goldenberg, Arndt, Hart, and Routledge (in press) applied these ideas to understand women's reluctance to perform the vital behavior of breast self-examination (BSE). This work reveals that part of this reluctance may stem from concerns about one's physical, and thus ultimately mortal, nature. Across three studies, priming thoughts of the physicality of the body decreased BSE intentions after MS; and when participants were dealing with a more realistic BSE confrontation that itself served to increase death thought accessibility, rendering salient concerns with creatureliness reduced actual BSE behavior (among both college women and at-risk women with ages > 35). Furthermore, this research utilized a classic misattribution of arousal paradigm to show that concerns with creatureliness decreased BSE behavior by increasing existential discomfort with the exam procedure. Consistent with this analysis, Goldenberg and colleagues also found that priming the physicality of the body increased reported discomfort among women actually attending a mammogram clinic. Taken together, these studies may constitute the most troubling evidence to date that mortality concerns can lead to behavior that is ironically contrary to the goal of staying alive.

## Fatal Distractions: The Role of Terror Management in Mental Health

Another current line of empirical inquiry is examining the role of terror management in mental health. Yalom (1980) contended that all psychopathology is (at least in part) the result of ineffective terror management. Based on this perspective, we have proposed that phobias, compulsive behaviors, and dissociation from a coherent self all reflect maladaptive strategies for coping with the fear of death. Thus we hypothesized in two sets of studies that MS would increase symptomatology in people suffering from phobias, compulsions, and dissociations. In phobias and compulsions, people are engaging in what we call *terror focalization*; they are displacing their fears concerning death onto more narrow threats such as spiders or germs. With dissociation, people may be avoiding their fear by disconnecting from the everyday view of the self as a tangible and coherent, but transient, being.

To provide preliminary empirical support for this "terror mismanagement" conception of psychopathology, Strachan and colleagues (in press, Study 1) compared avoidance and threat reactions of spider-phobic and non-spider-phobic participants following either an MS or control induction. Specifically, participants (under the guise of a cognitive processing task) viewed a series of pictures of spiders and flowers. Participants advanced through the pictures at their own pace and then rated how likely it was that the spiders they viewed were dangerous to humans and might attack humans if close enough to do so. In accord with our predictions, MS decreased the time spider-phobic participants spent viewing the spider pictures and increased their perceptions of danger of spiders to humans.

In a second experiment, Strachan and colleagues (in press) selected participants based on their responses to the Contamination Obsessions and Washing Compulsions subscale of the Padua Inventory—Washington State University Revision (Burns, Keortge, Formea, & Sternberger, 1996) to take part in an ostensible study of physiological responses. Mortality-salient and control participants were then connected to a physiograph machine, and electrode cream was used on their fingers. After a brief period of supposedly measuring physiological responses, participants were disconnected from the physiograph, told that the study was over, and brought to a sink to wash their hands. The length of time each participant spent washing his or her hands served as the primary dependent measure. Consistent with the previous study and with predictions, those high in compulsive hand washing spent more time washing their hands after an MS induction than did either those low in compulsive hand washing or control induction participants.

Additional research by Kosloff and colleagues (in press) examined the causal role of MS in dissociative reactions to trauma, consistent with a theoretical model advanced by Gershuny and Thayer (1999) suggesting a relationship among fears of death, psychological dissociation, and posttraumatic stress disorder (PTSD). According to this model, concerns about death engender psychological dissociation, which is in turn highly predictive of the severity of PTSD symptoms. Consequently, following an MS or control induction, Kosloff and colleagues had participants complete a modified version of the Peritraumatic Dissociative Experiences Questionnaire (Marshall, Orlando, Jaycox, Foy, & Belzberg, 2002) while reflecting on their reactions to the events of 9/11. As expected, mortality-salient participants reported greater psychological dissociation than exam-salient control participants. In addition, this MS-induced increase in dissociation was found to lead to an increase in anxiety sensitivity, a variable associated with proneness to anxiety disorders (Reiss, Peterson, Gursky, & McNally, 1986). Taken together, this body of work suggests that certain forms of anxiety-related psychological disorders serve as substitutes for more constructive forms of terror management.

## TMT and Legal Decision Making

TMT also offers insights into various other applied domains of social behavior. For example, TMT provides a vehicle for understanding how extraneous psychological factors can influence jurors' decision making and thus undermine the presumption of fairness that is at the heart of legal intent. Indeed, the first study assessing the MS hypothesis was conducted with municipal court judges as subjects and found that judges reminded of their mortality subsequently rendered much higher bail recommendations for an alleged prostitute than judges who were not reminded of their mortality

(Rosenblatt et al., 1989). In recent years, trial attorneys have begun to consider the pertinence of these ideas for understanding bias and other factors in courtroom proceedings, especially as various elements of a case (e.g., charges, punishment, testimony) can serve to activate thoughts of death. Furthermore, given that the legal system is designed to allow for the application and regulation of cultural guidelines, and that mortality concerns have pervasive effects on people's affirmation of cultural beliefs, it is perhaps not surprising that a growing empirical TMT literature reveals that the awareness of death can have wide-ranging and predictable effects on legal decision making (see Arndt, Lieberman, Cook, & Solomon 2005, for a review).

MS has been found to increase punitive legal judgments of perpetrators who violate one's worldview with respect to a wide array of crimes (e.g., assault, burglary, prostitution). However, MS does not simply exacerbate punitive judgments against legal transgressors. In fact, when the victim of a crime represents a worldview threat, adopting a favorable perception of a defendant's law-breaking action may actually serve a worldview-defensive purpose. Supporting this variability of outcome perspective, Lieberman, Arndt, Personius, and Cook (2001) found that reminders of mortality led participants to increase their disdain for hate crimes when abstract views on such crimes were solicited (Study 1). However, if a specific victim was identified in a hate crime attack and represented a worldview threat to perceivers, then after MS mock jurors were more lenient in their judgments of hate crime perpetrators (Study 2). Similarly, Greenberg, Schimel, Martens, Solomon, and Pyszczynski (2001) found that white mock jurors after MS were more tolerant of a white employer facing charges of discriminatory hiring practices against blacks.

In addition, MS effects have also been observed in the context of fair process proceedings (e.g., van den Bos & Miedema, 2000) and compliance with judicial admonitions (Cook, Arndt, & Lieberman, 2004). In this latter research, Cook and colleagues (2004) built on van den Bos and Miedema's (2000) work to reason that part of the punitive reaction motivated by MS may stem from participants' supporting a worldview that prescribes what are believed to be fair and just laws. Thus Cook and colleagues found that whereas persons prone to follow their own sense of justice (rather than the substantive definition of the law) may be particularly likely to show what is known as the *backfire effect* (in which judicial instructions to ignore incriminating evidence actually backfire), MS, by increasing tendencies to adhere to admonitions about inadmissible evidence, attenuates this effect.

Thus the emerging research begins to reveal that MS may produce complex reactions depending on the motivations of the offenders and important aspects of the worldviews of those who pass judgment. Given that extant theories do not consider the role of death awareness and the motivations it provokes in legal decision making, TMT is in a unique position to offer novel insights into understanding the nature and causes of legal bias.

### Fatal Attractions: The Effect of MS on Evaluations of Charismatic Leaders

One final new line of research we'd like to describe here concerns a particularly topical matter: the role of terror management concerns in political preferences for charismatic leaders. Max Weber (1925/1968) proposed that attachment to, and enthusiasm for, charismatic leaders is amplified by psychological distress. Similarly, Fromm (1941) maintained that loyalty to charismatic leaders results from a defensive need; relinquishing individual freedom to a larger-than-life leader serves as a source of meaning and self-worth. Becker (1973), referring to examples ranging from Hitler to Gandhi, proposed that when existing bases of meaning and self-worth are lacking, the fear of death motivates devotion to supremely confident leaders who promote grand worldviews, in which life is richly meaningful and each individual can be an enduringly significant contributor to a quest for heroic triumph over evil.

Based on these ideas, Cohen, Solomon, Maxfield, Pyszczynski, and Greenberg (2004) conducted an experiment to determine if affection for charismatic leadership increases when terror management needs are activated by a reminder of mortality. After an MS or control induction, participants were exposed to short campaign statements by political candidates with different leadership styles: charismatic (portrayed as having high expectations of followers, expressing confidence in the followers' abilities, engaging in risky but calculated behavior, and emphasizing the importance of the overarching vision and identity of the group as a whole); task-oriented (characterized as setting high yet achievable goals, and effectively achieving those goals by efficient allocation of resources and delegation of responsibilities); or relationship-oriented (treating followers compassionately and respectfully, placing emphasis on communication by listening to followers, showing followers trust and confidence, and acknowledging followers with recognition and appreciation). It was predicted and found that MS produced more positive evaluations and more votes for the charismatic candidate, and more negative evaluations and fewer votes for the relationship-oriented leader. As Becker (1973) argued, for terror management purposes, people need a supremely confident leader with a grand vision who can provide self-worth through identification with the leader and the leader's vision. By emphasizing his or her own humanity and an egalitarian approach in which everyone participates, the relationship-oriented leader demystifies government; however, for terror management purposes, mystification is precisely what people desire (Becker, 1973, 1975).

Landau, Solomon, and colleagues (2004) subsequently assessed the extent to which reminders of death and vulnerability might be (at least in part) responsible for George W. Bush's striking popularity after the attacks on the Pentagon and World Trade Center in 2001. As late as September 9, 2001, President Bush was perceived by members of his party as stilted, indecisive, and lacking a commanding presence as a leader. Yet by October 2001, after he declared that God had chosen him to rid the world of evil, President Bush's approval ratings reached unprecedented levels. To determine the extent to which Bush's popularity was a terror-induced inflation, participants in two studies were asked to read a pro-Bush statement after either a typical MS induction; a parallel set of questions about the events of 9/11 ("Please describe the emotions that the thought of the terrorist attacks on September 11, 2001 arouses in you," "Write down, as specifically as you can, what happened during the terrorist attacks on September 11, 2001"; note that even subliminal presentations of 9/11 increased death thought accessibility); or an exam salience control induction. The pro-Bush statement included the following:

> . . . We need to stand behind our President and not be distracted by citizens who are less than patriotic. Ever since the attack on our country on September 11, 2001, Mr. Bush has been a source of strength and inspiration to us all. God bless him and God bless America.

Participants then rated their agreement with the statement. Consistent with the results of the charisma study, control participants were not especially enthusiastic about President Bush; however, reminders of either death or the events of 9/11 produced substantially higher support for Bush, and in a fourth study they also reduced support for the 2004 Democratic presidential nominee, John Kerry. These are ominous findings that do not bode well for the rational democracy envisioned by the Founding Fathers. They also suggest a need for further research into the role of terror management needs in the attraction of particular leaders.

## SUMMARY AND CONCLUSION

We have briefly reviewed TMT and an extensive body of research indicating that the motivation to control the potential for anxiety inherent in the awareness of mortality plays a role in self-esteem striving and defense, nationalism, prejudice, prosocial behavior, norm following, and close relationships. We have then considered three issues that have been raised regarding this work. Finally, we have presented six recent lines of research indicating a role of terror management in preference for meaning, creativity, physical health, mental health, the law, and politics. Although each of these new lines of work requires additional development, we hope that readers have found them not only provocative, but indicative of the range of relevance of terror management motivation and the value of examining motivations stemming from core existential concerns such as terror management.

To place this value in the broader context of motivation science, we conclude by returning to the question from our opening hypothetical example: Why did the businessman tie his shoes? From a TMT perspective, he did so to help him play out a role within a meaningful cultural drama that allows him to feel that he is a significant being—a person of enduring stature and value—rather than an animal product of a purposeless process of evolution fated only to the oblivion of death. This existential-level answer to this question is often not the most useful way to understand such concrete-level behavior. However, we think that the research we have reviewed shows that terror management motivation plays a role nonetheless, and that this motivation is very useful for understanding, for example, his reactions if a potentially important client notes that his shoe has come untied at a critical meeting—or, more generally, for understanding the businessman's level of creativity at work and his reactions to an economic downturn affecting his company, to rival companies, to rivals for his position in the firm, or to being laid off. When important matters such as these arise, TMT is a valuable supplement to other motivation science perspectives focused on understanding human behavior.

## REFERENCES


Arndt, J., Allen, J. J. B., & Greenberg, J. (2001). Traces of terror: Subliminal death primes and facial electromyographic indices of affect. *Motivation and Emotion, 25*, 253–277.

Arndt, J., Cook, A., Goldenberg, J. L., & Cox, C. R. (2007). Cancer and the threat of death: The cognitive dynamics of death thought suppression and its impact on behavioral health intentions. *Journal of Personality and Social Psychology, 92*, 12–29.

Arndt, J., Cook, A., & Routledge, C. (2004). The blueprint of terror management: Understanding the cognitive architecture of psychological defense against death-related thought. In J. Greenberg, S. Koole, & T. Pyszczynski (Eds.), *Handbook of empirical existential psychology* (pp. 35–53). New York: Guilford Press.

Arndt, J., Cox, C. R., Cohen, F., Goldenberg, J. L., & Routledge, C. (2007). *The effects of mortality salience, malleable standards for attractiveness, and bases of self-worth on tanning intentions.* Manuscript under review.

Arndt, J., & Greenberg, J. (1999). The effects of a self-esteem boost and mortality salience on responses to boost relevant and irrelevant worldview threats. *Personality and Social Psychology Bulletin, 25*, 1331–1341.

Arndt, J., Greenberg, J., & Cook, A. (2002). MS and the spreading activation of worldview-relevant constructs: Exploring the cognitive architecture of terror management. *Journal of Experimental Psychology: General, 131*, 307–324.

Arndt, J., Greenberg, J., Pyszczynski, T., & Solomon, S. (1997). Subliminal exposure to death-related stimuli increases defense of the cultural worldview. *Psychological Science, 8*, 379–385.

Arndt, J., Greenberg, J., Schimel, J., Pyszczynski, T., & Solomon, S. (2002). To belong or not to belong, that is the question: Terror management and identification with gender and ethnicity. *Journal of Personality and Social Psychology, 83*, 26–43.

Arndt, J., Greenberg, J., Solomon, S., Pyszczynski, T., & Schimel, J. (1999). Creativity and terror management: Evidence that creative activity increases guilt and social projection following MS. *Journal of Personality and Social Psychology, 77*, 19–32.

Arndt, J., Greenberg, J., Solomon, S., Pyszczynski, T., & Simon, L. (1997). Suppression, accessibility of death-related thoughts, and cultural worldview defense: Exploring the psychodynamics of terror management. *Journal of Personality and Social Psychology, 73*, 5–18.

Arndt, J., Lieberman, J. D., Cook, A., & Solomon, S. (2005). Terror management in the courtroom: Exploring the effects of mortality salience on legal decision-making. *Psychology, Public Policy, and Law, 11*, 407–438.

Arndt, J., Routledge, C., & Goldenberg, J. L. (2006). Predicting proximal health responses to reminders of death: The influence of coping style and health optimism. *Psychology and Health, 21*, 593–614.

Arndt, J., Routledge, C., Greenberg, J., & Sheldon, K. M. (2005). Illuminating the dark side of creative expression: Assimilation needs and the consequences of creative action following mortality salience. *Personality and Social Psychology Bulletin, 31*, 1327–1339.

Arndt, J., Routledge, C., & Vess, M. (2007). *The effect of mortality salience on creativity.* Manuscript in preparation, University of Missouri.

Arndt, J., Schimel, J., & Goldenberg, J. L. (2003). Death can be good for your health: Fitness intentions as proximal and distal defense against MS. *Journal of Applied Social Psychology, 33*, 1726–1746.

Aron, A., & Aron, E. N. (1994). Love. In A. L. Weber & J. H. Harvey (Eds.), *Perspectives on close relationships* (pp. 131–152). Boston: Allyn & Bacon.

Aronson, E., & Carlsmith, J. M. (1963). Effect of severity of threat on the devaluation of forbidden behaviour. *Journal of Abnormal and Social Behavior, 66*, 584–588.

Bargh, J. A., & Chartrand, T. L. (1999). The unbearable automaticity of being. *American Psychologist, 54*, 462–479.

Becker, E. (1971). *The birth and death of meaning* (2nd ed.). New York: Free Press.

Becker, E. (1973). *The denial of death.* New York: Academic Press.

Becker, E. (1975). *Escape from evil.* New York: Free Press.

Brehm, J. W. (1956). Postdecisional changes in the desirability of alternatives. *Journal of Abnormal and Social Psychology, 52*, 384–389.

Bruner, J. (1996). Foreword. In B. Shore, *Culture in mind: Cognition, culture and problem of meaning* (p. xv). New York: Oxford University Press.

Burns, G. L., Keortge, S. G., Formea, G. M., & Sternberger, L. G. (1996). Revision of the Padua Inventory of obsessive compulsive disorder symptoms: Distinctions between worry obsessions, and compulsions. *Behaviour Research and Therapy, 34*, 163–173.

Carver, C. S., & Scheier, M. F. (1981). *Attention and self-regulation: A control theory approach to human behavior.* New York: Springer-Verlag.

Cesario, J., Plaks, J. E., & Higgins, E. T. (2006). Automatic social behavior as motivated preparation to interact. *Journal of Personality and Social Psychology, 90*(6), 893–910.

Chaudary, N., Tison, J., & Solomon, S. (2002). *What's death got to do with it?: The role of psychological uncertainty on implicit death thoughts.* Paper presented at the annual meeting of the American Psychological Society, New Orleans, LA.

Cohen, F., Solomon, S., Maxfield, M., Pyszczynski, T., & Greenberg, J. (2004). Fatal attraction: The effects of mortality salience on evaluations of charismatic, task-oriented, and relationship-oriented leaders. *Psychological Science, 15*, 846–851.

Cook, A., Arndt, J., & Lieberman, J. D. (2004). Backing off the backfire effect: The role of mortality salience and nullification beliefs on the influence of inadmissible evidence. *Law and Human Behavior, 28*, 389–410.

Cox, C. R., Arndt, J., Pyszczynski, T., Greenberg, J., & Solomon, S. (2007). *Terror management and adults' attachment to their parents: The safe haven remains.* Unpublished manuscript, University of Missouri, Columbia.

Cox, C. R., Goldenberg, J. L., Arndt, J., & Pyszczynski, T. (2007). Mother's milk?: The influence of mortality salience on reactions to breastfeeding. *Personality and Social Psychology Bulletin, 33*, 110–122.

Deacon, T. (1997). *The symbolic species: The co-evolution of language and the brain.* New York: Norton.

Dechesne, M., Janssen, J., & van Knippenberg, A. (2000). Defense and distancing as terror management strategies: The moderating role of need for structure and permeability of group boundaries. *Journal of Personality and Social Psychology, 79*, 923–932.

Deci, E. L., & Ryan, R. M. (2002). *Handbook of self-determination research.* Rochester, NY: University of Rochester Press.

Donald, M. (1991). *Origins of the modern mind: Three stages in the evolution of culture and cognition.* Cambridge, MA: Harvard University Press.

Florian, V., & Mikulincer, M. (2004). A multifaceted perspective on the existential meanings, manifestations, and consequences of the fear of personal death. In J. Greenberg, S. L. Koole, & T. Pyszczynski (Eds.), *Handbook of experimental existential psychology* (pp. 54–70). New York: Guilford Press.

Fromm, E. (1941). *Escape from freedom.* New York: Holt.

Gershuny, B. S., & Thayer, J. F. (1999). Relations among psychological trauma, dissociative phenomena, and trauma-related distress: A review and integration. *Clinical Psychology Review, 19*(5), 631–657.

Goldenberg, J. L., Arndt, J., Hart, J., & Brown, M. (2005). Dying to be thin: The effects of mortality salience and body-mass-index on restricted eating among women. *Personality and Social Psychology Bulletin, 31*, 1400–1412.

Goldenberg, J. L., Arndt, J., Hart, J., & Routledge, C. (in press). Uncovering an existential barrier to breast self-exam behavior. *Journal of Experimental Social Psychology.*

Goldenberg, J. L., McCoy, S. K., Pyszczynski, T., Greenberg, J., & Solomon, S. (2000). The body as a source of self-esteem: The effects of mortality salience on identification with one's body, interest in sex, and appearance monitoring. *Journal of Personality and Social Psychology, 79*, 118–130.

Goldenberg, J. L., Pyszczynski, T., Greenberg, J., & Solomon, S. (2000). Fleeing the body: A terror management perspective on the problem of human corporeality. *Personality and Social Psychology Review, 4*, 200–218.

Greenberg, J., Arndt, J., Simon, L., Pyszczynski, T., & Solomon, S. (2000). Proximal and distal defenses in response to reminders of one's mortality: Evidence of a temporal sequence. *Personality and Social Psychology Bulletin, 26*, 91–99.

Greenberg, J., Kosloff, S., Solomon, S., & Cohen, F. (2007). *Star light, star bright: The effect of mortality salience on the appeal of fame and celebrity.* Manuscript submitted for publication.

Greenberg, J., Martens, A., Jonas, E., Eisenstadt, D., Pyszczynski, T., & Solomon, S. (2003). Detoxifying thoughts of death: Eliminating the potential for anxiety eliminates the effects of mortality salience on worldview defense. *Psychological Science, 14*, 516–519.

Greenberg, J., Pyszczynski, T., & Solomon, S. (1995). Toward a dual-motive depth psychology of self and human behavior. In M. H. Kernis (Ed.), *Efficacy, agency, and self-esteem* (pp. 73–99). New York: Plenum Press.

Greenberg, J., Pyszczynski, T., Solomon, S., Pinel, E., Simon, L., & Jordan, K. (1993). Effects of self-esteem on vulnerability-denying defensive distortions: Further evidence of an anxiety-buffering function of self-esteem. *Journal of Experimental Social Psychology, 29*, 229–251.

Greenberg, J., Pyszczynski, T., Solomon, S., Simon, L., & Breus, M. (1994). Role of consciousness and accessibility of death-related thoughts in mortality salience effects. *Journal of Personality and Social Psychology, 67*, 627–637.

Greenberg, J., Schimel, J., Martens, A., Solomon, S., & Pyszcznyski, T. (2001). Sympathy for the devil: Evidence that reminding whites of their mortality promotes more favorable reactions to white racists. *Motivation and Emotion, 25*, 113–133.

Greenberg, J., Solomon, S., & Pyszczynski, T. (1997). Terror management theory of self-esteem and social behavior: Empirical assessments and conceptual refinements. In M. P. Zanna (Ed.), *Advances in experimental social psychology* (Vol. 29, pp. 61–139). San Diego, CA: Academic Press.

Greenberg, J., Solomon, S., Pyszczynski, T., Rosenblatt, A., Burling, J., Lyon, D., et al. (1992). Assessing the terror management analysis of self-esteem: Converging evidence of an anxiety-buffering function.

*Journal of Personality and Social Psychology, 63*, 913–922.

Harmon-Jones, E., Simon, L., Greenberg, J., Pyszczynski, T., Solomon, S., & McGregor, H. (1997). Terror management theory and self-esteem: Evidence that increased self-esteem reduces mortality salience effects. *Journal of Personality and Social Psychology, 72*, 24–36.

Harris, M. (1979). *Cultural materialism: The struggle for a science of culture*. New York: Random House.

Helmuth, L. (2001). New route to big brains. *Science, 293*, 1746–1747.

Hirschberger, G. (2006). Terror management and attribution of blame to innocent victims: Reconciling compassionate and defensive responses. *Journal of Personality and Social Psychology, 91*, 832–844.

James, K., & Greenberg, J. (1989). Ingroup salience, intergroup comparison, individual performance and self-esteem. *Personality and Social Psychology Bulletin, 15*, 604–616.

Jonas, E., & Greenberg, J. (2004). Terror management and political attitudes: The influence of mortality salience on Germans' defence of the German reunification. *European Journal of Social Psychology, 34*, 1–9.

Jonas, E., Martens, A., Johns, M., Greenberg, J., & Reiss, L. (2007). *Focus theory of normative conduct and terror management theory: The interactive impact of mortality salience and salient norms on social judgment and behavior.* Unpublished manuscript, Salzburg, Austria.

Jonas, E., Schimel, J., Greenberg, J., & Pyszczynski, T. (2002). The Scrooge effect: Evidence that mortality salience increases prosocial attitudes and behavior. *Personality and Social Psychology Bulletin, 28*, 1342–1353.

Kanazawa, S. (2004). General intelligence as a domain-specific adaptation. *Psychological Review, 111*, 512–523.

Kosloff, S., Solomon, S., Greenberg, J., Cohen, F., Gershuny, B., Routledge, C., et al. (In press). Fatal distraction: The impact of mortality salience on dissociative responses to 9/11 and subsequent anxiety sensitivity. *Basic and Applied Social Psychology.*

Kunda, Z. (1990). The case for motivated reasoning. *Psychological Bulletin, 108*, 480–496.

Landau, M., Greenberg, J., Pyszczynski, T., Solomon, S., & Martens, A. (2007). *Death, structure, and complexity of the self-concept*. Unpublished manuscript, University of Arizona.

Landau, M. J., Greenberg, J., Arndt, J., & Routledge, C. (2006). *Marking time: Managing mortality through meaningful conceptions of time and the self in time.* Manuscript submitted for publication.

Landau, M. J., Greenberg, J., Solomon, S., Pyszczynski, T., & Martens, A. (2006). Windows into nothingness: Terror management, meaninglessness, and negative reactions to modern art. *Journal of Personality and Social Psychology, 90*, 879–892.

Landau, M. J., Johns, M., Greenberg, J., Pyszczynski, T., Solomon, S., & Martens, A. (2004). A function of form: Terror management and structuring of the social world. *Journal of Personality and Social Psychology, 87*, 190–210.

Landau, M. J., Solomon, S., Greenberg, J., Cohen, F., Pyszczynski, T., Arndt, J., et al. (2004). Deliver us from evil: The effects of mortality salience and reminders of 9/11 on support for President George W. Bush. *Personality and Social Psychology Bulletin, 30*, 1136–1150.

Langer, S. K. (1975). *Mind: An essay on human feeling* (Vol. 1). Baltimore: Johns Hopkins University Press.

Lieberman, J. D., Arndt, J., Personius, J., & Cook, A. (2001). Vicarious annihilation: The effect of MS on perceptions of hate crimes. *Law and Human Behavior, 25*, 547–566.

Lifton, R. J. (1968). *Revolutionary immortality.* New York: Random House.

Marshall, G. N., Orlando, M., Jaycox, L. H., Foy, D. W., & Belzberg, H. (2002). Development and validation of a modified version of the Peritraumatic Dissociative Experiences Questionnaire. *Psychological Assessment, 14*(2), 123–134.

Maslow, A. H. (1970). *Motivation and personality* (2nd ed.). New York: Harper & Row.

McGregor, I., Zanna, M. P., Holmes, J. G., & Spencer, S. J. (2001). Compensatory conviction in the face of personal uncertainty: Going to extremes and being oneself. *Journal of Personality and Social Psychology, 80*, 472–488.

McKoon, G., & Ratcliff, R. (1992). Spreading activation versus compound cue accounts of priming: Mediated priming revisited. *Journal of Experimental Psychology: Learning, Memory, and Cognition, 18*, 1155–1172.

Mikulincer, M., & Florian, V. (2002). The effect of mortality salience on self-serving attributions: Evidence for the function of self-esteem as a terror management mechanism. *Basic and Applied Social Psychology, 24*, 261–271.

Mikulincer, M., Florian, V., & Hirschberger, G. (2003). The existential function of close relationships: Introducing death into the science of love. *Personality and Social Psychology Review, 7*, 20–40.

Nisbett, R. E., & Wilson, T. D. (1977). Telling more than we can know: Verbal reports on mental processes. *Psychological Review, 84*, 231–259.

Peters, H. J., Greenberg, J., Williams, J. M., & Schneider, N. R. (2005). Applying terror management theory to performance: Can reminding individuals of their mortality increase strength output? *Journal of Sport and Exercise Psychology, 27*, 111–116.

Powers, W. T. (1973). *Behavior: The control of perception.* Chicago: Aldine.

Powers, W. T. (1978). Quantitative analysis of purposive systems: Some spadework at foundations of scientific psychology. *Psychological Review, 85*, 417–435.

Pyszczynski, T., Abdollahi, A., Solomon, S., Greenberg, J., Cohen, F., & Weise, D. (2006). Mortality salience, martyrdom, and military might: The Great Satan versus the Axis of Evil. *Personality and Social Psychology Bulletin, 32*, 525–537.

Pyszczynski, T., & Greenberg, J. (1992). *Hanging on and letting go: Understanding the onset, progression, and remission of depression.* New York: Springer-Verlag.

Pyszczynski, T., Greenberg, J., & Goldenberg, J. L. (2003). Freedom versus fear: On the defense, growth, and expansion of the self. In M. R. Leary & J. P. Tangney (Eds.) *Handbook of self and identity* (pp. 314–343). New York: Guilford Press.

Pyszczynski, T., Greenberg, J., & Solomon, S. (1997). Why do we need what we need?: A terror management perspective on the roots of human social motivation. *Psychological Inquiry, 8*, 1–21.

Pyszczynski, T., Greenberg, J., & Solomon, S. (1999). A dual-process model of defense against conscious and unconscious death-related thoughts: An extension of terror management theory. *Psychological Bulletin, 106*, 835–845.

Pyszczynski, T., Greenberg, J., Solomon, S., Arndt, J., & Schimel, J. (2004). Why do people need self-esteem?: A theoretical and empirical review. *Psychological Bulletin, 130*, 435–468.

Pyszczynski, T., Greenberg, J., Solomon, S., & Maxfield, M. (in press). On the unique psychological import of the human awareness of mortality: Theme and variations. *Psychological Inquiry.*

Pyszczynski, T., Solomon, S., & Greenberg, J. (2003). *In the wake of 9/11: The psychology of terror.* Washington, DC: American Psychological Association.

Rank, O. (1941). *Beyond psychology.* New York: Dover.

Reiss, S., Peterson, R. A., Gursky, D. M., & McNally, R. J. (1986). Anxiety sensitivity, anxiety frequency, and predictions of fearfulness. *Behaviour Research and Therapy, 24*, 1–8.

Rosenblatt, A., Greenberg, J., Solomon, S., Pyszczynski, T., & Lyon, D. (1989). Evidence for terror management theory: I. The effects of MS on reactions to those who violate or uphold cultural values. *Journal of Personality and Social Psychology, 57*, 681–690.

Routledge, C., & Arndt, J. (2007). *Self-sacrifice as self-defense: Mortality salience increases efforts to affirm a symbolic immortal self at the expense of the physical self.* Manuscript submitted for publication.

Routledge, C., Arndt, J., & Goldenberg, J. L. (2004). A time to tan: Proximal and distal effects of mortality salience on sun exposure intentions. *Personality and Social Psychology Bulletin, 30*, 1347–1358.

Routledge, C., Arndt, J., & Sheldon, K. M. (2004). Task engagement after mortality salience: The effects of creativity, conformity, and connectedness on worldview defense. *European Journal of Social Psychology, 34*, 477–487.

Schimel, J., Hayes, J., Williams, T., & Jahrig, J. (2007). Is death really the worm at the core?: Converging evidence that worldview threat increases death-thought accessibility. *Journal of Personality and Social Psychology, 92*, 789–803.

Schimel, J., Simon, L., Greenberg, J., Pyszczynski, T., Solomon, S., Waxmonski, J., et al. (1999). Support for a functional perspective on stereotypes: Evidence that mortality salience enhances stereotypic thinking and preferences. *Journal of Personality and Social Psychology, 77*, 905–926.

Simon, L., Arndt, J., Greenberg, J., Solomon, S., & Pyszczynski, T. (1998). Terror management and meaning: Evidence that the opportunity to defend the worldview in response to mortality salience increases the meaningfulness of life in the mildly depressed. *Journal of Personality, 66*, 359–382.

Simon, L., Greenberg, J., Arndt, J., Pyszczynski, T., Clement, R., & Solomon, S. (1997). Perceived consensus, uniqueness, and terror management: Compensatory responses to threats to inclusion and distinctiveness following mortality salience. *Personality and Social Psychology Bulletin, 23*, 1055–1065.

Simon, L., Greenberg, J., Harmon-Jones, E., Solomon, S., Pyszczynski, T., Arndt, J., et al. (1997). Cognitive–experiential self-theory and terror management theory: Evidence that terror management occurs in the experiential system. *Journal of Personality and Social Psychology, 72*, 1132–1146.

Solomon, S., Greenberg, J., & Pyszczynski, T. (1997). Return of the living dead. *Psychological Inquiry, 8*, 59–71.

Strachan, E., Arndt, J., Schimel, J., Solomon, S., Pyszczynski, T., & Greenberg, J. (In press). Evidence that mortality salience intensifies phobic and compulsive behavior: Terror mismanagement. *Personality and Social Psychology Bulletin.*

Taubman Ben-Ari, O., Florian, V., & Mikulincer, M. (1999). The impact of mortality salience on reckless driving: A test of terror management mechanisms. *Journal of Personality and Social Psychology, 76*, 35–45.

Vallacher, R. R., & Wegner, D. M. (1987). What do people think they're doing?: Action identification and human behavior. *Psychological Review, 94*, 3–15.

van den Bos, K., & Miedema, J. (2000). Toward understanding why fairness matters: The influence of MS on reactions to procedural fairness. *Journal of Personality and Social Psychology, 79*, 355–366.

Weber, M. (1968). The types of legitimate domination. In G. Roth & C. Wittich (Eds.), *Economy and society: An outline of interpretive sociology* (pp. 212–301). New York: Bedminster Press. (Original work published 1925)

Wegner, D. M. (1992). You can't always think what you want: Problems in the suppression of unwanted thoughts. In M. P. Zanna (Ed.), *Advances in experimental social psychology* (Vol. 25, pp. 193–225). San Diego, CA: Academic Press.

Wegner, D. M., & Smart, L. (1997). Deep cognitive activation: A new approach to the unconscious. *Journal of Consulting and Clinical Psychology, 65*, 984–995.

Yalom, I. (1980). *Existential psychotherapy.* New York: Basic Books.

Chapter 9

# Prosocial Motivation

C. Daniel Batson
Nadia Ahmad
Adam A. Powell
E. L. Stocks

At times, people can do spectacular things for others. Soldiers have been known to throw themselves on live grenades to protect their comrades. Mother Teresa dedicated her life to the dying of Calcutta, the poorest of the poor, and brought care and comfort to thousands. Rescuers of Jews in Nazi Europe, such as Miep Gies (who helped hide Anne Frank and her parents), Oskar Schindler, and Raoul Wallenberg, risked their own lives—and often the lives of their loved ones—day after day for months, even years.

## THE QUESTION OF PROSOCIAL MOTIVATION: WHY DO WE HELP OTHERS?

Such examples are heartwarming, even inspiring. For the social psychologist, they are also puzzling. They raise the question of prosocial motivation—the question of why we humans do what we do for others. This question is not about the magnitude or intensity of prosocial motivation; it is about the nature. Clearly, we humans can and do act to benefit others. But why? Do we help simply because in some more or less subtle way it promotes our own self-interest? Or can we be motivated to promote the interests of others too? If so, which others—our immediate family, our friends, our nation, all humanity? Can we be motivated to be moral? Answers to these questions tell us something about how truly social we humans really are, or are capable of becoming. Behind the question of prosocial motivation is, then, an even more fundamental question of human nature.

In the past three decades, a number of social psychologists have begun a serious attempt to provide answers to such questions. These social psychologists have drawn heavily on general theories of motivation, especially those stemming from the work of Sigmund Freud, Clark Hull, and various social learning theorists (e.g.,

Dollard & Miller; Bandura). But they have been most importantly influenced by the motivational theories of Kurt Lewin.

## MOTIVES AS GOAL-DIRECTED FORCES TO OBTAIN OR MAINTAIN VALUED STATES

Following Lewin (1951), social psychologists seeking to address the question of prosocial motivation have typically viewed motives as goal-directed forces to obtain or maintain valued states. If a negative discrepancy is perceived between a current or anticipated state and a valued (desired, preferred) state, then obtaining or maintaining the valued state is likely to become a goal.

### Ultimate Goals, Instrumental Goals, and Unintended Consequences

It is possible—and important—to distinguish among ultimate goals, instrumental goals, and unintended consequences (see Heider, 1958; Lewin, 1951). *Ultimate goals* are the valued states the individual is seeking to reach. *Ultimate* does not here mean "cosmic" or "most important"; it simply refers to the state or states a person is seeking at a given time. It is the ultimate goal that defines a motive; each different motive has a unique ultimate goal evoked by an opportunity to obtain or maintain some valued state.

*Instrumental goals* are sought because they are steppingstones to ultimate goals. When the ultimate goal can be reached more efficiently by other means, an instrumental goal is likely to be bypassed. Pursuit of a goal, whether instrumental or ultimate, may produce effects—sometimes dramatic—that are not themselves a goal. These are *unintended consequences*. It is possible to benefit others as an unintended consequence of pursuing some other goal, such as some form of self-benefit. (For further discussion of the relations among valued states, goals, and motives, see Batson, 1991, 1994.)

A major implication that both Lewin (1951) and Heider (1958) wished to draw from the distinctions among ultimate goals, instrumental goals, and unintended consequences was the importance of focusing on motives rather than on behavior or consequences, even if one's goal is to understand the occurrence of some behavior, such as helping others. Behavior is highly variable. Whether a given behavior will occur in a given situation depends on the strength of some motive that might evoke that behavior, as well as on (1) the strength of complementary and competing motives, if any; (2) how the behavior relates to each of these motives; and (3) the other behavioral options available in the situation at the time. The more directly a given behavior promotes an ultimate goal, and the more uniquely it does so among the behavioral options available, the more likely it is to occur. Behavior that promotes an instrumental goal can easily change if the causal association between the instrumental and ultimate goal changes, or if behavioral pathways to the ultimate goal arise that bypass the instrumental goal. Unintended consequences can easily change as the behavioral options change, unless these consequences are a product of some behavior that directly and uniquely promotes the ultimate goal. Invariance (and explanatory stability) is found not in behavior or consequences, but in the link of a given motive to its ultimate goal (Lewin, 1951).

### Multiple Motives: Cooperation, Conflict, and Change

An individual often has more than one ultimate goal at a time, and so more than one motive. When this occurs, these motives may cooperate or conflict. Moreover, a person's motives can change over time, often quickly. The value placed on some states is relatively stable, producing enduring motives. The value placed on other states is more changeable; opportunities to obtain or maintain these states elicit motives only in certain situations.

### Motives as Situational Forces, Not Dispositions or Needs

This Lewinian perspective on motivation can be contrasted with the perspective of another pioneer in research on motivation, Henry Murray. Lewin (1951) treated goals as force fields within the current life space of the individual; he treated motives as goal-directed forces in these fields; and he treated valued states as power fields that could, under the appropriate circumstances, activate motivational forces. These motivational forces could in turn produce behavior, or movement within the life space. Murray (1938) and his followers treated motives as relatively stable dispositions or needs (e.g., achievement motivation), similar to valued states rather than to motives in Lewin's framework. As noted, Lewin made much of the distinction among instrumental goals, ultimate goals, and unintended consequences; Murray gave little attention to these distinctions. For Lewin, the list of potential motives is endless; it is as rich and varied as one's preferences. Murray and his followers attempted to identify a relatively small number of primary motives.

In the pages that follow, we wish to consider four possible ultimate goals of acting to benefit someone else: self-benefit (*egoism*), benefiting another individual (*altruism*), benefiting a group (*collectivism*), and upholding a moral principle (*principlism*). These goals are not mutually exclusive; any or all might be ultimate goals of acting to benefit another person. The four ultimate goals define four distinct forms of prosocial motivation.

## FOUR ANSWERS TO THE QUESTION OF WHY WE HELP OTHERS

### Egoism: Benefiting Another as a Means to Benefit Oneself

Humans are clearly capable of benefiting others as a means of benefiting themselves. When the ultimate goal is self-benefit, the motivation is egoistic. This is true no matter how beneficial to others or how noble the helping behavior may be.

The list of self-benefits that can motivate helping is long. Table 9.1 lists those self-benefits for which there is clear empirical evidence (for reviews, see Batson, 1998; Dovidio, Piliavin, Schroeder, & Penner, 2006). The list is organized into three general categories, reflecting three fundamental forms of egoistic motivation: (1) to gain material, social, or self-rewards (the entries in Table 9.1 are organized in rough order of material, then social, then self-rewards); (2) to avoid material, social, and self-punishments (again, in rough order); and (3) to reduce aversive arousal. In each case, benefiting another is an instrumental goal that is sought as a means to reach the ultimate goal specified.

**TABLE 9.1. Possible Self-Benefits from Benefiting Another**

| | |
|---|---|
| 1. Receiving material, social, and self-rewards | |
| Payment | Praise |
| Gifts | Honor |
| Reciprocity credit | Enhanced self-image |
| Thanks | Mood enhancement (maintenance) |
| Esteem | Empathic joy |
| Heaven | |
| 2. Avoiding material, social, and self-punishments | |
| Fines/imprisonment | Recrimination |
| Attack | Sanctions for norm violation |
| Hell | Shame |
| Censure | Guilt |
| 3. Reducing aversive arousal | |
| Escape from distressing situation | |
| Escape from discrepant situation | |
| Escape from unjust situation | |

#### Gaining Rewards

Among the rewards that a helper may seek, perhaps the only three that need any explanation are reciprocity credit, mood enhancement (maintenance), and empathic joy.

*Reciprocity Credit.* Reciprocity credit is the self-benefit of knowing that the person you have benefited owes you a favor. Sociologist Alvin Gouldner (1960) identified what he called the "universal norm of reciprocity"—the norm that for a benefit received, an equivalent benefit ought eventually to be returned. After reviewing the evidence, Gouldner concluded that "a norm of reciprocity is, I suspect, no less universal and important an element of culture than the incest taboo" (1960, p. 171). Gouldner assumed that this norm is instilled through socialization, but evolutionary biologist Robert Trivers (1971) suggested that it may have a genetic base.

Reciprocity credit can lead us to look for an opportunity to help someone from whom we want some reward in the future, as occurs with ingratiation (Jones, 1964). It may also lead at least some of us to help others whom we know cannot reciprocate. We may help them because of belief in generalized reciprocity—that we get in equal measure to what we give to the world in general (Zuckerman, 1975). Or it may lead us to help to establish a reputation as trustworthy that will encourage others to help us in the future (Frank, 1988).

*Mood Enhancement (Maintenance).* Mood enhancement can also be a reason for helping.

Cialdini, Darby, and Vincent (1973) proposed that we are more likely to help someone when we feel bad because we know that we can give ourselves a pat on the back when we do something nice like helping, and this will make us feel better. Consistent with this *negative-state relief model*, Cialdini and colleagues found that people who felt bad because they had accidentally harmed someone—or had seen another person harm someone—were more likely to volunteer to make phone calls for a worthy cause than were people who did not feel bad. But when people who felt bad had their negative state relieved by receiving praise or a dollar before being given the chance to volunteer, they did not help more.

Not only does helping have reward value for a person feeling bad, but it also seems to be rewarding for persons who feel good. Indeed, the effect seems even stronger when people are in a good mood. Alice Isen and her associates used a number of clever techniques to enhance people's moods—having them succeed at a task, giving them a cookie while they studied in the library, having them find a coin in the return slot of a public telephone. She found that each of these experiences increased the likelihood of a person's giving help to good causes (Isen, 1970; Isen & Levin, 1972).

What accounts for this pervasive reward value of helping for people in a good mood? One possibility is desire for good-mood maintenance. Seeing another person in need can throw a wet blanket on a good mood, so one may help in order to shed this blanket and maintain the mood (Isen & Levin, 1972; Wegener & Petty, 1994). Isen (1987; Isen, Shalker, Clark, & Karp, 1978) has also suggested a second possibility: Being in a good mood may bias one's memory about the positive and negative aspects of various activities, including helping. Isen has suggested that people in a good mood are more likely to recall and attend to positive rather than negative aspects of their lives. Applied to helping, this makes such people more likely to remember and attend to the positive, rewarding features, and less likely to attend to the negative features, such as the costs involved (see also Berkowitz, 1987; Clark & Waddell, 1983; Cunningham, Shaffer, Barbee, Wolff, & Kelley, 1990).

*Empathic Joy.* Empathic joy is the vicarious feeling of pleasure one has at seeing a person in need experience relief. As Hoffman (1981) described it, "When the victim shows visible signs of relief or joy after being helped, the helper may actually feel empathic joy. Having experienced empathic joy, he or she may subsequently be motivated to help in order to experience it again" (p. 135). At the time Hoffman wrote, there was no empirical evidence for the existence of such a motive; now there is (Batson et al., 1991; Smith, Keating, & Stotland, 1989). Interestingly, the evidence suggests that seeking empathic joy is a motive among individuals feeling little empathic concern for the person in need, but is not a motive among individuals feeling a lot of concern.

### Avoiding Punishments

Probably the only punishments listed in Table 9.1 that need explanation are fines/imprisonment and sanctions for norm violation.

*Fines/Imprisonment.* In some countries, especially in Europe, there are Good Samaritan laws. If people fail to offer aid when (1) someone else's life is in danger, (2) there is no serious risk for them, and (3) no one better qualified is available, then they are liable for a fine or a jail sentence. The reason for these laws is, of course, to motivate people to help in order to avoid these penalties.

*Sanctions for Norm Violation.* A number of social norms apply to helping. They dictate that we should help people in need—at least some people under some circumstances—lest we suffer socially administered or self-administered sanctions. One norm already mentioned is the norm of reciprocity. In addition to leading us to expect repayment when we help, this norm dictates that we should help those who help us. Although Gouldner (1960) believed that the norm of reciprocity is universal, he also believed that the pressure on us to help in return depends on the circumstances under which we received help: (1) how badly we needed help; (2) our perception of how much the other person gave us, relative to his or her total resources; (3) our perception of the other person's motives for helping (e.g., was it a bribe?); and (4) whether the other person helped voluntarily or was pressured into it. Research supports each of Gouldner's beliefs (see, e.g., Gergen, Ellsworth, Maslach, & Seipel, 1975; Pruitt, 1968; Wilke & Lanzetta, 1970).

A second norm that psychologists have suggested motivates helping is the norm of social responsibility. This norm tells us that we should help when a person in need is dependent upon us—that is, when no one else is available to help and so the person is counting specifically on us. Although such a norm does seem to exist, its effect has been surprisingly difficult to demonstrate. After over a decade of research, Berkowitz (1972) concluded, "The findings do not provide any clear-cut support for the normative analysis of help-giving. . . . The potency of the conjectured 'social responsibility norm' was greatly exaggerated" (pp. 68, 77).

Why has evidence that the norm of social responsibility motivates helping been so hard to find? Darley and Latané (1970) suggested that this norm may be at once too general and too specific. The norm may be too general in that everyone in our society adheres to it. If this is true, then it cannot account for why one person helps and another does not. The norm may also be too specific in that along with it comes a complex pattern of exceptions—situations in which an individual may feel exempt from acting in accordance with the norm. The norm may be characterized not simply by a rule that says, "If someone is dependent on you for help, then help," but by a more complex rule that says, "If someone is dependent on you for help, then help, *except when* . . . " Exceptions may vary for different individuals and social situations.

Other researchers have suggested that the problem with social norms may lie in our focus of attention. Only when our attention is focused on a particular norm as a standard for our behavior is concern about violating it likely to motivate our behavior (Cialdini, Kallgren, & Reno, 1991). Consistent with this suggestion, Gibbons and Wicklund (1982) found that if standards of helpfulness were salient, then focusing on oneself increased helping. However, in the absence of salient standards for helpfulness, people who were self-focused were *less* helpful than people who were not self-focused.

### *Reducing Aversive Arousal*

The three self-benefits under "Reducing aversive arousal" in Table 9.1 may be less familiar than the self-benefits under rewards and punishments. The general idea of aversive-arousal reduction is that it is upsetting to see someone else suffer, and people prefer not to be upset. To eliminate this aversive arousal, one option is to relieve the other person's suffering because it is the stimulus causing one's own suffering. Once again, the prosocial aspect of this motivation is instrumental, not ultimate; the ultimate goal is the self-benefit of having one's own discomfort go away.

Each of the three self-benefits listed in this category in Table 9.1 is based on the assumption that witnessing another in distress is aversive; yet each specifies a different form of aversive arousal.

*Escaping One's Own Distress.* Most straightforward is the possibility suggested by Piliavin, Dovidio, Gaertner, and Clark (1981); Hoffman (1981); and Dovidio, Piliavin, Gaertner, Schroeder, and Clark (1991), among others. They propose that the witness's vicarious distress has much the same character as the victim's distress; both are aversive, and the witness is motivated to escape his or her own distress. One way to escape is to help, because helping terminates the stimulus causing the distress. Of course, running away may enable the witness to escape just as well and at less cost, as long as the principle "out of sight, out of mind" works.

*Escaping Discrepancy.* Janusz Reykowski (1982) proposed a quite different source of prosocial motivation, but still one that involves reduction of an aversive tension state: "The sheer discrepancy between information about the real or possible state of an object and standards of its normal or desirable state will evoke motivation" (p. 361). Reykowski applied this general psychological principle—which is closely akin to cognitive dissonance (Festinger, 1957)—to prosocial motivation as follows: If a person perceives a discrepancy between the current state and the expected or ideal state of another person (i.e., perceives the other to be in need), then this will produce cognitive inconsistency and motivation to reduce this uncomfortable inconsistency. Relieving the other's need by helping is one way to remove the inconsistency and escape the discrepant situation. Another, less prosocial way is to change one's perception and decide that the other's suffering is acceptable, even desirable. This has been called "blaming the victim" (Ryan, 1971).

*Escaping Injustice.* Melvin Lerner's (1980) just-world hypothesis led him to a similar but more specific view. If one believes in a just world—a world in which people get what they deserve and deserve what they get—then witnessing an innocent victim suffer should be upsetting because it threatens this belief. In order to reduce the discomfort produced by this threat, one may help the victim. Once again, however, there is an alternative way to escape the aversive arousal. It is possible to derogate or blame the victim; if the victim is a less deserving person, then his or her suffering is more just and less upsetting. Consistent with Lerner's analysis, research suggests that if people can easily help in order to relieve the suffering of an innocent victim, they are likely to do so, but if they cannot easily help, they are likely to derogate the victim (Lerner & Simmons, 1966; Mills & Egger, 1972).

## Altruism: Benefiting Another as an Ultimate Goal

Both for philosophers through the ages and for behavioral and social scientists today, the most intriguing and the most controversial form of prosocial motivation is altruism. Is it really possible for one person to have another person's welfare as an ultimate goal, rather than simply as an instrumental means of reaching the ultimate goal of one or another form of self-benefit?

One response to this question needs to be laid to rest at the outset. It goes like this: Even if it were possible for a person to be motivated to increase another's welfare, such a person would be pleased by attaining this desired goal, so even this apparent altruism would actually be a product of egoism. This argument, based on the general principle of *psychological hedonism*, is, in the words of Edward Tolman's (1923) well-turned epithet, "more brilliant than cogent" (p. 203). Philosophers have pointed out that it involves a confusion between two different forms of hedonism. The *strong* form of psychological hedonism asserts that attainment of personal pleasure is always the goal of human action; the *weak* form asserts only that goal attainment always brings pleasure. The weak form is not inconsistent with the possibility of altruism (i.e., that one can have an ultimate goal to benefit another rather than to benefit oneself); the pleasure obtained can be a consequence of reaching the goal without being the goal itself. The strong form of psychological hedonism is inconsistent with the possibility of altruism, but to affirm this form of hedonism is simply to assert that altruism does not exist. It is an empirical assertion that may or may not be true. (See MacIntyre, 1967, and Sober & Wilson, 1998, for discussions of these philosophical arguments.)

Advocates of universal egoism argue for the strong form of psychological hedonism. They assert that some self-benefit is always the ultimate goal of helping; benefiting the other is simply an instrumental goal on the way to one or another ultimately self-serving end. They remind us of all the self-benefits of helping, such as those listed in Table 9.1. Advocates of altruism argue back that simply to show that self-benefits follow from benefiting someone does not prove that the self-benefits were the ultimate goal. It is at least logically possible that the self-benefits are unintended consequences of reaching the ultimate goal of benefiting the other. If so, then the motivation is altruistic, not egoistic.

Advocates of altruism claim more than logical possibility, of course. They claim that altruistic motivation is an empirical reality, that at least some people under some circumstances act with an ultimate goal of increasing another person's welfare. They claim that people can want another person to be happy and free of distress, not because it is upsetting to them if he or she is not (although it may be upsetting), but because they care about the other's welfare as an end in itself.

### *The Empathy–Altruism Hypothesis*

Over the centuries, the most frequently proposed source of altruistic motivation has been an other-oriented emotional response congruent with the perceived welfare of another person—today usually called *empathy* (Batson, 1987) or *sympathy* (Wispé, 1986). If another person is in need, then empathic feelings include sympathy, compassion, tenderness, and the like. These feelings appear to be a product not only of perceiving the other as in need, but also of valuing the other's welfare (Batson, Eklund, Chermok, Hoyt, & Ortiz, 2007; Batson, Turk, Shaw, & Klein, 1995). The *empathy–altruism hypothesis* claims that these other-oriented feelings produce motivation with an ultimate goal of relieving the valued other's need—that is, altruistic motivation. Various forms of this hypothesis have been espoused by Thomas Aquinas, David Hume,

Adam Smith, Charles Darwin, Herbert Spencer, and William McDougall, and in contemporary psychology by Hoffman (1975), Krebs (1975), and Batson (1987).

Considerable evidence supports the idea that feeling empathy for a person in need leads to increased helping of that person (Coke, Batson, & McDavis, 1978; Dovidio, Allen, & Schroeder, 1990; Krebs, 1975; for reviews, see Batson, 1991; Eisenberg & Miller, 1987). To observe an empathy–helping relationship, however, tells us nothing about the nature of the motivation that underlies this relationship. Relieving the other person's need could be (1) an ultimate goal, producing self-benefits as unintended consequences; (2) an instrumental goal sought as a means to reach the ultimate goal of gaining one or more self-benefits; or (3) both. That is, the motivation could be altruistic, egoistic, or both.

### *Egoistic Alternatives to the Empathy–Altruism Hypothesis*

Self-benefits in each of the three general classes listed in Table 9.1 can result from helping a person for whom one feels empathy. Such help can (1) reduce one's empathic arousal, which may be experienced as aversive; (2) enable one to avoid possible social and self-punishments for failing to help; and (3) enable one to gain social and self-rewards for doing what is good and right. The empathy–altruism hypothesis does not deny that these self-benefits of empathy-induced helping exist, but it claims that they are unintended consequences of acting on the altruistic motivation produced by empathy. Proponents of egoistic alternatives to the empathy–altruism hypothesis disagree; they claim that one or more of these self-benefits is the ultimate goal of empathy-induced motivation.

*Aversive-Arousal Reduction.* The most frequently proposed egoistic explanation of the empathy–helping relationship is aversive-arousal reduction. This explanation claims that feeling empathy for someone who is suffering is unpleasant, and the motivation produced by empathy is directed toward benefiting oneself by eliminating these empathic feelings. Helping is simply a means to this self-serving end.

Over half a dozen experiments have tested the aversive-arousal reduction explanation against the empathy–altruism hypothesis by varying the ease of escaping further exposure to a suffering victim without helping. Because empathic arousal is a result of witnessing the victim's suffering, either terminating this suffering by helping or terminating exposure to it by escaping should reduce one's own aversive arousal. Escape does not, however, enable one to reach the altruistic goal of relieving the victim's distress. Therefore, the aversive-arousal explanation predicts elimination of the empathy–helping relationship when escape is easy; the empathy–altruism hypothesis does not. Results of experiments have consistently shown patterns predicted by the empathy–altruism hypothesis and not the aversive-arousal reduction explanation, casting doubt on this popular egoistic account (see Batson, 1991, for a review).

*Empathy-Specific Punishment.* A second egoistic explanation claims that people learn through socialization that additional obligation to help, and thus additional shame and guilt for failure to help, are attendant on feeling empathy for someone in need. As a result, when people feel empathy, they are faced with impending social or self-censure beyond any general punishment associated with not helping. They say to themselves, "What will others think [or what will I think of myself] if I don't help when I feel like this?" They then help out of an egoistic desire to avoid these empathy-specific punishments. Once again, experiments designed to test this explanation have consistently failed to support it; results have consistently supported the empathy–altruism hypothesis instead (Batson, 1991).

*Empathy-Specific Reward.* The third major egoistic explanation claims that people learn through socialization that special rewards in the form of praise, honor, and pride are attendant on helping a person for whom they feel empathy. As a result, when people feel empathy, they think of these rewards and help out of an egoistic desire to gain them.

The general form of this explanation has been tested in several experiments and has received no support (Batson et al., 1988, Studies 1 & 5; Batson & Weeks, 1996), but there are two variations for which at least some support has been claimed. Best known of these is the negative-state relief explanation proposed by Cialdini and colleagues (1987), who suggested that the empathy experienced when witnessing another person's suffering is a negative affective state—a state of temporary sadness or sorrow—and the person feeling empathy helps in order to gain mood-enhancing rewards.

Although this egoistic alternative received some initial support (Cialdini et al., 1987; Schaller & Cialdini, 1988), subsequent research revealed that the initial support was probably due to procedural artifacts. Experiments avoiding these artifacts have not provided support for the negative-state relief explanation, but have instead supported the empathy–altruism hypothesis (Batson et al., 1989; Dovidio et al., 1990; Schroeder, Dovidio, Sibicky, Matthews, & Allen, 1988). It now seems clear that the motivation produced by empathy is not directed toward the egoistic goal of negative-state relief.

A second interesting variation on the empathy-specific reward explanation was proposed by Smith and colleagues (1989). They claimed that, rather than helping in order to gain the rewards of seeing oneself or being seen by others as a helpful person, empathically aroused individuals help in order to feel joy at the needy individual's relief: "It is proposed that the prospect of empathic joy, conveyed by feedback from the help recipient, is essential to the special tendency of empathic witnesses to help. . . . The empathically concerned witness to the distress of others helps in order to be happy" (Smith et al., 1989, p. 641).

Some early self-report data were supportive of this empathic-joy hypothesis (Smith et al., 1989), but more rigorous experimental evidence has failed to provide support. Experimental results have instead consistently supported the empathy–altruism hypothesis (Batson et al., 1991; Smith et al., 1989). The empathic-joy hypothesis, like other versions of the empathy-specific reward explanation, seems unable to account for the empathy–helping relationship.

### *A Tentative Conclusion*

Reviewing the empathy–altruism research, as well as recent literature in sociology, economics, political science, and biology, Piliavin and Charng (1990) concluded:

> There appears to be a "paradigm shift" away from the earlier position that behavior that appears to be altruistic must, under closer scrutiny, be revealed as reflecting egoistic motives. Rather, theory and data now being advanced are more compatible with the view that true altruism—acting with the goal of benefiting another—does exist and is a part of human nature. (p. 27)

Pending new evidence or a plausible new egoistic explanation of the existing evidence, this conclusion seems correct. It appears that the empathy–altruism hypothesis should (tentatively) be accepted as true.

### *Implications of the Empathy–Altruism Hypothesis*

If the empathy–altruism hypothesis is true, the implications are wide-ranging. Universal egoism—the assumption that all human behavior is motivated by self-benefit—has long dominated not only psychology, but other social and behavioral sciences as well (Campbell, 1975; Mansbridge, 1990; Wallach & Wallach, 1983). If empathy can produce motivation with the ultimate goal of increasing the welfare of another, then the assumption of universal egoism must be replaced by a more complex view of motivation that allows for altruism as well as egoism. Such a shift in our view of motivation requires, in turn, a revision of our underlying assumptions about human nature and human potential. It implies that we humans may be more social than we have thought: Other people can be more to us than sources of information, stimulation, and reward as we each ultimately seek our own welfare. We can care about them for their sakes, not only for ours.

The empathy–altruism hypothesis also may have wide-ranging practical implications (Batson, Ahmad, & Stocks, 2004). Knowing that empathic feelings produce altruistic motivation, people may at times wish to suppress or avoid these feelings. Suppressing or avoiding empathy for clients may be a factor, possibly a central one, in the experience of burnout among caseworkers in the helping professions (Maslach, 1982). Aware of the extreme effort involved in helping or of the impossibility of helping effectively, these caseworkers—or nurses caring for terminal patients, or even pedestrians confronted by homeless persons—may try to avoid feeling empathy in order to avoid the resulting altruistic motivation (Shaw, Batson, & Todd, 1994; Stotland, Mathews, Sherman, Hansson, & Richardson, 1978). Empathy avoidance is an egoistic motive to avoid an altruistic motive.

More positively, experiments have tested the possibility that empathy-induced altruism can be used to improve attitudes toward stigmatized outgroups. Thus far, results look quite encouraging. Inducing empathy has improved racial attitudes, as well as attitudes toward people with AIDS, homeless persons, and even convicted murderers (Batson, Polycarpou, et al., 1997; Dovidio, Gaertner, & Johnson, 1999). Empathy-induced altruism has also been found to increase cooperation in a competitive situation (a Prisoner's Dilemma), even when one knows that the person for whom one feels empathy has acted competitively rather than cooperatively (Batson & Ahmad, 2001; Batson & Moran, 1999).

### *Other Possible Sources of Altruistic Motivation*

Might there be sources of altruistic motivation other than empathic emotion? Several have been proposed, including an "altruistic personality" (Oliner & Oliner, 1988), principled moral reasoning (Kohlberg, 1976), and internalized prosocial values (Staub, 1974). There is some evidence that each of these potential sources is associated with increased prosocial motivation, but as yet it is not clear that this motivation is altruistic. It may be, or it may be an instrumental means to the egoistic ultimate goals of (1) maintaining a positive self-concept or (2) avoiding guilt (Batson, 1991; Batson, Bolen, Cross, & Neuringer-Benefiel, 1986; Carlo, Eisenberg, Troyer, Switzer, & Speer, 1991; Eisenberg et al., 1989). More research exploring these possibilities is needed.

Thinking even more broadly, beyond the egoism–altruism debate that has been a focus of attention and contention for the past three decades, might there be other forms of prosocial motivation—forms in which the ultimate goal is neither to benefit self nor to benefit another individual? Two seem especially worthy of consideration.

## Collectivism: Benefiting Another to Benefit a Group

*Collectivism* is motivation to benefit a valued group as a whole. The ultimate goal is not to increase one's own welfare or the welfare of the specific others who are benefited; the ultimate goal is to increase the welfare of the group. Robyn Dawes and his colleagues put it succinctly: "Not me or thee but we" (Dawes, van de Kragt, & Orbell, 1988). They suggested that collectivist motivation is a product of group identity (Brewer & Kramer, 1986; Tajfel, 1981; Turner, 1987) and may be especially important in addressing social dilemmas. A social dilemma arises when (1) individuals in a group or collective have a choice about how to allocate personally held scarce resources (e.g., money, time, energy); and (2) allocation to the group provides more benefit for the group as a whole than does allocation to any single individual (e.g., oneself), but allocation to a single individual provides that individual with more benefit than does allocation to the group as a whole (Dawes, 1980). It has often been assumed that when people act to benefit the group in a social dilemma, they are motivated by collectivism.

But, as with altruism, what looks like collectivism may actually be a subtle form of egoism. Perhaps attention to group welfare is simply an expression of enlightened self-interest. If one recognizes that ignoring group needs in a headlong pursuit of self-benefit will only lead to less self-benefit in the long run, then one may decide to benefit the group as a means to maximize long-term self-benefit. Appeals to enlightened self-interest are commonly used by politicians and social activists to encourage response to societal needs: They warn us of the long-term consequences for ourselves and our children of pollution and squandering natural resources; they remind us that if the plight of the poor becomes too severe, the well-off may face revolution. Such appeals assume that collectivism is simply a form of egoism. Enlightened self-interest also underlies strategies for collective action based on (1) reciprocity (e.g., "Tit for Tat"—see Axelrod, 1984; Komorita & Parks, 1995) or (2) sanctions that punish those who seek to "hitch a free ride" on the contributions of other group members (Hardin, 1977; Yamagishi, 1986).

The most direct evidence that collectivism is independent of egoism comes from research by Dawes, van de Kragt, and Orbell (1990). They examined the responses of individuals who had been given a choice between allocating money to themselves or to a group when allocation to oneself maximized individual but not group profit, whereas allocation to the group maximized collective but not individual profit. Dawes and colleagues found that if individuals faced with this dilemma made their allocation after discussing it with other members of the group, they gave more to the group than if they had had no prior discussion. Moreover, this effect was specific to the ingroup with whom the discussion occurred; allocation to an outgroup was not enhanced.

Based on this research, Dawes and colleagues (1990) claimed evidence for collectivist motivation independent of egoism, arguing that their procedure ruled out the two most plausible egoistic explanations: (1) enlightened self-interest and (2) socially instilled conscience based on a norm to share. However, there is reason to doubt that their procedure effectively ruled out all self-rewards and self-punishments associated with conscience. The research on norms reviewed earlier suggests that norms can be more refined than the one Dawes and colleagues addressed. The operative norm in their research may have been "share with your buddies" rather than simply "share." So, although this research is important and suggestive, more and better evidence is needed to justify the conclusion that collectivist motivation is not reducible to egoism.

## Principlism: Benefiting Another to Uphold a Moral Principle

Most moral philosophers have argued for the importance of a prosocial motive other than egoism. Most since Immanuel Kant have argued for a motive other than altruism or collectivism as well. They reject appeals to altruism, especially empathy-induced altruism, because feelings of empathy, sympathy, and compassion are too fickle and too circumscribed. Empathy is not felt for everyone in need, at least not to the same degree. They reject appeals to collectivism because group interest is bounded by the limits of the group; it not only permits, but may even encourage, doing harm to those outside the group. Given these problems with altruism and collectivism, moral philosophers have typically advocated prosocial motivation with an ultimate goal of upholding a universal and impartial moral principle, such as justice (Rawls, 1971). We call this motive *principlism*.

Is acting with an ultimate goal of upholding a valued moral principle really possible? When Kant (1785/1889) briefly shifted from his analysis of what ought to be to what is, he admitted that even concern for others that appears to be prompted by duty to principle may actually be prompted by self-love (pp. 23–24). The goal of upholding a moral principle may be an instrumental goal pursued as a means to reach the ultimate goal of self-benefit. If this is true, then principle-based motivation is a form of egoism.

The self-benefits of upholding a moral principle are conspicuous. One can gain the social and self-rewards of being seen and seeing oneself as a good person. One can also avoid the social and self-punishments of shame and guilt for failing to do the right thing. As Freud (1930) suggested, society may inculcate such principles in the young in order to bridle their antisocial impulses by making it in their best personal interest to act morally (see also Campbell, 1975). Perhaps, however, through internalization (Staub, 1989) or development of moral reasoning (Gilligan, 1982; Kohlberg, 1976), principles may come to be valued in their own right and not simply as instrumental means to self-serving ends.

The issue here is the same we faced with altruism and collectivism. Once again, we need to know the nature of a prosocial motive. Is the desire to uphold justice (or some other moral principle) an instrumental goal on the way to the ultimate goal of self-benefit? If so, then this desire is a subtle and sophisticated form of egoism. Alternatively, is upholding the principle an ultimate goal, with the ensuing self-benefits unintended consequences? If so, then principlism is a fourth type of prosocial motivation, independent of egoism, altruism, and collectivism.

Recent research suggests that people are often motivated to appear moral while, if possible, avoiding the cost of actually being moral. This motive has been called *moral hypocrisy* (Batson, Kobrynowicz, Dinnerstein, Kampf, & Wilson, 1997; Batson, Thompson, & Chen, 2002; Batson, Thompson, Seuferling, Whitney, & Strongman, 1999). The research also suggests that if principlism exists, it is often overpowered by self-interest. Many of us are, it seems, quite adept at moral rationalization. We are good at justifying to ourselves (if not to others) why a situation that benefits us or those we care about does not violate our moral principles: why we have the right to a disproportionate share of the world's natural resources; why dumping our nuclear waste in someone else's backyard is fair; why attacks by our enemies are atrocities, but attacks by our side are necessary. The abstractness of most moral principles, and their multiplicity, make rationalization easy (Bandura, 1999; Bersoff, 1999).

But this may be only part of the story. Perhaps, at least for some people under some circumstances, upholding a moral principle *can* serve as an ultimate goal, defining a form of prosocial motivation independent of egoism. If so, then principlism provides a motive for responding to the needs of others that transcends reliance on self-interest or on vested interest in and feeling for the welfare of certain other individuals or groups. This is quite an *if*, but it seems well worth conducting research to find out.

## CONFLICT AND COOPERATION OF PROSOCIAL MOTIVES

Recognizing the range of possible prosocial motives makes available more resources to those seeking to produce a more humane, caring society. At the same time, a multiplicity of prosocial motives complicates matters. These different motives for helping others do not always work in harmony. They can undercut and compete with one another.

Well-intentioned appeals to extended or enlightened self-interest can backfire by undermining other prosocial motives. Providing people with money or other incentives for showing concern may lead people to interpret their motivation as egoistic even when it is not (Batson, Coke, Jasnoski, & Hanson, 1978; Stukas, Snyder, & Clary, 1999). In this way, the assumption that there is only one answer to the question of why we act for the common good—egoism—may become a self-fulfilling prophecy (Batson, Fultz, Schoenrade, & Paduano, 1987). It may create a self-perpetuating norm of self-interest (Miller, 1999).

Nor do the other three prosocial motives (assuming that each exists) always work in harmony. They can conflict with one another. For example, altruism may conflict with collectivism or principlism. We may ignore the larger social good, or we may compromise our principles—not only to benefit ourselves, but also to benefit those individuals about whom we especially care (Batson, Batson, et al., 1995; Batson, Klein, Highberger, & Shaw, 1995). Indeed, whereas there are clear social sanctions against unbridled self-interest, there are not clear sanctions against altruism. As a result, Batson, Ahmad, and colleagues (1999) found that at times, altruism can be a greater threat to the common good than is egoism.

Each of the four prosocial motives that we have identified has its strengths. Each also has its weaknesses. The potential for the greatest good may come from strategies that orchestrate prosocial motives so that the strengths of one can overcome weaknesses of another. Strategies that combine appeals to either altruism or collectivism with appeals to principle seem especially promising. For example, think about the principle of justice. It may be universal and impartial, but motivation to uphold justice seems to be vulnerable to rationalization and easily co-opted. Empathy-induced altruism and collectivism seem less vulnerable, but they are limited in scope and produce partiality—special concern for particular persons or groups. Perhaps if we can lead people to feel empathy for the victims of injustice or to perceive themselves in a common group with them, then we can get these motives working together rather than at odds. Desire for justice may provide perspective and reason; empathy-induced altruism or collectivism may provide emotional fire and a force directed specifically toward seeing the victims' suffering end, preventing rationalization.

Something of this sort occurred, we believe, in a number of rescuers of Jews in Nazi Europe. A careful look at data collected by the Oliners and their colleagues (Oliner & Oliner, 1988) suggests that involvement in rescue activity frequently began with concern for a specific individual or individuals for whom compassion was felt—often individuals known previously. This initial involvement subsequently led to further contacts and rescue activity, and to a concern for justice that extended well beyond the bounds of the initial empathic concern. Something of this sort also lay at the heart of Gandhi's and Martin Luther King's practice of nonviolent protest. The sight on the TV news of a small black child in Birmingham being rolled down the street by water from a fire hose under the direction of Police Chief Bull Connor, and the emotions this sight evoked, seemed to do more to arouse concern for racial equality and justice than hours of reasoned argument about civil rights.

## SUMMARY AND CONCLUSION

Why do people help others, even at considerable cost to themselves? What does this behavior tell us about the human capacity to care, about the degree of interconnectedness among us, about how social we humans really are? These classic philosophical questions have resurfaced in the behavioral and social sciences in the past several decades. Social psychologists have begun to address the question of the nature of prosocial motivation by drawing on (1) Kurt Lewin's ideas about goal-directed motivation and the resulting distinctions among instrumental goals, ultimate goals, and unintended consequences; and (2) the experimental research methods introduced by Lewin that have become the trademark of social psychology over the past 50 years.

Specifically, social psychological research has first added to and documented a long list of self-benefits that may serve as the ultimate goal of egoistic prosocial motives. This list includes material, social, and self-rewards to be obtained; material, social, and self-punishments to be avoided; and three forms of aversive arousal to be reduced.

Social psychological research has also been used to test the claim that altruistic motives—motives with the ultimate goal of increasing another's welfare—exist that are independent of and irreducible to egoistic motives. Results of over 30 experiments designed to test the empathy–altruism hypothesis against egoistic alternatives have proved remarkably supportive of this hypothesis, leading to the tentative conclusion that feeling empathy for a person in need produces altruistic motivation to relieve the need. Sources of altruistic motivation other than empathy have also been proposed, but as yet there is not compelling research evidence to support these proposals.

Beyond the egoism–altruism debate, two additional forms of prosocial motivation seem especially worthy of consideration: collectivism and principlism. Collectivism—motivation with the ultimate goal of benefiting some group or collective as a whole—has been claimed to result from group identity and to account for prosocial responses to social dilemmas. Principlism—motivation with the ultimate goal of upholding some moral principle—has long been advocated by religious teachers and moral philosophers. Whether either is a separate form of motivation, independent of and irreducible to egoism, is not yet clear. The research done to test whether empathy-induced altruism is independent of egoism could serve as a useful model for future research assessing the independent status of collectivism and principlism.

More is known now than 50 years ago about why people help others. As a result, more is known about human motivation, and even about human nature. These are substantial gains. Still, many questions remain about the motivational resources we can tap in trying to build a more caring, humane society. Fortunately, the legacy from Lewin—both his rich conceptual framework for understanding motivation, and his use of laboratory experiments to isolate and identify complex social motives—places social psychologists in an ideal position to provide further answers. A lot may rest on their ability to do so.

## REFERENCES

Axelrod, R. (1984). *The evolution of cooperation*. New York: Basic Books.

Bandura, A. (1999). Moral disengagement in the perpetration of inhumanities. *Personality and Social Psychology Review, 3*, 193–209.

Batson, C. D. (1987). Prosocial motivation: Is it ever truly altruistic? In L. Berkowitz (Ed.), *Advances in experimental social psychology* (Vol. 20, pp. 65–122). New York: Academic Press.

Batson, C. D. (1991). *The altruism question: Toward a social-psychological answer.* Hillsdale, NJ: Erlbaum.

Batson, C. D. (1994). Why act for the public good?: Four answers. *Personality and Social Psychology Bulletin, 20*, 603–610.

Batson, C. D. (1995). Prosocial motivation: Why do we help others? In A. Tesser (Ed.), *Advanced social psychology* (pp. 333–381). New York: McGraw-Hill.

Batson, C. D. (1998). Altruism and prosocial behavior. In D. T. Gilbert, S. T. Fiske, & G. Lindzey (Eds.), *The handbook of social psychology* (4th ed., Vol. 2, pp. 282–316). New York: McGraw-Hill.

Batson, C. D., & Ahmad, N. (2001). Empathy-induced altruism in a Prisoner's Dilemma II: What if the target of empathy has defected? *European Journal of Social Psychology, 31*, 25–36.

Batson, C. D., Ahmad, N., & Stocks, E. L. (2004). Benefits and liabilities of empathy-induced altruism. In A. G. Miller (Ed.), *The social psychology of good and evil* (pp. 359–385). New York: Guilford Press.

Batson, C. D., Ahmad, N., Yin, J., Bedell, S. J., Johnson, J. W., Templin, C. M., et al. (1999). Two threats to the common good: Self-interested egoism and empathy-induced altruism. *Personality and Social Psychology Bulletin, 25*, 3–16.

Batson, C. D., Batson, J. G., Griffitt, C. A., Barrientos, S., Brandt, J. R., Sprengelmeyer, P., et al. (1989). Negative-state relief and the empathy–altruism hypothesis. *Journal of Personality and Social Psychology, 56*, 922–933.

Batson, C. D., Batson, J. G., Slingsby, J. K., Harrell, K. L., Peekna, H. M., & Todd, R. M. (1991). Empathic joy and the empathy–altruism hypothesis. *Journal of Personality and Social Psychology, 61*, 413–426.

Batson, C. D., Batson, J. G., Todd, R. M., Brummett, B.

H., Shaw, L. L., & Aldeguer, C. M. R. (1995). Empathy and the collective good: Caring for one of the others in a social dilemma. *Journal of Personality and Social Psychology, 68*, 619–631.

Batson, C. D., Bolen, M. H., Cross, J. A., & Neuringer-Benefiel, H. E. (1986). Where is the altruism in the altruistic personality? *Journal of Personality and Social Psychology, 50*, 212–220.

Batson, C. D., Coke, J. S., Jasnoski, M. L., & Hanson, M. (1978). Buying kindness: Effect of an extrinsic incentive for helping on perceived altruism. *Personality and Social Psychology Bulletin, 4*, 86–91.

Batson, C. D., Dyck, J. L., Brandt, J. R., Batson, J. G., Powell, A. L., McMaster, M. R., et al. (1988). Five studies testing two new egoistic alternatives to the empathy–altruism hypothesis. *Journal of Personality and Social Psychology, 55*, 52–77.

Batson, C. D., Eklund, J. H., Chermok, V. L., Hoyt, J. L., & Ortiz, B. G. (2007). An additional antecedent of empathic concern: Valuing the welfare of the person in need. *Journal of Personality and Social Psychology, 93*, 65–74.

Batson, C. D., Fultz, J., Schoenrade, P. A., & Paduano, A. (1987). Critical self-reflection and self-perceived altruism: When self-reward fails. *Journal of Personality and Social Psychology, 53*, 594–602.

Batson, C. D., Klein, T. R., Highberger, L., & Shaw, L. L. (1995). Immorality from empathy-induced altruism: When compassion and justice conflict. *Journal of Personality and Social Psychology, 68*, 1042–1054.

Batson, C. D., Kobrynowicz, D., Dinnerstein, J. L., Kampf, H. C., & Wilson, A. D. (1997). In a very different voice: Unmasking moral hypocrisy. *Journal of Personality and Social Psychology, 72*, 1335–1348.

Batson, C. D., & Moran, T. (1999). Empathy-induced altruism in a Prisoner's Dilemma. *European Journal of Social Psychology, 29*, 909–924.

Batson, C. D., Polycarpou, M. P., Harmon-Jones, E., Imhoff, H. J., Mitchener, E. C., Bednar, L. L., et al. (1997). Empathy and attitudes: Can feeling for a member of a stigmatized group improve feelings toward the group? *Journal of Personality and Social Psychology, 72*, 105–118.

Batson, C. D., Thompson, E. R., & Chen, H. (2002). Moral hypocrisy: Addressing some alternatives. *Journal of Personality and Social Psychology, 83*, 330–339.

Batson, C. D., Thompson, E. R., Seuferling, G., Whitney, H., & Strongman, J. (1999). Moral hypocrisy: Appearing moral to oneself without being so. *Journal of Personality and Social Psychology, 77*, 525–537.

Batson, C. D., Turk, C. L., Shaw, L. L. , & Klein, T. R. (1995). Information function of empathic emotion: Learning that we value the other's welfare. *Journal of Personality and Social Psychology, 68*, 300–313.

Batson, C. D., & Weeks, J. L. (1996). Mood effects of unsuccessful helping: Another test of the empathy–altruism hypothesis. *Personality and Social Psychology Bulletin, 22*, 148–157.

Berkowitz, L. (1972). Social norms, feelings, and other factors affecting helping and altruism. In L. Berkowitz (Ed.), *Advances in experimental social psychology* (Vol. 6, pp. 63–108). New York: Academic Press.

Berkowitz, L. (1987). Mood, self-awareness, and willingness to help. *Journal of Personality and Social Psychology, 52*, 721–729.

Bersoff, D. M. (1999). Why good people sometimes do bad things: Motivated reasoning and unethical behavior. *Personality and Social Psychology Bulletin, 25*, 28–39.

Brewer, M. B., & Kramer, R. M. (1986). Choice behavior in social dilemmas: Effects of social identity, group size, and decision framing. *Journal of Personality and Social Psychology, 50*, 543–549.

Campbell, D. T. (1975). On the conflicts between biological and social evolution and between psychology and moral tradition. *American Psychologist, 30*, 1103–1126.

Carlo, G., Eisenberg, N., Troyer, D., Switzer, G., & Speer, A. L. (1991). The altruistic personality: In what contexts is it apparent? *Journal of Personality and Social Psychology, 61*, 450–458.

Cialdini, R. B., Darby, B. L., & Vincent, J. E. (1973). Transgression and altruism: A case for hedonism. *Journal of Experimental Social Psychology, 9*, 502–516.

Cialdini, R. B., Kallgren, C. A., & Reno, R. R. (1991). A focus theory of normative conduct: A theoretical refinement and reevaluation of the role of norms in human behavior. In M. P. Zanna (Ed.), *Advances in experimental social psychology* (Vol. 24, pp. 201–234). Orlando, FL: Academic Press.

Cialdini, R. B., Schaller, M., Houlihan, D., Arps, K., Fultz, J., & Beaman, A. L. (1987). Empathy-based helping: Is it selflessly or selfishly motivated? *Journal of Personality and Social Psychology, 52*, 749–758.

Clark, M. S., & Waddell, B. A. (1983). Effect of moods on thoughts about helping, attraction, and information acquisition. *Social Psychology Quarterly, 46*, 31–35.

Coke, J. S., Batson, C. D., & McDavis, K. (1978). Empathic mediation of helping: A two-stage model. *Journal of Personality and Social Psychology, 36*, 752–766.

Cunningham, M. R., Shaffer, D. R., Barbee, A. P., Wolff, P. L., & Kelley, D. J. (1990). Separate processes in the relation of elation and depression to helping: Social versus personal concerns. *Journal of Experimental Social Psychology, 26*, 13–33.

Darley, J. M., & Latané, B. (1970). Norms and normative behavior: Field studies of social interdependence. In J. Macaulay & L. Berkowitz (Eds.), *Altruism and helping behavior* (pp. 83–101). New York: Academic Press.

Dawes, R. M. (1980). Social dilemmas. *Annual Review of Psychology, 31*, 169–193.

Dawes, R. M., van de Kragt, A. J. C., & Orbell, J. M. (1988). Not me or thee but we—the importance of group identity in eliciting cooperation in dilemma situations: Experimental manipulations. *Acta Psychologica, 68*, 83–97.

Dawes, R. M., van de Kragt, A. J. C., & Orbell, J. M. (1990). Cooperation for the benefit of us—not me, or my conscience. In J. J. Mansbridge (Ed.), *Beyond self-interest* (pp. 97–110). Chicago: University of Chicago Press.

Dovidio, J. F., Allen, J. L., & Schroeder, D. A. (1990). The specificity of empathy-induced helping: Evidence for altruistic motivation. *Journal of Personality and Social Psychology, 59*, 249–260.

Dovidio, J. F., Gaertner, S. L., & Johnson, J. D. (1999, October). *New directions in prejudice and prejudice reduction: The role of cognitive representations and affect.* Paper presented at the annual meeting of the Society of Experimental Social Psychology, St. Louis, MO.

Dovidio, J. F., Piliavin, J. A., Gaertner, S. L., Schroeder, D. A., & Clark, R. D., III. (1991). The arousal:cost–reward model and the process of intervention: A review of the evidence. In M. S. Clark (Ed.), *Prosocial behavior* (pp. 86–118). Newbury Park, CA: Sage.

Dovidio, J. F., Piliavin, J. A., Schroeder, D. A., & Penner, L. A. (2006). *The social psychology of prosocial behavior.* Mahwah, NJ: Erlbaum.

Eisenberg, N., & Miller, P. (1987). Empathy and prosocial behavior. *Psychological Bulletin, 101*, 91–119.

Eisenberg, N., Miller, P. A., Schaller, M., Fabes, R. A., Fultz, J., Shell, R., et al. (1989). The role of sympathy and altruistic personality traits in helping: A reexamination. *Journal of Personality, 57*, 41–67.

Festinger, L. (1957). *A theory of cognitive dissonance.* Stanford, CA: Stanford University Press.

Frank, R. H. (1988). *Passions within reason: The strategic role of the emotions.* New York: Norton.

Freud, S. (1930). *Civilization and its discontents* (J. Riviere, Trans.). London: Hogarth Press.

Gergen, K. J., Ellsworth, P., Maslach, C., & Seipel, M. (1975). Obligation, donor resources, and reactions to aid in three cultures. *Journal of Personality and Social Psychology, 31*, 390–400.

Gibbons, F. X., & Wicklund, R. A. (1982). Self-focused attention and helping behavior. *Journal of Personality and Social Psychology, 43*, 462–474.

Gilligan, C. (1982). *In a different voice: Psychological theory and women's development.* Cambridge, MA: Harvard University Press.

Gouldner, A. W. (1960). The norm of reciprocity: A preliminary statement. *American Sociological Review, 25*, 161–179.

Hardin, G. (1977). *The limits of altruism: An ecologist's view of survival.* Bloomington: Indiana University Press.

Heider, F. (1958). *The psychology of interpersonal relations.* New York: Wiley.

Hoffman, M. L. (1975). Developmental synthesis of affect and cognition and its implications for altruistic motivation. *Developmental Psychology, 11*, 607–622.

Hoffman, M. L. (1981). Is altruism part of human nature? *Journal of Personality and Social Psychology, 40*, 121–137.

Isen, A. M. (1970). Success, failure, attention and reaction to others: The warm glow of success. *Journal of Personality and Social Psychology, 15*, 294–301.

Isen, A. M. (1987). Positive affect, cognitive organization, and social behavior. In L. Berkowitz (Ed.), *Advances in experimental social psychology* (Vol. 20, pp. 203–253). New York: Academic Press.

Isen, A. M., & Levin, P. F. (1972). Effect of feeling good on helping: Cookies and kindness. *Journal of Personality and Social Psychology, 21*, 344–348.

Isen, A. M., Shalker, T. E., Clark, M., & Karp, L. (1978). Affect, accessibility of material in memory, and behavior: A cognitive loop? *Journal of Personality and Social Psychology, 36*, 1–13.

Jones, E. E. (1964). *Ingratiation.* New York: Appleton-Century-Crofts.

Kant, I. (1889). *Kant's critique of practical reason and other works on the theory of ethics* (4th ed.) (T. K. Abbott, Trans.). New York: Longmans, Green. (Original work published 1785)

Kohlberg, L. (1976). Moral stages and moralization: The cognitive-developmental approach. In T. Lickona (Ed.), *Moral development and behavior: Theory, research, and social issues* (pp. 31–53). New York: Holt, Rinehart & Winston.

Komorita, S. S., & Parks, C. D. (1995). Interpersonal relations: Mixed-motive interaction. *Annual Review of Psychology, 46*, 183–207.

Krebs, D. L. (1975). Empathy and altruism. *Journal of Personality and Social Psychology, 32*, 1134–1146.

Lerner, M. J. (1980). *The belief in a just world: A fundamental delusion.* New York: Plenum Press.

Lerner, M. J., & Simmons, C. H. (1966). Observer's reaction to the "innocent victim": Compassion or rejection? *Journal of Personality and Social Psychology, 4*, 203–210.

Lewin, K. (1951). *Field theory in social science.* New York: Harper.

MacIntyre, A. (1967). Egoism and altruism. In P. Edwards (Ed.), *The encyclopedia of philosophy* (Vol. 2, pp. 462–466). New York: Macmillan.

Mansbridge, J. J. (Ed.). (1990). *Beyond self-interest.* Chicago: University of Chicago Press.

Maslach, C. (1982). *Burnout: The cost of caring.* Englewood Cliffs, NJ: Prentice Hall.

Miller, D. T. (1999). The norm of self-interest. *American Psychologist, 54*, 1053–1060.

Mills, J., & Egger, R. (1972). Effect on derogation of a victim of choosing to reduce his stress. *Journal of Personality and Social Psychology, 23*, 405–408.

Murray, H. A. (1938). *Explorations in personality.* New York: Oxford University Press.

Oliner, S. P., & Oliner, P. M. (1988). *The altruistic personality: Rescuers of Jews in Nazi Europe.* New York: Free Press.

Piliavin, J. A., & Charng, H.-W. (1990). Altruism: A review of recent theory and research. *American Sociological Review, 16*, 27–65.

Piliavin, J. A., Dovidio, J. F., Gaertner, S. L., & Clark, R. D., III. (1981). *Emergency intervention*. New York: Academic Press.

Pruitt, D. G. (1968). Reciprocity and credit building in a laboratory dyad. *Journal of Personality and Social Psychology, 8*, 143–147.

Rawls, J. (1971). *A theory of justice*. Cambridge, MA: Harvard University Press.

Reykowski, J. (1982). Motivation of prosocial behavior. In V. J. Derlega & J. Grzelak (Eds.), *Cooperation and helping behavior: Theories and research* (pp. 352–375). New York: Academic Press.

Ryan, W. (1971). *Blaming the victim*. New York: Random House.

Schaller, M., & Cialdini, R. B. (1988). The economics of empathic helping: Support for a mood-management motive. *Journal of Experimental Social Psychology, 24*, 163–181.

Schroeder, D. A., Dovidio, J. F., Sibicky, M. E., Matthews, L. L., & Allen, J. L. (1988). Empathy and helping behavior: Egoism or altruism? *Journal of Experimental Social Psychology, 24*, 333–353.

Shaw, L. L., Batson, C. D., & Todd, R. M. (1994). Empathy avoidance: Forestalling feeling for another in order to escape the motivational consequences. *Journal of Personality and Social Psychology, 67*, 879–887.

Smith, K. D., Keating, J. P., & Stotland, E. (1989). Altruism reconsidered: The effect of denying feedback on a victim's status to empathic witnesses. *Journal of Personality and Social Psychology, 57*, 641–650.

Sober, E., & Wilson, D. S. (1998). *Unto others: The evolution and psychology of unselfish behavior*. Cambridge, MA: Harvard University Press.

Staub, E. (1974). Helping a distressed person: Social, personality, and stimulus determinants. In L. Berkowitz (Ed.), *Advances in experimental social psychology* (Vol. 7, pp. 293–341). New York: Academic Press.

Staub, E. (1989). Individual and societal (group) values in a motivational perspective and their role in benevolence and harmdoing. In N. Eisenberg, J. Reykowski, & E. Staub (Eds.), *Social and moral values: Individual and societal perspectives* (pp. 45–61). Hillsdale, NJ: Erlbaum.

Stotland, E., Mathews, K. E., Sherman, S. E., Hansson, R. O., & Richardson, B. Z. (1978). *Empathy, fantasy, and helping*. Beverly Hills, CA: Sage.

Stukas, A. A., Snyder, M., & Clary, E. G. (1999). The effects of "mandatory volunteerism" on intentions to volunteer. *Psychological Science, 10*, 59–64.

Tajfel, H. (1981). *Human groups and social categories: Studies in social psychology*. Cambridge, UK: Cambridge University Press.

Tolman, E. C. (1923). The nature of instinct. *Psychological Bulletin, 20*, 200–218.

Trivers, R. L. (1971). The evolution of reciprocal altruism. *Quarterly Review of Biology, 46*, 35–57.

Turner, J. C. (1987). *Rediscovering the social group: A self-categorization theory*. Oxford, UK: Blackwell.

Wallach, M. A., & Wallach, L. (1983). *Psychology's sanction for selfishness: The error of egoism in theory and therapy*. San Francisco: Freeman.

Wegener, D. T., & Petty, R. E. (1994). Mood management across affective states: The hedonic contingency hypothesis. *Journal of Personality and Social Psychology, 66*, 1034–1048.

Wilke, H., & Lanzetta, J. T. (1970). The obligation to help: The effects of amount of prior help on subsequent helping behavior. *Journal of Experimental Social Psychology, 6*, 483–493.

Wispé, L. (1986). The distinction between sympathy and empathy: To call forth a concept a word is needed. *Journal of Personality and Social Psychology, 50*, 314–321.

Yamagishi, T. (1986). The provision of a sanctioning system as a public good. *Journal of Personality and Social Psychology, 51*, 110–116.

Zuckerman, M. (1975). Belief in a just world and altruistic behavior. *Journal of Personality and Social Psychology, 31*, 972–976.

Chapter 10

# Implicit Motivation

## PAST, PRESENT, AND FUTURE

**Melissa J. Ferguson**
**Ran Hassin**
**John A. Bargh**

Why do people behave as they do? Although scholars across a wide array of disciplines and schools of thought have wrestled with this fundamental question from many perspectives, the lion's share of both historical and contemporary research in social psychology on this topic centers on a person's conscious and reportable experiences of intention and motivation. Specifically, much of this work examines the characteristics of a person's conscious intention to achieve various goals, and the relationship between those characteristics and the actual ways in which the person pursues those goals (e.g., Bandura, 1986; Carver & Scheier, 1998; Deci & Ryan, 1985; Gollwitzer, 1990; Locke & Latham, 1990; see also Mischel, Cantor, & Feldman, 1996, for a review). In particular, this research addresses the development, content, organization, and operation of people's conscious goals, and the influence of such goals on people's (conscious) judgments, feelings, plans, and behaviors.

Some of the research on motivation over the last two decades, however, has diverged from this tradition and can perhaps be termed research on *implicit motivation*, in that much of it focuses on how goals operate in implicit or nonconscious ways. The scope of this area of research is broad. It does not focus exclusively on whether goals can be activated nonconsciously, for instance, but rather on the complex ways in which both consciously and nonconsciously instigated goals operate based on a variety of implicit mechanisms (e.g., Aarts & Dijksterhuis, 2000; Aarts, Gollwitzer, & Hassin, 2004; Bargh, 1990; Bargh & Ferguson, 2000; Bargh, Gollwitzer, Lee-Chai, Barndollar, & Troetschel, 2001; Chartrand & Bargh, 1996; Custers & Aarts, 2005; Ferguson, in press; Ferguson & Bargh, 2004; Fishbach & Ferguson, 2007; Fishbach, Friedman, & Kruglanski, 2003; Fitzsimons & Bargh, 2003; Glaser & Banaji, 1999; Glaser & Kihlstrom, 2005; Hassin, 2005; Hassin, Uleman, & Bargh,

2005; Kruglanski, 1996; Moskowitz, Li, & Kirk, 2004; Shah, 2003; Shah, Friedman, & Kruglanski, 2002; Shah & Kruglanski, 2002, 2003).

This relatively new area of motivation science reflects the influence of two major research trends within the field of social psychology over the last quarter of the 20th century, and it provides a somewhat different framework within which motivation can be studied, compared to the traditional reliance on reportable wants, needs, and urges. One trend is the increasingly adopted social cognitive approach to theory and methodology concerning classic social psychological phenomena (e.g., Abelson, 1994; Devine, Hamilton, & Ostrom, 1994; Fiske, 1992; Fiske & Taylor, 1984, 1991; Isen & Hastorf, 1982; Jones, 1998; Kunda, 1999; Sherman, Judd, & Park, 1989; Wegner & Bargh, 1998; Zajonc, 1980b). The other trend is the growing interest in the analysis of behavior according to conscious versus nonconscious processes (e.g., e.g., Bargh & Ferguson, 2000; Greenwald & Banaji, 1995; Hassin et al., 2005). Although one trend represents an approach to research, while the other reflects the popularity of a research question, we argue that they have each influenced the study of motivation over the last two decades, and have ultimately stimulated the new area of implicit motivation.

In this chapter we briefly review the research and theory that exemplify the influence of these two trends on the area of motivation, and then present recent findings in research on implicit motivation. The first group of new findings concerns the qualities that potentially differentiate between consciously and nonconsciously activated and pursued goals (Hassin & Bargh, 2004). In particular, this work suggests that *flexibility*—one of the widely assumed hallmarks of conscious goal pursuit (Ajzen, 1991; Bandura, 1986; Deci & Ryan, 1985; Locke & Latham, 1990)—also characterizes nonconscious goal pursuit. These findings are thus in harmony with the notion that goal pursuit operates in the same way, regardless of whether the goal is activated with or without conscious intent (see Bargh et al., 2001; Lewin, 1926). This research also challenges traditional conceptions concerning the function of consciousness in goal choice and pursuit by demonstrating that flexibility is not uniquely conscious.

The second area of recent research addresses the implicit ways in which motivation may operate. Specifically, much research now suggests that a perceiver's current (either conscious or nonconscious) motivational concerns implicitly influence the accessibility in memory of goal-relevant knowledge, and that such changes in accessibility have an impact on the effectiveness of the perceiver's goal pursuit (e.g., Aarts, Dijksterhuis, & De Vries, 2001; Fishbach et al., 2003; Moskowitz, 2002; Moskowitz et al., 2004; Shah et al., 2002). The greater accessibility of goal-relevant knowledge is certainly functional, in that it helps the perceiver to notice and recognize goal-relevant objects in the environment. Moreover, additional recent evidence suggests that the functionality of implicit goal pursuit may extend to the way in which goal-relevant knowledge is appraised or evaluated (Ferguson, in press; Ferguson & Bargh, 2004).

Together, these new lines of work take the idea of implicit motivation one step further by suggesting that it is inherently functional and adaptive. First, we argue that the system(s) involved in motivation allow people to automatically adapt their goal pursuit to changing external environments and the associated relevant demands and constraints. Second, these systems also allow people to automatically adapt evaluations to their goals; that is, automatic evaluations are sensitive to and contingent on *internal* environments (i.e., what people want or are trying to do at the moment). This work reflects a theme that has emerged in recent research on implicit social cognition in general—namely, a growing interest in the functional and adaptive nature of automatic processes (e.g., see Bargh, 1997; Greenwald & Banaji, 1995; Moskowitz et al., 2004).

We turn now to a brief review of the influence of social cognition and automaticity on motivation research, and then proceed to a description of the aforementioned new findings related to implicit motivation. We discuss in the section on recent findings various directions for future research in this area, some of which are comprehensively addressed in other chapters in the current volume.

## MOTIVATION AND THE SOCIAL COGNITIVE PERSPECTIVE

The social cognitive approach to understanding human social behavior was developed in the 1970s and consists chiefly of applying methods from cognitive psychology to the study of the perceptual and cognitive mechanisms underlying traditional social psychological phenomena, such as impression formation, the attitude–behavior relationship, and the self (e.g., Abelson, 1994; Devine et al., 1994; Fiske, 1992; Fiske & Taylor, 1984, 1991; Isen & Hastorf, 1982; Jones, 1998; Kunda, 1999; Moskowitz et al., 2004; Sherman et al., 1989; Zajonc & Markus, 1985). It should be noted that social psychology had been cognitive in its approach to many phenomena long before the emergence of the field of social cognition (see Zajonc, 1980a), such as in the early study of internal attitudes and beliefs (e.g., Thurstone, 1930), the role of motivation and values in perceptual processes (Allport, 1955; Greenwald, 1992), and Festinger's (1957) theory of cognitive dissonance. Instead, the difference between the social cognitive approach and traditional social psychology lies in the *degree* of attention paid to cognitive processes and mechanisms.

Motivational variables have been included in social cognitive analyses of phenomena, mainly as moderators of basic cognitive effects. For example, researchers have asserted that different levels and types of motivation influence how people process information. Much research suggests that people's goals influence the elements of a situation to which they pay attention, as well as how they then process information about those elements (e.g., Anderson & Pichert, 1978; Cacioppo, Petty, Kao, & Rodriguez, 1986; Chaiken, Liberman, & Eagly, 1989; Fiske, 1992; Kruglanski, 1989; Srull & Wyer, 1986). A perceiver who is motivated to be accurate, for instance, may spend more time and effort in understanding a persuasive appeal than someone who is less motivated may (e.g., Chen & Chaiken, 1999).

Most recently, researchers have focused on the cognitive nature of motivational phenomena—that is, the specific ways in which goals may be represented in memory and operate according to the standard characteristics of information processing (e.g., Aarts & Dijksterhuis, 2000; Aarts, Dijksterhuis, & De Vries, 2001; Bargh, 1990; Bargh et al., 2001; Baumeister & Vohs, 2004; Fishbach et al., 2003; Fishbach & Ferguson, 2007; Goschke & Kuhl, 1993; Hassin, 2005; Higgins, 1997, 1998; Kruglanski, 1996; Liberman & Trope, 1996; Moskowitz, 2002; Shah et al., 2002; Shah & Kruglanski, 2002, 2003; Trope & Ferguson, 2000). This social cognitive approach to the nature of motivational influences is evidenced by the attention devoted to the ways in which goals are structured in memory, and to whether they operate according to principles such as the accessibility of knowledge (e.g., Bruner, 1957; Förster, Liberman, & Higgins, 2005; Higgins, 1996b; Liberman, Förster, & Higgins, in press).

Higgins and colleagues, for example, have demonstrated how basic motivational orientations and strategies are associated with certain patterns of knowledge accessibility (Higgins, 1987, 1997, 1998). For instance, for people who most often compare their current selves with their ideal selves, information about this discrepancy may be chronically more accessible in memory than information concerning a discrepancy with their ought selves may be. And, importantly, the accessibility of the discrepancy can predict a range of emotional and behavioral outcomes. The more accessible an ideal–actual discrepancy is to a person, for example, the more that person is likely to focus on the presence or absence of positive versus negative things, and the more that person is likely to experience emotions such as sadness rather than anxiety. The work by Higgins and colleagues more generally shows how the nature of chronically accessible information will likely guide not only the type of goals that people choose, but also the way that they pursue those goals (e.g., promotion vs. prevention self-regulatory focus) and the emotional consequences of those pursuits (see also Higgins, Shah, & Friedman, 1997). This research exemplifies the social cognitive approach through its emphasis on the mediational role played by the structure and operation of relevant information in memory.

As another example, researchers have studied how the particular ways in which goals are represented in memory may influence an individual's goal pursuit (Kruglanski, 1996; Shah et al., 2002). Kruglanski and colleagues have argued that research on how goals are represented and operate in memory can advance an understanding of mechanisms of goal pursuit and self-regulation more generally (e.g., Kruglanski, 1996). In their *goal systems theory*, they conceptualize goals as networks of cognitive associations (Shah et al., 2002). Although from this perspective goals are conceptualized as cognitive knowledge structures in memory, they are nevertheless thought to be distinct in certain ways from other cognitive structures. For example, the activation of goal structures involves affective consequences that are not necessarily implicated in non-goal structures (see Fishbach & Ferguson, 2007; Shah et al. 2002).

These examples illustrate the increased attention that motivation researchers have devoted to the representational structure and format of goal knowledge, as well as to the cognitive-based mechanisms underlying phenomena of interest more generally. This research represents a shift in emphasis within motivation research and is thus an important forerunner of the contemporary work on the operation of implicit motivation.

## MOTIVATION AND AUTOMATICITY RESEARCH

The second trend that has influenced the study of motivation concerns the nonconscious nature of many of the processes underlying higher-order cognitive processes, affect, decision making, and behavior. Since the 1970s, researchers in both cognitive (e.g., Neely, 1976; Neisser, 1967; Posner & Snyder, 1975; Shiffrin & Schneider, 1977) and social (e.g., Bargh & Ferguson, 2000; Greenwald & Banaji, 1995; Hassin et al., 2005) psychology have demonstrated how much of human psychological processing proceeds without the conscious guidance and intention once assumed to be necessary elements. In line with this trend, in the past decade researchers have systematically examined whether goals and motivation also similarly involve automatic processes. These studies have revealed that goals can indeed be activated nonconsciously, and can then operate without conscious choice or guidance (e.g., Aarts & Dijksterhuis, 2000; Aarts et al., 2004; Bargh, 1990; Bargh & Gollwitzer, 1994; Bargh et al., 2001; Chartrand & Bargh, 1996, 2002; Fishbach, Friedman, & Kruglanski, 2003; Fitzsimons & Bargh, 2003; Glaser & Kihlstrom, 2005; Gollwitzer, Bayer, & McCulloch, 2005; Hassin, 2005; Hassin et al., 2005; Shah, 2002, 2003).

In the first empirical paper to address this possibility (Chartrand & Bargh, 1996), the authors replicated two classic studies in social cognition concerning the influence of conscious goals on the organization in memory of information about persons. Chartrand and Bargh tested whether the same effects would emerge even if the goals were covertly activated and then operated without participants' awareness. In particular, they sought to demonstrate that the goal to understand another person's behaviors can be nonconsciously activated from simply reading related words (such as *interpret*, *judge*, and *impression*) in the context of an ostensible test of verbal ability. Both of the earlier studies were in fact replicated, demonstrating for the first time that goals can be invoked nonconsciously and influence how people interpret and organize information about other people, just as when they are pursued consciously.

Since then, researchers have demonstrated how goals activated without a person's conscious intention or choice can then influence how the person behaves in social situations (Aarts & Dijksterhuis, 2000; Bargh et al., 2001; Fitzsimons & Bargh, 2003). For instance, Bargh et al. (2001) demonstrated that a nonconsciously activated achievement goal caused experimental participants to work longer and harder on the assigned word puzzles; in fact, the majority of the goal-primed participants continued working on the puzzles even after they were supposed to stop, illustrating their concern with achieving the highest score possible on the puzzles.

That people can pursue goals and objectives without constant conscious monitoring and guidance makes sense from an economy-of-effort standpoint (e.g., Bargh, 1990, 1994; Baumeister, Heatherton, & Tice, 1994; Fiske & Taylor, 1991; James, 1890; Kahneman, 1973). Assuming that people possess multiple goals and objectives within and across situations, the system(s) responsible for such pursuit would be severely strained if constant attention was required for their operation. Indeed, much research demonstrates the severe limitations of a person's conscious regulatory capacity, in that the ability to consciously and effortfully regulate behavior can be quickly and easily exhausted (e.g., Baumeister, 2000, 2001; Baumeister, Bratslavsky, Muraven, & Tice, 1998; Muraven & Baumeister, 2000; Schmeichel, Vohs, & Baumeister, 2003). This research suggests the adaptive benefit of being able to negotiate the social environment according to important objectives in a relatively automatic fashion, without the necessity of conscious deliberation at every turn.

The work on the automatic activation and operation of goals is inherently in harmony with the social cognitive approach to studying motivation. Most of the work described above is based on the assumption that goals are represented in memory as structures that follow some (or all) of the same processing constraints as do stereotypes and attitudes, for example (see Bargh, 1990; Bargh et al., 2001). In addition, this research typically employs the types of priming methods that have become fixtures in social cognitive research. However, these studies also suggest that a person's complex *sequence* or pattern of choices over time—rather than just single, static choices or movements—can be determined by an implicitly operating goal (Bargh et al., 2001). This area of research thus belongs squarely within the framework of implicit motivation science.

## RECENT ADVANCES IN IMPLICIT MOTIVATION RESEARCH

Researchers working on implicit motivation assume that once a goal has been repeatedly linked with a certain situation and with specific behaviors, the situation can itself activate the goal without the person's intention or awareness, and this activation can influence the perceiver's subsequent choices and actions (e.g., Bargh, 1990). Recent research suggests that the interaction of that activated knowledge with the dynamic, unfolding situation is more adaptive and flexible than previously suspected.

### Flexibility and Goal Pursuit

As argued above, goal choice and pursuit are traditionally considered to be conscious, intentional, and effortful activities—that is, controlled processes. One of the main virtues of controlled processes is their ability to adapt to novel and changing circumstances. Such flexibility is crucial for successful goal pursuit. In adopting a goal, one fixes a future end-state toward which one strives. If the means one usually uses to achieve similar goals are available, then goal pursuit can proceed rigidly or habitually. Flexibility becomes advantageous when new means, which happen to be more efficient than those that one usually uses, become available. It becomes a necessary condition for goal achievement when one's habitual means are either unavailable or they stop working; without flexibility, the road to goal achievement is simply blocked in these cases. Because physical and social environments frequently change, and with them the appropriateness and effectiveness of means, flexibility seems to be highly important for successful goal pursuit.

Previous research has shown that nonconscious goal pursuit produces the same outcomes as does conscious goal pursuit (Chartrand & Bargh, 2002). Moreover, the two modes of goal pursuit also possess similar qualities or operating characteristics, such as tenacity in the face of obstacles and persistence over time (e.g., Bargh et al., 2001). In the studies reported in this section of the chapter, we examine whether automatic goal pursuit is similar to controlled goal pursuit in another important respect—that is, in the capacity to be flexible when faced with changes in the current situation.

At the outset, there would seem to be two alternatives. One is that controlled goal pursuit is flexible, but automatic goal pursuit is rigid. This hypothesis is reminiscent of many dual-process models in social psychology, which suggest and find consistent differences between these two modes of operation (see Chaiken & Trope, 1999). The competing hypothesis is that both controlled and automatic goal pursuit are (potentially) flexible. This option would represent a rather marked shift in thinking, as automatic processes have long been characterized as inflexible (e.g., Logan, 1988; Robinson, 1996; Schneider, Dumais, & Shiffrin, 1984; Wegner & Bargh, 1998; but see Stapel & Blanton, 2004).

Yet it is this latter alternative that seems the more plausible from an economy-of-mental-resources point of view. We assume that goal pursuit, in its various forms and levels, is ubiquitous in our lives. Given that mental resources to conduct effortful controlled processes are quite limited (e.g., Bargh, 1994; Baumeister et al., 1994; Kahneman, 1973), it seems reasonable to assume that a considerable proportion of our daily goal pursuits operate automatically. But if automatic goal pursuit is handicapped by rigidity, then goals that are automatically pursued should frequently fail. And this obviously would not be a very adaptive arrangement.

We do not suggest that automatic goal pursuit should always lead to enhanced flexibility. Rather, the flexibility of an automatic goal should manifest itself when (1) flexibility is a means of attaining that goal or (2) flexibility itself *is* the goal. Below, we describe the results of studies that examined the flexibility of automatic goal pursuit under these two conditions (Hassin, 2005; Hassin & Bargh, 2004).

### Examining Automatic Flexibility

Before we go on to describe the studies, a definitional note is in order. The concept of *flexibility* is complex, and the term has been used to refer to a family of related phenomena. For our current purposes, we have adopted the definition of the *Oxford English Dictionary*, according to which flexibility is the "capacity for ready adaptation to various purposes or conditions."

### The Wisconsin Card Sorting Test

The first three studies used the Wisconsin Card Sorting Test (WCST) to measure flexibility. The WCST was originally developed to assess abstract reasoning and the ability to shift cognitive strategies in response to changing environmental contingencies (Berg, 1948; Heaton, Chelune, Talley, Kay, & Curtiss, 1993). It consists of four response cards and 128 stimulus cards that depict figures of varying colors (red, blue, yellow, or green), forms (stars, triangles, circles, or crosses), and numbers (one, two, three, or four). In the computerized version of the WCST, four response cards—one red triangle, two green stars, three yellow crosses, and four blue circles—appear at the bottom of the computer screen. Participants see one stimulus card at a time, and their task is to match the stimulus card with one of the response cards. The sorting rules refer to color, form, or number, and are controlled by the software. Participants are given feedback about the accuracy of each sorting ("right" vs. "wrong"), but never about the sorting rule. After 10 consecutive correct sortings the rule is changed without prior warning, requiring the participants to use the negative feedback to realize that the sorting rule has changed and that a new rule should be found. In the version we used, the test continues until participants finish sorting all 128 cards.

Several subscores of the WCST are discussed here. First, *overall correct* is defined as the number of correctly sorted cards. Errors can be of two kinds. When a participant persists in sorting according to a rule that is no longer valid, his or her errors are scored as *perseverative errors* (there are a number of criteria for perseverance; see Heaton et al., 1993). These errors constitute a widely accepted measure of flexibility (e.g., Miyake, Friedman, Emerson, Witzki, & Howerter, 2000): The more one perseveres in using a strategy that is no longer working, the less flexible one is. Finally, errors that do not match the perseverance principle are called *nonperseverative errors*.

The WCST is particularly suitable for examining mental flexibility for a few reasons. First, because one of the motivations for its development was to assess flexibility in thinking, it captures the *essence* of flexible adaptation to changing environments (e.g., Berg, 1948; Demakis, 2003). The logic is simple: Physical and social environments suggest behavioral rules that, if followed, lead to (better) survival. Changes in environments often entail changes in these rules, and at the heart of (better) survival is rapid adaptation to these new rules. As the description above makes clear, the structure of the WCST reflects this logic: The rules that govern sorting change without a prior warning, and participants need to look for a new rule and follow it, without recourse to the previous rule.

Second, a recent latent-variable analysis concluded that "the results from the perseveration measure [of the WCST] . . . support the conclusion that the Shifting ability is a crucial component of perseverative errors in the WCST" (Miyake et al., 2000, p. 75). As the ability to shift (strategies, attention, rules, approaches, tasks, etc.) is an important component of flexibility, these results suggest that flexibility is a crucial factor underlying successful performance in the WCST.

### Automatic Goal Pursuit and the WCST

All of the studies described below used goal priming to look at flexibility of automatic goal pursuit. The priming manipulation was carried out in what was allegedly a first experiment, in which participants were asked to complete a word search puzzle. In each of the two forms of the puzzle, a $10 \times 10$ matrix of letters was presented, below which was a list of 13 words that were embedded in the matrix. Each list contained the same set of six neutral words to be found, with the remaining seven words relevant (or not) to the concept of high performance. After they had completed the word search task, participants were asked to do the WCST, and they were then thoroughly debriefed. All of the results reported herein are from subjects who did not show any signs of awareness of being primed.

We hypothesized that subjects primed for the automatic pursuit of an achievement goal should do better on the WCST. Furthermore, since flexibility is a strategy for good performance of the WCST, we hypothesized that primed subjects should be more flexible than control subjects. In the context of the WCST, enhanced flexibility means that priming should result in fewer perseverative errors.

The results of the first study supported both hypotheses. Replicating previous findings regarding the behavioral results of automatic achievement pursuit, primed participants correctly sorted significantly more cards than did nonprimed participants. Crucially, primed participants also made fewer perseverative errors than did control participants. That is, primed participants were more flexible than nonprimed participants.

In order to provide a replication of these results, a second study was run, to which two new dependent variables of awareness were added. The first was a simple measure of goal commitment—"How important was it for you to succeed in this task?"—that was accompanied by a 9-point scale ranging from "not at all" to "very important." Another question asked participants, "What do you think one should do in order to succeed in this task?" If priming enhances the conscious importance of flexibility, or conscious intentions to be flexible, then participants' responses on these new measures should reflect it.

The results of the second study replicated those of the first: Primed participants scored higher than did control participants, and they were also more flexible (i.e., they made fewer perseverative errors). Notably, the goal commitment ratings of participants in the two conditions did not differ significantly from each other, and there were also no differences in the responses to the second question described above.

The first two studies show that automatic goal priming may lead to better adaptation to one's surroundings. However, these studies enhanced flexibility indirectly, by priming the achievement goal. In the third study we sought to increase flexibility directly, by priming the goal of being flexible. This study was identical in design to the first two studies, except that the experimental version of the word search task primed flexibility instead of achievement (using concepts such as *flexible, elastic change, [to] adapt*, and *[to become] accustomed*).[1] In addition, we again measured participants' commitment to the goal of being flexible.

The results showed that the two conditions significantly differed in terms of their perseverative errors, with the primed group making fewer errors. The two groups did not significantly differ in terms of their overall success, although the means suggested that primed participants fared better than controls. Importantly, the two groups did not differ in terms of their reported commitment to the goal of being flexible.

### *Flexibility as Open-Mindedness*

The next study employed a different measure of flexibility. In this study we presented participants with a scenario, in which the protagonist, who served as a senior secretary to a company's chief executive officer, got up in the middle of an important meeting and left the room. Embedded in the scenario were cues that could be used to form an explanation of this behavior. Thus, for example, the text subtly suggested that the secretary might have been romantically involved with one of the colleagues in the meeting, that it was getting too late for her, that her child was waiting in the other room, and so forth. Participants had been either primed with a flexibility goal or not, and were then asked to read the story and answer questions regarding the secretary's behavior. Specifically, participants were asked to assess, on a 9-point scale, "How likely it is that the secretary left the room because of *X*?" in which *X* stands for a possible reason for her behavior (e.g., "How likely it is that the secretary left the room because her child was waiting in the other room?"). Participants were asked eight such questions.

This study extended the research in two ways. First, it examined a different aspect of flexibility, in a task differing from those used in the previous studies. Second, it examined flexibility in a situation where no explicit feedback was available. We hypothesized that flexibility should be manifested here in the degree of acceptance of the different reasons. That is, the more flexible and open-minded participants were, the more they should be willing to accept multiple reasons for a behavior. And, conversely, the more rigid and one-track-minded participants were, the less they should be willing to accept different causes.

The results corroborated our hypothesis. The two groups showed identical levels of reported commitment to the goal of being flexible and open-minded. Nevertheless, primed subjects were more willing than control subjects to accept numerous reasons for the secretary's behavior. That is, primed subjects were significantly more flexible than control subjects.

### *From Flexibility to Sensitivity*

Recall that according to our definition, flexibility is the "capacity for ready adaptation to various purposes or conditions." In order for adaptation to take place, though, one has to know what to *adapt to*. That is, one has to know (understand, grasp) the state of the world at time $T_1$, and sense the changes that occur thereafter. In its widest sense, then, flexibility is inherently interwoven with learning in general, and with learning the structure of the environment in particular. The WCST studies suggest that automatically pursued goals make people more responsive to changes in the environment. However, these studies do not speak to the issue of sensitivity to the structure of the environment.

Recently we began to address this issue by examining the effects of automatically pursued goals on implicit learning (Eitam, Hassin, & Schul, 2004). If automatically pursued goals do indeed increase sensitivity to relevant structures in the environment, then, *ceteris paribus*, goal-primed subjects should be better at implicit learning than are control subjects (to the extent that learning serves the pursued goals). To test this hypothesis, we used an implicit learning paradigm developed by Berry and Broadbent (e.g., 1984, 1988). In this task, participants are asked to control the production of a sugar factory, and to keep it at a certain level (e.g., 9,000 tons a month). In each trial, participants are required to enter the size of the workforce they choose (ranging from 1,000 to 12,000), and they then receive the resulting production. Unbeknownst to them, there is a rule that relates their input and the factory's production, such that the production at the $n$th trial is a function of the workforce ($W_n$), the production at the ($n$ – 1)th trial, and random noise. Importantly, this rule comes from a class of systems described in engineering science as requiring *adaptive control* (Berry & Broadbent, 1984, p. 211). Despite behavioral evidence showing that participants learn these rules, they are typically unaware of having learned anything (e.g., Berry & Broadbent, 1984, 1988).

In one experiment (Eitam et al., 2004, Experiment 1), we gave participants the sugar factory task either after having been primed with a performance goal, or following a control (word search) task. The results supported our hypothesis: Primed participants implicitly learned the production rule faster, and reached higher levels of performance at the end of the experiment (after two blocks of 30 trials). Importantly, there were no differences in their explicit knowledge of the rules or in their goal commitment.

### *Summary*

We have begun this section with a presentation of two competing hypotheses. One is in line with the traditional view of automaticity: Automatic processes are inflexible and rigid. The second hypothesis, derived from the principle of economy of mental resources, suggests that automatic goal pursuit should be flexible. Evidence from five studies, involving three different paradigms, has favored the latter view: Automatic goal pursuit can enhance sensitivity to relevant aspects of the environment, and it can enhance cognitive and behavioral flexibility of related processes.

These results draw automatic and controlled goal pursuit a little closer. Specifically, they show that one of the central characteristics of controlled goal pursuit, flexibility, may also describe automatic goal pursuit. And this, we suggest, is good news: If they were not flexible, automatic goal pursuits would frequently fail, and thus so would we.

## Automatic Evaluative Processes and Goal Pursuit

Beyond the findings on nonconscious goal activation and pursuit, researchers have also been exploring the low level, implicit ways in which even conscious goals might operate. Various findings suggest that the activation of a goal in memory, whether by conscious or nonconscious means, implicitly influences how the person sees and acts in the world. Moreover, these effects have been characterized as functional in that they seem to foster the success of the person's goal pursuit. We review below some recent research demonstrating such implicit effects.

### *Effects of Goals on Knowledge Accessibility*

There is a long history in psychology of theorists asserting a fundamental relationship between a perceiver's motivational priorities and the accessibility of memories relevant to those priorities (e.g., Ach, 1935; Bargh, 1990; Bruner, 1957; Gollwitzer, 1996; Jones & Thibaut, 1958; Klinger, 1996; Kruglanski, 1996; Kuhl, 1983; Lewin, 1926; McClelland & Atkinson, 1948). Bruner (1957), for instance, argued that one determinant of heightened accessibility of particular memories is the relevance of those memories to what the perceiver is trying to do at the moment. His argument was that the relationship between knowledge accessibility and goal pursuit is *functional*, in that the perceiver whose attention is directed at goal-helpful objects as a consequence of that heightened accessibility should be more likely to attain the goal.

Research in social cognition since 2000 has provided strong empirical support for this theoretical connection between motivational states and knowledge accessibility (e.g., Aarts & Dijksterhuis, 2000; Aarts, Dijksterhuis, et al., 2001; Ferguson & Bargh, 2004; Fishbach & Ferguson, 2007; Fishbach et al., 2003; Förster et al., 2005; Liberman et al., 2005; Moskowitz, 2002; Moskowitz et al., 2004; Shah et al., 2002; Sherman, Rose, Koch, Presson, & Chassin, 2003). Specifically, these findings suggest that knowledge concerning objects that are relevant for a currently active goal becomes more accessible in memory (Moskowitz, 2002), which in turn can make the perceiver more likely to notice goal-helpful objects in the environment (Aarts et al., 2001).

For example, Aarts, Dijksterhuis, and De Vries (2001) found that participants who were induced into a thirsty state responded significantly faster to words related to beverages (e.g., *water*), as well as words for drinking objects (e.g., *bottle*), compared with those who were not thirsty. This effect suggests that knowledge related to objects that could satisfy thirst was more accessible in memory for thirsty than for nonthirsty participants. In addition, Aarts and colleagues also found that thirsty participants were more likely to spontaneously recall drinking-related objects (e.g., a soda can) in a room in which they had previously been waiting, compared to those who were not thirsty. This suggests that increased accessibility of goal-relevant knowledge leads to relatively more attention spontaneously directed toward goal-relevant objects in the environment, just as theories on knowledge accessibility and attention would predict (e.g., Higgins, 1996; Moskowitz, 2002).

This work establishes a clear link between what a perceiver is trying to do at the moment and the accessibility of knowledge in memory related to the perceiver's pragmatic concerns. As such, these findings are consistent with a long tradition of conceptualizing thinking as in the ultimate service of action (Bruner, 1957; Fiske, 1992; Glenberg, 1997; James, 1890; Lewin, 1935; Roskos-Ewoldsen & Fazio, 1992; Schwarz, 2002; Smith & Semin, 2004). In other words, a perceiver's current goals provide limitations and constraints on the types of knowledge that are accessible in memory, and this drives the perceiver's attention toward certain elements within the environment and away from others. Assuming that the heightened accessibility of goal-relevant objects makes the perceiver more likely to attend to those objects in the environment and thus to approach them (or avoid them, depending on the goal), this research suggests that the ability to effectively pursue a goal is facilitated by implicit changes in the accessibility of knowledge relevant to the goal.

### *Effects of Goals on Knowledge Inhibition*

Researchers have also demonstrated that during active goal pursuit, knowledge concerning objects or activities that could disrupt the focal goal implicitly becomes more inhibited than when the goal is not active in memory (e.g., Fishbach et al., 2003; Liberman et al., 2005; Shah et al., 2002; Trope & Fishbach, 2000). Fishbach and colleagues (2003), for example, showed that the perception of words related to academic achievement (e.g., *graduate, grades*) resulted in the immediate inhibition of knowledge related to tempting alternative, but less important, goals (e.g., watching TV, talking on the phone). Importantly, Fishbach and colleagues also demonstrated that the aforementioned effect emerged only for those who were successful in the goal domain of academic achievement, and not for those who were less successful. These results suggest that successful self-regulation may rely in part on active goal states implicitly inhibiting alternative goals (see also Mischel, Shoda, & Rodriguez, 1989). In particular, the more tempting alternatives are inhibited in memory during a focal goal pursuit, the less likely perceivers will be to stray from their focal goal trajectory.

These findings are also in accord with research in cognitive psychology in the area of prospective memory concerning the *intention superiority effect* (Goschke & Kuhl, 1993; Marsh, Hicks, & Bryan, 1999). This work suggests that an intention to perform some action in the future enjoys a heightened state of activation in memory before it is performed, and that once the intention has been carried out, it becomes inhibited in memory for a brief amount of time. Together, these findings highlight the ways in which motivation (e.g., goal states, intentions) implicitly influences the accessibility and inhibition of relevant knowledge in memory.

### *Effects of Goals on the Accessibility of Evaluations*

Recent research has expanded on the work described above by examining how goal states influence knowledge accessibility according to the *evaluative* characteristics of that knowledge (Ferguson & Bargh, 2004; Sherman et al., 2003). These findings suggest that active goal pursuit may not simply render more accessible all knowledge about goal-helpful objects; instead, goal states seem to influence the accessibility of knowledge in memory in a more selective manner. In particular, goal states seem to render *accessible* the evaluatively *positive* aspects of goal-helpful objects, and actively *inhibit* the evaluatively *negative* aspects of those same objects. In this way, goal pursuit automatically renders goal-helpful objects *approach-friendly.*

For example, in the studies by Ferguson and Bargh (2004), the implicit accessibility of positively versus negatively valenced knowledge about objects was measured via a sequential affective priming paradigm (Fazio, Sanbonmatsu, Powell, & Kardes, 1986). In the traditional version of the paradigm, primes that represent various objects (e.g., *puppy, bugs*) are paired with positive and negative adjectives (e.g., *terrific, repulsive*) across many trials. Within a particular trial, the presentation of a prime is quickly followed by the presentation of an adjective, which participants are usually asked to classify as either positive or negative in meaning. The central dependent measure in this paradigm is the speed with which participants respond to the adjectives, as a function of the valence of the preceding prime. A substantial literature on evaluative priming has demonstrated that responses to the target adjectives are facilitated when the preceding primes are of congruent (vs. incongruent) valence (e.g., for reviews, see Fazio, 2001; Ferguson, 2007a; Musch & Klauer, 2003).

Importantly, given this well-established effect that positively valenced primes facilitate responses to positive target adjectives, and negatively valenced primes facilitate responses to negative target adjectives, it is possible to use this paradigm to measure participants' idiosyncratic automatic evaluation of a particular object (or set of objects). This can be done by examining whether the object facilitates participants' responding to positive over negative adjectives, relative to a control comparison object or to a comparison group of other participants (e.g., Fazio, Jackson, Dunton, & Williams, 1995; see Wittenbrink & Schwarz, 2007). Such an evaluation is inherently relative, and can be based on either faster responses to positive adjectives in the goal versus control condition, or slower responses to negative adjectives in the goal versus control condition, or both. Either outcome would ostensibly make the object more likely to be approached for those in the goal condition.

This paradigm is regarded as implicit because participants are not asked to evaluate the prime objects (only the targets), and also show no awareness during debriefing that their evaluations have been measured (e.g., Bargh, Chaiken, Govender, & Pratto, 1992; Fazio et al., 1986; Greenwald & Banaji, 1995). The assumption that the evaluations measured by this paradigm are made automatically is also based on previous research (Neely, 1976, 1977) suggesting that the short time delay (300 milliseconds) between the presentation of the objects and the presentation of the adjectives is too brief to allow strategic, intentional processing to occur. This measure therefore allows an assessment of how goal states *unintentionally* influence the accessibility of evaluative information about objects, suggesting the low-level (i.e., not prompted by the perceiver's conscious intentions or strategic processing) operation of an evaluative self-regulatory mechanism.

In one experiment (Ferguson & Bargh, 2004), participants were induced into a thirsty or nonthirsty state. They then completed an evaluative priming paradigm in which some of the primes represented objects or activities that were relevant to sating their thirst (e.g., *water, juice, drinking*). As indicated by their response latencies from the priming paradigms, the positive aspects of those objects that could satisfy thirst were significantly more accessible in memory for thirsty than for nonthirsty participants. Furthermore, this effect for thirsty participants only emerged in response to those objects or activities that had been previously rated in a separate pilot study as thirst-quenching (e.g., *water, juice, drinking*) and not for objects that were rated as less relevant (e.g., *coffee*) or completely irrelevant (e.g., *chair, phone*). This finding demonstrates that implicit goal-driven evaluative processes are sensitive to the *degree* to which objects can satisfy an active goal.

In another experiment, participants' active goal states rendered negative information about goal-relevant objects relatively more *inhibited* than for those who had just completed the goal, as well as those who were never pursuing the goal. Participants played a word game and were told either that the task would measure their verbal intelligence (goal condition) or that the task was being developed for future use in experiments (control condition). Crucially, participants completed the evaluative priming paradigm at varying points during the experiment. One group of participants completed the paradigm while they were still playing the word game (unfinished condition), while the other group completed the paradigm after they had finished the word game (finished condition). The evaluative priming paradigm contained objects that were considered helpful to game performance (e.g., *words*). Those who were in the goal condition and unfinished condition exhibited significantly greater inhibition of negativity associated with objects that were helpful to task performance. In this case, then, participants' approach-friendly automatic evaluations were caused by the inhibition of negative information about goal-helpful objects. Those in the other three conditions did not differ in the speed of their responses to positive versus negative adjectives.

The results from this series of experiments therefore suggest that participants who were actively involved in an important goal pursuit exhibited more *approach-friendly* automatic evaluations of objects that could facilitate the goal. That is, active goal states implicitly facilitated knowledge about the positive aspects of goal-helpful objects, or else inhibited knowledge about the negative aspects of goal-helpful objects (or both). It is important to note that these effects occurred only for those who were still actively engaged in goal pursuit, and not for those who were not involved in goal pursuit or who had just completed the goal.

These goal-dependent, approach-friendly automatic evaluations represent *functional* consequences of the goal state, because such implicit evaluations are likely to make the goal-helpful objects more desirable and thus more likely to be approached. Indeed, research suggests that automatic evaluations of objects influence subsequent behavior and judgments toward those objects, as well as toward other objects of the same valence (e.g., Chen & Bargh, 1999; Fazio et al., 1995; Ferguson, 2006, in press; Ferguson & Bargh, 2002; Ferguson, Bargh, & Nayak, 2005; McConnell & Leibold, 2001; Nosek, Banaji, & Greenwald, 2002).

Do goal states also influence how goal-*harmful* objects are automatically evaluated? That is, are such objects more likely to be evaluated in an avoidance-inducing fashion while a perceiver is engaged in an important goal pursuit? Recent findings suggest that the answer to this is yes (Ferguson, 2007b). Furthermore, these findings suggest that such effects are contingent on the person's skill at the goal. Across the experiments, an evaluative priming paradigm was again used to measure the implicit effects of goal states on positive versus negative object information. It was hypothesized that avoidance-inducing (i.e., relatively negative) evaluations would emerge if the object facilitated negative adjectives over positive adjectives to a greater degree in the goal versus control condition. The negativity of such evaluations would again be inherently relative, and could mean that the object led to faster response times to negative adjectives in the goal condition relative to the control condition, or to slower responses to positive adjectives in the goal condition versus the control condition, or both. The former case would suggest that negative object information was particularly accessible for those in the goal (vs. control) condition, whereas the latter case would suggest that positive object information was more inhibited for those in the goal (vs. control) condition. Either outcome would mean that such repelling evaluations would ostensibly make the object more likely to be avoided by those in the goal condition.

In one experiment, participants' automatic evaluations of distractions from or hindrances to the goal of academic achievement (e.g., TV) were assessed as a function of participants' success at the goal (those with a relatively high grade point average [GPA] were classified as high-success, and those with a lower GPA were classified as low-success) and of whether the academic goal was nonconscioulsy activated at the time of the evaluative priming paradigm. The results showed that high-success participants who had been subliminally primed with words related to the achievement goal (e.g., *graduate, homework*) automatically evaluated distractions from the academic goal as significantly more avoidance-inducing (i.e., relatively negative) than did all other participants. Moreover, as predicted, those who were more successful in the goal domain implicitly evaluated distractions to the goal as more negative when the goal had been automatically activated than when it had not been. In other words, these results show that those high in academic success do not walk around with chronically negative automatic evaluations of activities that might disrupt their goal. Rather, their negative evaluations of such distractions are turned on only when the particular higher-order goal has been activated. Such a pattern of findings suggests that goal-relevant automatic evaluations are highly sensitive to the perceiver's current motivational context.

### *Conclusions*

The recent work on the goal dependence of automatic evaluations shows that the ways in which people automatically evaluate objects, other people, and possibly even themselves are contingent on what they happen to be trying to do at that moment (Fazio, 1989; Ferguson & Bargh, 2002; Roskos-Ewoldsen & Fazio, 1992); this conclusion is in line with classic theorizing in psychology (Lewin, 1926, 1935). In this way, these findings add to the growing evidence for the contextual dependence of automatically activated evaluations and attitudes (e.g., Blair, 2002; Dasgupta & Greenwald, 2001; Mitchell, Nosek, & Banaji, 2003; Wittenbrink, Judd, & Park, 2001). However, it should be noted that the research on the goal dependence of automatic evaluations shows that they are not simply (or solely) contingent on the nature (i.e., valence) of recent experiences with the corresponding attitude objects, as in other work (e.g., Dasgupta & Greenwald, 2001). That is, participants who were still engaged in active goal pursuit exhibited more positive automatic evaluations of goal-relevant objects than even those who had just successfully completed the goal (Ferguson & Bargh, 2004). This means that automatic evaluations sometimes reflect desired *future* experiences with the attitude objects, rather than *recent* experiences with them. In other words, the content of these types of evaluations can be *prospective*, in that they reflect a goal yet to be attained rather than a goal effectively completed.

This work not only speaks to the goal-dependent nature of automatic evaluation; it also demonstrates that implicit evaluative processing is an integral component of conscious and nonconscious goal pursuit (see also Custers & Aarts, 2005; Moors & De Houwer, 2001; Moors, De Houwer, Hermans, & Eelen, 2005). As such, these findings suggest that *automatic evaluation* is an important addition to the emerging cognitive model of goal development, representation, and operation (e.g., for reviews, see Fishbach & Ferguson, 2007; Kruglanski, 1996). Such an inclusion would be in line with the historically close ties in research and theory among motivation, affect, and behavior (e.g., Arnold, 1960; Custers & Aarts, 2005; de Rivera, 1977; Frijda, 1986, 1993; Lazarus, 1991a, 1991b; Omdahl, 1995; Ortony, Clore, & Collins, 1988; Scherer, Schorr, & Johnstone, 2001; Smith & Ellsworth, 1985; Weiner, 1985).

## GENERAL CONCLUSIONS

We have argued that a new area of motivation science, termed *implicit motivation*, has evolved over the last two decades. Researchers in this area focus on the cognitive representation and operation of goal pursuit and self-regulation, and the implicit processes underlying that operation. We have described new findings that address the functional aspects of implicit motivation—the characteristics of automatic goal pursuit, as well as the implicit processes underlying conscious goal pursuit. These new findings therefore reflect both the broad scope of implicit motivation research, and also an increasing emphasis on the functionality of the underlying processes and mechanisms of automatic processes in general.

## ACKNOWLEDGMENTS

Preparation of this chapter was supported in part by National Institute of Mental Health (NIMH) Grant No. R03-MH067877 to Melissa J. Ferguson, Israeli Science Foundation Grant No. 846/03 to Ran Hassin, and NIMH Grant No. R01-MH60707 to John A. Bargh.

## NOTE

1. In Hebrew, both *[to] adapt* and *[to become] accustomed* are one-word verbs.

## REFERENCES

Aarts, H., & Dijksterhuis, A. (2000). Habits as knowledge structures: Automaticity in goal-directed behavior. *Journal of Personality and Social Psychology, 78*, 53–63.

Aarts, H., Dijksterhuis, A., & De Vries, P. (2001). On the psychology of drinking: Being thirsty and perceptually ready. *British Journal of Psychology, 92*, 631–642.

Aarts, H., Gollwitzer, P. M., & Hassin, R. (2004). Goal contagion: Perceiving is for pursuing. *Journal of Personality and Social Psychology, 87*, 23–37.

Abelson, R. P. (1994). A personal perspective on social cognition. In P. G. Devine, D. L. Hamilton, & T. M. Ostrom (Eds.), *Social cognition: Impact on social psychology* (pp. 15–37). San Diego, CA: Academic Press.

Ach, N. (1935). Analyse des willens [Analysis of the will]. In E. Abderhalden (Ed.), *Handbuch der biolagishen arbeitsmethoden* (Vol. 6, Part E). Berlin: Urban & Schwarzenberg.

Ajzen, I. (1991). The theory of planned behavior. *Organizational Behavior and Human Decision Processes, 50*(2), 179–211.

Allport, F. H. (1955). *Theories of perception and the concept of structure: A review and critical analysis with an introduction to a dynamic-structural theory of behavior.* New York: Wiley.

Anderson, R. C., & Pichert, J. W. (1978). Recall of previously unrecallable information following a change in perspective. *Journal of Verbal Learning and Verbal Behavior, 17*, 1–12.

Arnold, M. B. (1960). *Emotion and personality.* New York: Columbia University Press.

Bandura, A. (1986). *Social foundations of thought and action: A social cognitive theory.* Englewood Cliffs, NJ: Prentice Hall.

Bargh, J. A. (1990). Auto-motives: Preconscious determinants of social interaction. In E. T. Higgins & R. M. Sorrentino (Eds.), *Handbook of motivation and cognition: Foundations of social behavior* (Vol. 2, pp. 93–130). New York: Guilford Press.

Bargh, J. A. (1994). The four horsemen of automaticity: Awareness, intention, efficiency, and control in social cognition. In R. S. Wyer, Jr. & T. K. Srull (Eds.), *Handbook of social cognition* (pp. 1–40). Hillsdale, NJ: Erlbaum.

Bargh, J. A. (1997). The automaticity of everyday life. In R. S. Wyer, Jr. (Ed.), *Advances in social cognition* (Vol. 10, pp. 1–61). Mahwah, NJ: Erlbaum.

Bargh, J. A., Chaiken, S., Govender, R., & Pratto, F. (1992). The generality of the automatic attitude activation effect. *Journal of Personality and Social Psychology, 62*, 893–912.

Bargh, J. A., & Ferguson, M. J. (2000). Beyond behaviorism: On the automaticity of higher mental processes. *Psychological Bulletin, 126*, 925–945.

Bargh, J. A., & Gollwitzer, P. M. (1994). Environmental control of goal-directed action: Automatic and strategic contingencies between situations and behavior. In W. D. Spaulding (Ed.), *Nebraska Symposium on Motivation* (Vol. 41, pp. 71–124). Lincoln: University of Nebraska Press.

Bargh, J. A., Gollwitzer, P. M., Lee-Chai, A., Barndollar, K., & Troetschel, R. (2001). The automated will: Nonconscious activation and pursuit of behavioral goals. *Journal of Personality and Social Psychology, 81*, 1014–1027.

Baumeister, R. F. (2000). Ego-depletion and the self's executive function. In A. Tesser, R. B. Felson, & J. M. Suls (Eds.), *Psychological perspectives on self and identity* (pp. 9–33). Washington, DC: American Psychological Association.

Baumeister, R. F. (Ed.). (2001). *Social psychology and human sexuality.* New York: Psychology Press.

Baumeister, R. F., Bratslavsky, E., Muraven, M., & Tice, D. M. (1998). Ego depletion: Is the active self a limited resource? *Journal of Personality and Social Psychology, 74*(5), 1252–1265.

Baumeister, R. F., Heatherton, T. F., & Tice, D. M. (1994). *Losing control: How and why people fail at self-regulation.* San Diego, CA: Academic Press.

Baumeister, R. F., & Vohs, K. D. (Eds.). (2004). *Handbook of self-regulation: Research, theory, and applications.* New York: Guilford Press.

Berg, E. A. (1948). A simple objective test for measuring flexibility in thinking. *Journal of General Psychology, 39*, 15–22.

Berry, D. C., & Broadbent, D. E. (1984). On the relationship between task performance and associated verbalizable knowledge. *Quarterly Journal of Experimental Psychology, 36A*, 209–231.

Berry, D. C., & Broadbent, D. E. (1988). Interactive tasks and the implicit–explicit distinction. *British Journal of Psychology, 79*, 251–272

Blair, I. (2002). The malleability of automatic stereotypes and prejudice. *Personality and Social Psychological Review, 6*, 242–261.

Bruner, J. S. (1957). On perceptual readiness. *Psychological Review, 64*, 123–152.

Chaiken, S., Liberman, A., & Eagly, A. H. (1989). Heuristic and systematic information processing within and beyond the persuasion context. In J. S. Uleman & J. A. Bargh (Eds.), *Unintended thought: Limits of awareness, attention, and control* (pp. 212–252). New York: Guilford Press.

Chaiken, S., & Trope, Y. (Eds.). (1999). *Dual-process theories in social psychology.* New York: Guilford Press.

Chartrand, T. L., & Bargh, J. A. (1996). Automatic activation of impression formation and memorization goals: Nonconscious goal priming reproduces effects of explicit task instructions. *Journal of Personality and Social Psychology, 71*, 464–478.

Chartrand, T. L., & Bargh, J. A. (2002). Nonconscious motivations: Their activation, operation, and consequences. In A. Tesser & D. Stapel (Eds.), *Self and motivation: Emerging psychological perspectives* (pp. 13–41). Washington, DC: American Psychological Association.

Chen, M., & Bargh, J. A. (1999). Consequences of automatic evaluation: Immediate Behavioral predispositions to approach and avoid the stimulus. *Personality and Social Psychology Bulletin, 25*, 215–224.

Chen, S., & Chaiken, S. (1999). The heuristic-systematic model in its broader context. In S. Chaiken & Y. Trope (Eds.), *Dual-process theories in social psychology* (pp. 73–96). New York: Guilford Press.

Custers, R., & Aarts, H. (2005). Positive affect as implicit motivator: On the nonconscious operation of behavioral goals. *Journal of Personality and Social Psychology, 89*(2), 129–142.

Dasgupta, N., & Greenwald, A. G. (2001). On the malleability of automatic attitudes: Combating automatic prejudice with images of liked and disliked individuals. *Journal of Personality and Social Psychology, 81*, 800–814.

Deci, E. L., & Ryan, R. M. (1985). The general causality orientations scale: Self-determination in personality. *Journal of Research in Personality, 19*(2), 109–134.

Demakis, G. J. (2003). A meta-analytic review of the sensitivity of the Wisconsin Card Sorting Test to frontal and lateralized frontal brain damage. *Neuropsychology, 17*(2), 255—264.

de Rivera, J. (1977). A structural theory of the emotions. *Psychological Issues, 10*(No. 4, Monograph 40). New York: International University Press.

Devine, P. G., Hamilton, D. L., & Ostrom, T. M. (1994). *Social cognition: Impact on social psychology.* San Diego, CA: Academic Press.

Eitam, B., Hassin, R. R., & Schul, Y. (2004). *Implicit motivation for implicit learning.* Unpublished manuscript, The Hebrew University.

Fazio, R. H. (1989). On the power and functionality of attitudes: The role of attitude accessibility. In A. R. Pratkanis, S. J. Breckler, & A. G. Greenwald (Eds.), *Attitude structure and function* (pp. 153–180). Hillsdale, NJ: Erlbaum.

Fazio, R. H. (2001). On the automatic activation of associated evaluations: An overview. *Cognition and Emotion, 14*, 1–27.

Fazio, R. H., Jackson, J. R., Dunton, B. C., & Williams, C. J. (1995). Variability in automatic activation as an unobtrusive measure of racial attitudes: A bona fide pipeline? *Journal of Personality and Social Psychology, 69*, 1013–1027.

Fazio, R. H., Sanbonmatsu, D. M., Powell, M. C., & Kardes, F. R. (1986). On thc automatic activation of attitudes. *Journal of Personality and Social Psychology, 50*, 229–238.

Ferguson, M. J. (2006). *Effects of automatic evaluations on self-regulation.* Unpublished manuscript, Cornell University.

Ferguson, M. J. (2007a). The automaticity of evaluation. In J. A. Bargh (Ed.), *Social psychology and the unconscious: The automaticity of higher mental processes* (pp. 219–264). Hove, UK: Psychology Press.

Ferguson, M. J. (2007b). *The effect of goals on implicit evaluations of temptations and distractions.* Unpublished manuscript, Cornell University.

Ferguson, M. J. (in press). On the automatic evaluation of end-states. *Journal of Personality and Social Psychology.*

Ferguson, M. J., & Bargh, J. A. (2002). Sensitivity and flexibility: Exploring the knowledge function of automatic attitudes. In L. F. Barrett & P. Salovey (Eds.), *The wisdom in feeling: Psychological processes in emotional intelligence* (pp. 383–405). New York: Guilford Press.

Ferguson, M. J., & Bargh, J. A. (2004). Liking is for doing: The effects of goal pursuit on automatic evaluation. *Journal of Personality and Social Psychology, 87*(5), 557–572.

Ferguson, M. J., Bargh, J. A., & Nayak, D. (2005). After-affects: How automatic evaluations influence the interpretation of unrelated, subsequent stimuli. *Journal of Experimental Social Psychology, 41*, 182–191.

Festinger, L. (1957). *A theory of cognitive dissonance.* Evanston, IL: Row, Peterson.

Fishbach, A., & Ferguson, M. J. (2007). The goal construct in social psychology. In A. W. Kruglanski & E. T. Higgins (Eds.), *Social psychology: Handbook of basic principles* (pp. 490–515). New York: Guilford Press.

Fishbach, A., Friedman, R., & Kruglanski, A. W. (2003). Leading us not unto temptation: Momentary allurements elicit automatic goal activation. *Journal of Personality and Social Psychology, 84*, 296–309.

Fiske, S., & Taylor, S. (1984). *Social cognition.* Reading, MA: Addison-Wesley.

Fiske, S., & Taylor, S. (1991). *Social cognition* (2nd ed.). New York: McGraw-Hill.

Fiske, S. T. (1992). Thinking is for doing: Portraits of social cognition from Daguerreotype to laserphoto. *Journal of Personality and Social Psychology, 63*, 877–889.

Fitzsimons, G. M., & Bargh, J. A. (2003). Thinking of you: Nonconscious pursuit of interpersonal goals associated with relationship partners. *Journal of Personality and Social Psychology, 84*(1), 148–163.

Förster, J., Liberman, N., & Higgins, E. T. (2005). Accessibility from active and fulfilled goals. *Journal of Experimental Social Psychology, 41*(3), 220–239.

Frijda, N. (1986). *The emotions*. Cambridge, UK: Cambridge University Press.

Frijda, N. H. (1993). Mood, emotion episodes, and emotions. In M. Lewis & J. M. Haviland (Ed.), *Handbook of emotions* (pp. 381–403). New York: Guilford Press.

Glaser, J., & Banaji, M. R. (1999). When fair is foul and foul is fair: Reverse priming in automatic evaluation. *Journal of Personality and Social Psychology, 77*, 669–687.

Glaser, J., & Kihlstrom, J. F. (2005). Compensatory automaticity: Unconscious volition is not an oxymoron. In R. Hassin, J. S. Uleman, & J. A. Bargh (Eds.), *The new unconscious* (pp. 171–195). Oxford, UK: Oxford University Press.

Glenberg, A. M. (1997). What memory is for. *Behavioral and Brain Sciences, 20*, 1–55.

Gollwitzer, P. M. (1990). Action phases and mind-sets. In E. T. Higgins & R. M. Sorrentino (Eds.), *Handbook of motivation and cognition: Vol. 2. Foundations of social behavior* (pp. 53–92). New York: Guilford Press.

Gollwitzer, P. M. (1996). The volitional benefits of planning. In P. M. Gollwitzer & J. A. Bargh (Eds.), *The psychology of action: Linking cognition and motivation to behavior* (pp. 287–312). New York: Guilford Press.

Gollwitzer, P. M., Bayer, U., & McCullouch, K. (2005). The control of the unwanted. In R. Hassin, J. S. Uleman, & J. A. Bargh (Eds.), *The new unconscious* (pp. 485–515). Oxford, UK: Oxford University Press.

Goschke, T., & Kuhl, J. (1993). Representation of intentions: Persisting activation in memory. *Journal of Experimental Psychology: Learning, Memory, and Cognition, 19*, 1211–1226.

Greenwald, A. G. (1992). New Look 3: Reclaiming unconscious cognition. *American Psychologist, 47*, 766–779.

Greenwald, A. G., & Banaji, M. R. (1995). Implicit social cognition: Attitudes, self-esteem, and stereotypes. *Psychological Review, 102*, 4–27.

Hassin, R. R. (2005). Non-conscious control and implicit working memory. In R. R. Hassin, J. S. Uleman, & J. A. Bargh (Eds.), *The new unconscious* (pp. 196–224). New York: Oxford University press.

Hassin, R. R., & Bargh, J. A. (2004). *Automatic but flexible: Evidence from goal pursuit*. Unpublished manuscript, The Hebrew University.

Hassin, R. R., Uleman, J. S., & Bargh, J. A. (Eds.). (2005). *The new unconscious*. New York: Oxford University Press.

Heaton, R. K., Chelune, G. J., Talley, J. L., Kay, G. G., & Curtiss, G. (1993). *Wisconsin Card Sorting Test manual* (revised and expanded). Odessa, FL: Psychological Assessment Resources.

Higgins, E. T. (1987). Self-discrepancy: A theory relating self and affect. *Psychological Review, 94*, 319–340.

Higgins, E. T. (1996a). Ideals, oughts, and regulatory focus: Affect and motivation from distinct pains and pleasures. In P. M. Gollwitzer & J. A. Bargh (Eds.), *The psychology of action: Linking cognition and motivation to behavior* (pp. 91–114). New York: Guilford Press.

Higgins, E. T. (1996b). Knowledge activation: Accessibility, applicability, and salience. In E. T. Higgins & A. W. Kruglanski (Eds.), *Social psychology: Handbook of basic principles* (pp. 133–168). New York: Guilford Press.

Higgins, E. T. (1997). Beyond pleasure and pain. *American Psychologist, 52*, 1280–1300.

Higgins, E. T. (1998). Promotion and prevention: Regulatory focus as a motivational principle. In M. P. Zanna (Ed.), *Advances in experimental social psychology* (Vol. 30, pp. 1–46). San Diego, CA: Academic Press.

Higgins, E. T., Shah, J., & Friedman, R. (1997). Emotional responses to goal attainment: Strength of regulatory focus as moderator. *Journal of Personality and Social Psychology, 72*, 515–525.

Isen, A. M., & Hastorf, A. H. (1982). Some perspectives on cognitive social psychology. In A. H. Hastorf & A. M. Isen (Eds.), *Cognitive social psychology*. New York: Elsevier North-Holland.

James, W. (1890). *The principles of psychology* (2 vols.). New York: Holt.

Jones, E. E. (1998). Major developments in five decades of social psychology. In D. T. Gilbert, S. T. Fiske, & G. Lindzey (Eds.), *The handbook of social psychology* (4th ed., Vol. 1, pp. 3–57). Boston: McGraw-Hill.

Jones, E. E., & Thibaut, J. W. (1958). Interaction goals as bases of inference in interpersonal perception. In L. Petrullo & R. Tagiuri (Eds.), *Person perception and interpersonal behavior* (pp. 151–178). Stanford, CA: Stanford University Press.

Kahneman, D. (1973). *Attention and effort*. Englewood Cliffs, NJ: Prentice Hall.

Kruglanski, A. W. (1989). *Lay epistemic and human knowledge: Cognitive and motivational biases*. New York: Plenum Press.

Kruglanski, A. W. (1996). Goals as knowledge structures. In P. M. Gollwitzer & J. A. Bargh (Eds.), *The psychology of action: Linking cognition and motivation to behavior* (pp. 599–618). New York: Guilford Press.

Kuhl, P. K. (1983). Perception of auditory equivalence classes for speech in early infancy. *Infant Behavior and Development, 70*, 263–285.

Kunda, Z. (1999). *Social cognition: Making sense of people*. Cambridge, MA: MIT Press.

Lazarus, R. S. (1991a). *Emotion and adaptation*. New York: Oxford University Press.

Lazarus, R. S. (1991b). Progress on a cognitive-motivational-relational theory of emotion. *American Psychologist, 46*, 819–834.

Lewin, K. (1926). Vorsatz, Wille, und Bedürfnis [Intention, will, and need]. *Psychologische Forschung, 7*, 330–385.

Lewin, K. (1935). *A dynamic theory of personality*. New York: McGraw-Hill.

Liberman, N., Förster, J., & Higgins, E. T. (in press). Completed vs. interrupted priming: Reduced accessibility from post-fulfillment inhibition. *Journal of Experimental Social Psychology*.

Liberman, A., & Trope, Y. (1996). Social hypothesis testing: Cognitive and motivational mechanisms. In E. T. Higgins & A. W. Kruglanski (Eds.), *Social psychology: Handbook of basic principles* (pp. 239–270). New York: Guilford Press.

Locke, E. A., & Latham, G. P. (1990). *A theory of goal setting and task performance*. Englewood Cliffs, NJ: Prentice Hall.

Logan, G. D. (1988). Toward an instance theory of automatization. *Psychological Review, 95*(4), 492–527.

Marsh, R. L., Hicks, J. L., & Bryan, E. S. (1999). The activation of unrelated and canceled intentions. *Memory and Cognition, 27*, 320–327.

McClelland, D. C., & Atkinson, J. W. (1948). The projective expression of needs, I: The effect of different intensities of the hunger drive on perception. *Journal of Psychology, 25*, 205–232.

McConnell, A. R., & Leibold, J. M. (2001). Relations among the Implicit Association Test, discriminatory behavior, and explicit measures of racial attitudes. *Journal of Experimental Social Psychology, 37*, 435–442.

Mischel, W., Cantor, N., & Feldman, S. (1996). Principles of self-regulation: The nature of willpower and self-control. In E. T. Higgins & A. W. Kruglanski (Eds.), *Social psychology: Handbook of basic principles* (pp. 329–360). New York: Guilford Press.

Mischel, W., Shoda, Y., & Rodriguez, M. L. (1989). Delay of gratification in children. *Science, 244*, 933–938.

Mitchell, J. P., Nosek, B. A., & Banaji, M. R. (2003). Contextual variations in implicit evaluation. *Journal of Experimental Psychology: General, 132*, 455–469.

Miyake, A., Friedman, N. P., Emerson, M. J., Witzki, A. A., & Howerter, A. (2000). The unity and diversity of executive functions and their contributions to complex "frontal lobe" tasks: A latent variable analysis. *Cognitive Psychology, 41*, 49–100.

Moors, A., & De Houwer, J. (2001). Automatic appraisal of motivational valence: Motivational affective priming and Simon effects. *Cognition and Emotion, 15*, 749–766.

Moors, A., De Houwer, J., Hermans, D., & Eelen, P. (2005). Unintentional processing of motivational valence. *Quarterly Journal of Experimental Psychology: A, 58A*, 1043–1063.

Moskowitz, G. B. (2002). Preconscious effects of temporary goals on attention. *Journal of Experimental Social Psychology, 38*, 397–404.

Moskowitz, G. B., Li, P., & Kirk, E. R. (2004). The implicit volition model: On the preconscious regulation of temporarily adopted goals. In M. P. Zanna (Ed.), *Advances in experimental social psychology* (Vol. 36, pp. 317–404). New York: Academic Press.

Muraven, M., & Baumeister, R. F. (2000). Self-regulation and depletion of limited resources: Does self-control resemble a muscle? *Psychological Bulletin, 126*(2), 247–259.

Musch, J., & Klauer, K. C. (2003). *The psychology of evaluation: Affective processes in cognition and emotion*. Mahwah, NJ: Erlbaum.

Neely, J. H. (1976). Semantic priming and retrieval from lexical memory: Evidence for faciliatory and inhibitory processes. *Memory and Cognition, 4*, 648–654.

Neely, J. H. (1977). Semantic priming and retrieval from lexical memory: Roles of inhibitionless spreading activation and limited-capacity attention. *Journal of Experimental Psychology: General, 106*, 225–254.

Neisser, U. (1967). *Cognitive psychology*. New York: Appleton-Century-Crofts.

Nosek, B. A., Banaji, M. R., & Greenwald, A. G. (2002). Math = male, me = female, therefore math = me. *Journal of Personality and Social Psychology, 83*, 44–59.

Omdahl, B. L. (1995). *Cognitive appraisal, emotional, and empathy*. Mahwah, NJ: Erlbaum.

Ortony, A., Clore, G. L., & Collins, A. (1988). *The cognitive structure of emotions*. New York: Cambridge University Press.

Posner, M. I., & Snyder, C. R. R. (1975). Attention and cognitive control. In R. L. Solso (Ed.), *Information processing and cognition: The Loyola Symposium* (pp. 55–85). Hillsdale, NJ: Erlbaum.

Robinson, M. D. (1996). Running from William James' bear: A review of preattentive mechanisms and their contributions to emotional experience. *Cognition and Emotion, 12*(5), 667–696.

Roskos-Ewoldsen, D. R., & Fazio, R. H. (1992). On the orienting value of attitudes: Attitude accessibility as a determinant of an object's attraction of visual attention. *Journal of Personality and Social Psychology, 63*, 198–211.

Scherer, K. R., Schorr, A., & Johnstone, T. (Eds.). (2001). *Appraisal processes in emotion: Theory, methods, research*. New York: Oxford University Press.

Schmeichel, B. J., Vohs, K. D., & Baumeister, R. F. (2003). Intellectual performance and ego depletion: Role of the self in logical reasoning and other information processing. *Journal of Personality and Social Psychology, 85*, 33–46.

Schneider, W., Dumais, S. T., & Shiffrin, R. M. (1984). Automatic and controlled processing and attention. In R. Parasuraman & D. Davies (Eds.), *Varieties of attention* (pp. 1–17). New York: Academic Press.

Schwarz, N. (2002). Situated cognition and the wisdom of feelings: Cognitive tuning. In L. F. Barrett & P. Salovey (Eds.), *The wisdom in feeling: Psychological processes in emotional intelligence* (pp. 144–166). New York: Guilford Press.

Shah, J. (2003). The motivational looking glass: How significant others implicitly affect goal appraisals. *Journal of Personality and Social Psychology, 85*(3), 424–439.

Shah, J. Y., Friedman, R., & Kruglanski, A. W. (2002). Forgetting all else: On the antecedents and consequences of goal shielding. *Journal of Personality and Social Psychology, 83*, 1261–1280.

Shah, J. Y., & Kruglanski, A. W. (2002). Priming against your will: How goal pursuit is affected by accessible alternatives. *Journal of Experimental Social Psychology, 38*, 368–382.

Shah, J. Y., & Kruglanski, A. W. (2003). When opportunity knocks: Bottom-up priming of goals by means and its effects on self-regulation. *Journal of Personality and Social Psychology, 84*, 1109–1122.

Sherman, S. J., Judd, C. M., & Park, B. (1989). Social cognition. *Annual Review of Psychology, 40*, 281–326.

Sherman, S. J., Rose, J. S., Koch, K., Presson, C. C., & Chassin, L. (2003). Implicit and explicit attitudes toward cigarette smoking: The effects of context and motivation. *Journal of Social and Clinical Psychology, 22*(1), 13–39.

Shiffrin, R. M., & Schneider, W. (1977). Controlled and automatic human information processing. *Psychological Review, 84*, 127–190.

Smith, C. A., & Ellsworth, P. C. (1985). Patterns of cognitive appraisal in emotion. *Journal of Personality and Social Psychology, 48*, 813–838.

Smith, E. R., & Semin, G. R. (2004). Socially situated cognition: Cognition in its social context. In M. P. Zanna (Ed.), *Advances in experimental social psychology* (Vol. 36, pp. 53–117). San Diego, CA: Academic Press.

Srull, T. K., & Wyer, R. S., Jr. (1986). The role of chronic and temporary goals in social information processing. In R. M. Sorrentino & E. T. Higgins (Eds.), *Handbook of motivation and cognition: Vol. 1. Foundations of social behavior* (pp. 503–549). New York: Guilford Press.

Stapel, D. A., & Blanton, H. (2004). From seeing to being: Subliminal social comparisons affect implicit and explicit self-evaluations. *Journal of Personality and Social Psychology, 87*, 468–481.

Thurstone, L. L. (1930). The learning function. *Journal of General Psychology, 3*, 469–493.

Trope, Y., & Ferguson, M. J. (2000). How and when preferences influence inferences. In J. Bargh & D. K. Apsley (Eds.), *Unraveling the complexities of social life: A festschrift in honor of Robert B. Zajonc* (pp. 111–132). Washington, DC: American Psychological Association.

Trope, Y., & Fishbach, A. (2000). Counteractive self-control in overcoming temptation. *Journal of Personality and Social Psychology, 79*, 493–506.

Wegner, D. M., & Bargh, J. A. (1998). Control and automaticity in social life. In D. T. Gilbert, S. T. Fiske, & G. Lindzey (Eds.), *Handbook of social psychology* (4th ed., Vol. 1, pp. 446–496). Boston: McGraw-Hill.

Weiner, B. (1985). Attribution theory of achievement motivation and emotion. *Psychological Review, 92*, 548–573.

Wittenbrink, B., Judd, C. M., & Park, B. (2001). Spontaneous prejudice in context: Variability in automatically activated attitudes. *Journal of Personality and Social Psychology, 81*, 815–827.

Wittenbrink, B., & Schwarz, N. (Eds.). (2007). *Implicit measures of attitudes*. New York: Guilford Press.

Zajonc, R. B. (1980a). Cognition and social cognition: A historical perspective. In L. Festinger (Ed.), *Retrospections on social psychology* (pp. 180–204). New York: Oxford University Press.

Zajonc, R. B. (1980b). Thinking and feeling: Preferences need no inferences. *American Psychologist, 35*, 151–175.

Zajonc, R. B., & Markus, H. (1985). Must all affect be mediated by cognition? *Journal of Consumer Research, 12*, 363–364.

# MOTIVATIONAL SYSTEMS

Chapter 11

# Motivations for Promotion and Prevention

**Daniel C. Molden**
**Angela Y. Lee**
**E. Tory Higgins**

From the beginning, the study of psychology has been intimately associated with the study of motivation (e.g., Triplett, 1898). Early pioneers in clinical (Freud, 1905/1953), personality (Murray, 1938), behavioral (Lewin, 1935), and even perceptual (Bruner & Postman, 1947) research fully embraced the importance of understanding people's motives, needs, desires, and goals for explaining their thoughts and actions. As exemplified by this handbook, contemporary psychologists continue to embrace the importance of these concepts and are busy employing them to derive basic motivational distinctions that could potentially integrate many areas of study.

What are some fundamental distinctions that have been identified? Examples discussed throughout the current volume include differences between needs and goals that are pursued consciously versus unconsciously (Chartrand, Dalton, & Cheng, Chapter 22; Ferguson, Hassin, & Bargh, Chapter 10), that are concerned with approaching desired outcomes versus avoiding undesired outcomes (Elliot & Fryer, Chapter 15; Gable & Strachman, Chapter 37), or that originate in a focus on oneself as a lone individual versus oneself as part of a larger social entity (Batson, Ahmad, Powell, & Stocks, Chapter 9; Finkel & Rusbult, Chapter 36; Leary & Cox, Chapter 2). In this chapter, we explore a separate motivational distinction that we believe is equally fundamental: needs or goals that are concerned with growth and advancement versus safety and security (cf. Bowlby, 1969; Maslow, 1955).

We begin our discussion of advancement (i.e., *promotion*) versus security (i.e., *prevention*) motivations with a basic characterization of these motivations from the perspective of regulatory focus theory (Higgins, 1997). Following this, we review some general consequences of promotion or prevention concerns for (1) sensitivities during evaluation, (2) strategies of judgment and reasoning, and (3) basic goal pursuit processes; we then describe the implications of these consequences for a variety of important social phenomena. We conclude by taking a broad perspective on this body of work and considering the unique costs and benefits of an emphasis on promotion or prevention.

## REGULATORY FOCUS THEORY: PROMOTION AND PREVENTION MOTIVATIONS

People are motivated to fulfill a variety of basic needs that are central to their survival within both physical and social environments. In considering such needs, researchers have frequently differentiated those concerned with advancement (i.e., nourishment, growth, and development) from those concerned with security (i.e., shelter, safety, and protection; see Bowlby, 1969; Maslow, 1955). Building upon this differentiation, regulatory focus theory (Higgins, 1997) proposes that beyond originating in different needs, motivations for advancement and security also foster different modes of goal pursuit. That is, this theory suggests that people represent and experience basic needs for advancement (*promotion concerns*) in an entirely different fashion than they do basic needs for security (*prevention concerns*).

### Representing the Pursuit of Promotion versus Prevention Concerns

When pursuing promotion concerns, people are focused on gains. That is, they view themselves as striving toward the presence of positive outcomes (i.e., *gains*) and striving to avoid the absence of positive outcomes (i.e., unrealized opportunities, or *non-gains*). For example, people with a promotion focus on improving their relationships with others would represent this goal as strengthening social connections and avoiding missed social opportunities. In contrast, when pursuing prevention concerns, people are focused on losses. That is, they view themselves as striving toward the absence of negative outcomes (i.e., protection from threats, or *non-losses*) and as striving to avoid the presence of negative outcomes (i.e., *losses*). For example, people with a prevention focus on protecting their relationships with others would represent this goal as eliminating anything that might threaten social connections and avoiding social exclusion (see Higgins, 1997).

### Experiencing Promotion- versus Prevention-Focused Outcomes

In addition to differing in how they are represented, promotion and prevention concerns differ in how they are experienced in the course of goal pursuit. Although perceived gains following success at promotion-focused goals and perceived non-losses following success at prevention-focused goals are both pleasurable, these experiences vary in the type of pleasure that occurs. Because gains are experienced as the presence of positive outcomes, promotion-related success elicits emotions reflecting this pleasurable presence, such as elation and cheerfulness. However, because non-losses are represented as the absence (i.e., elimination) of negative outcomes, prevention-related success elicits emotions reflecting this pleasurable absence, such as relaxation and quiescence (Higgins, 1987, 1997).

Similarly, although perceived non-gains following failure at promotion-focused goals and perceived losses following failure at prevention-focused goals are both painful, these experiences vary in the type of pain that occurs. Because non-gains are experienced as the absence of (i.e., unrealized) positive outcomes, promotion-related failure elicits emotions reflecting this painful absence, such as sadness and dejection. However, because losses are represented as the presence of negative outcomes, prevention-related failure elicits emotions reflecting this painful presence, such as nervousness and agitation (Higgins, 1987, 1997).

Beyond varying in the *type* of pleasure or pain elicited, experiences of successfully pursuing promotion or prevention concerns also vary in the *intensity* of this pleasure or pain (Idson, Liberman, & Higgins, 2000; Liberman, Idson, & Higgins, 2005). Because elation involves high motivational arousal (i.e., high eagerness; cf. Barrett & Russell, 1999), successful promotion evokes relatively intense positive feelings. In contrast, because relaxation involves low motivational arousal (i.e., low vigilance; cf. Barrett & Russell, 1999), successful prevention evokes less intense positive feelings. Thus, in the earlier examples, the happiness of people who are able to improve their social relationships should feel more intense than the calmness of people who are able to protect such relationships from harm.

Because dejection involves low motivational arousal (i.e., low eagerness; cf. Barrett & Russell, 1999), however, failed promotion evokes relatively less intense negative feelings. In contrast, because agitation involves high motivational arousal (i.e., high vigilance: cf. Barrett & Russell, 1999), failed prevention evokes more intense negative feelings. Thus, to use the earlier examples again, the sadness of people who fail to improve their social relationships should feel less intense than the anxiety of people who fail to protect such relationships from harm. (For more extensive discussions of the experience of promotion vs. prevention concerns, see Higgins, 1987, 2000.)

## Distinguishing Promotion–Prevention Concerns from Approach–Avoidance Motivations

Although promotion concerns relate to the presence and absence of gains, and prevention concerns relate to the presence and absence of losses, it is important to note that the distinction between these concerns is *not* simply equivalent to the distinction between motivations to approach desired (i.e., positive) end-states and to avoid undesired (i.e., negative) end-states (e.g., Carver, 2004; Elliot & Fryer, Chapter 15, this volume). Instead, concerns with promotion or prevention describe separate and distinct contexts in which more general desires for approaching positives or avoiding negatives can arise (Higgins, 1997). For example, imagine two students in an upper-level college course. Both are highly motivated to earn an A, which clearly involves approaching a positive end-state; however, the first views this as an opportunity to improve his or her class rank, whereas the second views this as a necessity for protecting his or her good standing in the premedical program. Thus, although both students have approach motivations, for the first these motivations would relate more to promotion concerns, whereas for the second they would relate more to prevention concerns. Moreover, in both cases the students' motivations are clearly distinct from those of a hypothetical third student who is highly motivated to avoid earning an F.

This separation of promotion versus prevention and approach versus avoidance motivations is shown in Figure 11.1. The top half illustrates

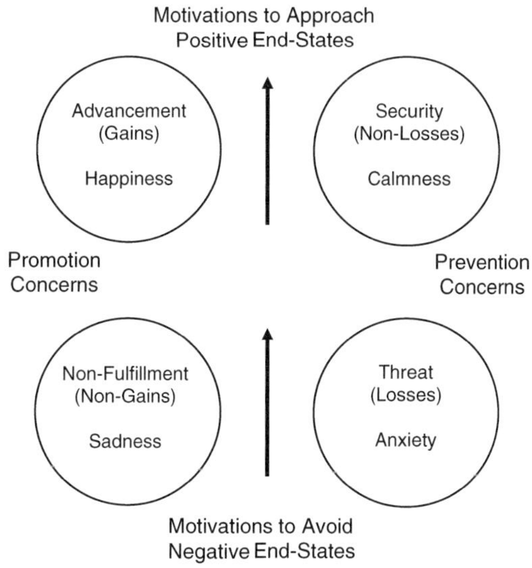


**FIGURE 11.1.** An illustration of the separation between promotion versus prevention concerns and motivations to approach positive end states versus avoid negative end states. Note that motivations for approach (the top half of the figure) and avoidance (the bottom half of the figure) each involve both promotion (the left half of the figure) and prevention (the right half of the figure) concerns, and that promotion and prevention concerns each include both motivations for approach and avoidance.

how motivations to approach positive end-states (e.g., earning an A) can involve either promotion or prevention concerns. When focused on promotion, approach motivation reflects desires for advancement and anticipations of happiness, whereas when focused on prevention, it reflects desires for security and anticipations of calmness. The bottom half illustrates how motivations to avoid negative end-states (e.g., earning an F) can also involve either promotion or prevention concerns. When focused on promotion, avoidance motivation reflects desires to avoid nonfulfillment and anticipations of sadness, whereas when focused on prevention, it reflects desires to avoid threat and anticipations of anxiety. Comparing the top and bottom halves of Figure 11.1 thus distinguishes between motivations for approaching positive end-states versus avoiding negative end-states (see Carver, 2004; Elliot & Fryer, Chapter 15, this volume), whereas comparing the left and right halves distinguishes between a promotion focus on advancement versus a prevention focus on security (see Higgins, 1997).

Another important point illustrated by Figure 11.1 is the ambiguity that arises when simple comparisons are made between desires to approach gains and desires to avoid losses (e.g., Kahneman & Tversky, 1979; Lockwood, Jordan, & Kunda, 2002). As can be seen by comparing the upper left and lower right portions of Figure 11.1, this contrast confounds promotion concerns with general approach motivations and prevention concerns with general avoidance motivations. Therefore, researchers testing hypotheses uniquely tied to motivations for promotion or prevention should take extra care to ensure that their measurements or manipulations focus on only a single common end-state (i.e., either a positive end-state that everyone approaches or a negative end-state that everyone avoids; see, e.g., Molden & Higgins, 2004; Roese, Hur, & Pennington, 1999). Another effective strategy would be to utilize experimental conditions representing all four of the promotion–prevention × approach–avoid conditions displayed in Figure 11.1 (e.g., Idson et al., 2000; Lee, Aaker, & Gardner, 2000, Studies 2 and 4; Shah & Higgins, 1997). This latter methodology allows both types of motivational distinctions to be examined simultaneously and independently.[1]

## Activating Promotion and Prevention Motivations

Given the important differences between promotion and prevention motivations we have described thus far, one question that immediately arises is this: What determines when each of these motivations is activated? As mentioned, everyone possess both advancement and security needs. However, certain circumstances may highlight one of these needs over the other and lead people to temporarily view whatever goal they are currently pursuing primarily in terms of promotion or prevention. What are some of these circumstances?

Because promotion and prevention concerns are each associated with unique representations and experiences, situations that evoke such representations or experiences can activate these concerns. For example, when goals involve gain-focused incentives (success brings rewards and failure brings the absence of rewards), pursuit of these goals should evoke promotion motivations. In contrast, when goals involve loss-focused incentives (success eliminates penalties and failure brings penalties), pursuit of these goals should evoke prevention motivations (e.g., Crowe & Higgins, 1997; Idson et al., 2000; Shah & Higgins, 1997). Similarly, circumstances that cue elated or dejected experiences should implicitly signal the possibility of promotion-relevant outcomes and activate these motivations. In contrast, circumstances that cue relaxed or agitated experiences should signal the possibility of prevention-relevant outcomes and activate these motivations (e.g., Roese et al., 1999; see Higgins, 2000; cf. LeDoux, 1996).

Other situations that can activate promotion and prevention motivations in a similar manner are those calling to mind personal standards that are particularly relevant to such motivations. Previous research on self-discrepancy theory (Higgins, 1987) has shown that when considering self-standards involving hopes and aspirations (i.e., their *ideals*), people view meeting these standards in terms of gaining or not gaining positive outcomes, which then leads to elation or dejection, respectively. Thus circumstances that bring attention to ideal self-standards should also activate promotion motivations. In contrast, research has also shown that when considering self-standards involving duties and obligations (i.e., their *oughts*), people view meeting these standards in terms of eliminating or failing to eliminate negative outcomes, which then leads to relaxation or agitation, respectively. Thus circumstances that bring attention to ought self-standards should also activate prevention motivations (e.g., Higgins et al., 1994; Idson & Higgins, 2000; Molden & Higgins, 2004, 2006).

Although the circumstances activating promotion versus prevention concerns discussed thus far involve specific incentives, emotions, or self-representations, there are many more general ways in which such circumstances can arise. For example, situations that highlight people's uniqueness and positive distinctiveness from others (i.e., create *independent self-construals*) can increase attention to ideal self-standards, whereas those that highlight social harmony and duties toward others (i.e., create *interdependent self-construals*) can increase attention to ought self-standards (Lee et al., 2000). Also, situations that lead people to represent their goals abstractly and project them into the distant future can inspire thoughts about how such goals might advance important ideals, whereas those that lead people to represent their goals concretely and project them only into the near future can inspire thoughts about how such goals might secure the fulfillment of important obligations (Förster & Higgins, 2005; Pennington & Roese, 2003). Furthermore, situations where people are targets of stereotypes involving expectations of high performance (e.g., "Women are good at verbal tasks") can create a diffuse promotion focus on the potential for gains, whereas situations where people are targets of stereotypes involving expectations of low performance (e.g., "Women are bad at math") can create a diffuse prevention focus on the potential for losses (Seibt & Förster, 2004). Finally, the lost social connections that occur when one is actively rejected or cast out by others can inspire prevention-oriented strategies of protecting oneself against further loss, whereas the missed opportunities for social gains that occur when one is more passively ignored or excluded by others can inspire promotion-oriented strategies of pursuing missed gains (Molden, Lucas, Gardner, Dean, & Knowles, 2006).

Thus, as summarized in Figure 11.2, many different types of circumstances can selectively activate promotion versus prevention motivations; this makes an understanding of

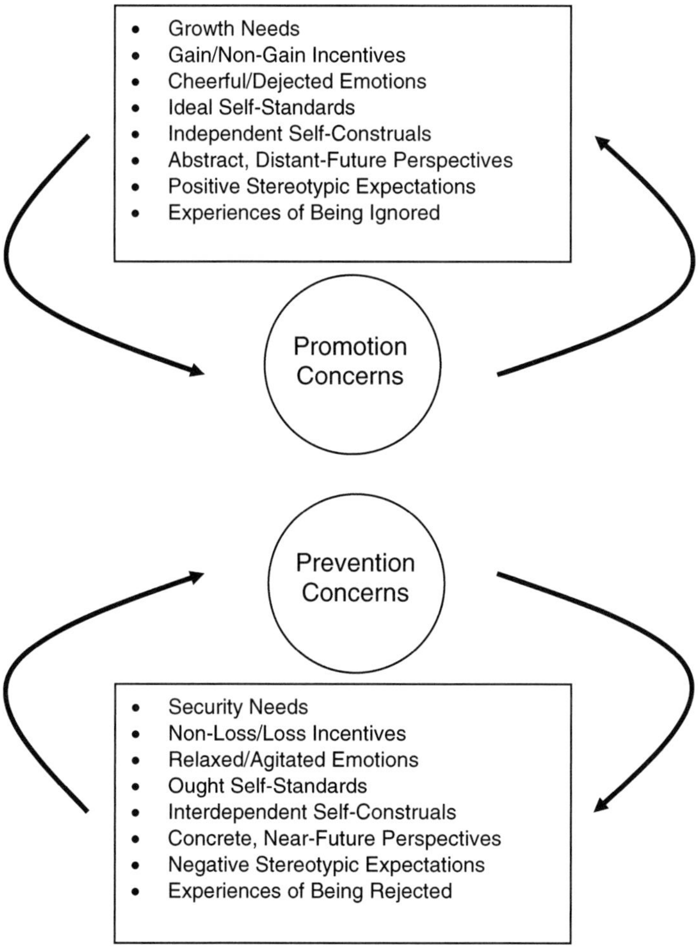


**FIGURE 11.2.** Circumstances that activate promotion or prevention concerns. Note that although the presence of any one of these psychological situations may be sufficient to activate such concerns, these concerns, once activated, may subsequently bring aspects of the remaining constellation of related psychological situations to mind as well.

such motivations important for a wide range of behaviors. Furthermore, this figure also illustrates that although any one of these circumstances may be sufficient to activate promotion or prevention concerns, such concerns, once activated, may subsequently bring aspects of the remaining motivationally relevant circumstances to mind as well. For example, goals perceived as involving independent self-construals have been shown to be generally associated with sensitivities for gain versus non-gain incentives, ideal self-standards, and elated or dejected reactions, whereas goals perceived as involving interdependent self-construals have been shown to be generally associated with sensitivities for non-loss versus loss incentives, ought self-standards, and relaxed or agitated reactions (Aaker & Lee, 2001; Lee et al., 2000; see also Seibt & Förster, 2004). It may well be that independent or interdependent goals also differentially activate abstract or concrete perspectives and positive or negative self-stereotypes as well, and further explorations of the reciprocal relationships between the antecedents of promotion or prevention motivations could be an interesting topic for future research.

One final point that should be made about the activation of promotion and prevention motivations is that just as certain circumstances can create a temporary focus on advancement or security needs, so too can prolonged exposure to similar circumstances create a more chronic focus on one of these needs. That is, just as situations that evoke temporary concerns with independence versus interdependence or ideal versus ought self-standards can generally place people in a promotion versus prevention focus, so too can a social upbringing that continually emphasizes independent accomplishments or meeting ideal self-standards versus interdependent responsibilities or meeting ought self-standards lead to the development of chronically promotion- or prevention-focused individuals (see Higgins, Shah, & Friedman, 1997; Higgins & Silberman, 1998; Lee et al., 2000; Manian, Strauman, & Denney, 1998). Thus, as is illustrated in the following sections, differences between promotion and prevention motivations are relevant for understanding both individual personalities and the general demands of different tasks and situations.[2]

## PSYCHOLOGICAL CONSEQUENCES OF PROMOTION VERSUS PREVENTION MOTIVATIONS

Having discussed the basic distinctions between promotion versus prevention motivations, and the different circumstances responsible for producing each, we now review research that illustrates the primary consequences of these separate motivations on people's evaluative processes, their judgment and decision making, and the way in which they pursue their goals.

### Promotion- and Prevention-Focused Evaluative Sensitivities

#### *Sensing Possibilities for Advancement versus Security*

One fundamental distinction we have drawn between promotion and prevention motivation is that promotion concerns are rooted in advancement needs, whereas prevention concerns are rooted in security needs. Therefore, those focused on promotion versus prevention should show a special interest in, and sensitivity to, information that is particularly relevant for advancement versus security (cf. Kunda, 1990). In one demonstration of this effect, Evans and Petty (2003) exposed people to persuasive messages portraying a product as helping to fulfill their advancement or security needs. When presented with a convincing advancement-oriented message, individuals with chronic promotion concerns processed it more thoroughly, and liked the product more, than did individuals with chronic prevention concerns. However, when presented with a convincing security-oriented message, the reverse was true (see also Aaker & Lee, 2001; Kim, 2006; Quinn & Olson, 2006).

Additional research by Freitas, Travers, Azizian, and Berry (2004) has shown that such differential evaluation of advancement- or security-relevant information can also occur at a less conscious level as well. Many studies have suggested that people feel more positive about stimuli that are easily processed, because this provides implicit information that such stimuli have been frequently encountered and do not threaten one's security (see Zajonc, 2001). If this is correct, then processing ease should be a stronger evaluative cue for those with a prevention versus a promotion focus. Consistent with this,

Freitas and colleagues found that manipulating the ease with which a series of pictures were processed had a greater effect on people's positive feelings about the pictures following the temporary activation of their prevention rather than promotion concerns.

### Sensing Gains versus Losses

A second fundamental distinction between promotion and prevention motivation described above is a primary focus on gains versus losses, respectively. Therefore, those concerned with promotion should be more sensitive to gain-related information that involves the presence or absence of positive outcomes, whereas those concerned with prevention should be more sensitive to loss-related information that involves the presence or absence of negative outcomes. In one study supporting this proposal, Markman, Baldwin, and Maddox (2005) had people perform a difficult category-learning task with visual stimuli. Some were given incentives for learning that involved gaining points for entry into a raffle for correct responses and not gaining points for incorrect responses, whereas others were given incentives that involved not losing points or losing points. When provided with gain or non-gain incentives, those for whom promotion concerns had been temporarily activated made more optimal discriminations between the visual categories than those for whom prevention concerns had been temporarily activated. However, when performing with non-loss or loss incentives, the reverse was true.

In another study demonstrating this effect, people read about the events of several days in the life of a hypothetical student and later recalled these events (Higgins & Tykocinski, 1992). Some of the events described the presence or absence of positive outcomes (e.g., finding $20 on the street, or missing a planned date at the movies, respectively), whereas others described the presence or absence of negative outcomes (e.g., being stuck in a crowded subway, or having a hard day of classes canceled, respectively). Promotion-focused individuals were found to recall more events involving both the presence and absence of positives rather than negatives, but the opposite was true for prevention-focused individuals (see also Higgins et al., 1994; Jain, Agrawal, & Maheswaran, 2006).

### Sensing Elation and Dejection versus Relaxation and Agitation

The third fundamental distinction between promotion and prevention motivation described earlier is the greater frequency of emotional experiences involving elation and dejection versus relaxation and agitation, respectively. Given this frequency, those focused on promotion should be more sensitive to affective evaluations of elation versus dejection, whereas those focused on prevention should be more sensitive to affective evaluations of relaxation versus agitation. Such effects were clearly demonstrated in a series of studies by Shah and Higgins (2001; see also Strauman, 1990). Across five separate experiments, they found that those who were promotion-focused were faster to evaluate experiences in terms of elation or dejection, whereas those who were prevention-focused were faster to evaluate experiences in terms of relaxation or agitation. Moreover, these findings occurred (1) both when promotion versus prevention concerns were measured individually and when they were experimentally induced; (2) for people's reports of how frequently they had felt these emotions over the past week, as well as how intensely they were currently experiencing them; and (3) both when people were making self-focused emotional appraisals and when they were reacting to common emotionally laden objects (e.g., cockroaches, money, flowers, etc.).

### Neurological Correlates of Promotion versus Prevention Evaluative Sensitivities

A particularly striking finding that broadly relates promotion and prevention motivations to all three of these different sensitivities comes from a recent study by Amodio, Shah, Sigelman, Brazy, and Harmon-Jones (2004). Much research on asymmetries in the activity of the brain's frontal cortex has shown that such asymmetries are related to specific motivational and emotional processes (see Davidson & Irwin, 1999). Gain-oriented motivations and emotions are associated with relatively greater left-hemisphere activity in this region, whereas loss-oriented motivations and emotions are associated with relatively greater right-hemisphere activity (but see Friedman & Förster, 2005). Amodio and colleagues showed that chronically promotion-focused individuals showed increased baseline activity in the left frontal cortex and decreased baseline activity in the right frontal cortex, whereas chronically prevention-focused individuals showed increased baseline activity in the right frontal cortex and decreased baseline activity in the left frontal cortex. As the authors note, this indicates that promotion and prevention motivations create different "pre-goal states" that alter their sensitivities, and reveals that such differences can even be detected at the neurological as well as the behavioral level.

## Promotion- and Prevention-Focused Judgments and Decisions

In addition to influencing the outcomes to which people are most sensitive (i.e., advancement or security, gains or losses), promotion or prevention motivations can also affect the judgment strategies people use when considering such outcomes (see Higgins & Molden, 2003; Molden & Higgins, 2004, 2005; see also Higgins, Chapter 23, this volume). Because promotion concerns center on gains, such concerns create preferences for *eager* judgment strategies. To borrow the terminology of signal detection theory (Tanner & Swets, 1954), this involves seeking *hits* (i.e., ensuring the addition of positive outcomes) and avoiding *errors of omission* (i.e., ensuring against overlooking positive outcomes). In contrast, because prevention concerns center on losses, such concerns create preferences for *vigilant* judgment strategies. To borrow signal detection terminology again, this involves seeking *correct rejections* (i.e., ensuring the elimination of negative outcomes) and avoiding *errors of commission* (i.e., ensuring against accepting negative outcomes).

An initial demonstration of this association between promotion versus prevention motivations and eager versus vigilant judgment strategies, respectively, comes from a study by Crowe and Higgins (1997). People viewed a list of nonsense words and were later given a recognition test including both words from the original list and new words not on the original list (see also Friedman & Förster, 2001). During the test, they were asked to respond "yes" if they had seen a word before and "no" if they had not seen the word before. In such tests, people may have a bias for responding "yes" in order to ensure that they identify all of the original words and to guard against errors of omission, which reflects an eager strategy, or they may have a bias for responding "no" in order to ensure that they eliminate all of the words they have not seen before and to guard against errors of commission, which reflects a vigilant strategy. When task incentives evoked promotion concerns, people were indeed biased toward "yes" responses, whereas when task incentives evoked prevention concerns, people were indeed biased toward "no" responses.

Another early study demonstrating that eager judgment strategies are linked to promotion concerns and that vigilant judgment strategies are linked to prevention concerns had people solve anagrams while their eagerness or vigilance was measured implicitly (Förster et al., 1998). On half of the problems, the force with which people pulled toward themselves on a scale (i.e., their arm flexion pressure) was used as an index for their eagerness, whereas on the other half, the force with which they pushed away from themselves on a scale (i.e., their arm extension pressure) was used as an index for their vigilance (cf. Cacioppo, Priester, & Berntson, 1993). It has long been known that as people move closer to goal completion, their overall motivational strength increases (the "goal looms larger" effect; Lewin, 1935). The results of this study revealed, however, that as people approached the end of the anagram set, those with chronic or temporarily induced promotion concerns showed greater increases in eagerness than vigilance (i.e., the strength of their pull vs. their push on the scale), whereas the reverse was true for those with chronic or temporarily induced prevention concerns.

### *Strategies for Considering Alternative Hypotheses*

Several more recent lines of research have explored the larger implications of promotion versus prevention judgment strategies for a variety of judgment processes. One of these processes is the consideration of alternative hypotheses. In general, an eager, promotion-focused strategy of considering alternatives should involve being open to many possibilities and setting lower thresholds for accepting potentially relevant information; this strategy increases the chance of identifying correct hypotheses and of avoiding the omission of any information that might be important. When one is using this strategy, it is thus better to endorse a hypothesis that might be correct (and risk being wrong) than to fail to endorse the hypothesis (and possibly miss being right). However, a vigilant, prevention-focused strategy of considering alternatives should involve narrowing in on what seems most certain and setting higher thresholds for accepting potentially relevant information; this strategy increases the chance of rejecting incorrect hypotheses and avoiding commitment to alternatives that are mistaken. When one is using this strategy, it is thus better to fail to endorse a hypothesis that might be correct (and possibly miss being right) than to endorse the hypothesis (and risk being wrong). Overall, those with promotion concerns should therefore typically endorse more alternative hypotheses during judgment than those with prevention concerns.

Several studies by Liberman, Molden, Idson, and Higgins (2001) tested this possibility by examining the hypotheses people form about others' actions. Participants read about a target person's helpful behavior and then evaluated several explanations for this behavior. Whether promotion versus prevention concerns were measured individually or induced experimentally, results confirmed that although participants did not differ on which explanation they rated as most likely, those with promotion concerns clearly endorsed more explanations than did those with prevention concerns. Furthermore, this difference was found to have important consequences for the subsequent impressions people formed of the target. Following their explanations, participants also predicted how helpfully the target person might behave in the future. Because they had endorsed a greater number of different explanations for the helpful behavior, and therefore presumably formed less certain impressions of the person who performed it (see Kelley, 1973), those with promotion concerns also made less certain predictions about the target's future helpfulness than did those with prevention concerns.

Additional research by Molden and Higgins (2004, 2006) has recently demonstrated similar influences of promotion versus prevention judgment strategies on the hypotheses people consider during social categorization and self-perception. Overall, as is consistent with previous findings, those with either chronic or temporarily induced promotion concerns (1) used more trait categories to label others' behaviors, and (2) endorsed more explanations for their own intellectual performance, than did those with chronic or induced prevention concerns. Furthermore, those with promotion concerns again seemed to form less certain impressions than those with prevention concerns and made less certain predictions about their own future intellectual performance.

Effects of promotion and prevention motivations on the strategic consideration of alternative hypotheses are not, however, limited to the domains of attribution and social perception. Friedman and Förster (2001) have also examined such effects in the area of insight and creative thought. They reasoned that because promotion concerns eagerly enhance the more open consideration of alternative hypotheses, they could also generally facilitate a more "exploratory" processing style and boost creativity. In contrast, because prevention concerns vigilantly narrow the consideration of alternate hypotheses, they could generally initiate a more "cautious" processing style and inhibit creativity. Consistent with this hypothesis, several studies revealed that, compared to those with chronic or induced prevention concerns, those with chronic or induced promotion concerns (1) solved more insight problems; (2) generated a higher quantity and quality of innovative uses for common, everyday objects; and (3) overcame previous associations in memory to produce more novel responses on word completion problems (see also Crowe & Higgins, 1997). Combined with the findings discussed above, this suggests that promotion and prevention judgment strategies have far-reaching influences on people's consideration of alternative hypotheses during reasoning.

### *Strategies for Decision Making*

Another implication of promotion versus prevention strategic preferences for basic judgment processes involves the relative weight given to particular considerations during decision making. Those with promotion concerns may adopt eager decision strategies that focus on the possibility for gains whereas those with prevention concerns may adopt more vigilant decision strategies that focus on the possibility for losses. These motivations may then affect people's vulnerabilities to classic decision biases (e.g., Kahneman & Tversky, 1979).

One set of studies that supports this proposal examined two different types of decisions (Higgins et al., 2001). The first decision involved choosing between two different (nonrefundable) trips that had accidentally been scheduled on the same day. One trip cost $50 and the other cost $100, but the $50 trip was expected to be more enjoyable. Since all of the money had already been spent, it would be a mistake to choose based on which trip avoided the greatest financial loss (i.e., the greater *sunk cost* of the $100 option) rather than on which trip promised the greatest personal gain (i.e., the greater enjoyment of the $50 option). Although this type of sunk-cost mistake is quite common, because of their preference for gain-focused decision strategies, promotion-focused individuals were less likely to make this type of error than prevention-focused individuals. The second decision involved imagining that one was the president of a company that had invested heavily in a product that was only 90% ready, but had already been made obsolete by the competition. The choice was between investing additional resources to finish the product or abandoning the project altogether. Since the product was unlikely to be successful, here it would be a mistake to choose based on the hope that an unexpected gain might justify continuing to add to the money already spent (i.e., the sunk cost of the original investment) rather than on the probability of losing additional resources on an already failed project. Although this type of mistake is also common, because of their preference for vigilant decision strategies, prevention-focused individuals were less likely to make this type of error than promotion-focused individuals.

Another example of differences in the types of decision errors influenced by promotion or prevention motivations was observed in a study by Brockner, Paruchuri, Idson, and Higgins (2002). People tend to overestimate the probability of *conjunctive* events, which require the joint presence of many separate occurrences. That is, people often do not recognize that no matter how likely each occurrence is individually, if any one fails to materialize, then the entire event will not happen (Bar-Hillel, 1973). Prevention concerns, however, create vigilant decision strategies focused on how losses could occur unless *all* necessary steps have been taken to eliminate them. These concerns should thus produce greater understanding of conjunctive events and lead to more accurate estimates of their occurrence, which is what Brockner and colleagues found. In contrast, people tend to underestimate the probability of *disjunctive* events, which merely require the singular presence of one of several separate occurrences. That is, people often do not recognize that no matter how *un*likely each occurrence is individually, only one must materialize for the event to happen (Bar-Hillel, 1973). Promotion concerns, however, create eager decision strategies focused on how gains can often be obtained by many possible means, *any* of which could suffice. These concerns should thus produce greater understanding of disjunctive events and lead to more accurate estimates of their occurrence, which is also what Brockner and colleagues found.

Differences in the decision strategies favored by those with promotion versus prevention motivations are not only relevant for predicting errors in judgment, however. They may also predict how people prioritize particular features of their choice options. For example, Raghunathan and Pham (1999) induced either a dejected or an agitated mood, and then had people choose between the option of a high-salary job with low security or an average-salary job with high security. Those whose promotion concerns were activated by their dejected mood displayed a gain-focused decision strategy and favored the high-salary job despite its low security. In contrast, participants whose prevention concerns were activated by their agitated mood displayed a loss-focused decision strategy and favored the high-security job despite its lesser rewards.[3]

Finally, in addition to influencing the strategies they employ during decision making, promotion and prevention motivations can affect people's strategies for coping with the consequences of their decisions. When decisions turn out poorly, people often generate *counterfactuals*, which involve mentally undoing these decisions and imagining alternate realities (Roese, 1997). Sometimes counterfactuals reverse a mistaken inaction (e.g., "If only I had done more research . . . "), whereas sometimes they reverse a mistaken action (e.g., "If only I hadn't listened to my colleague . . . "). Because mentally reversing inactions allows one to imagine correcting errors of omission, this represents an eager strategy of counterfactual thinking and should be seen more in those with promotion concerns. In contrast, because mentally reversing actions allows one to imagine correcting errors of commission, this represents a vigilant strategy of counterfactual thinking and should be seen more in those with prevention concerns. Roese and colleagues (1999) confirmed this pattern of results in several studies, in which people both considered hypothetical scenarios and described particular instances of their own behavior.

## Promotion- and Prevention-Focused Goal Pursuit

Given their effects on evaluation and judgment, it is not surprising that promotion and prevention motivations can also have profound effects on goal pursuit (see Higgins & Spiegel, 2004). Below, we trace such effects across people's choices of what goals to pursue, their initiation of goal directed action, their priorities during goal pursuit, and their reactions following successful or unsuccessful goal completion.

### *Choosing among Goals*

Many traditional accounts of goal pursuit recognize two primary factors influencing which goals people choose: (1) expectations for success, and (2) the value placed on this success (see Feather, 1982). Moreover, these *expectancy–value* accounts also include an interactive component between these factors, such that although everyone should prefer either goals on which they expect to succeed or goals that they value highly, as the value of a goal increases, expectations of success should become increasingly important in choosing this goal over others.

Shah and Higgins (1997) proposed, however, that this interactive effect on goal choice should differ for those with promotion versus prevention motivations. People with promotion concerns want to maximize advancement, which can best be done by choosing goals that are both highly valuable and have high likelihood for advancement. Thus promotion-focused individuals should show the typical expectancy × value interaction in their choice of goals: The more valuable the goal, the more expectations of success should influence their decision to pursue it. Consistent with this hypothesis, Shah and Higgins found that for students who were chronically or temporarily promotion-focused, the more valuable a hypothetical course was to them (i.e., the greater relevance a high grade had for acceptance into an honors society), the more influence expectations for success (i.e., receiving a high grade) had on their desire to enroll in the course.

In contrast, people with prevention concerns emphasize security, which can best be done by choosing the goals that have high security value, regardless of how likely it is that this security can be attained. That is, the larger a threat to security, the more necessary it is to prevent this threat, and the less expectations for success should determine one's attempts to do so (i.e., one must try no matter what the odds). Thus prevention-focused individuals should show a different expectancy × value interaction in their choice of goals: The more valuable the goal, the *less* expectations of success should influence their decision to pursue it. Consistent with this hypothesis, Shah and Higgins (1997) also found that for students who were chronically or temporarily prevention-focused, the more valuable a hypothetical college course was to them, the less influence expectations for success had on their desire to enroll in the course.

Beyond expectancy–value considerations, another factor that can determine what goals people choose is whether these goals maintain some currently stable (and desirable) situation or whether they bring about some new desirable situation. Typically, people display a *status quo bias* in their goal choice and focus on maintenance over attainment (Kahneman, Knetsch, & Thaler, 1991). However, since maintaining a desirable situation primarily concerns security, whereas attaining something new primarily concerns advancement, this status quo bias may also differ for those with promotion versus prevention motivations. Liberman, Idson, Camacho, and Higgins (1999) confirmed this possibility by giving people a choice between working to maintain an old prize they had already received or to attain an equally attractive new prize. Chronically and temporarily prevention-focused individuals displayed the standard status quo bias (across studies, only 19–29% of them chose to work for the new prize), whereas chronically and temporarily promotion-focused individuals did not and were equally likely to choose to work for the old or the new prize (cf. Lerner et al., 2004).

### *Initiating Goal-Directed Action*

Having chosen one or more goals to pursue, people must then decide when they need to begin acting to address these goals. Several classic theories of self-regulation (e.g., Maslow, 1955) suggest that perceived deficits (or *minimal* goals involving necessary outcomes) take priority over perceived opportunities for growth (or *maximal* goals involving ideal outcomes). Freitas, Liberman, Salovey, and Higgins (2002) thus hypothesized that because prevention motivations involve fulfilling minimum standards to avoid deficits (i.e., losses), and promotion motivations involve pursuing maximum standards for ideal growth (i.e., gains), people may typically act to address prevention concerns before promotion concerns. Supporting this hypothesis, when participants were solving anagrams where half of the problems were paired with promotion incentives (i.e., correct solutions were rewarded with monetary gains) and half were paired with prevention incentives (i.e., correct solutions protected against monetary losses), they were more likely to attempt the prevention-oriented problems before the promotion-oriented problems.

### Emphasizing Speed versus Accuracy in Goal Completion

Once people have initiated action toward their goals, another decision they soon face is whether to prioritize speed or accuracy in completing these goals (see Sanders, 1998). Prioritizing speed is a "riskier" strategy focused on maximizing potential gains over time. People should therefore be more likely to utilize this strategy when pursuing promotion concerns. In contrast, prioritizing accuracy is a more "cautious" strategy focused on minimizing potential losses over time. People should therefore be more likely to utilize this strategy when pursuing prevention concerns. Förster, Higgins, and Bianco (2003) examined this possibility by having people draw connections between sequentially numbered points (i.e., "connect the dots") to form several pictures. Speed was assessed by the number of points people connected by the end of a specified time period, and accuracy was assessed by the number of points they skipped while making the connections. Across three studies in which promotion or prevention concerns were both individually measured and experimentally induced, promotion-focused individuals did indeed produce faster (i.e., a higher quantity of) responses, whereas prevention-focused individuals did indeed produce more accurate responses (i.e., fewer mistakes). Moreover, as in other studies discussed earlier, preferences for promotion- or prevention-oriented pursuit priorities intensified toward the end of the task, as goal completion "loomed larger" (see Förster et al., 1998).

### Responding to Success and Failure Feedback

During goal pursuit, people often receive feedback regarding their progress toward achieving their goal, which then often influences their continued progress (Carver, 2004; Lewin, 1935). Success feedback typically increases approach motivations and focuses people on the positive end-state they are pursuing, whereas failure feedback typically increases avoidance motivations and focuses people on the negative end-state from which they wish to distance themselves. However, recent research suggests that these effects may be more or less prevalent, depending on whether such feedback addresses promotion or prevention concerns (Förster, Grant, Idson, & Higgins, 2001; Idson & Higgins, 2000).

Fulfilling promotion concerns produces elation and high motivational intensity (Idson et al., 2000; Liberman et al., 2005). When focused on promotion, success feedback should therefore be highly motivating and increase commitment toward approaching further success. In contrast, fulfilling prevention concerns produces relaxation and low motivational intensity. When focused on prevention, success feedback should therefore be less motivating and lead to smaller increases in commitment toward approaching further success. To test this possibility, Förster and colleagues (2001) gave people anagram problems that were framed in terms of opportunities for either promotion (i.e., gaining points) or prevention (i.e., preventing lost points). Halfway through the problems, some people were told that they were doing well, and their eager, approach motivations were implicitly assessed during the second half by measuring their arm flexion pressure, as described earlier. Those working on promotion-focused problems showed greater increases in their approach motivations, as well as greater persistence and performance on these problems, than did those working on prevention-focused problems.

Furthermore, failing to fulfill prevention concerns produces agitation and high motivational intensity (Idson et al., 2000; Liberman et al., 2005). When focused on prevention, failure feedback should therefore be highly motivating and increase commitment toward avoiding further failure. In contrast, failing to fulfill promotion concerns produces dejection and low motivational intensity. When focused on promotion, failure feedback should therefore be less motivating and lead to smaller increases in commitment toward avoiding further failure. To test this possibility, halfway through a set of promotion- or prevention-focused anagram problems, some people were told that they were not doing well, and their vigilant, avoidance motivations were implicitly assessed during the second half by measuring their arm extension pressure, as described earlier (Förster et al., 2001). Those working on prevention-focused problems showed greater increases in their avoidance motivations, as well as greater persistence and performance on these problems, than did those working on promotion-focused problems. Thus, success feedback increased motivation and performance more for those with promotion concerns, whereas failure feedback increased motivation and performance more for those with prevention concerns (see also Idson & Higgins, 2000).

### *Retaining Information Following Goal Completion*

Once people complete their goals, information tied to these goals often fades quickly from memory (Lewin, 1935). This fading serves a functional purpose and frees people's limited cognitive resources for the demands of new objectives. Yet it could also be functional in these circumstances to retain goal-relevant information, since this could facilitate the reinitiation of the goal if the need arises. Hedberg and Higgins (2006) recently proposed that people's promotion versus prevention motivations may influence the extent to which goal-relevant information fades or is retained following goal completion. Because they focus on gains, those with promotion concerns should show greater fading, to maximize the cognitive resources available for identifying new opportunities for gains. In contrast, because they focus on losses, those with prevention concerns should show greater retention, to minimize the chance that they will be caught off guard if previous goals reemerge. In a study supporting this hypothesis, people with chronic promotion or prevention concerns viewed a series of images and attempted to identify how many times pictures of eyeglasses were followed by pictures of scissors. The concept *eyeglasses* therefore signaled a possibility for goal completion, and should have been highly activated during the task, but this activation should then have faded when the task was over. As expected, those with promotion concerns indeed showed a marked decay in the activation of eyeglass-related concepts (assessed via a lexical decision task) as soon as 1 minute following the identification task. However, those with prevention concerns still showed increased activation of (and behavioral response to) these concepts up to 15 minutes later.

To summarize, the research reviewed thus far reveals a host of ways in which promotion and prevention motivations affect evaluation, judgment and decision making, and goal pursuit. Given these effects on such fundamental psychological processes, whether people are motivated by promotion or prevention has wide-reaching implications for how they conduct and experience many aspects of their lives. In the space remaining, we explore some of these implications for people's social interactions and social behavior.

## IMPLICATIONS OF PROMOTION VERSUS PREVENTION MOTIVATION FOR SOCIAL BEHAVIOR

Research on promotion and prevention motivations has recently begun to investigate how these motivations might influence many aspects of people's social lives. Here we consider these influences at several different levels of social interaction: relationships with intimate partners, relationships within groups, and intergroup relations.

### Promotion- and Prevention-Focused Relationships

Intimate relationships fulfill people's basic needs for acceptance, yet they can also be painful sources of rejection and betrayal. One important question when examining relationships, then, is this: How do people respond when rejection or betrayal does occur? Recent studies by Molden and Finkel (2006) have suggested that people's motivations for promotion or prevention can influence such responses by altering their focus on the perceived benefits of repairing a relationship versus the perceived cost of allowing the relationship to deteriorate.

Following both real and imagined betrayals by acquaintances, friends, and romantic partners, those with promotion concerns showed greater forgiveness in relationships where they trusted that future gains were still possible, whereas those with prevention concerns showed greater forgiveness in relationships where they were committed to protecting against losing their attachment to and investment in their partners.

Converging evidence for the greater attachment concerns shown by prevention-focused individuals comes from another study that more closely examined how promotion or prevention motivations affect people's reactions to rejection from close others (Ayduk, May, Downey, & Higgins, 2003). In this study, promotion- or prevention-focused individuals completed a daily diary with their dating partners. On days where the couples experienced conflict, prevention-focused individuals reported greater suppression of thoughts and feelings that might perpetuate this conflict; also, even when feeling highly rejected by their partners, they expressed their displeasure in more passive (e.g., distancing) than active (e.g., retaliating) ways. Thus prevention concerns also seem to lead people to guard against conflict that could damage their attachment to a close relationship partner, even when a compelling reason for this conflict does exist.

### Promotion- and Prevention-Focused Groups

Outside of intimate relationships, social interactions largely occur within a group context. Although group affiliations can be fleeting and arbitrary (e.g., riders on the uptown train) or lasting and meaningful (e.g., Red Sox or Yankees fans), such affiliations have important effects on social behavior (see Levine & Moreland, 1998). One well-established effect is that group members tend to converge on a unifying set of opinions and practices. Levine, Higgins, and Choi (2000) thus asked: (1) Do people form group affiliations based on shared promotion or prevention motivations, and (2) do such group members converge to display behaviors associated with such motivations?

To answer this, Levine and colleagues (2000) had three-person groups perform a recognition memory task (similar to that in Crowe & Higgins [1997], described above) and gave them either promotion- or prevention-focused incentives for overall group performance. Each group member reported his or her recognition judgment aloud, and over the course of the task, most groups (27 out of 34) did indeed develop a common response strategy. Furthermore, for promotion-focused groups, this strategy reflected eagerly ensuring hits and guarding against errors of omission, but for prevention-focused groups, it reflected vigilantly ensuring correct rejections and guarding against errors of commission. Thus not only can shared promotion or prevention concerns create common group norms, but they can influence group-level judgments and behaviors as well.

### Promotion- and Prevention-Focused Intergroup Relations

Besides convergence on shared norms, another well-established effect of affiliating with either meaningful or arbitrary groups is the favoritism that develops toward members of one's own ingroup over members of outgroups (Levine & Moreland, 1998). Might promotion or prevention motivations play a role in these types of group processes as well?

Two separate programs of research have investigated this question (Sassenberg, Kessler, & Mummendy, 2003; Shah et al., 2004). Each has shown that favoritism in rewarding and embracing ingroup members is driven by promotion concerns, because this eagerly develops ties to positively viewed groups, whereas favoritism in punishing and rejecting outgroup members is driven by prevention concerns, because this vigilantly eliminates ties to negatively viewed groups. In one study by Shah and colleagues (2004) illustrating this effect, people were assigned to teams competing on a word-matching task and were then asked about both their teammates and their competitors. Those for whom promotion concerns had been activated were more interested in getting to know their teammates than their competitors, and felt happier about meeting the former, whereas those for whom prevention concerns had been activated showed neither of these differences. However, those for whom prevention concerns had been activated were more interested in avoiding contact with their competitors than their teammates, and felt more anxious about meeting the former, whereas those for whom promotion concerns had been activated showed neither of these differences. A second study by Shah and colleagues showed similar effects when people's actual behaviors toward a perceived ingroup or outgroup member (i.e., how closely they sat next to this person) were assessed.

As these results show, promotion and prevention motivations may affect people's expressions of intergroup favoritism. Do these motivations influence how people experience favoritism shown by other groups as well? Experiencing discrimination from another group is clearly painful. However, if this discrimination is perceived as blocking opportunities for advancement, this pain may involve dejection and low motivational intensity, whereas if this discrimination is perceived as a threat to one's security, this pain may involve agitation and high motivational intensity. Thus, analogous to the differential effects of failure feedback discussed earlier (Förster et al., 2001; Idson & Higgins, 2000), people who experience discrimination as diminishing their security may be more motivated to act toward preventing such experiences than people who experience discrimination as diminishing their advancement.

Consistent with this hypothesis, Quinn and Olson (2006) demonstrated that in general, prevention-focused women report stronger intentions to engage in actions aimed at reducing discrimination toward women (e.g., participating in protests regarding women's issues), as well as a greater frequency of having previously performed such actions, than do promotion-focused women. However, as would be expected, Quinn and Olson also showed that in instances where such actions are explicitly framed as removing obstacles to advancement, promotion-focused women report stronger intentions to engage in these behaviors than do prevention-focused women. Taken together, the studies by Quinn and Olson (2006) and by Shah and colleagues (2004) therefore suggest that considering people's promotion versus prevention motivations in the context of intergroup relations could be important for understanding how people behave toward their ingroups and outgroups, and how they perceive and respond to behaviors by other members of these groups.

Overall, a growing body of research has shown that people's motivations for promotion and prevention have marked implications for many aspects of their social interactions. Therefore, in future explorations of social behavior, beyond considering people's larger motivations for affiliation and belonging (Leary & Cox, Chapter 2, this volume), it may also be fruitful to consider whether they are currently representing such motivations as promotion or prevention concerns (see Molden et al., 2006).

## SUMMARY AND CONCLUSIONS: COSTS AND BENEFITS OF PROMOTION OR PREVENTION

In this chapter, we have discussed a wide variety of ways in which promotion and prevention motivations have profound and distinct effects on thoughts, feelings, and behavior. Considering these effects as a whole, it may be tempting to ask, Is one motivational orientation "better" than the other? That is, are there greater benefits and fewer costs associated with a promotion or prevention focus?

At first glance, it may indeed seem that people motivated by promotion enjoy certain advantages over those motivated by prevention. Compared to the loss focus of prevention concerns, the gain focus of promotion concerns produces (1) more pleasurable responses to success and less painful responses to failure (Idson et al., 2000), (2) greater open-mindedness and creativity (Crowe & Higgins, 1997; Friedman & Förster, 2001; Liberman et al., 2001), and (3) greater flexibility and adaptiveness during goal pursuit (Liberman et al., 1999; Shah & Higgins, 1997). However, many of these qualities are not as universally advantageous as they seem. First, although the dejection arising from failed attempts at promotion can be less intense than the agitation arising from failed attempts at prevention (Idson et al., 2000), this dejection is also less motivating and results in less activity toward avoiding future failures (Förster et al., 2001; Idson & Higgins, 2000; Quinn & Olson, 2006). Indeed, in extreme cases, this reduced motivation can reach the point of having no interest in doing anything—a state associated with the extremely painful condition of clinical depression. Also, while promotion concerns allow a more open-minded consideration of alternatives during judgment, this can create greater uncertainty and indecision when these judgments must be applied or acted upon (Liberman et al., 2001; Molden & Higgins, 2004,

2006). Finally, whereas a promotion focus supports more flexibility in what goals are adopted and sustained, it also more readily allows important goals to be abandoned when success appears unlikely or when setbacks are encountered (Liberman et al., 1999; Shah & Higgins, 1997).

When one is comparing promotion and prevention motivations, it may therefore be more accurate to characterize such motivations as involving a series of complementary compromises. A promotion focus prioritizes flexibility, open-mindedness, and speedy, eager progress, but it does so by sacrificing commitment, certainty, and careful, vigilant analysis. A prevention focus reverses these priorities and sacrifices. Whatever one's emphasis, however, all of these qualities are important components of self-regulation and goal pursuit, and all are required for the successful execution of such processes. This is clearly illustrated in a study by Grant and Higgins (2003), which related people's histories of effectively regulating both their promotion and prevention concerns to their emotional and overall well-being. Although there were differences in what specific behaviors and emotions mediated the influences of effective promotion and effective prevention, results showed that both independently, and additively, predicted greater well-being. Thus the most crucial factor in comparing the advantages of promotion or prevention motivations in any given situation may be whether eagerness or vigilance best fits the demands of the current task at hand (see Higgins, Chapter 23, this volume).

To conclude, the research reviewed in this chapter has conclusively demonstrated that concerns with advancement (i.e., promoting gains) and concerns with security (i.e., preventing losses) are fundamentally distinct in how they are represented and experienced, and thus have fundamentally different effects on the processes of evaluation, judgment and decision making, and goal pursuit. What researchers are just beginning to explore are the implications of these various effects for how people navigate and interact with their social environments, as well as with the individuals that exist within those environments. Given the variety and importance of such interactions, continued research along these lines promises not only to expand our understanding of growth and security motivations, but also to provide greater insights into social behavior as a whole.

## NOTES

1. Indeed, findings from several studies using this methodology have shown separate main effects of both promotion versus prevention and approach versus avoidance manipulations on a variety of different measures (e.g., people's strategic focus during problem solving or in social situations, and their emotional well-being; see Carver, Lawrence, & Scheier, 1999; Förster, Higgins, & Idson 1998; Higgins, Roney, Crowe, & Hymes, 1994). This further illustrates the independence of these two motivational distinctions.

2. Several different methods have been developed for measuring and manipulating promotion versus prevention concerns (see Förster et al., 1998; Higgins et al., 1994, 1997, 2001; Roese et al., 1999; Shah, Brazy, & Higgins, 2004; Shah & Higgins, 1997). Space limitations preclude a detailed description or comparison of these methods in the studies presented in this chapter, however, and interested readers are encouraged to examine the original articles for more information on the specific operationalizations used in each study.

3. Raghunathan and Pham (1999) discussed these effects solely in terms of affective influences on decision making and did not relate them to larger promotion or prevention motivations. However, based on our earlier discussion of the emotional sensitivities associated with such motivations (see also Higgins, 2000; Roese et al., 1999), we suggest that by selectively inducing dejection or agitation, they did indeed activate more general promotion or prevention concerns (see also Lerner, Small, & Lowenstein, 2004).

## REFERENCES

Aaker, J. L., & Lee, A. Y. (2001). "I" seek pleasures and "we" avoid pains: The role of self-regulatory goals in information processing and persuasion. *Journal of Consumer Research, 28*, 33–49.

Amodio, D. M., Shah, J. Y., Sigelman, J., Brazy, P. C., & Harmon-Jones, E. (2004). Implicit regulatory focus associated with asymmetrical frontal cortical activity. *Journal of Experimental Social Psychology, 40*, 225–232.

Ayduk, O., May, D., Downey, G., & Higgins, E. T. (2003). Tactical differences in coping with rejection sensitivity: The role of prevention pride. *Personality and Social Psychology Bulletin, 29*, 435–448.

Bar-Hillel, M. (1973). On the subjective probability of compound events. *Organizational Behavior and Human Performance, 9*, 396–406.

Barrett, L. F., & Russell, J. A. (1999). The structure of current affect: Controversies and emerging consensus. *Current Directions in Psychological Science, 8*, 10–14.

Bowlby, J. (1969). *Attachment and loss: Vol. 1. Attachment.* New York: Basic Books.

Brockner, J., Paruchuri, S., Idson, L. C., & Higgins, E. T. (2002). Regulatory focus and the probability estimates of conjunctive and disjunctive events. *Organizational Behavior and Human Decision Processes, 87*, 5–24.

Bruner, J., & Postman, L. (1947). Tension and tension release as organizing factors in perception. *Journal of Personality, 15*, 300–308.

Cacioppo, J. T., Priester, J. R., & Berntson, G. G. (1993). Rudimentary determinants of attitudes: II. Arm flexion and extension have differential effects on attitudes. *Journal of Personality and Social Psychology, 65*, 5–17.

Carver, C. S. (2004). Self-regulation of action and affect. In R. F. Baumeister & K. D. Vohs (Eds.), *Handbook of self-regulation: Research, theory, and applications* (pp. 13–39). New York: Guilford Press.

Carver, C. S., Lawrence, J. W., & Scheier, M. F. (1999). Self-discrepancies and affect: Incorporating the role of feared selves. *Personality and Social Psychology Bulletin, 25*, 783–792.

Crowe, E., & Higgins, E. T. (1997). Regulatory focus and strategic inclinations: Promotion and prevention in decision-making. *Organizational Behavior and Human Decision Processes, 69*, 117–132.

Davidson, R. J., & Irwin, W. (1999). The functional neuroanatomy of emotion and affective style. *Trends Cognitive Sciences, 3*, 11–21.

Evans, L. M., & Petty, R. E. (2003). Self-guide framing and persuasion: Responsibly increasing message processing to ideal levels. *Personality and Social Psychology Bulletin, 29*, 313–324.

Feather, N. T. (Ed.). (1982). *Expectations and actions: Expectancy–value models in psychology.* Hillsdale, NJ: Erlbaum.

Förster, J., Grant, H., Idson, L. C., & Higgins, E. T. (2001). Success/failure feedback, expectancies, and approach/avoidance motivation: How regulatory focus moderates classic relations. *Journal of Experimental Social Psychology, 37*, 253–260.

Förster, J., & Higgins, E. T. (2005). How global versus local perception fits regulatory focus. *Psychological Science, 16*, 631–636.

Förster, J., Higgins, E. T., & Bianco, A. T. (2003). Speed/accuracy decisions in task performance: Built in trade-off of separate strategic concerns. *Organization Behavior and Human Decision Processes, 90*, 148–164.

Förster, J., Higgins, E. T., & Idson, L. C. (1998). Approach and avoidance strength during goal attainment: Regulatory focus and the "goal looms larger" effect. *Journal of Personality and Social Psychology, 75*, 1115–1131.

Freitas, A. L., Liberman, N., Salovey, P., & Higgins, E. T. (2002). When to begin?: Regulatory focus and initiating goal pursuit. *Personality and Social Psychology Bulletin, 28*, 121–130.

Freitas, A. L., Travers, S., Azizian, A., & Berry, S. (2004). The evaluative connotation of processing fluency: Inherently positive or moderated by motivational context? *Journal of Experimental Social Psychology, 41*, 636–644.

Freud, S. (1953). Fragments of an analysis of a case of hysteria. In J. Strachey (Ed. & Trans.), *The standard edition of the complete psychological works of Sigmund Freud* (Vol. 7, pp. 1–122). London: Hogarth Press. (Original work published 1905)

Friedman, R. S., & Förster, J. (2001). The effects of promotion and prevention cues on creativity. *Journal of Personality and Social Psychology, 81*, 1001–1013.

Friedman, R. S., & Förster, J. (2005). Effects of motivational cues on perceptual asymmetry: Implications for creativity and analytical problem solving. *Journal of Personality and Social Psychology, 88*, 263–275.

Grant, H., & Higgins, E. T. (2003). Optimism, promotion pride, and prevention pride as predictors of quality of life. *Personality and Social Psychology Bulletin, 29*, 1521–1532.

Hedberg, P. H., & Higgins, E. T. (2006). *Decay in concept accessibility as motivated cognition.* Unpublished manuscript.

Higgins, E. T. (1987). Self-discrepancy: A theory relating self and affect. *Psychological Review, 94*, 319–340.

Higgins, E. T. (1997). Beyond pleasure and pain. *American Psychologist, 52*, 1280–1300.

Higgins, E. T. (2000). Promotion and prevention experiences: Relating emotions to non-emotional motivational states. In J. P. Forgas (Ed.), *Handbook of affect and social cognition* (pp. 186–211). Mahwah, NJ: Erlbaum.

Higgins, E. T., Friedman, R. S., Harlow, R. E., Idson, L. C., Ayduk, O. N., & Taylor, A. (2001). Achievement orientations from subjective histories of success: Promotion pride versus prevention pride. *European Journal of Social Psychology, 31*, 3–23.

Higgins, E. T., & Molden, D. C. (2003). How strategies for making judgments and decisions affect cognition: Motivated cognition revisited. In G. V. Bodenhausen & A. J. Lambert (Eds.), *Foundations of social cognition: A festschrift in honor of Robert S. Wyer, Jr.* (pp. 211–236). Mahwah, NJ: Erlbaum.

Higgins, E. T., Roney, C., Crowe, E., & Hymes, C. (1994). Ideal versus ought predilections for approach and avoidance: Distinct self-regulatory systems. *Journal of Personality and Social Psychology, 66*, 276–286.

Higgins, E. T., Shah, J., & Friedman, R. (1997). Emotional responses to goal attainment: Strength of regulatory focus as moderator. *Journal of Personality and Social Psychology, 72*, 515–525.

Higgins, E. T., & Silberman, I. (1998). Development of regulatory focus: Promotion and prevention as ways of living. In J. Heckhausen & C. S. Dweck (Eds.), *Motivation and self-regulation across the life span* (pp. 78–113). New York: Cambridge University Press.

Higgins, E. T., & Spiegel, S. (2004). Promotion and prevention strategies for self-regulation: A motivated cognition perspective. In R. F. Baumeister & K. D. Vohs (Eds.), *Handbook of self-regulation: Research, theory, and applications* (pp. 171–187). New York: Guilford Press.

Higgins, E. T., & Tykocinski, O. (1992). Self-discrepancies and biographical memory: Personality and cognition at the level of psychological situations. *Personality and Social Psychology Bulletin, 18*, 527–535.

Idson, L. C., & Higgins, E. T. (2000). How current feedback and chronic effectiveness influence motivation: Everything to gain versus everything to lose. *European Journal of Social Psychology, 30*, 583–592.

Idson, L. C., Liberman, N., & Higgins, E. T. (2000). Distinguishing gains from non-losses and losses from non-gains: A regulatory focus perspective on hedonic intensity. *Journal of Experimental Social Psychology, 36*, 252–274.

Jain, S. P., Agrawal, N., & Maheswaran, D. (2006). When more may be less: The effects of regulatory focus on responses to different comparative frames, *Journal of Consumer Research, 33*, 91–98.

Kahneman, D., Knetsch, J. L., & Thaler, R. (1991). The endowment effect, loss aversion, and status quo bias. *Journal of Economic Perspectives, 5*, 193–206.

Kahneman, D., & Tversky, A. (1979). Prospect theory: An analysis of decision under risk. *Econometrica, 47*, 263–291.

Kelley, H. H. (1973). The process of causal attribution. *American Psychologist, 28*, 107–128.

Kim, Y. J. (2006). The role of regulatory focus in message framing in antismoking advertisements for adolescents. *Journal of Advertising, 35*, 143–151.

Kunda, Z. (1990). The case for motivated reasoning. *Psychological Bulletin, 108*, 480–498.

LeDoux, J. E. (1996). *The emotional brain*. New York: Simon & Schuster.

Lee, A. Y., Aaker, J. L., & Gardner, W. L. (2000). The pleasures and pains of distinct self-construals: The role of interdependence in regulatory focus. *Journal of Personality and Social Psychology, 78*, 1122–1134.

Lerner, J. S., Small, D. A., & Lowenstein, G. (2004). Heart strings and purse strings: Carryover effects of emotions on economic decisions. *Psychological Science, 15*, 337–341.

Levine, J. M., Higgins, E. T., & Choi, H. S. (2000). Development of strategic norms in groups. *Organizational Behavior and Human Decision Processes, 82*, 88–101.

Levine, J. M., & Moreland, R. L. (1998). Small groups. In D. T. Gilbert, S. T. Fiske, & G. Lindzey (Eds.), *The handbook of social psychology* (4th ed., Vol. 2, pp. 415–469). New York: McGraw-Hill.

Lewin, K. (1935). *A dynamic theory of personality*. New York: McGraw-Hill.

Liberman, N., Idson, L. C., Camacho, C. J., & Higgins, E. T. (1999). Promotion and prevention choices between stability and change. *Journal of Personality and Social Psychology, 77*, 1135–1145.

Liberman, N. Idson, L. C., & Higgins, E. T. (2005). Predicting the intensity of losses vs. non-gains and non-losses vs. gains in judging fairness and value: A test of the loss aversion explanation. *Journal of Experimental Social Psychology, 41*, 527–534.

Liberman, N., Molden, D. C., Idson, L. C., & Higgins, E. T. (2001). Promotion and prevention focus on alternative hypotheses: Implications for attributional functions. *Journal of Personality and Social Psychology, 80*, 5–18.

Lockwood, P., Jordan, C. H., & Kunda, Z. (2002). Motivation by positive or negative role models: Regulatory focus determines who will best inspire us. *Journal of Personality and Social Psychology, 83*, 854–864.

Manian, N., Strauman, T. J., & Denney, N. (1998). Temperament, recalled parenting styles, and self-regulation: Testing the developmental postulates of self-discrepancy theory. *Journal of Personality and Social Psychology, 75*, 1321–1332.

Markman, A. B., Baldwin, G. C., & Maddox, W. T. (2005). The interaction of payoff structure and regulatory focus in classification. *Psychological Science, 16*, 852–855.

Maslow, A. (1955). Deficiency motivation and growth motivation. In M. Jones (Ed.), *Nebraska Symposium on Motivation: Vol. 3. 1955* (pp. 1–30). Lincoln: University of Nebraska Press.

Molden, D. C., & Finkel, E. J. (2006). *Motivations for interpersonal forgiveness: Promoting gains in trust versus preventing losses of commitment*. Unpublished manuscript.

Molden, D. C., & Higgins, E. T. (2004). Categorization under uncertainty: Resolving vagueness and ambiguity with eager versus vigilant strategies. *Social Cognition, 22*, 248–277.

Molden, D. C., & Higgins, E. T. (2005). Motivated thinking. In K. Holyoak & R. G. Morrison (Eds.), *Cambridge handbook of thinking and reasoning* (pp. 295–317). New York: Cambridge University Press.

Molden, D. C., & Higgins, E. T. (2006). *Effects of preferences for eager versus vigilant judgment strategies on the pursuit of self-serving judgment outcomes*. Unpublished manuscript, Northwestern University.

Molden, D. C., Lucas, G. M., Gardner, W. L., Dean, K., & Knowles, M. (2006). *Distinct self-regulation following distinct social threats: Responding to rejection versus exclusion*. Unpublished manuscript, Northwestern University.

Murray, H. A. (1938). *Explorations in personality*. New York: Oxford University Press.

Pennington, G. L., & Roese, N. J. (2003). Regulatory focus and temporal distance. *Journal of Experimental Social Psychology, 39*, 563–576.

Quinn, K. A., & Olson, J. M. (2006). *Regulatory framing and collective action: The interplay of individual self-regulation and group behavior.* Unpublished manuscript.

Raghunathan, R., & Pham, M. T. (1999). All negative moods are not equal: Motivational influences of anxiety and sadness on decision making. *Organizational Behavior and Human Decision Processes, 79*, 56–77.

Roese, N. J. (1997). Counterfactual thinking. *Psychological Bulletin, 121*, 133–148.

Roese, N. J., Hur, T., & Pennington, G. L. (1999). Counterfactual thinking and regulatory focus: Implications for action versus inaction and sufficiency versus necessity. *Journal of Personality and Social Psychology, 77*, 1109–1120.

Sanders, A. F. (1998). *Elements of human performance: Reaction processes and attention in human skill.* Mahwah, NJ: Erlbaum.

Sassenberg, K., Kessler, T., & Mummendy, A. (2003). Less negative = more positive? Social discrimination as avoidance or approach. *Journal of Experimental Social Psychology, 39*, 48–58.

Seibt, B., & Förster, J. (2004). Stereotype-threat and performance: How self-stereotypes influence processing by inducing regulatory foci. *Journal of Personality and Social Psychology, 87*, 36–58.

Shah, J., Brazy, P. C., & Higgins, E. T. (2004). Promoting us or preventing them: Regulatory focus and manifestations of intergroup bias. *Personality and Social Psychology Bulletin, 30*, 433–446.

Shah, J., & Higgins, E. T. (1997). Expectancy × value effects: Regulatory focus as a determinant of magnitude and direction. *Journal of Personality and Social Psychology, 73*, 447–458.

Shah, J., & Higgins, E. T. (2001). Regulatory concerns and appraisal efficiency: The general impact of promotion and prevention. *Journal of Personality and Social Psychology, 80*, 693–705.

Strauman, T. J. (1990). Self-discrepancies and childhood memories: A study of retrieval efficiency and negative emotional content. *Journal of Personality and Social Psychology, 59*, 869–880.

Tanner, W. P., Jr., & Swets, J. A. (1954). A decision-making theory of visual detection. *Psychological Review, 61*, 401–409.

Triplett, N. (1898). The dynamogenic factors in pacemaking and competition. *American Journal of Psychology, 9*, 507–533.

Zajonc, R. B. (2001). Mere exposure: A gateway to the subliminal. *Current Directions in Psychological Science, 10*, 224–228.

Chapter 12

# The Neuroevolution of Motivation

**Gary G. Berntson**
**John T. Cacioppo**

Man with all his noble qualities still bears in his bodily frame the indelible stamp of his lowly origin.
—CHARLES DARWIN

Motivational concepts have been central to systematic psychological, behavioral, and social psychological theories over the past century (Berridge, 2004; Cofer & Appley, 1964; Higgins, 1997). Motivational theories have been highly diverse in their nature and focus, but for the most part they have been developed largely from psychological or behavioral data and concepts. This is true even for homeostatic motives, such as hunger and thirst, which have reasonably well-documented neural substrates. Although this single-level approach to theory building is perfectly appropriate, the question arises as to whether a multilevel, interdisciplinary approach to neurobehavioral organization may offer meaningful insights into, or constraints on, motivational concepts and theories (Berntson & Cacioppo, 2004; Cacioppo & Berntson, 1992). The present chapter considers some aspects of evolutionary neurodevelopment and neuraxial organization that offer a beginning framework for integrative neurobehavioral and neuropsychological models of motivation. We then consider the implications of this general approach for understanding social processes and behavior.

## LEVELS OF ORGANIZATION IN THE NERVOUS SYSTEM

### Neural Hierarchies

In his essay "Evolution and Dissolution of the Nervous System," the noted 19th-century neurologist John Hughlings Jackson emphasized a multilevel perspective on brain organization and function (Jackson, 1958). In contrast to the view that the evolutionary emergence of higher levels of the neuraxis functionally replaces lower-level organizations, Jackson noted that evolution results in a progressive layering of functional levels within the neuraxis. This yields what he termed a *re-representation* of function throughout the neuraxis, wherein higher levels are characterized by elaborated networks with progressively greater flexibility and functional sophistication. Rather than replacing lower mechanisms, however, higher systems critically depend on these lower substrates for informational inputs and for achieving motor outputs in a hierarchical-like fashion.

There is now ample documentation of a hierarchical dimension of organization across the neuraxis, with relatively simple, reflex-like organizations characteristic of the lowest levels, such as the spinal cord, and more complex, integrative substrates at higher levels (Figure 12.1; for reviews, see Berntson, Boysen, & Cacioppo, 1993; Berntson & Cacioppo, 2000; Berridge, 2004). The vertical gradients in Figure 12.1 illustrate important characteristics of different levels of organization in neural hierarchies. Lower-level substrates, such as reflex networks, are composed of relatively simple circuits, in the limit consisting of a single central synapse (e.g., monosynpatic stretch reflex). Although reflexes can and do interact, the basic circuits are organized in parallel, with limited inputs and outputs, allowing for rapid, efficient processing (Sherrington, 1906). The cost of this efficiency, however, is that lower-level systems have limited integrative capacity. In contrast, higher-level elements receive a much broader array of inputs, which requires more substantive processing, in addition to the need to relate this information associative networks and executive systems for strategic responding. Because of inherent processing capacity limits even in complex circuits, higher-level systems may be subject to a processing bottleneck that necessitates a less efficient, serial mode of information processing.

As illustrated in Figure 12.1, lower-level organizations in neural hierarchies are crucial, as they represent the basic output elements that allow higher-level systems to achieve motor expression. Moreover, lower-level systems represent the initial perceptual processing stages that transmit processed information to higher levels. In addition to these input and output functions, which are essentially in the service of higher integrative substrates, lower-level substrates have an inherent functional capability. Indeed, the distinct advantages and disadvantages associated with higher-level (integrative, flexible, but capacity-limited) and lower-level (rapid, efficient, but rigid) processing was a likely source of evolutionary pressure for the preservation of lower-level substates despite higher-level elaborations and rerepresentations. The ability to strategically

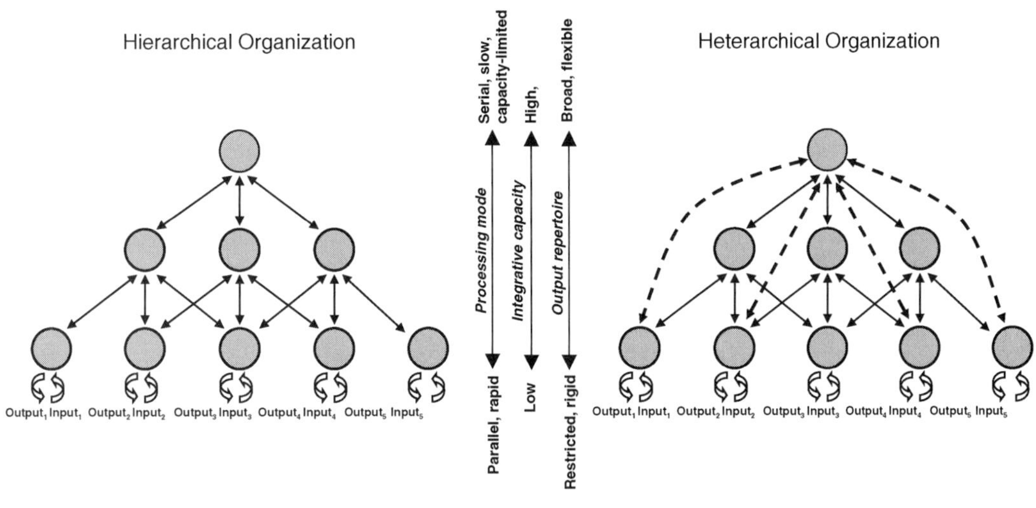


**FIGURE 12.1.** Hierarchical and heterarchical organizations. A heterarchy differs from a hierarchy in the existence of long ascending and descending pathways that span intermediate levels. Properties of the levels in both classes of organizations lie along the illustrated continuua of *processing mode*, *integrative capacity*, and *output repertoire*. Heterarchical organizations, however, have greater integrative capacity and output flexibility, as the long ascending and descending projections provide inputs and outputs that are not constrained by intermediate levels.

avoid potential danger based on memory and reasoning would confer tremendous adaptive advantage. At the same time, rapid low-level processing (e.g., pain withdrawal reflexes) may serve to sustain survival in the short term, so that higher-level strategies can develop.

Hierarchical dimensions of central nervous system organization are clearly established, and can be demonstrated anatomically as well as functionally (see Berntson et al., 1993). The simple hierarchy depicted in Figure 12.1, however, belies the true complexity of neurobehavioral substrates.

## Neural Heterarchies

It is now recognized that additional complexities exist in neural organizations, as long ascending and descending pathways can bypass intermediate levels of hierarchical organization and interconnect across widely separated neural levels. Much behavioral output entails higher-level operations on intermediate hierarchical levels of motor organization, which then translate descending neural commands into patterned actions, freeing higher-level substrates from the demands of coordinating individual response elements into adaptively meaningful behavioral outputs. Cortical motor neurons, however, have been shown to project not only to intermediate-level somatomotor networks, but also directly onto spinal motor neurons through long descending pathways (Edgley, Eyre, Lemon, & Miller, 1997; Porter, 1987). Similarly, while lower autonomic substrates can organize autonomic outflows into adaptive homeostatic reflexes, higher-level systems can bypass these intermediary substrates and yield nonhomeostatic or antihomeostatic effects via relatively direct actions on lower autonomic source nuclei (Berntson & Cacioppo, 2000).

The long ascending and descending pathways in neural hierarchies, which span hierarchical levels, together with the existence of lateral interactions within levels, yield an organizational plan that has been termed a *neural heterarchy* (see Berntson et al., 1993; Berntson & Cacioppo, 2000). One important distinction between a hierarchical organization and a heterarchical system is that the outputs of the former are coherent, as all pass through the same intermediary regulatory levels before accessing lower output mechanisms. In contrast, higher-level systems in a neural heterarchy (see Figure 12.1, right side) can directly access lower output substrates in parallel with intermediary levels. The existence of multiple, rerepresentative levels of organization at which stimuli can be processed and responses generated raises the possibility of functional conflicts between higher- and lower-level systems in regulating behavioral outputs. We will return to this issue below, but we first consider some features and implications of the evolutionary rerepresentation of function across levels of organization.

## Levels of Function

### *Lower Levels and Premotivational Functions*

The lowest and most primitive levels of organization within the central nervous system can be seen in spinal reflex networks. Evolution of the nervous system proceeded in parallel with the evolutionary increase in complexity and tissue differentiation within organisms, and the associated need to integrate internal functions and motor actions. Within the ventral horn of the spinal cord reside all lower motor neurons controlling the skeletal muscles of the trunk and limbs, and all somatosensory information from the these structures enters the nervous system at the level of the cord. In addition to serving as the final common pathway for central influences on the musculature, primitive integrative organizations are also present at the level of the cord. These reflex networks regulate simple stimulus–response relations, and represent the lowest levels in the central neural heterarchy.

Although spinal networks may have limited functions, they offer considerable advantages for the study of neurobehavioral relations, precisely because of their simplicity. Spinal circuits may have limited direct relevance for higher-level motivations, but they reveal the basic functional architecture that characterizes neural organizations at all levels of the neuraxis (for a historical introduction, see Sherrington, 1906). Neural networks evidence similar organizational schemes and adhere to common functional principles at all levels, but these schemes and principles may be more difficult to discern in view of the increasing complexities at higher levels.

Of particular relevance to the study of motivation and its origins in neural systems are the spinal reflexes of cutaneous origin, which represent basic patterns of response to the environment. One general class of spinal reflexes consists of the flexor (pain) withdrawal reflexes to noxious stimuli. Flexor withdrawal reflexes are among the most salient, the earliest to develop, and the most resistant to disruption. These attributes reflect an important functional manifestation of central neural systems: Powerful mechanisms exist at all levels of the neuraxis to protect the organism from danger by fostering escape and/or avoidance from potentially injurious stimuli or contexts. The potency of these protective organizations is readily apparent in the compelling motivational effects of pain and the powerful aversive reactions to threatening contexts, which arise from higher neuraxial levels. We will return to this topic below.

Although spinal flexor withdrawal reflexes would not be considered motivational, they represent primitive premotivational dispositions or response biases away from certain classes of stimuli. Flexor reflexes contrast with another class, the extensor reflexes. The latter foster limb approach-like extension reactions to moderate cutaneous stimulation of the plantar surface of the foot, which serve as an important substrate for locomotion and ultimately exploration.

The opposing flexor and extensor reflexes are reminiscent of elementary approach–withdrawal reflexes of simple invertebrates having only a primitive nervous system, and illustrate a general pattern of opponent organization in lower-level circuits. This opponent organization is not simply attributable to the fact that flexor and extensor reflexes control opposing muscles and hence are physically constrained to an opponent organization. Rather, there exist explicit inhibitory interneurons that exert mutual reciprocal inhibition between flexor and extensor motor neurons—a principle of neural organization that Sherrington termed the *principle of reciprocal innervation* (Sherrington, 1906). An increase in flexor outflow not only increases tension in flexor muscles and physically opposes extensor movements, but also results in a neural inhibition of extensor motor neurons.

Although there is a qualitative symmetry in the spinal flexor–extensor opponent organization, this does not imply a quantitative equivalence. As discussed above, flexor reflexes are generally more potent than extensor reflexes and can readily overpower extensor responses. The precedence of flexor reflexes is apparent in recovery of spinal reflexes after spinal cord transection, where the more rapid and potent recovery of flexor reflexes can seize the patient in a chronic state of paraplegia or quadriplegia in flexion. There is a similar quantitative asymmetry in higher-level approach–withdrawal systems, where powerful aversive reactions to proximal stimuli can overwhelm approach dispositions. This has obvious adaptive advantages and would be expected to lead to a selective evolutionary pressure. It would be far more important for an organism to avoid a predator, and thus survive, than to approach food in the vicinity of the predator. This illustrates an additional neuro-organizational principle termed the *negativity bias* (Cacioppo & Berntson, 1999; Cacioppo, Larsen, Smith, & Berntson, 2004), to which we return below.

Despite this negativity bias, flexor withdrawal reflexes do not always take precedence over extensor approach reflexes, as extensor approach reflexes may dominate at low levels of cutaneous stimuli. It is only with more intense stimuli that one sees the predominance of withdrawal responses. This illustrates an additional neuro-organizational principle also apparent in higher-level approach–withdrawal systems. This principle, termed the *positivity offset* (Cacioppo & Berntson, 1999; Cacioppo et al., 2004), describes the greater neurobehavioral dispositions observed toward extension approach with low levels of activation (or greater distances), which ultimately gives way to avoidance or withdrawal (negativity bias) at higher levels of activation (or shorter distances).

The general organizational features and their functional manifestations of spinal approach–withdrawal reflexes are illustrated in Figure 12.2. Note that despite separate and distinct circuits for flexor and extensor reflexes, the behavioral output of these spinal circuits lies along a bipolar axis from flexion to extension. This bipolar axis is constrained by the physical incompatibility of concurrent flexion and extension. Note also, however, that the functional neural output of spinal circuits is less constrained. Although the limb position can be described along a single continuum from flexion to extension, increases in flexor and extensor motorneuron activity and associated muscle tension can occur concurrently. As illustrated in Figure 12.2, however, this concurrent activity is also constrained—not by physical structures, but by the pattern of reciprocal

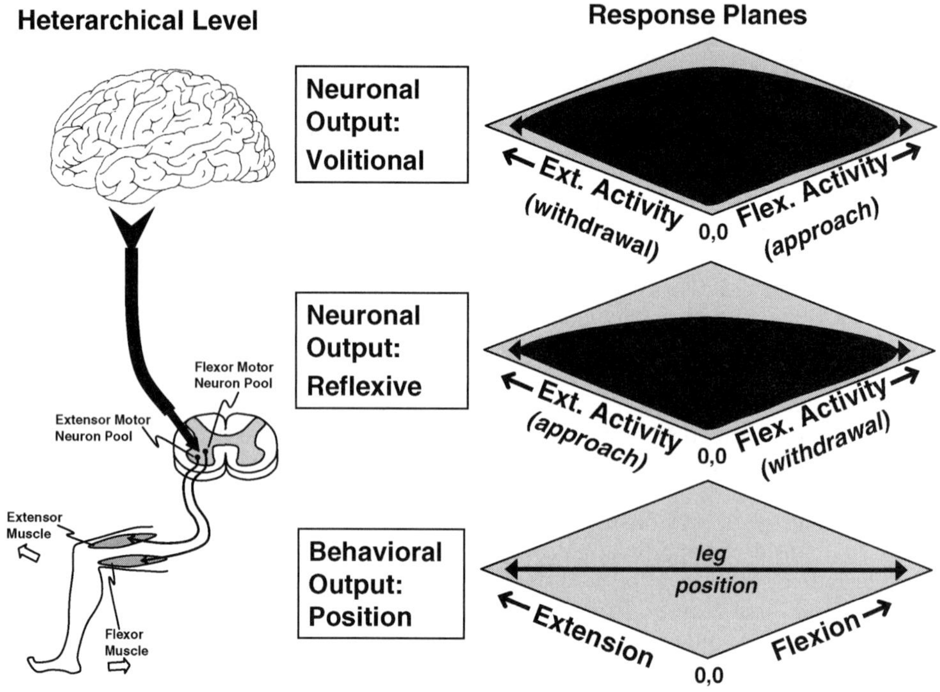


**FIGURE 12.2.** Illustrative output features of levels of organization in heterarchical systems. Left: Levels of organization in systems regulating flexion and extension. Somatomotor systems are depicted at the bottom, spinal flexion/extension reflexes at a lower level in heterarchical control systems (intermediate), and the higher volitional level at the top. Right: Potential outputs are depicted on response planes. At the bottom (behavioral or motor output), physical constraints limit outputs along a single continuum from extension to flexion. At a reflexive level, extensor and flexor reflex activity (motor neuron firing) can be independently activated, so outputs are broader at the neuronal level than at the motor output level. Extensor and flexor reflexes do evidence some mutual inhibition, which reduces the maximum concurrent activity. Consequently, potential patterns of reflex activity are limited to the blackened region of the response plane. At the highest levels, systems underlying volitional processes can exert even a broader range of control over extensor and flexor activity via heterarchical controls that directly impinge on motor neuron pools. The parenthetical *approach–withdrawal* designations along the axes illustrate the fact that similar behavioral outputs may reflect different motivation states at different levels of organization.

innervation and related mutual inhibition in flexor and extensor reflex circuits. Moreover, we humans can also volitionally increase muscle tension in both the flexors and extensors, increasing tension and stiffening the leg, even without limb movement. In fact, through volitional control, the development of tremendous tension in both muscles is possible because the spinal reciprocal inhibition resides in the reflex circuits, which can be bypassed by direct heterarchical control of motor neuron pools during volitional actions. This is illustrated in Figure 12.2, and the general trend in expansion of flexibility and breath of control with higher neuraxial levels is depicted in the *output repertoire* gradient of Figure 12.1.

Motivation is not a property of the nervous system; it is a construct designed to organize or account for complex psychological and behavioral manifestations or outputs of neural systems. Because spinal reflexes can be reasonably accounted for in terms of their eliciting stimuli and neural circuitry, there is little need for invoking motivational accounts of reflex dispositions. But this is not to suggest that the neurobehavioral organizations and operations that underlie motivationally relevant processes are fundamentally different from spinal reflex circuits. They are not, and the principles of neurobehavioral organization derived from lower-level systems offer a starting framework for studies and concepts of higher-level processes. Functional organizations across levels of the neuraxis are not identical, but they often follow similar principles. Moreover, evolution of organizational differences and trends as one proceeds across neuraxial levels may be as informative as commonalities in understanding neurobehavioral relations. From this vantage, we briefly consider higher-level organization.

### *Higher-Level Re-Representations*

As one progresses beyond the primitive organizations of the spinal cord, the progressive evolutionary re-representation and elaboration of functions are clearly apparent. *Decerebrate* animals and humans, whose state results from the tragic conditions of anencephaly and hydranencephaly, have no functional nervous tissue above the level of the brainstem (e.g., see Berntson & Micco, 1976; Tuber, Berntson, Bachman, & Allen, 1980). Decerebrates can show rather remarkable functional capacities, despite their limited nervous system. Indeed, decerebrate animals have dramatically expanded neurological and behavioral repertoires, compared to spinally transected animals. They can stand, locomote, and display many typical species-characteristic behaviors such as grooming and ingestive responses.

Of relevance is the expansion and elaboration of substrates for evaluative processes and approach–withdrawal reactions. As noted by Jackson (1958), higher-level re-representations do not come to replace lower-level processes, and decerebrate organisms as well as intact organisms continue to show pain withdrawal flexor reflexes. In addition, however, decerebrate organisms display a more generalized aversive reaction entailing crying or vocalization, and more organized and integrated withdrawal reactions that include locomotion away from the stimulus source and/or defensive responses (e.g., biting) if escape is not possible. This expanded repertoire of adaptive behavior, relative to simple pain withdrawal reflexes, entails a broader level of integration of bodily responses, as well as greater flexibility and adaptability in the face of aversive stimuli or contexts (see Berntson & Micco, 1976; Berntson et al., 1993).

Perhaps the best-studied example of opposing approach–avoidance responses in decerebrate organisms can be seen in the ingestive intake–rejection responses to hedonic stimuli (for reviews, see Berridge, 2004; Steiner, Glaser, Hawilo, & Berridge, 2001). Both animal and human decerebrates display stereotyped orofacial responses reflecting positive affective expression and ingestion (smiling, licking, swallowing) to palatable sucrose solutions. In contrast, bitter or other unpalatable tastes evoke aversive-like facial expressions and ejection responses (e.g., gaping). Similar responses can be seen in intact human and animal neonates, indicating an early ontological development of the neural circuits that provide the basic neurological substrates for positive and negative hedonic reactions to taste qualities (Steiner et al., 2001). It is interesting to note that although these positive and negative responses reflect opposite intake–rejection responses, their basic neural substrates appear to be independent, rather than converging on a single hedonic integrator (Berridge & Grill, 1984). Increasing the concentration of a bitter adulterant in an otherwise preferred sucrose solution, for example, can increase the probability of rejection responses without decreasing the probability of ingestive responses. Indeed, positive and negative responses may co-occur and/or display a rapid alternation. Equal taste preference (or consumption) therefore does not necessarily imply an equivalent hedonic state.

These findings indicate that basic affective reactions associated with motivationally relevant stimuli are organized at the level of the brainstem. Although decerebrate organisms display notable affective reactions, including approach and avoidance dispositions to environmental stimuli, they clearly lack other qualities of motivational states. In particular, the behavior of decerebrate animals is rather stimulus-bound. Although decerebrates display hedonic reactions to palatable stimuli and may spontaneously ingest food items they encounter adventitiously, they seem relatively indifferent to the absence of relevant goal stimuli, and they lack normal goal-directed striving when deprived of food (Berntson & Micco, 1976). Moreover, although decerebrates can learn simple conditioned aversive reactions and show organized escape responses, they do not display anticipatory avoidance behavior (see Berntson & Micco, 1976; Berntson et al., 1993). Rather, their responses are driven largely by immediate and proximal environmental stimuli impinging on body surface receptors. In the parlance of contemporary social psychology, the processes orchestrated by these neurobehavioral organizations are *implicit*, as they do not depend on conversant awareness, working memory, or voluntary (i.e., the pyramidal) motor outputs.

This is attributable to the fact that the visual and olfactory systems are more recent evolutionary developments that arise at more rostral levels of the neuraxis. Consequently, the somatosensory system dominates the sensorium of the brainstem and spinal cord. In this regard, the extensor–flexor approach–withdrawal reflexes of the cord, together with approach–withdrawal systems of the brainstem, provide basic adaptive reactions to these proximal stimuli. Note, too, that brainstem systems for aversive reactions do not supplant spinal pain withdrawal flexor reflexes, but rather come to *re-represent* and elaborate on the lower processes.

### *Higher Levels and the Elaboration of Motivational Processes*

Rerepresentation of function—and the emergence of explicit as well as implicit processes—become even more apparent with the evolutionary emergence of more rostral levels of the neuraxis. Affective and motivational systems are highly elaborated at the diencephalic level (the posterior part of the forebrain that connects the midbrain with the cerebral hemispheres, encloses the third ventricle, and contains the thalamus and hypothalamus) and the telencephalic level (the anterior portion of the forebrain, constituting of the cerebral hemispheres and related parts). Anatomical substrates associated with the amygdala, for example, play an important role in acquired aversive reactions (LeDoux, 2003) and in conferring the emotional coloring that guides behavior and choice (Bechara, Damasio, & Damasio, 2003; Berntson, Bechara, Damasio, Tranel, & Cacioppo, in press). Similarly, systems associated with the nucleus accumbens support not only the motivational "liking" reactions, as are also seen in the decerebrate, but the "wanting" processes that underlie incentive motivation and goal striving (Berridge, 2004). It is at the hypothalamic/diencephalic level, for example, that one sees the elaborated expression of hunger, which includes (1) a sensitivity to internal need states, (2) a broad repertoire of appetitive and consummatory reactions, (3) the capacity to learn about food sources and availability, (4) the ability to acquire novel behaviors in order to obtain a goal object, and (5) hedonic reward processes that support the appetitive behaviors.

The ultimate expression of neural rerepresentation is embodied in cerebral cortical systems (and their interactions with lower levels). It is the cortex that provides for the most sophisticated sensory and perceptual analyses, access to associative networks, attentional focus, conversant awareness, strategic planning, response selection, and outcome monitoring. These processes are critical to the strategic organization of behavior—for anticipatory planning (e.g., planting of food crops), mental simulations, and counterfactual reasoning; for the establishment of self awareness, actual–ideal self-discrepancies, and social alliances (e.g., for joint protection or support); and for adaptive, flexible, and creative responses to challenge.

Visual and olfactory systems contribute by conferring on these higher levels of organization a sensitivity to environmental stimuli remote from the organism, which allows the development of approach or avoidance reactions to distant stimuli or in anticipation of such stimuli. Moreover, the emergence of distance reception through the evolution of telereceptors (e.g., eyes, ears) can shift the valence of simple behavioral responses. Although a proximal pain stimulus at the body surface may elicit a lower-level flexor withdrawal response as an avoidance or protective reaction, the same flexor response may assist in the acquisition of a remote but visible food item by higher-level systems. Moreover, such a response would be reinforced by the acquisition of the food item and hence may assume a positive valence for higher-level systems. Conversely, an extensor thrust response to a remote aversive stimulus or organism may assist in avoidance or defense, and thereby can become an important component of a rejection response. Thus the association of flexor activation in the arm with a novel, neutral stimulus (e.g., a Chinese ideograph for a native speaker of English) may serve to promote liking for the stimulus, whereas the association of extensor activation in the arm may come to promote disliking through implicit associative processes (Cacioppo, Priester, & Berntson, 1993). As represented systems do not supplant lower systems, there is also the opportunity for conflicts among levels of organization. Such conflicts illustrate the multiple levels of organization and function within neurobehavioral systems, and the associated importance multiple levels of analysis in social psychology.

## MULTILEVEL ORGANIZATION AND CONFLICTS

Information is processed and responses are organized across multiple levels of the neuraxial heterarchy. Lower-level processing is rapid and efficient, as inputs and outputs are limited, and circuits are relatively rigidly organized for rapid response and parallel processing. Higher-level systems receive a wider array of inputs, are more complex and integrative, are linked with associative networks, and can support broader and more flexible outputs. Consequently, information-processing demands are considerably higher, and processing becomes more serialized, as processing resources are finite.

If the relations among levels were a strict hierarchy, the network would function as a supremely integrated system. There are costs to this integration, however. Upper levels of a hierarchy receive input only as processed by lower levels and exert outputs only by cascade through descending intermediary levels. The restricted analytical capacity of lower-level systems could limit or preclude higher-level perceptual processes. In addition to ascending somatosensory relays through intermediate levels, however, the somatosensory system has relatively direct projections to higher-level systems. Moreover, sophisticated sensory systems, such as the visual system, are directly linked with higher-level processing substrates. Thus different neuraxial levels "see" distinct aspects of or relations among environmental stimuli.

In a corresponding fashion, outputs are also distinct. The hierarchical features of neural organization allow higher-level systems to obtain access to lower response output mechanisms via connections to intermediary levels in the hierarchy. This would constrain outputs to the domain of lower-level organizations, although they may be spatially or temporally organized for specific purposes. The descending heterarchical features of the neuraxis, however, allow for much more flexible control over output substrates such as somatomotor neuron pools and autonomic source nuclei. Moreover, higher systems have unique sophisticated representational, integrative, and output systems (such as language).

Heterarchical systems thus support rapid, efficient, lower-level processing, which may be adequate for some functions, but they also provide for more integrated, elaborated processing and more adaptive, flexible outputs when necessary. A pain stimulus (such as a bite to the hand) may trigger a flexor withdrawal avoidance response while concurrently initiating an extensor thrust from higher-level systems (e.g., to repel the attacking agent). Similarly, a person may overcome lower-level pain-motivated escape behavior though a higher-level motivation to rescue a child from a burning building.

An example of the adaptive benefit offered by higher levels of neurobehavioral organization, along with the potential for conflict among levels of organization and function, comes from a study in nonhuman primates (Boysen, Berntson, Hannan, & Cacioppo, 1996). This study involved a chimpanzee that had been trained in the use of number symbols (Arabic numerals) as indicators of quantity, both receptively and productively. The task was to select (by pointing to) the smaller of two arrays of 1–6 candies, in order to obtain the larger, nonselected array as a reward. Despite considerable sophistication in prior laboratory tasks, this animal (and ultimately others) was unable to learn to select the smaller array over hundreds and hundreds of trials. In fact, the animal's response was not random; it consistently selected the larger array and thereby received the smaller reward. The basis of this inefficient performance became apparent when the candy selection arrays were replaced with Arabic numerals corresponding to the number of candies (candies, of course, continued to be used as the reward). On the very first trial, and significantly thereafter, the animal selected the smaller numeral and received the larger candy array as a reward. When candy arrays were reintroduced as stimuli, performance deteriorated immediately, and the animal again selected the larger array and received the smaller reward.

The optimal performance with Arabic numerals as stimuli clearly revealed that the animal had acquired knowledge concerning the rules of the task and the payoff contingencies. But this implicit knowledge could not be expressed when the task required the selection of a smaller quantity of candies. This probably reflected a multilevel conflict. Candies are highly valued by chimpanzees, and the lower-level approach disposition related to the perceptual features of the larger candy array clearly interfered with the adaptive performance based on a higher-level knowledge structure. When this interfering response disposition was removed through the use of symbolic stimuli, higher-level systems were able to organize a more adaptive response. In this case the lower-level, rather than the higher-level, organization prevailed when both were active.

## ELABORATION LIKELIHOOD MODEL: MULTILEVEL PROCESSING

The information-processing bottleneck at higher levels of neural organization imposes constraints on cognitive processing. Attentional systems minimize processing overload by focusing cognitive resources on selected stimuli, issues, or problems, to the exclusion of others. This is an active and effortful process that engages selected information and disregards or minimally regards nonselected information. If information (e.g., a particular aspect of a message) is not attended and processed by the highest levels of organization, however, it is not necessarily lost. Some degree of processing may occur at lower levels of the neural heterarchy. A pain withdrawal reflex can occur prior to the conscious perception of the pain stimulus, and well-practiced tasks such as driving or riding a bike can be performed in an automated fashion with minimal demands on cognitive resources.

The *elaboration likelihood model* (see Petty & Cacioppo, 1986) recognizes distinct levels of processing in attitudes and persuasion. The *central route* entails an effortful, thoughtful cognitive elaboration and evaluation of information, whereas the *peripheral route* represents a less elaborated, sometimes automated approach that capitalizes on more superficial heuristics, authority status, context, extant belief structures, and so forth. The peripheral route is less effortful, less demanding of higher cognitive resources, and in many cases may provide a "reasonable" attitude in many circumstances without the cost of effortful processing.

Recognition of the distinction between levels of processing allows a meaningful investigation of the determinants of whether, and to what extent, information is cognitively elaborated. The elaboration likelihood model offers a neurobiologically relevant framework for conceptualizing and investigating the determinants of attitude formation, including the availability of cognitive resources, the adequacy of available information, and the degree of personal involvement, among other factors.

Although different levels of processing are partly dissociable, they are not entirely independent. Descending heterarchical influences from higher substrates can modulate lower level processes. Simple classical aversive conditioning (with shock as an unconditioned stimulus), for example, is impeded by prior cognitive knowledge about the attitude stimulus or conditioned stimulus (words or pronounceable nonwords; Cacioppo, Marshall-Goodell, Tassinary, & Petty, 1992). Conversely, lower-level processes may also bias higher cognitive elaborations, such as the response decision making in the chimpanzee example above. Moreover, rudimentary processes associated with simple arm extension or flexion have been shown to bias attitude formation toward novel semantic stimuli (Priester, Cacioppo, & Petty, 1996) or ideographs (Cacioppo et al., 1993). Importantly, the elaboration likelihood model is not alone in proposing an elaborative and a more heuristic processing of information when one is forming a position, judgment, or decision, as dual-process theories depicting similar information-processing operations have now been proposed to account for a wide variety of social preferences and judgments (e.g., see review by Chaiken & Trope, 1999). Significant questions facing social psychologists include what the determinants of the processing levels are, how the multiple levels interact, and how they affect social and behavioral outputs.

## EVALUATIVE SPACE AND THE NEUROARCHITECTURE OF EVALUATIVE PROCESSES

Since Wundt (1896) and Thurstone (1931), it has been common to consider affective states or reactions to lie on a bipolar continuum extending from positive to negative (or happy to sad, liking to disliking, etc). In contrast, we have proposed a bivariate model of affect (see Figure 12.3), in which separable positive and negative dimensions exist (Cacioppo & Berntson, 1994; Cacioppo, Gardner, & Berntson,

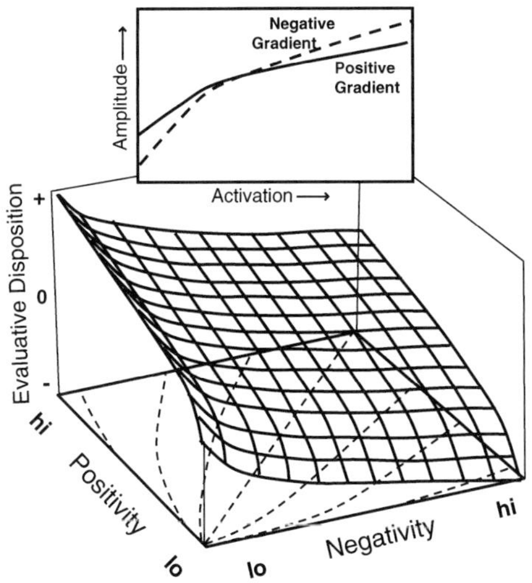


**FIGURE 12.3.** Evaluative space. Illustrative bivariate evaluative space and its associated affective response surface. This surface represents the net predisposition of an individual toward (+) or away from (–) the target stimulus. This net predisposition is expressed in relative units, and the axis dimensions are in relative units of activation. The point on the surface overlying the left axis intersection represents a maximally positive predisposition, and the point on the surface overlying the right axis intersection represents a maximally negative predisposition. Each of the points overlying the dashed diagonal extending from the back to the front axis intersections represents the same middling predisposition. The nonreciprocal diagonal on the evaluative plane—which represents different evaluative processes (e.g., neutral to ambivalence)—yields the same middling expression on the affective response surface. Dashed lines (including the coactivity diagonal) represent isocontours on the evaluative plane, which depict many-to-one mappings between the affective response surface and the underlying evaluative space. These isocontours are illustrative rather than exhaustive. Inset: The activation functions depicted separately for positivity and negativity. From Cacioppo and Berntson (1994). Copyright 1994 by the American Psychological Association. Adapted by permission of the authors.

1997; Cacioppo et al., 2004). This model subsumes the bipolar concept, but offers a more comprehensive account of affective states. Among other advantages, the evaluative space model can account for states of ambivalence or mixed feelings, and for the low correlation sometimes observed between positive and negative feelings (e.g., Larsen, McGraw, Mellers, & Cacioppo, 2004).

In this regard, an appreciation of neuroevolution and neuroarchitecture may inform our understanding and theories of emotional and motivational processes. As discussed above, basic principles of neuroarchitectural organization are often more apparent in the simpler circuits of lower levels of the neuraxis. Thus the extensor and flexor reflexes of the cord serve the distinct and opposing functions of approach and avoidance, and are embodied in distinct neural circuits. Reflected in what we termed the *cardinal principle of evaluative bivalence*, we (Berntson et al., 1993) presented evidence that the distinction between approach and avoidance (more generally, between positive and negative evaluative processes) is maintained throughout representative systems at higher levels of the neuraxis. Although these evaluative systems may and do interact, the basic substrates remain at least partially dissociable. Historically, the amygdala has been recognized as a primary integrative site for aversive reactions and negative affect, whereas the nucleus accumbens has been implicated in incentive motivation and positive affect (see Berntson et al., 1993). The contemporary picture is somewhat more complex than a simple dissociation between the amygdala and nucleus accumbens, however; the latter, for example, has now been implicated in both positive and negative affect. Nevertheless, the *microcircuitries* for these two classes of evaluative processes are distinct and bivalently organized within the nucleus accumbens (Reynolds & Berridge, 2002). Moreover, Reynolds and

Berridge (2002) demonstrated that a combination of positive and negative effects (e.g., positive appetitive eating and concurrent fear-like responses) could be evoked by pharmacological microinjections in intermediate areas of the accumbens.

It remains the case that behavioral outputs may evidence an output coupling between positive and negative, as there may be a final common pathway for behavioral output. Although the spinal neuronal circuits for flexion and extension are distinct, physical constraints prevent a limb from both flexing and extending at the same time. Similarly, one cannot walk toward and away from an object at the same time, although vacillation between approach and withdrawal responses is not uncommon. Moreover, when approach and avoidance responses are not incompatible, as with orofacial intake–rejection responses (see discussion above), both may be seen concurrently (Berridge & Grill, 1984).

In accord with Sherrington's (1906) principle of *reciprocal innervation*, there may be some inhibitory interaction between positive and negative substrates. This probably accounts for the fact that whereas positive and negative substrates can be coactivated, one does not generally observe strong concurrent positive and negative activations.

Additional insights into evaluative processes may be elucidated by considering neuroevolution of adaptive systems and the neuroarchitecture of basic lower-level systems. The separability of approach and avoidance substrates permits evolutionary pressures to adaptively sculpt these processes independently. Because avoiding negative stimuli may be more important to survival than approaching positive stimuli, at least in the short run, neural systems tend to show a bias toward avoidance. This can be seen at the level of spinal reflexes, where the prepotency of flexor reflexes is readily apparent. This *negativity bias* can also be seen in higher evaluative processes. In a series of studies in animals, Neal Miller and colleagues demonstrated that avoidance gradients in approach–avoidance conflict situations (e.g., food and shock in a runway maze) are steeper than approach gradients, as measured by the strength of pull against a tether (Miller, 1959, 1961). A similar negativity bias has been demonstrated in early stages of evaluative processing, as revealed by event-related potential studies (for a review, see Cacioppo et al., 2004). This negativity bias is reflected in the steeper slope of the negative function in Figure 12.3.

In addition to this negativity bias, Miller (1959, 1961) observed what has been termed a *positivity offset* in conflict paradigms, reflecting the fact that approach gradient becomes higher than the avoidance gradient as one moves further away from the goal. This, too, would have adaptive value for the organism and may reflect an adaptive feature of evolutionary development. Avoiding danger may be more adaptively important in the near term, especially when the threat is imminent. On the other hand, approach reactions and exploratory behavior are essential contributors to locating and acquiring food, water, and other life essentials. This positivity offset is apparent in the effect of mere exposure on attitude formation, where familiarity with a novel object tends to promote a positive attitude in the absence of explicit positive or negative manipulations. The positivity offset is depicted in Figure 12.3 by the higher intercept of the positivity function, despite the lower slope.

Higgins (1997) has questioned the bivariate structure of evaluative processes. He suggests that a further differentiation is necessary, in part because presentation of a positive stimulus and withdrawal of a negative stimulus may have different psychological and behavioral significance, even though both constitute reward. This is certainly true. The distinction between positive and negative reinforcement has been recognized for decades, but that does not necessitate more than two dimensions of the underlying substrates. It is further suggested by Förster, Higgins, and Idson (1998) that slopes of avoidance gradients are not necessarily steeper than those for approach, but vary depending on the regulatory focus. Appealing to the prior findings that volitional arm extension and flexion can bias higher-level evaluative processes, these researchers used spontaneous variations in flexion or extension force to index the degree of approach or avoidance, respectively (Förster et al., 1998). This is problematic, as the quantitative relation between force and motivational disposition is unknown. The fact that executing a flexor or extensor response can bias higher evaluative processes does not imply that variations in higher evaluative processes will be reflected in corresponding variations in flexor or extensor force (this is the logical flaw of *affirming the consequent*).

More importantly, it is important to note that Figure 12.3 depicts only one level of organization in the rerepresentative systems underlying evaluative processes. To fully conceptualize a heterarchical system, an additional dimension would be needed to depict the separate evaluative space functions for different levels of organization. As discussed above for flexion and extension (see Figure 12.2), the coupling between evaluative processes and behavioral outputs may differ across levels of organization. At the spinal level, for example, flexion is associated with avoidance, whereas at a higher cognitive level, flexion may be associated with approach. The relations between central states and flexion–extension responses thus depend on what level is manifesting in behavioral control, and this may change over time and across contexts. Indeed, one of the important questions raised by the evaluative space model is how different levels interact and achieve expression in behavior. The importance of the evaluative space model is that it provides a quantitative model whereby such issues can be addressed.

It is also important to note that the evaluative space model describes the structure and operating features of evaluative processes, not the factors that elicit positivity/appetition or negativity/aversion. Self-regulatory focus theory (Higgins, 1997) does not represent an alternative model, but rather distinguishes two ways people seek to approach pleasure and avoid pain. In the promotion focus, people attempt to achieve aspirations and meet their ideals. They are especially sensitive to information about gains versus non-gains and prefer approach procedures. In the prevention focus people try to live up to responsibilities and remain safe. They are especially sensitive to loss versus non-loss information and prefer avoidance procedures. The representation of aspirations and ideals are abstractions that depend on the highest level of neurobehavioral organization. As such, self-regulatory focus theory and the evaluative space model represent complementary rather than competing formulations, as the cognitive computations outlined in self-regulatory focus probably exert their effects through the modulation of the activity of processes delineated in the evaluative space model. Indeed, among the benefits of the multilevel approach to motivation articulated in this chapter are the potential syntheses that it offers.

## SUMMARY

Neuroscientifically relevant conceptualizations of social motivation are now feasible. Such models, grounded in solid evidence regarding genetic and neural organization and function, have the potential to improve the precision and verisimilitude of motivational concepts, resolve theoretical disputes, generate new and testable behavioral hypotheses, and broaden the scope and impact of social psychological theories of motivation. We have reviewed one such formulation, derived from evidence spanning three centuries of research, on the heterarchical organization of the central nervous system and its implications for implicit and explicit motivational processes underlying approach and withdrawal. This model illustrates the potential utility of neuroscientific perspectives for social psychological processes, and the broadened perspective that can arise from multilevel research and the integration of social psychology and neuroscience.

## REFERENCES


Bechara, A., Damasio, H., & Damasio, A. R. (2003). Role of the amygdala in decision-making. *Annals of the New York Academy of Science, 985*, 356–369.

Berntson, G. G., Bechara, A., Damasio, H., Tranel, D., & Cacioppo, J. T. (in press). Amygdala contributions to selective dimensions of emotion. *Social, Cognitive, and Affective Neuroscience.*

Berntson, G. G., Boysen, S. T., & Cacioppo, J. T. (1993). Neurobehavioral organization and the cardinal principle of evaluative bivalence. *Annals of the New York Academy of Sciences, 702*, 75–102.

Berntson, G. G., & Cacioppo, J. T. (2004). Multilevel analyses and reductionism: Why social psychologists should care about neuroscience and vice versa. In J. T. Cacioppo & G. G. Berntson (Eds.), *Essays in social neuroscience* (pp. 107–120). Cambridge, MA: MIT Press

Berntson, G. G., & Cacioppo, J. T. (2007). Integrative physiology: Homeostasis, allostasis and the orchestration of systemic physiology. In J. T. Cacioppo, L. G. Tassinary, & G. G. Berntson (Eds.), *Handbook of psychophysiology* (3rd ed., pp. 433–452). Cambridge, UK: Cambridge University Press.

Berntson, G. G., & Micco, D. J. (1976). Organization of brainstem behavioral systems. *Brain Research Bulletin, 1*, 471–483.

Berridge, K. C. (2004). Motivation concepts in behavioral neuroscience. *Physiology and Behavior, 81*, 179–209.

Berridge, K. C., & Grill, H. J. (1984). Idohedonic tastes

support a two-dimensional hypothesis of palatability. *Appetite, 5*, 221–231.

Boysen, S. T., Berntson, G. G., Hannan, M. B., & Cacioppo, J. T. (1996). Quantity-based interference and symbolic representations in chimpanzees (*Pan troglodytes*). *Journal of Experimental Psychology: Animal Behavior Processes, 22*, 76–86.

Cacioppo, J. T., & Berntson, G. G. (1992). Social psychological contributions to the decade of the brain: Doctrine of multilevel analysis. *American Psychologist, 47*, 1019–1028.

Cacioppo, J. T., & Berntson, G. G. (1994). Relationship between attitudes and evaluative space: A critical review with emphasis on the separability of positive and negative substrates. *Psychological Bulletin, 115*, 401–423.

Cacioppo, J. T., & Berntson, G. G. (1999). The affect system: Architecture and operating characteristics. *Current Directions in Psychological Science, 8*, 133–137.

Cacioppo, J. T., Gardner, W. L., & Berntson, G. G. (1997). Beyond bipolar conceptualizations and measures: The case of attitudes and evaluative space. *Personality and Social Psychology Review, 1*, 3–25.

Cacioppo, J. T., Larsen, J. T., Smith, N. K., & Berntson, G. G. (2004). The affect system: What lurks below the surface of feelings. In A. S. R. Manstead, N. Frijda, & A. Fischer (Eds.), *Feelings and emotions* (pp. 221–240). Cambridge, UK: Cambridge University Press.

Cacioppo, J. T., Marshall-Goodell, B. S., Tassinary, L. G., & Petty, R. E. (1992). Rudimentary determinants of attitudes: Classical conditioning is more effective when prior knowledge about the attitude stimulus is low than high. *Journal of Experimental Social Psychology, 28*, 207–233.

Cacioppo, J. T., Priester, J. R., & Berntson, G. G. (1993). Rudimentary determinants of attitudes: II. Arm flexion and extension have differential effects on attitudes. *Journal of Personality and Social Psychology, 65*, 5–17.

Chaiken, S., & Trope, Y. (Eds.). (1999). *Dual-process theories in social psychology.* New York: Guilford Press.

Cofer, C. N., & Appley, M. H. (1964). *Motivation: Theory and research.* New York: Wiley.

Edgley, S. A., Eyre, J. A., Lemon, R. N., & Miller, S. (1997). Comparison of activation of corticospinal neurons and spinal motor neurons by magnetic and electrical transcranial stimulation in the lumbosacral cord of the anaesthetized monkey. *Brain, 120*, 839–853.

Förster, J., Higgins, E. T., & Idson, L. C. (1998). Approach and avoidance strength during goal attainment: Regulatory focus and the "goal looms larger" effect. *Journal of Personality and Social Psychology, 75*, 1115–1131.

Higgins, E. T. (1997). Beyond pleasure and pain. *American Psychologist, 52*, 1280–1300.

Jackson, J. H. (1958). Evolution and dissolution of the nervous system. In J. Taylor (Ed.), *Selected writings of John Hughlings Jackson* (Vol. 2, pp. 3–92). New York: Basic Books.

Larsen, J. T., McGraw, A. P., Mellers, B. A., & Cacioppo, J. T. (2004). The agony of victory and the thrill of defeat: Mixed emotional reactions to disappointing wins and relieving losses. *Psychological Science, 15*, 325–330.

LeDoux, J. (2003). The emotional brain, fear, and the amygdala. *Cellular and Molecular Neurobiology, 23*, 727–738.

Miller, N. E. (1959). Liberalization of basic S-R concepts: Extensions to conflict behavior, motivation and social learning. In S. Koch (Ed.), *Psychology: A study of a science. Study 1* (pp. 198–292). New York: McGraw-Hill.

Miller, N. E. (1961). Some recent studies on conflict behavior and drugs. *American Psychologist, 16*, 12–24.

Petty, R. E., & Cacioppo, J. T. (1986). The elaboration likelihood model of persuasion. In L. Berkowitz (Ed.), *Advances in experimental social psychology* (Vol. 19, pp. 123–205). New York: Academic Press.

Porter, R. (1987). Functional studies of motor cortex. *Ciba Foundation Symposium, 132*, 83–97.

Priester, J. R., Cacioppo, J. T., & Petty, R. E. (1996). The influence of motor processes on attitudes toward novel versus familiar semantic stimuli. *Personality and Social Psychology Bulletin, 22*, 442–447.

Reynolds, S. M., & Berridge, K. C. (2002). Positive and negative motivation in nucleus accumbens shell: Bivalent rostrocaudal gradients for GABA-elicited eating, taste "liking"/"disliking" reactions, place preference/avoidance, and fear. *Journal of Neuroscience, 22*, 7308–7320.

Sherrington, C. S. (1906). *The integrative action of the nervous system.* New Haven, CT: Yale University Press.

Steiner, J. E., Glaser, D., Hawilo, M. E., & Berridge, K. C. (2001). Comparative expression of hedonic impact: Affective reactions to taste by human infants and other primates. *Neuroscience and Biobehavioral Reviews, 25*, 53–74.

Thurstone, L. L. (1931). The measurement of attitudes. *Journal of Abnormal Psychology, 26*, 249–269.

Tuber, D. S., Berntson, G. G., Bachman, D., & Allen, J. N. (1980). Associative learning in premature hydranencephalic and normal twins. *Science, 210*, 1035–1037.

Wundt, W. (1896). *Outlines of psychology.* Leipzig: Engelmann.

Chapter 13

# Contributions of Attachment Theory and Research to Motivation Science

Mario Mikulincer
Phillip R. Shaver

Attachment theory (Bowlby, 1969/1982, 1973) was a strongly motivational theory from the start. Beginning with his training in child psychiatry, Bowlby (1944) wondered what motivated juvenile thieves, many of whom had suffered from what he called *maternal deprivation* (e.g., loss of mother, separation from mother, inadequate mothering, disruptive experiences in foster or institutional care). Trained as a psychoanalyst, Bowlby assumed that the explanation of disordered behavior lay somewhere in childhood, especially in early social relationships; however, he was dissatisfied with the Freudian and object relations versions of psychoanalytic theory he encountered while training as a psychoanalyst. These theories tended to conceptualize human motivation in terms of *drives* and to view the mind as powered by *psychic energy*. They explained a child's ties to the mother in terms of benefits associated with feeding and other forms of drive reduction. They also based their conception of childhood relationships on theory-laden clinical conversations with adults.

Over a period of years, beginning around the end of World War II, Bowlby started to focus on the actual relations between infants and their mothers—observing them at the Tavistock Clinic in London, and participating in the making of films about children's reactions to separations from their mothers (often when a mother or child went alone to the hospital, which in those days entailed separation; see Robertson & Bowlby, 1952). Bowlby focused on the "making and breaking" of what he called *affectional bonds* between infants and mothers (Bowlby, 1979), and on the reasons for these bonds' seemingly profound effects on personality development and behavior in subsequent close relationships.

Bowlby was influenced by several scientific developments in the mid-20th century, especially control systems theory, cognitive developmental theory, and ethology. He created a *behavioral systems* model of motivation, according to which certain evolved behavioral systems, such as the attachment system, the caregiving system, the exploration system, and the sexual system, served particular functions critical to survival and reproduction. He viewed these systems as *goal-directed* and *goal-corrected*—that is, working like servomechanisms that were turned on or activated by certain stimuli or situations, and deactivated or terminated by other stimuli and situations (basically, by the attainment of what he called *set goals* and successful avoidance of feared dangers). After operating repeatedly in a particular environment, usually a home environment that included parental responses to behavioral system activation, a child was conceptualized as constructing *internal working models* of self, relationship partners, and the environment that altered the operating parameters of associated behavioral systems and provided expectations about possible access routes and barriers to goal attainment, and about the expected affective outcomes of goal attainment or goal obstruction.

According to Bowlby (1969/1982), this new conception of motivation rendered the Freudian notion of drives unnecessary. Goal-directed and goal-corrected behaviors were activated not by an accumulation of psychic energy or a desire to reduce the level of psychic energy to zero (notions associated with Freud), but by conditions within a person or the person's environment that activated behavior intended to achieve a certain goal state or avoid threats and dangers. Behavioral intensity was viewed as a function of the appraised effort needed to attain a targeted goal state, or of the overriding of one behavioral system by another, either when the set goal of the overridden system was attained or an alternative behavioral system was activated at a higher level. For example, when an infant of, say, 14 months of age encounters pain or environmental threats (a pin prick, unexpected noises, the appearance of a stranger, a frightening animal, sudden darkness), he or she terminates whatever activity is in progress (e.g., exploring the environment or affiliating with a peer) and searches visually for a caregiver—perhaps calling out to that person or beginning to cry, and, if possible, moving quickly to the person's side and signaling to be picked up, protected, or comforted. If the caregiver provides adequate comfort, the infant may quickly become interested once again in play or exploration and signal to be put down.

From the 1960s to the present, Bowlby's theory—especially as operationalized and elaborated by Ainsworth (e.g., Ainsworth, Blehar, Waters, & Wall, 1978)—has generated hundreds of studies of infant–caregiver attachment, parental caregiving (viewed as structured and guided by a caregiving behavioral system; George & Solomon, 1999), and short- and long-term social and personality sequelae in various age periods (see Cassidy & Shaver, 1999, for reviews of this extensive literature). Of most relevance here is the extension of the theory, first to the domain of romantic and marital relationships (Fraley & Shaver, 2000; Hazan & Shaver, 1987; Shaver & Clark, 1994), and then to the broader realm of social and intergroup relations (see the comprehensive reviews by Mikulincer & Shaver, 2003, 2007). In this chapter we focus on both the normative and individual difference aspects of Bowlby's theory, highlighting the *attachment behavioral system*—the control system that underlies activation and deactivation of attachment behavior in response to contextual threats and longer-term social experiences. We review evidence related to motivational aspects of attachment behavior, especially in adulthood; present new findings from our laboratories; and propose new ideas about the ways in which variations in attachment system functioning shape an adult's goals and goal pursuit, both generally and within particular interpersonal settings.

## BASIC CONCEPTS IN ATTACHMENT THEORY AND RESEARCH

Bowlby (1969/1982) claimed that the attachment behavioral system, a product of evolution, motivates infants (and older humans as well) to seek proximity to significant others (called *attachment figures*) when protection and care are needed. This system serves regulatory functions (protection from threats and alleviation of distress) in human beings of all ages, but is most directly observable during infancy (Bowlby, 1988). Bowlby (1973) also described important individual differences in attachment system functioning. Interactions with attachment figures who are reliably available and responsive in times of need promote optimal functioning of the attachment system, establish a relatively stable sense of security and safety, and heighten confidence in proximity seeking as a distress regulation strategy. When attachment figures are not reliably available and responsive, however, proximity seeking fails to relieve distress, a sense of security is not attained, and strategies of affect regulation other than proximity seeking (*secondary attachment strategies*, called *avoidance* and *anxiety*) are developed.

Empirical tests of Bowlby's ideas in studies of adults have generally focused on a person's *attachment style*—the systematic pattern of relational expectations, emotions, and behaviors that results from internalization of a particular history of attachment experiences (Fraley & Shaver, 2000). Research, beginning with Ainsworth and colleagues (1978) and continuing through recent studies by social and personality psychologists (reviewed by Shaver & Mikulincer, 2002, and Mikulincer & Shaver, 2007), indicates that individual differences in attachment style can be measured with self-report scales tapping two orthogonal dimensions corresponding to the two secondary strategies mentioned above, attachment-related anxiety and avoidance (Brennan, Clark, & Shaver, 1998). A person's position on the *avoidance* (or *avoidant attachment*) dimension indicates the extent to which he or she distrusts relationship partners' goodwill and strives to maintain behavioral independence and emotional distance from others. A person's position on the *anxiety* (or *anxious attachment*) dimension indicates the degree to which he or she worries that a partner will not be available and supportive in times of need. People who score low on both dimensions are said to be *secure*, to be *securely attached*, or to have a *secure attachment style*.

Based on an extensive literature review, we (Mikulincer & Shaver, 2003, 2007; Shaver & Mikulincer, 2002) have proposed a three-phase model of attachment system activation and dynamics in adulthood. Following Bowlby (1969/1982), we have assumed that relatively continuous monitoring of experiences and events results in attachment system activation when a potential or actual threat is detected. Once the attachment system is activated, an affirmative answer to the question "Is an attachment figure available and likely to be responsive to my needs?" results in a sense of security and facilitates the application of security-based strategies of affect regulation (Shaver & Mikulincer, 2002). These strategies are aimed at alleviating distress, maintaining comfortable and supportive intimate relationships, and increasing personal adjustment. They consist of optimistic beliefs about distress management, trust in others' goodwill, and a sense of self-efficacy about dealing with threats (Shaver & Hazan, 1993). These are the characteristics of securely attached individuals.

Perceived unavailability of an attachment figure results in attachment insecurity, which forces a decision about the viability of proximity seeking as a protective strategy. When proximity seeking is appraised as likely to be successful if sufficient effort is expended, a person tends to make very energetic, insistent attempts to attain proximity, love, and support. These intense efforts are called *hyperactivating strategies* (Cassidy & Kobak, 1988), because they involve strong activation of the attachment system until an attachment figure is perceived to be available and willing to provide safety and security. These strategies include attempts to elicit a partner's involvement through clinging and controlling responses, and overdependence on relationship partners as a source of protection (Shaver & Mikulincer, 2002). They also involve increased vigilance to threat-related cues, reduction in the threshold for detecting cues of attachment figures' unavailability, and maintenance of threat-related emotions and concerns in working memory—psychological maneuvers that keep the attachment system chronically activated (Shaver & Mikulincer, 2002). These concomitants of attachment system hyperactivation are characteristic of people who score high on attachment anxiety scales (Mikulincer & Shaver, 2003, 2007).

Appraising proximity seeking as unlikely to alleviate distress and perhaps even likely to exacerbate it results in inhibition of the quest for support and active attempts to handle distress alone. These secondary approaches to affect regulation are called *deactivating strategies* (Cassidy & Kobak, 1988), because their primary goal is to keep the attachment system deactivated so as to avoid the frustration and distress of continued attachment figure insensitivity or unavailability. These strategies involve denial of attachment needs, avoidance of emotional involvement and dependence in close relationships, suppression of threat- and attachment-related thoughts, and adoption of a self-reliant attitude. (Bowlby called this strategy *compulsive self-reliance*.). These aspects of deactivation are characteristic of people who score high on measures of avoidant attachment (Mikulincer & Shaver, 2003, 2007).

## THE MOTIVATIONAL IMPLICATIONS OF THE ATTACHMENT SYSTEM CONSTRUCT

When using the term *behavioral system*, Bowlby (1969/1982) referred to a species-universal, innate neural program that organizes an individual's behavior in ways that facilitate the satisfaction of fundamental human needs, and thereby increase the likelihood of survival, adaptation, and reproduction. As such, a behavioral system can be viewed as a motivational device that transforms what were originally neutral person–environment transactions into either desired *goal states* that facilitate need satisfaction, or aversive *anti-goal states* that interfere with or hinder need satisfaction. A behavioral system includes appetitive and aversive components that direct and organize intentional behavior. It can initiate approach tendencies that move a person toward desired goal states, or avoidance tendencies that move the person away from aversive anti-goal states. Behavioral systems also motivate a person to monitor, appraise, and evaluate goal-relevant internal and external cues, and to learn new means–end associations and stimulus–response contingencies that improve system functioning and facilitate need satisfaction.

In the case of the attachment behavioral system, Bowlby (1969/1982) focused on the fundamental need for care and protection, and the innate predisposition to search for and maintain proximity to protective and caring others in times of need. When this system is activated, it transforms proximity maintenance and the attainment of security, comfort, and protection into major goal states, and rejection, separation, and attachment figure unavailability into aversive anti-goal states. It also directs a person's cognitive processes and actions toward the attainment of proximity, love, and security, and the avoidance of or resistance to certain person–environment transactions (such as separation from attachment figures) that threaten the sense of security.

Bowlby's ideas about the motivational predisposition to seek proximity to others for the sake of care and protection have received extensive empirical support. In times of need, infants show a clear preference for their caregivers, engage in intense proximity seeking, and are soothed by a caregiver's presence and support (e.g., Ainsworth, 1973, 1991). Conceptually parallel research with adults has shown that people are likely to choose to affiliate with sympathetic others while awaiting a noxious event (see Shaver & Klinnert, 1982, for a review, and Fraley & Shaver, 1998, for a specific example of impending separation of attached romantic partners), and to turn to others for support while or immediately after encountering stressful events (see Lazarus & Folkman, 1984, for a review).

Recently, we (Mikulincer, Birnbaum, Woddis, & Nachmias, 2000; Mikulincer, Gillath, & Shaver, 2002) found that adults react to even minimal threat cues with activation of proximity-related thoughts and mental representations of security-providing attachment figures. In these studies, subliminal priming of a threat word (e.g., *illness, failure*) was found to heighten cognitive accessibility of attachment-related mental representations, indicated by faster lexical decision times for proximity-related words (e.g., *love, closeness*) and names of people nominated as providing protection and security (e.g., the name of a parent, spouse, or close friend). Interestingly, these effects were circumscribed to attachment-related representations and were not found for attachment-unrelated words or the names of people other than attachment figures, including family members who were not nominated as security-providing attachment figures.

There is also extensive evidence for the theoretical proposition that attachment figure unavailability is an aversive anti-goal state. Ethological observation of infants separated from their mothers (e.g., Heinicke & Westheimer, 1966; Robertson & Bowlby, 1952) reveals that inaccessibility or absence of an attachment figure evokes intense distress, anxiety, anger, protest, and yearning. In adulthood, bereavement research also indicates that attachment figure unavailability due to partner death is one of the most painful experiences a person can endure—one that typically elicits extreme distress, sorrow, despair, and painful longing for the deceased partner (see Fraley & Shaver, 1999, for a review). Similar emotional reactions have also been observed following the breakup of romantic relationships (e.g., Feeney & Noller, 1992; Simpson, 1990). Milder but still consequential forms of distress often occur even after separations from one's spouse (e.g., see Vormbrock, 1993, for a review of studies on wartime and job-related separations).

Adult attachment research has also provided information about the positive emotions associated with actual or symbolic reunions with attachment figures. For example, reunion with a spouse after a wartime or job-related separation is experienced as highly exciting and exhilarating (Vormbrock, 1993), as we often see in the news when troops return from service abroad and are greeted at the airport by their loved ones. In a series of studies (Mikulincer, Hirschberger, Nachmias, & Gillath, 2001; Mikulincer & Shaver, 2001), we found that a variety of experimental techniques can activate mental representations of internalized attachment figures and cause positive affective reactions similar to those produced by actual reunions. The Mikulincer and colleagues (2001) study found that these same techniques led to more positive evaluations of previously neutral stimuli, and did so even under threatening conditions, eliminating the usual negative effects of such situations on feelings about formerly neutral stimuli. In short, in line with theory, even the mere symbolic availability of an attachment figure has a measurably soothing effect.

According to Bowlby (1969/1982), behavioral systems operate in a complex goal-oriented and goal-corrected manner. The activation of a system instigates intentions and behaviors directed toward achieving a particular goal state and avoiding anti-goal states; it also initiates evaluative processes that assess progress toward the goal and induce corrective adjustments to make goal attainment more likely. One of Bowlby's most important observations, which increased his confidence in the notion of goal-corrected rather than merely habitual behavior, is that particular behavioral sequences get altered when necessary to put a person, even an infant, back on the track of goal attainment. In the case of the attachment system, this flexible, goal-directed, and goal-corrected adjustment of behavior requires monitoring and appraisal of threatening events and of one's inner states (e.g., distress, security); monitoring and appraisal of an attachment figure's responses to one's proximity-seeking attempts; and monitoring and appraisal of the effectiveness of the chosen behaviors in a given context. These cognitive and cybernetic operations organize intentional behavior aimed at attaining security and satisfying basic needs for care and protection.

Borrowing from more recent feedback control theories (e.g., Carver & Scheier, 1981, 1990; Carver, Sutton, & Scheier, 2000), our model of attachment system functioning involves self-regulatory feedback loops that shape the course and consequences of proximity-seeking efforts. While in the process of seeking affection, comfort, and protection, people either explicitly or implicitly compare their current state with the attachment system's reference values (goal and anti-goal states), adjust proximity-seeking efforts to reduce the distance to the goal state or increase the distance from anti-goal states, and decide whether to persist in or disengage from proximity-seeking efforts after discovering that they are unsuccessful. In other words, a choice is made between the aforementioned hyperactivating and deactivating strategies.

Beyond these general, normative features of the attachment behavioral system, there are, as already mentioned, important individual differences between security and insecurity and between attachment-related anxiety and avoidance. In the following sections, we consider the effects of these individual differences on (1) the goals people pursue in social interactions and close relationships, (2) the organization of personal goals, (3) the dynamic processes of goal engagement and disengagement, and (4) the balance between approach and avoidance motivational tendencies.

## Attachment Orientations and Interaction Goals

In our model, recurrent failure to attain a sense of safety and security, and the consolidation of a secondary attachment strategy (hyperactivating, deactivating, or some combination), lead to the endorsement of goals that radically affect the way people deal with threats and threat-related emotions. For anxious and avoidant individuals, proximity seeking for the sake of protection and care often gives way to the goal of managing attachment system activation and the pain caused by failing to achieve security. Whereas hyperactivating strategies lead anxiously attached people to keep their attachment system chronically activated, constantly on the alert for threats, slights, separations, and losses, deactivating strategies lead avoidant people to suppress the attachment system and inhibit proximity-seeking efforts. That is, each of the major secondary attachment strategies has a specific regulatory goal, and the resulting attachment orientation (anxious or avoidant) is warped in the direction of attaining this goal. These goals account for the ways in which people scoring high on measures of attachment anxiety or avoidance construe themselves, appraise relationship partners, cope with threats, and regulate distressing thoughts and memories (for reviews, see Fraley, Davis, & Shaver, 1998; Mikulincer & Shaver, 2003; Shaver & Mikulincer, 2002).

Variations in attachment history and attachment system functioning are important for understanding a person's goals in social interactions and close relationships. People who succeed in attaining a sense of security learn that proximity seeking is rewarding, and so tend to organize their interactions around the goals of interdependence, closeness, and intimacy. In contrast, reliance on hyperactivating strategies causes anxiously attached people to organize their interactions around an unquenchable need for security, and so to engage in clinging, controlling, and hypervigilant behaviors intended to assure a partner's love and attention but paradoxically often inciting anger, distancing, or abandonment. Reliance on deactivating strategies leads avoidant individuals to organize their interactions around desires for autonomy and control, and to perceive interdependence and closeness as aversive antigoal states. Research shows that these interaction goals can account for attachment style differences in interpersonal trust (e.g., Collins & Read, 1990; Mikulincer, 1998), patterns of self-disclosure (e.g., Keelan, Dion, & Dion, 1998; Mikulincer & Nachshon, 1991), excessive seeking of reassurance from a romantic partner (Shaver, Schachner, & Mikulincer, 2005), sexual behavior (Schachner & Shaver, 2002, 2004), and strategies for dealing with interpersonal conflicts (e.g., Scharfe & Bartholomew, 1995; Simpson, Rholes, & Phillips, 1996).

Two recent studies (Avihou, 2006; Raz, 2002) provide even more direct evidence concerning the hypothesized attachment style differences in interaction goals, based on coding the *core conflictual relationship themes* (CCRT; Luborsky & Crits-Christoph, 1998) in people's open-ended narratives. In Raz's (2002) study, participants completed a measure of attachment style (the Relationship Questionnaire; Bartholomew & Horowitz, 1991) and the Relationship Anecdotes Paradigm (Luborsky & Crits-Christoph, 1998). Specifically, participants were asked to recall three meaningful interactions with significant others and describe in each case what happened, including what they and their partner said and did. Two independent judges, who were unaware of participants' attachment scores, read the narratives and used the CCRT coding scheme to extract the underlying needs, motives, and intentions that were expressed in these narratives (the *wish* component of the CCRT). Raz found that self-reports of attachment anxiety were associated with wishes for security and for being loved and accepted by significant others—the major goal of hyperactivating strategies. Self-reports of attachment avoidance were associated with two major wishes: (1) to assert oneself and be independent, and (2) to retain interpersonal distance and avoid conflicts. These are the goals of deactivating strategies.

Raz's (2002) findings were conceptually replicated in Avihou's (2006) study of the thematic content of dreams. Fifty-five Israeli undergraduates completed the Experience in Close Relationships (ECR) scale (Brennan et al., 1998), tapping variations in dispositional attachment anxiety and avoidance. Then, for 30 consecutive days, participants completed a diary questionnaire each morning before going to school or work—a questionnaire in which they were asked to recall any memorable dreams or dream fragments from the previous night. If they had such memories, they were asked to write a detailed description of their dream(s). The number of reported dreams ranged from 7 to 27 across the month-long period and averaged 14 dreams. Two independent judges, who were unaware of participants' attachment scores, used the CCRT coding scheme to analyze each dream episode that contained a narrative of interpersonal interactions (1,152 dream episodes) and extracted the wishes expressed in each episode. For each participant, the pervasiveness of a wish was computed by dividing the number of dream episodes in which a wish occurred by the total number of dream episodes scored.

The findings indicated clearly that attachment-related interaction goals are manifested in dreams. On the one hand, the wishes expressed in the dreams of anxiously attached individuals reflected hyperactivation of the attachment system and the goals associated with hyperactivation. Specifically, self-reported attachment anxiety was associated with the pervasiveness of wishes to be loved and accepted by others and to be controlled by them, and inversely associated with the wish to help needy others. On the other hand, the wishes expressed in the dreams of avoidant individuals reflected deactivation of the attachment system. Self-reported avoidant attachment was associated with the pervasiveness of wishes to assert oneself and be independent, to oppose and control others, and to be distant and avoid interpersonal conflicts.

## Attachment Orientations and the Construal and Organization of Personal Goals

Theory and research on personal goals indicate that people differ not only in the goals they pursue, but also in the ways in which they cognitively appraise and organize their goals (e.g., Cantor & Langston, 1989; Emmons, 1986, 1997). In a review of research on *personal strivings*—the goals a person regularly tries to attain—Emmons (1992, 1997) specified four dimensions along which people vary in their construal of personal strivings. The first dimension is *degree of commitment*—the value and importance placed on personal goals and the effort invested in pursuing them. The second dimension is *anticipated outcome of goal pursuit*—the expectations of success and personal control in attaining one's habitual goals. The third dimension is *appraisal of threats/demands in goal pursuit*—the difficulties, obstacles, and problems people anticipate encountering as they strive toward their goals. The fourth dimension, *level of abstraction*, concerns the extent to which people frame their central goals in broad and abstract terms ("being a psychologist") versus narrow and concrete terms ("getting an A in a psychology course").

Beyond characterizing these properties of people's goal striving, Emmons (1997) discussed three dimensions along which people vary when organizing their strivings within a goal system. The first dimension is *level of inter-goal conflict*—the extent to which people believe that the pursuit or attainment of one goal interferes with the pursuit or attainment of another. The second dimension, *goal differentiation*, concerns the extent to which people perceive their goals as distinct, dissimilar, and unrelated to each other. The third dimension is *goal integration*—the extent to which people possess superordinate goal categories that connect different subordinate goals without eliminating their uniqueness and contradictions. Highly integrated people can compare different goals, appraise the interactions among the goals, evaluate tradeoffs, and view specific goals as alternative means for attaining superordinate goals or supporting personal meaning structures. Less integrated people have fragmented goal systems in which different goals are not coherently linked to an overarching, unifying goal or set of goals.

Variations in construal and organization of personal goals are important for understanding goal engagement and disengagement, as well as the affective states that accompany and follow goal pursuit (Emmons, 1986, 1997). For example, whereas positive expectations of anticipated outcomes can facilitate goal engagement and maintenance of positive affect during goal pursuit, high levels of threat appraisal and inter-goal conflict can hinder goal engagement and elicit negative affect. Research has shown that these variations have important implications for psychological and physical well-being (e.g., Emmons, 1986, 1992; Emmons & King, 1988). Whereas high levels of inter-goal conflict and a high level of abstraction in framing personal goals are associated with depression and distress, the tendency to frame personal goals in concrete and narrow terms is associated with physical disorders (Emmons, 1992; Emmons & King, 1988). Sheldon and Emmons (1995) also found that people characterized by a high degree of goal integration feel more committed to their personal strivings and more successful in attaining them than less integrated people.

This research led us to propose that variations in attachment system functioning should affect the way people construe and organize their personal strivings. On the one hand, anxious hyperactivating strategies should bias appraisals of anticipated outcomes and threats or demands during goal pursuit. According to our model, anxiously attached people tend to exaggerate threats and adversities as part of maintaining the attachment system in a chronically activated state. They also tend to appraise and present themselves as helpless and weak, hoping to elicit other people's compassion, love, and support. Such hyperactivating maneuvers may lead anxiously attached people to appraise threats and problems during goal pursuit in inflated terms, and to hold negative and pessimistic expectations about their ability to attain personal goals.

Hyperactivating strategies also interfere with the ability and willingness to pursue non-attachment-related goals before attachment security has been attained (Bowlby, 1969/1982; Mikulincer & Shaver, 2003). Anxiously attached people are so focused on the need for security that they have few resources left to engage in other kinds of goal-directed activities. Furthermore, they may perceive these activities as interfering with the pursuit of security, because they draw attention and effort away from security attainment. As a result, chronic reliance on hyperactivating strategies may lead to high levels of perceived conflict between goals and interfere with the formation of an integrated, coherent goal system.

On the other hand, avoidant, deactivating strategies promote disengagement from the pursuit of attachment security, and they may also discourage personal involvement in other kinds of demanding and challenging activities because these can easily generate frustration and pain, which naturally tend to reactivate the attachment system (Mikulincer & Shaver, 2003). These strategies may cause avoidant individuals to defensively reduce their degree of commitment to and investment in goal pursuit. Moreover, they may encourage avoidant individuals to frame their strivings in more concrete and narrower terms, because broader and more abstract strivings tend to require greater risk and investment, opening a person up to greater frustration and disappointment (Little, 1989).

This defensive stance may also encourage segregation of attachment-related goals from other kinds of goals in one's personal goal system (Bowlby, 1980). Deactivating strategies involve denial of attachment-related goals, suppression of thoughts related to these goals, and the establishment of accessibility barriers to attachment-related mental contents (Mikulincer & Shaver, 2003). This defensive exclusion of attachment-related goals can lead to fragmentation within the personal goal system and interfere with the formation of an integrated and coherent superordinate system.

We recently conducted a correlational study examining the hypothesized associations between attachment orientations and construal and organization of personal goals. In the first session of the study, 80 Israeli undergraduates (41 women, 39 men) completed a brief, 10-item scale tapping attachment anxiety and avoidance (Mikulincer, Florian, & Tolmacz, 1990), along with measures of trait anxiety and self-esteem. In the second session, conducted 3–4 weeks later, each participant was asked to generate a list of six personal strivings, which (following Emmons, 1986) were described as "goals that you are typically trying to accomplish or attain in your everyday behavior." Participants then rated each of the six goals on the Commitment, Anticipated Outcome, and Difficulty dimensions of the Striving Assessment Scale (Emmons, 1986). Specifically, participants appraised (1) how committed they felt to each goal, (2) the degree to which they had succeeded with each form of striving in the past, and (3) the difficulty each form of striving had caused them. All three dimensions were assessed using 6-point scales. Scores for each dimension were computed by averaging a participant's ratings for that dimension across all six goals. Cronbach alphas for the dimension scales were adequate, ranging from .76 to .84.

Participants were also asked to make three additional ratings. First, they provided ratings of inter-goal conflict in accordance with Emmons and King's (1988) procedure. They received a 6 × 6 matrix, the rows and columns of which were labeled with their six goals; compared each goal with every other goal (30 comparisons); and rated, using a 6-point scale, "how much being successful in one striving has a harmful effect on the other striving." For each participant, we computed an inter-goal conflict score by averaging the 30 conflict ratings (alpha = .93). Second, participants provided ratings of goal differentiation, using Sheldon and Emmons's (1995) procedure. Specifically, they received a 6 × 6 triangular grid on which they rated, using a 6-point scale, every possible pair of goals as to how dissimilar the two strivings were. For each participant, we averaged the resulting 15 ratings to form a global goal differentiation score (alpha = .74). Third, participants provided ratings of goal integration: They received another 6 × 6 triangular grid (identical to the one described above), and rated, using a 6-point scale, every possible pair of goals as to "how much you perceive the two strivings as being part of a single broader purpose in life." We then computed a global goal integration score for each participant by averaging the resulting 15 ratings (alpha = .89).

Two independent judges, who were unaware of participants' attachment scores, coded the strivings generated by each participant according to their level of breadth and abstraction. Following Emmons (1992), we defined *high-level strivings* as those that were abstract, reflective, or mentioned internal states. *Low-level strivings* were defined as those involving more behavioral descriptions and being more concrete and specific. Judges were instructed to read the six strivings a participant generated and to assign a single score on a 6-point scale, ranging from 1 (almost all low-level strivings) to 6 (almost all high-level strivings). Since the correlation between the two judges was high (.84), we averaged their ratings to form a single score for abstraction level.

The findings were consistent with our reasoning and hypotheses. Higher attachment anxiety was significantly associated with lower ratings of success in goal pursuit, $r(78) = -.40$, $p < .01$; higher ratings of difficulty in goal pursuit, $r(78) = .29$, $p < .01$; higher ratings of intergoal conflict, $r(78) = .35$, $p < .01$; and lower ratings of goal integration, $r(78) = -.34$, $p < .01$. Higher attachment avoidance was significantly associated with low ratings of commitment in goal pursuit, $r(78) = -.31$, $p < .01$; lower levels of abstraction in framing personal strivings, $r(78) = -.39$, $p < .01$; and lower ratings of goal integration, $r(78) = -.43$, $p < .01$. Importantly, these significant associations could not be explained by trait anxiety or self-esteem. That is, although these measures were significantly related to attachment scores, the associations between attachment scores and the various goal dimensions remained the same after trait anxiety and self-esteem were statistically controlled for.

Overall, the findings highlight the relevance of attachment system functioning for understanding how people construe and organize their personal goals. Whereas attachment anxiety favors a pessimistic appraisal of goal pursuit and a conflictual organization of one's goal system, attachment avoidance favors lack of commitment in goal pursuit and the framing of goals in narrow and concrete terms. Importantly, the two attachment orientations, which reflect nonoptimal functioning of the attachment system, are associated with a failure to integrate goals into superordinate meaning structures.

## Attachment Orientations and the Dynamics of Goal Disengagement

In the preceding section, we have focused on the influence of attachment orientations on the appraisal and organization of personal goals. In this section, we extend our discussion to the motivational relevance of attachment orientations to the dynamic process of self-regulation of goal-oriented behavior. We propose that hyperactivation and deactivation of the attachment system affect the decision to persist or disengage from goal pursuit following an encounter with external or internal obstacles to goal attainment. This decision is crucial for the adaptive regulation of goal-oriented behavior, and it has serious implications for psychological and physical well-being (e.g., Carver & Scheier, 1990, 1998).

According to feedback control theories such as Carver and Scheier's (1981, 1990, 1998), goal-oriented behavior proceeds smoothly until people encounter an obstacle that impedes progress. A person then stops the behavioral flow momentarily, assesses what can be done to attain the goal, and then decides whether to withdraw or persist in goal pursuit. In Carver and Scheier's model, successful adaptive self-regulation results from accurately assessing the opportunities for and constraints on goal attainment present in a given context. In such cases, people decide either to persist when there are opportunities to remove obstacles and attain the goal, or to disengage when external or internal constraints render the goal unattainable. Pursuing this sensible strategy, a person will rarely miss an opportunity to reach attainable goals, but will avoid recurrent failure when a goal is unobtainable. In contrast, maladaptive self-regulation involves premature disengagement—abandoning goal pursuit when there are still good opportunities to attain the goal—and failure to disengage from unattainable goals. Both common sense and empirical research indicate that these two nonoptimal courses of action have negative effects on physical and psychological well-being (e.g., Wrosch & Heckhausen, 1999; Wrosch, Scheier, Miller, Schultz, & Carver, 2003).

We suspected that the two major secondary, insecure attachment strategies of deactivation and hyperactivation would lead people to make poor decisions regarding goal persistence and disengagement, both in general and especially in interpersonal situations. The deactivating strategies favored by avoidant individuals should predispose them to disengage prematurely from objectively attainable goals. As reviewed in the preceding section, these strategies reduce commitment to and investment in challenging and demanding strivings that threaten to cause the kind of frustration and pain that can reactivate a deactivated attachment system. (Such frustration and disappointment naturally incline a person to seek comfort and support from other people, but exhibiting dependence on one's attachment figure is an anti-goal for avoidant individuals.) This tendency may be further exacerbated when an avoidant person encounters difficulties and impediments that demand renewed effort and threaten self-efficacy and self-reliance. Thus avoidant individuals should react to obstacles and difficulties defensively, withdrawing commitment and suspending effort. While allowing them to avoid potential failures, this reaction is likely to result in missed opportunities to reach attainable goals and overly cautious choices to engage in unchallenging activities.

In contrast, the hyperactivating strategies adopted by anxiously attached individuals predispose a person to continue pursuing unattainable goals. After all, their prototypical striving is for reassurance and commitment in a relationship that they perceive as inadequately reliable. This often generates a long chain of self-fulfilling, "oh-woe-is-me" experiences in troubled love relationships, including loss of romantic and marital partners to "poachers" (Schachner & Shaver, 2002, 2004). The payoff for this strategy, if there is one, is to continue to feel that one has suffered unduly and deserves more sympathy and support. It fits well with low and unstable self-esteem, and it emphasizes vulnerability and need.

Although adult attachment researchers have not yet systematically documented attachment style differences in premature disengagement from attainable goals and failure to disengage from unattainable goals, there is some evidence for the hypothesized effects of deactivating and hyperactivating strategies. For example, week-long diary studies in which participants completed the Rochester Interaction Record each time they engaged in a social interaction lasting 10 minutes or longer (e.g., Pietromonaco & Barrett, 1997; Tidwell, Reis, & Shaver, 1996) revealed that avoidant people felt bored and disengaged during many of their daily social interactions, suggesting a failure to pursue interesting, engaging interpersonal goals. In a different kind of study—of military training teams—Rom and Mikulincer (2003) found that avoidant trainees reported lower levels of personal involvement during group interactions, and saw fewer benefits and challenges in these interactions, than did more secure individuals. Interestingly, they also performed worse as team members (as assessed by other members of their team).

Another study provides evidence concerning goal disengagement following a marital breakup. Mikulincer and Florian (1996) examined patterns of ongoing involvement with ex-spouses among middle-aged divorced adults and found that anxiously attached people failed to disengage from their lost relationships; they reported the strongest continuing bonds with their ex-spouses (e.g., frequent contacts, high levels of perceived and expected intimacy). (See also Davis, Shaver, & Vernon, 2003, for evidence concerning anxiously attached individuals' use of sexual wiles to lure separated partners back into a relationship.) In contrast, avoidant people reported the strongest inclinations to disengage from and forget their ex-spouses. More secure individuals reported a relatively balanced pattern of engagement with and disengagement from their former partners. They tended to satisfy their attachment needs in other relationships without totally severing their previous emotional ties. This also seems to be the secure strategy for grieving following the death of an attachment figure—maintaining positive representations of the person and relationship, while reorganizing one's attachment strategies to get on with life in the absence of the deceased partner (Fraley & Shaver, 1999).

In a recent series of studies of investment escalation behavior, Jayson (2004) provided evidence concerning how attachment orientations affect patterns of goal disengagement even in attachment-irrelevant settings. In Jayson's first study, participants who had previously completed the ECR scale (Brennan et al., 1998) read about hypothetical scenarios in which they were asked to imagine that they were the research and development (R&D) manager of a pharmaceutical firm that had invested money in a new anti-cancer drug. They were then informed that development of the drug was not going well and in fact was causing the firm to lose money. The participants were given an amount of money to invest in R&D, and were asked to divide the money between further development of the questionable drug and working on an alternative product. The amount that participants chose to invest in the as-yet-unsuccessful drug was used as an index of continuing commitment to the original investment. In two subsequent studies, Jayson used similar scenarios to see what would happen when he experimentally manipulated participants' personal responsibility for having made the initial investment (high, low) and expectancies of success in further developing the questionable drug (low, high).

Jayson (2004) observed the expected inverse association between attachment avoidance and goal persistence: The higher a person's avoidance score, the less money he or she decided to allocate to the troubled project. However, this association was not significant in experimental conditions that minimized the participant's personal responsibility for the initial investment; this result supports our idea that avoidant individuals' disengagement from frustrating activities is a defensive maneuver aimed at preventing further damage to their sense of self-worth. When the activity has few or no negative repercussions for the self (as in the low-responsibility condition), avoidant individuals no longer seem motivated to disengage from goal pursuit.

Other findings supported our ideas concerning the difficulty experienced by anxiously attached individuals when they should abandon unattainable goals. When expectations about continuing to develop the original drug were experimentally manipulated to be favorable, attachment anxiety was not significantly associated with the amount of money invested in further development of the drug. However, when participants were led to believe that the goal of successful development was perhaps unattainable (they received pessimistic messages about the drug's prospects), attachment anxiety was significantly associated with a paradoxical escalation in the amount of money participants allocated to the losing investment. That is, anxiously attached people seemed to find it very difficult to withdraw commitment to an unattainable goal.

Following this line of research, we conducted a correlational study in which 60 Israeli undergraduates (40 women, 20 men) completed the ECR scale and Wrosch and colleagues' (2003) four-item goal disengagement scale, which assesses the ease with which participants are able to reduce effort and relinquish commitment to a goal (e.g., "It's easy for me to reduce my effort toward a goal," "It's easy for me to stop thinking about a goal and let it go"). Participants completed this brief scale twice. In one version, they were asked about goal disengagement after experiencing some unexpected problems that could be solved by investing further effort (attainable goal condition). In the other version, participants were asked about goal disengagement after experiencing recurrent failure over an extended period of time (unattainable goal condition).

We observed a significant positive association between attachment avoidance and goal disengagement in the attainable goal condition, $r(58) = .44$, $p < .01$, but not in the unattainable goal condition, $r(58) = .01$. That is, attachment avoidance was associated with goal disengagement when there were still opportunities to achieve the goal (a case of premature disengagement). As expected theoretically, attachment anxiety was inversely associated with goal disengagement in the unattainable goal condition, $r(58) = -.38$, $p < .01$, but not in the attainable goal condition, $r(58) = -.04$. In a conceptual replication of Jayson's (2004) findings, attachment anxiety interfered with disengagement from unattainable goals.

Overall, the findings reviewed above document the tendency of avoidant individuals to disengage prematurely from goals when goal pursuit is challenging and demands personal involvement. They also indicate, as expected, that anxiously attached individuals seem relatively unable or unwilling to disengage from unattainable goals. Hyperactivating strategies create a motivational trap in which a person is caught between negative feelings related to blocked progress toward a goal and inability to disengage from the goal. The inability to let go of unattainable goals may be a hallmark of anxious attachment.

### Attachment Anxiety and the Passage from Approach to Avoidance Motivation

As discussed earlier, the attachment system includes both a tendency to approach the goals of protection and security and a tendency to avoid the anti-goals of separation, rejection, and attachment figure unavailability. This kind of opposition between appetitive and aversive forces is common in motivational systems; it seems to be based in different neural substrates, and to have different effects on cognition and behavior (e.g., Carver & Scheier, 1990; Gable, Reis, & Elliot, 2003). Research has shown that individual differences in the relative strength of approach and avoidance tendencies affect emotional and cognitive reactions to positive and negative experiences, and tend to determine how these experiences contribute to well-being and life satisfaction (e.g., Carver & White, 1994; Updegraff, Gable, & Taylor, 2004). We suspect that anxiously attached individuals' reluctance to disengage from unattainable goals creates an imbalance between aversive and approach tendencies.

For anxious people, the experience of aversive anti-goal states is a common experience, because hyperactivation of the attachment system is often followed by failure to attain security. Moreover, due to their tendency to exaggerate the presence and seriousness of aversive states and to ruminate mentally on their meaning and consequences (Mikulincer & Shaver, 2003), attachment-anxious people become chronically preoccupied with failure and other distress-eliciting experiences. As a result, anxiously attached people may be highly attentive and sensitive to possible recurrences of anti-goal states (rejection, separations, loss, and attachment-unrelated failures and threats that might cause a person to need protection and support while not being certain of its availability). Their thoughts and actions may thus become mainly directed toward precluding aversive states rather than toward achieving positive goal states. When a person's motives are organized in this way, avoiding aversive states becomes the main source of satisfaction, which is likely not to be as beneficial in most respects as attaining positive goals (as is suggested by differences between the affective states of relief and happiness; Roseman & Evdokas, 2004).

Attachment research has provided extensive evidence that anxiously attached persons tend to be extremely sensitive and responsive to signs of attachment figure unavailability. For example, strong correlations have been found between attachment anxiety and measures of rejection sensitivity (e.g., Downey & Feldman, 1996). Moreover, studies examining emotional reactions to loss of a spouse (e.g., Field & Sundin, 2001; Wayment & Vierthaler, 2002), breakup of a dating relationship (e.g., Feeney & Noller, 1992; Simpson, 1990), and temporary separation from a romantic partner (e.g., Fraley & Shaver, 1998; Medway, Davis, Cafferty, & Chappell, 1995) indicate that anxiously attached people exhibit the most intense and pervasive distress reactions. Of course, one can alternatively interpret these findings as a reflection of undifferentiated strong affective responses rather than sensitivity to aversive events. However, findings from studies of emotional reactions to actual or symbolic reunion with an attachment figure (e.g., Cafferty, Davis, Medway, O'Hearn, & Chappell, 1995; McGowan, 2002) seem to rule out this alternative. For example, in Cafferty and colleagues' (1995) study of separation due to overseas deployment of husbands during a war, anxiously attached participants evinced less intense positive emotions upon reunion than securely attached participants.

In a series of three studies, Mikulincer, Florian, Birnbaum, and Malishkevich (2002) uncovered an interesting feature of anxiously attached participants' hypersensitivity to separation from an attachment figure. Across studies, people were asked to imagine being separated from a loved partner, and then to perform a word completion task that tapped accessibility of death-related thoughts. Participants who scored high on attachment anxiety reacted to separation reminders with heightened availability of death-related thoughts. When given partial words and asked to complete them, anxious individuals in the separation condition produced more death-related words. This tendency was particularly strong when the imagined separation was long-lasting or final, or when it involved a romantic partner. In other words, separation reminded anxious individuals of death, which is both the ultimate separation and also the event that Bowlby (1969/1982) thought the attachment behavioral system evolved to protect a person from. If attachment-anxious people's reactions to imagined separations sometimes seem extreme to their less anxious associates, the extremity of the reaction might be more understandable if the observers knew that the foreboding of actual death lay beneath it.

A recent diary study of marital relationships provided additional evidence concerning the focus of anxious individuals' concerns on aversive anti-goals (Mikulincer, Florian, & Hirschberger, 2002). In this study of 86 newlywed couples, husbands and wives independently completed the ECR scale and filled out a questionnaire every evening for a period of 21 days. Each day, participants provided ratings of marital satisfaction on that day; read a series of 8 possible positive partner behaviors (e.g., "My partner helped me solve a problem") and 10 possible negative partner behaviors (e.g., "My partner was cold and rejecting"); and marked whether each action had occurred on that day. Daily scores indicating the partner's positive and negative behaviors were computed by counting the number of such actions checked on a particular day.

For both women and men, attachment anxiety moderated the effects of partner behavior (positive and negative) on daily marital satisfaction. For participants scoring low on attachment anxiety, both kinds of partner behavior were significantly associated with ratings of marital satisfaction—the greater the number positive partner behaviors and the lower the number of negative partner behaviors on a given day, the higher the rated satisfaction on that day. However, among participants scoring high on attachment anxiety, daily marital satisfaction was more strongly tied to the number of negative partner behaviors than to the number of positive behaviors. In fact, only negative partner behaviors made a unique contribution to anxiously attached spouses' daily ratings of marital satisfaction. This indicates that anxiously attached individuals tend to overweight aversive interpersonal experiences and underweight or ignore their partners' positive behaviors—a sign of overemphasizing anti-goals rather than approach goals (Updegraff et al., 2004).

Research is also beginning to show that anxious individuals' tendency to organize their actions around aversive rather than pleasant events is observable even in attachment-unrelated contexts (Elliot & Reis, 2003; Kogot, 2002). In several studies, participants completed self-report measures tapping attachment orientations as well as approach and avoidance achievement-related goals in academic settings (e.g., learning new skills, attaining high grades, avoiding low grades). In these studies, attachment anxiety was more strongly associated with anti-goals than with approach goals.

## CONCLUDING REMARKS

In this chapter we have explained and illustrated ways in which Bowlby's central theoretical construct, the attachment behavioral system, is relevant to motivation science. Individual differences in attachment security, and in particular forms of insecurity (anxiety and avoidance), are associated with personal goals, the organization of those goals, and goal-related cognitions and behaviors in both attachment-related and attachment-unrelated contexts. This application of attachment theory to broad motivational issues encourages us to think that important psychodynamic issues—such as conflicts related to love, dependence, and security, and the defenses that arise when a person struggles to master or cope with these conflicts—underlie processes of goal engagement and disengagement as well as cognitive assessments of goal attainability or goal value. The theory also leads us to consider such issues as the evolution of certain goal-directed behaviors and the effects of a person's attachment history on goals, fears, and defenses. Because attachment theory is both an evolutionary theory and a theory of personality development, it suggests that motivation theorists and researchers need to pay attention to biological and developmental roots of people's goal systems and the ways in which these are shaped by interactions with attachment figures during infancy and childhood. As Bowlby (1969/1982) intended, attachment theory creates important bridges between still-useful psychoanalytic formulations and more recent cognitive and developmental theories of personality and motivation.

We hope that the ideas and findings presented in this chapter will stimulate other scholars to apply Bowlby's attachment theory to the study of human motivation. We also hope that future research will be directed at the normative and individual difference aspects of other behavioral systems (e.g., exploration, caregiving, sex, affiliation). Bowlby's ideas about the attachment behavioral system can be extended to provide guides to the investigation of other behavioral systems, each of which involve additional areas of striving, conflict, and defense. Moving beyond the almost exclusive emphasis on the attachment behavioral system that has characterized the field of attachment research, including our own work, would yield a much broader conception of human motivation—a conception that, when fully developed, might have a place among the "grand theories" of motivation and personality.

## REFERENCES


Ainsworth, M. D. S. (1973). The development of infant–mother attachment. In B. M. Caldwell & H. N. Ricciuti (Eds.), *Review of child development research* (Vol. 3, pp. 1–44). Chicago: University of Chicago Press.

Ainsworth, M. D. S. (1991). Attachment and other affectional bonds across the life cycle. In C. M. Parkes, J. Stevenson-Hinde, & P. Marris (Eds.), *Attachment across the life cycle* (pp. 33–51). New York: Routledge.

Ainsworth, M. D. S., Blehar, M. C., Waters, E., & Wall, S. (1978). *Patterns of attachment: A psychological study of the strange situation.* Hillsdale, NJ: Erlbaum.

Avihou, N. (2006). *Attachment orientations and dreaming: An examination of the unconscious components of the attachment system.* Unpublished doctoral dissertation, Bar-Ilan University.

Bartholomew, K., & Horowitz, L. M. (1991). Attachment styles among young adults: A test of a four-category model. *Journal of Personality and Social Psychology, 61*, 226–244.

Bowlby, J. (1944). Forty-four juvenile thieves: Their characters and home life. *International Journal of Psycho-Analysis, 25*, 19–52, 107–127.

Bowlby, J. (1969/1982). *Attachment and loss: Vol. 1. Attachment* (2nd ed.). New York: Basic Books.

Bowlby, J. (1973). *Attachment and loss: Vol. 2. Separation: Anxiety and anger.* New York: Basic Books.

Bowlby, J. (1979). *The making and breaking of affectional bonds.* London: Tavistock.

Bowlby, J. (1980). *Attachment and loss: Vol. 3. Loss: Sadness and depression.* New York: Basic Books.

Bowlby, J. (1988). *A secure base: Clinical applications of attachment theory.* London: Routledge.

Brennan, K. A., Clark, C. L., & Shaver, P. R. (1998). Self-report measurement of adult attachment: An integrative overview. In J. A. Simpson & W. S. Rholes (Eds.), *Attachment theory and close relationships* (pp. 46–76). New York: Guilford Press.

Cafferty, T. P., Davis, K. E., Medway, F. J., O'Hearn, R. E., & Chappell, K. D. (1994). Reunion dynamics among couples separated during Operation Desert Storm: An attachment theory analysis. In K. Bartholomew & D. Perlman (Eds.), *Attachment processes in adulthood* (pp. 309–330). London: Kingsley.

Cantor, N., & Langston, C. A. (1989). Ups and downs of life tasks in a life transition. In L. A. Pervin (Ed.), *Goal concepts in personality and social psychology* (pp. 87–126). Hillsdale, NJ: Erlbaum.

Carver, C. S., & Scheier, M. F. (1981). *Attention and self-regulation: A control-theory approach to human behavior.* New York: Springer-Verlag.

Carver, C. S., & Scheier, M. F. (1990). Origins and functions of positive and negative affect: A control-process view. *Psychological Review, 97*, 19–35.

Carver, C. S., & Scheier, M. F. (1998). *On the self-regulation of behavior.* New York: Cambridge University Press.

Carver, C. S., Sutton, S. K., & Scheier, M. F. (2000). Action, emotion, and personality: Emerging conceptual integration. *Personality and Social Psychology Bulletin, 26*, 741–751.

Carver, C. S., & White, T. L. (1994). Behavioral inhibition, behavioral activation, and affective responses to impending reward and punishment: The BIS/BAS scales. *Journal of Personality and Social Psychology, 67*, 319–333.

Cassidy, J., & Kobak, R. R. (1988). Avoidance and its relationship with other defensive processes. In J. Belsky & T. Nezworski (Eds.), *Clinical implications of attachment* (pp. 300–323). Hillsdale, NJ: Erlbaum.

Cassidy, J., & Shaver, P. R. (Eds.). (1999). *Handbook of attachment: Theory, research, and clinical applications.* New York: Guilford Press.

Collins, N. L., & Read, S. J. (1990). Adult attachment, working models, and relationship quality in dating couples. *Journal of Personality and Social Psychology, 58*, 644–663.

Davis, D., Shaver, P. R., & Vernon, M. L. (2003). Physical, emotional, and behavioral reactions to breaking up: The roles of gender, age, emotional involvement, and attachment style. *Personality and Social Psychology Bulletin, 29*, 871–884.

Downey, G., & Feldman, S. I. (1996). Implications of rejection sensitivity for intimate relationships. *Journal of Personality and Social Psychology, 70*, 1327–1343.

Elliot, A. J., & Reis, H. T. (2003). Attachment and exploration in adulthood. *Journal of Personality and Social Psychology, 85*, 317–331.

Emmons, R. A. (1986). Personal strivings: An approach to personality and subjective well-being. *Journal of Personality and Social Psychology, 51*, 1058–1068.

Emmons, R. A. (1992). Abstract versus concrete goals: Personal striving level, physical illness, and psychological well-being. *Journal of Personality and Social Psychology, 62*, 292–300.

Emmons, R. A. (1997). Motives and goals. In R. Hogan, J. Johnson, & S. Briggs (Eds.), *Handbook of personality psychology* (pp. 485–512). San Diego, CA: Academic Press.

Emmons, R. A., & King, L. (1988). Conflict among personal strivings: Immediate and long-term implications for psychological and physical well-being. *Journal of Personality and Social Psychology, 54*, 1040–1048.

Feeney, J. A., & Noller, P. (1992). Attachment style and romantic love: Relationship dissolution. *Australian Journal of Psychology, 44*, 69–74.

Field, N. P., & Sundin, E. C. (2001). Attachment style in adjustment to conjugal bereavement. *Journal of Social and Personal Relationships, 18*, 347–361.

Fraley, R. C., Davis, K. E., & Shaver, P. R. (1998). Dismissing avoidance and the defensive organization of emotion, cognition, and behavior. In J. A. Simpson &

W. S. Rholes (Eds.), *Attachment theory and close relationships* (pp. 249–279). New York: Guilford Press.

Fraley, R. C., & Shaver, P. R. (1998). Airport separations: A naturalistic study of adult attachment dynamics in separating couples. *Journal of Personality and Social Psychology, 75*, 1198–1212.

Fraley, R. C., & Shaver, P. R. (1999). Loss and bereavement: Attachment theory and recent controversies concerning grief work and the nature of detachment. In J. Cassidy & P. R. Shaver (Eds.), *Handbook of attachment: Theory, research, and clinical applications* (pp. 735–759). New York: Guilford Press.

Fraley, R. C., & Shaver, P. R. (2000). Adult romantic attachment: Theoretical developments, emerging controversies, and unanswered questions. *Review of General Psychology, 4*, 132–154.

Gable, S. L., Reis, H. T., & Elliot, A. J. (2003). Evidence for bivariate systems: An empirical test of appetition and aversion across domains. *Journal of Research in Personality, 37*, 349–372.

George, C., & Solomon, J. (1999). Attachment and caregiving: The caregiving behavioral system. In J. Cassidy & P. R. Shaver (Eds.), *Handbook of attachment: Theory, research, and clinical applications* (pp. 649–670). New York: Guilford Press.

Hazan, C., & Shaver, P. R. (1987). Romantic love conceptualized as an attachment process. *Journal of Personality and Social Psychology, 52*, 511–524.

Heinicke, C., & Westheimer, I. (1966). *Brief separations*. New York: International Universities Press.

Jayson, Y. (2004). *An attachment perspective to escalation of commitment*. Unpublished doctoral dissertation, Bar-Ilan University.

Keelan, J. P. R., Dion, K. K., & Dion, K. L. (1998). Attachment style and relationship satisfaction: Test of a self-disclosure explanation. *Canadian Journal of Behavioural Science, 30*, 24–35.

Kogot, E. (2002). *Adult attachment style and cognitions, affect, and behavior in achievement settings*. Unpublished doctoral dissertation, Bar-Ilan University.

Lazarus, R. S., & Folkman, S. (1984). *Stress, appraisal, and coping*. New York: Springer.

Little, B. R. (1989). Personal project analysis: Trivial pursuits, magnificent obsessions, and the search for coherence. In D. M. Buss & N. Cantor (Eds.), *Personality psychology: Recent trends and emerging directions* (pp. 15–31). New York: Springer-Verlag.

Luborsky, L., & Crits-Christoph, P. (1998). *Understanding transference: The core conflictual relationship theme method*. Washington, DC: American Psychological Association.

McGowan, S. (2002). Mental representations in stressful situations: The calming and distressing effects of significant others. *Journal of Experimental Social Psychology, 38*, 152–161.

Medway, F. J., Davis, K. E., Cafferty, T. P., & Chappell, K. D. (1995). Family disruption and adult attachment correlates of spouse and child reactions to separation and reunion due to Operation Desert Storm. *Journal of Social and Clinical Psychology, 14*, 97–118.

Mikulincer, M. (1998). Attachment working models and the sense of trust: An exploration of interaction goals and affect regulation. *Journal of Personality and Social Psychology, 74*, 1209–1224.

Mikulincer, M., Birnbaum, G., Woddis, D., & Nachmias, O. (2000). Stress and accessibility of proximity-related thoughts: Exploring the normative and intraindividual components of attachment theory. *Journal of Personality and Social Psychology, 78*, 509–523.

Mikulincer, M., & Florian, V. (1996). Emotional reactions to loss over the life span: An attachment perspective. In S. McFadden & C. Magai (Eds.), *Handbook of emotions, adult development, and aging* (pp. 269–285). San Diego, CA: Academic Press.

Mikulincer, M., Florian, V., Birnbaum, G., & Malishkevich, S. (2002). The death-anxiety buffering function of close relationships: Exploring the effects of separation reminders on death-thought accessibility. *Personality and Social Psychology Bulletin, 28*, 287–299.

Mikulincer, M., Florian, V., & Hirschberger, G. (2002, January). *The dynamic interplay of global, relationship-specific, and contextual representations of attachment security*. Paper presented at the annual meeting of the Society for Personality and Social Psychology, Savannah, GA.

Mikulincer, M., Florian, V., & Tolmacz, R. (1990). Attachment styles and fear of death: A case of affect regulation. *Journal of Personality and Social Psychology, 58*, 273–280.

Mikulincer, M., Gillath, O., & Shaver, P. R. (2002). Activation of the attachment system in adulthood: Threat-related primes increase the accessibility of mental representations of attachment figures. *Journal of Personality and Social Psychology, 83*, 881–895.

Mikulincer, M., Hirschberger, G., Nachmias, O., & Gillath, O. (2001). The affective component of the secure base schema: Affective priming with representations of attachment security. *Journal of Personality and Social Psychology, 81*, 305–321.

Mikulincer, M., & Nachshon, O. (1991). Attachment styles and patterns of self-disclosure. *Journal of Personality and Social Psychology, 61*, 321–331.

Mikulincer, M., & Shaver, P. R. (2001). Attachment theory and intergroup bias: Evidence that priming the secure base schema attenuates negative reactions to out-groups. *Journal of Personality and Social Psychology, 81*, 97–115.

Mikulincer, M., & Shaver, P. R. (2003). The attachment behavioral system in adulthood: Activation, psychodynamics, and interpersonal processes. In M. P. Zanna (Ed.), *Advances in experimental social psychology* (Vol. 35, pp. 53–152). San Diego, CA: Academic Press.

Mikulincer, M., & Shaver, P. R. (2007). *Attachment in*

*adulthood: Structure, dynamics, and change*. New York: Guilford Press.

Pietromonaco, P. R., & Barrett, L. F. (1997). Working models of attachment and daily social interactions. *Journal of Personality and Social Psychology, 73*, 1409–1423.

Raz, A. (2002). *Personality, core relationship themes, and interpersonal competence among young adults experiencing difficulties in establishing long-term relationships*. Unpublished doctoral dissertation, Haifa University.

Robertson, J., & Bowlby, J. (1952). Responses of young children to separation from their mothers. *Courier of the International Children's Center, Paris, 2*, 131–140.

Rom, E., & Mikulincer, M. (2003). Attachment theory and group processes: The association between attachment style and group-related representations, goals, memory, and functioning. *Journal of Personality and Social Psychology, 84*, 1220–1235.

Roseman, I. J., & Evdokas, A. (2004). Appraisals cause experienced emotions: Experimental evidence. *Cognition and Emotion, 18*, 1–28.

Schachner, D. A., & Shaver, P. R. (2002). Attachment style and human mate poaching. *New Review of Social Psychology, 1*, 122–129.

Schachner, D. A., & Shaver, P. R. (2004). Attachment dimensions and motives for sex. *Personal Relationships, 11*, 179–195.

Scharfe, E., & Bartholomew, K. (1995). Accommodation and attachment representations in young couples. *Journal of Social and Personal Relationships, 12*, 389–401.

Shaver, P. R., & Clark, C. L. (1994). The psychodynamics of adult romantic attachment. In J. M. Masling & R. F. Bornstein (Eds.), *Empirical studies of psychoanalytic theories: Vol. 5. Empirical perspectives on object relations theory* (pp. 105–156). Washington, DC: American Psychological Association.

Shaver, P. R., & Hazan, C. (1993). Adult romantic attachment: Theory and evidence. In D. Perlman & W. Jones (Eds.), *Advances in personal relationships* (Vol. 4, pp. 29–70). London: Kingsley.

Shaver, P. R., & Klinnert, M. (1982). Schachter's theories of affiliation and emotions: Implications of developmental research. In L. Wheeler (Ed.), *Review of personality and social psychology* (Vol. 3, pp. 37–71). Beverly Hills, CA: Sage.

Shaver, P. R., & Mikulincer, M. (2002). Attachment-related psychodynamics. *Attachment and Human Development, 4*, 133–161.

Shaver, P. R., Schachner, D. A., & Mikulincer, M. (2005). Attachment style, excessive reassurance seeking, relationship processes, and depression. *Personality and Social Psychology Bulletin, 31*, 343–359.

Sheldon, K. M., & Emmons, R. A. (1995). Comparing differentiation and integration within personal goal systems. *Personality and Individual Differences, 18*, 39–46.

Simpson, J. A. (1990). Influence of attachment styles on romantic relationships. *Journal of Personality and Social Psychology, 59*, 871–980.

Simpson, J. A., Rholes, W. S., & Phillips, D. (1996). Conflict in close relationships: An attachment perspective. *Journal of Personality and Social Psychology, 71*, 899–914.

Tidwell, M. C. O., Reis, H. T., & Shaver, P. R. (1996). Attachment, attractiveness, and social interaction: A diary study. *Journal of Personality and Social Psychology, 71*, 729–745.

Updegraff, J. A., Gable, S. L., & Taylor, S. E. (2004). What makes experiences satisfying?: The interaction of approach–avoidance motivations and emotions in well-being. *Journal of Personality and Social Psychology, 86*, 496–504.

Vormbrock, J. (1993). Attachment theory as applied to war-time and marital separation. *Psychological Bulletin, 114*, 122–144.

Wayment, H. A., & Vierthaler, J. (2002). Attachment style and bereavement reactions. *Journal of Loss and Trauma, 7*, 129–149.

Wrosch, C., & Heckhausen, J. (1999). Control processes before and after passing a developmental deadline: Activation and deactivation of intimate relationship goals. *Journal of Personality and Social Psychology, 77*, 415–427.

Wrosch, C., Scheier, M. F., Miller, G. E., Schultz, R., & Carver, C. S. (2003). Adaptive self-regulation of unattainable goals: Goal disengagement, goal reengagement, and subjective well-being. *Personality and Social Psychology Bulletin, 29*, 1494–1508.

Chapter 14

# Structural Dynamics

## THE CHALLENGE OF CHANGE IN GOAL SYSTEMS

**James Y. Shah**
**Arie W. Kruglanski**

Although goals have long been thought to play a vital role in effective self-regulation by linking needs to behavior and giving mental form and direction to our basic needs and desires (see Carver & Scheier, 1998; Higgins, 1997; Pervin, 1989), social psychologists have increasingly recognized the broader self-regulatory benefits of these mental representations. That is, in addition to articulating the specific manner in which needs can be addressed, goals may provide a broader "structural" benefit to self-regulation by helping us to organize, prioritize, and manage our often disparate motives. Indeed, as any student, parent, or busy professional will attest, everyday self-regulation inevitably involves the juggling of often very disparate goals, necessitating that they be both pursued individually and managed collectively. A complete understanding, then, of the role goals play in self-regulation must consider not only how goals are individually adopted and pursued, but how they are structured, prioritized, and managed with respect to each other and the general needs that gave rise to them. And these qualities take on even more significance in light of research suggesting that the general capacity for goal pursuit is limited and exhaustible (see Carver & Scheier, 1998; Emmons, 1986; Pervin, 1989; Baumeister & Vohs, 2004).

The present analysis, then, begins by assuming that goals are typically adopted and pursued not in motivational isolation, but rather in a regulatory context consisting of goals that best reflect an individual's current motivations, cognitions, and capacities, as well as the constraints and affordances provided by the immediate situation. Because regulatory context is defined by what the situation allows and what the pursuer currently wants, it is not simply a static representation of an individual's entire set of goals. Rather, it represents the subset of goals most relevant to the person's current needs and best fitting with his or her current capacities and immediate physical environment. Given the inevitable changes in our motivations, capacities, and environment, this "working set" of personal goals is inherently dynamic in nature. Yet this set is not without internal structure at any given moment. As will be discussed, associations among goals, means, and motives may play an important role in defining and constraining this context. Thus, after providing a more detailed definition of both the static and dynamic qualities of goal structure, the present analysis explores how this *structural dynamics* approach may help define the fundamental challenges in defining, pursuing, and managing goals over time. But before we discuss the potential theoretical utility of this approach for our understanding of optimal self-regulation, more precise definitions of goal structure and goal dynamics are required.

## MULTIPLE MOTIVES ON THE MOVE

The notion that goals are situated with respect to each other is certainly not a novel concept to the study of motivation and self-regulation. Indeed, it may immediately bring to mind Lewin's (1947) classic theorizing on the interaction of various environmental forces or *force fields*, and it is certainly reminiscent of Simon's (1967) conceptualization of a mental *queue* or waiting list of goals, which is revised and updated with every goal-related success and failure and every change in circumstance. It is also a fundamental assumption of more recent conceptualizations of hierarchical goal systems, as prominently detailed by Carver and Scheier (1998) (see also Kruglanski et al., 2002).

The present analysis builds on such classic theorizing, as well as important research on the individual nature of goals, in formulating a conception of regulatory context that is *structurally dynamic*—a context that can be detailed in terms of both the "hot" motivations and "cold" cognitions that provide the impetus for internal structure and the push for change over time. As described below, the present analysis assumes that the regulatory context in which goals are pursued is dynamically defined and redefined by the multiplicity of individuals' needs, and constrained by how these needs are represented cognitively (via goals) as well as by their own capacity for goal pursuit. It is further constrained and expanded by goal-related obstacles or affordances in the immediate environment.

As mentioned earlier, a fundamental assumption of the present analysis is that goals are pursued within a context of other, potentially competing goals, each arising to address fundamental (and sometimes correcting) motivations. Like individual goals, then, a regulatory context is fundamentally, if more complexly, motivational in nature, and its motivational qualities may importantly influence not only how the context changes over time (as needs and their corresponding goals are met or abandoned), but also how it is experienced and managed as a whole. Perhaps the most compelling support for this last assumption can be found in the extensive recent research on the regulatory focus of goals by Higgins and his colleagues (see Higgins, 1997). This work has extensively documented how differences in fundamental needs for promotion and prevention can significantly affect how even the same goal (e.g., doing well in school) is perceived, pursued, and experienced. Similarly, work on the instrinsicality of goal pursuit (see Deci & Ryan, 2000) and on achievement-related goals also suggests that the distinct motives giving rise to goals may have a significant impact on how they are pursued, experienced, and abandoned (Ames, 1992; Bandura, 1986; Dweck, 1999; Emmons, 1991; Harackiewicz, Manderlink, & Sansone, 1992; Klinger, 1977; Nicholls, 1989).

To suggest that regulatory contexts are motivated and dynamic is not to suggest that these contexts are without stability or structure over time. Indeed, it is assumed that the goals constituting any particular regulatory context have a particular relation to each other that reflects associations built up over time. The formation and configuration of goals within a regulatory context reflect not only goals' motivational underpinnings, but the cognitive qualities that goals share with other mental representations.

## GOAL ASSOCIATIONS

Like that of other mental representations, the accessibility of goals may vary dispositionally and situationally (see Shah & Kruglanski, 2000). They are also commonly thought to be organized hierarchically (see Bandura, 1997; Carver & Scheier, 1998; Shah & Kruglanski,

2000; Vallerand & Ratelle, 2002), with very general goals (e.g., achievement) giving rise to more concrete goals (e.g., success in school), which in turn give rise to even more specific intentions (e.g., getting an A in social psychology) and behaviors (e.g., studying). Such an arrangement highlights that within a given system or more specific context, goals are both (1) *end-states* for the more specific goals, intentions, or behaviors that they give rise to, and (2) *means* for the more general or abstract goals they serve (see also Carver & Scheier, 1998; Emmons, 1992; Hyland, 1988; Powers, 1973). Lateral connections between the entities are also possible, in light of the fact that a given goal may be associatively linked to other goals (e.g., because of their common link to a given context), and a given means may be associatively linked to other means (e.g., because of their common link to a particular goal). Finally, goals may differ in the number of associations they have with other goals and with specific behaviors. Indeed, even goals at the same general level may differ in their *equifinality*, or the number of different ways they can be pursued behaviorally.

## HOW GOALS KNOW EACH OTHER

And in addition to differing in their direction (upward vs. downward vs. lateral), goals' associations may also differ in *nature*. They may, for instance, both activate and inhibit other goals and means (see Read & Miller, 1998). Moreover, they may activate (or inhibit) other constructs for different reasons. Goal associations, for instance, may develop because goal pursuits facilitate each other or because goals fulfill the same underlying needs (and are thus potentially substitutable for each other).

## "GOOD FOR NOW": REGULATORY CONTEXT AS A WORKING GOAL SYSTEM

How do goals' cognitive qualities structure the dynamic motivational context in which they are pursued? If regulatory context can be seen as the currently active subset of an individual's larger collection of goals, the relative salience and structure of this subset will undoubtedly reflect the goals' chronic structural qualities. Goals that are generally more salient or more abstract, then, will typically be more salient and abstract in the moment, although the relative salience or level of abstraction may vary contextually. Moreover, the internal structure of a regulatory context may also come to influence how it changes over time. But whereas motivation may dictate when contexts change, associations among goals may influence how contexts change as goals are accomplished or abandoned. Thus not only may recently attained goals be dropped from an individual's regulatory context, but so might goals closely associated with this attainment. Alternatively, unattained goals may ultimately be replaced by closely associated goals that address the same underlying need. Therefore, although the dynamics of regulatory context may be driven by changes in need and environment, they may further be constrained by preexisting goal associations to each other and to behavior.

## "WILLING AND ABLE": CAPACITY IN CONTEXT

In addition to being structured by how goals may be mentally represented and associated with each other, the nature and dynamics of regulatory context may also be constrained by the pursuer's general capacity for engaging in goals. Indeed, various self-regulatory theories and models have assumed that goal-related effort involves the momentary mobilization of potentially exhaustible self-regulatory resources that are generally applicable to goal pursuits (e.g., Kahneman, 1973; Kanfer, Ackerman, Murtha, Dugdale, & Nelson, 1994). Such resources include (but are not limited to) physical and mental energy (Hockey, 1996; Wright & Brehm, 1989; Zijlstra, 1996) and various forms of executive functioning (e.g., impulse control and affect regulation; see Schmeichel & Baumeister, 2004), and they are generally understood to be limited, exhaustible, and not immediately replenished. Drawing from this work, the present analysis assumes that a pursuer's capacity for goal pursuit within his or her particular regulatory context is constrained by the various self-regulatory resources that collectively define it (a collection of resources that admittedly awaits further specification; see Zijlstra, 1996). Moreover, whereas attention and working memory also have their limits (Baddeley, 2003; Norman & Shallice, 1986), the capacity for goal-related effort can only be restored gradually, and sometimes even requires expending additional effort (analogous to the time and fuel one may occasionally waste trying to find a gas station). Given these potential limitations (see Mukhopadhayay & Johar, 2005), the difficulty in precisely assessing the limits of capacity, and the variety of goals that typically define the current regulatory context, it is assumed that goal-related effort must be regulated with respect not only to the goal at hand, but also to the other goals that constitute individuals' immediate regulatory context and to their anticipations regarding how this context will change. It is assumed, then, that participants' limited capacity for effort requires them to balance an immediate need to expend effort on a current pursuit with a more general need to conserve and restore their limited capacity, in anticipation of addressing upcoming goals and in hindsight of what they have already expended. This dynamic regulation will be discussed in greater detail later.

## THE RIGHT TIME AND PLACE: THE SETTING OF CONTEXT

As Lewin (1938) famously highlighted in his topological conceptualization of force fields, not only do goal pursuits vary as a function of situational forces, but such forces can take many forms. Indeed, there has been a long-standing emphasis in psychology on the ways in which we are influenced by both immediate and general social forces—by our families, friends, and colleagues, as well as by more abstract social forces such as our social groups and culture that may be brought to mind in the moment (e.g., Bowlby, 1969; Kelley, 1952; Sherif, 1948). Such forces may deliberately or automatically influence our regulatory context by influencing the goals that constitute them. Moreover, as long ago noted by Freud (1912/1958), such influence may also be quite automatic, requiring little if any conscious intent or awareness (see Glassman & Andersen, 1999). Accordingly, self-discrimination theory (Kuhl, 1992) articulates a process of self-infiltration through which a goal originally ascribed by others is mistakenly assumed to be one's own, with detrimental consequences for how it is pursued and experienced.

Evidence that regulatory context may be at least partially constructed from the situation can be seen in how readily goal pursuits can be primed by situational and social stimuli, with significant self-regulatory implications for behavior and emotional experience (see Austin & Vancouver, 2001; Carver & Scheier, 1998; Gollwitzer & Moskowitz, 1996; Higgins, 1997; Shah, 2003). Goals, for instance, may be activated by significant others (see Fitzsimons & Bargh, 2002; Shah, 2003) and by role models (Lockwood & Kunda, 2000). They may even be "caught" from others who are simply perceived to be pursuing a goal (Aarts, Gollwitzer, & Hassin, 2004).

Moreover, the situation can also change regulatory context from the bottom up by providing the means for pursuing other goals that may not otherwise have been active. Indeed, recent research on regulatory fit has found compelling evidence that individuals become sensitive to such opportunities as they come to value environments that traditionally best accommodate, or fit, their current need state (see Higgins, 2000). Regulatory context, then, is influenced not only by changes in goals' desirability but also by changes in their feasibility. Further support for this possibility is found in research suggesting that goals, unlike other mental representations, can be primed by environmental stimuli that typically serve as means for goal attainment, whether these stimuli are individuals, objects, or even settings, and regardless of their semantic relationship to the goal in question (Gollwitzer & Brandstätter, 1997; Shah & Kruglanski, 2000).

As summarized in Figure 14.1, then, the structural dynamics of goal systems are defined by how an individual's *working goal system* is structured in the moment and changes over time as different goals are recalled or adopted and abandoned or attained. This context is defined individually and situationally, and represents the ever-changing regulatory context in which each goal is adopted, pursued, and experienced—a context further constrained by the capacities of the pursuer and the situation.

## THE CHALLENGING CHOICES OF CHANGING CONTEXT

The fact that goals *are* pursued in such a dynamic context raises or highlights fundamental questions regarding how goals are adopted and defined, how they are pursued, and how they are maintained, as we describe below.

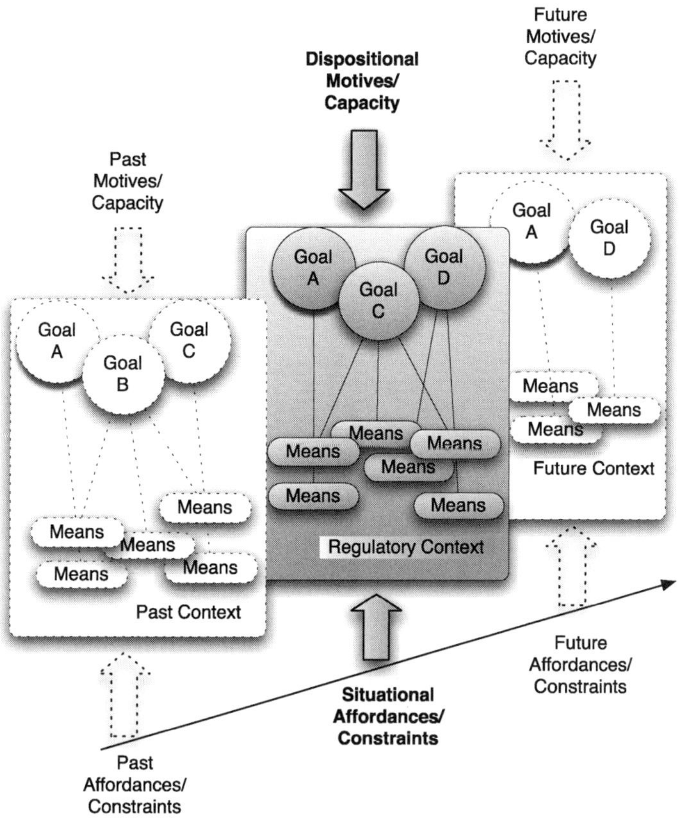


**FIGURE 14.1.** The structural dynamics of goal systems.

## Goal Adoption: How Many, How Much, and How Motivated?

### *How Many: Prioritizing Goals to Pursue*

The collective management of goals with limited and potentially exhaustible resources raises important issues regarding how and when goals are "taken on." The sheer number of goals that constitute a working goal system can have important implications for how goals are most effectively managed. Although the simultaneous pursuit of many (vs. few) goals may reflect fleeting situational affordances and may encourage productivity and effective multitasking, it also runs the risk of overly taxing the pursuer, especially when the size of a working goal system reflects the pursuer's inability to properly prioritize potential goal pursuits. Indeed, the fact that goals are formed in a regulatory context may encourage consideration of their relative utility, or utility in comparison to the possible alternatives within its present regulatory context. The notion that goals may be appraised on a "regulatory curve" raises the intriguing possibility that their perceived importance may change as a function of how it compares to the other goals the pursuer is currently juggling.

### *How Much: Specifying Goal Level*

In addition to prioritizing the number of goals one chooses to pursue at any given time, one must also often consider the level at which each individual goal should be set (in terms of performance). Certainly goal attainment may often be readily defined by the contents of the goal itself (as when an athlete strives for a gold medal) or the context in which it is pursued. Yet we often have considerable leeway in defining successful attainment, especially with regard to more general goals that are not tied to a specific settings, such as the abstract "be" goals that define who we are in a general sense (Carver & Scheier, 1998; Higgins, 1997; Lewin, Dembo, Festinger, & Sears, 1944;

Markus & Ruvolo, 1989). Two students, for instance, may be striving to do well academically during a given semester, but may differ dramatically in how they come to define this goal. Whereas one may decide that success would be a B average, the other might view anything less than a 4.0 grade point average as a failure.

Do such differences in goal setting matter? Undoubtedly such differences may come to affect how these students feel about their performance, and ultimately about themselves (e.g., Mento, Locke, & Klein, 1992). If the students described above take the same courses and receive the same mix of A's and B's, the student specifying a higher goal level may come to feel considerably less satisfied with his or her performance at semester's end (an issue we return to later). Yet, in extensive work on goal-setting theory, Locke and Latham (1990, 2002) have consistently demonstrated that individuals induced to adopt challenging and specific goals show greater goal-related performance than individuals adopting "do your best" goals. Goals that are relatively more challenging lead to greater performance than relatively easy goals, especially when these goals are quite specific, as will soon be discussed. In fact, the relationship between performance and goal challenge has been found to be quite robust, leveling off only at the limits of pursuers' ability and resources (Locke & Latham, 2002). At first glance, these findings appear to contradict those tenets of expectancy–value theory discussed earlier, positing that higher levels of expectancy should lead to greater goal commitment and, presumably, greater goal-related performance (Feather, 1982). This seeming contradiction can be resolved upon consideration of the distinction between choosing a goal and setting its level. Indeed, Locke, Motowidlo, and Bobko (1986) found that when goal level is constant (a general assumption of expectancy–value theories), higher expectancies lead to higher levels of performance. At any particular goal level, then, greater expectancy has a positive impact on performance.

A significant caveat to these compelling results, however, is a requirement that individuals accept a challenging goal. Such acceptance may depend on the regulatory context of the pursuers. Indeed, the differences in the demands posed by different regulatory contexts may significantly moderate individuals' receptiveness to challenges, as they may feel compelled to "save something for later." Such a possibility may also provide an explanation for why individuals do not frequently set higher performance standards, even when they know that these will lead to overall better performance. Not only may the effort put toward a challenging goal be diverted from other current pursuits, but the likelihood and distraction of failure may be particularly aversive if seen as detrimental to these other pursuits.

### *How Motivated: Juggling Motivationally Similar or Different Goals*

Another challenge of managing goals involves the relations of goals to each other. As suggested earlier, goals within a given context can vary in terms of (1) the degree to which they facilitate or hinder other goals, and (2) the degree to which they are redundant with, or substitutable for, other goals. In articulating his *personal striving* approach to personality, for instance, Emmons (1991) noted that one important way in which goals may vary is in the degree to which they are perceived to facilitate or conflict with each other—what Sheldon and Kasser (1995) later labeled *horizontal coherence*. Such facilitation can be examined at the goal level or at the level of the individual. At the goal level, any one goal (e.g., doing well in school) may be viewed as facilitating or hindering one's other goals (e.g., to be social, to work out), or may be viewed as unrelated to one's other pursuits. Commitment to any particular goal may be encouraged by the perception that its pursuit will have positive implications for other goals, as this provides both additional reasons for pursuing the goal (in that it will also help attain other pursuits) and, if the facilitation is bidirectional, additional reasons to believe that attainment is likely (since the pursuit of these alternatives will actually aid attainment of the goal in question). Moreover, such tight integration may have important implications for psychological health. Emmons and King (1988) examined the influence of such facilitation and conflict on psychological and physical well-being, and found that conflict among personal goals was associated not only with high levels of negative affect, depression, neuroticism, and psychosomatic complaints, but also with more frequent health center visits and illnesses over the course of an academic year. Interestingly, these results remained stable over a year. A separate study shed light on the processes underlying these effects, finding that participants were less likely to act on conflicting strivings, but more likely to ruminate about them. It follows that appraising a goal as potentially conflicting with other important pursuits can undermine commitment to this end-state, whereas perceiving a pursuit as potentially facilitating other goals provides yet another reason for pursuing it (see also Donahue, Robins, Roberts, & John, 1993).

Yet not all types of perceived similarity may actually encourage goal commitment. Just as goals may be seen as facilitating other goals, so might they be seen as redundant with (or substitutable for) these goals. Put another way, they may be perceived as fulfilling the same underlying need or motive. Although relatively little empirical work has examined goal substitutability directly, the significance of this goal quality has long been acknowledged in psychoanalytic theory (see Freud, 1923/1961). Similarly, Lewin (1935) noted that substitution of one goal for another is possible when both arise from the same tension system—that is, when both goals fulfill the same underlying need or motive. More recently, the work of Steele and Liu (1983) and Tesser, Martin, and Cornell (1996) has illustrated how various psychological phenomena, including cognitive dissonance and self-affirmation, may represent substitutable goals for maintaining a positive self-view.

What are the implications of substitutability? Whereas perceived facilitation and substitutability may often go hand in hand, they may have very different self-regulatory functions and consequences. Although the redundancy of goals may provide important alternative routes to need fulfillment if an initial goal proves too challenging, this redundancy also renders the goals involved less distinctly important, potentially limiting commitment to either one (see Shah, Friedman, & Kruglanski, 2002). For example, an individual may be particularly encouraged to run 5 miles when he or she believes that running facilitates another related goal, such as lifting weights. The individual may be discouraged from spending time in the gym, however, if he or she believes that the goals of running and working out are substitutable for each other.

Thus both similarity and distinction, albeit of a different sort, may encourage effective goal management. Individuals may more easily manage similar goals if these pursuits facilitate each other, but may be less driven to do so if these pursuits are perceived to be redundant.

## Goal Pursuit: How Fast, How Furious, How Far-Reaching?

Dynamic changes in what goals we are pursuing may also have important implications for *how* we pursue them. Specifically, managing a complex and changing collection of goals may often necessitate that each is pursued with maximum efficiency in regard to time and resources. Thus a need for efficiency may lead to goal-related behaviors that are relatively easy, enjoyable, or even automatic to employ (Aarts & Dijksterhuis, 2000; Sansone & Harackiewicz, 1996; Wood, Quinn, & Kashy, 2002), to help ensure that resources remain available for other pursuits and that the goal pursuit can completed as quickly as possible (and presumably to the benefit of subsequent pursuits).

The need for efficiency, then, may lead individuals to "automate" many common goal pursuits in order to limit the time and resources such pursuits require, even at the cost of potential flexibility (Dijksterhuis & Bongers, 2005). Indeed, as readily evidenced in the current volume, an ever-increasing body of research has found that goals, like other knowledge structures, can be automatically activated by the environmental context in which they are pursued, and that such activation can have significant self-regulatory implications for behavior and emotional experience (see Bargh, 1990; Bargh & Chartrand, 1999; Ferguson, Hassin, & Bargh, Chapter 10, this volume).

The structural dynamics of goal pursuits may also affect how "furiously" we pursue any particular goal and dictate that the effort we put forth in the moment be significantly influenced by both our immediately past and future pursuits. Undoubtedly, of course, the effort put forth toward a current goal will depend on the goal's own motivationally relevant qualities. The *energization* model (Wright & Brehm, 1989), for instance, asserts that the effort put toward a goal is a function of its perceived value and difficulty. Whereas the difficulty of goal attainment establishes how much effort is necessary, the perceived value of goal attainment specifies the amount of effort individuals are actually willing to commit. Thus increases in goal difficulty lead to increases in effort until the effort required exceeds the effort one is willing to expend. The present approach, however, suggests that effort will be regulated with respect not only to the qualities of the goal itself, but also to what effort has already been expended as well as what needs to be saved within the current regulatory context.

Consistent with this argument, research by Wright, Martin, and Bland (2003) demonstrated that effort regulation in the present was moderated by the goal-related effort individuals exerted in the immediate past. The depletion of participants' capacity for effort through an initially difficult task goal was found to affect their subsequent effort regulation on a mental arithmetic task goal, such that the depleted participants exerted less effort on this second task when given a difficult performance standard, in comparison to control participants who had not been initially depleted. An entirely different line of research by Muraven, Baumeister, and their colleagues on the phenomenon of *ego depletion* also suggests that goal-related effort regulation may depend on both past exertions and present pursuits. This work suggests that goal pursuits may deplete individuals' subsequent capacity for effort on unrelated goal pursuits and increase their tendency to regulate their effort, at least when such effort involves self-control (Muraven & Baumeister, 2000; Muraven, Tice, & Baumeister, 1998). Muraven and Baumeister (2000), found that the amount of self-control required to eat an unappetizing vegetable (a raw radish) decreased the subsequent effort put forth for completing an anagram task (as seen in participants' decreased performance). Similarly, Muraven and colleagues (1998) found that the regulation of thoughts or emotions decreased the subsequent physical effort that participants put forth in squeezing a handgrip. These depletion effects, however, also depend on the nature of the present goal pursuit. Muraven and Slessareva (2003) found that depleted individuals who were led to believe that a current task (or their efforts) would benefit others did not demonstrate the detriments typically associated with ego depletion, suggesting that the tendency to regulate effort after a previous exertion can be overridden by the general importance of a present pursuit.

Finally, in addition to regulatory hindsight regarding how much effort has recently been expended, effort regulation may importantly involve regulatory anticipation of what is required by upcoming pursuits—especially those coming up immediately, as such goals will draw from a depleted (rather than potentially restored) capacity. In examining various aspects of Shah's (2005) *supervisory hindsight and anticipation in regulatory exertion* (SHARE) model, Shah, Brazy, and Jungbluth (2004) sought to examine whether such regulatory anticipation may meaningfully influence the effort put toward a present pursuit and whether it may do so automatically, and thus not require much effort in the process. Across five studies, Shah and colleagues found that the effort participants intended to or actually put forth for the initial goal pursuit was automatically affected by the manipulated value and difficulty of an *upcoming* goal that was primed during an initial goal pursuit, especially when the upcoming goal was imminent and when participants were relatively high in their self-reported tendency to regulate their goal-related efforts. Moreover, these changes in effort were not accompanied by changes in how participants perceived a current goal, but were found even when the upcoming goal was subliminally primed; this suggested that the anticipation of future pursuits, and subsequent adjustment of effort upward or downward, may indeed require few resources, and thus may only increase the pervasiveness with which such anticipation influences goal-related effort.

The challenge of a changing regulatory context may also lead to another type of efficiency in pursuing goals. Behaviors may be chosen with respect not only to how little effort they require, but also to how they may ease the subsequent need for effort by simultaneously addressing a variety of different goals. This regulatory versatility has been labeled *multifinality*, as it pertains to a behavior's "far-reaching" potential for addressing other relevant goals (see Shah & Kruglanski, 2000). Such versatility may, of course, vary as a function of the regulatory context in which it is assessed, as the multifinality of any behavior is more apparent with respect to those goals most salient in the moment. Moreover, the desire for multipurpose behaviors may vary with the general challenge or complexity of a regulatory context: The more goals in a given context, the greater the need for multifinal (i.e., multipurpose) means.

### Goal Maintenance: How Protective and How Persistent?

We end our chapter by considering how the structural dynamics of goals may highlight fundamental issues regarding the maintenance of goals over time. The fact that goals are pursued in a regulatory context, for instance, suggests that goal maintenance must address how each pursuit can be "protected" from the ever-present temptation of other pursuits and how each will persist in the face of difficulties or setbacks. Maintaining goals over time, then, may involve both *goal support* and *goal shielding*: "pulling up" a pursuit that has momentarily stalled, and "pushing down" attractive alternatives that may arise as contexts change. Each may play an important and perhaps distinct role in maintaining goal pursuits—a possibility considered in more detail below.

### *Goal Shielding: Protection against Other Goals*

The notion that goals may need to be defended, or shielded from other goals, is not new. Albeit with little fanfare, this assumption has been made in several models of self-regulation. Ach (1935) suggested that the activation of an intention invokes a process of selective attention that both magnifies one's focus on information pertaining to a current concern, and diminishes the salience of information pertaining to alternative pursuits (see also Kuhl & Beckmann, 1994). More recently, Shallice (1972) has suggested that action systems (or general plans) may similarly struggle for conscious supremacy, causing each system, upon activation, to inhibit the others in order to maintain conscious dominance. The general significance of such everyday challenges is highlighted by classic motivational research demonstrating that the cognitive presence of alternative goals often creates an "approach–approach" conflict that hampers progress toward any of the involved objectives (Lewin, 1935, 1951; Zeigarnik, 1927/1938).

The models described above suggest that there may be significant volitional benefit from inhibiting alternative goals. To the extent that alternative goals are accessible, they may interfere with commitment to the original goal by competing with it for limited attentional and volitional resources. We (Shah et al., 2002) have explored the role of goal inhibition in self-regulation by examining how the activation of goals may inhibit the salience of other important intentions. In five studies, we found consistent evidence of such goal shielding, particularly when individuals were highly committed to an activated goal because of its perceived importance. We (Shah et al., 2002) also found evidence to suggest that goal shielding may depend on people's emotional states, in that the inhibition of alternative goals appears to be tied to participants' levels of anxiety and depression in different ways. Whereas depression seems to hinder inter-goal inhibition, anxiety appears to strengthen it. The results of these studies also suggest that such inhibition does not occur equally for all alternatives. Rather, we found that goal activation more readily inhibits alternatives that fulfill the same regulatory need (i.e., goals that are substitutable for each other). Thus, for some individuals, the goal of playing tennis may readily inhibit the goal of jogging, because both fulfill a higher-order need to get in shape. Alternatively, goal activation less readily inhibits alternatives whose attainment is viewed as facilitating the salient focal goal. For other individuals, the goal of playing tennis may not inhibit the goal of jogging, because the latter may help them attain the former. Finally, we (Shah et al., 2002) demonstrated that goal shielding may serve important self-regulatory functions, because it has distinct consequences for how intensely goals are pursued and how likely they are to be attained. This was evidenced in participants' persistence and performance in pursuing specific task goals.

### *Goal Support: Self-Control against Immediate Obstacles and Temptations*

When Henry Ford remarked that "obstacles are those frightful things you see when you take your eyes off your goals," he anticipated the rightful focus of goal researchers on issues of self-control: the ability to successfully defend a pursuit against momentary temptations and obstacles by refocusing on the goal at hand (see Mischel, 1996). Indeed, past research suggests that goals may be strengthened in response to tempting alternatives through adjustments in their salience, value, and expectancy, as well as in the resources devoted to their pursuit.

Like goals, temptations are attractive possibilities. In the language of goals, a *temptation* may be defined as an alternative goal, the pursuit of which would (1) hinder attainment of a focal goal, and (2) provide less important (though often more psychologically immediate) rewards than would attainment of the focal goal (see Trope & Fishbach, 2000; Trope & Liberman, 2003). This definition suggests the relative nature of temptations. Whereas in one motivational context (e.g., studying for finals) a particular desired end-state may be viewed as a temptation (e.g., watching a football game), in another (e.g., relieving stress) it may not. In fact, in a third context (e.g., being entertained) it may even represent the goal itself. Despite its relative status, however, some objects by their very nature and tenuous connection to long-term pursuits may be more often perceived as temptations across a variety of different motivational settings (e.g., eating chocolate, drinking beer). The rewards for these activities are immediate and short-lived, regardless of the long-term goal one is pursuing in the moment.

Not only may goals and temptations be distinguished conceptually, but they may also be primarily linked to different forms of goal defense. Whereas goal pursuits may be defended from alternative goals through shielding, the immediacy of temptations may make inhibition harder. Instead, effective self-regulators may react to the immediate threat of temptations by strengthening their focus on the goal at hand. Trope and Fishbach (2000), for instance, have suggested that when individuals perceive short-term temptations as a threat to their long-term (if more arduous) ambitions, they may counteract the threat of the temptation to discontinue goal pursuit by increasing the perceived importance of the goal. This may be especially likely if they are generally effective self-regulators. Individuals may also respond to the threat of temptations by simply increasing the salience of the goal that the temptations would hinder. In support of this, Fishbach, Friedman, and Kruglanski (2003) found that among effective self-regulators and those committed to a goal, activation of a temptation-related construct (via priming) automatically activated constructs related to the goal that the temptation would hinder. Moreover, consistent with the notion that this association was meant to prevent engagement in the temptation, this pattern of activation was unidirectional: Goal-related constructs showed a trend toward *inhibiting* temptation-related constructs.

## FUTURE DIRECTIONS: DYNAMIC DISENGAGEMENT

Finally, the present analysis of structural change suggests that effective goal management may frequently involve disengaging from pursuits that are not proceeding quickly enough. Considerable research has suggested that this process can be difficult and different from that of goal engagement, and can have distinct antecedents and consequences (see Kuhl & Kazen-Saad, 1988; Wrosch, Scheier, Carver, & Schulz, 2003). How disengagement may differ from engagement, and how various forms of disengagement may have distinct and dynamic self-regulatory benefits and costs, are questions warranting further research.

## CONCLUSION

In detailing the qualities and potential implications of goals' dynamic regulatory context, the present analysis has sought to provide a context of a different sort: one that provides a means of more completely integrating, and more effectively building on, the fundamental principles of goals and goal pursuit that have been so compellingly demonstrated by social, cognitive, and motivational scientists. Of course, much remains to be specified regarding both the static and dynamic qualities of goal systems, such as how they vary as a function of differences in the needs that give rise to them and how changes over time may vary situationally and individually. Our modest hope, however, is that the present analysis of structural dynamics in goal systems may form the beginnings of a broader theoretical basis for understanding the complex and dynamic managerial challenges that must be effectively handled in connecting need to action and optimally regulating the self.

## REFERENCES

Aarts, H., & Dijksterhuis, A. (2000). Habits as knowledge structures: Automaticity in goal-directed behavior. *Journal of Personality and Social Psychology, 78*, 53–63.

Aarts, H., Gollwitzer, P. M., & Hassin, R. R. (2004). Goal contagion: Perceiving is for pursuing. *Journal of Personality and Social Psychology, 87*, 23–37.

Ach, N. (1935). Analyse des Willens [An analysis of the will]. In E. Abderhalden (Ed.), *Handbuch der biologischen Arbeitsmethoden* [Handbook of biology research methods] (Vol. 6, pp. 1–460). Berlin: Urban & Schwarzenberg.

Ames, C. (1992). Achievement goals and the classroom motivational climate. In D. H. Schunk & J. L. Meece (Eds.), *Student perceptions in the classroom* (pp. 327–348). Hillsdale, NJ: Erlbaum.

Austin, J. T., & Vancouver, J. B. (2001). Goal constructs

in psychology: Structure, process, and content. *Psychological Bulletin, 120*, 338–375.

Baddeley, A. D. (2003). Working memory: Looking back and looking forward. *Nature Reviews Neuroscience, 4*, 829–839.

Bandura, A. (1986). *Social foundations of thought and action: A social cognitive theory.* Englewood Cliffs, NJ: Prentice Hall.

Bandura, A. (1997). *Self-efficacy: The exercise of control.* New York: Freeman.

Bargh, J. A. (1990). Auto-motives: Preconscious determinants of social interaction. In E. T. Higgins & R. M. Sorrentino (Eds.), *Handbook of motivation and cognition: Foundations of social behavior* (Vol. 2, pp. 93–130). New York: Guilford Press.

Bargh, J. A., & Chartrand, T. L. (1999). The unbearable automaticity of being. *American Psychologist, 54*, 462–479.

Baumeister, R. F., & Vohs, K. D. (Eds.). (2004). *Handbook of self-regulation: Research, theory, and applications.* New York: Guilford Press.

Bowlby, J. (1969). *Attachment and loss: Vol. 1. Attachment.* New York: Basic Books.

Carver, C. S., & Scheier, M. F. (1998). *On the self-regulation of behavior.* New York: Cambridge University Press.

Deci, E. L., & Ryan, R. M. (2000). The "what" and "why" of goal pursuits: Human needs and the self-determination of behavior. *Psychological Inquiry, 11*, 227–268.

Dijksterhuis, A., & Bongers, K. C. (2005). Conscious thought as a trouble shooting mechanism?: The role of consciousness in goal pursuit. In E. Morsella, J. Bargh, & P. Gollwitzer (Eds.), *The psychology of action: Vol. 2. Mechanisms of human action.* New York: Oxford University Press.

Donahue, E. M., Robins, R. W., Roberts, B. W., & John, O. P. (1993). The divided self: Concurrent and longitudinal effects of psychological adjustment and social roles on self-concept differentiation. *Journal of Personality and Social Psychology, 64*, 834–846.

Dweck, C. S. (1999). *Self-theories: Their role in motivation, personality, and development.* New York: Psychology Press.

Emmons, R. A. (1986). Personal strivings: An approach to personality and subjective well-being. *Journal of Personality and Social Psychology, 51*, 1058–1068.

Emmons, R. A. (1991). Personal strivings, daily life events, and psychological and physical well-being. *Journal of Personality, 59*, 453–472.

Emmons, R. A. (1992). Abstract versus concrete goals: Personal striving level, physical illness, and psychological well-being. *Journal of Personality and Social Psychology, 62*, 292–300.

Emmons, R. A., & King, L. A. (1988). Conflict among personal strivings: Immediate and long-term implications for psychological and physical well-being. *Journal of Personality and Social Psychology, 54*, 1040–1048.

Feather, N. T (1982). Actions in relation to expected consequences: An overview of a research program. In N. T. Feather (Ed.), *Expectations and actions: Expectancy–value models in psychology* (pp. 53–95). Hillsdale, NJ: Erlbaum.

Fishbach, A., Friedman, R. S., & Kruglanski, A. W. (2003). Leading us not into temptation: Momentary allurements elicit overriding goal activation. *Journal of Personality and Social Psychology, 84*, 296–309.

Fitzsimons, G. M., & Bargh, J. A. (2003). Thinking of you: Nonconscious pursuit of interpersonal goals associated with relationship partners. *Journal of Personality and Social Psychology, 84*, 148–163.

Freud, S. (1958).The dynamics of transference. In J. Strachey (Ed. & Trans.), *The standard edition of the complete psychological works of Sigmund Freud* (Vol. 12, pp. 97–108). London: Hogarth Press. (Original work published 1912)

Freud, S. (1961). The ego and the id. In J. Strachey (Ed. & Trans.), *The standard edition of the complete psychological works of Sigmund Freud* (Vol. 19, pp. 3–66). London: Hogarth Press. (Original work published in 1923)

Glassman, N. S., & Andersen, S. M. (1999). Activating transference without consciousness: Using significant-other representations to go beyond what is subliminally given. *Journal of Personality and Social Psychology, 77*, 1146–1162.

Gollwitzer, P. M., & Brandstätter, V. (1997). Implementation intentions and effective goal pursuit. *Journal of Personality and Social Psychology, 73*, 186–199.

Gollwitzer, P. M., & Moskowitz, G. B. (1996). Goal effects on action and cognition. In E. T. Higgins & A. W. Kruglanski (Eds.), *Social psychology: Handbook of basic principles* (pp. 361–399). New York: Guilford Press.

Harackiewicz, J. M., Manderlink, G., & Sansone, C. (1992). Competence processes and achievement motivation: Implications for intrinsic motivation. In A. K. Boggiano & T. S. Pittman (Eds.), *Achievement and motivation: A social-developmental perspective* (pp. 115–137). New York: Cambridge University Press.

Higgins, E. T. (1997). Beyond pleasure and pain. *American Psychologist, 52*, 1280–1300.

Higgins, E. T. (2000). Making a good decision: Value from fit. *American Psychologist, 55*, 1217–1230.

Hockey, G. R. J. (1996). Energetical-control processes in the regulation of human performance. In W. Battmann & S. Dutke (Eds.), *Processes of the molar regulation of behavior* (pp. 271–287). Lengerich, Germany: Pabst Science.

Hyland, M. E. (1988). Motivational control theory: An integrative framework. *Journal of Personality and Social Psychology, 55*, 642–651.

Kahneman, D. (1973). *Attention and effort.* Englewood Cliffs, NJ: Prentice Hall.

Kanfer, R., Ackerman, P. L., Murtha, T. C., Dugdale, B., & Nelson, L. (1994). Goal setting, conditions of practice, and task performance: A resource allocation perspective. *Journal of Applied Psychology, 79*, 826–835.

Kelley, H. H. (1952). Two functions of reference groups. In G. E. Swanson, T. M. Newcomb, & E. L. Hartley (Eds.), *Readings in social psychology* (2nd ed., pp. 410–420). New York: Holt, Rinehart & Winston.

Klinger, E. (1977). *Meaning and void: Inner experience and the incentives in people's lives*. Minneapolis: University of Minnesota Press.

Kruglanski, A. W., Shah, J. Y., Fishbach, A., Friedman, R., Chun, W. Y., & Sleeth-Keppler, D. (2002). A theory of goal systems. In M. P. Zanna (Ed.), *Advances in experimental social psychology* (Vol. 34, pp. 331–378). San Diego, CA: Academic Press.

Kuhl, J. (1992). A theory of self-regulation: Action versus state orientation, self-discrimination, and some applications. *Applied Psychology: An International Review, 41*, 97–129.

Kuhl, J., & Beckmann, J. (1994). *Volition and personality: Action versus state orientation*. Göttingen, Germany: Hogrefe.

Kuhl, J., & Kazen-Saad, M. (1988). A motivational approach to volition: Activation and de-activation of memory representations related to uncompleted intentions. In V. Hamilton, G. H. Bower, & N. H. Frijda (Eds.), *Cognitive perspectives on emotion and motivation* (pp. 63–85). New York: Kluwer Academic/Plenum.

Lewin, K. (1935). *A dynamic theory of personality: Selected papers*. New York: McGraw-Hill.

Lewin, K. (1938). *The conceptual representation and the measurement of psychological forces*. Durham, NC: Duke University Press.

Lewin, K. (1947). *A dynamic theory of personality: Selected papers* (D. E. Adams & K. E. Zener, Trans.). New York: McGraw-Hill.

Lewin, K. (1951). *Field theory in social science: Selected theoretical papers* (D. Cartwright, Ed.). Oxford, UK: Harpers.

Lewin, K. (1966). *Principles of topological psychology* (F. Heider & G. M. Heider, Trans.). Oxford, UK: Oxford University Press.

Lewin, K., Dembo, T., Festinger, L., & Sears, P. S. (1944). Level of aspiration. In J. M. Hunt (Ed.), *Personality and the behavioral disorders* (pp. 333–371) New York: Roland Press.

Locke, E. A., & Latham, G. P. (1990). *A theory of goal setting and task performance*. Englewood Cliffs, NJ: Prentice Hall.

Locke, E. A., & Latham, G. P. (2002). Building a practically useful theory of goal setting and task motivation: A 35-year odyssey. *American Psychologist, 57*, 705–717.

Locke, E. A., Motowidlo, S. J., & Bobko, P. (1986). Using self-efficacy theory to resolve the conflict between goal-setting theory and expectancy theory in organizational behavior and industrial/organizational psychology. *Journal of Social and Clinical Psychology, 4*, 328–338.

Lockwood, P., & Kunda, Z. (2000). Outstanding role models: Do they inspire or demoralize us? In A. Tesser, R. B. Felson, & J. M. Suls (Eds.), *Psychological perspectives on self and identity* (pp. 147–171). Washington, DC: American Psychological Association.

Markus, H., & Ruvolo, A. (1989). Possible selves: Personalized representations of goals. In L. A. Pervin (Ed.), *Goal concepts in personality and social psychology* (pp. 211–241). Hillsdale, NJ: Erlbaum.

Mento, A. J., Locke, E. A., & Klein, H. J. (1992). Relationship of goal level to valence and instrumentality. *Journal of Applied Psychology, 77*, 395–405.

Mischel, W. (1996). From good intentions to willpower. In P. M. Gollwitzer & J. A. Bargh (Eds.), *The psychology of action: Linking cognition and motivation to behavior* (pp. 197–218). New York: Guilford Press.

Mukhopadhayay, A., & Johar, G. (2005). *Where there is a will, is there a way?: Effects of lay theories of self-control on setting and keeping resolutions*. Manuscript submitted for publication.

Muraven, M., & Baumeister, R. F. (2000). Self-regulation and depletion of limited resources: Does self-control resemble a muscle? *Psychological Bulletin, 126*, 247–259.

Muraven, M., & Slessareva, E. (2003). Mechanism of self-control failure: Motivation and limited resources. *Personality and Social Psychology Bulletin, 29*, 894–906.

Muraven, M., Tice, D. M., & Baumeister, R. F. (1998). Self-control as a limited resource: Regulatory depletion patterns. *Journal of Personality and Social Psychology, 74*, 774–789.

Nicholls, J. G. (1989). *The competitive ethos and democratic education*. Cambridge, MA: Harvard University Press.

Norman, D. A., & Shallice, T. (1986). Attention to action: Willed and automatic control of behavior. In J. R. Davidson, G. E. Schwartz, & D. Shapiro (Eds.), *Consciousness and self-regulation: Advances in research and theory* (Vol. 4, pp. 1–18). New York: Plenum Press.

Pervin, L. A. (1989). Goal concepts in personality and social psychology: A historical introduction. In L. A. Pervin (Ed.), *Goal concepts in personality and social psychology* (pp. 1–17). Hillsdale, NJ: Erlbaum.

Powers, W. T. (1973). Feedback: Beyond behaviorism. *Science, 179*, 351–356.

Read, S. J., & Miller, L. C. (Eds.). (1998). *Connectionist models of social reasoning and social behavior.* Mahwah, NJ: Erlbaum.

Sansone, C., & Harackiewicz, J. M. (1996). "I don't feel like it": The function of interest in self-regulation. In L. L. Martin & A. Tesser (Eds.), *Striving and feeling:*

*Interactions among goals, affect, and self-regulation* (pp. 203–228). Hillsdale, NJ: Erlbaum.

Schmeichel, B. J., & Baumeister, R. F. (2004). Self-regulatory strength. In R. F. Baumeister & K. D. Vohs (Eds.), *Handbook of self-regulation: Research, theory, and applications* (pp. 84–98). New York: Guilford Press.

Shah, J. Y. (2003). The motivational looking glass: How significant others implicitly affect goal appraisals. *Journal of Personality and Social Psychology, 85*, 424–439.

Shah, J. Y. (2005). *Get the balance right: Optimal self-regulation and the tension of goal dialectics.* Manuscript in preparation.

Shah, J.Y., Brazy, P., & Jungbluth, N. (2004). *SAVE it for later: Implicit resource regulation and the self-regulatory anticipation of volitional effort.* Manuscript submitted for publication.

Shah, J. Y., Friedman, R., & Kruglanski, A. W. (2002). Forgetting all else: On the antecedents and consequences of goal shielding. *Journal of Personality and Social Psychology, 83*, 1261–1280.

Shah, J. Y., & Kruglanski, A. W. (2000). Aspects of goal networks: Implications for self-regulation. In M. Boekaerts, P. R. Pintrich, & M. Zeidner (Eds.), *Handbook of self-regulation* (pp. 85–110). San Diego, CA: Academic Press.

Shallice, T. (1972). Dual functions of consciousness. *Psychological Review, 79*, 383–393.

Sheldon, K. M., & Kasser, T. (1995). Coherence and congruence: Two aspects of personality integration. *Journal of Personality and Social Psychology, 68*, 531–543.

Sherif, M. (1948). *An outline of psychology.* New York: Harper.

Simon, H. A. (1967). Motivational and emotional controls of cognition. *Psychological Review, 74*, 29–39.

Steele, C. M., & Liu, T. J. (1983). Dissonance processes as self-affirmation. *Journal of Personality and Social Psychology, 45*, 5–19.

Tesser, A., Martin, L. L., & Cornell, D. P. (1996). On the substitutability of self-protective mechanisms. In P. M. Gollwitzer & J. A. Bargh (Eds.), *The psychology of action: Linking cognition and motivation to behavior* (pp. 48–68). New York: Guilford Press.

Trope, Y., & Fishbach, A. (2000). Counteractive self-control in overcoming temptation. *Journal of Personality and Social Psychology, 79*, 493–506.

Trope, Y., & Liberman, N. (2003). Temporal construal. *Psychological Review, 110*, 403–421.

Vallerand, R. J., & Ratelle, C. F. (2002). Intrinsic and extrinsic motivation: A hierarchical model. In E. L. Deci & R. M. Ryan (Eds.), *Handbook of self-determination research* (pp. 37–69). Rochester, NY: University of Rochester Press.

Wood, W., Quinn, J. M., & Kashy, D. (2002). Habits in everyday life: The thought and feel of action. *Journal of Personality and Social Psychology, 83*, 1281–1297.

Wright, R. A., & Brehm, J. W. (1989). Energization and goal attractiveness. In L. A. Pervin (Ed.), *Goal concepts in personality and social psychology* (pp. 169–210). Hillsdale, NJ: Erlbaum.

Wright, R. A., Martin, R. E., & Bland, J. L. (2003). Energy resource depletion, task difficulty, and cardiovascular response to a mental arithmetic challenge. *Psychophysiology, 40*, 98–105.

Wrosch, C., Scheier, M. F., Carver, C. S., & Schulz, R. (2003). The importance of goal disengagement in adaptive self-regulation: When giving up is beneficial. *Self and Identity, 2*, 1–20.

Zeigarnik, B. (1938). On finished and unfinished tasks. In W. D. Ellis (Ed.), *A source book of Gestalt psychology* (pp. 300–314). New York: Harcourt, Brace & World. (Original work published 1927)

Zijlstra, F. R. H. (1996). Effort as energy regulation. In W. Battmann & S. Dutke (Eds.), *Processes of the molar regulation of behavior* (pp. 219–235). Lengerich, Germany: Pabst Science.

# PART III

# Motivational Processes and Differences

# MOTIVATIONAL PROCESSES AND GOAL PURSUITS

Chapter 15

# The Goal Construct in Psychology

**Andrew J. Elliot**
**James W. Fryer**

The term *goal* has long been utilized in scientific accounts of motivation. The theoretical and empirical utility of goals has been richly documented over the years, and it is difficult to envision a complete account of motivation that does not take into consideration, implicitly or explicitly, the goal-directed nature of behavior. In fact, many theorists incorporate the goal construct into their very definition of *motivation* per se. Mitchell (1982), for example, defines *motivation* as "those psychological processes that cause the arousal, direction, and persistence of voluntary actions that are goal directed" (p. 81). Likewise, Phares and Chaplin (1997) define it as "the forces within us that activate our behavior and direct it toward one goal rather than another" (p. 434; see also Beck, 1978; Ford, 1992; Kleinginna & Kleinginna, 1981; Valenstein, 1973; Young, 1961).

Given the centrality of the goal construct in motivational science, and the widespread use of different types of goal constructs in contemporary psychology, it is surprising how little the precise nature of the term *goal* has been explicitly discussed in the literature. Goals typically occupy the "ground" rather than the "figure" in motivational analyses of behavior (Kruglanski, 1996), as researchers and theorists commonly neglect to offer a definition of *goal*, even as they use it extensively throughout their work. It seems that scholars take as a given that they and their readers share the same understanding of what is meant by the term *goal*. Unfortunately, this presumption cannot possibly be accurate, because *goal* takes on many different meanings in everyday language and in the language of psychology, and researchers and theorists use the term in many different ways. Simply put, consensual agreement on the definition and use of *goal* in the psychological literature does not exist.

In this chapter we overview some of the different ways that the term *goal* is defined and conceptualized in the contemporary literature, and identify problems that this variability poses for researchers and theorists. We then proceed to examine the roots of the term in common language, and offer a history of the development of the goal construct in psychological thought. We conclude by offering a definition and conceptualization of *goal*, based on our linguistic and historical analyses. Until we offer our precise definition, we use the term *goal* in the vague, general sense of "something involved in the direction of behavior."

## THE GOAL CONSTRUCT IN THE CONTEMPORARY PSYCHOLOGICAL LITERATURE

In 1985, Heckhausen and Kuhl described *goal* as a "notoriously ill-defined term" (p. 137), and little progress has been made in this regard over the past two decades. As noted above, a technical definition of *goal* is often not provided in theoretical and empirical work, and the definitions that are provided vary considerably. Some definitions include mention of an internal representation (Caprara & Cervone, 2000); others do not (Reeve, 1992). Some definitions include a focus on the future (e.g., Kruglanski, 1996); others do not (e.g., Austin & Vancouver, 1996). Some definitions include reference to an appetitive or desired possibility (Locke & Latham, 1990); others do not (e.g., Winter, 1996). Some definitions include reference to movement as well as an object that is the focal point of the movement (e.g., Ferguson, 2000); others do not (Bandura, 1986). Some definitions include mention of commitment (e.g., Deckers, 2001); others do not (e.g., Geen, 1995). Some definitions include a reference to affect (e.g., Lewis, 1990); others do not (e.g., Ford, 1992). Finally, some definitions are quite precise and specific, referring to several of the aforementioned characteristics (e.g., Pervin, 1983); others are quite vague and general (Maehr, 1989).

Researchers and theorists not only exhibit disagreement in their technical definitions of *goal*, but they also conceptualize goals in many different ways. Some equate goals with standards for behavior (Bandura, 1986); others do not (Boldero & Francis, 2002). Some equate goals with wishes or fantasies (Ford, 1992); others do not (Gollwitzer, 1990). Some collapse goals together with needs, motives, or drives (Pervin, 1983); others do not (Brunstein, Schultheiss, & Graessman, 1998). Some contend that goals energize as well as direct behavior (Pintrich & Schunk, 1996); others do not (Kuhl, 2000). Some apply *goal* to biological set points (e.g., Austin & Vancouver, 1996) and to vegetative acts such as a heartbeat or a flower turning toward the sun (Binswanger, 1986); others do not. Some view essentially all behavior as goal-directed (Beach, 1985); others do not (e.g., Ferguson, 2000).

Clearly, there is a great deal of disagreement in the literature as to how the term *goal* is best defined and conceptualized. We think that this lack of definitional and conceptual clarity has several deleterious implications for theoretical and empirical development.

First, this lack of clarity makes it difficult to establish the core aspect(s) of the goal construct, which hinders progress in empirical research. Construct operationalization is inherently grounded in construct definition; thus ambiguity with regard to the core definitional feature(s) of *goal* will produce variability in the way that goals are operationalized in the research process. This operational variability inevitably leads to empirical variability, which produces results that are difficult to interpret, and a cumulative yield that lacks coherence and a clear "take-home message."

Second, this lack of clarity makes it difficult to establish the conceptual boundaries of the goal construct—what should and should not be included under the *goal* rubric. Problems loom in both directions. If goals are conceptualized in an extremely narrow fashion, their predictive and theoretical utility will not be fully exploited, and parsimony will be sacrificed as more constructs are utilized than are necessary to account for the phenomena under consideration. Conversely, if goals are conceptualized in an extremely broad fashion, there is a danger that the term *goal* will become so overextended that it loses any precise psychological meaning.

Third, this lack of clarity makes it difficult to determine the functional properties best attributed to the goal construct. Without a clear sense of the explanatory role of goals, it is impossible to know what additional constructs are needed to fully account for motivated behavior, and what relationship the goal construct has to other constructs that are delineated. One of two things tends to happen as a result: Either the goal construct becomes meshed with other motivational constructs such as needs or motives (thereby losing its distinct identity), or the goal construct becomes artificially isolated from other constructs (thereby yielding a fragmented or incomplete analysis of motivation).

Fourth, this lack of clarity limits cross-talk and cross-fertilization among different researchers and theorists working on the goal construct. If *goal* means different things in different disciplines or literatures, and even different things to different scholars within the same discipline or literature, there is little common ground for sharing ideas, empirical results, and applications. As such, many opportunities for facilitated progress and knowledge integration are missed.

The achievement goal approach to achievement motivation may be used to illustrate these points. Achievement goal theorists seek to account for motivated behavior in competence-relevant settings such as school, sports, and work. The achievement goal literature has been in place for over two decades, but a consensual definition of the goal construct has not yet emerged. Three distinct definitions may be identified: (1) the purpose or reason for behavior (Maehr, 1989), (2) a network or integrated pattern of variables that create an orientation toward behavior (Ames, 1992), and (3) the aim of behavior (Elliot & Thrash, 2001). As might be expected, the achievement goal manipulations and measures that are utilized in this literature vary considerably, depending on which of these definitions they are (explicitly or, often, implicitly) based on. The empirical yield is likewise variable, and this empirical inconsistency has undoubtedly contributed to several recent debates and controversies in the literature regarding the nature and implications of achievement goals (see Harackiewicz, Barron, Pintrich, Elliot, & Thrash, 2002; Harwood, Hardy, & Swain, 2000; Midgley, Kaplan, & Middleton, 2001; Treasure, Duda, Hall, Roberts, & Ames, 2001). Furthermore, the functional role of the goal construct in the achievement goal approach is not clear. Some seem to view achievement goals as analogous to achievement motives and grant them energizational properties (Pintrich & Schunk, 1996), whereas others characterize them as emerging (in part) from conceptually independent achievement motives and argue that they serve a directional role in achievement behavior (Elliot & Church, 1997). Finally, the achievement goal literature is quite fragmented across disciplines, as research efforts in social personality and educational psychology proceed quite independently of those in sport and exercise psychology, and both of the aforementioned have little integrative contact with achievement goal work in industrial organizational psychology. Incorporation of ideas from other goal literatures (e.g., goal-setting theory—Locke & Latham, 1990; goal systems theory—Kruglanski et al., 2002) is very uncommon in achievement goal research; likewise, achievement goal ideas are rarely utilized by scholars working in other literatures or disciplines. Thus, despite the fact that the achievement goal literature has made important theoretical and empirical contributions in the area of achievement motivation, a lack of definitional and conceptual clarity has hampered progress in this literature, if not actually induced stagnation (Elliot, 2005). The specific travails of the achievement goal literature may be unique, but the general notion of encountering difficulty due to definitional and conceptual ambiguity surrounding the goal construct most certainly is not (see Geen, 1995; Heckhausen & Kuhl, 1985; McClelland, Koestner, & Weinberger, 1989; Weiss, 1925).

## THE ROOTS OF THE WORD *GOAL* IN COMMON LANGUAGE

Given the absence of a clear definition and conceptualization of *goal* in the contemporary psychological literature, we turn to linguistic and historical sources of information for assistance. First, we examine the roots of the word *goal* in common language. Then, in the following section, we overview the development of the goal construct in psychological thought.

Scientific psychology in general, and the scientific study of motivation specifically, emerged in large part in German- and English-speaking countries. As such, to examine the linguistic roots of the word *goal*, it is necessary to examine the terms used for the goal construct in both the German and English languages. These terms are *Ziel* and *goal* in German and English respectively.

### *Ziel*

The word *Ziel* initially appeared as *Zil* (also *Cil*) in Old High German around the year 800, and carried the meaning "boundary/limit," "specific end," or "destination" (*Deutsches*

*Wörterbuch*, 1992; *Etymologisches Wörterbuch des Deutschen*, 1989). *Zil* was uncommon in Old High German, but it became much more frequent during the Middle High German period between approximately 1000 and 1350. For example, the 13th-century poet Wolfram von Eschenbach used *Zil* regularly in his writings (e.g., "She was far above the *Zil* [limit] of desire," "the *Zil* [end] of this adventure") (see Grimm & Grimm, 1965, p. 1055). During the New High German period, *Zil* was lengthened to *Ziel*, and the two terms were used interchangeably. *Zil* and *Ziel* continued to be used with the meaning "end" (and related meanings) intact, but a new, figurative meaning—"what one is striving for"—was also added during this period (Grimm & Grimm, 1965). This figurative use of *Ziel* can be found in Martin Luther's translation of the Bible, which appeared in the early to mid-1500s (*Deutsches Wörterbuch*, 1992).

Etymologically, *Ziel* emerged from the Germanic language Gothic. Specifically, scholars have traced the origin of *Ziel* back to the Gothic–runic word *tilarids*, which meant "striving toward the target" (Grimm & Grimm, 1965).

### *Goal*

There have been many different renderings of the word *goal* in the English language, including *gol*, *gole*, and *goale*. The word first appeared in Middle English as *gol* in Shoreham's *Poems* in 1315 and was used to denote "boundary or limit" (*Oxford English Dictionary [OED]*, 1989). This is the only occurrence of this form of the word in English literature, and it did not appear again for over 200 years. In 1531, *gole* appeared in Elyot's *The Boke Named the Governour*, and was used to denote "the terminal point of a race; any object (as a pillar, mound, etc.) by which this is marked; a winning post or the like" (*OED*, 1989, p. 632). This second definition of *goal* became common soon thereafter, appearing many times throughout the middle and late 1500s (and beyond). In the early 1600s, this second definition began to be used in a figurative sense to denote "the object to which effort or ambition is directed" (*OED*, 1989). The first occurrence of this figurative usage is in Shakespeare's (1609/1964) *Pericles*: "Then Honour be but a Goale to my Will, This day Ile rise, or else adde ill to ill" (p. 21).

The etymology of the word *goal* is not altogether clear; the *OED* characterizes it as "difficult" and "insecure." However, the available evidence suggests that the Middle English *gol* as "boundary or limit" came from the Old English *gál*, which meant "barrier or obstacle" (Barnhart, 1988). The semantic development from "barrier" to "boundary" is straightforward, as is the development from the literal "terminal point of a race" to the figurative "object to which effort or ambition is directed." The development from "boundary" to "terminal point of a race" is less direct and is likely rooted in the Latin word *mēta*.

*Mēta* initially referred to the conical columns set in the ground at each end of the Roman Circus to mark the turning place in a race (Lewis & Short, 1879), and this reference was generalized to denote "a cone-shaped turning-post at either end of a race-track" (Glare, 1973). This denotation of a turning point or endpoint was generalized further over time, yielding a second definition of *mēta*: "boundary or limit" (Glare, 1973). Scholars have noted the similarities between the different meanings of *mēta* and the different meanings of *goal*, and have suggested that the semantic development from "boundary" to "terminal point of a race" for *goal* may have been patterned after the fact that *mēta* carried the meaning of "turning point" or "endpoint" as well as "boundary" (Lewis & Short, 1879).

In sum, in both German and English, the words *Zeil* and *goal* have literal and figurative usages that are deeply rooted in their respective languages. Both usages convey similar meanings in the two languages. The literal usage carries the meaning of a specific boundary or endpoint, whereas the figurative usage carries the meaning of something striven for that directs action.

## DEVELOPMENT OF THE GOAL CONSTRUCT IN PSYCHOLOGICAL THOUGHT

Goal-relevant concepts and constructs have been present throughout the history of psychological thought. Aristotle (384–322 B.C.E.) is often regarded as the first truly psychological thinker (Leahey, 1997; R. I. Watson, 1968), and his writings make clear reference to the directional nature of behavior. For Aristotle, behavior is always purposeful, and imagined end-states are viewed as having an important influence on human action (Brett, 1912). In *The Nicomachean Ethics*, he wrote that "the origin of action . . . is choice, and that of choice is desire and reasoning with a view to an end" (Aristotle, n.d., p. 139). Aristotle used the work of a sculptor creating a statue to illustrate this notion of purpose and directedness. Standing before a block of marble, the sculptor has an idea of what is wanted at the end of the sculpting process. It is this imagined end-state that is thought to determine the way that the marble is chiseled as the sculptor produces the statue.

Friedrich Herbart (1776–1841) is commonly viewed as the first scholar to advocate for a scientific psychology (Boring, 1957; Klein, 1970). Specifically, Herbart sought to establish a scientific analysis of the mechanics of mental representations, and in so doing he made use of dynamic explanations of behavior—including, on occasion, goal-relevant explanations. For example, in his *Psychologie als Wissenschaft* (1824–1825/1850), Herbart wrote of desire as a "movement of the mind" that is directed toward a particular "object." Herbart even used the word *goal* (*Ziel*) in this context; he stated that desire "has an object to which it is directed as to its goal (*Ziel*)" (see Mischel, 1967, p. 264).

Like Herbart, other psychologically oriented philosophers utilized the notion of direction toward an object or end in their writings. Herbart's contemporary James Mill wrote of "trains of the mind" that are "directed toward an end" (1829; see Mandler & Mandler, 1964, p. 115), and Hermann Lotze wrote of the "image of intended events" in his influential *Medicinsche Psychologie oder Physiologie der Seele* (1852, p. 301). Mill's successor, Alexander Bain (1873; see also J. S. Mill, 1868), discussed voluntary action in terms of movement toward an idea or end in the future. It should be noted that neither Herbart nor the aforementioned psychological philosophers who followed made extensive or systematic use of goal-relevant constructs. Their main interest was in detailing the nature of mental activity, and goal-relevant constructs were simply utilized sporadically in the process of discussing issues regarding the will, causality, and voluntary action.

In 1879 Wilhelm Wundt established the first psychological laboratory—an event that is often considered the beginning of experimental psychology (Hothersall, 1984). Wundt focused and wrote a great deal on issues of the will and volition, albeit primarily in the middle and later part of his career. He utilized goal-relevant constructs on occasion in his writing; *end* was the term he most frequently used, but *goal* (*Ziel*) itself appeared in his writing in several instances (e.g., see *Ethics*, 1892/1914, p. 88; *Grundzüge der Physiologischen Psychologie*, 1908, p. 91). However, Wundt's work on will and volition primarily addressed issues of motives, impulses, and actions, rather than the goal construct per se; and, as in the writings of Herbart and his other predecessors, goal-relevant concepts or constructs were not discussed in a central or systematic manner in his work.

In fact, goal-relevant concepts/constructs and the term *goal* (*Ziel*) continued to be relegated to the periphery of the psychological literature throughout the latter part of the 19th century and the (very) beginning of the 20th. When goal-relevant constructs did appear, the term *end* was typically utilized, as seen in the writings of Baldwin (1894), Bradley (1901), James (1890), Kulpe (1895), and Stout (1899); other terms such as *aim* or *object* were also used on occasion in this regard. *Goal* (*Ziel*) was used only sporadically, appearing in the published version of Brentano's 1876–1894 lectures (see Mayer-Hillebrand, 1952/1973), Dewey's (1886) *Psychology*, James's (1890) landmark *The Principles of Psychology*, and other psychological books and articles (see Pfänder, 1900/1967; Muirhead, 1897; Munsterberg, 1898; Shand, 1897; Thorndike, 1905; Ziehen, 1895). It was in the work of the Würzburg school that the goal construct came to the fore in psychological theorizing, and received sustained and primary conceptual and empirical attention.

Although the Würzburg school is of foremost interest herein, the advances made by this group are best seen as emerging from earlier research and theorizing on volition by other scholars. In the latter part of the 19th century, the standard account of thought and action focused exclusively on associations between stimuli and responses (Roelofs, 2004), but the sufficiency of this strict associationism was beginning to be called into question. In his analysis of volition, Wundt (1874) posited that a person's mental preparation impacts the way the person responds to stimuli. This was empirically documented in Wundt's lab by Ludwig Lange (1888) in what has been called "the first experiment in volitional psychology" (Heckhausen, 1991, p. 22). Lange demonstrated that subjects were faster to respond to a stimulus when they were instructed to attend to their anticipated response than when they were instructed to attend to the stimulus itself. Oswald Kulpe (1891) conceptually replicated Lange's work, and proposed that the instructions provided to subjects establish a specific predisposition that has an influence on the way subjects construe and respond to the task. Müller and colleagues' (Müller & Pilzecker, 1900; Müller & Schumann, 1889) work on "motor set" and "perseverative tendencies" further highlighted the need to consider extraassociationistic principles in accounting for thought and action (Mandler & Mandler, 1964).

In their research and theorizing, members of the Würzburg school, particularly James Watt and Narziss Ach, introduced the goal construct as a way of addressing the limitations that were becoming apparent in the standard associationism. Watt, in his dissertation work (completed in 1904, published in 1905), proposed that subjects' responses in reaction time experiments can be separated into four phases: (1) a preparatory period in which the subject readies him- or herself for the presentation of the stimulus, (2) presentation of the stimulus, (3) working on the response, and (4) the response. Watt contended that the volitional act takes place in the first, preparatory phase when the task instructions are given to the subject, and the subject prepares for action accordingly. These task instructions were labeled *Aufgaben*, and *Aufgaben* were viewed as establishing an *Einstellung* ("set") to respond in a particular way. Preparation following the *Aufgabe* during the first phase was presumed to be a conscious process, but Watt believed that the influence of the *Aufgabe* during the remaining phases took place outside of consciousness.

Watt's colleague, Narziss Ach, developed an analysis of volition fundamentally similar to that of Watt, only more elaborate and detailed. Ach began his initial work in 1900 at Göttingen, and finished it in 1904 (published in 1905) at Würzburg (Boring, 1957). Despite their shared conceptual viewpoint, Ach and Watt used different terminology to portray the goal construct. Whereas Watt used the term *Aufgaben*, Ach used *Zielvorstellung*, commonly translated as "goal image." Ach also utilized the term *determining tendency* rather than the more general term *Einstellung* when making reference to the consequences of a *Zielvorstellung*. For Ach (1905), "the *Zielvorstellung* . . . results in a determination in the sense of or in accordance with the meaning of th[e] *Zielvorstellung*. These determining tendencies form the basis of those psychical phenomena whose manifestations have been traditionally subsumed under the concept of volitional activity" (p. 197). Ach viewed the determining tendency as the crucial link between the *Zielvorstellung* and the emitted response, and he viewed this tendency as operating outside of conscious awareness. In addition to his 1905 book, Ach contributed a second book in 1910 that provided an even more elaborate explication of the role of *Zielverstellung* and determining tendencies in volitional activity.

It is interesting to note a subtle but important difference in the goal constructs used by Watt and Ach. Watt's (1905) *Aufgaben* literally meant "task" or "instruction," and referred specifically to the task instructions provided by the experimenter to the subject. Although Watt clearly presumed that subjects accepted and followed these externally provided task instructions, his *Aufgaben* construct did not refer to the task instructions as internally represented by the subject. Later scholars have tended to read this meaning into the term (G. W. Allport, 1935; Bolles, 1993; Roelofs, 2004), but this meaning was not a part of the original construct (see Boring, 1957). Ach's (1905) *Zielvorstellung* (goal image), on the other hand, explicitly carried the notion of the task instructions as mentally represented by the subject. Thus, relative to Watt, Ach may be seen as taking a bolder (or at least more explicit) step away from direct stimulus–response (S-R) associationism and toward mediation by mental representation.

Watt and Ach limited their analysis and examination of the goal concept to *Aufgaben* and *Zielvorstellung* elicited from external sources such as instructions, commands, or suggestions; intrapsychic sources of goals were not considered (Rapaport, 1951). In England, William McDougall took up this issue in *An Introduction to Social Psychology* (1908), in which he laid out the foundational elements of a fundamentally goal-directed account of behavior. McDougall posited instinct as the ultimate source of all behavior, and viewed goals as operating in the service of instincts. He defined *instincts* as innate, emotionally grounded dispositions that represent the springs or energizers of all thought and action. He did not explicitly define *goal* in the first edition of *An Introduction to Social Psychology*; rather, he simply used the term in a colloquial sense on a few occasions, and relied on the term *end* (p. 239) when referring to the goal concept. However, by the printing of the eighth edition of this groundbreaking work, McDougall (1914) repeatedly used the term *goal* in a technical sense to denote "desired object" (p. 365) and "end of action" (p. 358), and he stated that the function of a goal is "to guide the course of action" (p. 359). McDougall explicitly and emphatically characterized the behavior of all organisms as "purposive" in nature, by which he meant to convey "goal-directed."

Although McDougall's technical definition of *goal* was straightforward, it should be noted that he used the term in two different ways in his writing, each of which carried a somewhat different meaning. First, McDougall used the term to refer to an inherently valued, general end-state that forms the terminal guiding point of an instinct. Each instinct contains a natural goal of this sort, and there are a limited number of natural goals (and, therefore, a limited number of instincts). Used in this sense, the goal construct is inextricably tethered to the instinct construct; it is a component of the instinct construct, rather than a separate construct in and of itself. McDougall also used the goal construct to refer to the myriad variety of ends that individuals may seek as a function of learning, experience, and self-based processes. Although these other types of goals can emerge from various sources, they are ultimately seen as subgoals or means operating in the distal service of the natural goals of the instincts. McDougall focused less on and wrote less explicitly about goals of this later type.

McDougall's work, along with that of Watt and Ach, was highly influential at the beginning of the 20th century in establishing a central role for the goal construct in accounts of thought and action. In essence, the work of these theorists put the goal construct on the psychological map. However, despite the fact that specific goal constructs were being introduced to the psychological literature and the word *goal* (*Ziel*) was being utilized more regularly, the word remained rather uncommon as the second decade of the 20th century began. This point may be illustrated by the fact that Baldwin's (1911) authoritative and ostensibly comprehensive *Dictionary of Philosophy and Psychology* did not even contain an entry for *goal*. The terms *action*, *end*, *intention*, *motivation*, *objective*, *plan*, *purpose*, *volition*, and *will* were all included, but not *goal*. *End* was clearly the entry that was designated to cover the content of the goal construct.

Alfred Adler, like McDougall, proposed a thoroughly goal-based, future-oriented portrait of behavior. From Adler's perspective, "A person would not know what to do with himself were he not oriented toward some goal. We cannot think, feel, will, or act without the perception of some goal" (Adler, 1914; see Ansbacher & Ansbacher, 1956, p. 96). The term *goal* (*Ziel*) appeared in Adler's writings as early as 1908 (Adler, 1908a, 1908b), but he did not use it in a technical, systematic sense until 1912 in his book *The Neurotic Constitution*. In this work (Adler, 1912/1926; see also Adler, 1914), Adler did not offer a definition of *goal* per se; rather, he introduced a specific form of goal construct labeled *fictional final goal* (also termed *guiding self-ideal*). This fictional final goal was characterized as the person's subjectively perceived, uniquely conceived life ambition that gives direction and meaning to life. Adler believed that all human activity reflects a desire to overcome a deep sense of inferiority by striving for domination (or, as he articulated later, for perfection, superiority, and completeness), and that this striving takes its concrete form in the individual's fictional final goal. This goal was thought to be largely outside of the person's conscious awareness, and was characterized as the internal unifying principle and guiding cause of a person's actions. In his later work, Adler (1931) added that in daily life, this ultimate goal is served by myriad other idiographic strivings. For Adler, to truly understand a person, one must know the individual's fictional final goal, which lends coherence and stability to the self and personality.

In his 1915 *Instincts and Their Vicissitudes*, Freud made use of the goal construct in laying out his first systematic conceptualization of motivation. The focal construct in this conceptualization was *instinct*, which he portrayed as an internal, biologically based "drive" or "need." Freud delineated several different aspects of the instinct construct, one of which he labeled *Ziel* (which is typically translated as "aim" in the psychoanalytic literature). *Ziel* refers to the state that the instinct aims for, which is satisfaction in the form of the (complete and immediate) elimination of stimulation. Freud distinguished between two types of *Ziel*: "ultimate" *Ziel*, which is the aforementioned satisfaction of the instinct; and "intermediate" *Ziel*, which represents alternative ways and means of acquiring satisfaction. Overall, Freud's use of the goal concept was rather abstract and did not occupy a central place in his theorizing.

With the rise of behaviorism in the second decade of the 20th century, mentalistic concepts, including goal-relevant concepts, began to be seen as outside the purview of a scientific psychology. However, Robert Woodworth, in his influential textbook *Psychology: A Study of Mental Life* (1921), argued strongly that a strict S-R psychology could not sufficiently explain behavior. Specifically, he embraced the general S-R framework, but contended that the notion of purpose must additionally be given consideration:

> What persists, in purposive behavior, is the tendency towards some end or goal. The purposeful person wants something he has not yet got, and is striving towards some future result. Whereas a stimulus pushes him from behind, a goal beckons to him from ahead. This element of action directed towards some end is absent from the simple response to a stimulus. In short, we have to find room in our stimulus–response psychology for action persistently steered in a certain direction by some cause acting from within the individual. (1921, pp. 70–71)

Following this statement, Woodworth proceeded to present a diagram that put a T (for "inner tendencies," or states that "last for a time and direct action," p. 71) in between the S-R, thereby representing a S → T → R psychology. This S → T → R framework (which others would later generalize to S → O → R, with O denoting "organism") clearly retained an important role for mentalistic concepts such as goals in a scientific psychology.

Woodworth's declaration set the stage for a purposive behaviorism, with Edward Tolman serving as prominent spokesperson. Tolman, like Woodworth, remained convinced of the need to make reference to processes intervening between stimulus and response, such as *purpose* or *goal seeking* (terms he considered synonymous; Tolman, 1925b, p. 285), to adequately describe and understand behavior. As a behaviorist, Tolman sought to account for the seemingly goal-seeking nature of behavior by relying exclusively on objective descriptions of the observable actions of the organism. Specifically, he defined *goal seeking* in terms of the "persistence until" quality of behavior: "It is this purely *objective* fact of persistence until a certain type of goal-object is reached that we define as a *goal-seeking*. And as thus defined, a goal-seeking is a wholly objective and a wholly behavioristic phenomenon. There is nothing 'mentalistic' about it" (Tolman, 1925b, p. 286).

*Goal object* was Tolman's (1925a) goal construct, and it was defined as the object or situation toward which or away from which the organism moved. Tolman was an animal psychologist, so the goal objects that he typically focused on in his research and literature reviews were things such as food that an animal would strive to obtain or confinement from which an animal would struggle to escape. Tolman posited that the strength of the demand of a particular goal object varies as a function of both the inherent positive or negative value of the goal object (e.g., bread and milk are preferred to sunflower seeds; see Simmons, 1924) and the present physiological state of the organism (e.g., increased hunger produces increased demand; see Elliott, 1929). In his classic book *Purposive Behavior in Animals and Men*, Tolman (1932) proceeded to distinguish between two different types of goal objects: an ultimate goal object and a subordinate goal object. The ultimate goal object was defined as the state of physiological quiescence or disturbance that the animal persists to attain or eliminate, and the subordinate goal object was the aforementioned type of goal object that was now conceptualized as the means of getting to or from the ultimate goal object.

In his "molar" account of behavior, Tolman (1920) declared the broad adjustments and actions of the whole organism to be the focal unit of analysis, in contrast to J. B. Watson's (1913) "molecular" account, which focused on isolated muscle movements and glandular secretions. This molar level of analysis retained a central place for the goal construct in psychology, and demonstrated that behaviorism and a consideration of goals were not necessarily incompatible.

A contemporary of Tolman, Kurt Lewin, developed an elaborate, dynamic analysis of behavior that was unabashedly mentalistic and goal-based. In his initial work, Lewin (1922) followed in the tradition of Watt and Ach in attempting to account for the effects of task instructions on subjects' responses by using extraassociationistic constructs. From this starting point, Lewin (1926, 1935) proceeded to construct an extensive theoretical account of behavior that focused on the goals toward or away from which behavior is directed, and the various motivational forces that underlie goal direction. The term *goal* (*Ziel*) was both central to and ubiquitous in Lewin's theorizing, and the term appeared in myriad forms in his writing, including *concrete goal* (Lewin, 1926), *goals of will* (Lewin, 1926), *real goal* (Lewin, 1935), *ideal goal* (Lewin, 1936), *action goal* (Lewin, Dembo, Festinger, & Sears, 1944), *dream goal* (Lewin et al., 1944), *wish goal* (Lewin et al., 1944), *verbal goal* (Lewin et al., 1944), *true goal* (Lewin et al., 1944), and *inner goal* (Lewin et al., 1944). Given the clear importance of the goal concept in Lewin's work, it is surprising that he neglected to provide a precise, technical definition of the term. Indeed, the word *goal* (*Ziel*) was not even included in the extensive glossary of psychological concepts provided at the end of the 1936 overview of his theoretical concepts entitled *Principles of Topographical Psychology*. The closest Lewin came to defining *goal* in this work was to state, "It is not usually correct to designate the material object itself as the goal. The goal is usually an action or state, for instance the eating of an apple or the possessing of an object" (p. 110). Throughout his theorizing, Lewin seemed to presume that goals were so integrally interwoven into the fabric of behavior that their nature was obvious and not in need of precise delineation.

Two primary contexts in which Lewin made use of the goal construct may be identified. First in his topographical model, Lewin conceptualized goals as the positively or negatively "valenced" activities or objects that attract or repel the person (respectively), and he portrayed them as residing within a "region" of a person's perceived psychological "life space" (Lewin, 1926, 1935). Lewin focused on the goal as represented by the person in his theorizing, and viewed goals (or goal regions) as the endpoints of a complex dynamic of situation-specific "needs," "tensions," and "forces." Second, Lewin (see Hoppe, 1930; Lewin et al., 1944) conceptualized goals in terms of the specific targets or aspirations that individuals select and strive to attain in achievement situations. The level of a person's aspiration was posited to be a function of characteristics of the task itself and stable tendencies within the person (Lewin et al., 1944). Lewin's work on both the topographical model and on aspiration behavior had a widespread and lasting influence, and his explicit championing of the goal construct clearly helped to further anchor it as an important explanatory tool in scientific psychology.

By the 1930s, the goal construct had come into its own in the psychological literature. The word *goal* was commonplace, and was used as a scientific term to describe or explain psychological phenomena. Researchers and theorists addressing diverse issues and writing from diverse perspectives made use of goal constructs in their work. For example, Hull (1931, 1932) introduced the ideas of a *goal gradient* and a *fractional anticipatory goal response* in the early stages of developing his drive-based conceptualization of behavior. Mace (1935) conducted a series of experiments explicitly designed to examine goal setting as an independent variable. F. H. Allport (1937) coined the term *teleonomic trend* to describe the individual's dynamic and enduring attempts at goal striving throughout daily life. Murray (1938) portrayed needs as inner states of tension that impel the individual to strive for a certain goal. Dollard, Miller, Doob, Mowrer, and Sears (1939) placed goals at the center of their conceptualization of frustration and aggression. It is important to note, however, that many psychologists during this time, including B. F. Skinner (1938), argued strongly against positing intervening variables focused on purpose or goal direction in the scientific study of behavior.

From the 1930s onward, most of the goal constructs utilized in psychological research and theory had conceptual precedent in the work of the pioneers overviewed in the preceding discussion. Most subsequent work focused on introducing specific variants of goal constructs or applying the goal construct to the study of various motivational issues. One additional development is particularly noteworthy, however: the emergence of a cybernetic portrait of goal-directed behavior.

The notion that the functioning of machines may be described in terms of goal-directedness had been present in psychological thought as early as Loeb's theory of tropisms (Crozier, 1929; see also Lotka, 1925). However, it was Rosenblueth, Wiener, and Bigelow (1943; see also Wiener, 1948) who firmly established this idea by describing the "behavior" of machines in terms of goals and negative feedback (i.e., discrepancy reduction) processes. A thermostat, for example, contains a target temperature (a goal) and regulates its "behavior" according to this target. That is, a thermostat operates by comparing the current temperature to the target temperature, and if a discrepancy is detected, heat is turned on until the discrepancy is eliminated. Miller, Galanter, and Pribram (1960; see also Mowrer, 1960) adapted this cybernetic analysis to human behavior. They posited that people possess representations of standards (viewed as goals) for their behavior, and that these standards are part of a cognitive mechanism that is used to regulate their behavior. This cognitive mechanism was purported to operate like a thermostat. One's current behavior is compared to one's standard, and if a discrepancy is detected, action is enacted until the discrepancy is eliminated. Miller and colleagues' cognitively based analysis of goal-directed behavior was concordant with the increasingly cognitive emphasis in psychology, whereby the need, motive, and drive constructs with which goals were often thought to be associated were omitted from consideration (Pervin, 1989).

## *GOAL* DEFINED AND CONCEPTUALIZED

Our linguistic analysis of the word *goal* (*Ziel*) has taken us back to chariot races in the Roman Circus, and our historical analysis of the goal construct has taken us back to the psychological musings of the Greek philosopher Aristotle. From these ancient roots, the term and construct "goal" appeared in many different forms and variations, but a few themes may be identified.

First, at the time that psychology emerged as a scientific discipline, a figurative use of the word *goal* (*Ziel*) was firmly in place in the German and English languages. Both languages shared a common figurative sense, which was, in essence, "something striven for that directs action." Early use of goal and goal-relevant constructs in scientific psychology followed this figurative meaning.

Second, the term *goal* (*Ziel*) was not commonly used in the psychological literature until long after the establishment of psychology as a scientific discipline. *End* was the term usually used in reference to goals, even after goals began to be examined in rigorous, programmatic research. When *goal* (*Ziel*) did emerge as a common psychological term, it was often used without provision of a technical definition, and those scholars who did provide a definition tended to do so briefly and in passing. Thus a clear and consensual definition of *goal* was not present in the early literature on goal and goal-relevant constructs.

Third, the goal construct was used in different ways by different scholars as scientific psychology developed. Thus a consensual conceptualization of *goal* was not present in the literature, either. Nevertheless, it is possible to note some basic features of *goal* that appeared, implicitly or explicitly, in many early conceptualizations: (1) It is focused on an object, (2) it is used to direct or guide behavior, (3) it is focused on the future, (4) it is internally represented (only strict behaviorists disagreed with this point), and (5) it is something that the organism is committed to approach or avoid. Given the common utilization of these characteristics of *goal* in early conceptual work, it seems wise to incorporate them into a contemporary definition of the term. Accordingly, we offer the following definition: A *goal* is a cognitive representation of a future object that the organism is committed to approach or avoid.

In the following, we offer brief commentary on each primary aspect of our definition of *goal*. This commentary is not meant to be complete or to comprehensively address the myriad metatheoretical and philosophical issues raised by any goal definition. Rather, it is meant to more clearly and explicitly articulate the goal construct implicit in our definition. Furthermore, although we take a specific stand in our commentary on many issues relevant to the goal construct, in no way do we intend to wed our goal definition to any specific model or theory of goals, self-regulation, or motivation. Rather, we intend to provide a definition and explication of the goal construct that is applicable to and may be utilized within many different models and theories.

In large part, our definitional and conceptual efforts are guided by a sense that the term *goal* has been utilized in too vague and broad (if not all-encompassing) a fashion, both in the history of psychological thought and especially in recent years. Popular psychological constructs are sometimes applied so extensively that they end up with little precise meaning and little explanatory utility (see Locke, 1969, for examples), and we are concerned that the goal construct is in danger of this fate. As such, our aim, as much as anything, is to constrain—and in so doing hone—the goal construct.

## Cognitive Representation

A goal is a cognitive representation; this means that the goal construct is restricted to animate organisms that utilize a mental apparatus in the process of regulation. Some define *goal* in terms of an internal, rather than a cognitive representation (e.g., Austin & Vancouver, 1996), thereby allowing the goal construct to be incorporated within mechanical devices (see cybernetic and some control theories in this regard). We acknowledge that standard-based discrepancy reduction in a mechanical context shares some similarities to cognitively mediated goal striving in animate organisms, but we also contend that there are important differences between these two forms of regulation (see Bandura, 1986; Locke & Latham, 1990; Nuttin, 1984). Mechanical devices, for example, rely on an extrinsically supplied and invariant energy source for operation, and therefore afford a less flexible regulatory process than that observed in intrinsically and dynamically energized animate organisms (see Nuttin, 1984). As such, we think it is best to use terms such as *standard* and *reference value* rather than *goal* in mechanical models, and to consider negative feedback processes as analogous to rather than isomorphic with goal processes (see Carver & Scheier, 1998).

An important issue in the goal literature concerns the precise way in which goals are represented within the cognitive system. Bargh (1990), Kruglanski (1996), Shah (Shah & Kruglanski, 2003), and others have recently highlighted the fact that goals, as knowledge structures, operate according to general cognitive principles, and have documented several interesting and informative implications of this point. However, goal representations are also quite distinct from other, simpler cognitive representations, in that they contain additional features such as a specific commitment with regard to an object (Ach, 1935). Little is known at present about the nature of this complex form of representation and the *unique* cognitive principles by which it might operate (for speculation, see Herbart, 1824–1825/1850; Lewin, 1926; Wyer & Srull, 1986; for recent empirical work, see Bargh, Gollwitzer, Lee-Chai, Barndollar, & Trötschel, 2001; Förster, Liberman, & Higgins, 2005, Shah, Friedman, & Kruglanski, 2002).

## Future

A goal is focused on the future; it is a cognitive representation of something that is possible in the future. Goal-directed behavior is proactive, not reactive. It entails use of a future image as a guide to present behavior; it does not simply entail an immediate, unmediated response to a present stimulus (behavior of this latter type may be considered reflex-directed rather than goal-directed). Implicit in this conceptualization is that the mental image of the future possibility has a *causal* influence on present behavior.

In contrast to several theorists (Austin & Vancouver, 1996; Binswanger, 1986; Klinger, 1977; Locke, 1969), we do not consider the actions of plant life (e.g., the sunflower turning toward the sun) or simple organisms (e.g., the amoeba moving away from light) to involve goal direction. In these cases, the organism is simply reacting reflexively to an encountered stimulus; it is not responding with regard to an envisioned possibility. Likewise, and also in contrast to the aforementioned theorists, we do not view autonomic physiological functions such as digestion or blood circulation as goal-directed, in that these functions are carried out without any prevision or imaging of the future. Plants, simple organisms, and internal organs may carry out actions that outwardly mimic goal-directed behavior, but to attribute future-focused directionality in these instances is, in our view, fallacious.

## Object

The object of a goal (i.e., the *goal object*) is the hub or focal point of regulation. We use the term *object* broadly herein to refer to an entity, event, experience, characteristic, and so on that is the centerpiece of the goal. Objects may be of an infinite variety of content, and may be concrete or abstract, physical or psychological, observable or unobservable. Furthermore, objects may be classified in terms of valence: Some entities, events, experiences, characteristics, and so on are positively valenced, whereas others are negatively valenced.

Importantly, the object of the goal is not the goal itself. A goal encompasses both an object and some sort of approach or avoidance commitment with regard to the object. For example, in the goal "Develop a deeper relationship with my wife," "a deeper relationship with my wife" is the object, and "develop" is the (appetitive) commitment. Likewise, in the goal "avoid failing my calculus class," "failing my calculus class" is the object, and "avoid" is the (aversive) commitment. Both an object and an approach/avoidance commitment are necessary, conceptually separable components of a goal. This issue has been the source of much confusion over the years; as in many dictionary definitions and psychological conceptualizations, it is unclear whether *object* is meant to refer to the hub of regulation or to the goal itself.

## Committed To

A cognitive representation of a future object that the organism would like to approach or avoid is not a goal; it is a wish or fantasy (Gollwitzer, 1990; cf. Ford, 1992), an incentive (Klinger, 1977), or a goal candidate (Elliot & Friedman, 2005). It is only when an organism commits to some directional action with respect to a cognitively represented future object that a goal may be said to have been adopted. Degree of commitment may, of course, vary considerably, both within and between goals; this variability has important implications for effort, persistence, and absorption in the goal pursuit process.

By *commit*, we mean "consciously commit." We think it is best to restrict the term *goal* to commitments that have their origin in conscious acts of volition. Once in place in the cognitive system, goals may be activated and may operate in a thoroughly automatic, nonconscious fashion, as compellingly demonstrated by Bargh and colleagues (see Bargh & Ferguson, 2000; Chartrand & Bargh, 2002). From this perspective, goals are to be differentiated from needs and motives, in that needs and motives have their origin in inherent tendencies or nonconscious affective learning processes (McClelland, 1951; Murray, 1938). In addition, the nomothetic terminal point of a need or motive, which is sometimes referred to as *goal*, would seem best labeled something like *need object*, *motive object*, *satisfier*, or *end-state*. This separation of goals from needs and motives allows the two types of constructs to operate in concert in hierarchical fashion, with needs and motives functioning as energizers of behavior, and goals directing this energization in a way that flexibly (and idiographically) serves the needs and motives (Elliot & Church, 1997). In this way, the same need or motive may prompt the use of different goals, and different needs or motives may prompt use of the same goal. Importantly, needs and motives may at times affect behavior without goal mediation (McClelland, Koestner, & Weinberger, 1989); this raises interesting, and largely overlooked, questions about the different properties of need- and motive-oriented, relative to goal-directed, behavior. Furthermore, it should be noted that there are many antecedents of goal adoption besides needs and motives (e.g., self-beliefs and perceptions, relational histories, specific environmental affordances), some of which may derive from or be associated with needs and motives, and others of which may be completely independent (see Elliot, 1999; Kuhl, 2000; Shah, 2003).

## Approach or Avoid

*Approach–avoidance* is a basic psychological distinction that is applicable to all forms of goals (Elliot & Covington, 2001). By *approach* we mean "move toward or maintain a positively valenced object," and by *avoid* we mean "move or stay away from a negatively valenced object." Approach and avoidance movement may entail actual physical activity (e.g., "Go on a date with Julie") or psychological activity (e.g., "Develop a better relationship with Julie").

As implied above, approach and avoidance take on different manifestations as a function of the current presence or absence of the goal object. If a positively valenced object is currently absent, approach entails trying to move toward the object, whereas if a positively valenced object is currently present, approach entails trying to maintain the object. In similar fashion, if a negatively valenced object is currently absent, avoidance entails trying to keep away from the object, whereas if a negatively valenced object is currently present, avoidance entails trying to get away from the object (see Lewin, 1938; Mowrer, 1960). Within each of these manifestations of approach and avoidance are myriad idiographic possibilities.

## SUMMARY STATEMENT

The goal construct is clearly integral to motivational analyses of behavior, and it is surprising how little definitional and conceptual work has been done on goals, given their prominence in the literature. Our aim in this chapter has been to highlight the need for explicit attention to this issue, and to glean insights from common language and the history of psychological thought in the process of crafting a precise definition and conceptualization of *goal*. We carry no illusions that our definition and conceptualization will please all. Any attempt to pursue precision in this arena is fraught with difficulty, as it inevitably raises many age-old metatheoretical and philosophical questions, and runs the risk of stepping on scholarly toes. Nevertheless, it is our hope that our attempt at precision will generate dialogue and thoughtful consideration about this simple yet profound psychological construct, and that the result will be a more clear and judicious use of the term *goal* in contemporary theory and research on motivation.

## ACKNOWLEDGMENTS

Preparation of this chapter was facilitated by support from the William T. Grant Foundation (Grant No. 2565) and a Friedrich Wilhelm Bessel Research Award from the Alexander von Humboldt Foundation.

## REFERENCES

Ach, N. (1905). *Über die Willenstätigkeit und das Denken* [*Willing and thinking*]. Göttingen, Germany: Vandenhoeck & Ruprecht.

Ach, N. (1910). *Über den Willensakt und das Temperament* [*Temperament and the act of willing*]. Leipzig: Quelle & Meyer.

Ach, N. (1935). *Analyse des Willens* [*The analysis of willing*]. Berlin: Urban & Schwarzenberg.

Adler, A. (1908a). Der Aggressionstrieb im Leben und in der Neurose. *Fortschritte der Medizin*, *26*, 577–584.

Adler, A. (1908b). Das Zärtlichkeitsbedürfnis des Kindes. *Monatshefte für Pädagogik und Schulpolitik*, *1*, 7–9.

Adler, A. (1914). Die Individualpsychologie, ihre Voraussetzungen und Ergebnisse [Individual psychology, its assumptions and results]. *Scientia*, *16*, 74–87.

Adler, A. (1926). *The neurotic constitution* (B. Glueck & J. Lind, Trans.). New York: Dodd, Mead. (Original work published 1912)

Adler, A. (1931). *What life should mean to you*. Boston: Little, Brown.

Allport, F. H. (1937). Teleonomic description in the study of personality. *Character and Personality*, *5*, 202–214.

Allport, G. W. (1935). Attitudes. In C. Murchison (Ed.), *A handbook of social psychology* (pp. 798–844). Worcester, MA: Clark University Press.

Ames, C. (1992). Classrooms: Goals, structures, and student motivation. *Journal of Educational Psychology*, *84*, 261–271.

Ansbacher, H. L., & Ansbacher, R. R. (Eds.). (1956). *The individual psychology of Alfred Adler*. New York: Basic Books.

Aristotle. (n.d.). *The Nicomachean ethics* (D. Ross, W. D. Ross, J. L. Ackrill, & J. O. Urmson, Trans.). Oxford, UK: Oxford University Press.

Austin, J., & Vancouver, J. (1996). Goal constructs in psychology: Structure, process, and content. *Psychological Bulletin*, *120*, 338–375.

Bain, A. (1873). *Mind and body*. New York: Appleton.

Baldwin, J. M. (1894). *Handbook of psychology*. New York: Holt.

Baldwin, J. M. (Ed.). (1911). *Dictionary of philosophy and psychology*. New York: Macmillan.

Bandura, A. (1986). *Social foundations of thought and action*. Englewood Cliffs, NJ: Prentice Hall.

Bargh, J. A. (1990). Auto-motives: Preconscious determinants of social interaction. In E. T. Higgins & R. M. Sorrentino (Eds.), *Handbook of motivation and cognition: Foundations of social behavior* (Vol. 2, pp. 93–130). New York: Guilford Press.

Bargh, J. A., & Ferguson, M. J. (2000). Beyond behaviorism: On the automaticity of higher mental processes. *Psychological Bulletin*, *126*, 925–945.

Bargh, J. A., Gollwitzer, P., Lee-Chai, A., Barndollar, K.. & Trötschel, R. (2001). The automated will: Nonconscious activation and pursuit of behavioral goals. *Journal of Personality and Social Psychology*, *81*, 1014–1027.

Barnhart, R. K. (Ed.). (1988). *The Barnhart dictionary of etymology*. New York: Wilson.

Beach, L. R. (1985). Action: Decision-implementation strategies and tactics. In M. Frese & J. Sabini (Eds.), *Goal directed behavior: The concept of action in psychology* (pp. 123–131). Hillsdale, NJ: Erlbaum.

Beck, R. C. (1978). *Motivation: Theories and principles*. Englewood Cliffs, NJ: Prentice Hall.

Binswanger, H. (1986). The goal-directedness of living action. *The Objectivist Forum*, *7*, 1–10.

Boldero, J., & Francis, J. (2002). Goals, standards, and the self: Reference values serving different functions. *Personality and Social Psychology Review*, *6*, 232–241.

Bolles, R. C. (1993). *The story of psychology: A thematic history*. Pacific Grove, CA: Brooks/Cole.

Boring, E. G. (1957). *A history of experimental psychology* (2nd ed.). New York: Appleton-Century-Crofts.

Bradley, F. H. (1901). Some remarks on conation. *Mind, 40*, 437–454.

Brett, G. S. (1912). *A history of psychology, ancient and patristic*. Oxford, UK: Allen.

Brunstein, J. C., Schultheiss, O. C., & Graessman, R. (1998). Personal goals and emotional well-being: The moderating role of motive dispositions. *Journal of Personality and Social Psychology, 75*, 494–508.

Caprara, G. V., & Cervone, D. (2000). *Personality: Determinants, dynamics, and potentials*. New York: Cambridge University Press.

Carver, C. S., & Scheier, M. F. (1998). *On the self-regulation of behavior*. New York: Cambridge University Press.

Chartrand, T. L., & Bargh, J. A. (2002). Nonconscious motivations: Their activation, operation, and consequences. In A. Tesser & D. A. Stipek (Eds.), *Self and motivation: Emerging psychological perspectives* (pp. 13–41). Washington, DC: American Psychological Association.

Crozier, W. J. (1929). The study of living organisms. In C. Murchison (Ed.), *The foundations of experimental psychology* (pp. 45–127). Worcester, MA: Clark University Press.

Deckers, L. (2001). *Motivation: Biological, psychological, and environmental*. Boston: Allyn & Bacon.

*Deutsches Wörterbuch*. (1992). Tübingen, Germany: Niemeyer.

Dewey, J. (1886). *Psychology*. New York: American Book.

Dollard, J., Miller, N. E., Doob, L. W., Mowrer, O. H., & Sears, R. R. (1939). *Frustration and aggression*. New Haven, CT: Yale University Press.

Elliot, A. J. (1999). Approach and avoidance motivation and goals. *Educational Psychologist, 34*, 169–189.

Elliot, A. J. (2005). A conceptual history of the achievement goal construct. In A. Elliot & C. Dweck (Eds.), *Handbook of competence and motivation* (pp. 52–72). New York: Guilford Press.

Elliot, A. J., & Church, M. A. (1997). A hierarchical model of approach and avoidance achievement motivation. *Journal of Personality and Social Psychology, 72*, 218–232.

Elliot, A. J., & Covington, M. V. (2001). Approach and avoidance motivation. *Educational Psychology Review, 12*, 73–92.

Elliot, A. J., & Friedman, R. (2005). Approach and avoidance personal goals. In B. Little, K. Salmela-Aro, J. Nurmi, & S. Phillips (Eds.), *Personal project pursuit: Goals, action, and human flourishing* (pp. 97–116). Mahwah, NJ: Erlbaum.

Elliot, A. J., & Thrash, T. M. (2001). Achievement goals and the hierarchical model of achievement motivation. *Educational Psychology Review, 12*, 139–156.

Elliott, M. H. (1929). The effect of change of reward on the maze performance of rats. *University of California Publications in Psychology, 4*, 19–30.

*Etymologisches Wörterbuch des Deutschen*. (1989). Berlin: Akademie-Verlag.

Ferguson, E. D. (2000). *Motivation: A biosocial and cognitive integration of motivation and emotion*. London: Oxford University Press.

Ford, M. E. (1992). *Motivating humans: Goals, emotions, and personal agency beliefs*. Thousand Oaks, CA: Sage.

Förster, J., Liberman, N., & Higgins, E. T. (2005). Accessibility from active and fulfilled goals. *Journal of Experimental Social Psychology, 41*, 220–239.

Freud, S. (1959). Instincts and their vicissitudes. In J. Riviere (Trans.), *Collected papers* (Vol. 4, pp. 60–83). New York: Basic Books. (Original work published 1915)

Geen, R. G. (1995). *Human motivation*. Belmont, CA: Brooks/Cole.

Glare, P. (Ed.). (1973). *Oxford Latin dictionary*. Oxford, UK: Clarendon Press.

Gollwitzer, P. M. (1990). Action phases and mind-sets. In E. T. Higgins & R. M. Sorrentino (Eds.), *Handbook of motivation and cognition: Foundations of social behavior* (Vol. 2, pp. 53–92). New York: Guilford Press.

Grimm, J., & Grimm, W. (1965). *Deutsches Wörterbuch*. Leipzig: Hirzel.

Harackiewicz, J. M., Barron, K. E., Pintrich, P. R., Elliot, A. J., & Thrash, T. M. (2002). Revision of achievement goal theory: Necessary and illuminating. *Journal of Educational Psychology, 94*, 638–645.

Harwood, C., Hardy, L., & Swain, A. (2000). Achievement goals in sport: A critique of conceptual and measurement issues. *Journal of Sport and Exercise Psychology, 22*, 235–255.

Heckhausen, H. (1991). *Motivation and action* (P. Leppman, Trans.). New York: Springer-Verlag.

Heckhausen, H., & Kuhl, J. (1985). From wishes to action: The dead ends and short cuts on the long way to action. In M. Frese & J. Sabini (Eds.), *Goal directed behavior: The concept of action in psychology* (pp. 134–159). Hillsdale, NJ: Erlbaum.

Herbart, J. F. (1850). Psychologie als Wissenschaft. In G. Hartenstein (Ed.), *Sämmtliche Werke* (Vol. 5, pp. 191–514). Leipzig: Voss. (Original work published 1824–1825)

Hoppe, F. (1930). Untersuchungen zur handlungs-und affektpsychologie: IV. Erfolg and Misserfolg [Studies on the psychology of action and emotion: IV. Success and failure]. *Psychologische Forschung, 14*, 1–63.

Hothersall, D. (1984). *History of psychology*. New York: Random House.

Hull, C. L. (1931). Goal attraction and directing ideas conceived as habit phenomena. *Psychological Review, 38*, 487–506.

Hull, C. L. (1932). The goal-gradient hypothesis and maze learning. *Psychological Review, 39*, 25–43.

James, W. (1890). *The principles of psychology* (2 vols.). New York: Holt.

Klein, D. B. (1970). *A history of scientific psychology: Its origins and philosophical backgrounds*. New York: Basic Books.

Kleinginna, P. R., & Kleinginna, A. M. (1981). A categorized list of motivation definitions, with a suggestion for a consensual definition. *Motivation and Emotion, 5*, 263–291.

Klinger, E. (1977). *Meaning and void: Inner experience and the incentives in people's lives.* Minneapolis: University of Minnesota Press.

Kruglanski, A. W. (1996). Goals as knowledge structures. In P. M. Gollwitzer & J. A. Bargh (Eds.), *The psychology of action: Linking cognition and motivation to behavior* (pp. 599–618). New York: Guilford Press.

Kruglanski, A. W., Shah, J. Y., Fishbach, A., Friedman, R., Chun, W. Y., & Sleeth-Keppler, D. (2002). A theory of goal systems. In M. P. Zanna (Ed.), *Advances in experimental social psychology* (Vol. 34. pp. 331–378). San Diego, CA: Academic Press.

Kuhl, J. (2000). A functional-design approach to motivation and self-regulation: The dynamics of personality systems and interactions. In M. Boekaerts & P. R. Pintrich (Eds.), *Handbook of self-regulation* (pp. 111–169). San Diego, CA: Academic Press.

Kulpe, O. (1891). Uber die Gleichzeitigkeit und Ungleichzeitigkeit von Bewegungen. *Philosophische Studien, 6*, 514–535.

Kulpe, O. (1895). *Outlines of psychology* (E. B. Titchener, Trans.). London: Sonnenschein.

Lange, L. (1888). Neue Experimente über den Vorgang der einfachen Reaction auf Sinneseindrücke [New experiments on the process of simple reaction to sensory impressions]. *Philosophische Studien, 4*, 497–510.

Leahey, T. H. (1997). *A history of psychology* (4th ed.). Upper Saddle River, NJ: Prentice Hall.

Lewin, K. (1922). Das Problem der Willensmessung und das Grundgesetz der Assoziation: I und II. *Psychologische Forschung, 1*, 191–302; *2*, 65–140.

Lewin, K. (1926). Vorsatz, wille und bedürfnis [Intention, will, and need]. *Psychologische Forschung, 7*, 330–385.

Lewin, K. (1935). *A dynamic theory of personality.* New York: McGraw-Hill.

Lewin, K. (1936). *Principles of topological psychology* (F. Heider & G. M. Heider, Trans.). New York: McGraw-Hill.

Lewin, K. (1938). *The conceptual representation and the measurement of psychological forces.* Durham, NC: Duke University Press.

Lewin, K., Dembo, T., Festinger, L., & Sears, P. S. (1944). Level of aspiration. In J. McV. Hunt (Ed.), *Personality and the behavior disorders* (Vol. 1, pp. 333–378). New York: Ronald Press.

Lewis, C., & Short, C. (Eds.). (1879). *A Latin dictionary.* Oxford, UK: Clarendon Press.

Lewis, M. (1990). The development of intentionality and the role of consciousness. *Psychological Inquiry, 1*, 231–247.

Locke, E. A. (1969). Purpose without consciousness: A contradiction. *Psychological Reports, 25*, 991–1009.

Locke, E. A., & Latham, G. P. (1990). *A theory of goal setting and task performance.* Englewood Cliffs, NJ: Prentice Hall.

Lotka, A. J. (1925). *Elements of physical biology.* Baltimore: Williams & Wilkins.

Lotze, H. (1852). *Medicinische Psychologie oder Physiologie der Seele.* Leipzig: Weidmann.

Mace, C. A. (1935). *Incentives: Some experimental studies* (Report No. 72). London: Industrial Health Residency Board.

Maehr, M. L. (1989). Thoughts about motivation. In C. Ames & R. Ames (Eds.), *Research on motivation in education: Goals and cognitions* (Vol. 3, pp. 299–315). San Diego, CA: Academic Press.

Mandler, J. M., & Mandler, G. (Eds.). (1964). *Thinking: From association to Gestalt.* New York: Wiley.

Mayer-Hillebrand, F. (1973). *The foundation and construction of ethics* (E. Schneewind, Ed. & Trans.). New York: Humanities Press. (Original work published 1952)

McClelland, D. C. (1951). *Personality.* Oxford, UK: Sloane.

McClelland, D. C., Koestner, R., & Weinberger, J. (1989). How do self-attributed and implicit motives differ? *Psychological Review, 96*, 690–702.

McDougall, W. (1908). *An introduction to social psychology.* Boston: Luce.

McDougall, W. (1914). *An introduction to social psychology* (8th ed.). Boston: Luce.

Midgley, C., Kaplan, A., & Middleton, M. (2001). Performance–approach goals: Good for what, for whom, under what circumstances, and at what cost? *Journal of Educational Psychology, 93*, 77–86.

Mill, J. (1829). *Analysis of the phenomena of the human mind.* London: Baldwin & Cradock.

Mill, J. S. (1868). *Dissertations and discussions: Political, philosophical, and historical* (Vol. 4). Boston: Spencer.

Miller, G. A., Galanter, E., & Pribram, K. H. (1960). *Plans and the structure of behavior.* New York: Holt.

Mischel, T. (1967). Affective concepts in the psychology of J. F. Herbart. *Journal of the History of the Behavioral Sciences, 3*, 262–268.

Mitchell, T. R. (1982). Motivation: New directions for theory, research, and practice. *Academy of Management Review, 7*, 80–88.

Mowrer, O. H. (1960). *Learning theory and the symbolic processes.* New York: Wiley.

Muirhead, J. H. (1897). The goal of knowledge. *Mind, 6*, 476–492.

Müller, G. E., & Pilzecker, A. (1900). *Experimentelle beiträge zur lehre vom gedächtniss* [*Experimental contributions on the theory of memory*]. Leipzig: Barth.

Müller, G. E., & Schumann, F. (1889). Uber die psychologischen Grundlagen der Vergleichung gehobener Gewichte [On the psychological foundations of the comparison of lifted weights]. *Pflügers Archiv für die Gesamte Physiologie, 45*, 37–112.

Munsterberg, H. (1898). The psychology of the will. *Psychological Review, 5*, 639–645.

Murray, H. A. (1938). *Explorations in personality.* New York: Oxford University Press.

Nuttin, J. (1984). *Motivation, planning, and action: A relational theory of behavior dynamics* (R. P. Lorion & J. E. Dumas, Trans.). Hillsdale, NJ: Erlbaum.

*Oxford English Dictionary* (*OED*) (2nd ed.). (1989). Oxford: Clarendon Press.

Pervin, L. A. (1983). The stasis and flow of behavior: Toward a theory of goals. In M. M. Page (Ed.), *Nebraska Symposium on Motivation: Vol. 30. Personality: Current theory and research* (pp. 1–53). Lincoln: University of Nebraska Press.

Pervin, L. A. (Ed.). (1989). *Goal concepts in personality and social psychology.* Hillsdale, NJ: Erlbaum.

Pfänder, A. (1967). *Phenomenology of willing and motivation and other phenomenologica* (H. Spiegelberg, Trans.). Evanston, IL: Northwestern University Press. (Original work published 1900)

Phares, J. E., & Chaplin, W. F. (1997). *Introduction to personality* (4th ed.). New York: Addison Wesley Longman.

Pintrich, P. R., & Schunk, D. H. (1996). *Motivation in education: Theory, research, and applications.* Upper Saddle River, NJ: Merrill.

Rapaport, D. (Ed.). (1951). *Organization and pathology of thought.* New York: Columbia University Press.

Reeve, J. (1992). *Understanding motivation and emotion.* Fort Worth, TX: Harcourt Brace Jovanovich.

Roelofs, A. (2004). The seduced speaker: Modeling of cognitive control. In A. Belz, R. Evans, & P. Piwek (Eds.), *Natural language generation* (pp. 1–10). Berlin: Springer-Verlag.

Rosenblueth, A., Wiener, N., & Bigelow, J. (1943). Behavior, purpose and teleology. *Philosophy of Science, 10,* 18–24.

Shah, J. Y. (2003). Automatic for the people: How representations of significant others implicitly affect goal pursuit. *Journal of Personality and Social Psychology, 84,* 661–681.

Shah, J. Y., Friedman, R., & Kruglanski, A. W. (2002). Forgetting all else: On the antecedents and consequences of goal shielding. *Journal of Personality and Social Psychology, 83,* 1261–1280.

Shah, J. Y., & Kruglanski, A. W. (2003). When opportunity knocks: Bottom-up priming of goals by means and its effects on self-regulation. *Journal of Personality and Social Psychology, 84,* 1109–1122.

Shakespeare, W. (1964). *Pericles.* London: University Microfilms Limited. (Original work published 1609)

Shand, A. F. (1897). Types of will. *Mind, 23,* 289–326.

Simmons, R. (1924). The relative effectiveness of certain incentives in animal learning. *Comparative Psychology Monographs, 2,* 1–79.

Skinner, B. F. (1938). *The behavior of organisms.* New York: Appleton-Century-Crofts.

Stout, G. F. (1899). *A manual of psychology.* London: Clive.

Thorndike, E. L. (1905). *The elements of psychology.* New York: Mason Press.

Tolman, E. C. (1920). A new formula for behaviorism. *Psychological Review, 29,* 44–53.

Tolman, E. C. (1925a). Behaviorism and purpose. *Journal of Philosophy, 22,* 36–41.

Tolman, E. C. (1925b). Purpose and cognition: The determiners of animal learning. *Psychological Review, 32,* 285–297.

Tolman, E. C. (1932). *Purposive behavior in animals and men.* London: Century.

Treasure, D. C., Duda, J. L., Hall, H. K., Roberts, G. C., & Ames, C. (2001). Clarifying misconceptions and misrepresentations in achievement goal research in sport. A response to Harwood, Hardy, and Swain. *Journal of Sport and Exercise Psychology, 23,* 317–329.

Valenstein, E. S. (Ed.). (1973). *Brain stimulation and motivation: Research and commentary.* Glenview, IL: Scott, Foresman.

Watson, J. B. (1913). Psychology as the behaviorist views it. *Psychological Review, 20,* 158–177.

Watson, R. I. (1968). *The great psychologists* (2nd ed.). Philadelphia: Lippincott.

Watt, H. J. (1905). Experimental contribution to a theory of thinking. *Journal of Anatomy and Physiology, 40,* 257–266.

Wiener, N. (1948). *Cybernetics: Control and communication in the animal and the machine.* New York: Wiley.

Weiss, A. P. (1925). Purposive striving as a fundamental category of psychology. *Psychological Review, 32,* 171–177.

Winter, D. G. (1996). *Personality: Analysis and interpretation of lives.* New York: McGraw-Hill.

Woodworth, R. S. (1921). *Psychology: A study of mental life.* New York: Holt.

Wundt, W. (1874). *Grundzüge der Physiologischen Psychologie* [*Principles of physiological psychology*] (Vols. 1–2). Leipzig: Englemann.

Wundt, W. (1908). *Grundzüge der Physiologischen Psychologie* [*Principles of physiological psychology*] (6th ed., Vol. 1). Leipzig: Englemann.

Wundt, W. (1914). The principles of morality and the departments of the moral life. In M. Washburn (Trans.), *Ethics* (3rd ed., Vol. 3). London: Allen. (Original work published 1892)

Wyer, R. S., Jr., & Srull, T. K. (1986). Human cognition in its social context. *Psychological Review, 93,* 322–359.

Young, P. T. (1961). *Motivation and emotion.* New York: Wiley.

Ziehen, T. (1895). *Introduction to physiological psychology* (C. C. Van Liew & O. W. Beyer, Trans.). New York: Macmillan.

Chapter 16

# The Impact of Social Comparisons on Motivation

**Penelope Lockwood**
**Rebecca T. Pinkus**

Traditionally, social comparison research has focused largely on the impact of better- and worse-off others on individuals' self-esteem and affect (for reviews, see Collins, 1996; Wood, 1989), rather than on the motivational consequences of such comparisons. Upward comparisons, for example, can have a positive or negative impact on one's affect and self-perceptions. One might feel pleased and proud if one has a close connection to a superior other, and can bask in the reflected glory of the other's achievements (Cialdini et al., 1976); if one's brother is a football star, and football is not a domain in which one has personal ambitions, then one may derive pleasure from one's association with the star sibling (Tesser, 1988). If, on the other hand, the comparison domain is highly self-relevant, the achievements of a close other may be distressing, highlighting one's personal inferiority. For example, finding out that a peer is outperforming one at school may have a negative impact on one's self-esteem (e.g., Lockwood & Kunda, 1999).

Downward comparisons can also have both positive and negative effects on the self. Exposure to a worse-off other can buoy one's self-image, providing evidence that one is superior to another person in a cherished domain. Such comparisons can have an especially positive impact to the extent that one has recently received a threat to the self (Wills, 1981). However, if one recognizes that one is vulnerable to the fate of the other, one may be discouraged by the prospect of a similarly dismal future (Aspinwall, Hill, & Leaf, 2002; Lockwood, 2002).

Recent evidence suggests that comparisons can influence not only affect and self-perceptions, but also individuals' motivation to change their behaviors (Aspinwall et al., 2002; Lockwood & Kunda, 2000; Markman & McMullen, 2003). Comparisons can influence motivation through the activation of *alternative selves*—representations of a self that differs in some way from one's current self (cf. Markman & McMullen, 2003). Upward comparisons can encourage one to develop a more positive future self; the superior other functions as a positive role model, providing an example of the kinds of achievements for which one can strive, and serving as a guide for how one might go about attaining such goals. For example, when Joan encounters a highly successful graduate from her program, she may be inspired; provided that she perceives the other's success to be attainable, she may picture herself achieving similar academic glory, and so decide to work harder in her studies (Lockwood & Kunda, 1997, 1999). Downward comparisons, in contrast, can activate feared selves; the unsuccessful other functions as a negative role model, providing an example of the kinds of pitfalls that may lie ahead, and illustrating the behaviors that one should avoid if one is to escape such a negative fate. For example, if John encounters someone who dropped out of his program as a result of poor grades, he may be motivated to work harder; to the extent that he perceives the other's fate to be a plausible future outcome for himself, he may be alarmed at the possibility that he might fail, and so decide to spend more time at the library (Lockwood, 2002). Social comparisons thus can serve as representations of the selves that one hopes or fears one might become in the future. Upward comparison targets can serve as positive role models, inspiring individuals to approach more positive alternative selves; downward comparison targets can serve as negative role models, motivating individuals to avoid more negative alternative selves.

## MOTIVATION ARISING FROM POSSIBLE SELVES

Considerable evidence suggests that highlighting alternative selves can motivate individuals to change their behavior. The literature on possible selves indicates that the self-concept can include a number of alternatives to one's current self, including desirable selves that one hopes to become, and undesirable selves that one fears one might become (Markus & Nurius, 1986). When a hoped-for self is activated, individuals are motivated to approach this desirable outcome. When a feared self is activated, individuals are motivated to avoid this undesirable outcome. Indeed, the presence of positive and negative achievement-related possible selves together is associated with increased persistence and success in school, suggesting that these hoped-for and feared selves do indeed affect individuals' motivation to achieve success (Oyserman, Gant, & Ager, 1995). For example, African American students who took part in an intervention that activated positive possible selves (i.e., they were encouraged to develop perceptions of themselves as successful adults) became more concerned with doing well in school, more likely to attend classes, and less likely to get into trouble (Oyserman, Terry, & Bybee, 2002).

## MOTIVATION ARISING FROM COUNTERFACTUAL SELVES

Further evidence regarding the potential for alternative selves to influence motivation comes from the literature on counterfactual thinking. Upward counterfactuals—thoughts about how a situation might have turned out better—can be demoralizing if one simply focuses on one's less optimal actual outcome. However, such thoughts can also be motivating if one believes that one may face similar situations in the future: A student who narrowly misses achieving an A on a midterm exam may experience the close counterfactual of an alternative self who achieved the better grade, and consequently may be motivated to study harder for the next test and so achieve the desirable alternative. In one study, for example, students who generated upward counterfactuals regarding a poor test score reported greater intentions to engage in activities aimed at improving their academic standing (Roese, 1994, Study 2). Similarly, students who generated upward counterfactuals regarding their performance on an anagram task showed enhanced performance, relative to those who generated downward counterfactuals, when the task was administered a second time (Roese, 1994, Study 3). The thoughts about how they might have done better on the first task served a preparative function, encouraging the participants to consider strategies for future improvement.

More recent evidence suggests that downward counterfactuals—thoughts about how a situation might have turned out worse—also have motivating potential. An individual who narrowly escapes failing a course may experience relief that a dreaded outcome did not occur. However, to the extent that he or she focuses on this negative outcome, rather than simply contrasting it with his or her current circumstances, he or she may be motivated to avert such undesirable situations in the future. In one study, for example, students who had just received a midterm grade were asked to consider a worse grade that they might have received; those students who focused on this worse grade reported greater intentions to work hard and study for future tests than did students who simply contrasted the worse grade with their actual grade, or those who did not consider a counterfactual self at all (McMullen & Markman, 2000). Thus counterfactuals involve thoughts about more positive selves that one just missed becoming or more negative selves that one just managed to avoid becoming. These alternative selves can in turn motivate individuals to pursue more desirable or avoid less desirable outcomes in the future.

## MOTIVATION ARISING FROM SOCIAL COMPARISON

To the extent that social comparison targets, like possible selves and counterfactual outcomes, represent alternatives to one's current self, they have the potential to motivate behavior change. To date, social comparison researchers have focused largely on the possible motivational effects of upward comparisons, noting that superior others can serve a self-improvement function (Taylor & Lobel, 1989; Wood, 1989). For example, couples in distressed marriages may benefit from exposure to more satisfied couples, because such examples provide them with information about how they can improve their own relationships (Buunk, Collins, Taylor, Van Yperen, & Dakof, 1990). A number of studies from the literature on social comparison and health have examined how individuals can use upward comparisons as exemplars of how to cope with physical and psychological distress associated with illness (e.g., Blalock, Afifi, DeVellis, Holt, & DeVellis, 1990; DeVellis et al., 1991; Giorgino et al., 1994; Llewellyn-Thomas, Thiel, & McGreal, 1992; Taylor, Aspinwall, Giuliano, Dakof, & Reardon, 1993; Van der Zee, Oldersma, Buunk, & Bos, 1998; Wood, Taylor, & Lichtman, 1985). However, because these studies typically focused on the self-reported impact of comparisons on ability to cope with illness, it remains unclear how such comparisons might alter individuals' motivation to change their behaviors.

Additional evidence regarding the motivating impact of upward comparisons comes from longitudinal studies assessing the effect of social comparison direction on academic performance. Blanton, Buunk, Gibbons, and Kuyper (1999) found that students who compared themselves to more successful peers were more likely to perform well in school. However, other research suggests that students in a high-achieving cohort tend to develop more negative self-perceptions over time than those who start with a similar performance level but are in a less successful cohort; those who are "small fish" in "big ponds" are faced with more demoralizing upward comparisons, and consequently have less positive academic self-concepts (Marsh & Hau, 2003; Marsh, Hau, & Craven, 2004; Marsh & Parker, 1984). These less positive self-concepts may in turn lead to diminished academic performance over time (Guay, Marsh, & Boivin, 2003). Thus, although there is some evidence that upward comparisons can be motivating, this may not always be the case. Moreover, research to date has given little attention to the motivating potential of downward comparisons. Overall, it is unclear when upward and downward comparisons will be most effective in motivating individuals to change their behavior.

## REGULATORY FOCUS DETERMINES MOTIVATION BY ROLE MODELS

In a series of studies, we have examined the degree to which both upward and downward comparisons affected individuals' intentions to work hard, and the circumstances under which each form of comparison was most influential. We have proposed that individuals should be most motivated by social comparisons when the comparisons match their regulatory orientations—the extent to which they are focused on promoting positive outcomes or preventing negative outcomes. Specifically, individuals may be most likely to be motivated by upward comparisons to targets that represent desired alternative selves when they are focused on promoting successful outcomes, and by downward comparisons to targets that represent undesirable alternative selves when they are focused on preventing unsuccessful outcomes.

These hypotheses were based on the theory of regulatory focus developed by Higgins and his colleagues (Higgins, 1997, 1998). Higgins has argued that individuals can be characterized by two forms of regulatory orientation: *promotion* or *prevention*. Promotion-focused individuals pursue a strategy aimed at achieving their ideal selves, the desirable selves that they hope to become. They are therefore especially attuned to the presence or absence of positive outcomes, and adopt a strategy aimed at pursuing gains and successes. They are especially likely to attend to and recall information involving the pursuit of success by others (Higgins & Tykocinski, 1992). In addition, their performance tends to be enhanced when task incentives are framed in terms of achieving gains rather than avoiding losses (Shah, Higgins, & Friedman, 1998). Moreover, their motivational strength in completing a task tends to be maintained more vigorously when the task is framed in terms of approaching gains (Förster, Higgins, & Idson, 1998). Promotion-focused individuals' motivation is also strongest when benefits of compliance rather than costs of noncompliance with a persuasive message are emphasized (Spiegel, Grant-Pillow, & Higgins, 2004). We therefore reasoned that individuals with strong promotion orientations should be most motivated by upward comparisons to positive role models (Lockwood, Jordan, & Kunda, 2002). Positive models highlight a strategy of pursuing a desirable end-state, illustrating the benefits of success, and thus fit with the strategic approach inclinations of promotion-focused individuals.

Prevention-focused individuals, in contrast, are especially attuned to the presence or absence of negative outcomes, and adopt a strategy aimed at avoiding losses and failures. They are especially likely to attend to and recall information pertaining to prevention of failures rather than the pursuit of success by others (Higgins & Tykocinski, 1992), and their performance tends to be enhanced when task incentives are framed in terms of avoiding losses rather than achieving gains (Shah et al., 1998). Moreover, their motivational strength in completing a task tends to be maintained more vigorously when the task is framed in terms of avoiding losses (Förster et al., 1998). Prevention-focused individuals' motivation is also strongest when costs of noncompliance rather than benefits of compliance with a persuasive message are emphasized (Spiegel et al., 2004). We therefore reasoned that individuals with strong prevention orientations should be most motivated by downward comparisons to negative role models. Negative models highlight a strategy of avoiding negative outcomes, illustrating the costs of failure, and thus fit with the strategic avoidance inclinations of prevention-focused individuals.

### Study 1: Priming Academic Strategies Determines Motivation by Role Models

In a first set of studies (Lockwood et al., 2002), we examined the degree to which individuals' regulatory orientation would determine their responses to upward and downward comparisons. Although individuals differ in their chronic regulatory focus, situational cues can also activate promotion or prevention orientations (e.g., Brendl, Higgins, & Lemm, 1995; Roney, Higgins, & Shah, 1995). We first assessed whether temporarily activated regulatory focus would determine responses to role models. In one study, participants first completed a priming task in which they described either a situation in which they had successfully promoted a positive academic outcome (promotion prime) or successfully averted a negative academic outcome (prevention prime). Participants then read about either a positive or negative role model. The positive model was a recent graduate who had achieved high grades in his or her academic program, had been accepted to the graduate or professional program of his or her choice, and had also been offered a number of prestigious jobs. The negative model was a recent graduate whose grades had become increasingly poor throughout his or her college career, who had not been accepted to the postgraduate program of his or her choice, and who was currently working in a fast food restaurant. After reading about the role model, participants completed a measure assessing their motivation to engage in activities such as studying, spending time at the library, participating in classes, and keeping up with assignments. A control group of participants completed this measure without first reading about a role model. As predicted, participants were most motivated by role models who matched their primed regulatory focus: Promotion-primed participants were motivated only by the outstanding recent graduate; prevention-primed participants were motivated only by the abysmally unsuccessful recent graduate. Thus individuals were motivated by role models who highlighted strategies that were congruent with their own regulatory goals.

### Study 2: Primed Regulatory Focus Determines Motivation by Role Models

In Study 1, we primed specific academic promotion and prevention strategies. In a second study, we attempted to replicate our findings, using a more general regulatory focus prime (Lockwood et al., 2002, Study 2). Participants were asked to sort a list of 36 words into three categories. Two categories were neutral, and involved words relating to cooking and children, respectively; the third category comprised 12 target words that were associated with either promotion (e.g., *seek*, *gain*, *pursue*) or prevention (e.g., *avert*, *avoid*, *prevent*). By exposing participants to these target words, we sought to temporarily prime their promotion or prevention orientations. After completing the sorting task, participants read about the same role models and completed the same motivation measure as in Study 1. Once again, those participants primed with promotion were motivated only by positive models, whereas those primed with prevention were motivated only by negative models.

### Study 3: Regulatory Focus Determines Choice of Role Models in Everyday Life

In Studies 1 and 2, we assessed the impact of temporarily activated regulatory strategies on the motivating effect of role models. We reasoned that individuals' chronic promotion and prevention strategies might also influence the kinds of role models that they would attend to and seize upon when attempting to maintain their motivation to achieve goals on an ongoing basis. Accordingly, we next examined whether participants' chronic regulatory orientation would influence their choice of role models in everyday life (Lockwood et al., 2002, Study 3). We predicted that promotion-focused individuals would be most likely to select positive models, and that prevention-focused individuals would be most likely to select negative models.

Participants completed an 18-item measure of regulatory orientation. Nine items assessed promotion focus (e.g., "I frequently imagine how I will achieve my hopes and aspirations"), and nine items assessed prevention focus (e.g., "I frequently think about how I can prevent failures in my life"). Then, in an ostensibly unrelated questionnaire, participants were asked to describe someone who had motivated them to work harder in the past, either by setting a positive example that they hoped to emulate or a negative example that they hoped to avoid.

Overall, participants tended to report stronger promotion than prevention orientations, and were more likely to describe being motivated by positive (73%) than by negative models. However, consistent with our predictions, results of a logistic regression analysis revealed that promotion orientation was associated with nominating positive models; prevention orientation, in contrast, was associated with nominating negative models. Thus chronic regulatory orientation appears to play a role in determining the kinds of role models that individuals seize upon to harness their motivation in everyday life: Individuals use role models who match their regulatory strategies.

## CULTURAL DIFFERENCES IN RESPONSES TO ROLE MODELS

To the extent that regulatory orientations influence motivation by role models, it seems likely that groups that differ in their focus on promotion relative to prevention will show similar patterns of responses to role models. Recent evidence suggests that cultural groups differ in their regulatory orientations (Lee, Aaker, & Gardner, 2000). Members of individualistic cultures tend to have especially strong independent self-construals. They view the self as a distinct, unique individual (for reviews, see Heine, Lehman, Markus, & Kitayama, 1999; Markus & Kitayama, 1991; Triandis, 1989). Individuals with highly independent self-construals are motivated to stand out from others by being exceptionally successful, and thus tend to focus on the personal attainments and ambitions they hope to achieve (Markus & Kitayama, 1991). Such individuals view information about personal successes as more relevant to their self-esteem than information about personal failures (Kitayama, Markus, Matsumoto, & Norasakkunkit, 1997).

This concern with personal achievement and self-enhancement appears to be associated with an emphasis on promotion strategies. North Americans, who are typically characterized by strongly independent self-construals, view events framed in terms of winning as more important than events framed in terms of losing; they also report especially strong emotional reactions to gains relative to losses (Lee et al., 2000). North Americans also tend to persist on tasks following success rather than failure experiences, indicating a focus on the pursuit of success rather than the correction of mistakes (Heine et al., 2001). Indeed, North Americans tend to report greater strivings for approach relative to avoidance goals (Elliot, Chirkov, Kim, & Sheldon, 2001). For such individuals, positive role models may be especially relevant: The successful other exemplifies the achievements for which one can strive, illustrating the strategies through which one can attain such successes. Thus positive role models highlight a strategy that may be particularly relevant to the regulatory focus of North Americans. Indeed, in Study 3 above, the North American participants in our sample were more likely to remember a positive than a negative role model.

In contrast, members of collectivistic cultures tend to have stronger interdependent self-construals, viewing the self as part of a complex web of social relationships (Heine et al., 1999; Markus & Kitayama, 1991; Triandis, 1989). Individuals with strongly interdependent selves are motivated to fit in with their social groups; they tend to focus on their obligations and duties to others, and try to avoid behaviors that could create social discord or cause distress to significant others in their lives (Heine et al., 1999). Among such individuals, special emphasis is placed on the correction of faults rather than on the achievement of successes (Heine, Takata, & Lehman, 2000).

This concern with self-criticism and personal obligations appears to be associated with an emphasis on prevention strategies. Members of East Asian cultures, who tend to have strong interdependent relative to independent self-construals, view events framed in terms of losing as more important than events framed in terms of winning (Lee et al., 2000). They tend to persist longer at a task after failure than after success, suggesting that they are motivated to avoid similar failures in the future (Heine et al., 2001). Members of East Asian cultures also report especially strong avoidance relative to approach goals (Elliot et al., 2001). For such individuals, negative role models may be particularly relevant: The unsuccessful other highlights the failures that they seek to avoid, illustrating the strategies that can be used to prevent such undesirable outcomes in the future.

In sum, to the extent that cultures differ in their emphasis on promotion or prevention, we might expect to find corresponding cross-cultural differences in responses to positive and negative role models. Specifically, members of individualistic cultures, which emphasize promotion, may be more motivated by positive than negative role models; members of collectivistic cultures, which emphasize prevention, may be more motivated by negative than positive role models.

### Study 4: Cultural Differences in Perceived Motivation by Role Models

To assess our hypotheses, we selected undergraduate participants who described their cultural background as either Western European or East Asian, and examined their beliefs about the kinds of role models that would motivate them (Lockwood, Marshall, & Sadler, 2005). All participants were residing in Canada at the time of the study. Participants completed measures assessing their self-construals (Singelis, 1994) and regulatory focus (Lockwood et al., 2002). They then rated the extent to which they would be motivated to work harder by a series of six positive and six negative academic role models. The positive models had achieved successful outcomes, such as attaining an A+ average or getting an excellent job following graduation; the negative models had experienced unsuccessful outcomes, such as being placed on academic probation due to poor grades or failing to find a job following graduation.

Results indicated that East Asian Canadians reported stronger interdependent self-construals, which were associated with stronger prevention orientations. Moreover, these stronger prevention orientations predicted motivation by negative role models. In contrast, Western European Canadians reported marginally stronger independent self-construals, which in turn tended to be associated with stronger promotion orientations; furthermore, promotion was strongly associated with greater motivation by positive models. The effects of culture on motivation by positive and negative role models were partially mediated by self-construals and regulatory focus.

### Study 5: Cultural Differences in the Impact of Role Models on Motivation

In an additional study, we examined the relation between culture and responses to role models, this time preselecting East Asians who had lived in Canada for fewer than 10 years. In addition, rather than assessing beliefs about the motivating effects of role models, we measured the impact of role models on participants' intentions to work hard.

Participants were first-year undergraduate students who described their cultural background as East Asian or Western European. Participants first read a one-page self-description, ostensibly written by a previous participant in the study. In one condition, the target described increasingly positive academic experiences, culminating in an award for academic achievement. In another condition, the target described increasingly negative academic experiences, and finished by noting that he or she had been placed on academic probation at the end of the year due to poor performance. After reading about the role model, participants rated their motivation to work hard at their own academic pursuits, using the same scale described in Study 1. Control participants rated themselves on these motivation items without first reading about a role model.

As predicted, participants were motivated only by role models who emphasized a regulatory strategy congruent with that favored by their cultural group. That is, participants from Western European backgrounds, whom we would expect to have stronger promotion orientations, were motivated only by positive models; participants from East Asian backgrounds, whom we would expect to have stronger prevention orientations, were motivated only by negative models. Role models who highlighted strategies that were incongruent with participants' culturally emphasized regulatory orientation had no impact on motivation: Western European participants were unaffected by negative models, and East Asian participants were unaffected by positive models.

Taken together, these two studies suggest that cultural differences in regulatory orientation have an impact on how individuals respond to role models. Members of cultures that emphasize independent self-construals tend to favor promotion strategies, and so are most likely to be motivated by positive models. Individuals with strong independent selves are especially concerned with promoting self-enhancement and achieving success. An outstanding role model provides an example of success, and highlights strategies needed to attain similar achievements. Members of cultures that emphasize interdependent self-construals, in contrast, tend to favor prevention strategies, and so are most likely to be motivated by negative models. Individuals with strong interdependent selves are especially concerned with preventing failure and avoiding situations that might bring shame to themselves and those close to them. A model who has experienced a failure provides an example of the situation that they are striving to avoid, and highlights strategies needed to avert such an outcome in the future.

## MOTIVATION BY ROLE MODELS ACROSS THE ADULT LIFESPAN

Although Studies 4 and 5 suggest that North Americans will typically be more motivated by positive than by negative models, we note that this tendency should be weakened or reversed in domains for which individuals have especially strong prevention concerns. For example, in the domain of health, we might expect to find age differences in regulatory orientation that in turn affect reactions to role models. Older adults tend to perceive greater stability in their development than do younger adults; they expect fewer changes in desirable and undesirable attributes (Heckhausen & Krueger, 1993), and reporting fewer hoped-for and feared selves (Cross & Markus, 1991). To the extent that they are anticipating little change in the near future, older adults may place less emphasis on approaching gains and avoiding losses than do younger adults. However, although older adults report fewer possible selves overall, they report more possible selves, and more feared selves in particular, in the domain of health than do younger adults (Cross & Markus, 1991). Thus, although older adults' general regulatory goals may be attenuated, their specific focus on avoiding health problems may be enhanced. Consequently, in health domains, older adults may have especially strong prevention orientations.

We predicted that young adults, who are generally expecting positive health outcomes and are not anticipating health problems in their near futures, would be especially promotion-oriented with respect to health, focusing on gains that they hope to pursue. Older adults, who have had more experience with health problems and have less positive expectations about their future health, should be more prevention-oriented with respect to health, focusing on losses that they hope to avoid. They may continue to hope for positive health outcomes, but this hope may be balanced by the recognition that health problems may lie ahead. Thus we expected that young adults would be especially motivated by examples of fit, healthy individuals, who highlight their strategy of pursuing health gains. In contrast, older adults would be motivated not only by examples of healthy individuals, but also by examples of individuals who are experiencing health problems as a result of their behaviors, and who thus highlight a strategy of avoiding losses.

### Study 6: The Impact of Health-Related Role Models on Young and Older Adults

To test this possibility, we examined both general and health-related regulatory focus among young (ages 18–25) and older (ages 60–75) adults (Lockwood, Chasteen, & Wong, 2005). On a general regulatory focus measure (Lockwood et al., 2002), older adults scored lower on both promotion and prevention goals than did younger adults, possibly reflecting the greater stability that older adults perceive in their lives. However, on a modified version of the regulatory focus measure consisting of six health-related promotion items (e.g., "My major health-related goal right now is to increase my level of physical fitness") and six health-related prevention items (e.g., "My major health-related goal right now is to avoid experiencing health problems"), older adults reported stronger health-related prevention orientations than did younger adults; health-related promotion orientations did not differ across the two groups.

Participants also rated the extent to which they would be motivated by a series of 12 role models: Six were positive (e.g., "a person my age who is trim and fit," "a very athletic person my age," "a person my age in excellent physical condition"), and six were negative (e.g., "a person my age in poor physical condition," "a very unathletic person my age," "a person my age who is overweight"). As expected, older adults perceived the negative models to be more motivating than did the young adults. Older and younger adults did not differ in their perceptions of the motivating impact of positive models. Moreover, the difference in motivation by negative role models among young and older adults was mediated by health-related prevention focus. This difference was independent of any perceived differences in participants' health; older adults were not simply more influenced by the negative role models because they were already experiencing poor health, and so viewed the negative model to be more relevant. Rather, older adults were more motivated by models of poor health than were younger adults because of their stronger focus on averting negative health outcomes. Thus, in any domain in which individuals are attuned to avoiding losses rather than simply focused on accruing gains, negative role models may be especially effective.

## ROLE MODEL PREFERENCES AND FIT WITH THE DESIRED BEHAVIOR CHANGE

Up to this point, we have discussed the characteristics of individuals, their regulatory strategies, and the degree to which these characteristics will determine the motivating impact of positive and negative role models. However, it is also possible that the effectiveness of role models may be determined in part by the nature of the behavior change that the role model is expected to elicit. Specifically, role models may be most motivating when they highlight a strategy that is congruent with the desired behavior change. Additive behavior changes involve starting a new activity with potentially beneficial consequences; for example, individuals may decide to join a fitness club or start an exercise program. Subtractive behavior changes involve abstaining from or cutting back on an activity with potentially injurious consequences; for example, individuals may decide to refrain from smoking or reduce their intake of high-fat foods. Individuals' receptiveness to making such additive and subtractive behavior changes may depend on the degree to which incentives for the changes are framed in promotion or prevention terms. Promotion involves a concern with avoiding errors of omission—with making sure that one engages in the activities that will lead one to a desirable end-state (Higgins, 1997). When one is faced with an incentive framed in terms of achieving gains, a promotion stimulus, one may be especially likely to engage in additive behaviors; by adopting behaviors with potentially beneficial consequences, one can increase one's likelihood of approaching the desirable end-state. Prevention involves a concern with errors of commission—averting activities that could lead to unpleasant outcomes (Higgins, 1997). When one is faced with an incentive framed in terms of avoiding losses, a prevention stimulus, one may be especially likely to engage in subtractive behaviors; by cutting back on a potentially deleterious activity, one can prevent an undesirable end-state.

Support for this possibility comes from research on counterfactual thinking, which suggests that the kinds of behaviors (additive or subtractive) that individuals select when trying to mentally undo an event are influenced by whether the event is framed in promotion or prevention terms. For example, in one study (Roese, Hur, & Pennington, 1999), when individuals were encouraged to make prevention counterfactuals about how negative situations could have been avoided, they tended to select subtractive behaviors: They mentally deleted actions that produced the unpleasant outcomes. In contrast, when individuals were encouraged to make promotion counterfactuals about how positive situations might have been achieved, they tended to select additive behaviors: They mentally adopted actions that could have produced a more desirable outcome. Thus, when situations were framed as losses that could have been avoided, the resulting counterfactuals involved subtractive behaviors, whereas when situations were framed as gains that could have been achieved, the resulting counterfactuals involved additive behaviors.

We expected to find a similar congruence between behavior changes and role model preferences. When individuals are considering engaging in an additive behavior, such as studying harder, they may be most motivated by a positive role model, such as someone who is academically successful. The positive model represents the gains that such a behavior change can lead to, and so may be most effective among individuals seeking to boost their motivation to study. When individuals are considering engaging in a subtractive behavior, such as procrastinating less or watching less TV, they may be most motivated by a negative model, such as a poorly coping student. The unfortunate other represents the losses that such undesirable behaviors can lead to, and so will likely be most effective among individuals seeking to cut back on their bad habits. Thus individuals may show a preference for models that are congruent with the behavior change that they are seeking to make: By maximizing the fit between the behavior and the strategy highlighted by the model, individuals can attempt to boost the motivation that they draw from the model. We conducted an additional set of studies to examine this possibility (Lockwood, Sadler, Fyman, & Tuck, 2004).

### Study 7: Preferences for Positive and Negative Academic Role Models

We first examined preferences for positive and negative academic role models among individuals contemplating additive and subtractive behavior changes. Introductory psychology students were asked to consider a set of six additive behaviors (e.g., develop better study habits, spend more time studying, try to get more A's) and six subtractive behaviors (e.g., spend less time partying with friends, procrastinate less, stop falling behind in readings). For each behavior, participants rated the degree to which they would be motivated by a positive relative to a negative model (e.g., "someone who is on academic probation for poor performance" vs. "someone who has won an award for academic achievement"; "someone from your program who has been unemployed since graduating last year" vs. "someone from your program who landed a great job after graduating last year"). Ratings were made on a 7-point scale ranging from –3 (greater motivation by negative model) to +3 (greater motivation by positive model). As we predicted, participants' preference for positive relative to negative models was stronger for additive ($M$ = 1.71) than for subtractive ($M$ = 0.48) behaviors.

We also considered the possibility that participants' regulatory focus would influence role model preferences. Promotion focus and additive behaviors are both associated with a strategy of accruing gains. We therefore expected that promotion would be associated with a preference for positive models, who represent such gains; moreover, we expected that this effect would be strongest for individuals considering additive behaviors. In contrast, prevention focus and subtractive behaviors are both associated with a strategy of avoiding losses. We therefore expected that prevention would be associated with a preference for negative models, who illustrate such losses, and that this effect would be strongest among individuals considering subtractive behaviors. Thus an individual's regulatory focus should be most influential in determining role model preferences when there is a good fit (Higgins, 2000) between regulatory focus and behavior type.

As expected, role model preferences among individuals considering additive behaviors were predicted by promotion but not prevention focus. Also as expected, role model preferences among individuals considering subtractive behaviors were predicted by prevention focus.

Unexpectedly, however, promotion focus also predicted role model preferences among individuals considering subtractive behaviors. It is possible that students typically consider academic activities in promotion rather than prevention terms. These first-year college students had been high achievers in high school; they may not have been accustomed to thinking about avoiding academic failure, because they may have had little past experience with such failures. Accordingly, in an additional study, we examined role model preferences in a domain in which individuals tend to have more evenhanded perceptions of possible positive and negative outcomes. Most individuals have at one time or another felt uncomfortable with their body shape and fitness levels; therefore, in this domain, individuals may have goals to prevent an unhealthy body image as well as to promote a healthy body image. We thus examined preferences for physical fitness role models (Lockwood et al., 2004, Study 2).

### Study 8: Preferences for Positive and Negative Health-Related Role Models

Participants rated the degree to which they would be motivated by a series of positive models (e.g., someone in great physical condition) versus negative models (e.g., someone in terrible shape) when considering a set of additive (e.g., joining a gym) and subtractive (e.g., cutting back on dietary fat) health-related behaviors. They also completed a measure of their health-related promotion and prevention orientations, as described in Study 6.

As in Study 7, participants considering additive behaviors ($M$ = 2.12) were more likely to select positive relative to negative models than were participants considering subtractive behaviors ($M$ = 1.09). Moreover, role model preferences among individuals considering additive health behaviors were predicted by health-related promotion but not prevention orientation; in contrast, role model preferences among individuals considering subtractive health behaviors were predicted by health-related prevention but not promotion orientation.

Taken together, these two studies suggest that the perceived effectiveness of role models is influenced by both the type of behavior change involved (additive or subtractive) and by regulatory focus (promotion or prevention). Positive role models are most likely to be perceived as effective by individuals with strong promotion orientations who are harnessing their motivation to make additive behavior changes. Negative role models are most likely to be perceived as effective by individuals with strong prevention orientations who are harnessing their motivation to make subtractive behavior changes.

## CONCLUSION

Overall, the impact of social comparisons on motivation will be influenced by the degree of fit among the direction of the comparison, an individual's regulatory focus and culture, and the nature of the behavior change involved. Upward comparisons are most likely to be motivating among individuals with strong chronic or temporarily activated promotion orientations, and among individuals from cultures that emphasize promotion concerns. Such comparisons, moreover, will be preferred by individuals who are attempting to harness their motivation to make additive behavior changes. Downward comparisons, in contrast, are most likely to be motivating among individuals with strong chronic or temporarily activated prevention orientations, and may be especially effective among individuals from cultures that emphasize prevention concerns. Such comparisons, moreover will be preferred by individuals who are attempting to boost their motivation to make subtractive behavior changes.

In this chapter we have focused on the degree to which the fit among regulatory focus, role models, and behaviors will determine motivation. We note that several other variables are also likely to moderate the impact of social comparisons on motivation. For example, Aspinwall and her colleagues have argued that individuals are likely to change their behavior in response to comparisons only when there is sufficient time available to make proactive changes (Aspinwall, 1997; Aspinwall et al., 2002). For example, if one encounters a stylish and well-dressed competitor for a job, one is only likely to attempt to improve one's own appearance if one has the opportunity to do so; encountering the elegant competitor just before one's own interview begins is likely to be stressful and demoralizing rather than motivating.

In addition, a number of researchers have noted that perceived control over the comparison dimension plays an important role in determining comparison outcomes (Buunk et al., 1990; Major, Testa, & Bylsma, 1991; Testa & Major, 1990). When individuals are faced with a more successful other, but believe they have little control over their own ability to achieve success, they are unlikely to find this comparison to be inspiring, and instead may simply be demoralized (Aspinwall, 1997). When individuals believe that they are vulnerable to the outcome experienced by a worse-off other, but believe that they have little ability to control their own fate, they may find such a comparison to be discouraging rather than motivating. For example, patients with cancer may find it distressing to encounter patients experiencing more serious symptoms if they believe that they can do little to avert a similar outcome for themselves (Wood & Van der Zee, 1997). Similarly, in our own past research, we have argued that the attainability of upward comparisons, and perceived vulnerability to downward comparisons, will be important in determining the impact of such comparisons on motivation (Lockwood, 2002; Lockwood & Kunda, 1997, 1999). If one has no hope of becoming like a more successful other, or no fear of becoming like an unsuccessful other, then one is unlikely to change one's behavior in response to a comparison. One's regulatory focus will moderate comparison effects only to the degree that the comparison target represents a plausible alternative self (Lockwood, 2002).

In the present chapter, we have discussed the motivating influence of upward and downward comparisons, rather than the effects of such comparisons on self-perceptions and affect. Nevertheless, it seems likely that these effects will often be interrelated (Markman & McMullen, 2003). An upward comparison that activates a more positive future self and so inspires one to work harder is also likely to result in a boost to one's current affect. A downward comparison that activates an undesirable future self and so frightens one into working harder is also likely to result in more negative affect. However, there may be circumstances under which affective or self-evaluative responses are not associated with any corresponding effects on motivation. For example, if individuals come to construe a superior other as similar to themselves, such comparisons may not in fact be motivating; to the extent that one is "almost as good" as a highly successful other, a comparison to the other may enhance one's self-evaluations without activating goals for self-improvement (Collins, 1996). In addition, if an upward comparison leads one to fantasize about a more positive or negative self without actually activating one's more specific achievement goals, one's behavior may be unaffected (Oettingen & Mayer, 2002). If one simply indulges in wishful thinking about future stardom in response to an upward comparison, or wallows in abject depression in response to a downward comparison, one's affect may be boosted or dampened, but one is unlikely to change one's behavior.

Indeed, individuals are most likely to be motivated by possible future selves that include self-regulatory information. For example, students whose achievement-related possible selves included information on how to achieve those selves showed greater engagement in school than did students whose achievement-related selves lacked this regulatory component (Oyserman, Bybee, Terry, & Hart-Johnson, 2004). Social comparisons are therefore most likely to lead to behavior changes when they not only activate alternative selves, but also encourage individuals to consider the means by which they can approach or avoid those selves. An individual is thus most likely to be motivated by comparisons that highlight a strategy congruent with the individual's regulatory focus; such comparisons are most likely to be relevant to the individual's regulatory goals, providing "roadmaps" (Oyserman et al., 2004) for achieving those goals.

Comparisons may also influence affect and self-esteem without a corresponding change in motivation when one views the target's identity as overlapping with one's own. For example, when one compares oneself to one's spouse or child, one may experience empathetic responses to the comparison (Beach et al., 1998; McFarland, Buehler, & MacKay, 2001) that have no implications for one's motivation. Rather than seeing the comparison other as an alternative self, one may actually view the other as part of one's own identity, and so experience the other's outcomes as one's own. One may be positively affected by a more successful close other, enjoying his or her success, and negatively affected by a less successful other, feeling sympathy for his or her failure, without being motivated to work any harder oneself. In future research, it will be important to consider more carefully the interrelationships among self-evaluations, affect, and motivation in response to social comparisons.

In this chapter, we have discussed the impact of social comparisons—comparisons to other people—on motivation to change behavior. We note that temporal comparisons—comparisons to past or future selves—may also affect motivation to change behaviors. For example, an individual struggling to become more physically fit might remind him- or herself that a few short years ago he or she was able to run 10 miles, and use this upward temporal comparison as an incentive to exercise more in the present. Comparing one's current self to a past self who experienced smoking-related health problems, a downward temporal comparison, might motivate one to maintain one's current status as a nonsmoker. Of course, more distant past selves may not be motivating; memories of one's active and healthy self at age 12 are unlikely to be perceived as relevant to one's fitness at age 40. Research on temporal comparisons has to date focused largely on the self-enhancement and self-assessment function of these comparisons (for a review, see Wilson & Ross, 2000). It will be useful to assess whether temporal comparisons can, like social comparisons, motivate behavior change.

The research described in this chapter focuses on individuals' intentions to make behavior changes. Of course, even with the best of intentions, individuals do not always make the changes that they contemplate. Nevertheless, by identifying circumstances under which motivation to change behavior is boosted, these studies take an important step toward determining how actual behaviors will be affected by social comparisons. When social comparisons activate desired or undesired future selves, they have the potential to influence not only individuals' emotions and self-perceptions, but also their goals and activities. It may be that positive and negative role models can be used on a day-to-day basis to keep alive complex and challenging goals, such as improving one's long-term health or achieving success in one's career. Such social comparisons may assist individuals in maintaining their motivation as they attempt to make ongoing behavior changes.

## REFERENCES

Aspinwall, L. (1997). Future-oriented aspects of social comparison: A framework for studying health-related comparison activity. In B. P. Buunk & F. X. Gibbons (Eds.), *Health, coping, and well-being: Perspectives from social comparison theory* (pp. 125–165). Hillsdale, NJ: Erlbaum.

Aspinwall, L. G., Hill, D. L., & Leaf, S. L. (2002). Prospects, pitfalls, and plans: A proactive perspective on social comparison activity. *European Review of Social Psychology, 12*, 267–298.

Beach, S. R. H., Tesser, A., Fincham, F. D., Jones, D. J., Johnson, D., & Whitaker, D. J. (1998). Pleasure and pain in doing well, together: An investigation of performance-related affect in close relationships. *Journal of Personality and Social Psychology, 74*, 923–938.

Blalock, S. J., Afifi, R. A., DeVellis, B. M., Holt, K., & DeVellis, R. F. (1990). Adjustment to rheumatoid arthritis. *Journal of Applied Social Psychology, 19*, 665–680.

Blanton, H., Buunk, B. P., Gibbons, F. X., & Kuyper, H. (1999). When better-than-others compare upward: Choice of comparison and comparative evaluation as independent predictors of academic performance. *Journal of Personality and Social Psychology, 76*, 420–430.

Brendl, C. M., Higgins, E. T., & Lemm, K. M. (1995). Sensitivity to varying gains and losses: The role of self-discrepancies and event framing. *Journal of Personality and Social Psychology, 69*, 1028–1051.

Buunk, B. P., Collins, R. L., Taylor, S. E., Van Yperen, N. W., & Dakof, G. A. (1990). The affective consequences of social comparison: Either direction has its ups and downs. *Journal of Personality and Social Psychology, 59*, 1238–1249.

Cialdini, R. B., Borden, R. J., Thorne, A., Walker, M. R., Freeman, S., & Sloan, L. R. (1976). Basking in reflected glory: Three (football) field studies. *Journal of Personality and Social Psychology, 34*, 366–375.

Collins, R. L. (1996). For better or worse: The impact of

upward social comparison on self-evaluation. *Psychological Bulletin, 119*, 51–69.

Cross, S., & Markus, H. (1991). Possible selves across the life span. *Human Development, 34*, 230–255.

DeVellis, R. F., Blalock, S. J., Holt, K., Renner, B. R., Blanchard, L. W., & Klotz, M. L. (1991). Arthritis patients' reactions to unavoidable social comparisons. *Personality and Social Psychology Bulletin, 17*, 392–399.

Elliot, A. J., Chirkov, V. I., Kim, Y., & Sheldon, K. M. (2001). A cross cultural analysis of avoidance (relative to approach) personal goals. *Psychological Science, 12*, 505–510.

Förster, J., Higgins, E. T., & Idson, L. C. (1998). Approach and avoidance strength during goal attainment: Regulatory focus and the "goal looms larger" effect. *Journal of Personality and Social Psychology, 75*, 1115–1131.

Giorgino, K. B., Blalock, S. J., DeVellis, R. F., DeVellis, B. M., Keefe, F. J., & Jordan, J. M. (1994). Appraisal of and coping with arthritis-related problems in household activities, leisure activities, and pain management. *Arthritis Care and Research, 7*, 20–28.

Guay, F., Marsh, H. W., & Boivin, M. (2003). Academic self-concept and academic achievement: Developmental perspectives on their causal ordering. *Journal of Educational Psychology, 95*, 124–136.

Heckhausen, J., & Krueger, J. (1993). Developmental expectations for the self and most other people: Age grading in three functions of social comparison. *Developmental Psychology, 29*, 539–548.

Heine, S. J., Kitayama, S., Lehman, D. R., Takata, T., Ide, E., Leung, C., et al. (2001). Divergent consequences of success and failure in Japan and North America: An investigation of self-improving motivation and malleable selves. *Journal of Personality and Social Psychology, 81*, 599–615.

Heine, S. J., Lehman, D. R., Markus, H. R., & Kitayama, S. (1999). Is there a universal need for positive self-regard? *Psychological Review, 106*, 766–794.

Heine, S. J., Takata, T. L., & Lehman, D. R. (2000). Beyond self-presentation: Evidence for self-criticism among Japanese. *Personality and Social Psychology Bulletin, 26*, 71–78.

Higgins, E. T. (1997). Beyond pleasure and pain. *American Psychologist, 52*, 1280–1300.

Higgins, E. T. (1998). Promotion and prevention: Regulatory focus as a motivational principle. In M. P. Zanna (Ed.), *Advances in experimental social psychology* (Vol. 30, pp. 1–46). San Diego, CA: Academic Press.

Higgins, E. T. (2000). Making a good decision: Value from fit. *American Psychologist, 55*, 1217–1230.

Higgins, E. T., & Tykocinski, O. (1992). Self-discrepancies and biographical memory: Personality and cognition at the level of psychological situation. *Personality and Social Psychology Bulletin, 18*, 527–535.

Kitayama, S., Markus, H. R., Matsumoto, H., & Norasakkunkit, V. (1997). Individual and collective processes of self-esteem management: Self-enhancement in the United States and self-depreciation in Japan. *Journal of Personality and Social Psychology, 72*, 1245–1267.

Lee, A. Y., Aaker, J. L., & Gardner, W. L. (2000). The pleasures and pains of distinct self-construal: The role of interdependence in regulatory focus. *Journal of Personality and Social Psychology, 78*, 1122–1134.

Llewellyn-Thomas, H. A., Thiel, E. C., & McGreal, M. J. (1992). Cancer patients' evaluations of their current health states: The influences of expectations, comparison, actual health status, and mood. *Medical Decision Making, 12*, 115–122.

Lockwood, P. (2002). Could it happen to you? Predicting the impact of downward comparisons on the self. *Journal of Personality and Social Psychology, 82*, 343–358.

Lockwood, P., Chasteen, A., & Wong, C. (2005). Age and regulatory focus determine preferences for health-related role models. *Psychology and Aging, 20*, 376–389.

Lockwood, P., Jordan, C. H., & Kunda, Z. (2002). Motivation by positive or negative role models: Regulatory focus determines who will best inspire us. *Journal of Personality and Social Psychology, 83*, 854–864.

Lockwood, P., & Kunda, Z. (1997). Superstars and me: Predicting the impact of role models on the self. *Journal of Personality and Social Psychology, 73*, 91–103.

Lockwood, P., & Kunda, Z. (1999). Salience of best selves undermines inspiration by outstanding role models. *Journal of Personality and Social Psychology, 76*, 214–228.

Lockwood, P., & Kunda, Z. (2000). Outstanding role models: Do they inspire or demoralize us? In A. Tesser, R. B. Felson, & J. M. Suls (Eds.), *Psychological perspectives on self and identity* (pp. 147–171). Washington, DC: American Psychological Association.

Lockwood, P., Marshall, T., & Sadler, P. (2005). Promoting success or preventing failure. Cultural differences in motivation by positive and negative role models. *Personality and Social Psychology Bulletin, 31*, 379–392.

Lockwood, P., Sadler, P., Fyman, K., & Tuck, S. (2004). To do or not to do: Using positive and negative role models to harness motivation. *Social Cognition, 22*, 422–450.

Major, B., Testa, M., & Bylsma, W. H. (1991). Responses to upward and downward social comparisons: The impact of esteem-relevance and perceived control. In J. Suls & T. A. Wills (Eds.), *Social comparison: Contemporary theory and research* (pp. 237–260). Hillsdale, NJ: Erlbaum.

Markman, K. D., & McMullen, M. N. (2003). A reflection and evaluation model of comparative thinking. *Personality and Social Psychology Review, 7*, 244–267.

Markus, H., & Nurius, P. (1986). Possible selves. *American Psychologist, 41*, 954–969.

Markus, H. R., & Kitayama, S. (1991). Culture and the self: Implications for cognition, emotion, and motivation. *Psychological Review, 98*, 224–253.

Marsh, H. W., & Hau, K. (2003). Big-fish–little-pond effect on academic self-concept: A cross-cultural (26-country) test of the negative effects of academically selective schools. *American Psychologist, 58*, 364–376.

Marsh, H. W., Hau, K., & Craven, R. (2004). The Big-fish–little-pond effect stands up to scrutiny. *American Psychologist, 59*, 269–271.

Marsh, H. W., & Parker, J. W. (1984). Determinants of student self-concept: Is it better to be a relatively large fish in a small pond even if you don't learn to swim as well? *Journal of Personality and Social Psychology, 47*, 213–231.

McFarland, C., Buehler, R., & MacKay, L. (2001). Affective responses to social comparisons with extremely close others. *Social Cognition, 19*, 547–586.

McMullen, M. N., & Markman, K. D. (2000). Downward counterfactuals and motivation: The wake-up call and the Pangloss effect. *Personality and Social Psychology Bulletin, 26*, 575–584.

Oettingen, G., & Mayer, D. (2002). The motivating function of thinking about the future: Expectations versus fantasies. *Journal of Personality and Social Psychology, 83*, 1198–1212.

Oyserman, D., Bybee, D., Terry, K., & Hart-Johnson, T. (2004). Possible selves as roadmaps. *Journal of Research in Personality, 38*, 130–149.

Oyserman, D., Gant, L., & Ager, J. (1995). A socially contextualized model of African American identity: Possible selves and school persistence. *Journal of Personality and Social Psychology, 69*, 1216–1232.

Oyserman, D., Terry, K., & Bybee, D. (2002). A possible selves intervention to enhance school involvement. *Journal of Adolescence, 25*, 313–326.

Roese, N. J. (1994). The functional basis of counterfactual thinking. *Journal of Personality and Social Psychology, 66*, 805–818.

Roese, N. J., Hur, T., & Pennington, G. L. (1999). Counterfactual thinking and regulatory focus: Implications for action versus inaction and sufficiency versus necessity. *Journal of Personality and Social Psychology, 77*, 1109–1120.

Roney, C. J. R., Higgins, E. T., & Shah, J. (1995). Goals and framing: How outcome focus influences motivation and emotion. *Personality and Social Psychology Bulletin, 21*, 1151–1160.

Shah, J., Higgins, E. T., & Friedman, R. S. (1998). Performance incentives and means: How regulatory focus influences goal attainment. *Journal of Personality and Social Psychology, 74*, 285–293.

Singelis, T. M. (1994). The measurement of independent and interdependent self-construals. *Personality and Social Psychology Bulletin, 20*, 580–591.

Spiegel, S., Grant-Pillow, H., & Higgins, E. T. (2004). How regulatory fit enhances motivational strength during goal pursuit. *European Journal of Social Psychology, 34*, 39–54.

Taylor, S. E., Aspinwall, L. G., Giuliano, T. A., Dakof, G. A., & Reardon, K. K. (1993). Storytelling and coping with stressful events. *Journal of Applied Social Psychology, 23*, 703–733.

Taylor, S. E., & Lobel, M. (1989). Social comparison activity under threat: Downward evaluation and upward contacts. *Psychological Review, 96*, 569–575.

Tesser, A. (1988). Toward a self-evaluation maintenance model of social behavior. In L. Berkowitz (Ed.), *Advances in experimental social psychology* (Vol. 21, pp. 181–227). San Diego, CA: Academic Press.

Testa, M., & Major, B. (1990). The impact of social comparisons after failure: The moderating effects of perceived control. *Basic and Applied Social Psychology, 11*, 205–218.

Triandis, H. C. (1989). The self and social behavior in differing cultural contexts. *Psychological Review, 96*, 506–520.

Van der Zee, K., Oldersma, F., Buunk, B. P., & Bos, D. (1998). Social comparison preferences among cancer patients as related to neuroticism and social comparison orientation. *Journal of Personality and Social Psychology, 75*, 801–810.

Wills, T. A. (1981). Downward comparison principles in social psychology. *Psychological Bulletin, 90*, 245–271.

Wilson, A. E., & Ross, M. (2000). The frequency of temporal-self and social comparisons in people's personal appraisals. *Journal of Personality and Social Psychology, 78*, 928–942.

Wood, J. V. (1989). Theory and research concerning social comparisons of personal attributes. *Psychological Bulletin, 106*, 231–248.

Wood, J. V., Taylor, S. E., & Lichtman, R. R. (1985). Social comparison in adjustment to breast cancer. *Journal of Personality and Social Psychology, 49*, 1169–1183.

Wood, J. V., & Van der Zee, K. (1997). Social comparisons among cancer patients: Under what conditions are comparisons upward and downward? In B. P. Buunk & F. X. Gibbons (Eds.), *Health, coping, and well-being: Perspectives from social comparison theory* (pp. 299–328). Mahwah, NJ: Erlbaum.

Chapter 17

# Goal Contagion

## INFERRING GOALS FROM OTHERS' ACTIONS—AND WHAT IT LEADS TO

**Henk Aarts**
**Ap Dijksterhuis**
**Giel Dik**

As social beings, humans attribute goals to other people's behaviors. Thinking about behaviors in terms of the goals they serve allows an understanding of how the same behaviors, conducted in different circumstances, may serve divergent intentions. Think, for example, about being offered a beer by a colleague in the hotel bar after a long sitting at a conference dinner table. Such an offer may serve the goal of collaborating, socializing, or seeking casual sex. For social animals like ourselves, it is important to know what *caused* the agent's behavior, and which one of the end-states the colleague views as *desired*. Importantly, in some circumstances answers to both questions—that is, what causes the behavior, and what are its desired states or outcomes—are based on an understanding of an agent's goals (e.g., Heider, 1958; Meltzoff & Moore, 1996). Comprehending the other's goals may prevent mistakes that could be embarrassing or even harmful.

Furthermore, perceiving other people's behavior in terms of goals may have important implications for one's own behavior. For instance, it has been argued that humans and great apes can use others' goals to represent, organize, and guide their own courses of goal-directed actions (Byrne & Russon, 1998; Tomasello, Kruger, & Ratner, 1993). Specifically, an appreciation of the goals motivating other people allows one to entertain similar goals and to try to attain them oneself. Knowing, for example, that someone's goal is to seek collaboration or casual sex may cause one to adopt these goals readily, provided that collaboration with others or seeking casual sex is a desired goal for oneself. Inferring these goals as potential causes of behavior, then, is important not only for a direct understanding of the intentions of people we interact with, but also for the successful pursuit of one's own needs and goals.

In this chapter we present a framework for the comprehension and examination of goal pursuit resulting from the perception of other people's actions. Specifically, we aim to advance the idea that individuals are capable of taking on the goals implied by other people's actions without conscious intent. The framework consists of two key components. First, we propose that people can automatically infer other people's goals from behavioral information. Second, we posit that these inferred goals can be automatically acted on by the perceivers. Thus we suggest that the perception of goal-implying behaviors may facilitate the perceivers' own achievement of the implied goals without the need for conscious assistance—an instance we have recently labeled *goal contagion* (Aarts, Gollwitzer, & Hassin, 2004; Aarts & Hassin, 2005).

Our framework builds on two major developments in social psychology research over the last 20 years or so. The first is rooted in the observation that people often go beyond the behavioral information given automatically, and recognizes that under certain circumstances, social (causal) inferences occur without conscious intent (e.g., Gilbert, 1989; Hassin, Bargh, & Uleman, 2002; Uleman, Newman, & Moskowitz, 1996). Such an ability allows a deeper understanding of the social world without the costs that are associated with conscious processes. The other development is the diversion from the traditional views that goal setting and adoption are accompanied by a conscious decision, and that goal striving (i.e., the initiation and maintenance of goal-directed action) is characterized by conscious intent (e.g., Ajzen, 1991; Bandura, 1986; Deci & Ryan, 1985; Locke & Latham, 1990). Instead, it has been proposed that the mere activation of representations of goals can also cause behavior directly, and that motivated social behavior can operate outside of conscious awareness (e.g., Aarts & Dijksterhuis, 2000; Bargh, 1990; Moskowitz, Li, & Kirk, 2004; see also Chartrand, Dalton, & Cheng, Chapter 22, this volume; Ferguson, Hassin, & Bargh, Chapter 10, this volume).

Remarkably, in these last two decades, these two developments have led relatively separate lives. Accordingly, the questions of whether, and if so how, social (goal) inferences affect behavior have hitherto received little theoretical analysis and empirical attention. The present chapter contributes to closing this gap and provides a perspective within which the automatic emergence of needs, desires, and goals in the presence of others in everyday life can be understood. We now turn to a review of research (partly based on our own recent work) that has addressed and empirically examined the issue of automatic social inferences, particularly automatic goal inferences, and their direct motivational implications for social behavior.

## AUTOMATIC SOCIAL INFERENCES

Originally, automatic processes were thought of as unintentional, nonconscious, ballistic, and effortless. This monolithic approach, however, gave way to a more flexible view, according to which these characteristics do not always co-occur, and some automatic processes may exhibit only a subset of them (e.g., Bargh, 1994; Gilbert, 1989). A large body of social psychological research on the automaticity of social inferences has examined a specific collection of these features—namely, *spontaneity.* An inference is said to be spontaneous if (1) it does not require explicit instructions, (2) people are unaware of their intentions to make it, and (3) people are usually unaware of the inference itself. Basically, this means that inferences can occur without conscious intent (Uleman, 1999).

### Trait Inferences

The empirical work on spontaneous inferences has mainly focused on examining trait inferences. Uleman and his colleagues (e.g., Uleman et al., 1996; Winter & Uleman, 1984) have convincingly argued and showed that trait inferences may sometimes be spontaneous. Thus, upon reading the sentence "While dancing the salsa, Jackson slapped his girlfriend in the face," readers may spontaneously infer the trait *clumsy.* These inferences do not require a conscious impression formation goal: They occur when participants are instructed to memorize sentences, as well as when they are just asked to familiarize themselves with them or to judge how interesting they are. Recently, it has been demonstrated that spontaneous trait inferences are linked in memory to the actor (Todorov & Uleman, 2002; Van Overwalle, Drenth, & Marsman, 1999), suggesting that, in line with Gilbert and his colleagues' model (e.g., Gilbert, Pelham, & Krull, 1988), dispositional attributions can occur automatically as well (e.g., readers of the sentence above automatically conclude that Jackson is a clumsy person).

### Causal Inferences

Lately it has been suggested that various types of spontaneous inferences described in the literature fit under the same conceptual umbrella, that of *automatic causal inferences* (the ACI framework—Hassin et al., 2002; see also Hassin, Aarts, & Ferguson, 2005). That is, spontaneous inferences of traits (Winter & Uleman, 1984), and predictable events (McKoon & Ratcliff, 1986) can be conceived of as instances of causal inferences—the former in terms of possible *reasons* for behavior, and the latter in terms of its expected *results*.

An interesting implication of the ACI framework suggested by Hassin and colleagues is that people should be able to automatically infer other social constructs that are perceived as serving a prominent role in the causal chain of behaviors. One such type of construct is that of *goals*: the representations of desired states that people aim to attain. The ability to infer goals offers an important extension to the understanding of others in terms of their traits, because unlike traits—which are relatively stable characteristics—goals are more flexible and context-dependent. As such, goals may help us understand why a person performs a variety of behaviors that may be less explicable in terms of traits (e.g., when we see someone running after a cab with a suitcase in his or her hand, it is usually not because the person is athletic).

It should be noted, though, that work on dispositional attribution of behavior suggests that goal and trait inferences can be interrelated. Specifically, contemporary stage models of attribution propose that trait inferences are usually preceded by a stage involving identification or categorization of the observed behavior (e.g., Gilbert et al., 1988; Trope, 1986). This stage is required to make sense of, and to assign meaning to, the perceived body movements that people orchestrate and exhibit in a given context or environment. This stage of information processing is so obvious that we usually forget that we do it. In their analysis of behavior identification, Jones and Davis (1965) emphasized that action is often identified by making an inference about another person's intention. Others have argued that humans have a natural tendency to represent and perceive overt behaviors in terms of the goals they serve (e.g., Heider, 1958; Vallacher & Wegner, 1987). Because observable action is often identified by ascribing goals or intentions to it, the behavioral categorization stage often involves making goal inferences. Thus, to the extent that the causes inferred from another's behavior (e.g., running after a cab) pertain to the accomplishment of desired states or outcomes (e.g., wanting to be on time), exposure to such behavior may induce the individual to categorize it in terms of the goal or motive causing the action (McClure, 2002).[1]

Furthermore, trait inferences (e.g., the individual running after the cab is a punctual person) sometimes require behaviors to be identified in terms of goals or motives. Accordingly, goal inferences can precede (and can be necessary for) the emergence of trait inferences. In line with this reasoning is work demonstrating that the extent to which a behavior is rated as typical of a certain trait is strongly predicted by its relatedness to the goal associated with that trait (Read, Jones, & Miller, 1990; Read & Miller, 1989). As Read and colleagues (1990) suggest, "inferring the goal for which an individual is striving is a central part of the trait inference process" (p. 1056). In short, goal inferences ("What is the person trying to do?") seem to occur first when dispositional trait inferences ("What is the person like?") cannot be drawn directly. Important for the present argument is the idea that when goals are perceived as causes for behavior, people should be able to infer them automatically.

## AUTOMATIC GOAL INFERENCES

Classic social theories on consciousness propose that conscious awareness or intent allows social animals to understand each other's goals through insight in the motivational causes of each other's behaviors (see e.g., Humphrey, 1978). Although conscious intent may aid the comprehension of goal-directed behavior, it may not be a prerequisite to encoding others' goals. The idea that social animals naturally and automatically infer the goals that guide others' behaviors has interested researchers in several areas in psychology. In general, two areas of research have empirically focused on the question whether goal inferences can occur automatically: (1) research on animated movements of physical objects, which conceives of goal inferences as a perceptual process, and examines the attribution of mental states to moving objects by adults, babies, and even chimps; and (2) research on text comprehension, which attests to the occurrence of goal inferences in making sense of other people's actions expressed through language.

## Animated Movements and Automatic Goal Inferences

### *Research on Adults*

One of the first demonstrations of the emergence of goal inferences is Heider and Simmel's (1944) animated movie study on causality and social perception. In a nutshell, Heider and Simmel showed that adults readily attribute mental properties (such as goals) to geometric shapes, as long as they move in a particular interactive or "social" way. As an illustrative sample of the movie, participants saw a scene in which a small triangle and a small ball left a rectangle by opening a door, but were directly and hastily followed by a larger triangle that was also inside that rectangle. When participants were asked to report their thoughts as to what they believed the larger triangle was trying to do, they came up with answers such as "He wants to separate the small triangle from the ball" or "He chases the small triangle and ball"—answers that clearly referred to goal-directedness and specific social aims. These findings point to the human tendency to perceive functional properties in simple displays that are found objectively in neither the actual events themselves nor one's retinal projections (see also Michotte, 1963).

For a long time, Heider and Simmel's work enjoyed an anecdotal status, and their evidence for goal inferences was mostly taken for granted. Fortunately, subsequent studies conducted by other research groups replicated their findings with a wide range of different stimuli and movements, which corroborated the notion that people uncover the causal and social structures of the world by inferring properties such as agency, intentionality, desires, or goals (for overviews, see Kassin, 1982; Scholl & Tremoulet, 2000). Most of the research in this area seems to assume that goal inferences occur immediately and effortlessly, and that goal inferences are default responses of our human mental system. However, it should be noted that participants in these kinds of studies are usually *explicitly* asked to think in terms of goals, to reflect retrospectively on the observed movements, or to provide goal ratings. Evidence gathered in these studies is thus not conclusive with regard to the automaticity of goal inference upon exposure to animated movements of physical objects.

### *Research on Babies and Chimps*

Stronger evidence that pertains to the automaticity of goal inferences comes from studies on the ability of very young infants and chimpanzees to encode animated movements of physical objects in terms of goals (Csibra, Gergely, Biro, Koos, & Brockbank, 1999; Gergely, Nadasdy, Csibra, & Biro, 1995; Hauser, 1999; Premack, 1990; Uller & Nichols, 2000). For example, some research suggests that babies use different aspects of biological motion, such as self-propelled movement, to assign a sense of agency to inanimate objects (Premack, 1990; Premack & Premack, 1997).

Furthermore, babies seem to employ principles of rationality at a very young age to infer desires or goals from animated movements of objects. For instance, in one study (Csibra et al., 1999), 6- and 9-month-old babies were habituated to a computerized scene in which a ball "tried to meet" another ball. Since the balls were separated by a barrier, one of the balls "jumped" over it in order to meet the other ball. In the subsequent test phase, the babies were shown one of two scenarios in which there was no barrier. In one such scenario, the ball, in its "attempt to meet" the other ball, still "jumped" over the now nonexistent barrier; in the other scenario, the ball simply moved in a straight line. Despite the fact that the motion in the second condition was novel, and that babies generally look longer at novel events, the 9-month-olds looked longer at the first event than at the second (this was not the case with the 6-month-olds). The results from a control group showed that the effects with the 9-month-olds were attributable neither to novelty per se, nor to the illogical nature of jumping over a nonexistent barrier. The data suggest that these very young children used an efficiency principle in understanding the intention of the moving object. In other words, they perceived the ball's behavior as goal-oriented—it simply "wanted" to meet the other ball—and the babies somehow realized that it did not make sense to accomplish this by jumping over a barrier that did not exist. Similar findings have been reported for chimpanzees.

These findings are interpreted as indicating that primates, humans included, have an early-developed system for ascribing unobservable mental states to an agent (a desire or goal to produce a state) on the basis of contextual information of actions or movements performed by this agent (see Frith & Frith, 2003, for a possible neuroscientific account of this system). More importantly, they suggest that goal inferences can occur in the absence of fully developed capacity for higher cognitive reasoning and processing, and hence in the absence of full-blown human conscious processes (Gergely, 1994; MacPhail, 1998; Zeman, 2001). Thus they support the suggestion that goal inferences, at least under certain circumstances, may be automatic.

## Text Comprehension and Automatic Goal Inferences

Goal inferences have also been extensively studied in research on text comprehension. Most researchers in this field consider the understanding of protagonists' goals as central to narrative comprehension. Accordingly, the consensus seems to be that readers make goal-relevant inferences when they are actively trying to understand information about scripted behavior (e.g., Graesser, Singer, & Trabasso, 1994; McClure, 2002; McKoon & Ratcliff, 1992; Trabasso & van den Broek, 1985). However, for many text comprehension researchers, the distinction between automatic and controlled inferences is less important than that between online and offline inferences—that is, inferences that occur during initial comprehension of text or after it, respectively. There are a few exceptions, though.

In proposing their *logic of the minimalist* hypothesis, McKoon and Ratcliff (e.g., 1992) suggest that under certain circumstances goal inferences may occur automatically. Specifically, they posit that inferences automatically emerge during reading to the extent that they are necessary for local coherence (e.g., understanding the connection between two successive sentences in a text) or can be based on easily available general knowledge (e.g., typical or clear inferences). To date, however, they have not examined the full implication of their theory.

Furthermore, Long and Golding (1993; see also Long, Golding, & Graesser, 1992) examined the automaticity of online inferences of goals. In their study, participants were asked to read a short story including all kind of actions that could be identified in terms of superordinate goals or subordinate goals (the "why" and "how" of the action, respectively; cf. the action identification framework proposed by Vallacher & Wegner, 1987). For example, participants read a story about "the Czar and his daughters" that included sentences such as "One day the daughters went walking in the woods" (superordinate goal of *exercising* and subordinate goal of *strolling*) and "A dragon kidnapped the three daughters" (superordinate goal of *eating* and subordinate goal of *grasping*). A lexical decision task was used to assess the accessibility of these two types of goals to determine which inference participants made from each action while trying to comprehend the story. They showed that superordinate goal words were more accessible than subordinate goal words, suggesting that goals were indeed automatically inferred from the text. Several concerns, however, cast doubt on the conclusiveness of these studies. Critically, the researchers did not examine whether these processes met various criteria for automaticity (i.e., they did not check whether subjects intended to infer goals and whether they were aware of such inferences).

To further explore this issue in a more systematic way, Hassin and colleagues (2005) conducted a series of studies that included offline as well as online measurement for the examination of automatic goal inferences. In a first study, they used a surprise cued-recall paradigm to demonstrate offline inferences. Participants read short pilot-tested sentences under instructions to rate "how interesting they are." The sentences described a behavior performed to attain a specific goal (e.g., "The student is cycling to the campus as fast as he can" implied the goal of attending a lecture), or a similar behavior that did not imply this goal (e.g., "The student is cycling away from the campus as fast as he can"). After completing a filler task for 5 minutes, they were presented with a surprise cued-recall task for the sentences. The cues were either the implied goals (goal cue condition) or a word taken from the sentences (repetition cue condition). Results showed that only goal cues (and not repetition cues) helped in retrieving goal-implying sentences more than control sentences, even though the two types of sentences shared all the words that were semantically related to the cue. In a second study, goal cues facilitated the retrieval of goal-implying sentences even when the road to successful achievement of the goal was blocked and the expected goal attainment thus should not have occurred (e.g., the front tire of the bicycle went flat because of a stray nail), suggesting that goals are inferred from actions even when they do not predict future events (cf. the concept of *predictive inferences*; McKoon & Ratcliff, 1986, 1992).

The inferences obtained in the surprise cued-recall paradigm result from retrieval processes, and thus tell us something about the long-term representations of inferred goals. However, do people rely on these representations to infer goals during perception of actions? That is, do goal inferences also occur automatically online, at encoding? In two further studies, Hassin and colleagues (2005, Studies 3 and 4) examined this issue by employing a probe recognition task and a lexical decision task. As in the previous studies, participants read goal-implying sentences and control sentences within a very short amount of time, and each sentence was immediately followed by the goal word. To disguise the critical trials, the goal-implying and control trials (i.e., sentence and corresponding goal word) were embedded in a large number of fillers. In the probe recognition study, participants' task was to decide whether the word had appeared in the previous sentence or not (a "no" response should take longer if the goal-implying sentences would enhance the accessibility of the goal). In the lexical decision study, they had to indicate whether the string of letters following the sentences was an existing word or not (a "yes" response should go faster in the case of enhanced accessibility of the goal). Both studies established that goal-implying sentences did enhance the accessibility of the goal representation, showing that goals were inferred online. Altogether, then, these findings provide strong evidence for the notion that people automatically infer other people's goals from descriptions of behaviors.

## The Role of Perceived Effort in Automatic Goal Inferences

The research on automatic goal inferences discussed so far suggests that the human mental system is well tuned toward inferring goals from observed specific pattern of actions performed by inanimate objects in a movie or by a person described in a short script. We have recently begun to examine the operation of this system more closely, to better understand the basic features that signal the pursuit of goals in a given behavioral context and affect the strength of goal inferences. Specifically, in a series of studies, we investigated the role of behavioral effort exerted by an actor as a cue to the incentive value or goal of motivating the actor's behavior (Dik & Aarts, in press). Effort is one of the hallmarks of motivation and goal pursuit; it tells an organism that the (different) actions performed by someone else in response to the situation at hand may serve a goal (Geen, 1995; Pervin, 1989; Toates, 1986). In addition, recent research suggests that perceptions of effort are readily used to infer the incentive value or goal of a produced item or behavior (Kruger, Wirtz, Van Boven, & Altermatt, 2004). Thus the more an agent reinitiates his or her behavior, using different but related actions, the more strongly that agent's behavior is perceived in terms of the desired goal driven by the behavior in the given context (Heider, 1958; Jones, 2001). In other words, the representation of a goal may increase in accessibility (because of inferring the goal) when more behavioral effort is perceived.

To investigate this idea, we exploited animated movie technology, which enabled us to experimentally test the effects of the amount of effort displayed by a physical object on the occurrence of inferences about the goal of helping (Dik & Aarts, in press, Studies 1 and 2). Participants were asked to watch a computerized movie that was allegedly a pilot for future research. The scene consisted of houses and trees, and in one of the trees a kite that "belonged" to a small ball was stuck in the twigs. The small ball was waiting under the tree until the kite would fall out (thereby indicating the need for help). Subsequently a large ball appeared on the scene, moving in the direction of a house that had four different doors and contained a ladder. The ladder could serve as a means to help the small ball get the kite out of the tree. To manipulate the perceived effort, the large ball "tried to open" no doors, one door, two different doors, or all four doors. The moving speed of the large ball was fixed, and the whole movie took about 10 seconds. The rationale here, then, was that "trying to open" more different doors would more strongly imply the desire or goal to help.

To assess whether automatic goal inferences had occurred, in one study a lexical decision task was used to unobtrusively measure the accessibility of the goal of helping after exposure to the movie (faster lexical decisions to help-related words would indicate higher accessibility of the helping goal). In another study, the accessibility measure consisted of a word completion task, in which participants had to provide as many words as possible with the letter H (higher accessibility of the helping goal would thus be shown when participants provided the word *helping* more often or earlier in the list of words). As predicted, the results of both studies showed a linear effect of the perceived amount of effort on the accessibility of the goal of helping. Awareness ratings further showed that participants were unaware of these effects.

These findings demonstrate that individuals more strongly impute unobservable social motivational causes (in this case, the goal to help) to a moving inanimate object when that object displays more effort in the movement. These findings extend previous work on automatic goal inferences, which demonstrated that people infer the content of goals from behavior performed by inanimate objects or human actors without explicit instructions or conscious intent to do so, by showing that perceived effort may play a key role in the inference process. Thus goal inferences result from a rather sophisticated system that allows us to easily detect, assess, and combine behavioral information into a goal representation to grasp the goals of others—a magnificent piece of "mind work" that can be handled by, and delegated to, the unconsciousness (Nørretranders, 1998; Wilson, 2002).

## GOAL CONTAGION: AUTOMATIC GOAL PURSUIT UPON INFERRING GOALS

As we have argued in the opening paragraphs of this chapter, automatic goal inferences do not only provide a direct understanding of the intentions of other people. In addition, they may directly promote the successful pursuit of one's own needs and goals without the need for conscious guidance. Indeed, human beings are capable of initiating and pursuing the goals they infer from other people's actions automatically, and hence exhibit goal contagion. Before we discuss the evidence supporting the goal contagion hypothesis, however, we briefly address some general issues pertaining to the conceptualization of automatic goal pursuit, and the recent interest in the activation of goals to understand the direct behavioral effects of inferred goals on one's own goal-directed behavior.

### Automatic Goal Pursuit

A growing number of studies show that goal pursuit can be elicited by mental processes that are put into motion by features of the social environment, and that goal pursuit can subsequently operate outside of conscious awareness (for overviews, see Custers & Aarts, 2005a; Chartrand et al., Chapter 22, this volume; Ferguson et al., Chapter 10, this volume; Moskowitz et al., 2004). Central to the idea of automatic goal pursuit is the assumption that goals are mentally represented as desired states that may pertain to behavior (e.g., performing well, helping other people) or to an outcome (e.g., earning money, being proud of oneself; see also the distinction between "do" and "be" goals, as described by Carver & Scheier, 1998). Although often implicitly assumed, conceptualizing goals as representations of desired states suggests the operation of two informational features (Custers & Aarts, 2005a, 2005b): (1) a cognitive one, which provides the knowledge of the state that has to be met; and (2) an affective/motivational one, which signals the individual that the state has incentive value and is worth pursuing. Thus activation of the goal representation directs as well as energizes activity that is instrumental in attaining the goal (Geen, 1995; Hyland, 1988; Pervin, 1989; Wright, 1996).

Furthermore, goals are assumed to be part of mental structures including situations, the goals themselves, and actions that may aid goal pursuit. This implies that goals can be primed by situational cues (Aarts & Dijksterhuis, 2000; Bargh & Gollwitzer, 1994; Kruglanski et al., 2002). Importantly, goal-priming effects are more pronounced when there is a current need or desire making it more pertinent to attain a goal. For instance, priming people with the goal of drinking and quenching thirst only enhances the accessibility and selection of thirst-reducing items if participants are indeed already thirsty (Aarts, Dijksterhuis, & De Vries, 2001; Strahan, Spencer, & Zanna, 2002). A nonconsciously activated goal, then, is likely to operate if the goal already exists as a desired state in the mind of the individual

(Fitzsimons & Bargh, 2004; see also Lewin, 1951). In other words, one can only prime goals when they are there.

Previous empirical work used conceptual priming procedures to test whether goals can be activated and pursued automatically (Bargh, Gollwitzer, Lee-Chai, Barndollar, & Trötschel, 2001; Chartrand & Bargh, 1996; Hassin, 2005). This research has established that direct priming of goals via exposure to words that are closely related to them exerts an unconscious influence on action in a subsequent goal-relevant situation. For instance, Bargh and colleagues (2001) unobtrusively exposed participants to words such as *strive* and *succeed* to prime the achievement goal (a goal held by most students, although not always in operation), and then gave them the opportunity to perform well (finding as many words as possible in an anagram puzzle task). Results indicated that participants who were primed with the achievement goal outperformed those who were not primed with the goal. In a recent line of experimentation, we replicated these goal-priming effects in the realm of social stereotypes, showing that people automatically pursue the goals associated with social groups after mere exposure to these groups, such as the goals of helping and making money that are stereotypical for nurses and stockbrokers, respectively (Aarts et al., 2005). Moreover, it has been demonstrated that this goal priming leads to qualities associated with motivational states or goal-directedness, such as persistence, flexibility, and increased effort in working for the goal, especially in the face of obstacles (when the road to successful goal attainment is hampered).

## Goal Imitation of Simple Actions on Objects

The research described above provides evidence that motivational, goal-directed behavior can be automatically put into motion if the representation of the goal is primed. Accordingly, inferring the goal motivating others' actions may directly affect one's own goal-directed behavior. Recently, researchers in developmental psychology have started to examine this topic to broaden the perspective on behavioral imitation. Specifically, they analyze the adoption as goals of actions on objects that young children perceive in a model's behavior. The common view about the mechanism underlying behavioral imitation is that observing an action performed by another person activates a matching motor program by direct perceptual–motor mapping. This way, people do what they see other people do. This view has stimulated a tremendous amount of research in different fields of psychology to investigate the neurological and perceptual–motor processes involved in basic action imitation (see reviews by Dijksterhuis, Chartrand, & Aarts, 2006; Meltzoff & Prinz, 2002).

Several observations of imitation, however, indicate that a direct mapping between perception and action does not fully capture the complexity of human behavior that results from the perception of other individuals' behavior. For instance, pairing positive affect with the representation of behaviors increases the probability of imitating the behaviors (De Houwer, Thomas, & Baeyens, 2001). Thus, when children observe another person displaying a positive facial expression while performing a specific action, they are more likely to perform that action themselves. This suggests that observed behaviors that become attached to positive affect form an incentive or desired goal state, for which one mobilizes more effort or energy in order to engage in it (Custers & Aarts, 2005b). In taking this idea one step further, Carpenter, Akhtar, and Tomasello (1998) showed that infants (between 14 and 18 months old) engaged in simple actions on an object more readily when the models' actions were marked vocally as desired and goal-directed ("There!") than when these actions were marked vocally as accidental ("Whoops!"). In short, behaviors that represent an incentive or goal are more likely to be imitated than behaviors that do not reflect a goal.

Earlier we have presented evidence for the idea that great apes and humans (even very young ones) go beyond the behavioral information given to infer the goals that may guide the simple movements exhibited by physical objects or other persons. When individuals pursue (and thus imitate) such an inferred goal, they seem to be capable of effectively orchestrating and performing the relevant actions leading to this goal, even though they have not seen the resulting goal or end-state at issue. Research in developmental psychology provides initial support for this hypothesis.

In a line of experimentation on the imitation of simple goal-directed action patterns, Meltzoff (1995; see also Bellagamba & Tomasello, 1999) investigated whether preverbal infants who watched an adult perform a series of acts on an object would reenact what the adult actually did (or tried to do). For example, an adult female experimenter first showed a hollow plastic square and a stick and then tried to put the hollow square over the stick. In one condition the experimenter succeeded, whereas in the other she never did. The 18-month-old participants were then given the same objects, and the question was what they would do with these objects. Interestingly, the toddlers who saw the unsuccessful experimenter were as likely to complete the target action as the toddlers from the successful group. This effect was not observed in a control group (in which the model displayed random movements with the objects). The interesting finding here, then, is that the infants produced a target behavior that they did not perceive. Rather than imitating the behavior, they tried to attain the goal they inferred. These findings suggest that the children adopted the goal they inferred from the model's behavior.

It should be noted, though, that several issues have been raised that may disqualify this conclusion. For instance, the infants' behavior may have been attributable to an understanding of the causal structure of the task (e.g., they simply discovered or knew the beginning and ending positions of the objects), rather than to an understanding of the goal guiding the observed actions. Accordingly, the behavioral effects do not necessarily require the observation of a model's actions in order to occur. Additionally, because the young participants were given exactly the same objects and means in the same setting, it is not clear whether they simply relied on motor activity available in their behavioral repertoire to directly imitate the target action, or whether the inferred goal was an incentive they were motivated to strive for by themselves (for discussions of these topics, see, e.g., Gergely, Bekkering, & Király, 2002; Heyes & Ray, 2002; Huang, Heyes, & Charman, 2002). In other words, the findings do not allow us to conclude firmly that humans are capable of initiating and pursuing the goals they infer from other people's actions automatically, and therefore that the goals of others are contagious.

## On the Contagion of Social Goals

The idea that people automatically act on the goals they infer from other individuals' actions has also been investigated recently in social psychological research. In this research, some of the concerns with the goal imitation studies addressed above have been solved by using an different experimental paradigm. In this paradigm, goal inferences are assumed to be made on the basis of a protagonist's actions in a specific setting described in a written scenario. However, goal striving among the perceivers is subsequently tested in a different setting that requires a different behavior from the one displayed by the protagonist. Of importance, the goals used in these studies have clear incentive value and thus should act as motivators for most people, such as the goals of ingratiating, being accurate, helping others, seeking sex, or earning money (for a taxonomy of social goals, see Chulef, Read, & Walsh, 2001).

Preliminary evidence supporting the suggestion that an individual may automatically pursue the social goals (and resultant actions) he or she is currently perceiving in another person was obtained by Chaiken and colleagues (Chaiken, Giner-Sorolla, & Chen, 1996; Chen, Schechter, & Chaiken, 1996). They examined whether goals that result from thinking about concrete behaviors can alter the expression of attitudes. Participants in their study were asked, for 12 minutes, to take the perspective of another person performing several behaviors related to either the goal to be accurate (e.g., a reporter seeking the objective facts) or the goal to provide a favorable impression (e.g., a person on a blind date with a close friend's cousin). Subsequently, participants engaged in a discussion with another person. As predicted, participants who had been exposed to the ingratiation goal scenarios were more likely than those exposed to the accuracy goal scenarios to express attitudes that were consistent with the discussion partner's opinion. Suspicion probes showed that participants were not aware of these effects. These results point to the emergence of goal contagion. It should be noted, however, that this study used explicit perspective-taking instructions and devoted a relatively large amount of time to having participants imagine themselves in another's position. Therefore, it is unclear whether such findings occur upon the mere exposure to another's behavior, or whether they require a much more elaborated and effortful process (Albrecht, O'Brien, Mason, & Myers, 1995). Furthermore, the behavioral effects were not tested for features of goal-directedness.

Aarts, Gollwitzer, and Hassin (2004) directly tested the emergence of automatic pursuit of social goals after mere (and brief) exposure to behavioral information. One of their aims was to demonstrate goal contagion by examining whether the behavioral effects of goal contagion show features of goal-directedness (e.g., Bargh et al., 2001; Gollwitzer & Moskowitz, 1996; Toates, 1986; Tolman, 1925). For example, in one of their studies, they investigated whether the behavioral effects of an implied goal of making money are more pronounced when a preexisting need for money feeds the desire for that goal (e.g., for students lacking the necessary income to run their daily lives). Participants (undergraduate students) read a short behavioral script in which a student plans a vacation with friends. After planning the vacation, the student either (1) goes to a farm to work as an assistant for a month (a pretest showed that our sample of students—either high or low in need for money—encoded this behavior in terms of the goal of making money) or (2) goes to a community center to do volunteer work for a month (control condition). Each of these scripts was briefly (for 30 seconds) presented on a computer screen, just long enough for participants to read it. Participants were then told that the study was almost completed, but that they had to perform a short task on the computer. Crucially, participants were told that if enough time was left at the end of the session, they would be able to engage in a lottery in which they could win money. Participants' pace of working on the computer task served as a measure of goal-directed activity: The faster they worked on it, the stronger was their motivation to get to the last part of the session, where they could earn money.

Results showed that participants who were exposed to the behavior implying the goal of earning money worked faster than those in the control condition. However, these behavioral differences only emerged when participants had a high need for money, suggesting that the implied goal was contagious when that goal already existed as a desired state in the perceivers' minds. Importantly, thorough debriefing and awareness ratings indicated that participants were unaware of these effects.

In two other studies, Aarts and colleagues (2004) replicated these goal contagion effects for the goal of seeking casual sex. In these studies, heterosexual male students in all conditions read a short story about a man who meets a former female friend at a bar and spends a few hours with her. In the condition implying the casual sex goal—but not in the control condition—the man asks the woman whether he can come with her to her apartment (see also Clark & Hatfield, 1989). Next, all participants were asked to help a female or male experimenter by providing feedback on a task they performed earlier on in the study. Previous findings showed that heterosexual men know that offering help can be instrumental in attaining (casual) sex with women, and that men behave accordingly (Buss, 1988; Canary, Emmers-Sommer, & Faulkner, 1997). Thus goal contagion should lead participants to be more helpful. Indeed, male participants exerted more effort in helping the female experimenter in the sex goal condition than in the control condition. These behavioral changes did not ensue if participants were asked to provide feedback to the male experimenter, indicating the quality of goal appropriateness (i.e., participants made use of good opportunities to reach the goal and shunned bad ones). Furthermore, the goal contagion effects were even manifested after a 5-minute delay, showing some degree of persistence.

In short, then, the studies presented above indicate that humans are keen to act on the goals of other social beings that are implied in behavioral scenarios or scripts. However, it may be argued that goal contagion occurred because participants could identify or compare with the agents in the scripts. After all, both the actors and the participants were persons, and thus belonged to the same group: humans. There is research to suggest that subjective variables pertaining to relational aspects (such as the level of social identification and significance) may influence how individuals appreciate the goals that are implied by those other persons (e.g., Andersen, Reznik, & Manzella, 1996; Shah, 2003). For instance, people who are primed with the name of a significant other seem to adjust their perceived value of a task goal to the goal value associated with the significant other (Shah, 2003). However, these findings do not mean that the emergence of automatic goal pursuit upon perception of behavior requires for its occurrence a human actor as a necessary condition. According to the goal contagion hypothesis, it should not matter whether a target is human or not, as long as the movements of the target allow for goal inferences that are represented as desired states in a perceiver's mind.[2]

To investigate this hypothesis, Dik and Aarts (in press, Study 3) used the animated movie described earlier. As described earlier, this task was used successfully in demonstrating that people are more prone to automatically infer the goal of helping implied by the movements of a physical object when that object puts more effort into its goal pursuits. Because it was demonstrated that the mental representation of the goal to help was rendered more accessible when more effort was perceived, we expected that this heightened accessibility would lead to more goal-directed behavior, aimed at the achievement of this very same goal. Participants were instructed to watch the computerized movie in which a large ball tried to help a little ball get a kite out of a tree by obtaining access to a ladder in a house. The large ball tried to open no doors, one door, two doors, or four doors to enter the house; thus the amount of effort to help was experimentally varied. Dik and Aarts found that the increased effort displayed by the large ball in the animated movie produced more willingness to help the experimenter by volunteering for follow-up research, showing indeed that the inferred goal of helping was contagious. These findings, then, show that people act on implied goals, even if these goals are inferred from movements of nonhuman objects. This suggests that goal contagion is a basic process put in motion by the enhanced accessibility of the goal one infers from movements of agents to understand the potential cause and desired outcome of the observed movements.

## The Ceasing of Goal Contagion: Perceiving Goal Pursuits in a Negative Light

It is important to note that in the studies discussed so far, participants were favorable toward the implied goal in general. Goal contagion occurred because the goal already existed as a desired state in the mind of most of the perceivers upon observing the goal-implying behaviors (e.g., because of a current or chronic need). Given this general "desirability" of the implied goal, it may be questioned whether people always take on the goals they perceive in other people's action. In our own research, we have started to address this issue by examining whether an observed goal pursuit (e.g., seeking casual sex) that unfolds in a socially unacceptable or negative way (e.g., is associated with being unfaithful) fails to be contagious, even though the person is favorable toward the goal in general. But why would this be the case? Why should people not act on a goal representation that becomes attached to negative information?

It is known that humans show hypersensitivity to negative social and behavioral information (e.g., Dijksterhuis & Aarts, 2003; Pratto & John, 1991). Exposing people to negative goal-related cues can easily spoil the appreciation of a given goal (Rozin & Royzman, 2001). Research on evaluative conditioning further suggests that goal stimuli can easily become less attractive when these stimuli are paired with negative information (De Houwer et al., 2001). In a recent empirical demonstration of this idea, Aarts, Custers, and Holland (2007) used the evaluative conditioning paradigm to unobtrusively link the goal of socializing and partying (a goal most of our students perceive as a desired state; see also Sheeran et al., 2005) to negatively valenced words, and tested effects of this affective shaping treatment on the motivation to work at the goal in a subsequent goal-relevant task (the speed of a mouse-clicking task that gave access to a lottery game in which one could win tickets for a popular student party). They found that participants were less motivated to strive for the goal when the goal was linked to negative information (compared to conditions in which the goal was not primed or not directly linked to negative information). These findings suggest that the incentive value of a goal decreases when the goal is coactivated with negative affect. Importantly, these effects occurred outside of participants' awareness, indicating that if activated goals become attached to negative affect, then this can lead to nonconscious cessation of motivation.

The previous findings may have important implications for the emergence of goal contagion. Specifically, they suggest that the perception of another person's goal-implying behaviors will not always lead to goal contagion; when the goal pursuit is perceived as negative, goal contagion may be less likely to occur. To examine this issue, Aarts and colleagues (2004) exposed heterosexual male students to the behavioral script implying either the goal of seeking casual sex or not. In one version of the sex goal, it was made clear that the protagonist was already engaged in a serious relationship (this should render the goal pursuit of casual sex unacceptable and thus put it in a negative light; Margolin, 1989). Participants were then given the opportunity to help a female experimenter, and the question was how much effort they would expend to help (as a means for goal achievement). The results indicated that goal contagion vanished when the situation in the behavioral script rendered the implied goal unacceptable. Further experimentation revealed that perceiving others pursuing a goal under unacceptable conditions made the goal less desirable for the perceivers, even though it was generally favorable. Importantly, the fact that goals that were pursued improperly were not contagious did not result from a competition with other goals evoked by the situation described in the behavioral script. These data, then, support the contention that people do not automatically adopt goals that are pursued in the context of socially unacceptable, negative circumstances.

These findings further establish the important point that people do not always automatically adopt the goals of others, even though the goal is activated in the mind of the perceiver. Negative information that co-occurs with an inferred goal seems to be an important moderator of goal contagion. Such negative information may derive from the way or context in which an actor pursues the implied goal, but also from properties of the actor itself—an issue that certainly requires further research. The bottom line is that as soon as a goal is linked to negative affect or categorized as unattractive, that goal no longer operates as an incentive or state one desires to attain, and thus is not capable of directly shaping goal-directed activity. As the Aarts and colleagues (2004, 2007) studies showed, however, people do not have to be aware of these behavioral effects; the reduced desire in itself may suffice to moderate goal contagion. This raises the possibility that individuals have an effortless protection or blocking mechanism that make them immune, so to speak, against taking and acting on goals that are rendered unattractive. This idea concurs well with the literature on goal assignment illustrating the difficulty of talking people into adopting new or impersonal goals if these are not presented in the most positive light possible (Locke & Latham, 1990; Oettingen & Gollwitzer, 2001).

## GENERAL CONCLUSIONS

In this chapter we have expanded on the progress researchers have made in two separate major developments in social psychology research (i.e., work on social causal inferences and on automatic goal pursuit) to analyze the human ability to automatically infer and adopt goals from actions performed by someone else. Our review of recent empirical research on the topic demonstrates that individuals have a natural ability to automatically infer goals from others' behaviors, and that these inferred goals can be automatically pursued by the perceivers—a phenomenon we have termed *goal contagion*. These new findings show that (causal) goal inferences do not only help people to directly understand and predict the behaviors of others in the situation at hand. Goal inferences may also directly promote the successful pursuit of individuals' own needs, desires, and goals. By adopting the goals of others, people may become more similar in what they desire and strive for in the current social situation, without much conscious thought. We believe that the notion of goal contagion in general, and further explorations of this process in particular, may improve our understanding of how people orchestrate their goals and behaviors in everyday life.

## ACKNOWLEDGMENTS

The writing of this chapter was supported by grants from the Netherlands Organization for Scientific Research (VIDI; Grant No. 452-02-047) and from Vernieuwingsimpuls (Grant No. 016-025-030).

## NOTES

1. More recent models also take unintentionality into account when making causal explanations of behavior (Malle, 1999; Malle & Knobe, 1997). However, because the present line of argument pertains to goals as causes of behavior, we only consider behavior that signals intentionality to a perceiver.

2. More recent models also take unintentionality into account when making causal explanations of behavior (Malle, 1999; Malle & Knobe, 1997). However, because the present line of argument pertains to goals as

causes of behavior, we only consider behavior that signals intentionality to a perceiver.. In fact, research on the animated movie technology has established that the attribution of goals to inanimate or nonhuman objects renders these objects animate and social. More generally, this tendency to anthropomorphize is quite common among human beings, and it may constitute the core feature that allows us to establish some sort of social bonding with nonhuman objects, such as pets, computers, cars, blow-up dolls, and so on (Mitchell, Thompson, & Miles, 1997).

## REFERENCES


Aarts, H., Chartrand, T. L., Custers, R., Danner, U., Dik, G., Jefferis, V., et al. (2005). Social Stereotypes and automatic goal pursuit. *Social Cognition, 23*, 464–489.

Aarts, H., Custers, R., & Holland, R. (2007). On the cessation of nonconscious goal pursuit: When goals and negative affect are co-activated. *Journal of Personality and Social Psychology, 92*, 165–178.

Aarts, H., & Dijksterhuis, A. (2000). Habits as knowledge structures: Automaticity in goal-directed behavior. *Journal of Personality and Social Psychology, 78*, 53–63.

Aarts, H., Dijksterhuis, A., & De Vries, P. (2001). The psychology of drinking: Being thirsty and perceptually ready. *British Journal of Psychology, 92*, 631–642.

Aarts, H., Gollwitzer, P., & Hassin, R. (2004). Goal contagion: Perceiving is for pursuing. *Journal of Personality and Social Psychology, 87*, 23–37.

Aarts, H., & Hassin, R. (2005). Automatic goal inferences and contagion: On pursuing goals one perceives in other people's behavior. In J. P. Forgas, K. D. Williams, & S. M. Laham (Eds.), *Social motivation: Conscious and unconscious processes* (pp. 153–167). New York: Cambridge University Press.

Ajzen, I. (1991). The theory of planned behavior. *Organizational Behavior and Human Decision Processes, 50*, 179–211.

Albrecht, J. E., O'Brien, E. J., Mason, R. A., & Myers, J. L. (1995). The role of perspective in the accessibility of goals during reading. *Journal of Experimental Psychology: Learning, Memory, and Cognition, 21*, 364–372.

Andersen, S. M., Reznik, I., & Manzella, L. M. (1996). Eliciting facial affect, motivation, and expectancies in transference: Significant-other representations in social relations. *Journal of Personality and Social Psychology, 71*, 1108–1129.

Bandura, A. (1986). *Social foundations of thought and action: A social-cognitive theory.* Englewood Cliffs, NJ: Prentice Hall.

Bargh, J. A. (1990). Auto-motives: Preconscious determinants of social interaction. In E. T. Higgins & R. M. Sorrentino (Eds.), *Handbook of motivation and cognition: Foundations of social behavior* (Vol. 2, pp. 93–130). New York: Guilford Press.

Bargh, J. A. (1994). The four horsemen of automaticity: Awareness, intention, efficiency and control in social cognition. In R. S. Wyer, Jr., & T. K. Srull (Eds.), *Handbook of social cognition* (Vol. 2, pp. 1–40). Hillsdale, NJ: Erlbaum.

Bargh, J. A., & Gollwitzer, P. M. (1994). Environmental control of goal-directed action: Automatic and strategic contingencies between situations and behavior. In D. Spaulding (Ed.), *Nebraska Symposium on Motivation* (Vol. 41, pp. 71–124). Lincoln: University of Nebraska Press.

Bargh, J. A., Gollwitzer, P. M., Lee-Chai, A., Barndollar, K., & Trötschel, R. (2001). The automated will: Nonconscious activation and pursuit of behavioral goals. *Journal of Personality and Social Psychology, 81*, 1014–1027.

Bellagamba, F., & Tomasello, M. (1999). Reenacting intended acts: Comparing 12- and 18-month-olds. *Infant Behavior and Development, 22*, 277–282.

Buss, D. M. (1988). The evolution of human intrasexual competition: Tactics of mate attraction. *Journal of Personality and Social Psychology, 54*, 616–628.

Byrne, R. W., & Russon, A. E. (1998). Learning by imitation: A hierarchical approach. *Behavioral and Brain Sciences, 21*, 667–721.

Canary, D. J., Emmers-Sommer, T. M., & Faulkner, S. (1997). *Sex and gender differences in personal relationships.* New York: Guilford Press.

Carpenter, M., Akhtar, N., & Tomasello, M. (1998). Fourteen- through 18-month-old infants differentially imitate intentional and accidental actions. *Infant Behavior and Development, 21*, 315–330.

Carver, C. S., & Scheier, M. F. (1998). *On the self-regulation of behavior.* New York: Cambridge University Press.

Chaiken, S., Giner-Sorolla, R., & Chen, S. (1996). Beyond accuracy defense and impression motives in heuristic and systematic information processing. In P. M. Gollwitzer & J. A. Bargh (Eds.), *The psychology of action* (pp. 553–578). New York: Guilford Press.

Chartrand, T. L., & Bargh, J. A. (1996). Automatic activation of impression formation and memorization goals: Nonconscious goal priming reproduces effects of explicit task instructions. *Journal of Personality and Social Psychology, 71*, 464–478.

Chen, S., Schechter, D., & Chaiken, S. (1996). Getting at the truth or getting along: Accuracy- versus impression-motivated heuristic and systematic processing. *Journal of Personality and Social Psychology, 71*, 262–275.

Chulef, A. S., Read, S. J., & Walsh, D. A. (2001). A hierarchical taxonomy of human goals. *Motivation and Emotion, 25*, 191–232.

Clark, R. D., & Hatfield, E. (1989). Gender differences in receptivity to sexual offers. *Journal of Personality and Human Sexuality, 2*, 39–55.

Csibra, G., Gergely, G., Biro, S., Koos, O., &

Brockbank, M. (1999). Goal attribution without agency cues: The perception of "pure reason" in infancy. *Cognition*, *72*, 237–267.

Custers, R., & Aarts, H. (2005a). Beyond accessibility: The role of affect and goal-discrepancies in implicit processes of motivation and goal-pursuit. *European Review of Social Psychology*, *16*, 257–300.

Custers, R., & Aarts, H. (2005b). Positive affect as implicit motivator: On the nonconscious operation of behavioral goals. *Journal of Personality and Social Psychology*, *89*, 129–142.

Deci, E. L., & Ryan, R. M. (1985). *Intrinsic motivation and self-determination in human behavior.* New York: Plenum Press.

De Houwer, J., Thomas, S., & Baeyens, F. (2001). Association learning of likes and dislikes: A review of 25 years of research on human evaluative conditioning. *Psychological Bulletin*, *127*, 853–869.

Dijksterhuis, A., & Aarts, H. (2003). On wildebeest and human beings: The detection of positive and negative information. *Psychological Science*, *14*, 14–18.

Dijksterhuis, A., Chartrand, T. L., & Aarts, H. (2007). Effects of priming and perception on social behavior and goal pursuit. In J. A. Bargh (Ed.), *Social psychology and the unconscious: The automaticity of higher mental processes* (pp. 51–131). New York: Psychology Press.

Dik, G., & Aarts, H. (in press). Behavioral cues to others' motivation and goal-pursuit: The perception of effort facilitates goal inference and contagion. *Journal of Experimental Social Psychology.*

Fitzsimons, G. M., & Bargh, J. A. (2004). Automatic self-regulation. In K. D. Vohs & R. F. Baumeister (Eds.), *Handbook of self-regulation: Research, theory, and applications* (pp. 151–170). New York: Guilford Press.

Frith, U., & Frith, C. D. (2003). Development and neurophysiology of mentalizing. *Philosophical Transactions of the Royal Society of London, Series B*, *358*, 459–473.

Geen, R. G. (1995). *Human motivation: A social psychological approach*. Pacific Grove, CA: Brooks/Cole.

Gergely, G. (1994). From self-recognition to theory of mind. In S. T. Parker, R. W. Mitchell, & M. L. Boccia (Eds.), *Self-awareness in animals and humans: Developmental perspectives* (pp. 51–60). New York: Cambridge University Press.

Gergely, G., Bekkering, H., & Király, I. (2002). Rational imitation in preverbal infants. *Nature*, *415*, 755.

Gergely, G., Nadasdy, Z., Csibra, G., & Biro, S. (1995). Taking the intentional stance at 12 months of age. *Cognition*, *56*, 165–193.

Gilbert, D. T. (1989). Thinking lightly about others: Automatic components of the social inference process. In J. S. Uleman & J. A. Bargh (Eds.), *Unintended thought* (pp. 189–211). New York: Guilford Press.

Gilbert, T. D., Pelham, W. B., & Krull, S. D. (1988). On cognitive busyness when person perceivers meet persons perceived. *Journal of Personality and Social Psychology*, *54*, 733–740.

Gollwitzer, P. M., & Moskowitz, G. B. (1996). Goal effects on action and cognition. In E. Higgins & A. W. Kruglanski (Eds.), *Social psychology: Handbook of basic principles* (pp. 361–399). New York: Guilford Press.

Graesser, C. A., Singer, M., & Trabasso, T. (1994). Constructing inferences during narrative text comprehension. *Psychological Review*, *101*(3), 371–395.

Hassin, R., Aarts, H., & Ferguson, M. (2005). Automatic goal inferences. *Journal of Experimental Social Psychology*, *41*, 129–140.

Hassin R., Bargh, J. A., & Uleman, J. S. (2002). Spontaneous causal inferences. *Journal of Experimental Social Psychology*, *38*, 515–522.

Hassin, R. R. (2005). Non-conscious control and implicit working memory. In R. R. Hassin, J. S. Uleman, & J. A. Bargh (Eds.), *The new unconscious* (pp. 196–224). New York: Oxford University Press.

Hauser, M. D. (1999). Primate representations and expectations: Mental tools for navigating in a social world. In P. D. Zelazo, J. W. Astington, & D. R. Olson (Eds.), *Developing theories of intention: Social understanding and self-control* (pp. 169–194). Mahwah, NJ: Erlbaum.

Heider, F. (1958). *The psychology of interpersonal relations*. New York: Wiley.

Heider, F., & Simmel, M. (1944). An experimental study of apparent behavior. *American Journal of Psychology*, *57*, 243–259.

Heyes, C. M., & Ray, E. D. (2002). Distinguishing intention-sensitive from outcome sensitive imitation. *Developmental Science*, *5*, 34–36.

Huang, C, Heyes, C. M., & Charman, T. (2002). Infants' behavioral reenactment of failed attempts: Exploring the roles of emulation learning, stimulus enhancement, and understanding of intentions. *Developmental Psychology*, *38*, 840–855.

Humphrey, N. (1978). Nature's psychologists. *New Scientist*, *78*, 900–903.

Hyland, M. E. (1988). Motivational control-theory: An integrative framework. *Journal of Personality and Social Psychology*, *55*, 642–651.

Jones, E. E., & Davis, K. E. (1965). From acts to dispositions: The attribution process in person perception. In L. Berkowitz (Ed.), *Advances in experimental social psychology* (Vol. 2, pp. 219–266). New York: Academic Press.

Jones, E. F. (2001). The influence of goal-related action and goal information on children's perceptions of trying and wanting: An action-perception approach. *Journal of Genetic Psychology*, *156*, 153–166.

Kassin, S. (1982). Heider and Simmel revisited: Causal attribution and the animated film technique. *Review of Personality and Social Psychology*, *3*, 145–169.

Kruger, J., Wirtz, D., Van Boven, L., & Altermatt, T. W. (2004). The effort heuristic. *Journal of Experimental Social Psychology*, *40*, 91–98.

Kruglanski, A. W., Shah, J. Y., Fishbach, A., Friedman, R., Chun, W. Y., & Sleeth-Keppler, D. (2002). A theory of goal systems. In M. Zanna (Ed.), *Advances in experimental social psychology* (pp. 331–378). San Diego, CA: Academic Press.

Lewin, K. (1951). *Field theory in social science*. Chicago: University of Chicago Press.

Locke, E. A., & Latham, G. P. (1990). *A theory of goal-setting and task performance*. Englewood Cliffs, NJ: Prentice Hall.

Long, D. L., & Golding, J. M. (1993). Superordinate goal inferences: Are they automatically generated during comprehension? *Discourse Processes, 16*, 55–73.

Long, D. L., Golding, J. M., & Graesser, C. A. (1992). A test of on-line status of goal-related inferences. *Journal of Memory and Language, 31*, 634–647.

MacPhail, E. (1998). *The evolution of consciousness*. London: Oxford University Press.

Malle, B. F. (1999). How people explain behavior: A new theoretical framework. *Personality and Social Psychology Review, 3*, 23–48.

Malle, B. F., & Knobe, J. (1997). The folk concept of intentionality. *Journal of Experimental Social Psychology, 33*, 101–121.

Margolin, L. (1989). Gender and the prerogatives of dating and marriage: An experimental assessment of a sample of college students. *Sex Roles, 20*, 91–102.

McClure, J. L. (2002). Goal-based explanations of actions and outcomes. *European Review of Social Psychology, 12*, 201–236.

McKoon, G., & Ratcliff, R. (1986). Inferences about predictable events. *Journal of Experimental Psychology: Learning, Memory, and Cognition, 12*(1), 82–91.

McKoon, G., & Ratcliff, R. (1992). Inference during reading. *Psychological Review, 99*(3), 440–466.

Meltzoff, A. N. (1995). Understanding the intentions of others: Re-enactment of intended acts by 18-months-old children. *Developmental Psychology, 31*, 838–850.

Meltzoff, A. N., & Moore, M. K. (1996). Infants' understanding of people and things: From body imitation to folk psychology. In J. L. Bermúdez, A. Marcel, & N. Eilan (Eds.), *The body and the self* (pp. 43–69). Cambridge, MA: MIT Press.

Meltzoff, A. N., & Prinz, W. (2002). *The imitative mind: Development, evolution, and brain bases*. Berlin: Springer-Verlag.

Michotte, A. (1963). *The perception of causality* (T. R. Miles & E. Miles, Trans.). New York: Basic Books.

Mitchell, R. W., Thompson, N. S., & Miles, H. L. (1997). *Anthropomorphism, anecdotes, and animals*. Albany: State University of New York Press.

Moskowitz, G. B., Li, P., & Kirk, E. R. (2004). The implicit volition model: On the preconscious regulation of temporarily adopted goals. In M. Zanna (Ed.), *Advances in experimental social psychology*. San Diego, CA: Academic Press.

Nørretranders, T. (1998). *The user illusion: Cutting consciousness down to size*. New York: Viking.

Oettingen, G., & Gollwitzer, P. M. (2001). Goal setting and goal striving. In A. Tesser & N. Schwarz (Eds.), *Blackwell handbook of social psychology* (pp. 329–347). Oxford, UK: Blackwell.

Pervin, L. A. (Ed.). (1989). *Goal concepts in personality and social psychology*. Hillsdale, NJ: Erlbaum.

Pratto, F., & John, O. P. (1991). Automatic vigilance: The attention-grabbing power of negative social information. *Journal of Personality and Social Psychology, 63*, 380–391.

Premack, D. (1990). The infant's theory of self-propelled objects. *Cognition, 36*, 1–16.

Premack, D., & Premack, A. J. (1997). Infants attribute value? to the goal-directed actions of self-propelled objects. *Journal of Cognitive Neuroscience, 9*, 848–856.

Read, S. J., Jones, D. K., & Miller, L. C. (1990). Traits as goal-based categories: The importance of goals in the coherence of dispositional categories. *Journal of Personality and Social Psychology, 58*, 1048–1061.

Read, S. J., & Miller, L. C. (1989). Inter-personalism: Toward a goal-based theory of persons in relationships. In L. A. Pervin (Ed.), *Goal concepts in personality and social psychology* (pp. 413–472). Hillsdale, NJ: Erlbaum.

Rozin, P., & Royzman, E. B. (2001). Negativity bias, negativity dominance, and contagion. *Personality and Social Psychology Review, 5*, 296–320.

Scholl, B. J., & Tremoulet, P. D. (2000). Perceptual causality and animacy. *Trends in Cognitive Sciences, 4*, 299–309.

Shah, J. Y. (2003). The motivational looking glass: How significant others implicitly affect goal appraisals. *Journal of Personality and Social Psychology, 85*, 424–439.

Sheeran, P., Aarts, H., Custers, R., Webb, T. L., Cooke, R., & Rivis, A. J. (2005). The goal-dependent automaticity of drinking habits. *British Journal of Social Psychology, 44*, 47–63.

Strahan, E. J., Spencer, S. J., & Zanna, M. P. (2002). Subliminal priming and persuasion: Striking while the iron is hot. *Journal of Experimental Social Psychology, 38*, 556–568.

Toates, F. (1986). *Motivational systems*. Cambridge, UK: Cambridge University Press.

Tolman, E. C. (1925). Purpose and cognition: The determinants of animal learning. *Psychological Review, 32*, 285–297.

Todorov, A., & Uleman, J. S. (2002). Spontaneous trait inferences are bound to actors' faces: Evidence from a false recognition paradigm. *Journal of Personality and Social Psychology, 83*(5), 1051–1065.

Tomasello, M., Kruger, A. C., & Ratner, H. H. (1993). Cultural learning. *Behavioral and Brain Sciences, 16*, 495–552.

Trabasso, T., & van den Broek, P. (1985). Causal thinking and the representation of narrative events. *Journal of Memory and Language*, *24*, 612–630.

Trope, Y. (1986). Identification and inferential processes in dispositional attribution. *Psychological Review*, *93*, 239–257.

Uleman, J. S. (1999). Spontaneous versus intentional inferences in impression formation. In S. Chaiken & Y. Trope (Eds.), *Dual-process theories in social psychology* (pp. 141–160). New York: Guilford Press.

Uleman, J. S., Newman, S. L., & Moskowitz, G. B. (1996). People as flexible interpreters: Evidence and issues from spontaneous trait inference. In M. P. Zanna (Ed.), *Advances in experimental social psychology* (Vol. 28, pp. 211–279). San Diego, CA: Academic Press.

Uller, C., & Nichols, S. (2000). Goal attribution in chimpanzees. *Cognition*, *76*, 27–34.

Van Overwalle, F., Drenth, T., & Marsman, G. (1999). Spontaneous trait inferences: Are they linked to the actor or to the action? *Personality and Social Psychology Bulletin*, *25*, 450–462.

Vallacher, R. R., & Wegner, D. M. (1987). What do people think they're doing?: Action identification and human behavior. *Psychological Review*, *94*, 3–15.

Wilson, T. D. (2002). *Strangers to ourselves: Discovering the adaptive unconscious*. Cambridge, MA: Harvard University Press.

Winter, L., & Uleman, J. S. (1984). When are social judgments made?: Evidence for the spontaneousness of trait inferences. *Journal of Personality and Social Psychology*, *47*, 237–252.

Wright, R. A. (1996). Brehm's theory of motivation as a model of effort and cardiovascular response. In P. M. Gollwitzer & J. A. Bargh (Eds.), *The psychology of action: Linking cognition and motivation to behavior* (pp. 424–453). New York: Guilford Press.

Zeman, A. (2001). Consciousness. *Brain*, *124*, 1263–1289.

Chapter 18

# Implicit and Explicit Counteractive Self-Control

**Ayelet Fishbach**
**Yaacov Trope**

Individuals face a self-control problem when the attainment of their overriding long-term interests comes at the expense of short-term but influential outcomes. For example, the boredom that is often associated with studying long hours is a price students have to pay in order to attain academic success, and the discomfort that is often associated with dieting or undergoing a medical checkup is a price people often have to pay in order to maintain good health. In many cases, individuals fail to pursue their goals because those goals do not seem sufficiently important, or because they feel they lack the means that are required to achieve those goals. Self-control problems represent a special type of motivational conflict. Individuals may want to pursue their goals. They may also have the prerequisite knowledge, skill, and opportunity. Nevertheless, short-term outcomes may tempt those individuals to act against their long-term interests. For example, a dieter may want to losc weight and know what is required to achieve this goal. Nevertheless, the smell of baking cake may lead this person to break the diet. Similarly, a student may want to study for an important exam, know how to study for the exam, and possess the required materials. Nevertheless, a beautiful spring day may be sufficiently tempting to prevent the student from studying for the exam and achieving the academic goals he or she has set. As these examples demonstrate, self-control problems arise when the pursuit of high-order goals with long-term benefits does not coincide with the pursuit of low-order goals (i.e., desires and temptations) with short-term benefits.

Self-control phenomena have been studied by theoreticians and researchers across different behavioral science disciplines, including economics (e.g., Becker, 1960; O'Donoghue & Rabin, 2000; Thaler & Shefrin, 1981), political science (e.g., Elster, 1977; Schelling, 1984), and psychology (e.g., Ainslie, 2001; Baumeister &

Vohs, 2004; Kuhl & Beckmann, 1985; Mischel & Patterson, 1976; Rachlin, 2000). In recent years, there has been an upsurge in interest in self-control failures, the antecedents of such failures, and their maladaptive psychological consequences (e.g., Baumeister, Bratslavsky, Muraven, & Tice, 1998; Baumeister & Heatherton, 1996; Baumeister, Heatherton, & Tice, 1994; Loewenstein, 1996). Surprisingly, there has been a relatively small amount of research on the strategies individuals employ to overcome temptation. Walter Mischel's seminal research on delay of gratification has demonstrated that the cognitive strategies children employ when facing a conflict between immediate and delayed rewards (e.g., distraction, abstract representation of the immediate reward) determine their ability to wait for the larger delayed reward (Metcalfe & Mischel, 1999; Mischel, 1974; Mischel, Shoda, & Rodriguez, 1989). However, beyond the delay-of-gratification paradigm, there has been little systematic research on self-control strategies, the conditions that give rise to the use of those strategies, and the consequences of their use for the pursuit of one's goals.

To address these issues, we have conducted a program of research on *counteractive control*—namely, on how people protect their high-order goals against the influence of low-order temptations. Based on *counteractive control theory* (CCT—Fishbach & Trope, 2005; Trope & Fishbach, 2000), this research assumes that when low-order temptations threaten the attainment of high-order goals, people proactively employ counteractive control designed to offset the influence of low-order temptations on their behavior. Counteractive control is often an intentional process of committing to high-order goals and eliminating tempting alternatives. For example, dieters may deliberately plan to impose real and mental sanctions on themselves for failure to follow their self-imposed dietary constraints. Counteractive control may also be an unconscious process. For example, the temptation to have fatty food may automatically bring to mind thoughts about the goal to lose weight, which in turn may alter the dieter's motivation to order this food in a restaurant. The present chapter describes a program of research on these deliberative and implicit counteractive control processes. We start with a general description of the process of counteractive control. Next, we describe research on specific counteractive control strategies, what activates them, and how they help people overcome temptation. We end with a review of research bearing on the goal-directedness and flexibility of counteractive control processes.

## COUNTERACTIVE CONTROL

In order to accomplish high-order goals, individuals need to resist the momentarily salient, yet lower-priority, desires or temptations with which these goals are in conflict. CCT assumes that temptations are defined within a given situation and with respect to the overriding goals at hand. This context-specific definition of temptations suggests that any personal goal can potentially constitute an interfering temptation with respect to another higher-level goal. For example, while "working out" may be perceived as interfering with the pursuit of higher-order academic objectives, this activity may in itself represent a goal that is disrupted by other low-order enticements, such as the consumption of unhealthy food. Thus the immediate cost of studying is that one has to give up on a workout, whereas the immediate cost of keeping in shape is that one has to give up on one's favorite foods.

In response to temptations, individuals engage in self-control operations designed to protect their long-term interests (Dhar & Wertenbroch, 2000; Gollwitzer, 1999; Kivetz & Simonson, 2002; Kuhl, 1986; Metcalfe & Mischel, 1999; Muraven & Baumeister, 2000; Trope & Fishbach, 2000). Specifically, the presence of temptations influences behavior in two opposite directions. Directly, temptations act to decrease the likelihood of acting according to high-order goals. However indirectly, temptations elicit counteractive control operations, which in turn act to increase the likelihood of acting in line with goals. For example, an invitation to go out on the night before an important exam directly decreases the likelihood of studying, but it may further set into action counteractive bolstering of the value of studying, which increases the likelihood of engaging in this activity. On a cold winter night, the perceived attractiveness of going out is small, and little or no counteractive control will be exercised. However, on a beautiful spring night, the greater threat to studying may elicit more intensive counteractive control efforts. As a result, a student who is tempted to go out on a beautiful spring night may study at least as much as a student who is not tempted to go out on a cold winter night. In itself, the attractiveness of going out acts to diminish the motivation to study. However, the counteractive control efforts elicited by the anticipated pleasure of this activity may prevent the anticipated pleasure from actually affecting the time that a student devotes to studying.

CCT assumes that counteractive control is a flexible, goal-directed process. Counteractive control therefore depends on the value of the high-order goal and on the absence of alternative means of overcoming temptation and shielding one's long-term interests. It is only when low-order motives are expected to interfere with the attainment of important goals, and when external controls over one's behaviors are absent, that counteractive control processes are set into action and determine the attainment of high-order objectives.

Self-control dilemmas are often experienced as an internal conflict that is resolved by employing a variety of metacognitive strategies such as precommitments (Green & Rachlin, 1996; Rachlin & Green, 1972; Thaler, 1991), self-imposed penalties and rewards (Ainslie, 1975; Becker, 1960), and the formation of implementation intentions (Gollwitzer, 1990; Gollwitzer & Brandstätter, 1997). CCT acknowledges the contribution of these high-level self-control strategies to the resolution of self-control dilemmas. However, CCT further proposes that self-control dilemmas may be resolved outside of conscious awareness and without intentional planning. In this respect, CCT is consistent with past research on automatic goal pursuit (e.g., Aarts & Dijksterhuis, 2000; Bargh & Chartrand, 1999; Bargh & Ferguson, 2000; Bargh, Gollwitzer, Lee-Chai, Barndollar, & Troetschel, 2001; Moskowitz, Gollwitzer, Wasel, & Schaal, 1999; Shah & Kruglanski, 2003), which has demonstrated that individuals are sometimes unaware of the origins of their goals, their choice of means, and the actual pursuit of these goals. CCT goes beyond this research by proposing that implicit counteractive control may be elicited by situational cues and at the same time may act to offset the influence of these cues on behavior (e.g., Fishbach, Friedman, & Kruglanski, 2003; Fishbach & Shah, 2006; Gollwitzer, Bayer, & McCulloch, 2005; Moskowitz et al., 1999). In what follows, we describe some of the deliberate and implicit counteractive control strategies our research has explored.

## Deliberate Counteractive Control

### *Self-Imposed Penalties*

Individuals may attempt to ensure that they pursue their high-order interests by imposing on themselves penalties ("side bets") for failing to do so (Ainslie, 1975; Becker, 1960). These self-imposed penalties may then actually prevent individuals from deviating from their goal pursuits. We investigated this strategy in a study that manipulated the short-term costs of undertaking an activity that had long-term benefits. The question we addressed in this study was how short-term costs affect the magnitude of self-imposed penalties (Trope & Fishbach, 2000, Study 1). We offered participants an opportunity to take a diagnostic test that required abstinence from food containing glucose for either a short period of time (6 hours) or a long period of time (3 days). The period of abstinence manipulated the costs of completing the test. Participants were then asked to indicate the amount of money they would be willing to pay as a penalty for failing to complete the test. In line with CCT, they chose to set higher penalties for failure to complete a long period of abstinence than a short period of abstinence. Since in itself, a long period of abstinence increases the likelihood of failure and thus the likelihood of having to pay the monetary penalty, we concluded that participants used the penalties to ensure that the abstinence did not prevent them from attaining the useful feedback.

### *Self-Imposed Reward Contingencies*

Individuals may change choice situations by making a reward contingent on performing an activity. We examined this strategy by assessing participants' interest in making a bonus contingent upon completing a test (Trope & Fishbach, 2000, Study 2). Participants were offered an opportunity to take part in a study on the risk of heart disease that included a cardiovascular test, which was said to be highly diagnostic but to involve either a low or high degree of physical discomfort. The participants were also offered an extra course credit for undergoing the test, and were asked to indicate whether they preferred to receive the credit before or after completing the test. Delaying the bonus made it contingent on completing the test. As predicted, those who expected the more painful test showed a greater preference to receive the bonus after the test—that is, to make the bonus contingent on actual completion of the test. By self-imposing this contingency, participants risked losing the bonus, but they also motivated themselves to complete the more painful cardiovascular test.

Self-imposed penalties and self-imposed contingencies for receiving a reward change the choice situation. By adopting these strategies, individuals precommit themselves to acting according to their long-term interests (Brickman, 1987). Individuals may precommit themselves more directly by eliminating action alternatives and thus making their decision to act irreversible (Ainslie, 1975; Green & Rachlin, 1996; Rachlin & Green, 1972; Schelling, 1978, 1984; Strotz, 1956; Thaler, 1991; Thaler & Shefrin, 1981). For example, people may choose to eliminate the presence of cigarettes, alcohol, or high-calorie food in order to increase the likelihood of pursuing a healthy lifestyle. By adopting this strategy, people eliminate their future freedom of choice, which they ordinarily seek to maintain (Brehm, 1966), in order to secure the attainment of high-order interests.

### *Bolstering the Value of an Activity*

Other counteractive control strategies change the meaning of choice alternatives. People may selectively process information about these alternatives in order to increase the value of adhering to high-order goals and decrease the value of low-order temptations (e.g., Kuhl, 1986; Mischel, 1984). The value of high-order goals is increased by linking the attainment of these goals to self-standards. Failure to pursue these goals is then construed as a violation of important values and a threat to people's sense of self-worth (Bandura, 1989). In addition, people may bolster the value of attaining their goals by elaborating upon what makes attainment of these goals important and emotionally gratifying (Beckmann & Kuhl, 1985; Fishbach, Shah, & Kruglanski, 2004; Kuhl, 1984).

In a study that tested for counteractive evaluations (i.e., individuals' tendency to bolster the importance and perceived interest of an activity that serves a high-order goal but has immediate costs), participants were offered to take a test of the influence of glucose intake on their cognitive functioning (Trope & Fishbach, 2000, Study 3). As in our previous study, the test was described as requiring abstinence from food containing glucose for either a long or a short period (3 days vs. 6 hours). We then found that participants evaluated the test more positively when it required a long period of glucose abstinence than when it required a short period of abstinence. Furthermore, this study also assessed participants' intention to take the test. A series of path analyses conducted on behavioral intentions revealed that in itself, a long versus short period of abstinence directly decreased participants' interest in taking the test. But indirectly, a long versus short period of abstinence elicited bolstering of the value of the test, which in turn increased participants' interest in the test. These direct and indirect effects canceled each other out, suggesting that counteractive bolstering of the value of a costly test prevented the physical discomfort of the test from diminishing participants' interest in undergoing the test.

The counteractive control processes described thus far proactively change the motivational givens of choice situations, thereby increasing the likelihood of adhering to long-term interests. These processes are deliberate and may require some level of conscious awareness, intentionality, and processing resources. As such, they may depend on cognitive load, time pressure, mood, fatigue, and prior self-control efforts (see also Baumeister et al., 1998; Mischel, 1996; Muraven & Baumeister, 2000; Trope & Neter, 1994; Vohs & Heatherton, 2000). In the rest of this section, we explore the possibility that deliberate counteractive control strategies are supplemented and even supplanted by more implicit forms of counteractive control, which are elicited automatically and are less susceptible to depleted mental resources.

## Implicit Counteractive Control

Individuals may engage in counteractive control without realizing that they are trying to overcome temptation. They may be aware of the presence of a temptation and consciously try to bolster the value of their higher-order goal, without recognizing the relationship between the temptation and the bolstering responses. For instance, students may not fully recognize the relationship between an enhanced evaluation of an upcoming exam and the presence of their favorite television show, which poses a temptation to give up studying. Individuals may thus see their biased evaluations as reflecting the inherent value of different choice alternatives rather than as a mechanism that directs their choice among these alternatives. In these cases, the temptations and the overriding goals are processed consciously. It is possible, however, for the temptation to elicit counteractive control automatically without conscious awareness. The studies described below were designed to test this possibility.

### Implicit Counteractive Activation

CCT proposes that when a temptation is made salient, individuals may respond by directing their attention to the overriding goal. Consistent with this proposal, we found that students who were asked to describe their favorite social activities subsequently elaborated on the value of studying, and as a result were more likely to study for their exams (Trope & Fishbach, 2000, Study 5). A similar process of goal activation by temptation may take place more implicitly when people are unaware of the presentation of temptation-related primes. Moreover, not only temptations elicit automatic goal activation (i.e., greater goal accessibility); the presentation of goal-related primes can elicit inhibition of concepts related to temptations (i.e., weaker temptation accessibility) (Fishbach et al., 2003; Shah, Friedman, & Kruglanski, 2002).

These processes were explored in a series of studies that assessed (1) the activation level of a construct representing a potential goal after a subliminal presentation of a construct representing a potentially obstructive temptation, and (2) the activation of temptation constructs after presentation of goal constructs (Fishbach et al., 2003). These studies found that temptation-related concepts facilitated the activation level of goals (as indicated by faster lexical decision times), whereas goal-related concepts inhibited the activation of temptations (as indicated by slower lexical decision times). For example, one of these studies used participants' self-reported goals and temptations to obtain goal–temptation pairs such as *study–basketball* or *faithful–sex*. It was then found that goal-related keywords (e.g., *study*) were more quickly recognized following subliminal presentation of temptation-related keywords (e.g., *basketball*), whereas temptation recognition was inhibited by goal primes (Fishbach et al., 2003, Study 1). This was taken as evidence for implicit counteractive control, because participants were unaware of the subliminally presented goal and temptation stimuli.

Using a similar sequential priming procedure, another study (Fishbach et al., 2003, Study 2) found that this temptation-elicited goal activation was independent of cognitive load (memorizing a nine-digit number). Participants under cognitive load and participants under no load were equally likely to activate concepts representing a goal after being primed with concepts representing temptation, and they were also equally likely to inhibit concepts representing temptation after being primed with goal concepts. For example, independent of load conditions, temptation primes (e.g., *drugs*) facilitated the activation level of targets related to religious goals (e.g., *bible*), whereas religious primes inhibited the activation of targets related to temptations.

Other studies (Fishbach et al., 2003, Studies 4–5) found a direct link between implicit activation patterns of this sort and successful resolution of a self-control dilemma. These studies found, for example, that dieters activated concepts related to dieting in response to fatty food primes. As a result, after being exposed to food primes, dieters were more likely to choose a healthy snack over a fatty snack in a subsequent choice task. It seems likely, then, that as a result of counteractive control individuals associate temptations with concepts related to an overriding goal, and these associative patterns may then shield them against the detrimental effect of temptations.

### Implicit Counteractive Evaluation

Keeping an overriding goal at the forefront of attention diminishes the value of acting according to short-term preferences. However, people may also directly decrease the value of succumbing to a temptation by attending to its negative affective aspects and by attending to the positive aspects of an overriding goal. These counteractive evaluations may take an explicit form when, for instance, individuals elaborate upon what makes the attainment of some goals important and emotionally gratifying (Fishbach & Trope, 2005; Kuhl, 1984; Trope & Fishbach, 2000). They may also be expressed more implicitly in the form of an implicit evaluation.

We used an evaluative priming procedure to investigate implicit counteractive evaluations (e.g., Bargh, Chaiken, Govender, & Pratto, 1992; Fazio, Jackson, Dunton, & Williams, 1995; Fazio, Sanbonmatsu, Powell, & Kardes,

1986). We predicted that counteractive evaluations would produce asymmetrical shifts in subjective value: Accessible goal-related constructs would undermine the value of temptation, whereas accessible temptation-related constructs would augment the value of the goal.

In one study (Fishbach, Zhang, & Trope, 2007, Study 1), we manipulated goal accessibility by asking participants to unscramble sentences that included words related to achievement (e.g., *ambitious*, *excellent*) or not (Bargh & Chartrand, 2000; Srull & Wyer, 1979). We then measured the implicit evaluation of academic and nonacademic concepts in a second task that assessed the time for categorizing positive and negative target words after subliminal academic (e.g., *study*) and nonacademic (e.g., *movie*) primes. As expected, when achievement goals were accessible (vs. the control condition), subliminal nonacademic primes facilitated the categorization of negative targets, whereas subliminal academic primes facilitated the categorization of positive targets. For example, nonacademic primes facilitated categorization of *cancer*, whereas academic primes facilitated *love*.

Another study (Fishbach et al., 2007, Study 4) manipulated the accessibility of temptations, this time in the domain of healthy eating. Participants, who were all weight watchers, evaluated pictures depicting unhealthy food items (e.g., chocolate cake, ice cream) versus neutral pictures in the control condition. We then measured the implicit evaluation of unhealthy versus healthy food concepts (e.g., *pizza* vs. *salad*), using a similar evaluative priming procedure. In the condition of accessible temptations, we found a counteractive boost in the implicit value of healthy foods. Furthermore, a greater accessibility of unhealthy foods undermined the implicit value of these foods. These results further demonstrate that when faced with self-control conflicts, individuals engage in implicit counteractive evaluations that increase the value of the goal in response to temptation-related cues, and decrease the value of temptation in response to goal-related cues.

### *Implicit Dispositions toward Goals and away from Temptations*

While exercising self-control, individuals often choose to keep tempting objects out of sight and far from reach, while maintaining a close proximity to other objects that are more closely associated with their long-term objectives (Ainslie, 1992; Rachlin & Green, 1972; Schelling, 1984; Thaler & Shefrin, 1981; Wertenbroch, 1998). For example, foreseeing the self-control problems that the presence of cigarettes, alcohol, or culinary delights may induce, people sometimes choose to eliminate these objects from their houses; or, foreseeing the problems that a previous romantic partner may impose, a person sometimes moves to a different city or job.

A series of studies by Fishbach and Shah (2006) examined a more implicit form of these counteractive tactics. The method was based on the finding reported by Solarz (1960), and then by Bargh and his colleagues (Chen & Bargh, 1999; Duckworth, Bargh, Garcia, & Chaiken, 2002), that people are faster to pull a lever toward them to indicate an approach orientation and to pull a lever away from them to indicate an avoidance orientation. Fishbach and Shah found that while participants tended to automatically approach stimuli related to goals (through faster pulling responses), they avoided temptation stimuli (through faster pulling and pushing responses). Interestingly, the participants' tendency to avoid temptations increased in direct proportion to their explicit evaluation that these temptations were indeed attractive for them, and it had instrumental value in offsetting individuals' original tendency to approach tempting stimuli. For example, successful (vs. less successful) student participants responded faster with pulling (i.e., approaching) when presented with academic stimuli (e.g., *studying*), and with pushing (i.e., avoiding) when presented with nonacademic stimuli (e.g., *partying*). These tendencies increased with the perceived attractiveness of nonacademic temptations during a break in the academic schedule, when they did not pose a threat for goal attainment (Fishbach & Shah, 2006, Study 3).

Moreover, the tendency to automatically approach goals and avoid temptations facilitated the attainment of high-order interests. For example, in another study (Fishbach & Shah, 2006, Study 4), reaction times for pulling academic goals (e.g., *library*, *homework*) and pushing nonacademic temptations (e.g., *travel*, *party*) predicted student participants' grade point averages. Similarly, participants who were asked to pull (i.e., approach) in response to academic-related concepts, and to push (i.e., avoid) in response to nonacademic concepts, were planning to invest more time in their homework than were students who completed the opposite categorization task. These findings suggest that implicit approach and avoidance predispositions of this sort may play an important role in adhering to high-order goals.

Taken together, the studies described in this section shed light on the counteractive control strategies people employ when they anticipate situations that pit low-order temptations against high-order goals. These strategies change the motivational givens of the choice situation in order to secure the attainment of high-order goals. The greater the temptation to abandon the goals, the more likely people are to exercise counteractive control, and as a result to remain committed to pursuing their goals. The research described in this section further demonstrates that counteractive boosting of high-order goals and the resulting resistance to temptation may be implicit processes. These implicit operations are important, since they enable people to successfully implement their goals under conditions of depleted resources and whenever there is an advantage for responding quickly. Implicit counteractive control of this sort produces an implicit inoculation against situations that pose a threat to people's long-term objectives. This implicit inoculation mechanism may then free the individuals to set high-level goals without having to exert much effort in resisting immediate temptations.

## THE FLEXIBILITY OF COUNTERACTIVE CONTROL

CCT assumes that counteractive control is a flexible, goal-directed mechanism that is set into action when low-order temptations interfere with individuals' pursuit of their high-order interests. The research described in the earlier section supports this assumption by showing that counteractive control processes are contingent on exposure to low-order temptations that interfere with pursuing goals. In this section, we explore two additional hypotheses that follow the assumption that counteractive control is a flexible self-control process. The first is that *counteractive control is goal-dependent*. That is, individuals will exert more counteractive control when low-order desires threaten important rather than unimportant goals. Once a goal is achieved, counteractive control will cease. The second hypothesis is that *counteractive control is substitutable*. That is, counteractive control will be exerted when it is necessary for achieving goals. When other, external means of control are in place, counteractive control will cease.

### Goal-Dependent Counteractive Control

CCT assumes that counteractive control efforts are means to the end of attaining long-term interests. One could argue, however, that these efforts have intrinsic value—that overcoming temptations is challenging in and of itself (Atkinson & Feather, 1966; Brehm & Self, 1989; Brehm, Wright, Solomon, Silka, & Greenberg, 1983; Wright & Brehm, 1984). One could also argue that temptations activate counteractive evaluations inflexibly, regardless of people's goals. Our findings that counteractive control actually helps individuals attain their goals indirectly support the goal-directedness assumption of CCT. Several studies, described below, provide a more direct test of this assumption.

#### *Goal Importance*

If counteractive control is goal-dependent, then it should depend on the importance individuals place on the threatened high-order goal. This hypothesis was originally tested in the study on the self-imposed contingencies for receiving a reward (Trope & Fishbach, 2000). Recall that in that study, participants made a bonus contingent upon completion of a cardiovascular test when the test was described as physically painful. This study also assessed the importance participants placed on maintaining good health, before the information about the cardiovascular test was handed out. We found that only participants to whom maintaining good health was an important value preferred the bonus to be contingent on completing the painful test. The rest of the participants, to whom health was a less important value, tended to choose according to simple economic considerations—accepting the bonus before rather than after completing the test. It seems, then, that short-term costs do not elicit counteractive control unless they threaten central values.

### Goal Completion

If counteractive control is goal-dependent, then it should be employed before rather than after goal completion. We tested for this hypothesis by assessing counteractive bolstering of the value of studying for an important exam before and after the exam, and as a function of priming social motives that interfere with studying (Trope & Fishbach, 2000, Study 5). Before an exam, bolstering the value of studying may have instrumental value in helping students prepare for the exam. After the exam, studying is no longer a goal, and bolstering its value can only reduce the dissonance created by what the students had to sacrifice in order to pursue this activity (Aronson, 1997; Cooper & Fazio, 1984; Festinger, 1957; Shultz & Lepper, 1996).

Participants in this study were students 1 week before or after taking a midterm exam in an introductory psychology course. A temptation to abstain from studying was primed by asking half of the students to elaborate on their social lives. These questions were followed by questions regarding the value and importance of the exam, which assessed counteractive bolstering of studying. Consistent with our predictions, we found that priming of competing social motives led students to bolster the importance of studying before taking the exam, but not after taking it. After the exam, social priming had no effect on evaluations, which were generally low. Moreover, a series of path analyses indicated that evaluative bolstering enhanced students' performance on the upcoming exam. Specifically, before the exam, social priming directly impaired performance on the exam, but indirectly this priming manipulation led participants to bolster the value of studying, which in turn predicted relatively high grades on the exam. These opposite effects of social priming canceled each other out, so that overall counteractive control prevented social priming from impairing grades on the exam. This pattern of results was not obtained 1 week after the exam, when counteractive bolstering of the value of studying no longer had any instrumental value. Consistent with the goal-directedness assumption, these findings suggest that counteractive control is exercised only when there is an important goal at stake.

### Goal-Dependent Implicit Counteractive Control

Is implicit counteractive control goal-dependent? Does it depend on the importance of the overriding goal? Recent studies have found evidence for flexibility and goal dependency in automatic evaluations (e.g., Ferguson & Bargh, 2004; Mitchell, Nosek, & Banaji, 2003). Does this also hold true for implicit counteractive control? To address this question, we examined whether an implicit devaluation of temptations depends on the presence of an accessible goal (Fishbach et al., 2007); as indicated earlier, only those who were primed with an achievement goal expressed an implicit negative evaluation of nonacademic temptations along with an implicit positive evaluation of the goal.

In yet another study, we tested for individual differences in chronically holding a goal. We predicted that only committed individuals (e.g., committed dieters) would express an implicit negative evaluation of temptations (e.g., fattening foods). This study assessed commitment to dieting by using a subset of the Restrained Eating Scale (Polivy, Herman, & Warsh, 1978; Ruderman & Besbeas, 1992), and it used an evaluative priming task similar to that of Fazio and colleagues (1995): It assessed the speed of categorizing negative and positive targets following subliminal presentation of concepts related to high-calorie food versus weight-watching primes. In support of the goal dependency assumption, subliminal food primes (e.g., *candy, cake*) facilitated the categorization of negative (vs. positive) targets, and subliminal weight-watching primes (e.g., *diet, slim*) facilitated categorization of positive (vs. negative) targets, but only for committed dieters. These effects were not observed among participants who were not trying to lose weight and therefore did not exhibit an implicit negative evaluation of temptations and positive evaluation of goals. Another study examined the effect of commitment to dieting on participants' implicit dispositions toward approaching weight-watching concepts and avoiding food-related concepts (Fishbach & Shah, 2006, Study 2). As expected, participants showed faster response times for pulling (i.e., approaching) words related to weight watching, and pushing (i.e., avoiding) words related to high-calorie food, but only to the extent that they were concerned with watching their weight.

Commitment to dieting may also moderate the goal-activation-by-temptation effect. In a study that tested for this idea, participants completed a subliminal priming lexical decision task in which the targets were words related to dieting and the subliminal primes were either related to high-calorie food or not

(Fishbach et al., 2003, Study 4). Participants also indicated how important weight watching was for them, and how successful they were at watching their weight. It was then found that the more important weight watching was to participants, the faster successful (but not unsuccessful) self-regulators were to recognize diet-related targets following fattening food primes (but not control primes). In other words, only committed dieters who were successful at controlling their body weight associated food temptations with dieting. This pattern suggests that successful, more than unsuccessful, self-regulators developed implicit counteractive controls in direct proportion to their goal commitment.

In sum, the present studies on goal dependency provide consistent support for the assumption that counteractive control is a goal-directed process—a means to the end of securing the pursuit of long-term interests. Interestingly, both implicit and more deliberate forms of counteractive control show goal dependency. Individuals seem to exercise implicit or deliberate counteractive control only when important goals are at stake.

## The Substitutability of Self-Control

The assumption that counteractive controls are goal-directed suggests that they are substitutable—namely, that they are set into action only in the absence of alternative, external means of control. Such alternatives often take the form of social controls, such as family members, employers, and other social agents that impose incentives, social norms, and rules designed to help individuals overcome temptations. Media censorship, and laws prohibiting substance abuse and gambling, are common examples of externally imposed controls. Organizations may encourage and even require their members to maintain their health by refraining from cigarette smoking, engaging in physical exercise, and undergoing periodical medical checkups. At a more informal level, individuals sometime criticize their friends or family members for eating fattening food or overspending.

These external means of control may be sufficient to maintain a high probability of acting according to high-order goals, and may thus substitute for self-control. For example, the presence of social incentives to complete a boring drill may render counteractive bolstering of this activity unnecessary. In general, CCT predicts that in the absence of external control, counteractive self-control will be exercised, because it determines the likelihood of pursuing one's goals. However, in the presence of external control, counteractive self-control may become superfluous, as external control may be sufficient to maintain a high probability of acting according to high-order goals. External control may thus substitute for self-control.

Take, for instance, the effects of externally imposed controls on counteractive evaluation and actual choice of an option with long-term value. In the absence of externally imposed controls, self-control will be exercised and the option will be evaluated *more positively* when it is expected to have *higher short-term costs*. These prechoice counteractive evaluations in turn will offset the impact of the higher expected short-term costs on actual choice of the option. Thus, by eliciting greater counteractive control efforts, the higher expected short-term costs of an option should indirectly act to increase the likelihood of choosing the option. In contrast, in the presence of externally imposed controls, self-control efforts will not be exerted; as a result, the evaluation of the option will reflect its expected short-term costs. That is, in the presence of externally imposed controls, an option will be evaluated *more negatively* when it has *higher short-term costs*. However, externally imposed controls will prevent this evaluation from decreasing the likelihood of actually choosing the option. Thus, as is in the absence of externally imposed controls, the likelihood of choosing the option will not be diminished by its higher expected short-term costs.

These substitutability predictions were tested in a study that presented participants with an opportunity to take a diagnostic test of their cognitive functioning at night (Fishbach & Trope, 2005, Study 3). The immediate cost of taking the test was varied by scheduling the test either at a convenient early-night time (9:00 P.M.) or an inconvenient late-night time (1:00 A.M.). We further manipulated social control by either offering or not offering a large payment (approximately $20) for taking the test. Two forms of counteractive control were assessed. First, to assess self-imposed fines, participants were asked to indicate the amount of money they were prepared to pay as a cancellation fee if they failed to complete the test. Second, evaluative bolstering was assessed by the perceived value of the test. Finally, participants were asked to decide whether they actually intended to take the test.

Analysis of the self-imposed fines yielded the expected pattern, indicating that the fines unpaid participants imposed on themselves were higher when the test was scheduled at an inconvenient late-night time than when the test was scheduled at a convenient early-night time. In contrast, the fines paid participants imposed on themselves were unaffected by the time of the test. It appears that payment eliminated the need to use the fines as a self-control strategy. In other words, externally imposed control substituted for self-imposed penalties. Analysis of participants' evaluations of the test yielded a similar pattern. Unpaid participants evaluated the test more positively when it was scheduled at an inconvenient time, whereas paid participants evaluated the test more positively when it was scheduled at a convenient time. Unlike unpaid participants, the evaluations by paid participants showed a more conventional effect of temporary inconvenience—that is, a less positive evaluation of the inconvenient test than of the convenient test. Paid participants apparently allowed the inconvenience of the test to diminish their evaluation of the test. As with self-imposed penalties, the promised payment substituted for evaluative bolstering of the inconvenient test.

In another study, external controls were instituted via social monitoring (Fishbach & Trope, 2005, Study 1). The study offered participants the opportunity to take a diagnostic test of their reading skills and assessed their evaluation of the test. The immediate price of taking the test was manipulated by describing the test as involving reading boring versus interesting short paragraphs. Social monitoring was manipulated by having the experimenter present or absent while participants made their decision whether or not to complete the test. As expected, participants bolstered the value of the boring (rather than interesting) test only in the absence of an experimenter in the room. Similar results were obtained in a study that primed social controls (Fishbach & Trope, 2005, Study 2). Participants were either primed or not primed with representations of others who expected the participants to study (e.g., a parent or a teacher). In addition, participants were either primed or not primed with activities that would interfere with studying (e.g., watching television, going to movies). We found that when external controls were not primed, the priming (vs. no priming) of distracting activities elicited more positive evaluation of studying. In contrast, when external controls were primed, the priming of distracting activities elicited more negative evaluation of studying. Thus, consistent with the substitutability assumption, priming social controls eliminated counteractive bolstering of studying, so that studying seemed less attractive when its immediate costs came to mind.

Overall, the results of these studies are consistent with the idea that self-control and external control are substitutable. An immediate temptation steers people away from activities that serve an overriding goal. In the absence of external means of control, individuals exercise counteractive control in order to overcome this temptation. The presence of external controls (e.g., representations of others, social monitoring, and external rewards) secures the attainment of important goals regardless of immediate temptations. As a result, in the presence of external controls, individuals' evaluations of activities reflect, rather than counteract, the presence of those costs.

## CONCLUSIONS

The research reviewed in this chapter has important implications regarding goal activation and hedonic conceptions of human motivation. A simple goal activation rule would suggest that activating a goal promotes its pursuit and inhibits activation and pursuit of conflicting goals (see e.g., Bargh & Chartrand, 1999; Bargh & Ferguson, 2000; Kruglanski et al., 2002; Shah et al., 2002). By this rule, activating social goals (e.g., partying) should increase the pursuit of social goals and inhibit achievement goals (e.g., studying). The research reviewed in this chapter suggests that this is not always the case. For example, we found that priming social goals before an exam promoted rather than weakened students' commitment to studying and actually improved their performance on the exam (Trope & Fishbach, 2000, Study 5). It seems, then, that to predict how the activation of a goal affects behavior, it is necessary to take into account the relationship of that goal to one's high-order, overriding interests. When a given goal (partying) interferes with the attainment of one's high-order interests (doing well on an exam), activating the interfering goal promotes the pursuit of these interests rather than the interfering goal.

Similar considerations apply to hedonic conceptions of motivation. A simple hedonic rule would suggest that behavior is a function of the pleasure and pain with which it is associated. Attaching pleasurable outcomes to a behavior should increase its probability, and attaching negative outcomes to the behavior should decrease its probability. By this rule, nice weather should increase the likelihood that a student studying for an exam will abstain from studying. Similarly, the painfulness of a medical procedure should decrease the likelihood that it will actually be undertaken. The research on counteractive control suggests that behavior often violates this simple hedonic rule. For example, we found that describing a medical checkup as more painful increased participants' commitment to undergoing the checkup (Trope & Fishbach, 2000, Studies 1–3). Thus attaching pleasurable outcomes to a behavior may reduce its attractiveness when the behavior is in conflict with high-order goals, and attaching painful outcomes to a behavior may increase its appeal when the behavior serves high-order goals.

These seemingly paradoxical exceptions to simple goal activation and hedonic rules may reflect the same counteractive control logic. Without counteractive control, an action becomes less attractive when it is implicitly or explicitly associated with high short-term costs. The sacrifices that are associated with weight watching, undergoing medical checkups, or studying act to reduce the attractiveness of engaging in these activities. Counteractive control, in both its implicit and deliberate forms, serves to increase the attractiveness of such activities in direct proportion to their short-term costs. As a result, counteractive control helps maintain a high probability of pursuing high-order goals, despite the short-term costs this may entail. This enables people to set goals and formulate plans for achieving them, with a sense of assurance that they will not be tempted to deviate from their plans in a way that they will later regret.

Our research suggests that counteractive control is a flexible, goal-directed process. First, people seem to exercise counteractive control when situational temptations threaten their ability to pursue important rather than unimportant high-order goals. Second, counteractive control decreases following the pursuit of a goal-related activity. Before performing an activity, counteractive control can help people choose and carry out the activity, whereas after performing the activity, counteractive control has no instrumental value and can only reduce dissonance and regret (Aronson, 1997; Cooper & Fazio, 1984; Festinger, 1957). Third, counteractive control is substitutable. People exercise self-control when it is necessary for achieving their high-order goals. When other means of control are in place (e.g., social agents or material rewards), counteractive control becomes superfluous and ceases.

The flexibility of counteractive control processes does not mean that they are necessarily based on deliberate reasoning. Past self-control research has been primarily concerned with high-level evaluative processes (Baumeister et al., 1998; Beckmann & Kuhl, 1985; Gollwitzer, 1990; Gollwitzer & Brandstätter, 1997; Mischel, 1984; Mischel, Cantor, & Feldman, 1996). The present research adds to this work by demonstrating more implicit forms of counteractive control that, like deliberate counteractive controls, shield high-order goals from low-order temptations. We believe that counteractive controls, like any other mental operation, may become automatized after being repeatedly and successfully employed in resolving self-control problems. As a result, individuals may need to engage in very little conscious deliberation in carrying out some or all of the steps of counteractive control.

The research described in this chapter may help shed new light on the processes of counteractive control, but important questions regarding the origins of counteractive controls, the relationships among different kinds of counteractive controls, and their consequences remain unexplored. One such question is how implicit controls develop. It seems plausible to suggest that these controls develop over repeated experiences at deliberate self-control attempts. Alternatively, implicit and deliberative counteractive controls may develop in parallel, as two independent sets of distinctive control systems that complement each other. Another question concerns the relationship between different counteractive control strategies, and specifically between deliberate and implicit controls. It is possible that different counteractive control strategies can substitute for each other or serve as a "backup system" in relation to each other. Alternatively, it is also possible that only a combination of counteractive control strategies enables successful pursuit of long-term interests. We know very little about the operation and consequences of counteractive control when individuals are stressed, fatigued, or emotionally aroused. Does unavailability or underutilization of counteractive controls predict the self-control failures that have been documented in the self-control literature (see, e.g., Baumeister et al., 1994, 1998; Muraven & Baumeister, 2000)? We also know very little about how individuals assess their ability to control themselves, how perceived self-control is related to the availability and use of counteractive controls, and how perceived self-control affects specific outcome expectancies and individuals' general sense of self-efficacy. Future research addressing these questions would help advance our understanding of self-control as a unique facet of human motivation.

## REFERENCES

Aarts, H., & Dijksterhuis, A. (2000). Habits as knowledge structures: Automaticity in goal-directed behavior. *Journal of Personality and Social Psychology, 78*(1), 53–63.

Ainslie, G. (1975). Specious reward: A behavioral theory of impulsiveness and impulse control. *Psychological Bulletin, 82*(4), 463–496.

Ainslie, G. (1992). *Picoeconomics: The strategic interaction of successive motivational states within the person.* Cambridge, UK: Cambridge University Press.

Ainslie, G. (2001). *Breakdown of will.* New York: Cambridge University Press.

Aronson, E. (1997). The theory of cognitive dissonance: The evolution and vicissitudes of an idea. In C. McGarty & S. A. Haslam (Eds.), *The message of social psychology: Perspectives on mind in society* (pp. 20–35). Cambridge, MA: Blackwell.

Atkinson, J. W., & Feather, N. T. (1966). *A theory of achievement motivation.* New York: Wiley.

Bandura, A. (1989). Self-regulation of motivation and action through internal standards and goal systems. In L. A. Pervin (Ed.), *Goal concepts in personality and social psychology* (pp. 19–85). Hillsdale, NJ: Erlbaum.

Bargh, J. A., Chaiken, S., Govender, R., & Pratto, F. (1992). The generality of the automatic attitude activation effect. *Journal of Personality and Social Psychology, 62*(6), 893–912.

Bargh, J. A., & Chartrand, T. L. (1999). The unbearable automaticity of being. *American Psychologist, 54*(7), 462–479.

Bargh, J. A., & Chartrand, T. L. (2000). The mind in the middle: A practical guide to priming and automaticity research. In H. T. Reis & C. M. Judd (Eds.), *Handbook of research methods in social and personality psychology* (pp. 253–285). New York: Cambridge University Press.

Bargh, J. A., & Ferguson, M. J. (2000). Beyond behaviorism: On the automaticity of higher mental processes. *Psychological Bulletin, 126*(6), 925–945.

Bargh, J. A., Gollwitzer, P. M., Lee-Chai, A., Barndollar, K., & Troetschel, R. (2001). The automated will: Nonconscious activation and pursuit of behavioral goals. *Journal of Personality and Social Psychology, 81*(6), 1014–1027.

Baumeister, R. F., Bratslavsky, E., Muraven, M., & Tice, D. M. (1998). Ego depletion: Is the active self a limited resource? *Journal of Personality and Social Psychology, 74*(5), 1252–1265.

Baumeister, R. F., & Heatherton, T. F. (1996). Self-regulation failure: An overview. *Psychological Inquiry, 7*(1), 1–15.

Baumeister, R. F., Heatherton, T. F., & Tice, D. M. (1994). *Losing control: How and why people fail at self-regulation.* San Diego, CA: Academic Press.

Baumeister, R. F., & Vohs, K. D. (Eds.). (2004). *Handbook of self-regulation: Research, theory, and applications.* New York: Guilford Press.

Becker, H. S. (1960). Notes on the concept of commitment. *American Journal of Sociology, 66*, 32–40.

Beckmann, J., & Kuhl, J. (1985). *Action control: From cognition to behavior.* Berlin: Springer-Verlag.

Brehm, J. W. (1966). *A theory of psychological reactance.* New York: Academic Press.

Brehm, J. W., Wright, R. A., Solomon, S., Silka, L., & Greenberg, J. (1983). Perceived difficulty, energization, and the magnitude of goal valence. *Journal of Experimental Social Psychology, 19*(1), 21–48.

Brehm, J. W., & Self, E. A. (1989). The intensity of motivation. *Annual Review of Psychology, 40*, 109–131.

Brickman, P. (1987). *Commitment, conflict, and caring.* Englewood Cliffs, NJ: Prentice Hall.

Chen, M., & Bargh, J. A. (1999). Consequences of automatic evaluation: Immediate behavioral predispositions to approach or avoid the stimulus. *Personality and Social Psychology Bulletin, 25*(2), 215–224.

Cooper, J., & Fazio, R. H. (1984). A new look at dissonance theory. In L. Berkowitz (Ed.), *Advances in experimental social psychology* (Vol. 17, pp. 229–264). New York: Academic Press.

Dhar, R., & Wertenbroch, K. (2000). Consumer choice between hedonic and utilitarian goods. *Journal of Marketing Research, 37*(1), 60–71.

Duckworth, K. L., Bargh, J. A., Garcia, M., & Chaiken, S. (2002). The automatic evaluation of novel stimuli. *Psychological Science, 13*(6), 513–519.

Elster, J. (1977). *Ulysses and the sirens.* Cambridge, UK: Cambridge University Press.

Fazio, R. H., Jackson, J. R., Dunton, B. C., & Williams, C. J. (1995). Variability in automatic activation as an unobstrusive measure of racial attitudes: A bona fide pipeline? *Journal of Personality and Social Psychology, 69*(6), 1013–1027.

Fazio, R. H., Sanbonmatsu, D. M., Powell, M. C., &

Kardes, F. R. (1986). On the automatic activation of attitudes. *Journal of Personality and Social Psychology, 50*(2), 229–238.

Ferguson, M., & Bargh, J. A. (2004). Liking is for doing: The effects of goal pursuit on automatic evaluation. *Journal of Personality and Social Psychology, 87*(5), 557–572.

Festinger, L. (1957). *A theory of cognitive dissonance.* Evanston, IL: Row, Peterson.

Fishbach, A., Friedman, R. S., & Kruglanski, A. W. (2003). Leading us not unto temptation: Momentary allurements elicit overriding goal activation. *Journal of Personality and Social Psychology, 84*(2), 296–309.

Fishbach, A., & Shah, J. Y. (2006). Self-control in action: Implicit dispositions toward goals and away from temptations. *Journal of Personality and Social Psychology, 90*(5), 820–832.

Fishbach, A., Shah, J. Y., & Kruglanski, A. W. (2004). Emotional transfer in goal systems. *Journal of Experimental Social Psychology, 40*, 723–738.

Fishbach, A., & Trope, Y. (2005). The substitutability of external control and self-control. *Journal of Experimental Social Psychology, 41*(3), 256–270.

Fishbach, A., Zhang, Y., & Trope, Y. (2007). *Implicit counteractive evaluation.* Unpublished manuscript, University of Chicago.

Gollwitzer, P. M. (1990). Action phases and mind-sets. In E. T. Higgins & R. M. Sorrentino (Eds.), *Handbook of motivation and cognition: Foundations of social behavior* (Vol. 2, pp. 53–92). New York: Guilford Press.

Gollwitzer, P. M. (1999). Implementation intentions: Strong effects of simple plans. *American Psychologist, 54*(7), 493–503.

Gollwitzer, P. M., Bayer, U. C., & McCulloch, K. C. (2005). The control of the unwanted. In J. Uleman, R. Hassin, & J. A. Bargh (Eds.), *The new unconscious* (pp. 485–515). New York: Oxford University Press.

Gollwitzer, P. M., & Brandstätter, V. (1997). Implementation intentions and effective goal pursuit. *Journal of Personality and Social Psychology, 73*(1), 186–199.

Green, L., & Rachlin, H. (1996). Commitment using punishment. *Journal of the Experimental Analysis of Behavior, 65*(3), 593–601.

Kivetz, R., & Simonson, I. (2002). Self-control for the righteous: Toward a theory of precommitment to indulgence. *Journal of Consumer Research, 29*(2), 199–217.

Kruglanski, A. W., Shah, J. Y., Fishbach, A., Friedman, R., Chun, W. Y., & Sleeth-Keppler, D. (2002). A theory of goal systems. In M. P. Zanna (Ed.), *Advances in experimental social psychology* (Vol. 34, pp. 331–378). San Diego, CA: Academic Press.

Kuhl, J. (1984). Volitional aspects of achievement motivation and learned helplessness: Toward a comprehensive theory of action control. In B. A. Maher (Ed.), *Progress in experimental personality research* (Vol. 13, pp. 99–171). New York: Academic Press.

Kuhl, J. (1986). Motivation and information processing: A new look at decision making, dynamic change, and action control. In R. M. Sorrentino & E. T. Higgins (Eds.), *Handbook of motivation and cognition: Foundations of social behavior* (pp. 404–434). New York: Guilford Press.

Kuhl, J., & Beckmann, J. (1985). *Action control from cognition to behavior.* New York: Springer-Verlag.

Loewenstein, G. (1996). Out of control: Visceral influences on behavior. *Organizational Behavior and Human Decision Processes, 65*(3), 272–292.

Metcalfe, J., & Mischel, W. (1999). A hot/cool-system analysis of delay of gratification: Dynamics of willpower. *Psychological Review, 106*(1), 3–19.

Mischel, W. (1964). Personal constructs, rules, and the logic of clinical activity. *Psychological Review, 71*(3), 180–192.

Mischel, W. (1974). Processes in delay of gratification. In L. Berkowitz (Ed.), *Advances in experimental social psychology* (Vol. 7, pp. 249–292). San Diego, CA: Academic Press.

Mischel, W. (1984). Convergences and challenges in the search for consistency. *American Psychologist, 39*(4), 351–364.

Mischel, W. (1996). From good intentions to willpower. In P. M. Gollwitzer & J. A. Bargh (Eds.), *The psychology of action: Linking cognition and motivation to behavior* (pp. 197–218). New York: Guilford Press.

Mischel, W., Cantor, N., & Feldman, S. (1996). Principles of self-regulation: The nature of willpower and self-control. In E. T. Higgins & A. W. Kruglanski (Eds.), *Social psychology: Handbook of basic principles* (pp. 329–360). New York: Guilford Press.

Mischel, W., & Patterson, C. J. (1976). Substantive and structural elements of effective plans for self-control. *Journal of Personality and Social Psychology, 34*(5), 942–950.

Mischel, W., Shoda, Y., & Rodriguez, M. L. (1989). Delay of gratification in children. *Science, 244*, 933–938.

Mitchell, J. P., Nosek, B. A., & Banaji, M. R. (2003). Contextual variations in implicit evaluation. *Journal of Experimental Psychology: General, 132*(3), 455–469.

Moskowitz, G. B., Gollwitzer, P. M., Wasel, W., & Schaal, B. (1999). Preconscious control of stereotype activation through chronic egalitarian goals. *Journal of Personality and Social Psychology, 77*(1), 167–184.

Muraven, M., & Baumeister, R. F. (2000). Self-regulation and depletion of limited resources: Does self-control resemble a muscle? *Psychological Bulletin, 126*(2), 247–259.

O'Donoghue, T., & Rabin, M. (2000). The economics of immediate gratification. *Journal of Behavioral Decision Making, 13*, 233–250.

Polivy, J., Herman, C., & Warsh, S. (1978). Internal and external components of emotionality in restrained and unrestrained eaters. *Journal of Abnormal Psychology, 87*(5), 497–504.

Rachlin, H. (2000). *The science of self-control.* Cambridge, MA: Harvard University Press.

Rachlin, H., & Green, L. (1972). Commitment, choice and self-control. *Journal of the Experimental Analysis of Behavior, 17*, 15–22.

Ruderman, A. J., & Besbeas, M. (1992). Psychological characteristics of dieters and bulimics. *Journal of Abnormal Psychology, 101*(3), 383–390.

Schelling, T. C. (1978). Egonomics, or the art of self-management. *American Economic Review, 68*, 290–294.

Schelling, T. C. (1984). Self-command in practice, in policy, and in a theory of rational choice. *American Economic Review, 74*(2), 1–11.

Shah, J. Y., Friedman, R., & Kruglanski, A. W. (2002). Forgetting all else: On the antecedents and consequences of goal shielding. *Journal of Personality and Social Psychology, 83*(6), 1261–1280.

Shah, J. Y., & Kruglanski, A. W. (2003). When opportunity knocks: Bottom-up priming of goals by means and its effects on self-regulation. *Journal of Personality and Social Psychology, 84*(6), 1109–1122.

Shultz, T. R., & Lepper, M. R. (1996). Cognitive dissonance reduction as constraint satisfaction. *Psychological Review, 103*(2), 219–240.

Solarz, A. K. (1960). Latency of instrumental responses as a function of compatibility with the meaning of eliciting verbal signs. *Journal of Experimental Psychology, 59*, 239–245.

Srull, T. K., & Wyer, R. S., Jr. (1979). The role of category accessibility in the interpretation of information about persons: Some determinants and implications. *Journal of Personality and Social Psychology, 37*, 1660–1672.

Strotz, R. H. (1956). Myopia and inconsistency in dynamic utility maximization. *Review of Economic Studies, 23*, 166–180.

Thaler, R. H. (1991). *Quasi rational economics.* New York: Russell Sage Foundation.

Thaler, R. H., & Shefrin, H. M. (1981). An economic theory of self-control. *Journal of Political Economy, 89*, 392–406.

Trope, Y., & Fishbach, A. (2000). Counteractive self-control in overcoming temptation. *Journal of Personality and Social Psychology, 79*(4), 493–506.

Trope, Y., & Neter, E. (1994). Reconciling competing motives in self-evaluation: The role of self-control in feedback seeking. *Journal of Personality and Social Psychology, 66*(4), 646–657.

Vohs, K. D., & Heatherton, T. F. (2000). Self-regulatory failure: A resource-depletion approach. *Psychological Science, 11*(3), 249–254.

Wertenbroch, K. (1998). Consumption self control by rationing purchase quantities of virtue and vice. *Marketing Science, 17*, 317–337.

Wright, R. A., & Brehm, J. W. (1984). The impact of task difficulty upon perceptions of arousal and goal attractiveness in an avoidance paradigm. *Motivation and Emotion, 8*(2), 171–181.

Chapter 19

# Dealing with Unwanted Feelings

## THE ROLE OF AFFECT REGULATION IN VOLITIONAL ACTION CONTROL

**Sander L. Koole**
**Julius Kuhl**

On the road to successful goal achievement, people frequently have to endure frustrations, disappointments, and other forms of negative affect. Moderate amounts of negative affect can be adaptive, by promoting perceptual vigilance (Pratto & John, 1991), action readiness (Neumann, Förster, & Strack, 2003), and energy mobilization (Taylor, 1991). However, negative affect can become disruptive when it becomes a pervasive aspect of people's lives. Indeed, persistent negative affect interferes with effective self-regulation (Jostmann & Koole, 2006, in press; Kuhl, 1981), causes alienation from inner needs and emotional preferences (Kazén, Baumann, & Kuhl, 2003; Kuhl & Beckmann, 1994a), and undermines both physical and emotional health (Goleman, 1995; Gross & Muñoz, 1995; Kuhl, Kazén, & Koole, 2006a). Taken together, it seems crucial for people to develop effective strategies for *affect regulation*, which allow people to take charge of their own affective states.

Our aim in this chapter is to develop a theoretical framework for understanding the role of affect regulation in volitional action control. The principles that underlie this framework are based on *personality systems interactions* (PSI) theory (Kuhl, 2000; Kuhl & Koole, 2004), a new theoretical perspective on human motivation and personality functioning. In the following paragraphs, we begin by considering why affect regulation is needed to support volitional action. Next, we examine some of the cognitive processes that underlie effective affect regulation. Our analysis suggests that volitional action control is particularly served by *intuitive affect regulation* (Koole & Jostmann, 2004), a form of affect regulation that combines both automatic and controlled processes. We go on to discuss empirical evidence showing that action orientation is linked to intuitive affect regulation skills. Finally, we review our main conclusions and consider some avenues for future research.

## WHY REGULATE AFFECT?

People's ability to respond to the world in affective terms is incredibly useful. Affective reactions allow people to distinguish rapidly and reliably between hostile and hospitable stimuli. Positive affect informs people that the situation is benign, and prepares them for approach-oriented action; negative affect informs people that the situation is threatening, and prepares them for avoidance-related action (Cacioppo, Gardner, & Berntson, 1999; Neumann et al., 2003). These basic affective operations can be performed automatically and without conscious reflection (Berridge & Winkielman, 2003; Fazio, 2001; Zajonc, 1980), and they are grounded in innate biological processes (Öhman & Mineka, 2001; Peeters & Czapinsky, 1990). The affect system also interacts with more complex forms of information processing. Affective connotations underlie more than half of the semantic meanings of everyday language (Osgood, Suci, & Tannenbaum, 1957). Furthermore, affective input often guides and directs sophisticated decision-making processes (Damasio, Tranel, & Damasio, 1991; Martin & Stoner, 1996).

Despite the immense adaptive value of the affect system, people frequently tamper with their own affective states. Indeed, affect regulation research has identified numerous strategies through which people manipulate their initial affective reactions. These affect regulation strategies include suppression (Wenzlaff, Wegner, & Roper, 1988), repression (A. Freud, 1946; McGregor & Marigold, 2003), reappraisal (Gross, 1998), distraction (Wenzlaff et al., 1988), absorption (Erber & Tesser, 1992), projection (Jung, 1951/1959; Schimel, Pyszczynski, Greenberg, O'Mahen, & Arndt, 2000), denial (Greenberg et al., 1993), compartmentalization (Showers & Kling, 1996), and integration (Kuhl, 2000). This impressive arsenal of affect regulation strategies is applied across a host of different domains, such as social support seeking (Mikulincer, Shaver, & Pereg, 2004), impulse buying (Verplanken & Herabadi, 2001), food consumption (Vohs & Heatherton, 2000), religious practices (Wurff, 1996), medicine intake (Kuhl, 1983), drug abuse (Stiensmeier-Pelster & Schürmann, 1994), and environmental preference (Van den Berg, Koole, & Van der Wulp, 2003). In short, affect regulation is a very common and routine aspect of people's emotional lives.

One likely motive that explains the apparent popularity of affect regulation is *hedonism*. Hedonism, or the desire to maximize pleasure and to minimize pain, is a classic principle in motivational science (e.g., S. Freud, 1920/2003; Taylor, 1991; Tesser, 1988). According to a hedonistic account, people engage in affect regulation because this helps them to enhance pleasurable feelings and to avoid painful feelings. Consistent with a hedonistic account, affect regulation often helps people to get rid of aversive affect (Goleman, 1995; Gross, 1999). Hedonistic affect regulation can sometimes be so powerful as to interfere with other self-regulation processes (Tice, Bratslavsky, & Baumeister, 2001). Hedonistic motivation may thus form a powerful drive that underlies people's ubiquitous affect regulation efforts.

Although hedonism is important, it cannot account for all known forms of affect regulation. In everyday life, people frequently watch scary movies, listen to gloomy music, and engage in a variety of other activities that arouse aversive affect. Moreover, empirical research has documented affect regulation processes that lead people to suppress positive affect or amplify negative affect. For instance, people who anticipate a social interaction show a tendency to remain "cool and collected," and down-regulate both negative *and* positive moods before entering the interaction (Erber, Wegner, & Therriault, 1996). The anticipation of a demanding task appears to have a similar effect on affect regulation (Erber & Erber, 1994). Other research suggests that people may maintain negative affective states when they are ruminating and when their attention is focused inward (Kuhl, 1981; Pyszczynski & Greenberg, 1987). Indeed, chronic ruminators show a consistent tendency to stay away from enjoyable activities (Kuhl & Beckmann, 1994a; Lyubomirsky & Nolen-Hoeksema, 1993) and can be easily persuaded to engage in aversive activities (Kazén et al., 2003). In sum, many well-documented forms of affect regulation are difficult to reconcile with a strict hedonistic account.

Because the assumption of hedonism is deeply engrained in motivational theorizing, it is tempting to write off nonhedonistic forms of affect regulation as obscure or maladaptive. Nevertheless, nonhedonistic affect regulation is a common tendency among psychologically healthy individuals (Erber, 1996; Koole, Kuhl, Jostmann, & Vohs, 2005). Moreover, there are good reasons to believe that nonhedonistic affect regulation can be adaptive. As Erber (1994) noted, even happy moods may interfere with people's ongoing goal pursuits (see also Tice et al., 2001). Thus it may often be useful for people to strive for neutral rather than positive moods. Likewise, the ability to tolerate negative affect may be important in detecting threats and instigating proactive forms of coping (Aspinwall & Taylor, 1997). Taken together, the psychological functions of affect regulation appear more complex than has often been assumed. People often engage in affect regulation not to feel *good* but rather to feel *right*—that is, to bring their affective states in line with the demands of the situation.

If affect regulation allows people to feel right, then what determines whether people's feelings are wrong or right? In many situations, there exist *social constraints* on the appropriateness of people's affective states. Social constraints arise whenever social norms dictate which kinds of affective states are appropriate in a given situation. For instance, extreme positive or negative affective states are undesirable in mundane social interactions (Erber et al., 1996), and bearers of bad news are expected to suppress any signs of positive affect (Tesser, Rosen, & Waranch, 1973). There also exist *functional constraints* on the compatibility between affective states and the cognitive and behavioral tasks that people are performing (Erber & Tesser, 1992; Neumann et al., 2003; Schwarz & Bohner, 1996). Functional constraints arise when certain affective states are conducive to performing a given task. For instance, being in a positive mood facilitates creative problem solving (Ashby, Isen, & Turken, 1999). Functional constraints often operate along with social constraints. Nevertheless, functional constraints are important even in the absence of any social prescriptions concerning people's affective states. Thus, with respect to affect regulation, the significance of functional constraints seems more fundamental than that of social constraints.

PSI theory (Kuhl, 2000; Kuhl & Koole, 2004) further spells out which functional constraints operate on people's affective states. According to PSI theory, positive affect regulates how much people are disposed toward deliberation versus action. When positive affect is low, people are inclined to deliberate without acting (Goschke & Kuhl, 1993); when positive affect is high, people are inclined to act intuitively, without deliberation (Kuhl & Kazén, 1999). Regulation of positive affect is thus needed to coordinate the dynamic balance between deliberative and intuitive action systems. PSI theory further proposes that negative affect regulates how much people's experiences is oriented toward cognitive integration versus elementary perception. When negative affect is low, people are inclined to integrate their experiences into coherent wholes (Baumann & Kuhl, 2002; Bolte, Goschke, & Kuhl, 2003); when negative affect is high, people are more inclined to focus on isolated cognitive elements, without attending to the bigger picture (Kuhl, 1981). Regulation of negative affect is therefore needed to coordinate the dynamic balance between integrative and elementary cognitive systems.

Based on PSI theory, we can understand why affect regulation is fundamentally important to people. More specifically, people may use affect regulation to increase the compatibility between their own affective states and current task demands. Affect regulation may thus help people coordinate their affective states with the functional constraints that arise during their goal pursuits. In principle, this coordination problem is relevant to any goal that people pursue. Consequently, affect regulation may facilitate even goal pursuits that are unrelated or in opposition to hedonistic needs. Affect regulation is therefore an integral aspect of volitional action control. To the extent that people are effective in regulating their own affective states, *any* volitional activity will be facilitated. To the extent that people are ineffective in regulating their own affective states, any volitional activity will be impaired.

## INTUITIVE AFFECT REGULATION

To support volitional action control, the affect regulation process has to meet two basic requirements. First, affect regulation has to be *efficient*. Efficiency is important because the onset of the affect system is very rapid and automatic. Moreover, during volitional action control, people's attention is often focused on other tasks and goal pursuits. Affect regulation should thus ideally not require much attention. Second, affect regulation has to be *flexible*. Flexibility is important in two different ways. People's goal pursuits may change from situation to situation as certain opportunities arise and other opportunities are blocked. Therefore, affect regulation is ideally *context-sensitive*. In addition, many affective states are useful at moderate intensity levels, and only interfere with people's goal pursuits at high levels of intensity. For instance, although severe social anxiety can be extremely debilitating (Leary & Kowalski, 1995), some sensitivity to social disapproval is probably adaptive (Pickett, Gardner, & Knowles, 2004). To benefit optimally from potentially useful affective signals, a person should be able to tolerate even aversive affect as long as the affect does not become overwhelming. Thus affect regulation is ideally *nonrepressive*.

Can affect regulation be both flexible and efficient? So-called *dual-process models* (cf. Chaiken & Trope, 1999) have argued that human information processing is *either* flexible and inefficient (*controlled processing*) *or* inflexible and efficient (*automatic processing*). However, PSI theory suggests that flexible and efficient processing can be combined in some forms of volitional action control. The functional basis for flexible and efficient processing is provided by *extension memory*. Extension memory is a cognitive system that mediates an intelligent form of intuition (Baumann & Kuhl, 2002). Extension memory has access to extended cognitive networks that allow the system to acquire an overview of the person's motives and needs, as well as the broader meanings of the situation. Consequently, extension memory is capable of context-sensitive processing. Furthermore, extension memory operates by means of parallel-distributed information processing, which can handle vast amounts of complex information at speeds that greatly exceed the capacity of the conscious mind. In view of these considerations, extension memory seems ideally suited to support flexible and efficient affect regulation processes. To denote affect regulation processes that are under the control of extension memory, we use the term *intuitive affect regulation* (Koole & Jostmann, 2004).

The extent to which people engage in intuitive affect regulation will vary from situation to situation. Extreme stress may overwhelm most individuals, regardless of any individual differences in capacity for intuitive affect regulation. Alternatively, intuitive affect regulation may be primed by situational cues. Priming of intuitive affect regulation is possible when specific cues have become associated in memory with intuitive affect regulation (cf. Bargh & Barndollar, 1996). For instance, people often make a fist when they have overcome a negative experience (Schubert, 2004). Making a fist may thus become associated with intuitive affect regulation (Schubert & Koole, 2006). Intuitive affect regulation may similarly become associated with significant others (cf. Shah, 2003). For instance, Alex may have been encouraged many times by her good friend Agnes to use intuitive affect regulation. Through these repeated experiences, Alex may come to associate Agnes with the activation of intuitive affect regulation mechanisms. Therefore, the next time Alex meets or is reminded of Agnes, Alex may spontaneously activate intuitive affect regulation mechanisms (Kuhl, 2000). Through transference processes (Chen & Andersen, 1999), priming of intuitive affect regulation may even occur when Alex meets people who physically or psychologically resemble Agnes.

Intuitive affect regulation abilities may further vary among individuals. Intuitive affect regulation is a complex skill, which requires coordination between different psychological systems (i.e., extension memory and the affect systems). Thus practice is probably important for developing strong intuitive affect regulation skills. Interpersonal interactions may be crucial in this developmental process. This is because personal encounters can offer opportunities for self-affirmation that allow the person to confront painful experiences autonomously (Koole, Smeets, van Knippenberg, & Dijksterhuis, 1999; Schimel, Arndt, Pyszczynski, & Greenberg, 2001). When the social environment is autonomy-supportive, extension memory will develop strong connections with the affective systems (Baumann & Kuhl, 2005; Kuhl, 2000). By contrast, when the social environment is hostile, indifferent, or controlling, extension memory becomes inhibited and thus less able to connect with the affective systems. Given the natural variation in people's social environments, relatively stable individual differences in intuitive affect regulation skills may arise.

Like any other well-practiced skill, intuitive affect regulation is largely inaccessible to introspection. Fortunately, intuitive affect regulation skills may be measured indirectly. Although people cannot directly access the mental operations that underlie intuitive affect regulation, it is plausible that people can observe the behavioral consequences of intuitive affect regulation. Individuals with highly developed intuitive affect regulation skills will be able to pursue their goals in a highly efficient, unhesitating manner, even under highly stressful circumstances. Accordingly, strong intuitive affect regulation skills should go hand in hand with an *action-oriented* style of self-regulation. By contrast, individuals with weak intuitive affect regulation skills are vulnerable to uncontrollable ruminations and hesitation, especially under stressful circumstances. Weak intuitive affect regulation skills should thus be associated with a *state-oriented* style of self-regulation. Based on this logic, the Action Control Scale (ACS-90; Kuhl, 1994a) measures individual differences in action versus state orientation, and thus, indirectly, the strength of people's intuitive affect regulation skills. Illustrative items of the ACS-90 are provided in Table 19.1. Research indicates that the ACS-90 has good psychometric properties and has explanatory power over and above alternative personality constructs, such as the Big Five and self-esteem (Brunstein, 2001; Diefendorff, Hall, Lord, & Strean, 2000; Koole, 2004; Kuhl & Beckmann, 1994b).

**TABLE 19.1. Illustrative Items of the ACS-90 (Kuhl, 1994a)**

*Demand-Related Action Orientation*

- When I know I must finish something soon:
  A. I have to push myself to get started.
  B. I find it easy to get it over and done with.*
- When I am getting ready to tackle a difficult problem:
  A. It feels like I am facing a big mountain I don't think I can climb.
  B. I look for a way to approach the problem in a suitable manner.*
- When I have a boring assignment:
  A. I usually don't have a problem getting through it.*
  B. I sometimes just can't get moving on it.

*Threat-Related Action Orientation*

- When I have lost something that is very valuable to me and I can't find it anywhere:
  A. I have a hard time concentrating on anything else.
  B. I put it out of my mind after a little while.*
- If I've worked for weeks on a project and then everything goes completely wrong with the project:
  A. It takes me a long time to adjust myself to it.
  B. It bothers me for a while, but then I don't think about it any more.*
- When I am being told that my work is completely unsatisfactory:
  A. I don't let it bother me for too long.*
  B. I feel paralyzed.

*Note.* Action-oriented responses are marked with an asterisk.

## ACTION ORIENTATION AND INTUITIVE AFFECT REGULATION

According to PSI theory, action orientation is linked to strong intuitive affect regulation skills. Action-oriented individuals should therefore display flexible and efficient affect regulation. This prediction has been tested in a number of empirical investigations on individual differences in action orientation. Most of this research has focused on the effects of action orientation under negative conditions. This focus is consistent with a long tradition in motivation research to study coping with adversity. On a more theoretical level, volitional processes are especially likely to be invoked during difficult times, because this is when more routine forms of action control are unlikely to yield desired outcomes (Kuhl, 1984). Consequently, the association between action orientation and down-regulation of negative affect may be particularly strong and well rehearsed.

### Action Orientation and Efficient Affect Regulation

As noted earlier, a great deal of affective processing takes place on implicit levels. The onset of these implicit affective reactions typically occurs on a rapid time scale (Berridge & Winkielman, 2003). Thus, if affective reactions could be controlled on an implicit level, this would allow the person to intervene early in the affect generation process. Such a time advantage may be crucial for getting a grip on one's feelings (Gross, 2001). Thus, assuming that action orientation is linked to efficient affect regulation skills, we can expect action orientation to moderate implicit affective processes.

Koole and Jostmann (2004, Study 3) examined the effects of action orientation in a face discrimination task (Öhman, Lundqvist, & Esteves, 2001). The human face is a socially relevant stimulus that elicits strong implicit affective reactions (Murphy & Zajonc, 1993). Accordingly, the processing of facial affect provided a suitable context to gauge the efficiency of the affect regulation skills of action- versus state-oriented individuals. In the face discrimination task, participants were presented with crowds of faces with happy, angry, or neutral expressions. Among half of the crowds, there was one face with a different emotional expression. Participants' task was to locate these discrepant faces as quickly and accurately as possible. This task is relevant to affect regulation, because it requires switching attention from one affective valence (i.e., the emotional expression of the crowd) toward another affective valence (i.e., the emotional expression of the target). Thus, when action-oriented individuals are engaged in down-regulation of negative affect, their ability to detect happy faces among angry crowds may be enhanced. The results of Koole and Jostmann (2004) supported this reasoning. Action-oriented participants, unlike their state-oriented counterparts, were quicker to detect happy target faces among angry crowds. Notably, this effect only emerged under demanding conditions, which presumably trigger affect regulation among action-oriented individuals.

The effects of action orientation have been conceptually replicated with alternative measures of implicit affect, including an affective Simon task (Koole & Jostmann, 2004, Study 2), an implicit self-evaluation task (Koole, 2004), and an affective priming task (Koole & Coenen, in press; Koole & Fockenberg, 2006). Thus action orientation appears to regulate a variety of implicit affective processes. Even so, the aforementioned measures used affective stimuli that were consciously recognizable to participants. Jostmann, Koole, van der Wulp, and Fockenberg (2005) examined whether action orientation might regulate even affective reactions to stimuli that cannot be consciously recognized. In a parafoveal priming task, participants were subliminally primed with happy, angry, or neutral faces. Following this task, participants' implicit mood was assessed. Among state-oriented participants, subliminally presented angry faces led to more negative implicit moods, whereas subliminally presented happy faces led to more positive implicit moods. This mood-congruent pattern is consistent with previous research (Chartrand, van Baaren, & Bargh, 2006). Action-oriented individuals, however, displayed a mood-incongruent pattern as a function of subliminal priming, such that negative affective primes led to more positive implicit moods, whereas positive affective primes led to more negative implicit moods. Action orientation can thus regulate even subliminally induced affect.

Implicit affective reactions can evaporate within a single second (Murphy & Zajonc, 1993). Nevertheless, a consistent buildup of implicit affective reactions may translate into durable affective reactions (Chartrand et al., 2006). The effects of action orientation on implicit affect can thus potentially influence affective reactions that are unfolding over longer time periods, such as mood or physiological arousal. In line with this, action orientation is associated with substantially reduced amounts of pain (Kuhl, 1983) and depression (Rholes, Michas, & Shroff, 1989) in response to real-life stressors. Moreover, controlled laboratory studies have shown that action orientation is associated with less spontaneous expressions of negative affect (Brunstein & Olbrich, 1985), tension reduction (Koole & Jostmann, 2004), and reduced physiological arousal (Heckhausen & Strang, 1988) in response to threatening or demanding experimental manipulations. Taken together, these results indicate that action orientation is strongly related to efficiency at affect regulation, both on implicit and explicit levels of affective responding.

## Action Orientation and Flexible Affect Regulation

Action-oriented individuals certainly seem to be efficient affect regulators. But can action-oriented individuals also regulate their affective states in a flexible manner? One key aspect of flexibility is context sensitivity. Accordingly, the effects of action orientation should be responsive to contextual changes. Changes in affective context are particularly relevant for affect regulation, because such changes often introduce an imbalance between a person's affective states and the functional requirements of the situation. For instance, demanding conditions may give rise to aversive affect (e.g., frustration, tension, or dejection), which may disrupt the implementation of intended actions. Accordingly, an increase in affect regulation efforts is often useful under demanding conditions. In line with this reasoning, the aforementioned studies on action orientation and affect regulation efficiency found that action orientation only predicted down-regulation of aversive affect under demanding conditions (Koole, 2004; Koole & Fockenberg, 2006; Koole & Jostmann, 2004).

If there is no immediate need to act, aversive affect is less likely to interfere with volitional processes (Kuhl, 1994b). Aversive conditions may thus not invariably lead to down-regulation of negative affect among action-oriented individuals. Indeed, Van Dillen and Koole (2004) reasoned that action-oriented individuals may only down-regulate negative affect when negative affect could interfere with another ongoing task. To test this idea, the researchers exposed a group of action- versus state-oriented participants to a series of negative or neutral emotional pictures. Half of the pictures were followed by a difficult arithmetic sum. Next, participants rated their current moods. As might be expected, exposure to negative pictures led to more negative mood. However, this increase was moderated by an interaction between action orientation and the need to perform an arithmetic task. After participants had performed an arithmetic task, the negative pictures caused a smaller increase in negative mood among action- than among state-oriented participants. When participants had not performed an arithmetic task, action- and state-oriented participants displayed an equally large increase in negative mood upon viewing negative pictures. Thus the effects of action orientation on affect regulation were highly responsive to volitional demands. Only when volitional demands were high did action orientation moderate negative affective reactions.

A second aspect of flexibility is nonrepressiveness. Repression relies on avoidance strategies, and consequently interferes with vigilance for negative affect (Langens & Mörth, 2003). Therefore, if action orientation is indeed nonrepressive, it should facilitate down-regulation of negative affect without undermining vigilance for negative affect. This prediction was tested in the face discrimination study by Koole and Jostmann (2004, Study 3), discussed earlier. Recall that the face discrimination task measured affect regulation by looking at the speed with which participants could detect happy faces among angry crowds. Notably, the same task could be used to assess vigilance for negative affect. More specifically, vigilance for negative was indicated by participants' speed at detecting angry target faces among happy or neutral crowds (Öhman et al., 2001). The results showed that action orientation had no effect on detection of angry target faces among happy or neutral crowds, even though action orientation significantly moderated the detection of happy faces among angry crowds. Thus action orientation was associated with down-regulation of negative affect without suppressing vigilance for negative affect.

Vigilance for negative affect may even be enhanced by action orientation. Rosahl, Tennigkeit, Kuhl, and Haschke (1993) found evidence in event-related brain potentials that action-oriented individuals showed enhanced processing of the negative (compared to neutral) affective meaning of word stimuli at around 180 milliseconds, whereas state-oriented individuals showed enhanced processing of negative affective meaning much later during the processing sequence. Likewise, Koole and Fockenberg (2006) found that action-oriented individuals displayed enhanced activation of negative affect at very brief exposures to affective primes (i.e., less than 200 milliseconds), and inhibition of negative affect at somewhat longer exposures to affective primes (i.e., 300 milliseconds). In the same study, state-oriented individuals only displayed enhanced activation of negative affect at longer prime exposures (i.e., 300 milliseconds). Overall, the available evidence indicates that action orientation does not regulate negative affect through repression or avoidance mechanisms. Rather, action orientation appears to promote a highly dynamic form of affect regulation, in which unwanted affect only becomes down-regulated after it has been detected and processed by the affect system.

## VOLITIONAL BENEFITS OF ACTION ORIENTATION

Aided by their affect regulation skills, action-oriented individuals can control their emotional lives in a flexible and efficient manner. However, from the perspective of PSI theory, action-oriented individuals do not use their intuitive affect regulation skills for hedonistic purposes. Rather, intuitive affect regulation is aimed at improving the efficiency of volitional action control. Accordingly, the intuitive affect regulation skills of action-oriented individuals may become translated into significant volitional benefits. These volitional benefits should emerge especially under aversive conditions, because this is when well-developed affect regulation skills matter most.

Volition helps people to accomplish their goals, especially under difficult conditions (Kuhl, 1984). The ability to form and execute difficult intentions is thus a key component of volitional functioning. Research indicates that the formation of intentions is indeed more efficient among action- than among state-oriented individuals (Beckmann & Kuhl, 1984; Stiensmeier-Pelster, 1994). Research has further shown that action orientation facilitates the implementation of difficult intentions, especially under aversive conditions (Kuhl, 1984; Kuhl & Beckmann, 1994a). These effects of action orientation have recently been demonstrated for controlled laboratory tasks, including the classic Stroop color-naming task and established tests of working memory (Jostmann & Koole, 2006, in press).

Volition also has an experiential component that refers to the person's experience of autonomy, or sense of *self-determination* (Deci & Ryan, 2000). According to PSI theory, this subjective aspect of volition is mediated by cognitive integration processes (Kuhl, 2000). Several studies support the notion that action orientation fosters cognitive integration, particularly under aversive conditions (Baumann & Kuhl, 2002). Increased cognitive integration may also help a person to access his or her inner needs, even when these needs cannot be articulated on explicit levels. Consistent with this, action orientation is associated with improved access to one's own emotional preferences (Kuhl & Kazén, 1994), again especially under aversive conditions (Baumann & Kuhl, 2003). Finally, action orientation is associated with greater congruence between explicit goals and implicit needs, as assessed by the Thematic Apperception Test (Brunstein, 2001; cf. McClelland, Koestner, & Weinberger, 1989). The association between action orientation and goal–motive congruence again emerges mainly under aversive conditions (Baumann, Kaschel, & Kuhl, 2005). Notably, the tendency among action-oriented individuals to choose more motive-congruent goals is associated with improved physical and psychological health relative to state-oriented individuals (Baumann et al., 2005; Kuhl et al., 2006a).

Overall, action orientation is associated with considerable volitional benefits (for more extensive reviews, see Diefendorff et al., 2000; Koole, Kuhl, Kuhl, & Finkenauer, 2006; Koole et al., 2005; Kuhl & Beckmann, 1994b). Because these volitional benefits arise especially under aversive conditions, the volitional benefits of action orientation appear to derive from the intuitive affect regulation skills of action-oriented individuals. More direct studies would be desirable regarding the mediating role of intuitive affect regulation in the volitional benefits of action orientation (though for initial evidence, see Koole & Jostmann, 2004). Nevertheless, the available evidence supports the notion that strong intuitive affect regulation skills have significant volitional benefits.

## SUMMARY AND CONCLUSIONS

In this chapter we have highlighted the role of affect regulation in volitional action control. According to traditional views, affect regulation mainly serves to satisfy people's hedonistic needs. However, we believe that a strictly hedonistic account may underestimate the profound significance of affect regulation for people's goal pursuits. According to PSI theory (Kuhl, 2000; Kuhl & Koole, 2004), affect regulation is needed to support any action, including actions that are not directed at hedonistic need satisfaction. This fundamental role of affect regulation is based on the notion that affective changes modulate a person's cognitive and behavioral systems. Affect regulation is therefore needed to bring cognitive and behavioral systems in line with ongoing task demands. From this perspective, affect regulation represents an integral aspect of volitional action control.

To effectively support volitional action control, affect regulation should be flexible and efficient. Such flexible and efficient affect regulation—or *intuitive affect regulation* (Koole & Jostmann, 2004)—can be achieved with the help of extension memory, a powerful computational system that mediates an intelligent form of intuition. Intuitive affect regulation abilities may vary across situations and among individuals. Individual differences in action orientation (Kuhl, 1994b) are linked to well-developed intuitive affect regulation skills. Action orientation is associated with efficient affect regulation across a variety of implicit and explicit affective responses. In addition, action orientation is associated with context-sensitive and nonrepressive affect regulation. On the basis of PSI theory, well-developed intuitive affect regulation skills should become translated into improved volitional functioning. Consistent with this, action orientation is associated with important volitional benefits, such as efficiency at forming and enacting difficult intentions, and improved integration between implicit needs and explicit goals.

The role of affect regulation in volitional action control is complex. Understanding this role will therefore require much more theoretical and empirical work. One key area for future study is nonhedonistic affect regulation. Past research has already identified several instances of nonhedonistic affect regulation (Erber, 1996; Koole, 2006; Koole & Fockenberg, 2006). In view of the great theoretical interest in the topic, however, further research on nonhedonistic affect regulation is desirable. Nonhedonistic affect regulation may take the form of either inhibition of positive affect or amplification of negative affect. Based on PSI theory, inhibition of positive affect should be especially relevant to the formation and implementation of difficult intentions, whereas amplification of negative affect should be especially relevant to elementary perception. These ideas may be useful in guiding future research on nonhedonistic affect regulation.

Another important area for future study lies in the investigation of situational variations in action orientation. As our review has shown, research to date has focused primarily on individual differences. Although this focus is likely to remain important, it will be of great interest to look for situational determinants of action orientation. Theoretically, one can distinguish between short-term and long-term determinants of action orientation. Cues that have been associated with action orientation in the past (such as making a fist; Schubert & Koole, 2006) may prime temporary increases in action orientation. Autonomy-supportive social interactions may lead to chronic increases in action orientation, particularly when these social interactions occur repeatedly with significant others. There is some initial evidence that long-term changes in action orientation are socially transmitted. For instance, action orientation is significantly correlated with autonomy-supportive childrearing practices (Kuhl, 1994b), and action orientation can be raised through therapeutic interventions (Schulte, Hartung, & Wilke, 1997; Stiensmeier-Pelster et al., 1994). Future research along these lines will shed important new light on the development of individual differences in action orientation.

Motivation science and affect regulation research have traditionally developed as somewhat separate areas of investigation. Nevertheless, researchers in these two fields have much to learn from each other. Affect regulation research can bring a stronger process-oriented focus to motivation science, which has traditionally emphasized purpose over process (Kuhl, 2000). Conversely, motivation science can contribute a greater emphasis on the adaptive functions of affect regulation within human motivation and action control. Continued integration between motivation science and affect regulation research is also important for practical reasons (Kuhl, Kazén, & Koole, 2006b). So far, insights into action control and affect regulation processes have been useful in treating emotional disorders, such as depression, phobias, and compulsive behavior (Hartung & Schulte, 1994); coaching professional and nonprofessional athletes and sports teams (Beckmann & Kazén, 1994); and facilitating the work performance of students and employees (Boekaerts, 1994; Diefendorff et al., 2000). Further work on the role of affect regulation in volitional action control should greatly benefit these and other applied domains. Both in science and in everyday life, it is vital to understand how people are dealing with unwanted feelings.

## ACKNOWLEDGMENT

This research was facilitated by an Innovation Grant from the Netherlands Organization for Scientific Research to Sander L. Koole.

## REFERENCES

Ashby, F. G., Isen, A. M., & Turken, A. U. (1999). A neuropsychological theory of positive affect and its influence on cognition. *Psychological Review, 106*, 529–550.

Aspinwall, L. G., & Taylor, S. E. (1997). A stitch in time: Self-regulation and proactive coping. *Psychological Review, 121*, 417–436.

Bargh, J. A., & Barndollar, K. (1996). Automaticity in action: The unconscious as repository of chronic goals and motives. In P. M. Gollwitzer & J. A. Bargh (Eds.), *The psychology of action* (pp. 457–481). New York: Guilford Press.

Baumann, N., Kaschel, R., & Kuhl, J. (2005). Striving for unwanted goals: Stress-dependent discrepancies between explicit and implicit achievement motives reduce subjective well-being and increase psychosomatic symptoms. *Journal of Personality and Social Psychology, 89*, 781–799.

Baumann, N., & Kuhl, J. (2002). Intuition, affect and personality: Unconscious coherence judgments and self-regulation of negative affect. *Journal of Personality and Social Psychology, 83*, 1213–1223.

Baumann, N., & Kuhl, J. (2003). Self-infiltration: Confusing assigned tasks and self-selected in memory. *Personality and Social Psychology Bulletin, 29*, 487–498.

Baumann, N., & Kuhl, J. (2005). How to resist temptation: The effects of external control versus autonomy support on self-regulatory dynamics. *Journal of Personality, 73*, 443–470.

Beckmann, J., & Kazén, M. (1994). Action and state orientation and the performance of top athletes. In J. Kuhl & J. Beckmann (Eds.), *Volition and personality: Action versus state orientation* (pp. 439–451). Göttingen, Germany: Hogrefe & Huber.

Beckmann, J., & Kuhl, J. (1984). Altering information to gain action control: Functional aspects of human information processing in decision-making. *Journal of Research in Personality, 18*, 223–279.

Berridge, K. C., & Winkielman, P. (2003). What is an unconscious emotion? (the case for unconscious "liking"). *Cognition and Emotion, 17*, 181–211.

Boekaerts, M. (1994). Action control: How relevant is it for classroom learning? In J. Kuhl & J. Beckmann (Eds.), *Volition and personality: Action versus state orientation* (pp. 427–435). Göttingen, Germany: Hogrefe & Huber.

Bolte, A., Goschke, T., & Kuhl, J. (2003). Emotion and intuition: Effects of positive and negative mood on intuitive judgments of semantic coherence. *Psychological Science, 14*, 416–421.

Brunstein, J. C. (2001). Persönliche Ziele und Handlungs- versus Lageorientierung: Wer bindet sich an realistische und bedürfniskongruente Ziele? [Personal goals and action versus state orientation: Who builds a commitment to realistic and need-congruent goals?] *Zeitschrift für Differentielle und Diagnostische Psychologie, 22*, 1–12.

Brunstein, J. C., & Olbrich, E. (1985). Personal helplessness and action control: Analysis of achievement-related cognitions, self-assessments, and performance. *Journal of Personality and Social Psychology, 48*, 1540–1551.

Cacioppo, J. T., Gardner, W. L., & Berntson, G. G. (1999). The affect system has parallel and integrative processing components: Form follows function. *Journal of Personality and Social Psychology, 76*, 839–855.

Chaiken, S., & Trope, Y. (Eds.). (1999). *Dual-process models in social psychology.* New York: Guilford Press.

Chartrand, T. L., van Baaren, R., & Bargh, J. A. (2006). Linking automatic evaluation to mood and information processing style: Consequences for experienced affect, information processing, and stereotyping. *Journal of Experimental Psychology: General, 133*, 70–77.

Chen, S., & Andersen, S. M. (1999). Relationships from the past in the present: Significant-other representations and transference in interpersonal life. In M. P. Zanna (Ed.), *Advances in experimental social psychology* (Vol. 31, pp. 123–190). San Diego, CA: Academic Press.

Damasio, A. R., Tranel, D., & Damasio, H. C. (1991). Somatic markers and the guidance of behavior: Theory and preliminary testing. In H. S. Levin, H. M. Eisenberg, & A. L. Benton (Eds.), *Frontal lobe function and dysfunction* (pp. 230–255). Oxford, UK: Oxford University Press.

Deci, E. L., & Ryan, R. M. (2000). The "what" and "why" of goal pursuits: Human needs and the self-determination perspective. *Psychological Inquiry, 11*, 227–268.

Diefendorff, J. M., Hall, R. J., Lord, R. G., & Strean, M. L. (2000). Action-state orientation: Construct validity of a revised measure and its relationship to work-related variables. *Journal of Applied Psychology, 85*, 250–263.

Erber, R. (1996). The self-regulation of moods. In L. L. Martin & A. Tesser (Eds.), *Striving and feeling: Interactions among goals, affect, and self-regulation* (pp. 251–275). Hillsdale, NJ: Erlbaum.

Erber, R., & Erber, M. W. (1994). Beyond mood and social judgment: Mood incongruent recall and mood regulation. *European Journal of Social Psychology, 24*, 79–88.

Erber, R., & Tesser, A. (1992). Task effort and the regulation of mood: The absorption hypothesis. *Journal of Experimental Social Psychology, 28*, 339–359.

Erber, R., Wegner, D. M., & Therriault, N. (1996). On being cool and collected: Mood regulation in anticipation of social interaction. *Journal of Personality and Social Psychology, 70*, 757–766.

Fazio, R. H. (2001). On the automatic activation of associated evaluations: An overview. *Cognition and Emotion, 15*, 115–141.

Freud, A. (1946). *The ego and the mechanisms of defense.* New York: International Universities Press.

Freud, S. (2003). *Beyond the pleasure principle.* London: Penguin. (Original work published 1920)

Goleman, D. (1995). *Emotional intelligence: Why it can matter more than IQ.* London: Bloomsbury.

Goschke, T., & Kuhl, J. (1993). Representation of intentions: Persisting activation in memory. *Journal of Experimental Psychology: Learning, Memory, and Cognition, 19*, 1211–1226.

Greenberg, J., Pyszczynski, T., Solomon, S., Pinel, E., Simon, L., & Jordan, K. (1993). Effects of self-esteem on vulnerability-denying defensive distortions: Further evidence of an anxiety-buffering function of self-esteem. *Journal of Experimental Social Psychology, 29*, 229–251.

Gross, J. J. (1998). Antecedent- and response-focused emotion regulation: Divergent consequences for experience, expression, and physiology. *Journal of Personality and Social Psychology, 74*, 224–237.

Gross, J. J. (1999). Emotion regulation: Past, present, future. *Cognition and Emotion, 13*, 551–573.

Gross, J. J. (2001). Emotion regulation in adulthood: Timing is everything. *Current Directions in Psychological Science, 10*, 214–219.

Gross, J. J., & Muñoz, R. F. (1995). Emotion regulation and mental health. *Clinical Psychology: Science and Practice, 2*, 151–164.

Hartung, J., & Schulte, D. (1994). Action and state orientation during the treatment of phobic disorders. In J. Kuhl & J. Beckmann (Eds.), *Volition and personality: Action versus state orientation* (pp. 217–231). Göttingen, Germany: Hogrefe & Huber.

Heckhausen, H., & Strang, H. (1988). Efficiency under record performance demands: Exertion control—an individual difference variable? *Journal of Personality and Social Psychology, 55*, 489–498.

Jostmann, N., & Koole, S. L. (2006). On the waxing and waning of working memory: Action orientation moderates the impact of demanding relationship primes on working memory capacity. *Personality and Social Psychology Bulletin, 32*, 1716–1728.

Jostmann, N., & Koole, S. L. (in press). On the regulation of cognitive controls: Action orientation moderates the impact of high demands in Stroop interference tasks. *Journal of Experimental Psychology: General.*

Jostmann, N. B., Koole, S. L., van der Wulp, N., & Fockenberg, D. (2005). Subliminal affect regulation: The moderating role of action versus state orientation. *European Psychologist, 10*, 209–217.

Jung, C. G. (1959). Aion: Researches into the phenomenology of the self (R. F. C. Hull, Trans.). In H. Reed, M. Fordham, & G. Adler (Eds.), *The collected works of C. G. Jung* (Vol. 9, Part 2). Princeton, NJ: Princeton University Press. (Original work published 1951)

Kazén, M., Baumann, N., & Kuhl, J. (2003). Self-infiltration versus self-compatibility checking in dealing with unattractive tasks: The moderating influence of state versus action orientation. *Motivation and Emotion, 27*, 157–197.

Koole, S. L. (2004). Volitional shielding of the self: Effects of action orientation and external demands on implicit self-evaluation. *Social Cognition, 22*, 117–146.

Koole, S. L. (2006). [Volitional suppression of positive affect: The moderating role of action versus state orientation]. Unpublished raw data, Vrije Universiteit Amsterdam.

Koole, S. L., & Coenen, L. H. M. (in press). Implicit self and affect regulation: Effects of subliminal self-activation and action versus state orientation on affective priming. *Self and Identity.*

Koole, S. L., & Fockenberg, D. A. (2006). *Affective priming and affect regulation: The moderating role of action versus state orientation.* Manuscript submitted for publication.

Koole, S. L., & Jostmann, N. B. (2004). Getting a grip on your feelings: Effects of action orientation and external demands on intuitive affect regulation. *Journal of Personality and Social Psychology, 87*, 974–990.

Koole, S. L., Kuhl. J., Jostmann, N. B., & Finkenauer, C. (2006). Self-regulation in interpersonal relationships: The case of action versus state orientation. In K. D. Vohs & E. J. Finkel (Eds.), *Self and relationships: Connecting intrapersonal and interpersonal processes* (pp. 360–383). New York: Guilford Press.

Koole, S. L., Kuhl, J., Jostmann, N., & Vohs, K. D. (2005). On the hidden benefits of state orientation: Can people prosper without efficient affect regulation skills? In A. Tesser, J. Wood, & D. A. Stapel (Eds.), *On building, defending, and regulating the self: A psychological perspective* (pp. 217–243). London: Taylor & Francis.

Koole, S. L., Smeets, K., van Knippenberg, A., & Dijksterhuis, A. (1999). The cessation of rumination through self-affirmation. *Journal of Personality and Social Psychology, 77*, 111–125.

Kuhl, J. (1981). Motivational and functional helplessness: The moderating effect of state versus action orientation. *Journal of Personality and Social Psychology, 40*, 155–170.

Kuhl, J. (1983). Motivationstheoretische Aspekte der Depressionsgenese: Der Einfluss von Lageorientierung auf Schmerzempfinden, Medikamentenkonsum und Handlungskontrolle [Motivation-theoretical aspects of the development of depression: The influence of state orientation on the experience of pain, drug consumption and action control]. In M. Wolfersdorf, R. Staub, & G. Hole (Eds.), *Der depressiv Kranke in der psychiatrischen Klinik: Theorie und Praxis der Diagnostik und Therapie* (pp. 411–424). Weinheim, Germany: Beltz Verlag.

Kuhl, J. (1984). Volitional aspects of achievement motivation and learned helplessness: Toward a comprehensive theory of action-control. In B. A. Maher (Ed.), *Progress in experimental personality research* (Vol. 13, pp. 99–171). New York: Academic Press.

Kuhl, J. (1994a). Action versus state orientation: Psychometric properties of the Action Control Scale (ACS-90). In J. Kuhl & J. Beckmann (Eds.), *Volition and personality: Action versus state orientation* (pp. 47–59). Göttingen, Germany: Hogrefe & Huber.

Kuhl, J. (1994b). A theory of action and state orientations. In J. Kuhl & J. Beckmann (Eds.), *Volition and personality: Action versus state orientation* (pp. 9–46). Göttingen, Germany: Hogrefe & Huber.

Kuhl, J. (2000). A functional-design approach to motivation and self-regulation: The dynamics of personality systems interactions. In M. Boekaerts, P. R. Pintrich, & M. Zeidner (Eds.), *Handbook of self-regulation* (pp. 111–169). San Diego, CA: Academic Press.

Kuhl, J., & Beckmann, J. (1994a). Alienation: ignoring one's preferences. In J. Kuhl & J. Beckmann (Eds.), *Volition and personality: Action versus state orientation* (pp. 375–390). Göttingen, Germany: Hogrefe & Huber.

Kuhl, J., & Beckmann, J. (Eds.). (1994b). *Volition and personality: Action versus state orientation.* Göttingen, Germany: Hogrefe & Huber.

Kuhl, J., & Kazén, M. (1994). Self-discrimination and memory: State orientation and false self-ascription of assigned activities. *Journal of Personality and Social Psychology, 66,* 1103–1115.

Kuhl, J., & Kazén, M. (1999). Volitional facilitation of difficult intentions: Joint activation of intention memory and positive affect removes Stroop interference. *Journal of Experimental Psychology: General, 128,* 382–399.

Kuhl, J., Kazén, M., & Koole, S. L. (2006a). *Gaining wealth and maintaining your health: Effects of charming personality style and action orientation on sales performance and well-being.* Manuscript submitted for publication.

Kuhl, J., Kazén, M., & Koole, S. L. (2006b). Putting self-regulation theory into practice: A user's manual. *Applied Psychology: An International Review, 55,* 408–418.

Kuhl, J., & Koole, S. L. (2004). Workings of the will: A functional approach. In J. Greenberg, S. L. Koole, & T. Pyszczynski (Eds.), *Handbook of experimental existential psychology* (pp. 411–430). New York: Guilford Press.

Langens, T. A., & Mörth, S. (2003). Repressive coping and the use of passive and active coping strategies. *Personality and Individual Differences, 35,* 461–473.

Leary, M. R., & Kowalski, R. M. (1995). *Social anxiety.* New York: Guilford Press.

Lyubomirsky, S., & Nolen-Hoeksema, S. (1993). Self-perpetuating properties of dysphoric rumination. *Journal of Personality and Social Psychology, 65,* 339–349.

Martin, L. L., & Stoner, P. (1996). Mood as input: What we think about how we feel determines how we think. In L. L. Martin & A. Tesser (Eds.), *Striving and feeling: Interactions among goals, affect, and self-regulation* (pp. 279–301). Hillsdale, NJ: Erlbaum.

McClelland, D. C., Koestner, R., & Weinberger, J. (1989). How do self-attributed and implicit motives differ? *Psychological Review, 96,* 690–702.

McGregor, I., & Marigold, D. C. (2003). Defensive zeal and the uncertain self: What makes you so sure? *Journal of Personality and Social Psychology, 85,* 838–852.

Mikulincer, M., Shaver, P. R., & Pereg, D. (2003) Attachment theory and affect regulation: The dynamics, development, and cognitive consequences of attachment-related strategies. *Motivation and Emotion, 27,* 77–102.

Murphy, S. T., & Zajonc, R. B. (1993). Affect, cognition, and awareness: Affective priming with optimal and suboptimal stimulus exposures. *Journal of Personality and Social Psychology, 64,* 723–739.

Neumann, R., Förster, J., & Strack, F. (2003). Motor compatibility: The bidirectional link between behavior and evaluation. In J. Musch & K. C. Klauer (Eds.), *The psychology of evaluation: Affective processes in cognition and emotion* (pp. 371–391). Mahwah, NJ: Erlbaum.

Öhman, A., Lundqvist, D., & Esteves, F. (2000). The face in the crowd revisited: A threat advantage with schematic stimuli. *Journal of Personality and Social Psychology, 80,* 381–396.

Öhman, A., & Mineka, S. (2000). Fears, phobias, and preparedness: Toward an evolved module of fear and learning. *Psychological Review, 108,* 483–522.

Osgood, C. E., Suci, G. J., & Tannenbaum, P. H. (1957). *The measurement of meaning.* Urbana: University of Illinois Press.

Peeters, G., & Czapinsky, J. (1990). Positive–negative asymmetry in evaluations: The distinction between affective and informational negativity effects. In W. Stroebe & M. Hewstone (Eds.), *European review of social psychology* (Vol. 1, pp. 33–60). Chichester, UK: Wiley.

Pickett, C. L., Gardner, W. L., & Knowles, M. (2004). Getting a cue: The need to belong and enhanced sensitivity to social cues. *Personality and Social Psychology Bulletin, 30,* 1095–1107.

Pratto, F., & John, O. P. (1991). Automatic vigilance: The attention-grabbing power of negative social information. *Journal of Personality and Social Psychology, 61,* 380–391.

Pyszczynski, T., & Greenberg, J. (1987). Self-regulatory perseveration and the depressive self-focusing style: A self-awareness theory of reactive depression. *Psychological Bulletin, 102,* 122–138.

Rholes, W. S., Michas, L., & Shroff, J. (1989). Action control as a vulnerability factor in dysphoria. *Cognitive Therapy and Research, 13,* 263–274.

Rosahl, S. K., Tennigkeit, M., Kuhl, J., & Haschke, R. (1993). Handlungskontrolle und langsame Hirnpotentiale: Untersuchungen zum Einfluss subjectiv kritischer Wörter (Erste Ergebnisse) [Action control and slow brain potentials: Investigations on the influence of subjectively critical words (Preliminary findings)]. *Zeitschrift für Medizinische Psychologie, 2,* 1–8.

Schimel, J., Arndt, J., Pyszczynski, T., & Greenberg, J. (2001). Being accepted for who we are: Evidence that social validation of the intrinsic self reduces general defensiveness. *Journal of Personality and Social Psychology, 80,* 35–52.

Schimel, J., Pyszczynski, T., Greenberg, J., O'Mahen, H., & Arndt, J. (2000). Running from the shadow: Psychological distancing from others to deny characteristics people fear in themselves. *Journal of Personality and Social Psychology, 78,* 446–462.

Schubert, T. W. (2004). The power in your hand: Gender differences in bodily feedback from making a fist.

*Personality and Social Psychology Bulletin*, *30*, 757–769.

Schubert, T. W., & Koole, S. L. (2006). [Embodied autonomy: Making a fist enhances action orientation]. Unpublished raw data, Vrije Universiteit Amsterdam.

Schulte, D., Hartung, J., & Wilke, F. (1997). Handlungskontrolle der Angstbewältigung: Was macht Reizkonfrontationsverfahren so effektiv? *Zeitschrift für Klinische Psychologie*, *26*, 118–128.

Schwarz, N., & Bohner, G. (1996). Feelings and their motivational implications: Moods and the action sequence. In P. M. Gollwitzer & J. A. Bargh (Eds.), *The psychology of action* (pp. 119–145). New York: Guilford Press.

Shah, J. (2003). Automatic for the people: How representations of significant others implicitly affect goal pursuit. *Journal of Personality and Social Psychology*, *84*, 661–681.

Showers, C. J., & Kling, K. C. (1996). Organization of self-knowledge: Implications for recovery from sad mood. *Journal of Personality and Social Psychology*, *70*, 578–590.

Stiensmeier-Pelster, J. (1994). Choice of decision-making strategies and action versus state orientation. In J. Kuhl & J. Beckmann (Eds.), *Volition and personality: Action versus state orientation* (pp. 167–176). Göttingen, Germany: Hogrefe & Huber.

Stiensmeier-Pelster, J., & Schürmann, M. (1994). Antecedents and consequences of action- versus state orientation: Theoretical and empirical remarks. In J. Kuhl & J. Beckmann (Eds.), *Volition and personality: Action versus state orientation* (pp. 329–340). Göttingen, Germany: Hogrefe & Huber.

Taylor, S. E. (1991). Asymmetrical effects of positive and negative events: The mobilization-minimization hypothesis. *Psychological Bulletin*, *110*, 67–85.

Tesser, A. (1988). Toward a self-evaluation model of social behavior. In L. Berkowitz (Ed.), *Advances in experimental social psychology* (Vol. 21, pp. 181–227). New York: Academic Press.

Tesser, A., Rosen, S., & Waranch, E. (1973). Communicator mood and the reluctance to transmit bad news. *Journal of Communication*, *23*, 619–628.

Tice, D. M., Bratslavsky, E., & Baumeister, R. F. (2001). Emotional distress regulation takes precedence over impulse control: If you feel bad, do it! *Journal of Personality and Social Psychology*, *80*, 53–67.

Van den Berg, A. E., Koole, S. L., & Van der Wulp, N. (2003). Environmental preference and restoration: (How) are they related? *Journal of Environmental Psychology*, *23*, 135–146.

Van Dillen, L., & Koole, S. L. (2004). [How flexible is intuitive affect regulation? Dual task demands moderate the effects of action orientation on affect regulation]. Unpublished raw data, Vrije Universiteit Amsterdam.

Verplanken, B., & Herabadi, A. (2001). Individual differences in impulse buying tendency: Feeling and no thinking. *European Journal of Personality*, *15*, S71–S83.

Vohs, K. D., & Heatherton, T. F. (2000). Self-regulatory failure: A resource-depletion approach. *Psychological Science*, *11*, 249–254.

Wenzlaff, R. M., Wegner, D. M., & Roper, D. (1988). Depression and mental control: The resurgence of unwanted negative thoughts. *Journal of Personality and Social Psychology*, *55*, 882–892.

Wurff, D. M. (1996). *Psychology of religion: Classic and contemporary* (2nd ed.). New York: Wiley.

Zajonc, R. B. (1980). Feeling and thinking: Preferences need no inferences. *American Psychologist*, *35*, 151–175.

Chapter 20

# Feedback Processes in the Simultaneous Regulation of Action and Affect

**Charles S. Carver**
**Michael F. Scheier**

This chapter outlines the fundamentals of a viewpoint in which behavior reflects processes of feedback control. The particular version of this viewpoint that we describe here incorporates the idea that two layers of control manage two different aspects of behavior. We argue that these layers function together to permit people to handle multiple tasks across time. More specifically, they help transform simultaneous motives bearing on many different goals into a stream of actions that shifts repeatedly from one goal to another. This is not really a theory of motivation per se, but a viewpoint on some of the processes by which motives become manifest in action and affect.

The view described here has for a long time been identified with the term *self-regulation* (Carver & Scheier, 1981, 1990, 1998, 1999a, 1999b). This term means different things to different people, however. When we use it, we intend to convey the sense that the processes are purposive, that self-corrective adjustments are taking place as needed to stay on track for the purpose being served, and that the corrective adjustments originate within the person. These points converge in the view that behavior is a continuing process of moving toward (or sometimes away from) goal values, and that this movement embodies characteristics of feedback control. Although a number of people have recently ascribed to this term the additional quality of self-control—of overriding or restraining an impulse—we generally do not assume that quality here.

We want to make it clear at the outset that we are not arguing that the processes described in this chapter are the *only* processes involved in motivated action. Authors of other chapters in this volume examine aspects of motivation that differ substantially from the ideas we outline. We believe, however, that these principles are complementary to many of those other views.

## BEHAVIOR AS GOAL-DIRECTED AND FEEDBACK-CONTROLLED

An easy point of entry into the logic of control processes is the goal concept, which is central to several chapters in this volume. People have many goals at varying levels of abstraction and importance. Most goals can be reached in diverse ways, leading to the potential for vast complexity. And the fact that goals energize and guide activities qualifies the goal as a motivational construct.

### Feedback Processes

We have been interested for some time in the idea that moving toward a goal's attainment reflects the principle of feedback control. A *feedback loop* embodies four subfunctions (MacKay, 1966; Miller, Galanter, & Pribram, 1960; Powers, 1973; Wiener, 1948): an *input*, a *reference value*, a *comparison*, and an *output* (Figure 20.1). It is reasonable to think of the input as perception; it brings information into the system about present circumstances. A reference value can be thought of as equivalent to a goal. The input is compared to this reference value. A discrepancy detected in this comparison is often called an *error signal*. We will treat the output here as equivalent to behavior, but sometimes the behavior is internal. If the comparison detects no discrepancy, the output remains as it was. The effect of a discrepancy on output depends on what kind of loop it is.

In a *discrepancy-reducing loop* (also called a *negative feedback loop*, for negating), the output acts to reduce or eliminate any discrepancy noted between input and reference. In behavior, this is seen in attempts to reach a valued goal, maintain a desired condition, or conform to a standard. There also are *discrepancy-enlarging loops* (*positive feedback loops*), which avoid the reference value, rather than approach it. The value in this case is a threat or an *anti-goal*—for example, a feared or disliked possible self (Carver, Lawrence, & Scheier, 1999; Markus & Nurius, 1986; Ogilvie, 1987). A discrepancy-enlarging loop senses existing conditions, compares them to the anti-goal, and acts to enlarge the discrepancy. (For other theoretical views to which these principles can be linked, see the following chapters in this volume: Elliot & Fryer, Chapter 15; Gable & Strachman, Chapter 37; King, Chapter 34; and Molden, Lee, & Higgins, Chapter 11.)

The effects of discrepancy-enlarging processes in living systems are typically constrained by discrepancy-reducing processes. To put it differently, acts of avoidance often lead into other acts of approach. An avoidance loop tries to escape an anti-goal. But there may be a goal to approach that happens to keep the person distant from the anti-goal. If it is adopted, the tendency to avoid the anti-goal is joined by the tendency to approach that goal. The ap-

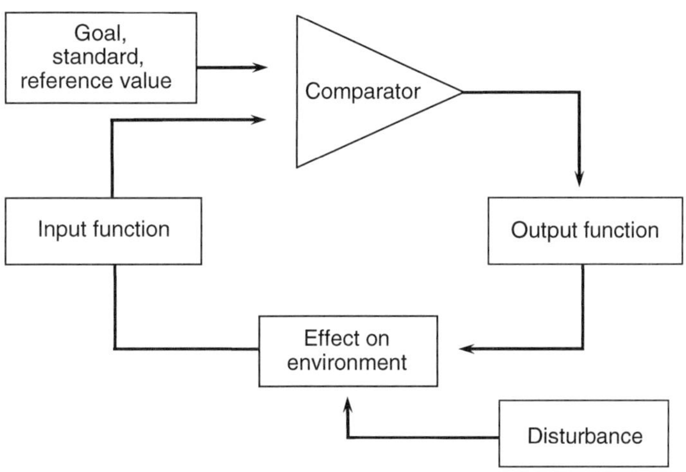


**FIGURE 20.1.** Schematic depiction of a feedback loop, the basic unit of cybernetic control. In a discrepancy-reducing loop, a sensed value is compared to a reference value or standard, and adjustments occur in an output function (if necessary) that shift the sensed value in the direction of the standard. In a discrepancy-enlarging loop, the output function moves the sensed value away from the standard.

proach loop pulls behavior into its orbit. This pattern of dual influence describes what occurs in situations that are referred to as *active avoidance*. An organism confronting a feared stimulus picks a relatively safe location to escape to, and approaches that location.

A few more points about this description are in order. It is easy to portray the elements of a feedback loop conceptually. In some instances of feedback control (e.g., in artificial electronic systems), it is also easy to point to each element. In other instances, doing so is harder. Some feedback processes have no explicit representation of a reference value. The system regulates around a value, but no value is represented as a goal (Berridge, 2004; Carver & Scheier, 2002).

We should also dispel a misconception about the nature of feedback processes. A common illustration of feedback processes is *homeostasis* (meaning "same state"). Because of the wide use of this illustration, some incorrectly infer that feedback loops act only to create and maintain steady states. Some reference values (and goals) *are* static end-states. But others are dynamic and evolving (e.g., the goal of taking a month's vacation, the goal of raising a child to become a good citizen). In such cases, the "goal" is the process of traversing the changing trajectory of the activity, not just reaching the endpoint. Feedback processes apply perfectly well to moving targets (Beer, 1995).

We also note that goals vary greatly in abstractness. You can have the goal of being a good citizen, but you can also have the goal of recycling refuse, a narrower goal that contributes to being a good citizen. To recycle entails concrete goals—for instance, placing newspapers into containers and moving them to a pickup location. Thus it is often said that goals form a hierarchy (Carver & Scheier, 1998, 1999a, 1999b, 2003; Powers, 1973; Vallacher & Wegner, 1987): Abstract goals are attained by the process of attaining concrete goals that help define them.

Finally, we note that although the goal concept is one place where the constructs of personality and social psychology intersect with the logic of feedback control, the intersection is actually much broader. The principle of discrepancy reduction has a long history in studies of conformity to norms (Asch, 1955) and in models of cognitive consistency (Festinger, 1957; Heider, 1946; Lecky, 1945). In effect, the feedback loop constitutes a metatheory or organizing framework for such phenomena.

## FEEDBACK PROCESSES AND AFFECT

Motivation is partly about behavior—the process of getting from here to there. There is more to motivation than that, however. Also involved is the degree of urgency behind the action. The sense of urgency or intensity suggests a role for affect—feelings—in the course of experience. What is *affect*? Where does it come from? It is widely held that affect pertains to one's desires and whether they are being met (Clore, 1994; Frijda, 1986, 1988; Ortony, Clore, & Collins, 1988). But what is the internal mechanism by which feelings arise?

Answers to these questions take several forms, ranging from neurobiological (e.g., Davidson, 1992) to cognitive (Ortony et al., 1988). We have posed a rather different kind of answer (Carver & Scheier, 1990, 1998, 1999a, 1999b), which focuses on what appear to be some of the functional properties of affect. We used feedback control once more as an organizing principle, but now the feedback control bears on a different quality than before.

We suggested that feelings arise as a consequence of a feedback process that operates simultaneously with the behavior-guiding process and in parallel to it. We regard its operation as automatic. The easiest characterization of what this second process is doing is that it is checking on how well the first process (the behavior loop) is doing. The input for this second loop thus is the *rate of discrepancy reduction in the action system over time*. (We limit ourselves at first to discrepancy-reducing loops, then turn to discrepancy-enlarging loops.)

Consider a physical analogy. Action implies change between states. Thus behavior is analogous to distance. If the action loop controls distance, and if the affect loop assesses the action loop's progress, then the affect loop is dealing with the psychological analogue of velocity, the first derivative of distance over time. To the degree that this analogy is meaningful, the perceptual input to the affect loop should be the first derivative over time of the input used by the action loop.

Input by itself does not create affect; a given rate of progress has different affective effects in different contexts. Our argument is that this input is compared to a reference value (cf. Frijda, 1986, 1988), as in other feedback systems. In this case, the reference is an acceptable or expected rate of behavioral discrepancy reduction. As in other feedback loops, the comparison checks for deviation from the standard. If there is a discrepancy, the output function changes.

We hold that the error signal in this loop is manifested phenomenologically as affect, a positive or negative valence. If the rate of progress is below the criterion, negative affect exists. If the rate is high enough to exceed the criterion, positive affect exists. If the rate is indistinguishable from the criterion, no affect exists. In essence, the argument is that feelings with a positive valence mean you are doing better at something than you need to, and feelings with a negative valence mean you are doing worse than you need to (for more detail, see Carver & Scheier, 1998, Chs. 8 and 9). The absence of affect means being neither ahead nor behind.

We should be clear here that we are not arguing for a thinking through of what the affect means. We assume that the meaning is intrinsic to the affect's valence. We also assume that this process occurs automatically.

One direct implication of this line of thought is that the affective valences that might potentially exist regarding any given action domain should fall on a bipolar dimension. That is, it should be the case that affect can be positive, neutral, or negative for any given goal-directed action, depending on how well or poorly the action seems to be attaining the goal.

Research in neuropsychology and related fields suggests the plausibility of this reasoning in two respects. One of them concerns the existence of timing devices in the nervous system. Our view is predicated on the existence of an ability to assess change over time. This requires some representation of time. Neural structures clearly do exist that represent time in some manner (e.g., Handy, Gazzaniga, & Ivry, 2003; Ivry & Spencer, 2004; Ivry & Richardson, 2002).

A second source of indirect support concerns the detection of discrepancies between actual and expected events. Our affect model assumes that discrepancies both above and below a velocity criterion are detected. Recent views of the function of dopamine appear to point to an analogous function. Specifically, dopaminergic neurons respond to rewards that are expected, but they respond more intensely when a reward occurs unexpectedly. Their responses diminish when an expected reward fails to occur (Schultz, 2000, 2006). This pattern appears to indicate that dopamine neurons are involved in detecting when things are going better than expected and worse than expected (see also Holroyd & Coles, 2002). Though this is not precisely the point of our theory (which deals with progress rather than outcome), it has a very strong parallelism to it.

What determines the criterion value for the velocity loop? There probably are many influences, and the orientation a person takes to an action can induce a different framing that may change the criterion (Brendl & Higgins, 1996). What is used as a criterion is probably quite flexible if the activity is unfamiliar. If the activity is familiar, however, the rate criterion is likely to reflect accumulated experience, in the form of an expected rate. Whether "expected" or "desired" or "needed" rate is more accurate as a depiction may depend greatly on the context.

Can the criterion change? Absolutely. We believe that change in rate criterion in a relatively familiar behavior domain occurs relatively slowly. Continuing overshoots result automatically in an upward drift; continuing undershoots result in a downward drift (see Carver & Scheier, 2000, for greater detail). A somewhat ironic consequence of such a recalibration would be to keep the balance of a person's affective experience (positive to negative, aggregated across a span of time) relatively similar, even when the rate criterion changes considerably.

## Two Kinds of Behavioral Loops, Two Dimensions of Affect

So far we have considered only approach loops. Now let us consider discrepancy-enlarging loops. The view just outlined is that positive feeling exists when a behavioral system is making rapid progress *doing what it is organized to do*. The systems addressed there are organized to reduce discrepancies. Yet there seems no obvious reason why the principle should not apply as well to systems that enlarge discrepancies. If such a system is making rapid progress attaining its ends, there should be positive affect. If it doing poorly, there should be negative affect.

That affects of both valences are possible seems applicable to both approach and avoidance. That is, both approach and avoidance have the potential to induce positive feelings (when doing well), and both have the potential to induce negative feelings (when doing poorly). But doing well at *approaching an incentive* is not quite the same as doing well at *moving away from a threat*. Thus there may be differences between the two positives and between the two negatives.

Based on this line of thought, and drawing on the work of Higgins (e.g., 1987, 1996) and his collaborators, we argue for two bipolar dimensions of affect—one bearing on approach, the other bearing on avoidance (Carver, 2001; Carver & Scheier, 1998). Approach-related affect includes such positive affects as elation, eagerness, and excitement, and such negative affects as frustration, anger, and sadness (Carver, 2004). Avoidance-related affect includes such positive affects as relief, serenity, and contentment, and such negative affects as fear, guilt, and anxiety. (For more discussion of the Higgins model, see Molden et al., Chapter 11, this volume. For discussion of the relevance of these ideas to social relationships in particular, see Gable & Strachman, Chapter 37, this volume; Laurenceau, Troy, & Carver, 2005.)

### Merging Affect and Action

This two-layered viewpoint implies a natural connection between affect and action. That is, if the input function of the affect loop is a sensed rate of progress in action, the output function of the affect loop must be a change in rate of that action. Thus the affect loop has a direct influence on what occurs in the action loop.

Some changes in rate output are straightforward. If you are lagging behind, you try harder. Some changes are less straightforward. The rates of many "behaviors" are defined not by a pace of physical action, but in terms of choices among potential actions (or entire programs of action). For example, increasing your rate of progress on a project at work may mean choosing to spend a weekend working rather than playing with family and friends. Increasing your rate of being kind means choosing to do an act that reflects kindness, when an opportunity arises. Thus, change in rate must often be translated into other terms, such as concentration, or allocation of time and effort.

The idea of two negative feedback systems functioning in concert is something that we more or less stumbled into. As it happens, however, this idea is quite common in control engineering (e.g., Clark, 1996). Engineers have long recognized that having two systems functioning together—one controlling position, one controlling velocity—permits the device they control to respond in a way that is both quick and stable, without overshoots and oscillations.

The combination of quickness and stability in responding is desirable in the kinds of devices that engineers deal with, but its value is not limited to such devices. It is also desirable in living beings. A person with very reactive emotions is prone to overreact and oscillate behaviorally. A person who is emotionally nonreactive is slow to respond even to urgent events. A person whose reactions are between those extremes responds quickly, but without overreaction and oscillation.

For biological entities, being able to respond quickly yet accurately confers a clear adaptive advantage. We believe that this combination of quick and stable responding is a consequence of having both behavior-managing and affect-managing control systems. Affect causes people's responses to be quicker (because this control system is time-sensitive); as long as the affective system is not overresponsive, the responses are also stable.

Our focus here is on how affects influence behavior, emphasizing the extent to which they are interwoven. However, note that the behavioral responses that are linked to the affects also lead to *reduction of the affects*. We thus would suggest that the affect system is, in a very basic sense, self-regulating (cf. Campos, Frankel, & Camras, 2004). It is undeniable that people also engage in voluntary efforts to regulate their emotions, but for the most part that is not our focus here (for discussion of that topic, see Koole & Kuhl, Chapter 19, this volume).

## DIVERGENT VIEW OF THE DIMENSIONAL STRUCTURE OF AFFECT

The ideas outlined up to this point have a certain degree of internal coherence, but there are ways in which this model differs from other theories bearing on motivation and emotion. At least two of the differences appear to have important implications.

One difference concerns the dimensional structure of affect (Carver, 2001). Some theories treat affects as aligned along dimensions (though not all theories do—cf. Izard, 1977;

Levenson, 1994, 1999). Our dimensional view holds that affect relating to approach has the potential to be either positive or negative, and that affect relating to avoidance has the potential to be either positive or negative. Most current dimensional models of affect, however, differ in that regard.

The idea that eagerness, excitement, and elation relate to approach is intuitive. It is also intuitive that fear and anxiety relate to avoidance. Both of these relations are noted commonly (Cacioppo, Gardner, & Berntson, 1999; Watson, Wiese, Vaidya, & Tellegen, 1999), and both are represented in neurobiological theories bearing on affect (Davidson, 1992, 1998; Depue & Collins, 1999; Gray, 1990, 1994a, 1994b). But on the opposite poles of these dimensions, the consensus breaks down. For example, Gray (e.g., 1990, 1994b) held that the inhibition (or avoidance) system is engaged by cues of punishment, and also by cues of frustrative nonreward. It thus is linked to negative feelings pertaining to approach as well as avoidance. Similarly, he held that the approach system is engaged by cues of reward, and also by cues of escape or avoidance of punishment. It thus is linked to positive feelings pertaining to avoidance as well as approach.

That view, then, is one in which each system is responsible for affect of one and only one hedonic tone (positive in one case, negative in the other). That theory yields two unipolar affective dimensions (running from neutral to negative and from neutral to positive), each linked to the functioning of a separate behavioral system. A similar position has been taken by Lang and colleagues (e.g., Lang, 1995; Lang, Bradley, & Cuthbert, 1990), by Cacioppo and colleagues (e.g., Cacioppo & Berntson, 1994; Cacioppo et al., 1999), and by Watson and colleagues (1999). In that respect, our version of a dimensional view is quite different from those that dominate today's discussions.

## Evidence of Bipolar Dimensions

Which view is more accurate? Consider first affect when people are "doing well" at threat avoidance. In one study bearing on this question (Higgins, Shah, & Friedman, 1997, Study 4), people took either an approach orientation to a laboratory task (trying to attain success) or an avoidance orientation to it (trying to avoid failing); they then experienced either goal attainment or nonattainment. After the task outcome (which was manipulated), feelings were assessed. Given an avoidance orientation, success caused elevation in calmness, and failure caused elevation in anxiety. Effects on these affects did not occur, however, among those with an approach orientation. This pattern suggests that calmness is linked to doing well at avoidance, rather than to doing well at approach.

A larger amount of evidence links certain kinds of negative affect to "doing poorly" in approaching incentives, and we review only a few sources of information. One source is the study by Higgins and colleagues (1997), just described. The conditions we focused on above were those that led to feelings of calmness and anxiety. However, the study also provided data on sadness. Among persons with an approach orientation, failure elevated sadness, and success elevated cheerfulness. These effects did not occur among participants with an avoidance orientation. The pattern suggests a link between sadness and doing poorly at approach, rather than doing poorly at avoidance.

Another source of evidence is a laboratory study (Carver, 2004) in which participants were led to believe they could obtain a desired reward if they performed well on a task. There was no penalty for doing poorly—only an opportunity of reward for doing well. Participants had been preassessed on the sensitivity of their approach and avoidance systems (Carver & White, 1994). All participants received feedback that they had not done well, and they thus failed to obtain the reward. Reports of sadness and discouragement at that point related to premeasured sensitivity of the approach system, but not to sensitivity of the avoidance system.

Yet another source of information is the literature of self-discrepancy theory. Several studies have shown that feelings of sadness relate uniquely (i.e., even when anxiety is controlled for) to discrepancies between people's actual selves and ideal selves (see Higgins, 1987, 1996, for reviews). Ideals are qualities a person intrinsically desires: aspirations, hopes, positive wishes for the self. There is evidence that pursuing an ideal is an approach process (Higgins, 1996). Thus this literature also suggests that sadness stems from a failure of approach.

There is also evidence linking the approach system to the negative affect of anger. Harmon-Jones and Allen (1998) studied individual differences in trait anger. Higher anger related to higher left frontal activity (and to lower right frontal activity). This suggests a link between anger and the approach system, because the approach system has been linked to activation of the left prefrontal cortex (e.g., Davidson, 1992). More recently, Harmon-Jones and Sigelman (2001) induced a state of anger in some persons but not others, and then examined cortical activity. They found elevations in left frontal activity, suggesting that anger relates to greater engagement of the approach system.

Further evidence pertaining to anger comes from research (Carver, 2004) in which people indicated the feelings they experienced in response to hypothetical events (Study 2) and after the destruction of the World Trade Center (Study 3). Participants had been preassessed on a self-report measure of the sensitivity of their approach and avoidance systems (Carver & White, 1994). Reports of anger related to premeasured sensitivity of the approach system, whereas reports of anxiety related instead to sensitivity of the avoidance system.

### Need for a Conceptual Mechanism

We have spent a good deal of space on this issue. Why? This issue matters a great deal, because it appears to have major implications for any attempt to identify a conceptual mechanism underlying affect. Theories that argue for two unipolar dimensions appear to assume that greater activation of a system translates directly into more affect of that valence (or greater potential for affect of that valence). If the approach system instead relates both to positive and to negative feelings, this direct transformation of system activation to affect is not tenable.

A conceptual mechanism is needed that naturally addresses both positive and negative feelings within the approach function (and, separately, the avoidance function). One such mechanism is the principle described here. There may be others as well, but this one has advantages. For example, its mechanism fits nicely with the fact that feelings occur continuously throughout the attempt to reach an incentive, not just at the point of its attainment. Indeed, feelings rise, wane, and change valence, as progress varies from time to time along the way forward.

## SOME COUNTERINTUITIVE IMPLICATIONS

A second important issue also differentiates this model from many other viewpoints on the meaning and consequences of affect. Recall our argument that affect reflects the error signal from a comparison in a feedback loop. This idea has some very counterintuitive implications—in particular, implications concerning positive affect (Carver, 2003).

As noted earlier, if affect reflects the error signal in a feedback loop, affect is a signal to adjust rate of progress. This would be true whether the rate is above the mark or below it—that is, whether affect is positive or negative. For negative feelings, this notion is not at all controversial; it is fully intuitive. The first response to negative feelings is usually to try harder. (For now we disregard the possibility of withdrawing effort and quitting, though that possibility clearly is important; we return to it later.) If the person tries harder—and if more effort (or better effort) increases the rate of intended movement—the negative affect diminishes or ceases.

What about positive feelings? Here prediction becomes counterintuitive. In this model, positive feelings arise when things are going better than they need to. But the feelings still reflect a discrepancy (albeit a positive one), and the function of a negative feedback loop is to minimize discrepancies. Such system is organized in such a way that it "wants" to see neither negative nor positive affect. Either quality (deviation from the standard in either direction) would represent an "error" and lead to changes in output that would eventually reduce it.

This view argues that people who exceed the criterion rate of progress (and who thus have positive feelings) will automatically tend to reduce subsequent effort in this domain. They will "coast" a little (cf. Frijda, 1994, p. 113)—not necessarily stop, but ease back, such that the subsequent rate of progress returns to the criterion. The impact on subjective affect would be that the positive feeling itself is not sustained for very long. It begins to fade.

We must be clear that expending greater effort to catch up when behind, and coasting when ahead, are both presumed to be specific to the goal domain to which the affect is attached. Usually this is the goal from which the affect arises in the first place (for exceptions, see Schwarz & Clore, 1983). We are not arguing that positive affect creates a tendency to coast *in general*, but rather that it creates a tendency to coast with respect to the specific activity producing the positive feelings.

This is a kind of "cruise control" model of the origins and consequences of affect. That is, a system of this sort would operate in the same way as a car's cruise control. If behavior is moving too slowly, negative affect arises. The person responds by increasing effort, trying to speed up. If the person is going faster than needed, positive affect arises, leading to coasting. A car's cruise control is very similar. Coming to a hill slows the car down; the cruise control responds by giving the engine more fuel, speeding back up. If the car comes across the crest of a hill and rolls downward too fast, the system cuts back the fuel, and the speed drags back down.

The analogy is intriguing partly because both sides have an asymmetry in the consequences of deviation from the reference point. That is, both in a car and in behavior, addressing the problem of going too slow requires adding resources. Addressing the problem of going too fast requires only reducing resources. The cruise control does not engage the brakes; it just reduces fuel. The car coasts back to the velocity set point. Thus the effect of the cruise control on a high rate of speed depends in part on external circumstances. If the hill is steep, the car may exceed the cruise control's set point all the way to the valley below.

In the same fashion, people usually do not react to positive affect by actively trying to make themselves feel less good (though there are exceptions). They just ease back a little on resources devoted to the domain in which the affect has arisen. The positive feelings may be sustained for a long time (depending on circumstances), as the person coasts down the subjective analogue of the hill. Eventually, though, the reduced resources would cause the positive affect to diminish. Generally, then, the system would act to prevent great amounts of pleasure as well as great amounts of pain (Carver, 2003; Carver & Scheier, 1998).

## Coasting

The idea that positive affect leads to coasting, which would eventually result in reduction of the positive affect, strikes some people as being very unlikely. Some believe that pleasure is a sign to continue what one is doing, or even to immerse oneself in it more deeply (cf. Fredrickson, 2001; Messinger, 2002). On the other hand, that view has a logical problem. If pleasure causes increase in engagement in the activity, leading thereby to more pleasure and thus more engagement, when and why would the person ever cease that activity? When would the person ever even slow down? The only reason for slowing would be the completion of the activity.

The idea that positive feelings induce coasting may seem unlikely, but we are not alone in having suggested it. In discussing joy, Izard (1977) wrote:

> If the kind of problem at hand requires a great deal of persistence and hard work, *joy may put the problem aside before it is solved*. . . . If your intellectual performance, whatever it may be, leads to joy, the joy will have the effect of *slowing down performance* and removing some of the concern for problem solving. This change in pace and concern may postpone or in some cases eliminate the possibility of an intellectual or creative achievement. . . . If excitement causes the "rushing" or "forcing" of intellectual activity, a *joy-elicited slowing down* may be exactly what is need to improve intellectual performance and creative endeavor. (p. 257; emphasis added)

More recently, Izard and Ackerman (2000) wrote, "Periodic joy provides *respite from the activity*" (p. 258; emphasis added).

Does positive affect lead to coasting? To test the idea, a study must assess coasting with respect to the same goal as underlies the affect. Many studies have created positive affect in one context and assessed its influence on another task (e.g., Isen, 1987, 2000; Schwarz & Bohner, 1996). However, that procedure does not test this question. Suggestive evidence has been reported by Mizruchi (1991) and Louro (2005), but the question remains relatively untested.

## Coasting and Multiple Concerns

One reason for skepticism about the idea that positive affect induces coasting is that it is hard to see why a process could possibly be built into the organism that limits positive feelings—indeed, dampens them. After all, a truism of life is that people supposedly are organized to seek pleasure and avoid pain. We believe that a basis for the adaptive value of the tendency to coast lies in the fact that people have multiple simultaneous concerns (Carver, 2003; Carver & Scheier, 1998; Frijda, 1994). Given multiple concerns, people do not optimize their outcome on any one of them, but rather *satisfice* (Simon, 1953)—that is, do a good enough job on each to deal with it satisfactorily.

A tendency to coast would virtually define satisficing regarding that particular goal. That is, any reduction in effort would prevent the best possible outcome on that goal from being attained. A tendency to coast would also foster satisficing on a broader set of several goals. That is, if progress in one domain exceeds current needs, a tendency to coast in that domain (satisficing) would make it easy to shift to another domain, at little or no cost. This would help ensure satisfactory goal attainment in the other domain and ultimately across multiple domains.

Continued pursuit of one goal without letup, in contrast, can have adverse effects. Continuing a rapid pace in one arena may sustain positive affect in that arena, but by diverting resources from other goals, it also increases the potential for problems elsewhere. This would be even more true of an effort to *intensify* the positive affect, because doing that would mean further diverting resources from other goals. Indeed, a single-minded pursuit of yet-more-positive feelings in one domain can even be lethal, if it causes the person to disregard threats looming elsewhere.

A pattern in which positive feelings lead to easing back, and an openness to shifting focus, would minimize such adverse effects. It is important to note that this view does not *require* that people with positive feelings shift goals. It simply holds that openness to a shift is a consequence—and a potential benefit—of the coasting tendency. This line of thought would, however, begin to account for why people do eventually turn away from what are clearly pleasurable activities.

A provocative finding, in this regard, is that smiling infants who are engaging in face-to-face interactions with their mothers periodically avert their gazes from their mothers, then stop smiling. Infants are more likely to do this (and to avert their gaze longer) when they are smiling intensely than when the smiles are less intense (Stifter & Moyer, 1991). This pattern hints that the infant's experience of happiness creates an openness to shifting focus, or at least a tendency to coast with respect to the interaction with the mother, letting the affect diminish before returning to the interaction.

## PRIORITY MANAGEMENT AS A CORE ISSUE IN SELF-REGULATION

This line of argument begins to implicate positive feelings in a broad function within the organism that deserves further consideration. This function is the shifting from one goal to another as focal in behavior (Dreisbach & Goschke, 2004; Shallice, 1978). This basic and very important phenomenon is often overlooked. Many goals are under pursuit simultaneously (cf. Atkinson & Birch, 1970; Murray, 1938), but only one can have top priority at a given moment. People need to shield and maintain the intentions being pursued (cf. Shah, Friedman, & Kruglanski, 2002), but they also need also to shift flexibly among goals.

The problem of priority management was addressed many years ago in a creative and influential article by Simon (1967). He pointed out that any entity with many goals needs a way to rank them for pursuit and a mechanism to change rankings as necessary. He argued as follows: Most of the goals people are pursuing are largely out of awareness at any given moment. Only the one with the highest priority has full access to consciousness. Sometimes events occur during the pursuit of that top-priority goal that create problems for a second goal, which now has a lower priority. Indeed, the mere passing of time can sometimes create a problem for the second goal, because the passing of time may be making its attainment less likely. If the second goal is also important, any emerging problem for its attainment needs to be registered and taken into account. If the situation evolves enough to seriously threaten the second goal, some mechanism is needed for changing priorities, so that the second goal replaces the first one as focal.

### Negative Feelings and Reprioritization

Simon (1967) reasoned that emotions are calls for reprioritization. He suggested that emotion arising with respect to a goal that is out of awareness eventually induces people to interrupt their behavior and give that goal a higher priority than it had. The stronger the emotion, the stronger is the claim being made that the unattended goal should have higher priority than the goal that is presently focal. The affect is what pulls the out-of-awareness into awareness. Simon did not address the negative affect that sometimes arises with respect to a goal that currently is focal, but the same principle seems to apply to this case as well. That is, negative affect in this case seems to be a call for an even greater investment of resources and effort in the focal goal than is now being made.

Simon's analysis is applied easily to negative feelings such as anxiety and frustration. If you promised your spouse you would go to the post office this afternoon and you've been too busy to go, the creeping of the clock toward closing time can cause an increase in frustration or anxiety (or both). Neither affect would pertain to the work you are doing, however. Frustration might arise from the issue of a potentially unmet obligation (a desired outcome that is slipping away); anxiety might arise from the issue of a potentially angry spouse (a threat that is coming closer). The greater the potential loss, the greater the frustration; the greater the threat, the stronger the anxiety. The stronger the affect, the more likely it is that the goal it stems from will rise in priority until it comes fully to awareness and becomes the focal reference point for behavior.

## Positive Feelings and Reprioritization

Simon's discussion of shifting priorities focused on cases in which a nonfocal goal demands a higher priority than it now has and *intrudes* on awareness. By strong implication, his discussion dealt only with negative affect. However, there is another way in which priority ordering can shift: The currently focal goal can *relinquish its place*. Simon noted this possibility obliquely; he noted that goal completion results in termination of pursuit of that goal. However, he did not address the possibility that an as-yet-unattained goal might also yield its place in line.

Consider the possibility that positive feelings represent a cue regarding reprioritization, but a cue to *reduce* the priority of the goal to which the feeling pertains. This appears consistent with the sense of Simon's analysis. It simply suggests that the function he asserted for affect is relevant to affects of both valences. Positive affect regarding an avoidance act (relief or tranquility) indicates that a threat has dissipated, no longer requires as much attention as it did, and can now assume a lower priority. Positive feelings regarding approach (happiness, joy) indicate that an incentive is being attained. If it *has* been attained, effort can cease, as Simon noted. If it is not yet attained, the affect is a signal that you could temporarily put this goal aside, because you are doing so well. That is, it is a sign that this goal can assume a lower priority (Carver, 2003).

If a focal goal diminishes in priority, what follows? This situation is less directive than the one in which a nonfocal goal demands an increase in priority (which is very specific about what goal should receive more attention). What happens in this case depends partly on what is waiting in line. It also depends partly on whether the context has changed in any important way while you were busy with the focal goal. That is, opportunities to attain incentives sometimes appear unexpectedly, and people put aside their plans to take advantage of such unanticipated opportunities (Hayes-Roth & Hayes-Roth, 1979; Payton, 1990). It seems reasonable that people with positive affect should be most prone to shift goals at this point if something else needs fixing or doing (regarding a next-in-line goal or a newly emergent goal), or if an unanticipated opportunity for gain has appeared.

Sometimes the next item in line is of fairly high priority in its own right. Sometimes the situation has changed and a new goal has emerged for consideration. On the other hand, sometimes neither of these conditions exists. In such a case, no change would occur, because the downgrade in priority of the focal goal does not make it lower than the priorities of the alternatives. Positive affect does not *require* a change in direction; it simply sets the stage for such a change to be more likely.

There is indirect support for this general line of reasoning from several sources. For one, the ideas have a good deal in common with ideas recently proposed about circumstances under which people do and do not engage in self-esteem-protective behavior. Maintaining self-esteem is an important goal (e.g., Tesser, 1988), but when people are in good moods, self-esteem enhancement becomes less likely (Tesser, Crepaz, Collins, Cornell, & Beach, 2000). Tesser and colleagues (2000) argued from this that self-esteem maintenance displays satisficing. That is, as long as the self-image is above a threshold of positivity, there is no effort to build it higher. Only if it falls below the threshold is effort engaged to prop it back up. A variety of other evidence also appears to fit the idea that positive feelings make people more open to taking up alternate goals, particularly desired goals that seem threatened (for a review, see Carver, 2003).

Effects such as these have contributed to the emergence of the view that positive experiences represent psychological resources. Trope and Pomerantz (1998) wrote that experiences such as a success or a positive mood serve as means to other ends, rather than as ends themselves. Reed and Aspinwall (1998) suggested that positive self-beliefs and self-affirmations act as resources that permit people to confront problematic situations such as health threats (see also Aspinwall, 1998; Isen, 2000; for broader resource models, see Gallo & Matthews, 2003; Hobfoll, 1989, 2002; Muraven & Baumeister, 2000). This line of thought is not quite the same as the one that underlies the position taken here, but some of its connotations are similar.

The idea that positive feelings act as psychological resources need not be limited to cases in which resources permit people to turn to problems. For example, secure infant attachment is widely seen as a resource that promotes exploration (Bowlby, 1988). Such a view also seems implicit in Fredrickson's (1998) position that positive feelings promote play. The idea that positive affect serves as a resource for exploration resembles in some ways the idea that positive feelings open people to noticing and taking advantage of emergent opportunities, to being distracted into enticing alternatives—in short, to opportunistic behavior.

Some evidence also fits this idea. Kahn and Isen (1993) gave people opportunities to try out choices within a food category. Those in whom positive affect had been induced switched among choice alternatives more than did controls. Isen (2000, p. 423) interpreted this as indicating that positive affect promotes "enjoyment of variety and a wide range of possibilities," which seems similar to opportunistic foraging. Dreisbach and Goschke (2004) similarly found that positive affect decreased perseveration on a task strategy and increased distractibility. Both of these are consistent with our reasoning.

We should make clear that we are not arguing that affect is the only source of shifts in goal reprioritization. Changes in context can also produce shifts, because different contexts have been linked in the past to different goals. The resulting associations in memory mean that a change in context can prompt the emergence of a different goal via those associations. Our argument is simply that affect is part of the prioritization process.

## Evading Automatic Functions of Affect

Our focus here has been primarily on what we construe as a set of automatic effects of emotions in priority management. However, it may also be useful to note briefly that people learn to intervene in these otherwise automatic effects, by regulating their own emotions in ways that go beyond goal-related action per se (see also Koole & Kuhl, Chapter 19, this volume).

For example, suppose you are an athlete trying to perform in an event that takes a particular period of time. Suppose you get ahead of your opponent quickly. By our reasoning, if you therefore feel happy, you may relax a little. Relaxing—becoming vulnerable to distraction—is not desirable in this situation, however. How can you prevent that from happening? A common strategy for athletes is to try to prevent feelings of pleasure from arising. This can be done by maintaining an extremely high level of aspiration, so that it could hardly ever be exceeded (and thus no positive affect could result). This is similar to the well-known principle that the highest performance comes from setting a goal that is just out of reach (Locke & Latham, 1990). Another strategy is to artificially generate anger, taking the place of any pleasure that exists in being ahead. Yet another strategy is to remind yourself that your lead is small and you are still vulnerable, or even to pretend that you are not really ahead at all.

The point more generally is that there often are ways to trick the automatic system of affective response by reframing the situation in various ways. If the affective reaction itself can be changed, the resulting impact on priority management should also change.

## Priority Management and Depressed Affect

One more aspect of priority management should be addressed here. It concerns the idea that there are some circumstances under which goals are not attainable and are better abandoned. We have long argued that sufficient doubt about goal attainment results in an impetus to disengage from efforts to reach the goal, and even to disengage from the goal itself (Carver & Scheier, 1981, 1998, 1999a, 1999b). This is certainly a kind of priority adjustment, in that the abandoned goal is now receiving an even lower priority than it had before. That is, no behavior is being directed to its attainment at all. How does this sort of reprioritization fit into the picture sketched up to here?

At first glance, the idea that doubt about goal attainment (and the negative feelings associated with that doubt) cause reduction in effort seems to contradict Simon's (1967) position that negative affect is a call for higher priority. However, there is an important distinction between two kinds of negative affective experiences associated with approach (Carver, 2003, 2004). (A parallel line of reasoning can be applied to avoidance, but we limit ourselves here to approach.) Some negative affects related to approach coalesce around frustration and anger. Others coalesce around sadness, depression, and dejection. The former relate to an increase in priority, the latter to a decrease.

## Integration

In describing our view on affect, we said that approach-related affects can be placed on a dimension. However, the dimension is not a simple straight line. The theory behind our work holds that falling behind—progress below the criterion—creates negative affect as the incentive slips away. Inadequate movement forward (or no movement, or reverse movement) gives rise to frustration, irritation, and anger. These feelings (or the mechanism that underlies them) function to engage effort more completely, in order to overcome obstacles and reverse the inadequacy of current progress. If the situation is one in which more effort (or better effort) can improve progress, such effort allows the person to move toward the incentive at an adequate rate, and attaining the incentive seems likely. This case fits the priority management model of Simon (1967).

Sometimes, however, continued efforts do not produce adequate movement forward. Indeed, if the situation involves loss, movement forward is precluded, because the incentive is gone. In a situation where failure seems (or is) assured, the feelings are sadness, depression, despondency, dejection, grief, and hopelessness (cf. Finlay-Jones & Brown, 1981). Accompanying behaviors also differ in this case. The person tends to disengage from—give up on—further effort toward the incentive (Klinger, 1975; Wortman & Brehm, 1975; for supporting evidence, see Lewis, Sullivan, Ramsay, & Allessandri, 1992; Mikulincer, 1988).

At least two published studies have obtained patterns of emotions consistent with this portrayal (Mikulincer, 1994; Pittman & Pittman, 1980). In each, participants received varying amounts of failure, and their emotional responses were assessed. In both cases, reports of anger were most intense after small amounts of failure and lower after larger amounts of failure. Reports of depression were low after small amounts of failure and intense after larger amounts of failure.

As just described, approach-related negative feelings in these two kinds of situations are presumed to link to two very different effects on ongoing action. Both effects have adaptive properties. In the first situation (when the person falls behind, but the goal is not seen as lost), feelings of frustration and anger accompany an *increase* in effort—a struggle to gain the incentive despite setbacks. Consistent with this view, Frijda (1986, p. 429) argued that anger implies having the hope that things can be set right (see also Harmon-Jones & Allen, 1998). This struggle is adaptive (and thus the affect is adaptive), because the struggle fosters goal attainment.

In the second situation (when effort appears futile), negative feelings of sadness and depression accompany *reduction* of effort. Sadness and despondency imply that things cannot be set right—that further effort is pointless. Reduction of effort in this circumstance can also have adaptive functions (Carver & Scheier, 2003; Wrosch, Scheier, Carver, & Schulz, 2003; Wrosch, Scheier, Miller, Schulz, & Carver, 2003). It serves to conserve energy rather than waste it in futile pursuit of the unattainable (Nesse, 2000). If reducing effort also helps diminish commitment to the goal (Klinger, 1975), it eventually readies the person to take up pursuit of other incentives in place of this one (see also King, Chapter 34, this volume).

The variations in effort described in the preceding paragraphs are portrayed in Figure 20.2. The left side portrays the hypothesized reduction in effort when velocity exceeds the criterion, discussed earlier. The right side por-

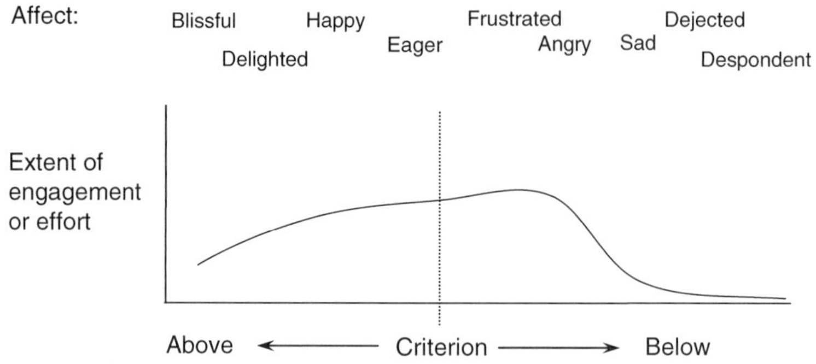


**FIGURE 20.2.** Hypothesized approach-related affects as a function of doing well versus doing poorly compared to a criterion velocity. A second (vertical) dimension indicates the degree of behavioral engagement posited to be associated with affects at different degrees of departure from neutral. Adapted from Carver (2004). Copyright 2004 by the American Psychological Association.

trays both the strong engagement that is implied by frustration and anger, and the disengagement of sadness and dejection.

Two additional points about the portion of Figure 20.2 to the right of the criterion line are worth noting. First, this part of the figure has much in common with several other depictions of variations in effort when difficulty in moving toward a goal gives way to loss of the goal (for greater detail, see Carver & Scheier, 1998, Ch. 11). Perhaps best known is Wortman and Brehm's (1975) integration of reactance and helplessness. They described a region of threat to control, in which there is enhanced effort to regain control, and a region of loss of control, in which efforts diminish. Indeed, the figure they used to illustrate those regions greatly resembles the right side of Figure 20.2.

Another point concerns the fact that the right side of Figure 20.2 is drawn with a rather abrupt shift from frustration to sadness. The degree of abruptness of the transition in this figure is arbitrary. There are probably cases in which the transition is abrupt, and also cases in which it is not. These two sets of cases may be distinguished by the relative importance of the goals involved. Importance as a variable has largely been ignored in this discussion, but it obviously must play a very large role in the intensity of affective and motivational experiences (cf. Pomerantz, Saxon, & Oishi, 2000). Although we cannot address this issue fully here, discussions of it can be found elsewhere (Carver & Scheier, 1998, 1999a, 1999b).

This aspect of Figure 20.2 also illustrates how these ideas can be linked to other ideas that are increasingly influencing psychology: the concepts of dynamic systems (Vallacher, Read, & Nowak, 2002). The transition from engagement to disengagement can be seen as gradual movement along a dimension, but it can also be seen as more of a qualitative shift, or a bifurcation (Carver & Scheier, 1998, Chs. 14–16). This is an idea that certainly deserves further examination.

## CONCLUDING COMMENT

We are painfully aware that the ideas outlined in this chapter do not provide a complete picture. They leave many questions unanswered. Indeed, they leave many questions *unasked.* For instance, what about will? What about self-determination? What about self-control and the overriding of impulses? Though these questions are important, they are beyond the scope of this chapter. Some of them are discussed in depth elsewhere (e.g., Bargh, 1997; Carver, 2005; Deci & Ryan, 2000; Ryan & Deci, 2001; Wegner, 2002). As we have said at the outset, however, in this chapter we can address only certain aspects of one particular way of thinking about motivation. To do a complete job discussing motivation would require, at the very least, an entire handbook.

## ACKNOWLEDGMENTS

Preparation of this chapter was facilitated by Grant Nos. CA64710, CA78995, and CA84944 from the National Cancer Institute and by additional funding to the Pittsburgh Mind–Body Center at the University of Pittsburgh and Carnegie Mellon University from the National Heart, Lung, and Blood Institute (Grant Nos. HL65111, HL65112, HL076852, and HL076858).

## REFERENCES


Asch, S. E. (1955). Opinions and social pressure. *Scientific American*, *193*, 31–35.

Aspinwall, L. G. (1998). Rethinking the role of positive affect in self-regulation. *Motivation and Emotion*, *22*, 1–32.

Atkinson, J. W., & Birch, D. (1970). *The dynamics of action*. New York: Wiley.

Bargh, J. A. (1997). The automaticity of everyday life. In R. S. Wyer, Jr. (Ed.), *Advances in social cognition* (Vol. 10, pp. 1–61). Mahwah, NJ: Erlbaum.

Beer, R. D. (1995). A dynamical systems perspective on agent–environment interaction. *Artificial Intelligence*, *72*, 173–215.

Berridge, K. C. (2004). Motivation concepts in behavioral neuroscience. *Physiology and Behavior*, *81*, 179–209.

Bowlby, J. (1988). *A secure base: Parent–child attachment and healthy human development*. New York: Basic Books.

Brendl, C. M., & Higgins, E. T. (1996). Principles of judging valence: What makes events positive or negative? In M. P. Zanna (Ed.), *Advances in experimental social psychology* (Vol. 28, pp. 95–160). San Diego, CA: Academic Press.

Cacioppo, J. T., & Berntson, G. G. (1994). Relationship between attitudes and evaluative space: A critical review, with emphasis on the separability of positive and negative substrates. *Psychological Bulletin*, *115*, 401–423.

Cacioppo, J. T., Gardner, W. L., & Berntson, G. G. (1999). The affect system has parallel and integrative processing components: Form follows function. *Journal of Personality and Social Psychology*, *76*, 839–855.

Campos, J. J., Frankel, C. B., & Camras, L. (2004). On the nature of emotion regulation. *Child Development*, *75*, 377–394.

Carver, C. S. (2001). Affect and the functional bases of behavior: On the dimensional structure of affective experience. *Personality and Social Psychology Review*, *5*, 345–356.

Carver, C. S. (2003). Pleasure as a sign you can attend to something else: Placing positive feelings within a general model of affect. *Cognition and Emotion*, *17*, 241–261.

Carver, C. S. (2004). Negative affects deriving from the behavioral approach system. *Emotion*, *4*, 3–22.

Carver, C. S. (2005). Impulse and constraint: Perspectives from personality psychology, convergence with theory in other areas, and potential for integration. *Personality and Social Psychology Review*, *9*, 312–333.

Carver, C. S., Lawrence, J. W., & Scheier, M. F. (1999). Self-discrepancies and affect: Incorporating the role of feared selves. *Personality and Social Psychology Bulletin*, *25*, 783–792.

Carver, C. S., & Scheier, M. F. (1981). *Attention and self-regulation: A control-theory approach to human behavior*. New York: Springer-Verlag.

Carver, C. S., & Scheier, M. F. (1990). Origins and functions of positive and negative affect: A control-process view. *Psychological Review*, *97*, 19–35.

Carver, C. S., & Scheier, M. F. (1998). *On the self-regulation of behavior*. New York: Cambridge University Press.

Carver, C. S., & Scheier, M. F. (1999a). Several more themes, a lot more issues: Commentary on the commentaries. In R. S. Wyer, Jr. (Ed.), *Advances in social cognition* (Vol. 12, pp. 261–302). Mahwah, NJ: Erlbaum.

Carver, C. S., & Scheier, M. F. (1999b). Themes and issues in the self-regulation of behavior. In R. S. Wyer, Jr. (Ed.), *Advances in social cognition* (Vol. 12, pp. 1–105). Mahwah, NJ: Erlbaum.

Carver, C. S., & Scheier, M. F. (2000). Scaling back goals and recalibration of the affect system are processes in normal adaptive self-regulation: Understanding "response shift" phenomena. *Social Science and Medicine*, *50*, 1715–1722.

Carver, C. S., & Scheier, M. F. (2002). Control processes and self-organization as complementary principles underlying behavior. *Personality and Social Psychology Review*, *6*, 304–315.

Carver, C. S., & Scheier, M. F. (2003). Three human strengths. In L. G. Aspinwall & U. M. Staudinger (Eds.), *A psychology of human strengths: Fundamental questions and future directions for a positive psychology* (pp. 87–102). Washington, DC: American Psychological Association.

Carver, C. S., & White, T. L. (1994). Behavioral inhibition, behavioral activation, and affective responses to impending reward and punishment: The BIS/BAS scales. *Journal of Personality and Social Psychology*, *67*, 319–333.

Clark, R. N. (1996). *Control system dynamics*. New York: Cambridge University Press.

Clore, G. C. (1994). Why emotions are felt. In P. Ekman & R. J. Davidson (Eds.), *The nature of emotion: Fundamental questions* (pp. 103–111). New York: Oxford University Press.

Davidson, R. J. (1992). Anterior cerebral asymmetry and the nature of emotion. *Brain and Cognition*, *20*, 125–151.

Davidson, R. J. (1998). Affective style and affective disorders: Perspectives from affective neuroscience. *Cognition and Emotion*, *12*, 307–330.

Deci, E. L., & Ryan, R. M. (2000). The "what" and "why" of goal pursuits: Human needs and the self-determination of behavior. *Psychological Inquiry*, *11*, 227–268.

Depue, R. A., & Collins, P. F. (1999). Neurobiology of the structure of personality: Dopamine, facilitation of incentive motivation, and extraversion. *Behavioral and Brain Sciences*, *22*, 491–517.

Dreisbach, G., & Goschke, T. (2004). How positive affect modulates cognitive control: Reduced perseveration at the cost of increased distractibility. *Journal of Experimental Psychology: Learning, Memory, and Cognition*, *30*, 343–353.

Festinger, L. (1957). *A theory of cognitive dissonance*. Evanston, IL: Row, Peterson.

Finlay-Jones, R., & Brown, G. W. (1981). Types of stressful life event and the onset of anxiety and depressive disorders. *Psychological Medicine*, *11*, 803–815.

Fredrickson, B. L. (1998). What good are positive emotions? *Review of General Psychology*, *2*, 300–319.

Fredrickson, B. L. (2001). The role of positive emotions in positive psychology: The broaden-and-build theory of positive emotions. *American Psychologist*, *56*, 218–226.

Frijda, N. H. (1986). *The emotions*. Cambridge, UK: Cambridge University Press.

Frijda, N. H. (1988). The laws of emotion. *American Psychologist*, *43*, 349–358.

Frijda, N. H. (1994). Emotions are functional, most of the time. In P. Ekman & R. J. Davidson (Eds.), *The nature of emotion: Fundamental questions* (pp. 112–126). New York: Oxford University Press.

Gallo, L. C., & Matthews, K. A. (2003). Understanding the association between socioeconomic status and physical health: Do negative emotions play a role? *Psychological Bulletin*, *129*, 10–51.

Gray, J. A. (1990). Brain systems that mediate both emotion and cognition. *Cognition and Emotion*, *4*, 269–288.

Gray, J. A. (1994a). Personality dimensions and emotion systems. In P. Ekman & R. J. Davidson (Eds.), *The nature of emotion: Fundamental questions* (pp. 329–331). New York: Oxford University Press.

Gray, J. A. (1994b). Three fundamental emotion systems. In P. Ekman & R. J. Davidson (Eds.), *The nature of emotion: Fundamental questions* (pp. 243–247). New York: Oxford University Press.

Handy, T., Gazzaniga, M., & Ivry, R. B. (2003). Cortical and subcortical contributions to the representation of temporal information. *Neuropsychologia*, *41*, 1461–1473.

Harmon-Jones, E., & Allen, J. J. B. (1998). Anger and frontal brain activity: Asymmetry consistent with approach motivation despite negative affective valence. *Journal of Personality and Social Psychology*, *74*, 1310–1316.

Harmon-Jones, E., & Sigelman, J. D. (2001). State anger and prefrontal brain activity: Evidence that insult-related relative left-prefrontal activation is associated with experienced anger and aggression. *Journal of Personality and Social Psychology*, *80*, 797–803.

Hayes-Roth, B., & Hayes-Roth, F. (1979). A cognitive model of planning. *Cognitive Science*, *3*, 275–310.

Heider, F. (1946). Attitudes and cognitive organization. *Journal of Psychology*, *21*, 107–112.

Higgins, E. T. (1987). Self-discrepancy: A theory relating self and affect. *Psychological Review*, *94*, 319–340.

Higgins, E. T. (1996). Ideals, oughts, and regulatory focus: Affect and motivation from distinct pains and pleasures. In P. M. Gollwitzer & J. A. Bargh (Eds.), *The psychology of action: Linking cognition and motivation to behavior* (pp. 91–114). New York: Guilford Press.

Higgins, E. T., Shah, J., & Friedman, R. (1997). Emotional responses to goal attainment: Strength of regulatory focus as moderator. *Journal of Personality and Social Psychology*, *72*, 515–525.

Hobfoll, S. E. (1989). Conservation of resources: A new attempt at conceptualizing stress. *American Psychologist*, *44*, 513–524.

Hobfoll, S. E. (2002). Social and psychological resources and adaptation. *Review of General Psychology*, *6*, 307–324.

Holroyd, C. B., & Coles, M. G. H. (2002). The neural basis of human error processing: Reinforcement learning, dopamine, and the error-related negativity. *Psychological Review*, *109*, 679–709.

Isen, A. M. (1987). Positive affect, cognitive processes, and social behavior. In L. Berkowitz (Ed.), *Advances in experimental social psychology* (Vol. 20, pp. 203–252). San Diego, CA: Academic Press.

Isen, A. M. (2000). Positive affect and decision making. In M. Lewis & J. M. Haviland-Jones (Eds.), *Handbook of emotions* (2nd ed., pp. 417–435). New York: Guilford Press.

Ivry, R. B., & Richardson, T. (2002). Temporal control and coordination: The multiple timer model. *Brain and Cognition*, *48*, 117–132.

Ivry, R. B., & Spencer, R. (2004). The neural representation of time. *Current Opinion in Neurobiology*, *14*, 225–232.

Izard, C. E. (1977). *Human emotions*. New York: Plenum Press.

Izard, C. E., & Ackerman, B. P. (2000). Motivational, organizational, and regulatory functions of discrete emotions. In M. Lewis & J. M. Haviland-Jones (Eds.), *Handbook of emotions* (2nd ed., pp. 253–264). New York: Guilford Press.

Kahn, B. E., & Isen, A. M. (1993). The influence of positive affect on variety-seeking among safe, enjoyable products. *Journal of Consumer Research*, *20*, 257–270.

Klinger, E. (1975). Consequences of commitment to and disengagement from incentives. *Psychological Review*, *82*, 1–25.

Lang, P. J. (1995). The emotion probe: Studies of motivation and attention. *American Psychologist*, *50*, 372–385.

Lang, P. J., Bradley, M. M., & Cuthbert, B. N. (1990). Emotion, attention, and the startle reflex. *Psychological Review*, *97*, 377–395.

Laurenceau, J.-P., Troy, A. B., & Carver, C. S. (2005). Two distinct emotional experiences in romantic relationships: Effects of perceptions regarding approach of intimacy and avoidance of conflict. *Personality and Social Psychology Bulletin*, *31*, 1123–1133.

Lecky, P. (1945). *Self-consistency: A theory of personality.* Washington, DC: Island Press.

Levenson, R. W. (1994). Human emotion: A functional view. In P. Ekman & R. Davidson (Eds.), *The nature of emotions: Fundamental questions* (pp. 123–126). New York: Oxford University Press.

Levenson, R. W. (1999). The intrapersonal functions of emotion. *Cognition and Emotion*, *13*, 481–504.

Lewis, M., Sullivan, M. W., Ramsay, D. S., & Allessandri, S. M. (1992). Individual differences in anger and sad expressions during extinction: Antecedents and consequences. *Infant Behavior and Development*, *15*, 443–452.

Locke, E. A., & Latham, G. P. (1990). *A theory of goal setting and task performance.* Englewood Cliffs, NJ: Prentice Hall.

Louro, M. J. (2005). *Leaving pleasure: Positive emotions and goal-directed behavior.* Unpublished doctoral dissertation, University of Tilburg, Tilburg, The Netherlands.

MacKay, D. M. (1966). Cerebral organization and the conscious control of action. In J. C. Eccles (Ed.), *Brain and conscious experience* (pp. 422–445). Berlin: Springer-Verlag.

Markus, H., & Nurius, P. (1986). Possible selves. *American Psychologist*, *41*, 954–969.

Messinger, D. S. (2002). Positive and negative: Infant facial expressions and emotions. *Current Directions in Psychological Science*, *11*, 1–6.

Mikulincer, M. (1988). Reactance and helplessness following exposure to learned helplessness following exposure to unsolvable problems: The effects of attributional style. *Journal of Personality and Social Psychology*, *54*, 679–686.

Mikulincer, M. (1994). *Human learned helplessness: A coping perspective.* New York: Plenum Press.

Miller, G. A., Galanter, E., & Pribram, K. H. (1960). *Plans and the structure of behavior.* New York: Holt, Rinehart & Winston.

Mizruchi, M. S. (1991). Urgency, motivation, and group performance: The effect of prior success on current success among professional basketball teams. *Social Psychology Quarterly*, *54*, 181–189.

Muraven, M., & Baumeister, R. F. (2000). Self-regulation and depletion of limited resources: Does self-control resemble a muscle? *Psychological Bulletin*, *126*, 247–259.

Murray, H. A. (1938). *Explorations in personality.* New York: Oxford University Press.

Nesse, R. M. (2000). Is depression an adaptation? *Archives of General Psychiatry*, *57*, 14–20.

Ogilvie, D. M. (1987). The undesired self: A neglected variable in personality research. *Journal of Personality and Social Psychology*, *52*, 379–385.

Ortony, A., Clore, G. L., & Collins, A. (1988). *The cognitive structure of emotions.* New York: Cambridge University Press.

Payton, D. W. (1990). Internalized plans: A representation for action resources. In P. Maes (Ed.), *Designing autonomous agents: Theory and practice from biology to engineering and back* (pp. 89–103). Cambridge, MA: MIT Press.

Pittman, T. S., & Pittman, N. L. (1980). Deprivation of control and the attribution process. *Journal of Personality and Social Psychology*, *39*, 377–389.

Pomerantz, E. M., Saxon, J. L., & Oishi, S. (2000). The psychological trade-offs of goal investment. *Journal of Personality and Social Psychology*, *79*, 617–630.

Powers, W. T. (1973). *Behavior: The control of perception.* Chicago: Aldine.

Reed, M. B., & Aspinwall, L. G. (1998). Self-affirmation reduces biased processing of health-risk information. *Motivation and Emotion*, *22*, 99–132.

Ryan, R. M., & Deci, E. L. (2001). On happiness and human potentials: A review of research on hedonic and eudaimonic well-being. *Annual Review of Psychology*, *52*, 141–166.

Schultz, W. (2000). Multiple reward signals in the brain. *Nature Reviews*, *1*, 199–207.

Schultz, W. (2006). Behavioral theories and the neurophysiology of reward. *Annual Review of Psychology*, *57*, 87–115.

Schwarz, N., & Bohner, G. (1996). Feelings and their motivational implications: Moods and the action sequence. In P. M. Gollwitzer & J. A. Bargh (Eds.), *The psychology of action: Linking cognition and motivation to behavior* (pp. 119–145). New York: Guilford Press.

Schwarz, N., & Clore, G. L. (1983). Mood, misattribution, and judgments of well-being: Informative and directive functions of affective states. *Journal of Personality and Social Psychology*, *45*, 513–523.

Shah, J. Y., Friedman, R., & Kruglanski, A. W. (2002). Forgetting all else: On the antecedents and consequences of goal shielding. *Journal of Personality and Social Psychology*, *83*, 1261–1280.

Shallice, T. (1978). The dominant action system: An information-processing approach to consciousness. In K. S. Pope & J. L. Singer (Eds.), *The stream of consciousness: Scientific investigations into the flow of human experience* (pp. 117–157). New York: Wiley.

Simon, H. A. (1953). *Models of man.* New York: Wiley.

Simon, H. A. (1967). Motivational and emotional controls of cognition. *Psychological Review*, *74*, 29–39.

Stifter, C. A., & Moyer, D. (1991). The regulation of positive affect: Gaze aversion activity during mother–infant interaction. *Infant Behavior and Development*, *14*, 111–123.

Tesser, A. (1988). Toward a self-evaluation maintenance model of social behavior. In L. Berkowitz (Ed.), *Advances in experimental social psychology* (Vol. 21, pp. 181–227). San Diego, CA: Academic Press.

Tesser, A., Crepaz, N., Collins, J. C., Cornell, D., &

Beach, S. R. H. (2000). Confluence of self-esteem regulation mechanisms: On integrating the self-zoo. *Personality and Social Psychology Bulletin, 26,* 1476–1489.

Trope, Y., & Pomerantz, E. M. (1998). Resolving conflicts among self-evaluative motives: Positive experiences as a resource for overcoming defensiveness. *Motivation and Emotion, 22,* 53–72.

Vallacher, R. R., Read, S. J., & Nowak, A. (Eds.). (2002). The dynamical perspective in personality and social psychology [Special issue]. *Personality and Social Psychology Review,* 6(4).

Vallacher, R. R., & Wegner, D. M. (1987). What do people think they're doing?: Action identification and human behavior. *Psychological Review, 94,* 3–15.

Watson, D., Wiese, D., Vaidya, J., & Tellegen, A. (1999). The two general activation systems of affect: Structural findings, evolutionary considerations, and psychobiological evidence. *Journal of Personality and Social Psychology, 76,* 820–838.

Wegner, D. M. (2002). *The illusion of conscious will.* Cambridge, MA: MIT Press.

Wiener, N. (1948). *Cybernetics: Control and communication in the animal and the machine.* Cambridge, MA: MIT Press.

Wortman, C. B., & Brehm, J. W. (1975). Responses to uncontrollable outcomes: An integration of reactance theory and the learned helplessness model. In L. Berkowitz (Ed.), *Advances in experimental social psychology* (Vol. 8, pp. 277–336). New York: Academic Press.

Wrosch, C., Scheier, M. F., Carver, C. S., & Schulz, R. (2003). The importance of goal disengagement in adaptive self-regulation: When giving up is beneficial. *Self and Identity, 2,* 1–20

Wrosch, C., Scheier, M. F., Miller, G. E., Schulz, R., & Carver, C. S. (2003). Adaptive self-regulation of unattainable goals: Goal disengagement, goal reengagement, and subjective well-being. *Personality and Social Psychology Bulletin, 29,* 1494–1508.

Chapter 21

# Flexible Tenacity in Goal Pursuit

**Peter M. Gollwitzer**
**Elizabeth J. Parks-Stamm**
**Alexander Jaudas**
**Paschal Sheeran**

Goal-directed behavior possesses various observable features (Gollwitzer & Moskowitz, 1996). First and foremost, it is characterized by persistent striving until the goal is reached. Second, goal-directedness expresses itself in energization when situations or means that can be used to reach the goal are encountered. And third, goal-directed organisms show appropriateness: If one route to goal attainment is blocked, another course of action to the same goal is taken. Alternatively, if the goal changes, the goal-directed individual readily adapts to these changes by performing different actions.

It is the aspect of appropriateness that is scrutinized in the present chapter. We assume that goal pursuits, conscious as well as nonconscious (Gollwitzer & Bargh, 2005), possess much flexibility. But we want to carry this issue one step further. We raise the question of whether very tenacious goal pursuits do still possess the feature of appropriateness, or whether such determined goal pursuits are characterized by rigidity. The kind of heightened tenacity we analyze is not that of increased energization, which is experienced in the face of difficulty (Wright, 1996). Rather, we focus on the tenacity that originates from planning out an intended goal pursuit in advance. As research on implementation intentions (i.e., if-then plans) has observed (see summaries by Gollwitzer, 1999; Gollwitzer, Bayer, & McCulloch, 2005; Gollwitzer & Sheeran, 2006), individuals who furnish their goals with implementation intentions achieve higher goal attainment rates than individuals who act on the basis of mere goals (or goal intentions). The question we want to answer first in the present chapter is therefore the following: Are the benefits of forming implementation intentions associated with costs in terms of reduced flexibility (appropriateness)? Once we have found an answer to this first question, we turn in the second part of the chapter to the possibility of using implementation intentions to achieve flexible tenacity. The second question raised is thus quite different: Can forming an implementation intention be used as an effective self-regulatory strategy to protect a focal goal pursuit from disruptions (i.e., spontaneous attention responses to distractions, bad habits, and detrimental self-states such as emotional experiences) that reduce flexibility in achieving the goal? In order to find answers to both of these questions, we first present an overview of research on the effects of implementation intentions and the psychological mechanisms on which these rest.

## PROMOTING GOAL ATTAINMENT BY FORMING IMPLEMENTATION INTENTIONS

An *implementation intention* is an if–then plan, in which an individual consciously specifies a goal-directed behavior to perform in response to an anticipated situational cue; an if–then plan is subordinate to its related goal intention (Gollwitzer, 1999). Whereas a goal intention specifies the desired event in the form of "I intend to perform Behavior *X* [e.g., to eat more vegetables] to reach Outcome *X* [e.g., to be slim]!", an implementation intention specifies an anticipated critical situation and a proper goal-directed response. Thus an implementation intention subordinate to the goal intention "to eat more vegetables" would follow the form "*If* Situation *Y* arises [e.g., I am handed a menu], *then* I will perform Behavior *Z* [e.g., look for a vegetarian meal]!" An implementation intention is therefore a consciously willed plan to enact a certain goal-relevant response in an expected situation. This response is initiated immediately and effortlessly upon contact with the specified situational cue without a second conscious act of will, just as a habitual response formed through repeated pairing with a critical situation is directly triggered by the situational cue. Unlike a habit, an implementation intention produces automaticity immediately through the willful act of creating an association between the critical situation and the goal-directed response. For this reason, implementation intentions are said to create *strategic automaticity* or *instant habits* (Gollwitzer, 1999; Gollwitzer & Schaal, 1998).

### How Do Implementation Intentions Affect Goal-Directed Behavior?

Implementation intentions are expected to facilitate goal attainment on the basis of psychological processes that relate to both the anticipated situation specified in the if-component and the intended behavior specified in the then-component. Each of these processes is analyzed separately in the following discussion.

#### *Mechanisms Related to the If-Component*

Because forming implementation intentions requires the selection of a critical future situation (i.e., a viable opportunity), it is proposed that the mental representation of this situation becomes highly activated, and hence more accessible (Gollwitzer, 1999). This heightened accessibility should make it easier to detect the critical situation in the surrounding environment, attend to it even when one is busy with other things, and recall it.

The accessibility hypothesis (i.e., the mental representation of the situation specified in the if-part of the implementation intention becomes highly activated) was tested in studies measuring how well participants holding implementation intentions attended to and recalled the critical situation (Achtziger, Bayer, & Gollwitzer, 2007) as compared to participants who had only formed goal intentions. In a study using a dichotic-listening paradigm, it was observed that words describing the anticipated critical situation were highly disruptive to focused attention in implementation intention participants as compared to goal intention participants (i.e., the shadowing performance of the attended material decreased). This finding implies that opportunities to act, as specified in implementation intentions, will not easily escape people's attention even when they focus on other things (e.g., listening to a stimulating conversation). In a further study, the heightened accessibility hypothesis was tested via a cued-recall procedure. Research participants had to form implementation intentions specifying when, where, and how they wanted to play prepared games from numerous predesigned options. Immediately, or 48 hours later, participants were given a surprise task to recall all of the situational cues they had been provided. Those cues specified in implementation intentions were recalled better than nonspecified cues, whether recall was tested immediately or at a later point. A study by Steller (1992) provides additional evidence that implementation intentions lead to high accessibility of the critical situation. This study used an embedded-figures test (Gottschaldt, 1926), where smaller a-figures were hidden within larger b-figures. Enhanced detection of the hidden a-figures was observed when participants had specified the a-figure in the if-part of an implementation intention (i.e., had made plans on how to create a traffic sign from the a-figure).

Further support for the accessibility notion comes from Aarts, Dijksterhuis, and Midden (1999; see also Webb & Sheeran, 2004, 2007). In the Aarts and colleagues (1999) study, all participants were given information about expected situational cues in which to achieve a goal. In a subsequent lexical decision task, faster response times for cue words were observed in those individuals who formed implementation intentions with these cues. In addition, the faster lexical decision responses to these critical words (i.e., their heightened accessibility) mediated the beneficial effects of implementation intentions on goal attainment. These results imply that some of the goal-promoting effects of implementation intentions are based on the heightened accessibility of selected critical situational cues.

How does the heightened accessibility of the cue specified in the if-portion of the implementation intention affect overall goal pursuit (i.e., goal pursuit by planned and unplanned routes to the goal)? If the if-component increases the accessibility of the critical situation relative to the cues in the surrounding environment, implementation intentions should lead to gains in the use of the planned situational cue at the expense of alternative cues. Parks-Stamm, Gollwitzer, and Oettingen (2007, Study 1) tested this hypothesis by creating a paradigm in which implementation intentions affected primarily the if-process (i.e., the identification of a goal-relevant situation). It was found that individuals with implementation intentions recognized more of the planned situational cues, but fewer of the alternative cues. These results lend further support to the claim that the if-component of implementation intentions facilitates planned routes to the goal by increasing the accessibility of the specified cue.

### *Mechanisms Related to the Then-Component*

It is also proposed that the mental act of linking a critical situation to an intended goal-directed behavior in the form of an if–then plan leads to automatic action initiation, in the sense that the planned response is immediate, is efficient, and does not require conscious intent once the critical situation is encountered. By forming implementation intentions, people can strategically switch from conscious and effortful action initiation (guided by goal intentions) to having their goal-directed actions effortlessly elicited by the specified situational cues. This postulated automatization of action initiation (also described as the strategic delegation of control to situational cues) has been supported by the results of various experiments that tested immediacy, efficiency, and the presence or absence of conscious intent of the planned response.

Gollwitzer and Brandstätter (1997, Study 3) demonstrated the immediacy of action initiation in a study wherein participants were induced to form implementation intentions that specified a plan to present counterarguments to a series of racist remarks made by a confederate. Participants with implementation intentions initiated the counterargument more quickly than the participants who had formed the mere goal intention to counterargue. The efficiency of action initiation has also been explored (Brandtstätter, Lengfelder, & Gollwitzer, 2001, Studies 3 and 4). Participants formed the goal intention to press a button as fast as possible if numbers appeared on the computer screen, but not if letters were presented (a go/no-go task). Participants in the implementation intention condition also made the plan to press the response button particularly fast if the number 3 was presented. This go/no-go task was then embedded as a secondary task in a dual-task paradigm. Implementation intention participants showed a substantial increase over control participants in speed of responding to the number 3, regardless of whether the simultaneously demanded primary task (a memorization task in Study 3 and a tracking task in Study 4) was either easy or difficult to perform. Apparently, the immediacy of responding induced by implementation intentions is also efficient, in the sense that it requires minimal cognitive resources (i.e., it can be performed even when a cognitively demanding activity is performed at the same time).

Bayer, Achtziger, Malzacher, Moskowitz, and Gollwitzer (2007) tested whether implementation intentions lead to action initiation without conscious intent once the critical situation is encountered. In these experiments, the critical situation was presented subliminally, and its facilitating influences on preparing for (Study 1) or performing (Study 2) the respective goal-directed behavior were assessed. In Study 1, the goal of asserting oneself against a rude experimenter was analyzed. Half of the participants were encouraged to set the goal of "telling her off" by pointing to her rude behavior (goal intention condition), while the other half planned this in the form of an implementation intention. Afterward, faces of either the rude experimenter or a neutral person were presented subliminally (primes), and the activation of knowledge relevant to rudeness (target words such as *offensive*, *mean*, *conceited*) was measured via reading latencies. Results indicated that after the subliminal presentation of the critical primes, implementation intention participants, but not participants who only had formed goals, showed faster reading times for words related to rudeness.

In Study 2, participants were asked to classify a series of geometrical figures (e.g., circles, ellipses, triangles, and squares) into rounded versus angular objects by left- versus right-button press responses. All participants formed the goal intention to classify the figures as quickly and accurately as possible. Implementation intention participants were asked in addition to make the following plan: "And if I see a triangle, then I will press the respective button particularly fast!" Participants worked on a set of 240 figures, presented in succession on a computer screen. Some of the figures were preceded by the subliminal presentation of the critical figure (i.e., a triangle), whereas others were preceded by a control prime (i.e., the % sign). In accord with the results of Study 1, participants in the implementation intention condition had faster classification responses for angular figures when the triangle instead of the % sign was presented as a subliminal prime; no such effect was observed with goal intention participants. The subliminal priming effects observed in the experiments reported by Bayer and colleagues (2007) suggest that the goal-directed behavior specified in an implementation intention is triggered by the anticipated situational cue without the need for further conscious intent.

How does the automation of the response specified in the then-portion of the implementation intention affect overall goal pursuit? If the then-component makes the planned response more immediate and efficient, implementation intentions should allow increased responding to the planned response without impeding alternative responses. Parks-Stamm and colleagues (2007, Study 2) tested this hypothesis by creating a paradigm in which implementation intentions affected primarily the then-process (i.e., the enactment of a goal-directed response). It was found that individuals with implementation intentions enacted more of the planned responses, without reductions in the enactment of alternative goal-directed responses. These results lend further support to the claim that the then-component of an implementation intention aids planned goal pursuit by automating the goal-directed response specified in the implementation intention.

Much like a habit, then, an implementation intention facilitates a planned response automatically when the anticipated situation is encountered. By creating strategic automaticity, implementation intentions allow attentional resources to be preserved for other goal-directed responses, mental activities, and concurrent goal pursuits. Forming an implementation intention to facilitate goal pursuit has been described as "passing the control of one's behavior on to the environment" (Gollwitzer, 1993, p. 173). After forming implementation intentions, one does not need to look consciously for an opportunity to act when one is busy with other thoughts, activities, or goal pursuits. A habit has been described as a final stage of goal pursuit in which one is no longer actively concerned about performing the specified goal-directed behavior or evaluating the outcomes of the behavior (Rothman, Hertel, Baldwin, & Bartels, Chapter 32, this volume). By forming an implementation intention, one can speed the attainment of this final stage in behavior adaptation. One can then effortlessly react to the anticipated situation with the predetermined behavior to work toward the goal automatically.

## Implementation Intentions and Effective Goal Attainment

Perhaps the most challenging problem of meeting one's goals is getting started with goal striving, and there are at least three reasons why this is so difficult. The first reason has to do with remembering one's goal intention (Einstein & McDaniel, 1996). When acting on a given goal is not part of one's routine, or when one must postpone acting on it, one can easily forget to initiate goal-directed behavior. Dealing with many things at once or becoming preoccupied by a particular task can make this even more likely, especially when the given goal is new or unfamiliar. For example, after forming the goal to begin performing breast self-examinations, 70% of inclined abstainers (i.e., those who had intended to perform the breast self-exams but did not) reported forgetting as the cause of their nonperformance (Milne, Orbell, & Sheeran, 2002; Orbell, Hodgkins, & Sheeran, 1997). Forgetting may also be responsible for the meta-analytic finding that the longer the time interval between measures of goal intentions and goal achievement, the less likely it is that intentions will be realized (Sheeran & Orbell, 1998). These findings suggest that remembering one's goal intentions can have negative outcomes for goal achievement.

Even if one remembers what one is supposed to do, a second problem needs to be solved in order to attain one's goal: seizing the opportunity at hand. This problem is especially acute when the opportunity to act is presented only briefly. In these circumstances, people may fail to initiate goal-directed responses because they fail to notice that a good time to get started has arrived, they are unsure how they should act when the moment presents itself, or they simply procrastinate in acting on it. For example, Oettingen, Hönig, and Gollwitzer (2000, Study 3) showed that failing to seize an available opportunity to act can occur even when people have formed strong goal intentions to perform a behavior at a particular time. Participants were provided with diskettes containing four concentration tasks, and formed goal intentions to perform these tasks on their computers at a particular time each Wednesday morning for the next 4 weeks. The program on the diskette recorded the times when participants started to work on the task from the clocks on participants' computers. Findings indicated that the mean deviation from the intended start time was 2 hours for each specified opportunity. Similar findings were obtained by Dholakia and Bagozzi (2003, Study 2), when participants' task was to evaluate a website that could be accessed only during a short time window. Here, only 37% of participants who formed a goal intention were successful at accomplishing the task. These two studies illustrate that people may not get started with goal pursuit because they fail to seize good opportunities to act.

There are also many instances where people remember their goal intentions (e.g., to order a low-fat meal) and recognize that an opportune moment is upon them (e.g., it is lunchtime at their usual restaurant), but nonetheless fail to initiate goal-directed behaviors because they start to reflect anew on the desirability of the goal intention (i.e., they start to have second thoughts). This problem, which requires overcoming a temporary reluctance to act, is likely to arise when people have decided to pursue a goal that involves a tradeoff between attractive long-term consequences and less attractive short-term consequences (Mischel, 1996). For example, a strong goal intention to order low-fat meals is commonly formed on the basis of long-term deliberative thinking, according to which eating low-fat food is perceived as highly desirable; however, once the critical situation is confronted, short-term desirability considerations are triggered that occupy cognitive resources at the moment of action (e.g., the low-fat meal is perceived as tasteless at the critical juncture). Such dilemmas should get in the way of readily acting on the goal in the face of good opportunities (Loewenstein, Weber, Hsee, & Welch, 2001; Metcalfe & Mischel, 1999; Trafimow & Sheeran, 2004). Rothman and colleagues (Chapter 32, this volume) have also found that short-term factors can be more powerful for behavior change than more serious long-term considerations. For example, they found that quitting smoking is easier when individuals focus on their present cough than when they focus on their long-term elevated risk of cancer. Short-term concerns are powerful, and when they run counter to long-term wishes, they can keep individuals from acting on their desired goal pursuit.

Various studies suggest that these different difficulties with getting started on a goal pursuit can be solved effectively by forming implementation intentions. For instance, Gollwitzer and Brandstätter (1997, Study 2) analyzed a goal intention (i.e., writing a report about how one spent Christmas Eve) that had to be performed at a given time (i.e., during the subsequent Christmas holiday) when people are commonly busy with other things. Similarly, Oettingen and colleagues (2000, Study 3) observed that implementation intentions helped people to act on their task goals on time (e.g., at 10:00 A.M. every Wednesday over the next 4 weeks). Other studies have examined the effects of implementation intentions on goal attainment rates with goal intentions that are somewhat unpleasant to perform. For instance, the goal intentions to perform regular breast self-examinations (Orbell et al., 1997), receive regular cervical cancer screenings (Sheeran &

Orbell, 2000), resume functional activity after joint replacement surgery (Orbell & Sheeran, 2000), and engage in physical exercise (Milne et al., 2002) were all more frequently acted upon when people had furnished these goals with implementation intentions. Moreover, implementation intentions have been found to facilitate the attainment of goal intentions in cases where it is easy to forget to act on them (e.g., regular intake of vitamin pills—Sheeran & Orbell, 1999; the signing of worksheets by elderly persons—Chasteen, Park, & Schwarz, 2001).

The overall results of these studies clearly indicate that the rate of goal attainment is increased by forming an implementation intention in advance—that is, an if–then plan for how one intends to act on one's goal. The various cognitive mechanisms triggered by if–then plans highlight one's chosen opportunities to act and automate action initiation, making it easier to begin working toward one's goals. This conclusion is also supported by the finding that the beneficial effects of implementation intentions are commonly more apparent with difficult-to-implement goals than with easy goals. For instance, implementation intentions were more effective in helping people to complete difficult as compared to easy personal projects during Christmas break (Gollwitzer & Brandstätter, 1997, Study 1). Forming implementation intentions were also more beneficial to patients with frontal lobe lesions, who typically have severe problems with executive control, than to college students (Lengfelder & Gollwitzer, 2001, Study 2).

## IS ACTION CONTROL BY IMPLEMENTATION INTENTIONS NECESSARILY RIGID?

Given that implementation intentions have strong effects on goal attainment, and that these effects are based on mechanisms that help to activate one situation at the expense of others and automate planned response initiation, we may wonder whether action control by if–then plans is associated with increased rigidity in keeping with the plan even when continued compliance is suboptimal. Do people with if–then plans behave rigidly in acting on their plans even when the superordinate goal is weak to begin with or has become weakened (i.e., do if–then plans ignore the strength of the goal intention)? Moreover, will people rigidly act on their plans even if the specified situation is encountered in a context that forbids acting on the superordinate goal (i.e., when the present situation does not activate this goal)? Will people fail to act on their goals in alternative situations (i.e., situations other than the one specified in the if-component of the implementation intention), even if these alternative situations qualify as better opportunities to move toward the goal than the specified situation? And finally, will people stick to their plans even when evidence indicates failure? Below, we review research that has begun to explore these issues empirically.

### The Goal Dependence of Implementation Intentions

Because implementation intentions are subordinate to goal intentions, they should operate in the service of meeting their superordinate goal intentions; they should not be mechanized as plans that influence behavior, regardless of the state of the superordinate goals. This means that implementation intentions should no longer affect behavior when the respective goals are not activated. In other words, implementation intentions should exhibit goal-dependent automaticity (Gollwitzer & Schaal, 1998), operating to bring about specified goal-directed responses only when the underlying goals are activated.

Sheeran, Webb, and Gollwitzer (2005, Study 2) investigated the impact of an implementation intention when the underlying goal was activated or not activated. All participants were given the task to be accurate in solving geometric puzzles. In a scrambled-sentences implicit priming procedure, they were exposed to words that activated a speed goal or to neutral words. An implementation intention then spelled out an if–then plan for how to be fast in solving the puzzles. Only when the superordinate goal of being fast was activated did this plan positively affect people's speed of solving the puzzles. This suggests that an implementation intention does not compulsorily affect behavior any time the critical situation specified in the if-part of the implementation intention is encountered. Rather, an implementation intention leads to action initiation only when the corresponding superordinate goal is also in a state of high activation. This implies that people do not have to worry that if–then plans will make them act on specified cues even if they appear in inappropriate contexts. For instance, imagine that Anne is a student with a goal to read a book in the library, who has formed an implementation intention to sit down immediately and read upon contact with that book. If Anne then finds the anticipated book in a bookstore, she need not worry that her plan will overtake her. She should still be able to carry the book to the register, buy it, and take it home to read.

If implementation intentions respect the activation state of their superordinate goals, they should also be sensitive to the immediate presence or absence of the superordinate goals. Seehausen, Bayer, and Gollwitzer (1994) found that when participants were told that they no longer needed to reach the goal at hand, the effect of the respective implementation intention disappeared. Once a person was no longer striving for the goal, the common implementation intention effect of enhanced memory for the critical situation specified in the if-part of the implementation intention could not be observed any longer. The implication of this finding is that an implementation intention should also loosen its grip on a person's behavior when the superordinate goal has been reached. People who plan out their goal pursuits in advance in the form of if–then statements thus do not have to worry about becoming restless strivers who will continually show goal-directed behaviors whenever the specified critical cues are encountered. Rather, this automatism will come to a halt as soon as the respective goal has been reached by one's own effort, has been achieved through the efforts of others, or has become obsolete for some other reason (e.g., one has disengaged from the goal because it is no longer desirable or feasible).

Finally, sensitivity of implementation intention effects to the superordinate goal also implies that the strength of the superordinate goal should moderate these effects. Implementation intention effects do indeed seem to reflect the strength of their respective goal intentions. For instance, Orbell and colleagues (1997) found that forming implementation intentions that specified when and where participants planned to perform a breast self-exam in the coming month resulted in an increased occurrence only in those participants who entertained a strong goal intention to perform a breast self-exam. Following up on this finding, Sheeran and colleagues (2005, Study 1) investigated the sensitivity of implementation intentions to the strength of the goal intention to engage in independent study (i.e., the number of hours per week a college student wanted to engage in this activity). They found a significant interaction between goal intention strength (i.e., number of intended study hours) and the effect of implementation intentions. When the goal intention was weak, the presence or absence of implementation intentions did not predict behavior; when it was moderate, implementation intentions increased their predictive validity; and when the goal intention was strong, the prediction of behavior by implementation intentions increased even more. Thus implementation intentions improved goal achievement more when the respective goal intention was stronger.

In sum, the reported findings strongly suggest that the automaticity created by implementation intentions is of the goal-dependent kind (Bargh, 1989). Implementation intentions are formed strategically (by an act of will) to enhance the attainment of their respective goals. It makes sense, therefore, that such an intention is sensitive not only to the state of activation of its superordinate goal, but also to whether a person still holds the goal and how strongly the person intends to reach the goal.

### Taking Advantage of Alternative Opportunities

If implementation intentions allow for flexibility, they should enable individuals to take advantage of viable alternative opportunities. This question was explored first by Häfner (2000) in an experiment where participants were instructed to work on a word-rating task at a computer. Participants were also asked to help another research assistant by filling out a questionnaire at the end of the experiment. All participants accepted this second goal ("Yes, I'll complete this questionnaire!"), and participants in the implementation intention condition additionally furnished this goal with an implementation intention ("Yes, I'll complete the questionnaire. And when the experiment is over, then I'll fill out the questionnaire!"). During the word-rating task, a bogus computer crash was staged. The experimenter informed participants that the computer was experiencing a known software problem, and asked them to wait about 5 minutes until the computer technician could come by to fix the problem. This unexpected break provided a good opportunity to fill out the questionnaire lying on the table next to the computer monitor. Significantly more participants in the goal intention condition used this unexpected opportunity than in the implementation intention condition (57% vs. 34%), demonstrating that the implementation intention hampered participants in their goal striving by binding them in their behavior to the specified opportunity. However, in a concluding questionnaire, even though 98% of participants responded that they noticed that the computer breakdown offered a good opportunity to complete the questionnaire, 38% reported that they felt that they were not allowed to complete it during that time (i.e., they felt an obligation toward the experimenter to wait until the end of the experiment). A new analysis excluding these latter participants revealed that within this sample, there was no longer a difference between the goal intention condition and the implementation intention condition. Apparently, it was not the implementation intention itself that led participants to miss the opportunity, but rather the feeling of obligation to achieve the goal at the time they agreed upon beforehand.

Jaudas and Gollwitzer (2004) therefore developed a choice reaction paradigm to get around the confound of social obligation. This paradigm consisted of two blocks of more than 100 trials each; in each trial a pair of objects was presented, and participants had to choose the one associated with the most points. In the first block, the cue (i.e., the original object) specified in the implementation intention was the best available object to act toward the goal. However, in the second block, an unexpected better alternative (i.e., a new object) was presented along with the original object specified in the implementation intention. This study tested whether participants would be able to make use of the new object, even if they had formed an implementation intention on the original object. Could participants with implementation intentions demonstrate flexibility by dropping their old plan (which was no longer functional) in order to take advantage of this new alternative?

More specifically, participants first memorized the value points associated with five different objects. Each score was between 10 and 50 points, with the flower icon worth the maximum 50 points. For each trial, two icons were presented on the computer screen side by side. The participant's goal was to maximize points by selecting the icons (objects) with the most points as quickly as possible within a given time frame. Participants were awarded the score of the selected object, plus up to 10 additional speed points depending on their response latency. Participants in the goal intention condition committed themselves to the goal: "I will try to get as many points as possible!" Those in the implementation intention condition additionally adopted an if–then plan: "And if the flower icon appears, then I will quickly snatch the 50 points!" Because participants in the goal-only condition also learned that the flower icon was the most valuable object, the implementation intention did not provide any additional information, but simply phrased the planned responding to the flower icon in terms of an if–then statement.

In the first block of trials, only the five icons (objects) introduced at the beginning of the experiment were presented. When faced with a choice between the flower and the other icons, participants in the implementation intention condition chose the flower icon faster than participants in the goal-only group, while there were no differences concerning the other icons. As there were no differences in error rates, participants in the implementation condition ended up earning more points than the goal intention participants. This effect was in line with the expectation that forming an implementation intention would facilitate task goal attainment, but what about associated costs in terms of rigidity when a new and better (i.e., a more valuable) object was presented?

Participants were informed that in the second block of trials new icons might appear, including a book icon worth 60 points. This new icon (object) was then paired exclusively with the flower icon. To succeed in these trials, participants had to select the new book icon over the flower icon. A costs-in-rigidity hypothesis would predict that implementation intention participants who had previously specified the flower icon in their plan should find it difficult to select the book icon, because the presentation of the flower icon would initiate an antagonistic selection response that required much effort to be controlled, leading to higher error rates and longer reaction times.

However, contrary to this pessimistic prediction, no differences were observed between the implementation intention participants and the goal intention participants when the (old) flower icon and the (new) book icon were presented together. Furthermore, when the flower icon was presented together with one of the four other old icons, participants in the implementation intention group still performed better than those in the goal intention group. Implementation intentions thus flexibly guided participants' task goal pursuit of making as many points as possible: When the flower icon was presented in combination with the new, more valuable icon, implementation intention participants managed to select the more valuable new icon (i.e., experienced no costs); when the flower icon was presented with one of the other four old icons, implementation intention participants effectively selected the flower icon (i.e., accrued benefits).

It appears, then, that the automaticity of responding associated with implementation intentions is high in terms of controllability, which is not surprising if one keeps in mind that implementation intentions operate in the service of their respective superordinate goals (in the present case, the earning of as many points as possible). These findings also support a theoretical conclusion drawn by Bargh (1994): Action control processes need not be conceived of as either automatic (i.e., possessing all of the four features of being unintentional, nonconscious, relatively effortless, and uncontrollable) or controlled (i.e., possessing none of these four features); rather, action control processes may possess any of these attributes to a greater or lesser degree. It is possible that action control by implementation intentions is highly efficient (i.e., it is effortless), but at the same time does not lack controllability (i.e., it still flexibly serves the respective superordinate goals).

## Flexible Modification of Ineffective Plans

As any other means to a given goal pursuit, plans may be faulty and thus fail to help people to move toward the goal at hand. Based on this consideration, Jaudas, Achtziger, and Gollwitzer (2006) focused on a different angle from which the theme of rigidity–flexibility of action control by if–then plans could be addressed. Jaudas and colleagues wondered whether people would be responsive to feedback that their if–then plans did not promote goal attainment, but instead hampered goal progress. If negative feedback on the instrumentality of an if–then plan was ignored by implementation intention participants, this would support the hypothesis that if–then plans favor rigid action control. If if–then plans allow for flexible action control, however, negative instrumentality feedback should instigate disengagement from the respective plans.

In a first study on this theme, participants played a computer game in which they had to navigate a figure (symbolizing a person) through 10 different mazes. The mazes were seen from a top view, and the figure was controlled by pressing one of four buttons, thus moving it left, right, up, or down. Participants were informed that in order to facilitate task performance, a green arrow would appear at some junctions suggesting a shortcut. In the goal intention condition, the participants' task goal was to find the shortest possible way through the various mazes ("I will try to find the shortest way through the mazes!"). In the implementation intention condition, participants had to add the following if–then plan: "And if the green arrow shows up, then I'll quickly press the respective button!"

In fact, the green arrow pointed to the shortest way in only 3 out of the 10 mazes. The plan adopted by the implementation intention participants actually had low instrumentality, so in order to perform well, implementation intention participants needed to disengage from their if–then plan. The study also manipulated whether participants received performance feedback about the instrumentality of their chosen paths. The dependent variable was the mean number of mazes in which participants actually found the shortest ways.

The results revealed an interesting interaction between implementation intentions and feedback. When no feedback was given on participants' performance, goal intention participants showed an advantage over implementation intention participants; the performance of implementation intention participants without performance feedback suffered because of the faulty if–then plan. However, when implementation intention participants received feedback and thus learned that following their if–then plan had little instrumentality in terms of finding the shortest ways, these participants performed as well as the goal intention participants. Apparently, the implementation intention participants disengaged from the if–then plan when they were provided evidence that this plan hindered rather than furthered task goal attainment.

## Summary

Concerns that gains produced by implementation intentions may be associated with costs in terms of increased rigidity of goal pursuit seem mostly unfounded. First, action control by an implementation intention reflects the quality of the superordinate goal, and this extends to its level of situational activation, the original strength of the goal, and the degree to which the goal is still held. Second, specifying a good opportunity to act in an implementation intention does not make a person oblivious to alternative better opportunities. The latter are used as effectively as they are by people who strive on the basis of mere goals. Most interestingly, this flexibility seems to come without any costs in terms of quickly using the originally specified opportunity when it arises. Third, people seem to be very responsive to the instrumentality of their if–then plans. If these plans are counterproductive, it is possible to disengage from them to operate on the respective goal intentions alone.

## GAINING FLEXIBILITY BY FORMING IMPLEMENTATION INTENTIONS

People set themselves goals to change a given status quo into a more desired future state, and these envisioned goals subsequently guide their thoughts, feelings, and actions toward goal attainment (Gollwitzer & Moskowitz, 1996). However, more often than not goal pursuit is disrupted when people spontaneously attend to distractive stimuli, fall prey to bad habits, or succumb to the negative influences of intrusive self-states (e.g., being upset). How can an individual avoid getting derailed by such disruptions, thus demonstrating flexible tenacity in pursuing the focal goal? We suggest that implementation intentions can be used to achieve this end. Over the years, we have explored the various ways in which implementation intentions may prevent people from compulsorily giving in to these disruptions.

### Blocking Spontaneous Attention Responses

The distraction of attention from a current goal pursuit can be successfully suppressed by using implementation intentions. In two studies, Gollwitzer and Schaal (1998) used implementation intentions to control the spontaneous diversion of attention from a primary task. Participants were instructed to concentrate on a boring mathematical task on a computer and to ignore the distracting commercials that would appear in a separate computer window. These award-winning commercials featured sound, music, beautiful people, and interesting activities; they were designed by professionals to be ultimately distracting. The performance of three groups on the arithmetic problems was compared: a goal intention group ("I will not let myself get distracted by the commercials!") and two implementation intention groups. Participants in the implementation intention groups were asked to form either a task-facilitating implementation intention to achieve their goal ("If I hear or see the commercials, then I will increase my efforts on the math task!") or a distraction-inhibiting implementation intention ("If I hear or see the commercials, then I will ignore them!"). When participants were highly motivated to do well on the task at hand, distraction-inhibiting implementation intentions consistently facilitated task performance. Thus implementation intentions designed to ignore the attractive distractions enabled participants to succeed in their primary task beyond even the strong intention not to be distracted. This is one way implementation intentions can be used as a tool to protect goal striving from outside forces that can reduce flexibility in achieving desired goals.

### The Suppression of Habitual Responses

Habitual responses acquired through consistent repetition may at times conflict with people's consciously chosen goals and thus may also derail goal pursuit. This is particularly true when people have set change goals, to overcome their usual ways of doing things. Can implementation intentions halt the habitual response (e.g., ordering tasty but unhealthy food in a restaurant) in favor of the effective pursuit of the newly set change goal (e.g., following a healthy diet)? Verplanken and Faes (1999) found that habitual eating behaviors and implementation intentions had an independent effect on subsequent healthy eating. That is, regardless of whether the old unhealthy eating habits were weak or strong, implementation intentions improved an individual's diet.

#### *Suppressing a Habitual Motor Response*

A critical test of whether implementation intentions can halt habitual behaviors has recently been performed by Cohen, Bayer, Jaudas, and Gollwitzer (in press, Study 2). This study used the *Simon task*, which takes advantage of a strong habitual response: Stimuli presented on the left side of a person are responded to by the left arm more effectively than stimuli presented on the right side, and vice versa. In the Simon task, tones are presented that simultaneously feature relevant (pitch) and irrelevant (location) attributes. For example, the participants must indicate whether a tone's pitch is low or high by pressing a key with their left or right hand, respectively. In this example, responses to low-pitch tones presented on the left side (and high-pitch tones presented on the right side) are typically faster than responses to high-pitch tones presented on the left side and low-pitch tones presented on the right side. This congruence effect on response times is termed the *Simon effect*.

The Simon effect is a robust phenomenon, which can be replicated for different stimuli and in different modalities (for an overview, see Lu & Proctor, 1995); it is commonly explained by so-called *two-route models*. One of the most frequently cited two-route models is the *dimensional overlap model* (Kornblum, Hasbroucq, & Osman, 1990). According to this model, the stimulus attributes (relevant and irrelevant) are processed along two different routes. The processing of the spatial location is habitual and thus immediately activates a respective response. The relevant stimulus attribute is processed by the slower, more controlled processes instigated by the task goal. If processing along both routes activates the same response, one finds shorter reaction times. On the other hand, when the responses activated by the two routes are different (or incongruent), then this results in a conflict that produces longer reaction times. This "race" between information processing along the habitual and task goal routes is supported by experiments investigating the temporal relationship between coding of the irrelevant stimulus attribute and coding of the relevant attribute (e.g., De Jong, Liang, & Lauber, 1994; Hommel, 1994).

Cohen and colleagues (in press, Study 2) attempted to help people achieve their task goal (i.e., classifying low and high tones) in the noncorresponding trials by automating the slower, controlled information-processing route with implementation intentions. Participants were asked to decide whether the pitch of the tone was low or high by pressing a left or a right key on the computer keyboard. The tones were presented by external loudspeakers placed at participants' left and right sides. Participants in the control group formed the following goal: "I'll respond to the tones by pressing the respective buttons as fast as possible!" Participants in the implementation intention condition fostered their pursuit of this goal with an additional implementation intention: "And if I hear the high tone on the left side, then I'll quickly press the right button!" This critical situation specified in the implementation intention was one of the two possible incongruent combinations of response type and spatial location.

The results were as follows: In the control (mere task goal) condition, the Simon effect was replicated for both incongruent combinations. In contrast, in the implementation intention condition, the Simon effect was found only for one incongruent combination; for the incongruent combination specified in the implementation intention, the Simon effect was eliminated. These results provide further evidence that implementation intentions can help to control unwanted habitual (automatic) responses, and in the present case this was achieved by vesting the slower but wanted response with heightened efficiency. Even a response so unquestionably habitual as responding to stimuli presented on one side with the matching hand failed to intrude on the task goal when it was furnished with a guiding implementation intention.

### Suppression of Chronic Fears

Not only do behaviors become habitual through consistent repetition; cognitions and emotions can be subjected to habitual control by this process as well. The pursuit of goals may thus not only be hampered by antagonistic behavioral habits, but also by antagonistic habitual ways of processing and evaluating information. Thus the question arises whether implementation intentions can be used to help people attain change goals that are geared toward overcoming these habitual cognitive and emotional responses.

The fearful responses to a frightening stimulus are a special case in point. When these responses are overly intense, as in individuals with phobias, the effective down-regulation of fear becomes important. Such individuals may form the change goal to stay calm in the face of threatening stimuli, and furnish this goal with respective implementation intentions. But do such if–then plans facilitate goal attainment? Schweiger Gallo, Keil, McCulloch, Rockstroh, and Gollwitzer (2006, Studies 2 & 3) investigated whether the emotional responses to spiders in participants with a spider phobia (arachnophobia) could be controlled by forming implementation intentions. Participants with arachnophobia were recruited to view images of spiders from the International Affective Picture System. There were three conditions: a control condition, a goal intention condition ("I will not get frightened!"), and an implementation intention condition ("And if I see a spider, then I will stay calm and relaxed!").

Immediately following the presentation of the spiders, valence, arousal, and dominance ratings were taken with the Self-Assessment Manikin scales. Spiders were presented for 100 milliseconds, followed by a random pattern mask; participants then made their evaluations within a time frame of 2 seconds (a short enough response window to prevent excessive deliberation). Whereas no differences between the control condition and the goal condition were observed, participants in the implementation intention condition reported feeling less negative, less aroused, and less out of control than participants in either of these other groups when viewing the spider pictures.

### *Suppressing Habitual Stereotypical and Prejudicial Responses*

The use of stereotypes in impression formation can be controlled effectively by effortful correctional strategies (Bodenhausen & Macrae, 1998; Brewer, 1988; Devine, 1989; Fiske & Neuberg, 1990). However, the activation of stereotypes carries features of automaticity, due to a long history of being repeatedly activated in the presence of members of the particular group (Bargh, 1999; Devine, 1989). Accordingly, stereotype activation should be more difficult to control than stereotype use, and the question arises as to whether people who have the goal of judging others fairly can protect themselves from the automatic activation of stereotypes by adding implementation intentions focused on the suppression of the "bad habit" of stereotyping others. If one applies a horse race metaphor, it seems possible that the response specified in the then-part of a fairness-oriented implementation intention can win out over the automatic activation of stereotypical beliefs.

Findings of priming studies using short SOAs (less than 300 milliseconds) suggest that forming implementation intentions does indeed inhibit the automatic activation of stereotypical beliefs (Gollwitzer & Schaal, 1998). When participants furnished their goal intentions of judging elderly people in a nonstereotypical manner with an implementation intention ("And if I see an old person, then I tell myself: Don't stereotype!"), the typical automatic activation of stereotypical beliefs (assessed through pronunciation speed in a semantic priming paradigm) was even reversed. Implementation intentions were also found to effectively suppress the automatic activation of gender stereotypes in a study where participants had to play the role of a personal manager in a simulated hiring situation. When participants had formed the goal intention to judge women applicants in a nonstereotypical way and furnished this goal intention with an implementation ("And if I see this person, then I will ignore her gender!"), no automatic activation of stereotypical beliefs about this particular woman (assessed through response latencies in a Stroop task using stereotypical words) was observed.

Implementation intentions were also observed to suppress the automatic activation of prejudicial feelings in a study on perceptions of homeless persons. When participants' goal intentions to judge homeless individuals in a nonprejudicial manner were furnished with implementation intentions ("And if I see a homeless person, then I will tell myself: No prejudice!" or "And if I see a homeless person, then I will ignore the fact that the person is homeless!"), automatic negative evaluation effects (assessed in an affect priming paradigm) vanished.

In Europe, one interesting stereotype concerns a certain group of individuals (primarily men) associated with negative attributes such as being disruptive and overly zealous: soccer fans. Recent work by Achtziger (2002) on prejudicial feelings toward soccer fans indicates that implementation intentions (e.g., "If I see a soccer fan, then I will not evaluate him negatively!") can block such negative feelings in a very flexible manner. In this study, a sequential priming paradigm was used, in which pictures of soccer fans served as primes and relevant person attributes (e.g., *rowdy*, *comradely*) served as targets that had to be read as quickly as possible. Half of the depicted soccer fans (primes) were cued with a signal tone, and the participants were told that the implementation intention would only apply to those soccer fans cued with the signal tone. Implementation intention effects (i.e., relevant positive attributes were read faster than negative attributes) were only observed when the depiction of soccer fans was accompanied with a signal tone.

In sum, it seems that the pursuit of goals to be nonstereotypical in one's judgments and nonprejudicial in one's evaluations of certain others can be protected from being derailed by habitual thoughts and feelings toward these persons. One only needs to form implementation intentions that are geared toward suppressing these habitual responses. Apparently, the horse race between the activation of the habitual response and the goal-directed response (i.e., to be fair toward others) is won by the latter, if this response is specified in the then-part of an implementation intention.

## Blocking the Influence of Intrusive Self-States

Goal pursuit becomes difficult when action control is hampered by a person's ongoing self-states, such as the activation of cognitive procedures or the experience of motivations and emotions that do not correspond with acting on the focal goal. We have recently explored whether spelling out the pursuit of the focal goal in advance by forming implementation intentions effectively protects the focal goal pursuit from getting derailed by such negative internal influences. Our hypothesis was that goal pursuits preprogrammed by implementation intentions should no longer be disrupted by the negative influences of adverse self-states, as the if–then preprogrammed persons are acting on automatic pilot.

### *Task Sets*

An easy-to-use paradigm to investigate the negative influence of activated adverse cognitive procedures on the performance of a focal task goal is the so-called *task switch paradigm*, in which participants repeatedly switch between simple but different cognitive tasks. When participants have to switch from one task to the next, they exhibit an increase in reaction times, labeled a *switch cost*. In other words, initially the immediately preceding task has a negative influence on pursuing the new task. The observation of such switch costs is a very robust finding that can be easily obtained in diverse experimental settings. In fact, it seems to be almost impossible to eliminate switch costs. For this reason, several theories have been advanced about the origins of switch costs, involving task sets, procedural priming, and memory retrieval (for a summary, see Kluwe, Lüer, & Röesler, 2003). The interesting question from the perspective of the present chapter is whether implementation intentions can be used to reduce switch costs.

In a recent experiment on this theme, Cohen and colleagues (in press, Study 1) used an alternating-run paradigm (Rogers & Monsell, 1995) in which participants switched between two simple cognitive tasks in a predictable sequence. In this study, a square separated into four smaller squares was presented on the computer screen. On each trial, a letter–number pair was presented in the center of one of the four squares (e.g., 7K). When the stimuli were presented in the two upper positions, participants had to decide whether the letter was a consonant or a vowel by pressing the respective button (thereby ignoring the number). When the stimuli were presented in the two lower positions, participants had to decide whether the number was odd or even (thereby ignoring the letter). The pairs predictably appeared in a clockwise pattern, resulting in the sequence AABBAABB . . . (i.e., A-switch, A-repetition, B-switch, B-repetition). Participants in the goal intention condition set themselves the following goal: "I will classify the letters and digits as fast as possible without making mistakes!" Participants in the implementation intention condition were also instructed to form this implementation intention: "And if an E appears in the upper row, then I'll quickly press the respective button!"

The results were as expected: Forming implementation intentions led to reduced reaction times for the critical stimulus (E). This benefit in reaction time was observed not only in the repetition trials, but also in the switch trials. Furthermore, results showed no cost in reaction times to numbers when these numbers were presented with the critical letter E. In sum, planning out the performance of a task goal (such as classifying letters) in advance by forming an implementation intention protects this goal from interferences stemming from the activation of procedures from an immediately preceding antagonistic task goal. As the ease of switching between task goals is a benchmark for flexibility in goal pursuit, forming implementation intentions qualifies as a very effective self-regulatory means to achieve flexibility in goal pursuit.

### *Self-Definitional Incompleteness*

One self-state that is detrimental to the pursuit of the social goal of demonstrating interpersonal sensitivity is *self-definitional incompleteness*. According to self-completion theory (Wicklund & Gollwitzer, 1982), individuals committed to an aspired-to identity (e.g., lawyer, musician) experience incompleteness when they receive negative feedback concerning their possession of a symbol of this identity. This state of incompleteness in turn motivates them to strive to regain a sense of completeness by talking or behaving in accordance with that coveted identity—a behavior pattern known as *self-symbolizing*. Self-symbolizing behavior can be antagonistic with the goal of being sensitive to the interests of others if these interests do not square with the orientation toward winning back self-definitional completeness (Gollwitzer & Wicklund, 1985).

In a self-completion experiment, Gollwitzer and Bayer (2000) either induced self-definitional incompleteness in male law students highly committed to becoming lawyers or left their sense of self-definitional completeness untouched. Then the law students were told that they would have a chance to get to know another person (i.e., a female student named Nadja), and they were assigned the interpersonal goal to take the other student's perspective during the upcoming conversation. Half of the participants formed the additional implementation intention: "And if my partner expresses a preference for a specific conversation topic, then I will turn the conversation around to it!" All participants finally read the potential conversation partner's chosen topics of interest, and were asked to list their own conversation preferences. The participants who had not formed implementation intentions showed the classic self-completion effect, in that the incomplete more than the complete participants preferred to talk about law- and lawyer-related issues (in spite of their partner's opposing preference to talk about vacations and movies). However, among those who had formed implementation intentions, this effect was completely eliminated: Incomplete as well as complete individuals were equally uninterested in law as a conversation topic. Apparently, the goal of taking the other person's perspective stayed unaffected by the self-state of incompleteness when acting on this goal was spelled out in advance by an implementation intention.

### *Moods*

A self-state known to impede the pursuit of egalitarian fairness-oriented goals is being in a positive mood. Research has demonstrated that a good mood can cause an individual to rely more heavily on general knowledge structures and heuristics, and thus the person may be more likely to stereotype others (e.g., Bless & Fiedler, 1995; Park & Banaji, 2000). Gollwitzer and Bayer (2000, Experiment 3) explored whether the pursuit of an egalitarian goal could be guaranteed even during a good mood when acting on the egalitarian goal was controlled by an appropriate implementation intention. Participants watched either a humorous video or an informational documentary, in order to put them in a positive or a neutral mood, respectively. One-third of the participants were not instructed to form a goal concerning a subsequent task involving person judgment. A second group set themselves the goal to make a nonstereotypical judgment, and the final group additionally furnished this goal with an implementation intention ("And if I start to evaluate a depicted character, then I will ignore the character's gender!").

All participants were then presented with a set of photographs and asked to choose a description of the depicted woman's actions from a list of presented options. These descriptions were selected beforehand to vary in stereotypicality. The control condition did show a significant effect of mood, such that participants in a good mood exhibited a higher level of stereotyping than those in a neutral mood. The goal-only condition showed similar results, indicating that being in a good mood severely hampered the attainment of the egalitarian goal. However, in the implementation intention condition, there was no effect of mood on the stereotypicality of the judgments made. Implementation intentions apparently managed to protect the goal to be egalitarian from the negative influences of being in a good mood.

### *Ego Depletion*

Another self-state that impedes one's ability to act on one's goals is *ego depletion* (e.g.,

Muraven & Baumeister, 2000; Muraven, Tice, & Baumeister, 1998). Ego depletion is a state experienced when one has drained one's regulatory resources by exercising self-control in a demanding first task. Muraven and colleagues showed in three studies that engaging in much self-regulation while performing a first task resulted in decreased performance on a second task that also required much self-regulation in order to be successful. For example, suppressing an emotional response while watching a movie subsequently resulted in less persistence in holding a handgrip; suppressing a prohibited thought resulted in less persistence in trying to solve difficult anagrams; and thought suppression resulted in a decreased ability to regulate one's emotions.

Webb and Sheeran (2003, Study 2) showed that implementation intentions could eliminate the effect of ego depletion on the performance of a subsequent task goal. After an ego-depleting first task, participants were asked to perform a demanding Stroop task. Half of the participants formed implementation intentions for the Stroop task, whereas the other half did not. Those with implementation intentions did not show an effect of ego depletion in their Stroop task performance; their Stroop performance was no different from that of the individuals who had not experienced the first ego-depleting task. These findings suggest that using implementation intentions to plan one's performance of a demanding task effectively protects meeting the task goal of performing well from the detrimental self-state of ego depletion. In other words, the performance-suppressing effect of ego depletion fails to unfold if the task is controlled by implementation intentions. The ability of implementation intentions to facilitate even tasks that are difficult to perform because of automatic interference (as is the case with the Stroop task) speaks to the power of self-regulation by if–then plans.

## SUMMARY AND CONCLUSION

Even though the self-regulation of goal pursuit by implementation intentions facilitates goal attainment, these benefits are not earned by paying a price in terms of reduced flexibility. People stay sensitive to the state of the goal, and this extends to the degree of situational activation of the goal, the degree to which a person is still striving for the goal, and the strength of the goal. Moreover, people are still able to seize alternative good opportunities to move toward attaining the goal. Finally, they readily disengage from if–then plans when these plans fail to be instrumental to goal attainment. All of these findings suggest that rigidity is not the price that must be paid for the more determined goal striving associated with implementation intentions.

Interestingly, implementation intentions can even be used to avoid rigidity in terms of readily giving in to spontaneous attentional responses to distractive stimuli, habitual responses, and detrimental self-states (e.g., activated disruptive cognitive procedures, the experience of disruptive emotional and motivational states). When a given focal goal pursuit is spelled out in advance by an if–then plan, such detrimental self-states no longer present a hindrance to the attainment of the focal goal. It appears, then, that furnishing goals with if–then plans not only allows for flexibility in the sense of staying sensitive to the state of the goals, alternative opportunities to act, and the instrumentality of the plans formed. By forming implementation intentions, people can also emancipate their goal pursuits from becoming easy prey to adverse self-states.

## REFERENCES

Aarts, H., Dijksterhuis, A., & Midden, C. (1999). To plan or not to plan?: Goal achievement or interrupting the performance of mundane behaviors. *European Journal of Social Psychology, 29*, 971–979.

Achtziger, A. (2002). *Sozial-, kognitions- und motivationspsychologische Determinanten des Eindrucksbildungsprozesses unter besonderer Berücksichtigung der Stereotypisierung. [Social-cognitive and motivational determinants of evaluating and judging others].* Unpublished doctoral dissertation, Universität Konstanz, Konstanz, Germany.

Achtziger, A., Bayer, U., & Gollwitzer, P. M. (2007). *Implementation intentions: The accessibility of cues for action.* Manuscript submitted for publication.

Bargh, J. A. (1989). Conditional automaticity: Varieties of automatic influence in social perception and cognition. In J. S. Uleman & J. A. Bargh (Eds.), *Unintended thought* (pp. 3–51). New York: Guilford Press.

Bargh, J. A. (1994). The four horsemen of automaticity: Awareness, intention, efficiency, and control. In R. S. Wyer, Jr. & T. K Srull (Eds.), *Handbook of social cognition* (Vol. 10, pp. 1–61). Hillsdale, NJ: Erlbaum.

Bargh, J. A. (1999). The cognitive monster: The case against the controllability of automatic stereotype effects. In S. Chaiken & Y. Trope (Eds.), *Dual-process theories in social psychology* (pp. 361–382). New York: Guilford Press.

Bayer, U. C., Achtziger, A., Malzacher, J. T., Moskowitz, G. B., & Gollwitzer, P. M. (2007). *Strategic automaticity by implementation intentions: Action initiation without conscious intent.* Manuscript submitted for publication.

Bless, H., & Fiedler, K. (1995). Affective states and the influence of activated general knowledge. *Personality and Social Psychology Bulletin, 21,* 766–778.

Bodenhausen, G. V., & Macrae, C. N. (1998). Stereotype activation and inhibition. In R. S. Wyer, Jr. (Ed.), *Stereotype activation and inhibition: Advances in social cognition* (pp. 1–52). Mahwah, NJ: Erlbaum.

Brandstätter, V., Lengfelder, A., & Gollwitzer, P. M. (2001). Implementation intentions and efficient action initiation. *Journal of Personality and Social Psychology, 81,* 946–960.

Brewer, M. B. (1988). A dual process model of impression formation. In T. K. Srull & R. S. Wyer, Jr. (Eds.), *Advances in social cognition* (pp. 1–36). Hillsdale, NJ: Erlbaum.

Chasteen, A. L., Park, D. C., & Schwarz, N. (2001). Implementation intentions and facilitation of prospective memory. *Psychological Science, 12,* 457–461.

Cohen, A.-L., Bayer, U. C., Jaudas, A., & Gollwitzer, P. M. (in press). Self-regulatory strategy and executive control: Implementation intentions modulate task switching and Simon task performance. *Psychological Research.*

De Jong, R., Liang, C.-C., & Lauber, E. (1994). Conditional and unconditional automaticity: A dual-process model of effects of spatial stimulus–response correspondence. *Journal of Experimental Psychology: Human Perception and Performance, 20,* 731–750.

Devine, P. G. (1989). Stereotypes and prejudice: Their automatic and controlled components. *Journal of Personality and Social Psychology, 56,* 5–18.

Dholakia, U. M., & Bagozzi, R. P. (2003). As time goes by: How goal and implementation intentions influence enactment of short-fuse behaviors. *Journal of Applied Social Psychology, 33,* 889–922.

Einstein, G. O., & McDaniel, M. A. (1996). Retrieval processes in prospective memory: Theoretical approaches and some new empirical findings. In M. Bradimonte, G. O. Einstein, & M. A. McDaniel (Eds.), *Prospective memory: Theory and applications* (pp. 115–141). Mahwah, NJ: Erlbaum.

Fiske, S. T., & Neuberg, S. L. (1990). A continuum of impression formation, from category-based to individuating processes: Influences of information and motivation on attention and interpretation. In M. P. Zanna (Ed.), *Advances in experimental social psychology* (Vol. 23, pp. 1–74). San Diego, CA: Academic Press.

Gollwitzer, P. M. (1993). Goal achievement: The role of intentions. *European Review of Social Psychology, 4,* 141–185.

Gollwitzer, P. M. (1999). Implementation intentions: Strong effects of simple plans. *American Psychologist, 54,* 493–503.

Gollwitzer, P. M., & Bargh, J. A. (2005). Automaticity in goal pursuit. In A. Elliot & C. Dweck (Eds.), *Handbook of competence and motivation* (pp. 624–646). New York: Guilford Press.

Gollwitzer, P. M., & Bayer, U. C. (2000). *Becoming a better person without changing the self.* Paper presented at the Self and Identity Preconference of the Annual Meeting of the Society of Experimental Social Psychology, Atlanta, GA.

Gollwitzer, P. M., Bayer, U. C., & McCulloch, K. C. (2005). The control of the unwanted. In R. R. Hassin, J. S. Uleman, & J. A. Bargh (Eds.), *The new unconscious* (pp. 485–515). New York: Oxford University Press.

Gollwitzer, P. M., & Brandstätter, V. (1997). Implementation intentions and effective goal pursuit. *Journal of Personality and Social Psychology, 73,* 186–199.

Gollwitzer, P. M., & Moskowitz, G. B. (1996). Goal effects on action and cognition. In E. T. Higgins & A. W. Kruglanski (Eds.), *Social psychology: Handbook of basic principles* (pp. 361–399). New York: Guilford Press.

Gollwitzer, P. M., & Schaal, B. (1998). Metacognition in action: The importance of implementation intentions. *Personality and Social Psychology Review, 2,* 124–136.

Gollwitzer, P. M., & Sheeran, P. (2006). Implementation intentions and goal achievement: A meta-analysis of effects and processes. In M. P. Zanna (Ed.), *Advances in experimental social psychology* (Vol. 38, pp. 69–119). San Diego, CA: Academic Press.

Gollwitzer, P. M., & Wicklund, R. A. (1985). Self-symbolizing and the neglect of others' perspectives. *Journal of Personality and Social Psychology, 56,* 531–715.

Gottschaldt, K. (1926). Über den Einfluß der Erfahrung auf die Wahrnehmung von Figuren [On the effects of familiarity on the perception of figures]. *Psychologische Forschung, 8,* 261–317.

Häfner, S. (2000). *Machen Vorsätze rigide? Eine experimentelle Studie zum Erkennen und Nutzen günstiger Handlungsgelegenheiten [Do implementation intentions make a person rigid?: An experimental study on seizing good opportunities to act].* Unpublished master's thesis, Universität Konstanz, Konstanz, Germany.

Hommel, B. (1994). Spontaneous decay of response-code activation. *Psychological Research, 56,* 261–268.

Jaudas, A., Achtziger, A., & Gollwitzer, P. M. (2006, March). *Bedingungen der effektiven Nutzung von Vorsätzen [Determinants of the effective use of implementation intentions].* Paper presented at the 48th Meeting of Experimental Psychologists, Mainz, Germany.

Jaudas, A., & Gollwitzer, P. M. (2004, April). Führen Vorsätze zu Rigidität im Zielstreben? [Do implementation intentions evoke rigidity in goal striving?]. In A. Achtziger & P. M. Gollwitzer (Chairs), *Recent developments in research on implementation inten-*

*tions*. Symposium conducted at the 46th Meeting of Experimental Psychologists, Giessen, Germany.

Kornblum, S., Hasbroucq, T., & Osman, A. (1990). Dimensional overlap: Cognitive basis for stimulus–response compatibility: A model and taxonomy. *Psychological Review, 97*, 253–270.

Kluwe, R. H., Lüer, G., & Rösler, F. (Eds.). (2003). *Principles of learning and memory*. Basel: Birkhäuser.

Lengfelder, A., & Gollwitzer, P. M. (2001). Reflective and reflexive action control in patients with frontal brain lesions. *Neuropsychology, 15*, 80–100.

Loewenstein, G. F., Weber, E. U., Hsee, C. K., & Welch, N. (2001). Risks as feelings. *Psychological Bulletin, 127*, 267–286.

Lu, C.-H., & Proctor, R. W. (1995). The influence of irrelevant location information on performance: A review of the Simon and spatial Stroop effects. *Psychonomic Bulletin and Review, 2*, 174–207.

Metcalfe, J., & Mischel, W. (1999). A hot/cool-system analysis of delay of gratification: dynamics of willpower. *Psychological Bulletin, 106*, 3–19.

Milne, S., Orbell, S., & Sheeran, P. (2002). Combining motivational and volitional interventions to promote exercise participation: Protection motivation theory and implementation intentions. *British Journal of Health Psychology, 7*, 163–184.

Mischel, W. (1996). From good intentions to willpower. In P. M. Gollwitzer & J. A. Bargh (Eds.), *The psychology of action: Linking cognition and motivation to behavior* (pp. 197–218). New York: Guilford Press.

Muraven, M., & Baumeister, R. F. (2000). Self-regulation and depletion of limited resources: Does self-control resemble a muscle? *Psychological Bulletin, 126*, 247–259.

Muraven, M., Tice, D. M., & Baumeister, R. F. (1998). Self-control as a limited resource: Regulatory depletion pattern. *Journal of Personality and Social Psychology, 74*, 774–789.

Oettingen, G., Hönig, G., & Gollwitzer, P. M. (2000). Effective self-regulation of goal attainment. *International Journal of Educational Research, 33*, 705–732.

Orbell, S., Hodgkins, S., & Sheeran, P. (1997). Implementation intentions and the theory of planned behavior. *Personality and Social Psychology Bulletin, 23*, 945–954.

Orbell, S., & Sheeran, P. (2000). Motivational and volitional processes in action initiation: A field study of the role of implementation intentions. *Journal of Applied Social Psychology, 30*, 780–797.

Park, J., & Banaji, M. R. (2000). Mood and heuristics: The influence of happy and sad states on sensitivity and bias in stereotyping. *Journal of Personality and Social Psychology, 78*, 1005–1023.

Parks-Stamm, E. J., Gollwitzer, P. M., & Oettingen, G. (2007). Action control by implementation intentions: Effective cue detection and efficient response initiation. *Social Cognition, 25*, 248–266.

Rogers, D., & Monsell, S. (1995). Costs of a predictable switch between simple cognitive tasks. *Journal of Experimental Psychology: General, 124*, 207–231.

Schweiger Gallo, I., Keil, A., McCulloch, K. C., Rockstroh, B., & Gollwitzer, P. M. (2006). *Strategic automation of emotion control*. Manuscript submitted for publication.

Seehausen, R., Bayer, U., & Gollwitzer, P. M. (1994, September). *Experimentelle Arbeiten zur "vorsaetzlichen" Handlungsregulation [Experimental studies on action control by implementation intentions]*. Paper presented at the Biennial Convention of the German Psychological Society, Hamburg, Germany.

Sheeran, P., & Orbell, S. (1998). Do intentions predict condom use?: A meta-analysis and examination of six moderator variables. *British Journal of Social Psychology, 37*, 231–250.

Sheeran, P., & Orbell, S. (1999). Implementation intentions and repeated behavior: Augmenting the predictive validity of the theory of planned behavior. *European Journal of Social Psychology, 29*, 349–369.

Sheeran, P., & Orbell, S. (2000). Using implementation intentions to increase attendance for cervical cancer screening. *Health Psychology, 19*, 283–289.

Sheeran, P., Webb, T. L., & Gollwitzer, P. M. (2005). The interplay between goal intentions and implementation intentions. *Personality and Social Psychology Bulletin, 31*, 87–98.

Steller, B. (1992). *Vorsätze und die Wahrnehmung günstiger Gelegenheiten [Implementation intentions and perceiving good opportunities to act]*. Munchen: Tuduv-Verlag.

Trafimow, D., & Sheeran, P. (2004). A theory about the translation of cognition into affect and behavior. In G. Haddock & R. Maio (Eds.), *Contemporary perspectives on the psychology of attitudes* (pp. 57–76). Hove, UK: Psychology Press.

Verplanken, B., & Faes, S. (1999). Good intentions, bad habits, and effects of forming implementation intentions on healthy eating. *European Journal of Social Psychology, 29*, 591–604.

Webb, T. L., & Sheeran, P. (2003). Can implementation intentions help to overcome ego-depletion? *Journal of Experimental Social Psychology, 39*, 279–286.

Webb, T. L., & Sheeran, P. (2004). Identifying good opportunities to act: Implementation intentions and cue discrimination. *European Journal of Social Psychology, 34*, 407–419.

Webb, T. L., & Sheeran, P. (2007). How do implementation intentions promote goal attainment?: A test of component processes. *Journal of Experimental and Social Psychology, 43*, 295–302.

Wicklund, R. A., & Gollwitzer, P. M. (1982). *Symbolic self-completion*. Hillsdale, NJ: Erlbaum.

Wright, R. A. (1996). Brehm's theory of motivation as a model of effort and cardiovascular response. In P. M. Gollwitzer & J. A. Bargh (Eds.), *The psychology of action: Linking cognition and motivation to behavior* (pp. 424–453). New York: Guilford Press.

Chapter 22

# The Antecedents and Consequences of Nonconscious Goal Pursuit

**Tanya L. Chartrand**
**Amy N. Dalton**
**Clara Michelle Cheng**

Traditional models of goal pursuit have long held deliberate choice and conscious guidance to be the fundamental drivers of the process. This certainly squares with intuition; we humans are often aware of choosing goals to pursue, deciding which behaviors and actions will help achieve those goals, engaging in these behaviors and actions, and evaluating our progress toward the goals. Certainly the goal pursuit process can and does often unfold in this manner. However, is it possible that goal pursuit can also occur outside of one's conscious intent and awareness?

At first the notion of nonconscious goal pursuit may seem like an oxymoron; goals are by definition intentional, so how could we engage in goal pursuit unintentionally? However, the last two decades or so have witnessed an explosion of research demonstrating the often automatic nature of goal pursuit. It seems that our goals can be automatically activated by features of the environment, and we then engage in behaviors that satisfy our chronic and temporary goals without being aware of doing so. In this way we are automatically pursuing our goals even when our cognitive resources are directed elsewhere. Nonconscious goals can enhance our sensitivity to goal-relevant environmental features and can even be flexible in some situations (see Ferguson, Hassin, & Bargh, Chapter 10, this volume). Automatic goal pursuit is adaptive, is functional, and serves us well in many situations (Bargh & Chartrand, 1999). Researchers exploring this phenomenon have also found that we succeed and fail at nonconsciously activated and pursued goals, and that there are downstream consequences of this for important outcomes (including mood, judgments of self and others, and behavior). In this chapter we review the history of nonconscious goal pursuit, including the initial evidence for the idea that goals can be activated outside awareness and intent, and then pursued as if the goals were consciously held. We then focus on the most recent research in this area, which has uncovered various real-world environmental triggers of nonconscious goals and downstream consequences that arise from succeeding and failing at them.

## THE FIRST ARGUMENT FOR NONCONSCIOUS GOAL PURSUIT

### The Auto-Motive Model

Bargh (1990) was the first to suggest in an influential paper that goals can be entirely activated and pursued outside of an individual's awareness and intent. He noted that evidence already existed that goals, once activated, are pursued automatically (e.g., once a goal to drive to work is in place, the actions necessary ensue without conscious intervention). He also argued that goals are likely to be represented just as other mental constructs are, and so should be capable of automatic activation by relevant features of the environment. Specifically, if a goal is consistently and frequently activated in a certain situation or environment, then the features of that environment should become linked in memory to the goal representation, and therefore the activation of one should activate the other. For instance, if an individual frequently and consistently chooses a self-presentational goal whenever he or she attends parties, eventually the features of the party environment (e.g., drinking, music, dancing) should automatically activate the self-presentational goal. Once activated, this goal should guide the person's behaviors as if it had been consciously chosen in the situation. Thus the individual may begin to monitor what he or she says or does more than usual, but may not be aware that he or she is engaging in a goal-directed activity that is serving chronically held goals.

Bargh's (1990) ideas were provocative, for he was going significantly beyond the argument that goal pursuit happens automatically once a person consciously decides to pursue a goal. He was arguing that the entire sequence—from automatic activation of the goal to pursuit of the goal via various strategies and plans of actions—can occur automatically, without the need for conscious intervention at any point in the sequence. To describe his theory, Bargh coined the phrase, "the auto-motive model."

### Initial Tests of Nonconscious Goal Activation and Pursuit

The initial studies testing the core tenets of the auto-motive model were based on the hypothesis that if goal activation and pursuit can occur nonconsciously, then researchers should be able to activate or "prime" goals in individuals without their awareness, and these individuals should then engage in goal-directed behaviors without intending to do so. The goal pursuit should occur as if the individuals had consciously chosen the goal. Thus the experimental paradigm in these initial studies was to prime a goal directly in the lab by using semantic associates of the goal. Both *supraliminal* (awareness of the semantic associates, but not of the pattern or goal that they activated) and *subliminal* (no awareness of exposure to the semantic associates) priming techniques were employed (see Bargh & Chartrand, 2000). After the priming manipulation, the extent to which individuals engaged in goal-directed action was measured. If goals can be activated and pursued outside of awareness, then individuals primed with a goal should engage in strategies and behaviors to achieve that goal, all without reporting conscious pursuit of that goal.

#### *Information-Processing Goals*

One of the earliest tests of nonconscious goal activation and pursuit was a conceptual replication of the classic effects of task instructions on information acquisition and memory organization. In the original study conducted by Hamilton, Katz, and Leirer (1980), participants were instructed either to memorize a series of behavioral predicates or to form an impression of the person who engaged in the behaviors. They found that participants who were given the impression formation "set" demonstrated better recall of the behaviors and more organization of the behaviors by trait category in memory than participants who were instructed to memorize the behaviors did. Chartrand and Bargh (1996) conceptually replicated this study, but whereas the task goals in the original study were given explicitly to participants, the task goals in the replication were given outside of participants' intent and conscious awareness (i.e., were primed). Specifically, Chartrand and Bargh used semantic associates in a scrambled-sentences task (Srull

& Wyer, 1979), in which participants rearrange sets of five words to form four-word sentences, to supraliminally prime information-processing goals and demonstrate that these nonconsciously activated goals are pursued in the same manner as consciously activated goals. The researchers primed participants either with an impression formation goal (by embedding words such as *evaluate* and *personality* in the sentences) or with a memorization goal (by embedding words such as *remember* and *retain* in the sentences).

In an ostensibly unrelated experiment, participants read a series of 24 behavioral predicates that described behaviors in four different trait categories. They were explicitly instructed to read the phrases carefully, because they would be asked questions about them later. No participants were told either to memorize the information or to form an impression of the person who would engage in the behaviors. The results closely replicated the original study, such that those primed with an impression formation goal recalled more behaviors than those primed with a memorization goal, and they showed greater "clustering" or organization of the material in memory. Follow-up questioning confirmed that Chartrand and Bargh's participants pursued these goals without realizing that they had them.

### Behavioral Goals

The Chartrand and Bargh studies examined cognitive (information-processing) goals. Social behavioral goals are also capable of automatic activation and pursuit. For instance, Bargh, Gollwitzer, Lee-Chai, Barndollar, and Trötschel (2001, Experiment 1) demonstrated that participants who completed a word search that included a number of achievement-related words showed superior performance on a subsequent intellectual task, compared to participants whose word search task included neutral words. Taken together, the Chartrand and Bargh (1996) and Bargh and colleagues (2001) studies supported the auto-motive theory's notion that nonconscious goals operate in the same manner and lead to the same outcomes as conscious goals.

Just as individuals differ in the goals that they consciously select and pursue, individuals also differ in the goals that they come to pursue nonconsciously. Individual differences in chronically pursued goals have been found to moderate the behavioral effects of semantic associate priming. For example, whereas primed affiliation or achievement goals direct immediate behavior, chronic affiliation or achievement goals direct behavior after a delay (Bargh & Gollwitzer, 1994). Participants supraliminally primed with an affiliation goal or an achievement goal immediately showed evidence of goal-directed behavior, with affiliation-primed participants performing down to the level of a confederate on a subsequent achievement task, and achievement-primed participants performing above the level of the confederate; however, after a delay, individual differences in chronic affiliation or achievement orientations had more influence on behavior.

### Presence of Motivational Properties

A critical component of the inference that priming can activate a motivational state is the demonstration that nonconsciously held goals exhibit the characteristic features of consciously held goals. The studies described above suggest that nonconsciously activated information-processing goals and behavioral goals will operate in much the same manner as consciously pursued goals. However, goal-directed behavior shows a number of specific properties that define these behaviors as motivational rather than cognitive in origin (e.g., Atkinson & Birch, 1970; Bandura, 1986; Gollwitzer, 1990; Lewin, 1951).

In a series of studies, Bargh and colleagues (2001) demonstrated the presence of uniquely motivational qualities during nonconscious goal pursuit. In one of these, they focused on dissociating motivational and perceptual priming effects. Specifically, motivational states increase in strength over time, and goal-directed individuals show persistence in spite of obstacles or interruptions (Atkinson & Birch, 1970). Cognitive states, such as those induced by perceptual priming effects, decrease in strength over time and as such do not result in task persistence (e.g., Higgins, Bargh, & Lombardi, 1985). Thus participants were either primed with achievement-related words or neutral words. Participants then completed either a goal-related task, which required them to form as many words as possible with a set of Scrabble letters, or a perceptual judgment task, which required them to read about and individual who behaves in an ambiguously achieving way (i.e., studying hard right before a test) and rate how achievement-oriented the individual was. Half the participants with the goal-related behavioral task completed the task immediately after the priming procedure, whereas the other half were given a 5-minute filler task in which they drew their family trees before completing the Scrabble task. Likewise, half the participants with the perceptual judgment task completed that task immediately, whereas the other half first completed the 5-minute filler task.

The results clearly demonstrated the differing effects of delay on motivational and perceptual priming effects (Bargh et al., 2001). Achievement-primed participants who completed the goal-related task showed significantly better performance than control participants, and this difference was significantly greater when the goal-related task was completed after a 5-minute delay than when it was completed immediately after priming. Achievement-primed participants who completed the perceptual judgment task exhibited a significant bias (compared to control participants) toward rating the ambiguously behaving individual as achievement-oriented, but only when the judgment task was completed immediately after the achievement prime. Consistent with the researchers' hypotheses, the achievement-related words activated a motivational state to achieve, and this goal strength increased in strength over time—one of the hallmarks of motivation (see Chartrand, Huber, Shiv, & Tanner, in press, for a similar finding using different goals).

In a subsequent study, Bargh and colleagues (2001) examined another uniquely motivational property of goal pursuit: persistence in the face of obstacles. The results demonstrated that achievement-primed participants showed persistence by continuing to work on a Scrabble task after receiving instructions over an intercom to stop. Participants in the control condition were less likely to continue to work after the signal to stop. In their final study, the researchers examined resumption of interrupted goal pursuits. Midway through an achievement-priming (or neutral) word search task, participants were interrupted by a staged power failure. When the power came back on and participants were given the choice of resuming the first task or proceeding to a second, more enjoyable task, achievement-primed participants were more likely to resume the interrupted task than were control participants.

Chartrand and colleagues (in press) focused on yet another quality of motivational states: Once satiated, they quickly dissipate. That is, if a nonconsciously activated goal has been satisfied through goal-directed activity, choice, or behavior, then the goal strength should be quickly reduced and should not affect subsequent behavior. To test this, the researchers used a scrambled-sentences task to prime participants with either a brand image or a value goal. Participants then made a choice between two options of crew socks valued at $6, one more brand-focused (one pair of Tommy Hilfiger) than the other (three pairs of Hanes). For some participants, the choice was real and they received the option they picked (real-choice condition). The other participants were told to pretend that their choice was real and that they would receive the option they picked (hypothetical-choice condition). Following the real or hypothetical choice, participants were told that by taking part in the study, they would automatically be entered into a drawing for a prize. Two winners would receive one of two prizes: either a Timex watch worth $25 plus $75 in cash, or a Guess watch worth $75 plus $25 in cash (pilot testing established these options as equally desirable). Participants were asked to select which of these two prizes they would like to receive, should they win the lottery.

Results revealed that participants' choices on the first task—whether real or hypothetical—were influenced by the goal prime, such that participants primed with value were more likely to choose the Hanes crew socks than those primed with brand image. However, on the second task, only participants who had made hypothetical choices on the first task were influenced by the primes. Participants who had made real choices satiated their nonconsciously activated goals, and no priming effects were found on the second task (Chartrand, Huber, et al., in press).

## A SEQUENTIAL PERSPECTIVE ON NONCONSCIOUS GOAL PURSUIT

Because the visual perception of a word automatically activates relevant and associated mental representations, initial research on nonconscious goal pursuit tested whether a goal can be automatically activated and pursued by using semantic associates to directly activate the goal outside of awareness. Findings from a number of studies indicated that even though individuals had no conscious awareness of having goals activated, they engaged in appropriate goal-directed behavior. Direct goal activation is one way to demonstrate that perceptual processes can act as triggers of motivational processes. The primary strength of direct goal activation is that the experimenter has a fair degree of control over the goal that is activated.

However, this technique constitutes an "artificial environment"; true environmental influences are not present, and therefore their effects cannot be unequivocally inferred. The auto-motive model (Bargh, 1990) posited that features of the current social situation activate goals nonconsciously. In naturalistic settings, individuals are typically primed not by semantic associates to a goal, but by situational triggers that activate a specific goal linked to that situation in memory. The contrived priming manipulations used in initial explorations were useful in reducing any extraneous variables and isolating the goal activation process in the lab, but once nonconscious goal activation and pursuit were established, researchers began exploring the ways in which goals are naturalistically triggered by the environment.

Moreover, researchers began speculating on potential consequences of this nonconscious version of goal pursuit. We humans succeed and fail at conscious goal pursuit all the time, and consequences ensue. We are disappointed after annoying someone whom we want to like us, and we are elated after finishing a marathon we have been training for. We succeed and fail at nonconscious goals just as we do conscious goals. The question is this: Are there consequences of nonconscious goal pursuit, and if so, in what ways are they similar to or different from the consequences of conscious goal pursuit?

To look at antecedents and consequences of nonconscious goal pursuit is to take a sequential perspective on the process (see Figure 22.1). Initial tests have primed goals directly with semantic associates (1b in the figure) and found evidence for goal activation (2) and pursuit (3). In the sections that follow, we review evidence examining the environmental features that activate goals (1a), and the consequences (5) that may arise from success or failure (4).

## ANTECEDENTS OF NONCONSCIOUS GOAL PURSUIT

There has been considerable recent research uncovering the antecedents of nonconscious goal pursuit, including social situations and norms, other people, and even inanimate objects. All of these triggers can elicit the motives that an individual has come to associate with those stimuli. It is to this research that we now turn.

### Social Situational Triggers

Social environments should automatically trigger goals in memory, provided that the goals have been repeatedly and consistently chosen in those environments in the past. Certain environments, in fact, should activate similar goals

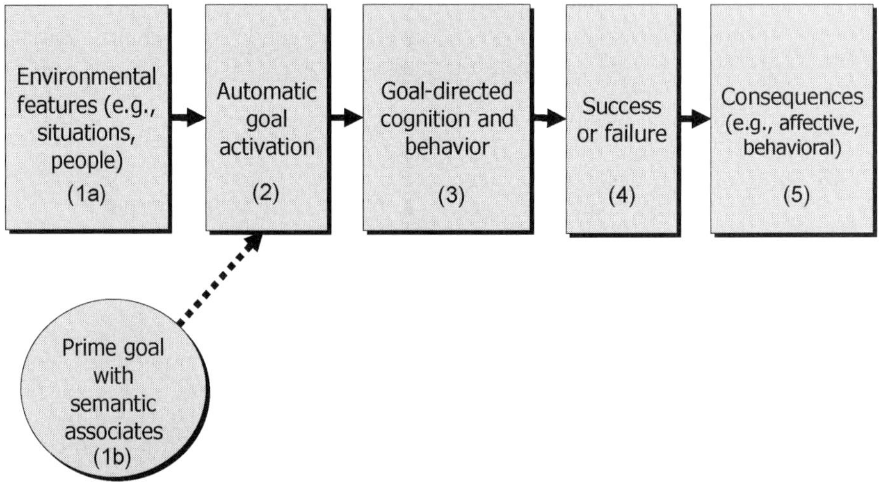


**FIGURE 22.1.** A sequential perspective on nonconscious goal pursuit.

across individuals. Situations of this sort presumably evoke culturally shared associative networks of cognitive, motivational, and behavioral responses.

### Ego Threat

One situation that has been found to trigger similar goals across individuals is ego threat. When a social situation is perceived as threatening to an individual's self-concept, that individual will engage in behaviors to enhance or maintain the self-concept. One behavior that people engage in to serve a self-enhancement goal is stereotyping (Fein & Spencer, 1997). In a study conducted by Spencer, Fein, Wolfe, Fong, and Dunn (1998), European American participants who received bogus negative feedback showed evidence of automatic stereotype activation when subliminally primed with drawings of an African American male face. Participants who did not receive negative feedback showed no such stereotype activation. The major implication of these results is that people with a threatened self-image are at higher risk of stereotyping members of minority groups in an unconscious attempt to satisfy a self-enhancement goal.

### Temptations

Another situation that may activate common goals across individuals is being faced with a temptation. Specifically, temptations may automatically activate the goal with which they typically interfere (see Fishbach & Trope, Chapter 18, this volume). Fishbach, Friedman, and Kruglanski (2003) examined the relationship between competing temptations and goals; they found an asymmetrical pattern of activation, such that temptations tended to activate competing goals, but goals did not activate competing temptations. Temptations also increased intentions and behavior congruent with the goal.

### Individual Differences in Situation–Goal Linkages

Although situations may often activate the same goal in most individuals, there are likely to be individual differences in situation–goal linkages. That is, a certain situation may be a trigger only for a certain type of person. This has been the focus of research by Bargh and colleagues. For instance, Bargh, Raymond, Pryor, and Strack (1995) examined individual differences in response to interpersonal power. Drawing on research showing that sexual harassers associate power with sex (e.g., Lisak & Roth, 1988; Pryor & Stoller, 1994), these researchers reasoned that perceived power would automatically activate sex-related goals in men exhibiting a high tendency toward sexual aggression, but not in men with no such tendency. Participants' tendency toward sexual aggression was assessed with the Attractiveness of Sexual Aggression (ASA) scale (Malamuth, 1989a, 1989b). The results supported the researchers' predictions.

A second experiment was conducted to examine the behavioral consequences of this automatic link between power and sex (Bargh et al., 1995). Again, the researchers examined male participants with high or low ASA scores. In this study, the participants completed the tasks in the presence of a female confederate who presented herself as another research participant. Participants first completed a word fragment completion task, which contained either power-related words or neutral words. The participant and confederate then worked individually on a "visual illusion" task, after which they were escorted into separate rooms. The participant was informed that the experiment was actually about the incidental impressions that people form of others with whom they interact only minimally, and was asked to provide ratings of the confederate on various scales. The critical ratings related to the confederate's attractiveness and to how much the participant would like to get to know her. Both ratings were higher for high-ASA males than for low-ASA males. These studies suggest that situational power is associated with sex in certain men, but not in others.

Chen, Lee-Chai, and Bargh (2001) also focused on situational power and the automatic activation of goals for certain individuals. Across three studies, they established that a situation of power elicits social responsibility goals in communally oriented people and self-interest goals in exchange-oriented people. This person $\times$ situation interaction was a key finding of this work, and of the work conducted on the relation between power and sex described above (Bargh et al., 1995), because it supports the notion that most environmental influences on behavior are likely to be moderated by individual differences—be they transient states (such as mood and drive) or long-lasting and potentially chronic motivations (such as interpersonal orientation or personality-related variables).

One of the compelling aspects of Chen and colleagues' (2001) research is its demonstration that naturally occurring cues in the environment can activate goals that are not directly or semantically related to the primed construct. For example, in their third experiment, power was primed in half the participants by seating them in a professor's chair to complete the experimental tasks, and a lack of power was primed in the other participants by seating them in a guest chair. This situational priming methodology probably parallels the manner in which goals are nonconsciously activated in the "real world," and thus provides persuasive evidence for the assertion that environmental cues can directly activate the goals people have chronically associated with those cues in the past.

## People as Triggers of Nonconscious Goals

Taken together, these studies demonstrate that specific situations can operate as triggers of nonconscious goals. The presence of other people in our social world is ubiquitous, and has recently been explored as another type of antecedent to nonconscious goal activation. A burgeoning area of research suggests that the presence of a person (actual or implied) can in fact be a powerful situational trigger of nonconscious goal pursuit. There are several ways in which people may activate nonconscious goals in others. For one, the perception of an individual pursuing a goal may be enough for others to "catch" the same goal and take it on themselves. Second, if a stereotype is activated, then goals frequently associated with members of that stereotyped group, or goals usually held when with members of the group, may be automatically activated. Finally, the presence of significant others with whom people have associated goals in various ways can automatically activate goals. This evidence is now reviewed.

### Goal Contagion

*Goal contagion* refers to the nonconscious perception and adoption of goals pursued by other people (see Aarts, Dijksterhuis, & Dik, Chapter 17, this volume). Aarts, Gollwitzer, and Hassin (2004) posited that individuals may automatically adopt and pursue a goal that is implied by another person's behavior. In several studies testing this notion, the researchers found that goal contagion occurred only when the goal was appropriate to the subsequent context and did not occur when goals were pursued in an unacceptable manner or under unacceptable conditions.

### Stereotype Activation

Moskowitz, Gollwitzer, Wasel, and Schall (1999) examined whether certain individuals are able to avoid stereotype activation by holding certain goals. They predicted that stereotype-related stimuli should lead to nonconscious goal activation for individuals with chronic egalitarian goals, and that this goal activation should cause these individuals to preconsciously inhibit related stereotypes. They found that stimuli associated with a stereotyped group member did in fact nonconsciously activate a chronic egalitarian goal in research participants for whom egalitarianism was a fundamental aspect of their value systems. Research participants for whom egalitarianism was not as important showed signs of stereotype activation. Note that this is consistent with the previously described research demonstrating individual differences in goal–situation linkages (Bargh et al., 1995; Chen et al., 2001).

After demonstrating that chronic egalitarian goals exist and that differences in stereotype activation occur between chronic and nonchronic egalitarians, the researchers aimed to demonstrate the underlying mechanism of the effect. Attribute words were presented following word and distracter primes, and response latencies to pronounce the attribute words were measured. Results showed that stereotypical distracters facilitated nonchronic egalitarians' response latencies to stereotypical attribute words, whereas stereotypical distracters inhibited chronic egalitarians' response latencies to stereotypical attribute words. These results strongly suggest that the mechanism underlying chronic egalitarians' control of stereotype activation is preconscious inhibition.

### Stereotype Activation and Goal Contagion

There is another mechanism by which stereotype activation may influence nonconscious goal pursuit. Members of stereotyped groups are associated with the pursuit of certain goals, and it is possible that these goals are automatically activated in the person encountering the stereotype. This would be consistent with the goal contagion findings of Aarts and colleagues (2004), but would suggest that people can "catch" goals that they perceive as operating on a group level rather than on the individual level.

Aarts and colleagues (2005) found that exposure to the names of social groups activated goals consistent with the group stereotype. In one study, participants were primed via a scrambled-sentences task with either social groups associated with the goal to make money (e.g., real estate agents, stockbrokers) or social groups not associated with this goal. Participants were told that they would have the opportunity to make money in a lottery game, but first had to do a mouse-clicking task. A time constraint was imposed on half of the participants, such that they would only do the lottery task if there was time at the end. The experimenters measured participants' speed during the mouse-clicking task. Their hypothesis was that participants primed with social groups thought to possess a money-making goal should work hard for the opportunity to make money, especially with an obstacle in their way (Bargh et al., 2001). The results showed significant differences in speed between the primed and control participants, but only under time constraints, suggesting that these participants put the most effort into overcoming the obstacle to making money.

### *Significant Others as Triggers of Nonconscious Goals*

Significant others (e.g., parents, best friends) elicit some of people's most strongly held goals. Can these goals become automatically activated by the mere presence of a significant other? Two types of significant-other goals have been explored thus far: goals that an individual normally has when with a significant other, and goals that the significant other has for the individual.

Fitzsimons and Bargh (2003) found that participants who volunteered to fill out a short questionnaire about a friend were more likely than participants who were asked questions about a coworker to volunteer to participate in a second study. This effect was hypothesized to occur because thinking about a friend activates a goal to be helpful more readily than does thinking about a coworker. Fitzsimons and Bargh also found that activating mental representations of significant others influenced participants' perceptions of a different target person's motives. Therefore, not only do significant others activate the goals people typically pursue in their presence, but people are also subsequently more likely to attribute these highly accessible goals associated with their significant others to different individuals.

Goals that a significant other has for an individual can also be automatically activated by the representation of the significant other. Shah (2003) found that participants primed with the name of a significant other who had a goal for them to do well persisted longer and performed better on a series of anagrams than those primed with a significant other who did not have such a goal for them. Changes in goal accessibility were found to mediate the significant-other priming effects on task performance and task persistence. Goal accessibility was determined to be a function of the importance of the task goal to the participants' significant others, as well as of the participants' closeness to their significant others.

Shah (2003) also investigated the extent to which significant others affected perceptions of goal difficulty. In one study, Shah examined the extent to which activating the representation of a significant other would affect the expectancy for goal attainment. In comparison to the control condition primed with a letter string, those primed with the names of significant others who would feel that the likelihood of the participants' goal attainment was high (low) rated their own likelihood of goal attainment higher (lower), persisted more (less) on an anagram task, and performed better (worse) on an anagram task.

### *Nonconscious Significant-Other Reactance*

Do individuals always assimilate automatically to the goals associated with significant others? Or can contrast (i.e., reactance) occur under some conditions, even at a nonconscious level? Chartrand, Dalton, and Fitzsimons (in press) explored whether nonconscious reactance can occur against significant others' goals for the self, and what the necessary conditions are for this to occur. In one experiment, they subliminally primed each participant with the name of a controlling significant other who had a goal for the participant either to work hard or to have fun. They found evidence for nonconscious reactance on a subsequent anagram task, such that those primed with the work-hard significant other did worse on the anagram task than those primed with the have-fun significant other. In a second experiment, Chartrand, Dalton, and Fitzsimons subliminally primed each participant with a string of letters (control prime condition) or with the name of a significant other who had a goal for the participant either to relax (relax prime condition) or to work hard (work-hard prime condition). On a subsequent anagram task, chronically low-reactance participants adopted their significant others' goal, replicating the assimilation effects found by Shah (2003). However, chronically high-reactance individuals demonstrated automatic reactance by pursuing the opposing goal. That is, those primed with the significant others who wanted them to work hard performed worse than those primed with the significant others who wanted them to relax, and vice versa. These studies are in line with other existing evidence (e.g., Fitzsimons & Bargh, 2003; Shah, 2003) for the inclusion of goal-related information in relational representations.

### Anthropomorphized Objects as Triggers of Nonconscious Goal Pursuit

Objects in the environment to which an individual has formed goal-related associations in memory may also be capable of nonconsciously and automatically influencing behavior. Chartrand, Fitzsimons, and Fitzsimons (in press) investigated this possibility vis-à-vis anthropomorphism (the attribution of humanlike characteristics to nonhuman entities). Their studies show that incidental exposure to a common object associated with human characteristics causes people to behave automatically in a manner that resembles the personality associated with the nonhuman object. In one study, participants were primed with images of cats or dogs in the context of a picture-ordering task. Subsequently, they responded to scenarios about interpersonal situations that were designed to assess loyalty in the face of transgressions by their friends. Results revealed that participants in the dog-primed condition responded more loyally than participants in the cat-primed conditions.

To determine the mechanism underlying the effect of anthropomorphized objects on behavior, Fitzsimons, Chartrand, and Fitzsimons (2007) borrowed the paradigm used by Bargh and colleagues (2001, Experiment 3) to distinguish between purely cognitive and motivational priming. Participants were first subliminally primed with either Apple (an anthropomorphized brand) or IBM logos. Some participants immediately engaged in a creativity task, in which they were asked to generate unusual uses for a brick, and other participants completed a 5-minute filler task before the unusual-uses task. Apple-primed participants were more creative and generated more uses on the unusual-uses task in the delay condition than in the no-delay condition. IBM-primed participants were less creative, they generated fewer uses, and their performance was not affected by the delay. These results suggest an involvement of motivational processes: The creativity observed in this study showed increasing strength over time, a hallmark of goal-directed behavior.

### Social Norms

A final antecedent of nonconscious goal activation was explored by Aarts and Dijksterhuis (2003), who tested whether social norms can serve as triggers of nonconscious goal pursuit. Participants were assigned to one of three conditions. They were exposed to a picture of a library (library prime condition) or a railway station (goal control prime condition) and told that they would have to visit the location in the picture after the experiment, or they were exposed to a picture of a library and asked to study the picture carefully (no-goal library prime condition). Next, participants were asked to do a word pronunciation task, which was purportedly helping in the design of a new communication system. As participants read aloud 10 words, the sound pressure level of their voices was measured. The results confirmed that voices of participants in the library prime condition were less loud than voices of participants in either the goal control prime condition or the no-goal library prime condition, which did not differ significantly. Controlling for mood, arousal, or frequency of past behavior did not influence the pattern of results. Therefore, this study suggests that normative behavior can be automatically activated when the relevant goal has been activated, and that this effect can occur regardless of the frequency of past experiences performing the normative behavior.

In sum, research exploring the antecedents of nonconscious goal pursuit has uncovered a number of triggers, including social situations such as power, ego threat, and temptation; stereotype activation; goal contagion; significant others; anthropomorphized objects; and social norms. Future research is likely to identify additional triggers and moderators of this nonconscious, unintentional type of goal pursuit.

## CONSEQUENCES OF NONCONSCIOUS GOAL PURSUIT

One might ask whether there are any implications for the idea that we humans are pursuing goals outside our awareness and conscious intent. Does it matter that we are often not aware of our goal pursuits and the guiding role that these motives play in our behavior? A number of recent studies have been exploring the downstream consequences of nonconscious goal pursuit in an attempt to answer this question. The findings from these studies suggest that the way we feel, perform, regulate our self-esteem and subsequent goal pursuits, and act toward others can be affected by pursuing a nonconscious goal—one that we are not aware of pursuing in the first place.

These consequences arise from success and failure at nonconscious goals (Chartrand & Bargh, 2002). Just as people succeed and fail at consciously chosen and held goals, they also succeed and fail at goals they are not aware of pursuing. There are consequences of succeeding and failing at consciously held goals for mood, self-evaluation, and behavior; are these consequences specific to consciously held goals, or do they ensue from success and failure at nonconsciously held goals as well? The fact that individuals are not aware of engaging in goal-directed behavior, and certainly not aware of having succeeded or failed at anything, suggests that perhaps the process is distinct and as a result may not lead to the same consequences. How can people feel bad if they are not aware of having failed at any goal? Is conscious awareness of the success or failure necessary for the consequences to follow, or would they follow in some form or another, regardless of whether the individuals were aware of pursuing the goal? The initial studies in this area examined the consequences of success and failure of nonconscious goal pursuit for mood.

### Consequences for Mood

We can all probably attest to the idea that conscious goal pursuit can influence our mood; succeeding at a goal makes us feel good, whereas failing at a goal makes us feel bad. Chartrand (2007) explored the idea that nonconscious goal pursuit can have similar effects on mood. She primed half of the participants with an achievement goal via a scrambled-sentences task. The other half of the participants were given a neutral version of the task, without the achievement-related words. Then participants were given an anagram task described as a "fun, filler task" that would take 2–3 minutes to complete. In fact, the anagram task served as the success–failure manipulation. Half of the participants were given an easy version of the task consisting of 8 items. The other half of the participants were given a 28-item version that was difficult to complete within 2–3 minutes. Thus participants given an easy anagram task were led to succeed at their goal to achieve, while those given a difficult anagram task were led to fail. Finally, participants' mood was assessed.

Chartrand (2007) found that participants who succeeded at the achievement goal reported being in a better mood, while participants who failed reported being in a worse mood, compared to those who had not been primed with a goal. Thus, just as in conscious goal pursuit, succeeding at a nonconscious goal can result in better mood, and failing at a nonconscious goal can lead to a worse mood. Interestingly, individuals reported not knowing why they were in the mood they were in. As a result, these were dubbed "mystery moods": The source of the mood was a "mystery" to participants, since they were not aware of having been pursuing a goal.

### Self-Enhancement

Thus failing at nonconscious goals puts people in a negative mystery mood. There is now evidence suggesting that being in a negative mystery mood as a result of failing at a nonconscious goal can have further downstream consequences for intrapersonal as well as interpersonal behaviors.

First, failing at a nonconscious goal can lead to self-enhancement. According to Steele, Spencer, and Lynch (1993), a blow to one's self-esteem can trigger the need to restore that self-image. Tesser and his colleagues (Tesser, 2000, 2001; Tesser, Crepaz, Collins, Cornell, & Beach, 2000; Tesser, Martin, & Cornell, 1996) have further suggested that because different self-enhancement mechanisms all serve the common purpose of maintaining self-esteem, they can substitute for one another. In other words, a self-esteem threat in one domain can be restored by enhancing oneself in another domain. Tesser and his colleagues posit, however, that this mechanism substitution is due to misattribution of affect, and can only occur if one is unaware of either the negative arousal triggered by the threat or the source of that negative arousal. The latter—being unaware of the source of a negative state generated by self-esteem threat—is exactly what a negative mystery mood is. Thus being in a negative mood of an unknown origin can lead to the use of an available self-enhancement strategy to maintain self-esteem.

Chartrand, Cheng, Tesser, and Dalton (2007) tested the hypothesis that the negative mystery mood resulting from failure at nonconscious goal pursuit can lead to self-enhancement. They primed one group of participants with an achievement goal via a scrambled-sentences task. A second group of participants was explicitly told to try to do the best they could on the next task. A third group did not receive a goal manipulation. Then all participants were led to fail by having them complete a difficult anagram task. Following the anagram task, participants were given a measure of self-serving attribution, taken from Dunning, Leuenberger, and Sherman (1995), which provided participants with an opportunity to engage in self-enhancement. In this measure, participants read about a target person who enjoyed a successful 25-year marriage, and about various attributes of this person (e.g., grew up in a big city, attended private school, etc.). Participants were then asked to indicate how important each attribute was in contributing to the successful marriage. Now imagine a participant who also grew up in a big city but went to a public school. If this person was trying to enhance his or her self-esteem, he or she would be likely to claim that having been raised in a big city (a shared attribute) was an important factor in the successful marriage, while the private school education (an unshared attribute) was not. In other words, people engaging in self-enhancement would tend to indicate that the attributes that they themselves possessed were more important in contributing to success than attributes they did not possess. Chartrand, Cheng, and colleagues found that participants who had failed at a nonconscious achievement goal were more likely to engage in this type of self-serving bias than those who failed at a conscious achievement goal and those who did not have an achievement goal. This effect of nonconscious goal failure on self-enhancement was also replicated with a different priming method (subliminal as opposed to supraliminal) as well as a different primed goal (impression formation).

While self-enhancement may take the form of mentally convincing oneself that one possesses success-related attributes, it can also take the form of more antisocial behaviors. In a follow-up study, Chartrand, Cheng, and colleagues (2007) found that failing at a nonconscious achievement goal also led to an increase in implicit stereotyping. In this case, participants who failed at a nonconscious goal were more likely to justify actions that were inconsistent with gender stereotypes.

## Aggression

Of course, one might argue that subtly stereotyping others may not be a terribly "antisocial" behavior. However, recent research has found that overt aggression can also be a consequence of failing at nonconscious goal pursuit (Jefferis & Chartrand, 2007). This is based on the idea that negative affect increases the likelihood of acting in an aggressive manner (Berkowitz, 1989). As noted earlier, nonconscious goal failure can result in negative affect. If negative affect causes aggressive behaviors, it follows that failing at a nonconscious goal can also lead to an increase in aggression. This idea was tested by Jefferis and Chartrand (2007). They primed participants with an impression formation goal via a scrambled-sentences task. Then participants read one of two versions of a short excerpt about a target person, Joe. In one version, Joe consistently behaved in an ungainly manner—spilling his coffee, bumping into a librarian, and so forth. This was meant to allow participants to succeed at the nonconscious goal, since participants could easily determine that Joe was a clumsy person. In the other version, Joe sometimes acted clumsily, but at other times he was graceful and agile (e.g., he avoided tripping over a toy). In this case, participants were led to fail at the nonconscious goal, because it was difficult for them to form an accurate impression of Joe. It was found that participants who were in the failure condition were subsequently more aggressive toward another, fictitious participant (purportedly completing the experiment in the next room) by giving this other participant a larger sample of hot sauce to taste—knowing full well that the other participant despised spicy foods.

These results were replicated with another behavioral measure of aggression, in which failed participants got significantly closer to a confederate walking head-on toward them before veering away to avoid a collision, as well as a projective measure of aggression, in which participants who failed at a nonconscious goal were more likely to provide an aggressive ending in a story completion task.

### Performance

Succeeding at conscious goal pursuit has been found to increase self-efficacy beliefs as well as persistence of goal-directed behavior, which then enhances performance on subsequent goal-relevant tasks (Bandura, 1997; Locke, Frederick, Lee, & Bobko, 1984). Conversely, failure at goal pursuit impairs subsequent performance. Chartrand (2007) examined whether this effect on subsequent performance would hold for nonconscious goals as well. She primed half of the participants with an achievement goal via a scrambled-sentences task, while the other half completed a neutral version of the task. Then participants were given the success–failure manipulation by having them complete an easy or difficult anagram task. The dependent measure was performance on a subsequent task consisting of questions from the verbal section of the Graduate Record Examination (GRE). Indeed, Chartrand found that success and failure at nonconscious goal pursuit affected participants' subsequent performance on a related task in much the same way as conscious goal pursuit would: Participants who had succeeded performed better on the GRE, while those who had failed performed worse, compared to participants who had not been primed with a goal.

Chartrand (2007) also demonstrated mediation of these performance effects by indirect self-efficacy beliefs. Individuals who succeeded at a nonconscious goal believed that they would do better at an immediate goal-relevant test (an indirect measure of self-efficacy), and they did. Conversely, individuals who failed at a nonconscious goal expected to perform more poorly, which in turn led to poorer performance. Direct measures of self-efficacy beliefs, which tapped into participants' stable beliefs about competence, failed to mediate the effects.

### Ego Depletion

The pursuit of nonconscious goals can affect performance on subsequent tasks not only by changing implicit efficacy beliefs, but also by draining resources that are needed to regulate the self. A growing literature suggests that all conscious regulatory efforts draw on a single, limited resource (e.g., Muraven & Baumeister, 2000). Deliberately performing a self-regulatory task depletes this resource, and performance on a second self-regulatory task will suffer as a consequence. Recently, Vohs (2007) has demonstrated that nonconscious goal pursuits also deplete self-regulatory resources and leave individuals less able to perform well on subsequent self-regulatory tasks. In one study, Vohs gave participants no task instructions (control group), explicit task instructions, or primed task instructions to suppress their emotions while watching a disgusting video. She then measured attentional control on a subsequent task as an index of resource availability.

The results showed that participants in the control group, who were free to express their emotions while viewing the video, showed the most attentional control on the second task. Participants who consciously suppressed their emotions showed the least attentional control, and participants who nonconsciously suppressed their emotions fell in between the conscious regulators (who were most depleted) and the nonregulating controls (who were least depleted). This finding is particularly interesting because it sheds light on an important theoretical issue: Does the automatic nature of nonconscious goal activation and pursuit mean that these goals do not use or drain capacity? Based on Vohs's research, the answer is a resounding "no." Although nonconscious self-regulation consumes fewer resources than conscious regulation, it is still depleting.

In sum, recent research has uncovered important consequences of succeeding and failing at nonconsciously activated and pursued goals. Some of these consequences are unique to nonconscious goal pursuit (e.g., self-enhancement, aggression), and some are similar to those arising from conscious goal pursuit (e.g., mood, performance, ego depletion). Future research can further explore the dissociations in the consequences of conscious versus nonconscious goal pursuit.

## CONCLUSION

Goal pursuit is not always a consciously driven and guided process. Sometimes we humans are pursuing goals outside of deliberate choice and conscious awareness. This is generally an adaptive process; we are able to pursue our goals without expending cognitive resources and energy to do so. This automatization of our goals may sometimes get us into trouble, but in general it serves us well. Research has been identifying the antecedents of nonconscious goals, and has uncovered a number of precursors that are notably ubiquitous in our environment. For example, we are almost always encountering significant others or anthropomorphized objects, or perceiving others who are pursing their own goals, or being faced with temptations or social norms. That these are all environmental triggers of nonconscious goals speaks to the considerable frequency with which we are pursing goals outside of our awareness and intention.

## REFERENCES


Aarts, H., Chartrand, T. L., Custers, R., Danner, U., Dik, G., Jefferis, V., et al. (2005). Social stereotype and automatic goal pursuit. *Social Cognition, 23*, 465–490.

Aarts, H., & Dijksterhuis, A. (2003). The silence of the library: Environment, situational norm, and social behavior. *Journal of Personality and Social Psychology, 84*, 18–28.

Aarts, H., Gollwitzer, P. M., & Hassin, R. R. (2004). Goal contagion: Perceiving Is for pursuing. *Journal of Personality and Social Psychology, 87*, 23–37.

Atkinson, J. W., & Birch, D. (1970). *The dynamics of action*. New York: Wiley.

Bandura, A. (1986). *Social foundations of thought and action: A social cognitive theory*. Englewood Cliffs, NJ: Prentice Hall.

Bandura, A. (1997). *Self-efficacy*. New York: Freeman.

Bargh, J. A. (1990). Auto-motives: Preconscious determinants of social interaction. In E. Higgins & R. M. Sorrentino (Eds.), *Handbook of motivation and cognition: Foundations of social behavior* (Vol. 2, pp. 93–130). New York: Guilford Press.

Bargh, J. A., & Chartrand, T. L. (1999). The unbearable automaticity of being. *American Psychologist, 54*, 462–479.

Bargh, J. A., & Chartrand, T. L. (2000). The mind in the middle: A practical guide to priming and automaticity research. In H. T. Reis & C. M. Judd (Eds.), *Handbook of research methods in social and personality psychology* (pp. 253–285). New York: Cambridge University Press.

Bargh, J. A., & Gollwitzer, P. M. (1994). Environmental control of goal-directed action. In W. Spaulding (Ed.), *Nebraska Symposium on Motivation: Integrative views of motivation, cognition, and emotion* (Vol. 41, pp. 71–124). Lincoln: University of Nebraska Press.

Bargh, J. A., Gollwitzer, P. M., Lee-Chai, A., Barndollar, K., & Trötschel, R. (2001). The automated will: Nonconscious activation and pursuit of behavioral goals. *Journal of Personality and Social Psychology, 81*, 1014–1027.

Bargh, J. A., Raymond, P., Pryor, J. B., & Strack, F. (1995). Attractiveness of the underling: An automatic power left-arrow sex association and its consequences for sexual harassment and aggression. *Journal of Personality and Social Psychology, 68*, 768–781.

Berkowitz, L. (1989). Frustration–aggression hypothesis: Examination and reformulation. *Psychological Bulletin, 106*, 59–73.

Chartrand, T. L. (2007). *Mystery moods and perplexing performance: Consequences of succeeding or failing at a nonconscious goal*. Working paper, Duke University.

Chartrand, T. L., & Bargh, J. A. (1996). Automatic activation of impression formation and memorization goals: Nonconscious goal priming reproduces effects of explicit task instructions. *Journal of Personality and Social Psychology, 71*, 464–478.

Chartrand, T. L., & Bargh, J. A. (2002). Nonconscious motivations: Their activation, operation, and consequences. In A. Tesser & D. A. Stapel (Eds.), *Self and motivation: Emerging psychological perspectives* (pp. 13–41). Washington, DC: American Psychological Association.

Chartrand, T. L., Cheng, C. M., Tesser, A., & Dalton, A. N. (2007). *Consequences of failing at nonconscious goals for self-enhancement and stereotyping*. Manuscript submitted for publication.

Chartrand, T. L., Dalton, A. N., & Fitzsimons, G. J. (in press). Nonconscious relationship reactance: When significant others prime opposing goals. *Journal of Experimental Social Psychology.*

Chartrand, T. L., Fitzsimons, G. M., & Fitzsimons, G. J. (in press). Automatic effects of anthropomorphized objects on behavior. *Social Cognition.*

Chartrand, T. L., Huber, J., Shiv, B., & Tanner, R. (in press). Nonconscious goals and consumer choice. *Journal of Consumer Research.*

Chen, S., Lee-Chai, A. Y., & Bargh, J. A. (2001). Relationship orientation as a moderator of the effects of social power. *Journal of Personality and Social Psychology, 80*, 173–187.

Dunning, D., Leuenberger, A., & Sherman, D. A. (1995). A new look at motivated inference: Are self-serving theories of success a product of motivational forces? *Journal of Personality and Social Psychology, 69*, 58–68.

Fein, S., & Spencer, S. J. (1997). Prejudice as self-image maintenance: Affirming the self through derogating others. *Journal of Personality and Social Psychology, 73*, 31–44.

Fishbach, A., Friedman, R. S., & Kruglanski, A. W. (2003). Leading us not into temptation: Momentary allurements elicit overriding goal activation. *Journal of Personality and Social Psychology, 84*, 296–309.

Fitzsimons, G. M., & Bargh, J. A. (2003). Thinking of you: Nonconscious pursuit of interpersonal goals associated with relationship partners. *Journal of Personality and Social Psychology, 84*, 148–163.

Fitzsimons, G. M., Chartrand, T. L., & Fitzsimons, G. J. (2007). *Automatic effects of brand exposure on behavior.* Manuscript submitted for publication.

Gollwitzer, P. M. (1990). Action phases and mind-sets. In E. Higgins & R. M. Sorrentino (Eds.), *Handbook of motivation and cognition: Foundations of social behavior* (Vol. 2, pp. 53–92). New York: Guilford Press.

Gollwitzer, P. M., & Bargh, J. A. (Eds.). (1996). *The psychology of action: Linking cognition and motivation to behavior.* New York: Guilford Press.

Hamilton, D. L., Katz, L. B., & Leirer, V. O. (1980). Cognitive representation of personality impressions: Organizational processes in first impression formation. *Journal of Personality and Social Psychology, 39*, 1050–1063.

Higgins, E., Bargh, J. A., & Lombardi, W. J. (1985). Nature of priming effects on categorization. *Journal of Experimental Psychology: Learning, Memory, and Cognition, 11*, 59–69.

Jefferis, V. E., & Chartrand, T. L. (2007). *Aggressive behavior and the role of nonconscious goal pursuit.* Manuscript in preparation, Ohio State University.

Lewin, K. (1951). Intention, will and need. In D. Rapaport (Ed.), *Organization and pathology of thought: Selected sources* (pp. 95–153). New York: Columbia University Press.

Lisak, D., & Roth, S. (1988). Motivational factors in nonincarcerated sexually aggressive men. *Journal of Personality and Social Psychology, 55*, 795–802.

Locke, E. A., Frederick, E., Lee, C., & Bobko, P. (1984). Effect of self-efficacy, goals, and task strategies on task performance. *Journal of Applied Psychology, 69*, 241–251.

Malamuth, N. M. (1989a). The Attraction to Sexual Aggression scale: I. *Journal of Sex Research, 26*, 324–354.

Malamuth, N. M. (1989b). The Attraction to Sexual Aggression scale: II. *Journal of Sex Research, 26*, 26–49.

Moskowitz, G. B., Gollwitzer, P. M., Wasel, W., & Schaal, B. (1999). Preconscious control of stereotype activation through chronic egalitarian goals. *Journal of Personality and Social Psychology, 77*, 167–184.

Muraven, M., & Baumeister, R. F. (2000). Self-regulation and depletion of limited resources: Does self-control resemble a muscle? *Psychological Bulletin, 126*, 247–259.

Pryor, J. B., & Stoller, L. M. (1994). Sexual cognition processes in men high in the likelihood to sexually harass. *Personality and Social Psychology Bulletin, 20*, 163–169.

Shah, J. (2003). The motivational looking glass: How significant others implicitly affect goal appraisals. *Journal of Personality and Social Psychology, 85*, 424–439.

Srull, T. K., & Wyer, R. S., Jr. (1979). The role of category accessibility in the interpretation of information about persons: Some determinants and implications. *Journal of Personality and Social Psychology, 37*, 1660–1672.

Spencer, S. J., Fein, S., Wolfe, C. T., Fong, C., & Dunn, M. A. (1998). Automatic activation of stereotypes: The role of self-image threat. *Personality and Social Psychology Bulletin, 24*, 1139–1152.

Steele, C. M., Spencer, S. J., & Lynch, M. (1993). Self-image resilience and dissonance: The role of affirmational resources. *Journal of Personality and Social Psychology, 64*, 885–896.

Tesser, A. (2000). On the confluence of self-esteem maintenance mechanisms. *Personality and Social Psychology Review, 4*, 290–299.

Tesser, A. (2001). On the plasticity of self-defense. *Current Directions in Psychological Science, 10*, 66–69.

Tesser, A., Crepaz, N., Collins, J. C., Cornell, D., & Beach, S. R. H. (2000). Confluence of self-esteem regulation mechanisms: On integrating the self-zoo. *Personality and Social Psychology Bulletin, 26*, 1476–1489.

Tesser, A., Martin, L. L., & Cornell, D. P. (1996). On the substitutability of self-protective mechanisms. In P. M. Gollwitzer & J. A. Bargh (Eds.), *The psychology of action: Linking cognition and motivation to behavior* (pp. 48–68). New York: Guilford Press.

Vohs, K. (2007). [Nonconscious goals and ego depletion]. Unpublished raw data, University of Minnesota.

Chapter 23

# Regulatory Fit

E. Tory Higgins

Broadly defined, *fit* has been of central interest to motivational scientists for over a century. Psychodynamic theories describe people's concerns with creating harmony between personal wishes and societal demands or standards (e.g., Adler, 1929/1964; Freud, 1923/1961; Horney, 1950; Sullivan, 1953). Cybernetic and control process models (e.g., Bandura, 1986; Carver & Scheier, 1981; Higgins, 1987; Miller, Galanter, & Pribram, 1960; Powers, 1973; Wiener, 1948) propose that people are motivated to have their current states match personally desired end-states. Social psychology's consistency theories have postulated that people want balance or congruence among their beliefs, attitudes, and behaviors (Abelson et al., 1968; Festinger, 1957; Heider, 1958). In organizational psychology, the notion of compatibility between an individual and a job, or "hiring the right type," has also existed for some time (Argyris, 1957; see also Fiedler, 1967, and Ostroff, 1993). As defined by *Webster's Ninth New Collegiate Dictionary* (1989), when two things fit with one another, they suit or agree with each other; they are in harmony. This captures the sense of *fit* as an adaptive regulatory process. In addition, when something is experienced as fitting, it feels correct, proper, or even just. This captures the sense of *fit* as an experience of feeling right about what is happening. These two senses of *fit* are both critical to the conceptualization of fit proposed in *regulatory fit theory* (Higgins, 2000). This chapter describes what is distinctive about the kind of fit proposed in regulatory fit theory, and reviews evidence of its motivational effects on performance and on value creation.

## REGULATORY FIT AS A DISTINCTIVE MOTIVATIONAL PRINCIPLE

When people pursue a goal, they begin with some motivational orientation—some concerns or interests that direct their goal pursuit. They also pursue the goal in some manner—some method or way of carrying out the goal pursuit. Finally, they experience or anticipate experiencing some consequences of their goal pursuit that are positive or negative. Historically, value from the manner of goal pursuit has been considered as deriving from its being a socially prescribed way to attain desired outcomes (e.g., value from procedural justice), an effective way (instrumental value), or an efficient way (low costs). Each of these sources of value from the manner of goal pursuit relates to the benefits or costs of the means for attaining outcomes. The value concerns the classic benefits–costs ratio for outcomes. This type of value from the manner of goal pursuit has received substantial attention in the literature. In contrast, value from the relation between the manner of goal pursuit and the actor's motivational orientation has received relatively little attention.

I have proposed in an earlier paper (Higgins, 2000) that people experience regulatory fit when the manner of their engagement in an activity *sustains* (vs. disrupts) their current regulatory orientation. It is notable that the term *sustains* has two separate meanings in the dictionary (e.g., *Webster's Ninth New Collegiate Dictionary*, 1989, p. 1189). One definition is "to hold up or prolong; to give support, sustenance, or nourishment." This first definition relates to the sense of fit as something that is adaptive by supplying what is needed to carry on. A second definition of *sustain* is "to allow or admit as valid; to confirm; to support as true, legal, or just." This second definition relates to the sense of *fit* as feeling right about something. Fit makes people engage more strongly in what they are doing and "feel right" about it.

Individuals, for example, can pursue (approach) the same goal with different orientations and in different ways. Consider, for instance, students in the same course who are working to attain an A. Some students have a *promotion focus* orientation toward an A, where a promotion focus represents goals as hopes and ideals. Others have a *prevention focus* orientation toward an A, where a prevention focus represents goals as responsibilities and oughts. With regard to how they pursue their goal, some students read material beyond the assigned readings as an *eager* way to attain an A, whereas others are careful to fulfill all course requirements as a *vigilant* way to attain an A. Previous studies have found that an eager manner fits a promotion focus better than a prevention focus, whereas the reverse is true for a vigilant manner (Higgins, 2000).

For all students, receiving an A in the course has certain outcome benefits, regardless of the orientation and manner of their goal pursuit. Independent of this outcome value, however, there is an additional experience from regulatory fit. Specifically, when people engage in goal pursuit in a manner that fits their orientation (e.g., promotion/eager or prevention/vigilant), they engage in that pursuit more strongly and have more intense evaluative reactions (Higgins, 2000). Regulatory fit makes them "feel right" about their positive reactions to what they are doing, or "feel right" about their negative reactions to what they are not doing (see Cesario, Grant, & Higgins, 2004; Higgins, 2005).

Regulatory fit can be distinguished from other motivational principles and experiences related to the general notion of *fit*. First, it can be distinguished conceptually from other *fit*-like concepts having to do with compatibility, concordance, relevance, and matching. Second, the regulatory fit value experience can itself be distinguished from other kinds of value experiences, such as hedonic outcome experiences (pleasure or pain) and moral process experiences. Third, regulatory fit can be distinguished as a distinctive source of good–bad evaluations. This section reviews evidence for each of these distinctions.

## Regulatory Fit as Distinct from Other *Fit*-Like Concepts

A long history of research has documented the importance of hierarchical relations between actions and goals, whereby specific actions are valued to the extent that they support attaining more abstract goals (e.g., Carver & Scheier, 1981; Miller et al., 1960; Powers, 1973; Shah & Kruglanski, 2000; Vallacher & Wegner, 1987; for a review, see Brendl & Higgins, 1996). In that research, *compatibility* refers to an action's instrumentality toward attaining a goal outcome. In distinguishing between *process* goals (or subgoals) and *purpose* goals, for instance, people more highly value those process goals (e.g., "making conversation") that are compatible with the attainment of their broader purpose goals (e.g., "achieving interpersonal closeness"; Harackiewicz & Sansone, 1991; Sansone & Harackiewicz, 1996; Tauer & Harackiewicz, 1999).

Consistent with the above-described findings on action–goal compatibility, recent work on *self-concordance* demonstrates that the relevance of one's day-to-day actions to one's broader aims increases the actions' value (e.g., Sheldon & Elliot, 1999). Unique to the concordance research, however, is an emphasis on the *contents* of one's broader aims. In an application of Deci and Ryan's (1985) theory of intrinsic motivation, self-concordance research categorizes people's abstract goals in terms of their degree of self-determination, whereby presumably self-determined goals (such as gaining autonomy and competence) are hypothesized to promote value experiences to a higher degree than are presumably other-determined goals (such as making money). Again, however, and most relevant to the current discussion, it is the instrumental relation of one's current actions to broader aims and outcomes that is hypothesized to influence action value.

In the persuasion literature, Millar and Tesser (1986) accounted for previously contradictory findings by showing how a match between the belief and behavior elements of attitudes increased the attitude–behavior correlation. More generally, there is considerable evidence that matching the content of a persuasive message to some characteristic of the message recipient's cognitive, motivational, or affective system can increase persuasion. The characteristics of the message recipient include the psychological functions served by the recipient's attitudes (e.g., Clary, Snyder, Ridge, Miene, & Haugen, 1994; Petty & Wegener, 1998; Petty, Wheeler, & Bizer, 2000), the recipient's culture (e.g., Han & Shavitt, 1994), the cognitive or affective basis of the recipient's attitude (e.g., Fabrigar & Petty, 1999), and the recipient's chronic self-guides (e.g., Evans & Petty, 2003). Recent message-matching work shows that matching the emotional implications of persuasive messages to participants' current moods increases agreement with the messages; importantly, this effect is mediated by the degree to which participants expect that the actions the messages describe will be instrumental in influencing the outcomes toward which the messages are focused (DeSteno, Petty, Rucker, Wegener, & Braverman, 2004).

In sum, although they cover a wide array of different phenomena and yield important conceptual divergences, studies on action–goal compatibility, self-concordance, and message matching converge in an important way. All specifically identify relations between actions and outcomes as important sources of action value. All relate to the instrumental value of the manner of goal pursuit for outcomes. Regulatory fit is different from this motivational principle, because the relation of concern is between the manner of goal pursuit and the actor's current orientation—independent of the efficiency (costs) or effectiveness (benefits) of the manner of goal pursuit (i.e., independent of outcomes). Indeed, there is evidence that regulatory fit is not related to actual or perceived efficiency or effectiveness of the goal pursuit (e.g., Higgins, Idson, Freitas, Spiegel, & Molden, 2003). In addition, the effect of regulatory fit on creating value is not dependent on the relation between manner of goal pursuit and outcome, as it is with action–goal compatibility and message-matching mechanisms. As an example, consider evidence for the effect of regulatory fit on persuasion. We (Cesario et al., 2004) reasoned that the most methodologically sound way to clearly distinguish a regulatory fit effect from a message-matching effect was to experimentally induce regulatory fit *prior to and independently of* the persuasion context. Their unique prediction was that participants would be more persuaded by an *identical* message if they had, versus had not, experienced regulatory fit prior to even receiving the message. This prediction was confirmed in a couple of studies.

## Regulatory Fit Experience as Distinct from Other Value-Related Experiences

What kind of value do people experience when they pursue goals? Once again, the classic answer has been couched in terms of outcomes or utility. People are motivated to pursue goals that produce positive outcomes. When making choices, for example, they want the alternative whose mix of pleasant or painful outcomes is the most positive. The same outcome can have different subjective value to different people or to the same person at different times. Historically, the critical insight to account for such variability is that the psychological value of an outcome is not simply its objective value (for reviews, see Abelson & Levi, 1985; Ajzen, 1996; Dawes, 1998). One of the great contributions of decision science in the last three decades has been to identify cognitive operations and representations that influence people's *experience* of outcome value (e.g., Kahneman,

Diener, & Schwarz, 1999; Kahneman & Tversky, 1979; for a recent review, see Thaler, 1999).

Goal pursuit, such as making a decision, has both outcome benefits and outcome costs. The means used to pursue goals can contribute to outcome benefits by, for instance, being enjoyable in themselves ("getting there is half the fun"). The means used can also contribute to outcome costs. For example, decision means can have high emotional costs (e.g., Janis & Mann, 1977) or high costs in cognitive effort or time (see, e.g., Payne, Bettman, & Johnson, 1993; Simon, 1955, 1967). The benefits or costs of the means used to pursue a goal are outcomes of the goal pursuit process itself and are weighed along with the positive and negative consequences of goal attainment in some kind of overall cost–benefit analysis.

People's experiences of outcome benefits and outcome costs have received the most attention in the literature. This emphasis on outcomes is natural, because outcomes concern whether a decision is experienced as "worthwhile" or "worth it." It makes intuitive sense that the value of a decision is related to its worth, because the decision science literature typically equates value with utility, and one sense of *utility* is "worth to some end" (*Webster's Ninth New Collegiate Dictionary*, 1989, p. 1300). However, *utility* has another sense—"fitness for some purpose" (*Webster's Ninth New Collegiate Dictionary*, 1989, p. 1300). The notion of value from regulatory fit concerns this additional sense of utility having to do with *how* a goal is pursued. In particular, I suggest that the central phenomenology underlying experiences of regulatory fit is, rather than a diffuse, global hedonic feeling of pleasure, a more particular sense of "feeling right" about what one is doing. Empirically supporting this prediction requires showing that fit effects on "feeling right" are obtained even when global hedonic feelings of pleasure are controlled for.

It is important to note, however, that value from regulatory fit is not the only value experience from the manner of goal pursuit that is independent of instrumentality. There is another such value experience from which regulatory fit must be distinguished—value from the use of proper means. It has been recognized for centuries that there is value from *how* a goal is pursued that is independent of the outcomes or consequences of the goal pursuit. This kind of value is captured in cultural maxims such as "It is not enough to do good; one must do it the right way," "The ends do not justify the means," and "Never good through evil." These maxims distinguish between value from the outcomes of goal pursuit and value from pursuing goals with proper means (see Merton, 1957). The literature has shown that people value the fairness of decision procedures apart from their instrumentality (e.g., Thibaut & Walker, 1975; Tyler & Lind, 1992), and that they value means providing a justification for their decision (e.g., Pennington & Hastie, 1988; Tetlock, 1991; Tversky & Shafir, 1992).

Value from proper means occurs when the manner of goal pursuit agrees with established rules and normative principles. The value derives from the manner being the right or proper way to attain outcomes according to established normative rules. In contrast, value from regulatory fit derives from the relation between the manner of goal pursuit and the current self-regulatory orientation of the person pursuing the goal. What matters for value from fit is not one's experience of pursuing goal outcomes in a manner that agrees with established rules (value from proper means). Instead, what matters is the experience of pursuing a goal in a manner that sustains one's own current self-regulatory orientation (see Higgins, 2000, 2002, 2006).

## Regulatory Fit's Distinctive Contribution to Good–Bad Evaluations

The psychological literature and dictionary definitions provide two predominant answers to the question "Where does value come from?"—value as need satisfaction, and value as shared beliefs about which means and which end-states are desirable. What is remarkable about these answers is their neglect of *value as experience* (for a more detailed discussion of both what value is and where it comes from, see Higgins, 2007). This is particularly curious, given the general emphasis historically on the hedonic principle of motivation—the notion that people are motivated to approach pleasure and avoid pain. From the ancient Greeks, through 17th- and 18th-century British philosophers, to 20th-century psychologists, this principle has dominated our understanding of people's motivation. But what are pleasure and pain if not subjective experiences? Moreover, success and failure to satisfy personal needs or to meet socialized standards produce pleasure and pain experiences. It is reasonable to begin with the (noncontroversial) assumption that the value of activities, objects, and choices must include the pleasures and pains that people experience from them. But these pleasure and pain feelings are not the only experiences that impart value to objects and activities. Specifically, regulatory fit theory assumes that under conditions of regulatory fit, feeling right about and engaging more strongly in what one is doing also contribute to value experiences.

When the value of an object, activity, or choice is considered in terms of experience, the experiences that have received the most attention historically have been the pleasures and pains of the outcomes associated with the object, activity, or choice. Perhaps the best-known and most highly developed model of pleasure and pain outcome experiences is *prospect theory* (Kahneman & Tversky, 1979), which describes differences in the intensity and form of pleasure experiences (in the domain of "gains") and pain experiences (in the domain of "losses"). In decision making, people imagine the pleasures and pains they will experience from the outcomes of different choices. It has been argued that the ability to imagine experiences resulting from future events is unique to humans (Taylor, Pham, Rivkin, & Armor, 1998). When deciding which of several actions to take, people are capable of envisioning not only the action outcomes, but also the experiences associated with these outcomes (Kahneman & Snell, 1990; Schwarz, 2000; Taylor et al., 1998).

How do people imagine what they would feel about making a particular choice? The most obvious answer to this question is that people anticipate the pleasure or pain of the outcomes that a particular choice will produce (e.g., Kahneman et al., 1999). People should imagine feeling good about a choice if they expect its outcome will be pleasant, and they should imagine feeling bad about a choice if they expect its outcome to be painful. In addition to this hedonic nature of the outcome, we (Idson, Liberman, & Higgins, 2004) proposed that people's feelings can also be affected by regulatory fit—specifically, by whether or not the imagined prospective outcome sustains their current regulatory state. We proposed that when an anticipated future outcome sustains or fits a person's current regulatory state, the motivation to engage in the approach or avoidance process that would make that outcome happen (if desirable) or not happen (if undesirable) increases in intensity.

We (Idson et al., 2004) tested this proposal within the framework of regulatory focus theory (Higgins, 1997; Higgins & Silberman, 1998). Regulatory focus theory assumes that self-regulation operates differently when serving fundamentally different needs, such as the distinct survival needs of nurturance (e.g., nourishment) and security (e.g., protection). Differences in socialization can produce chronic individual differences in regulatory focus (see Higgins & Silberman, 1998). Nurturant parenting engenders a *promotion focus*, in which self-regulation is concerned with accomplishments, hopes, and aspirations (i.e., ideals). It involves the presence of positive outcomes (e.g., "bolstering") and the absence of positive outcomes (e.g., "love withdrawal"). Security parenting engenders a *prevention focus*, in which self-regulation is concerned with safety, duties, and obligations (oughts). It involves the absence of negative outcomes (e.g., "safeguarding") and the presence of negative outcomes (e.g., "criticism").

Momentary situations are also capable of temporarily inducing either a promotion focus or a prevention focus. Just as the responses of caretakers to their children's actions communicate to the children about how to attain desired end-states, feedback from a boss to an employee or from a teacher to a student is a situation that can communicate *gain versus non-gain* information (promotion-related outcomes) or *non-loss versus loss* information (prevention-related outcomes). Task instructions that present task contingency or if–then rules concerning which actions produce which consequences can also communicate either gain versus non-gain (promotion) or non-loss versus loss (prevention) information. Thus the concept of regulatory focus is broader than just socialization of strong promotion focus ideals or prevention focus oughts. Regulatory focus can also be induced temporarily in momentary situations.

Regulatory focus theory also distinguishes between different strategic means of goal attainment. It distinguishes between an *eager strategy* and a *vigilant strategy* (see Crowe & Higgins, 1997; Higgins, 1997; Higgins & Silberman, 1998). Because an eager strategy ensures the presence of positive outcomes (searching for means of advancement) and ensures against the absence of positive outcomes (not closing off possibilities), it fits promotion focus concerns with the presence and absence of positive outcomes (gains and non-gains). Similarly, because a vigilant strategy ensures the absence of negative outcomes (being careful) and ensures against the presence of negative outcomes (avoiding mistakes), it fits prevention focus concerns with the absence and presence of negative outcomes (non-losses and losses) (see Crowe & Higgins, 1997; Higgins, 1997).

We (Idson et al., 2004) suggested that due to its effect on motivational intensity or strength of engagement, regulatory fit makes anticipated positive feelings about a prospective positive outcome even more positive, and anticipated negative feelings about a prospective negative outcome even more negative. We proposed that imagining making a desirable choice has higher regulatory fit for people in a promotion focus (because it maintains the eagerness that sustains their focus) than for people in a prevention focus (because it reduces the vigilance that sustains their focus). Therefore, when anticipating a prospective desirable choice, people in a promotion focus should be more strongly engaged in approach and thus should feel more intensely positive—that is, should experience a more intense force of attraction (Higgins, 2006)—than people in a prevention focus. In contrast, imagining making an undesirable choice has higher regulatory fit for people in a prevention focus (because it maintains the vigilance that sustains their focus) than for people in a promotion focus (because it reduces the eagerness that sustains their focus). Therefore, when anticipating a prospective undesirable choice, people in a prevention focus should be more strongly engaged in avoidance and thus should feel more intensely negative—that is, should experience a more intense force of repulsion (Higgins, 2006)—than people in a promotion focus.

To test these predictions, we (Idson et al., 2004) modified a well-known example from Thaler (1980). All participants were instructed to imagine that they were in a bookstore buying a book for a class. The orientation toward the buying decision was framed in two different ways—a promotion (gain vs. non-gain) framing and a prevention (non-loss vs. loss) framing—while keeping the desirable choice outcome (paying $60 for the book) and the undesirable choice outcome (paying $65 for the book) the same in both framing conditions. In both the promotion and prevention framing conditions, the participants were asked to imagine either how it would feel to make the desirable choice or how it would feel to make the undesirable choice on a scale ranging from "very bad" to "very good." As one would expect, the participants felt good when they imagined making the desirable choice and felt bad when they imagined making the undesirable choice. This is the classic outcome–valence effect. As predicted, however, there were also significant effects within the desirable choice condition and within the undesirable choice condition. In the desirable choice condition, the feeling better that participants imagined was more intense when they were in the promotion focus condition (fit) than in the prevention focus condition (non-fit). In the undesirable choice condition, the feeling worse that participants imagined was more intense when they were in the prevention focus condition (fit) than in the promotion focus condition (non-fit). These same findings were obtained in another study that experimentally primed either a promotion focus (ideal priming) or a prevention focus (ought priming).

The Idson and colleagues (2004) studies also examined whether the pleasure–pain hedonic experience and the motivational force experience make independent contributions to the value experience of attraction or repulsion. In addition to the measure of how good or bad participants felt about the imagined decision outcome, separate measures of pleasure–pain intensity and strength of motivational force were taken. The framing study and the priming study used slightly different measures to provide convergent validity. The priming study, for example, measured pleasure–pain intensity by asking the participants how pleasant the positive outcome would be or how painful the negative outcome would be, and it measured strength of motivational force by asking them how motivated they would be to make the positive outcome happen (in the positive outcome condition) or how motivated they would be to make the negative outcome not happen (in the negative outcome condition). Both studies found that pleasure–pain intensity and strength of motivational force each made significant *independent* contributions to the perceived value of the imagined outcome (i.e., its goodness–badness).

Several studies using different paradigms and different dependent measures have also found that fit effects are independent of pleasure–pain mood (e.g., Avnet & Higgins, 2003; Camacho, Higgins, & Luger, 2003; Cesario et al., 2004; Higgins, Idson, et al., 2003). For example, in an attitude change study (Cesario et al., 2004) discussed more fully below, fit was induced prior to participants' receiving a persuasive message by having them, ostensibly for a separate study, list either strategies for goal attainment that fit their personal goals (eager strategies/promotion goals, vigilant strategies/prevention goals) or did not fit (eager strategies/prevention goals, vigilant strategies/promotion goals). After reading the persuasive message, the participants were asked to rate how "happy," "pleased," "overjoyed," and "cheerful" they felt while reading the essay. The scores for these four items were combined to form an index of positive mood. It was found that higher positive mood predicted both higher perceived message persuasiveness and greater message effectiveness in changing opinions in the advocated direction. At the same time, fit had an independent effect of increasing both perceived message persuasiveness and message effectiveness. Thus regulatory fit and hedonic pleasure–pain mood each had independent effects on persuasion. This is further support for the conclusion that good–bad evaluations are not based solely on pleasure–pain experiences; regulatory fit experiences also play a role.

In sum, there is substantial evidence that regulatory fit is a distinctive motivational principle in several respects. It can be distinguished conceptually from other *fit*-like concepts having to do with compatibility, concordance, relevance, and matching. The regulatory fit motivational experience itself can be distinguished from other kinds of value-related experiences, including both hedonic outcome experiences (pleasure or pain) and moral process experiences. Finally, and especially significantly, regulatory fit can be distinguished as an independent source of good–bad evaluations. What then are the effects of this distinctive motivational principle? The next section reviews evidence for two major effects of regulatory fit—*performance* and *value creation*.

## HOW REGULATORY FIT AFFECTS PERFORMANCE AND VALUE CREATION

The effects of regulatory fit on performance and value creation derive from fit increasing strength of engagement (see Higgins, 2005, 2006). The fit effects on performance reviewed below provide indirect evidence that fit increases engagement strength, but there is also more direct evidence, which I briefly mention. One set of studies (Förster, Higgins, & Idson, 1998), for example, examined both chronic and situational instantiations of regulatory focus orientation. The participants performed an anagram task in either an eager or a vigilant manner. Performing the task in an eager versus vigilant manner was manipulated by using an arm pressure technique (Cacioppo, Priester, & Berntson, 1993). While performing the anagram task, the participants either pressed downward on the plate of a supposed skin conductance machine that was attached to the top of the table (a vigilance/avoidance-related movement of pushing away from oneself) or pressed upward on the plate attached to the bottom of the table (an eagerness/approach-related movement of pulling toward oneself). Participants' arm pressure while pressing downward or upward on the plate was recorded and served as the measure of engagement strength. On a measure of overall online arm pressure during task performance, strength of engagement was stronger when there was regulatory fit (i.e., promotion/eager, prevention/vigilant) than when there was non-fit (i.e., promotion/vigilant, prevention/eager). Another study in this series (Förster et al., 1998) used persistence as the measure of strength of engagement and found that persistence was greater when there was fit than when there was non-fit.

Using a similar paradigm as in the Förster and colleagues (1998) arm pressure studies, but one that also experimentally controlled for participants' outcome expectancies during task performance, we (Förster, Grant, Idson, & Higgins, 2001) replicated another Förster and colleagues (1998) finding: On a measure of the steepness of the arm pressure gradients (calculated over the recorded arm pressure values from the beginning to the end of the set of anagrams), the approach gradient (the recorded upward pressure values when the plate was attached to the bottom of the table) was steeper for participants in a promotion than in a prevention focus. In contrast, the avoidance gradient (the recorded downward pressure values when the plate was attached to the top of the table) was steeper for participants in a prevention than a promotion focus. We (Förster et al., 2001) also replicated the fit effect on persistence found by Förster and colleagues (1998). Importantly, the fit effects found in both the Förster and colleagues (1998, 2001) research were independent of participants' positive or negative feelings during the task performance. Additional evidence that regulatory fit increases strength of engagement is provided by the Idson and colleagues (2004) finding described earlier that participants in the regulatory fit conditions reported higher motivational intensity than participants in the non-fit conditions.

## Regulatory Fit and Performance

Given that regulatory fit increases strength of engagement, one would expect that fit would also influence performance. There is, indeed, considerable evidence that this is the case. In studies on anagram performance (Shah, Higgins, & Friedman, 1998), for example, participants' regulatory focus varied either chronically or through experimental induction, and either an eager or vigilant manner was manipulated by designating particular anagrams in vigilance terms (avoiding loss of payment by solving) or eagerness terms (gaining payment by solving). As predicted, anagram performance was better when there was regulatory fit (i.e., promotion focus/eager strategy, prevention focus/vigilant strategy) than when there was non-fit. In the Förster and colleagues (1998) studies described earlier, there was also evidence that anagram performance was better when there was regulatory fit (i.e., promotion focus/eager strategy, prevention focus/vigilant strategy) than when there was non-fit (i.e., promotion/vigilant, prevention/eager). Another study (Freitas, Liberman, & Higgins, 2002) found that prevention focus participants did better than promotion focus participants on a task that required vigilance against a tempting distractor.

In other research, we (Bianco, Higgins, & Klem, 2003) investigated another way in which regulatory fit can enhance performance. We examined how performance is affected by the fit between people's implicit theories of a given task's being either fun or important, and task instructions to engage that task in either a fun or important way. On tasks of predictive learning, paired-associate learning, and free recall of movie scenes, we found that performance was enhanced when there was a fit (vs. a non-fit) between participants' implicit theories and task instructions regarding the fun and importance of the task. Interestingly, in one study where participants' implicit theory of the academic activity was that it was important but not fun, instructing participants that doing the task would be high in both importance *and* fun (a non-fit) actually undermined performance compared to high-importance/low-fun instructions (a fit).

There is evidence of yet another way that regulatory fit can influence performance. Previous researchers have suggested that the mental simulation of steps needed to implement goal completion facilitates goal achievement (e.g., Gollwitzer, 1996). Given promotion-focused people's tactical preference for eagerly approaching matches to desired end-states, rather than vigilantly avoiding mismatches to desired end-states, we (Spiegel, Grant-Pillow, & Higgins, 2004) predicted that promotion-focused people would perform better at a task if they prepared by eagerly simulating and developing approach-oriented plans rather than avoidance-oriented plans, and that the reverse would be true for prevention-focused people. In one study, participants were asked to write a report on how they would spend their upcoming Saturday, and to turn it in by a certain deadline, in order to receive a cash payment. Before they left the lab, all participants were asked to imagine certain implementation steps that they might take in writing the report (i.e., simulations related to *when*, *where*, and *how* to do the report), and the steps were framed to represent either eager/approach means or vigilant/avoidance means. It was found that participants in the fit conditions were almost 50% more likely to turn in their reports than participants in the non-fit conditions.

As demonstrated by the Bianco and colleagues (2003) studies, regulatory fit effects on performance are not restricted to regulatory focus orientations. Further evidence of the generalizability of regulatory fit effects on performance is provided by some recent studies examining the impact on leadership effectiveness of the fit between leadership style and the regulatory mode orientation of the followers. Most goal pursuit activities involve two essential self-regulatory modes: a mode of *assessment* and a mode of *locomotion*. Assessment is the aspect of self-regulation that is concerned with critically evaluating entities or states, such as goals or means, in relation to alternatives in order to judge relative quality (Higgins, Kruglanski, & Pierro, 2003; Kruglanski et al., 2000). Individuals with strong assessment concerns want to compare all options and search for new possibilities before making a decision, even if that means waiting. They relate past and future actions to critical standards. They want to choose the option that has the best attributes overall compared to the alternative options; they want to make the correct choice (Higgins, Kruglanski, et al., 2003; Kruglanski et al., 2000). By contrast, the locomotion mode is the aspect of self-regulation that is concerned with movement from state to state. Individuals with strong locomotion concerns want to take action, to get started, even if that means not considering all the options fully. Once the task is initiated, they want to maintain it and complete it without undue disruptions or delays (Higgins, Kruglanski, et al., 2003; Kruglanski et al., 2000). They want to make steady progress.

Research (see Higgins, Kruglanski, et al., 2003; Kruglanski et al., 2000) has shown that locomotion and assessment may be differentially emphasized by different individuals. In the Kruglanski and colleagues (2000) research, two separate scales were developed to measure chronic individual differences in assessment and locomotion. A comprehensive series of studies demonstrated the unidimensionality, internal consistency, and temporal stability of each scale. It was found that locomotion and assessment tendencies are essentially uncorrelated with each other (i.e., a person can be high or low on both, or high on one and low on the other, etc.); that each type is needed for self-regulatory success; and that each relates to a distinct task orientation and motivational emphasis.

A recent study (Kruglanski, Pierro, & Higgins, in press) examined leadership effectiveness in diverse organizational contexts. Specifically, it compared the effectiveness of two leadership styles: (1) a *forceful* leadership style, represented by coercive, legitimate, and directive kinds of strategic influence; and (2) an *advisory* leadership style, represented by expert, referent, and participative kinds of strategic influence. A forceful leadership style fits individuals high in locomotion more than an advisory leadership style, because the former pushes for moving a task ahead, whereas the latter waits to allow reflection before moving ahead. In contrast, an advisory leadership style fits individuals high in assessment more than a forceful leadership style, because the former allows for critical comparison of alternatives, whereas the latter dictates one course of action (the leader's). Consistent with regulatory fit predictions, it was found that subordinates who were high in locomotion preferred and reported greater job satisfaction for forceful than advisory leadership, whereas the reverse was true for subordinates who where high in assessment. Benjamin and Flynn (in press) have also recently found, using both experiments and data collected from a survey of executives, that the effectiveness of transformational leadership depends on followers' regulatory mode. They hypothesized that transformational leadership would be more effective (e.g., increasing motivation, eliciting positive evaluations) when followers had a locomotion orientation than an assessment orientation, because transformational leaders emphasize movement and change through their strong sense of purpose, perseverance, and direction. The results supported their prediction.

## Regulatory Fit and Value Creation

The increase in engagement strength from regulatory fit not only influences performance. Perhaps even more significant is its impact on value creation. In another paper (Higgins, 2006), I have proposed that value derives not only from the hedonic experience of pleasure and pain, but also from strength of engagement. More specifically, I extend Lewin's (1951) ideas about valence by postulating a *force experience* that has direction and strength. Experiencing something as having positive value corresponds to experiencing attraction toward it (e.g., trying to move toward it), and experiencing something as having negative value corresponds to experiencing repulsion from it (e.g., trying to move away from it). Value experiences vary in intensity, so that the experience of attraction toward something can have relatively high or low intensity (high or low positive value), and the experience of repulsion from something can have relatively high or low intensity (high or low negative value).

I believe that the classic hedonic valence experiences of being attracted to pleasure and repulsed from pain is critical to the force experience, because it provides direction as well as strength. Although critical to the value experience, strength of valence is not enough. Value is not just an experience of pleasure or pain. Instead, I have proposed (Higgins, 2006) that value is essentially an experience of *motivational force*—the force of attraction toward or repulsion away from something—and that there can be contributions to the value force experience that are independent of the pleasure–pain valence experience per se.

The motivational force experience is an experience of how motivated one is to make something happen. Within pleasure or within pain, one can have high or low motivation to make something happen. Pleasure or pain is one source of the experience of motivational force, but it is not the only source. I have proposed (Higgins, 2006) that an additional contributor to the intensity experience of motivational force is *strength of engagement*. The state of being strongly engaged with some object or activity is to be involved with, occupied with, interested in, and attentive to it—in other words, being absorbed in or engrossed with it. Strength of engagement does not have direction. Strength of engagement alone does not make something attractive or repulsive. It is experienced valence that determines direction, that determines whether something is basically attractive or repulsive. Instead, strength of engagement contributes to *how* positively or *how* negatively something is experienced. Central to my proposal is the existence of sources of engagement strength that are beyond the pleasure–pain experiences produced by the value target's properties. One such source is regulatory fit. Research testing regulatory fit theory (Higgins, 2000) provides evidence that this source of engagement strength can change the value of an object, an activity, or even a public policy, independently of hedonic pleasure–pain experiences. Such value creation from regulatory fit has been demonstrated in a variety of fit-inducing contexts, including decision-making contexts, achievement contexts, and persuasive communication contexts.

### *Value Creation from Fit Induced in a Decision-Making Context*

Several studies using different paradigms and types of relations between actors' orientations and manner of goal pursuit have found that value can be created in judgment and decision-making contexts. For example, in one set of studies (Higgins, Idson, et al., 2003), participants' chronic promotion and prevention orientations were measured, and then they were told that over and above their usual payment for participating, they could choose between a coffee mug and a pen as a gift. (Pretesting indicated that the mug was clearly preferred.) The means of making the decision was manipulated through framing. Half of the participants were told to think about what they would gain by choosing the mug or the pen (an *eager manner* of making the decision), and the other half were told to think about what they would lose by not choosing the mug or the pen (a *vigilant manner* of making the decision). Note that both eager and vigilant participants were directed to consider the positive qualities of the mug and the pen. As expected, almost all participants chose the coffee mug. These participants were then asked either to assess the price of the chosen mug or were given the opportunity to actually buy the mug. Participants in the fit conditions (promotion/eager, prevention/vigilant) gave a much higher price for the mug than participants in the non-fit conditions (40–60% higher).

In one of the Higgins, Idson, and colleagues (2003) mug and pen studies, the participants' pleasure–pain mood was also measured at about the same time as the price measure was collected. The mood items prompted participants to indicate how they felt currently with respect to each of several emotions, including happy, dejected (reverse-scored), relaxed, tense (reverse-scored), and content. These items were summed to form an index of positive mood. As predicted, it was found that the fit effect on price of the mug was independent of the participants' pleasure–pain mood.

A recent study (Förster & Higgins, 2005) replicated these findings, using an indirect method of experimentally manipulating regulatory focus. Participants carried out either the global or local version of the Navon (1977) task, in which larger figures (e.g., large letters) are constructed by suitable arrangements of smaller figures (e.g., smaller letters). They were asked to decide whether either a global letter or a local letter was presented on the screen, thereby priming either global/promotion or local/prevention processing between participants. They then began a second "unrelated" task in which they made a decision between a mug and a pen in either an eager or vigilant manner, as in the Higgins, Idson, and colleagues (2003) studies described above. The participants later assigned a higher price to the mug if they had been in the fit conditions (global/eager, local/vigilant).

Another recent study (Avnet & Higgins, 2006) manipulated regulatory focus fit in yet another way. Participants were selected as being chronically promotion- or prevention-oriented as a function of whether they were more effective in meeting their personal ideals than their personal oughts (chronic promotion) or were more effective in meeting their personal oughts than their personal ideals (chronic prevention). They decided how much money they were willing to pay for a chosen type of white-out fluid after either considering their feelings about alternative white-out products or their reasons for wanting alternative white-out products. The results from earlier research (Pham & Avnet, 2004) suggested that considering feelings would have a better fit with a promotion orientation and considering reasons would have a better fit with a prevention orientation. The Avnet and Higgins study found that participants were willing to pay more money for the selected white-out when there was regulatory fit (promotion/feelings, prevention/reasons) than when there was non-fit (promotion/reasons, prevention/feelings).

The aforementioned studies demonstrate that regulatory fit can influence the monetary value of a chosen object. In these studies, it was the fit between promotion versus prevention orientations and eager versus vigilant strategies that yielded the fit effect. As discussed earlier for fit effects on task performance, however, the impact of fit on value creation is not restricted to regulatory focus variables. Yet another study (Avnet & Higgins, 2003), for example, experimentally induced either a locomotion orientation or an assessment orientation in the study participants. The participants then chose a book light from among a set of different book lights, using either a progressive elimination strategy (i.e., eliminating the worst alternative at each phase until only one alternative remained) or a full evaluation strategy (i.e., making comparisons among all of the alternatives for all of the attributes, and then choosing the one with the best attributes overall). The participants offered more of their own money to buy the same chosen book light in the fit conditions (assessment/full evaluation, locomotion/progressive elimination) than in the non-fit conditions (assessment/progressive elimination, locomotion/full evaluation). In addition, once again, this fit effect was independent of the participants' pleasant or painful mood at the time that they offered to buy the book light.

Value creation from regulatory fit in the context of decision making is not restricted to monetary value. In another study reported in the Higgins, Idson, and colleagues (2003) paper, for example, participants were asked to think about things that might improve the transition from elementary school to middle school (i.e., junior high school). The participants could list as many or as few suggestions as they wished. To manipulate regulatory fit, the strategic nature of the improvements that participants were asked to generate was varied. Half of the participants were given an eager strategy of making improvements by instructing them to think about what should be *added* to middle school, to ensure that students would gain as many positive experiences as possible during this transition. The other half were given a vigilant strategy by instructing them to think about what should be *eliminated* from middle school, to ensure that students would avoid as many negative experiences as possible during this transition. Once participants finished listing their suggested improvements, they were asked to judge the importance of middle school experiences. Consistent with the findings reported earlier on how regulatory fit affects motivational intensity, participants generated more strategies in the fit than in the non-fit conditions. Moreover, participants judged middle school experiences themselves to be more important in the fit than in the non-fit conditions.

### *Value Creation from Fit Induced in an Achievement Context*

Regulatory fit in achievement contexts can also create value. In an early regulatory fit study (Freitas & Higgins, 2002), for example, participants initially described either their hopes and aspirations in life or their beliefs about their duties and obligations in life, to induce either a promotion or a prevention orientation, respectively. The participants then began the supposed next study, in which they were to perform a task where the goal was to find as many four-sided objects as possible among dozens of multiply shaped objects on a sheet of paper. The task was introduced as being about scientists who were working with organic material, and the four-sided objects were the critical objects they needed to find. Half of the participants were instructed that the way to do well on the task was to be eager and to try to maximize the helpful four-sided objects. The other half were instructed that the way to do well on the task was to be vigilant and to try to eliminate the harmful four-sided objects. Thus all participants had the same goal of searching for and noting as many four-sided objects as possible, but they were induced to pursue this goal in an eager or vigilant way. It was found that the participants, regardless of their actual success on the task, valued the task activity more in the fit conditions (promotion orientation/eager approach to task, prevention orientation/vigilant approach to task) than in the non-fit conditions (promotion orientation/vigilant approach to task, prevention orientation/eager approach to task).

In more recent studies (Brodscholl, Kober, & Higgins, in press), participants varied chronically or situationally in their promotion and prevention orientations. All participants earned tokens by solving anagrams, and they were all motivated to end up with enough tokens to win a coffee mug as a prize. However, half of the participants began with no tokens and needed to solve anagrams to add enough tokens to reach criterion (the token *attainment* condition), whereas the other half began with tokens and needed to solve the anagrams to stop enough tokens from being subtracted to reach criterion (the token *maintenance* condition). The strategic "addition" in the attainment condition fits promotion, whereas the strategic "stop subtraction" in the maintenance condition fits prevention. All participants successfully reached the criterion and won the prize mug. They were then asked to assign a monetary price to it. Participants in the fit conditions (promotion/attainment, prevention/maintenance) assigned a higher monetary price than participants in the non-fit conditions (promotion/maintenance, prevention/attainment).

A study by Higgins, Idson, and colleagues (2003) induced fit in a different kind of achievement context and was designed to show that the fit effect on value can occur even when there is a complete separation of the activity producing the fit from the object being evaluated. Participants in this study were asked to list either two personal promotion goals (i.e., two of their personal hopes or aspirations) or two personal prevention goals (i.e., two of their duties or obligations). Then they listed for each of their goals either eager means of pursuit (i.e., strategies they could use to make sure everything would go right) or vigilant means (strategies they could use to avoid anything that could go wrong). Promotion goals/eager means and prevention goals/vigilant means were the regulatory fit conditions. In an "unrelated studies" paradigm, the participants were later asked to rate photographs of three dogs on "good-naturedness," supposedly as part of a general project to establish average ratings of various stimuli. The study found that the participants in the fit conditions rated the dogs as more "good-natured" overall than did participants in the non-fit conditions.

A recent study (Higgins, Pittman, & Spiegel, 2006) induced fit in a very different kind of achievement context that extended the Bianco and colleagues (2003) research described earlier. Undergraduate participants engaged in an activity for which they had either an inherently *fun* orientation (playing a "Shoot the Moon" game; see Pittman, Cooper, & Smith, 1977) or an inherently *important* orientation (a "Financial Duties"activity; see Bianco et al., 2003). For each of these activities, both the reward situation surrounding the focal activity and a later free-choice situation that measured subsequent interest in the activity were independently manipulated to be either *enjoyable* or *serious*. For the reward situation surrounding the focal activity, all participants were offered the chance to win an attractive ballpoint pen contingent on their performance, but the reward was framed as being enjoyable or serious. In the enjoyable reward condition, participants were told that the reward had been added to make the game more enjoyable, and that they should think of the game as being like something they would play at a carnival, where the game is even more fun because they can win a prize at the end. In the serious reward condition, the participants were told that the reward had been added to make the task more serious, and that they should think of the task as being like a real-life work situation, which is serious because they are paid a salary at the end.

For the later free-choice situation (the dependent measure of activity value), all of the participants could choose how much to engage in several different activities during a 5-minute period while the experimenter was away (with the target activity being one choice), but this free-choice situation was framed as being enjoyable or serious. In the enjoyable choice condition, participants were told that this was the "free-time" portion of the experiment, so they should feel free to do anything at all they wanted to do. In the serious choice condition, the participants were told that this was the "time management" portion of the experiment, so it was important that they use the time wisely and manage it in an appropriate and prudent manner. As predicted, the study found that participants chose to spend much more time doing the target activity again during the free-choice period—that is, they were more attracted to the focal activity—in the fit conditions (fun activity/enjoyable reward/enjoyable free-choice situations, important activity/serious reward/serious free-choice situations) than in the non-fit conditions (fun activity/serious reward/serious free-choice situations, important activity/enjoyable reward/enjoyable free-choice situations)—over five times as much!

### *Value Creation from Fit Induced in a Persuasive Communication Context*

The same type of "personal goals/type of means for goal attainment" paradigm used in the Higgins, Idson, and colleagues (2003) research described earlier was used in the Cesario and colleagues (2004) research to examine people's attitude toward a newly proposed public program. In the first part of the study, participants were asked to list either promotion goals or prevention goals, and then to list for each of their goals either eager or vigilant means of pursuit. Promotion goals/eager means and prevention goals/vigilant means were the regulatory fit conditions. After the participants had completed this supposed first study on personal goal achievement, they began the supposed second study, in which they all received exactly the same information about a new after-school program that was being proposed. They found that participants had more positive attitudes toward the proposed program when regulatory fit (vs. non-fit) was induced prior to reading the material. We (Cesario et al., 2004) used the same fit induction in another study, which measured participants' positive and negative thought reactions to the material they read. It was found that the fit effect on creating a positive attitude toward the new program occurred only for participants who had positive thoughts about the material. For participants who had negative thoughts about the material, fit had the opposite effect: It created more *negative* attitudes toward the new program. Thus it is not just that fit makes people "feel right" about an object or event per se. Rather, fit can make people "feel right" about, and engage more strongly in, whatever their response is to an object or event, which intensifies positivity if the response is positive and intensifies negativity if the response is negative.

In the Cesario and colleagues (2004) studies just described, regulatory fit was induced prior to the participants' receiving the persuasive message. It is also possible for the persuasive message itself to have properties that induce regulatory fit and then create value. In another study in this series (Cesario et al., 2004), for example, participants who varied chronically in the strength of their promotion or prevention focus read an article eliciting support for a new city tax to create an after-school program that would help elementary and high school students in their personal and academic lives. The structure, content, and primary goal of the article were identical for both versions. The only difference was the strategic framing used in the message to advocate the policy. For example, the eager-framed article said that "the primary reason for supporting this program is because it will advance children's education and support more children to succeed," whereas the vigilant-framed article said that "the primary reason for supporting this program is because it will secure children's education and prevent more children from failing." The study found that the message was perceived as more persuasive and was more effective in changing attitudes when there was a fit between its manner of presentation and participants' chronic focus orientation (eager/promotion, vigilant/prevention) than when there was a non-fit (eager/prevention, vigilant/promotion). In addition, this fit effect was independent of participants' positive or negative mood.

Lee and Aaker (2004) also found that fit induced in a persuasive communication context increased the value of the message. They found that advertising appeals to drink Welch's Grape Juice or use a new sun treatment lotion were more effective when promotion advertising appeals (e.g., energy creation, enjoyment of life) emphasized the benefits of compliance (eager gain framing) rather than the costs of noncompliance (vigilant loss framing), whereas the reverse was true for prevention advertising appeals (e.g., cancer and heart disease prevention, sunburn prevention). In subsequent studies, Lee and Aaker examined the relation among regulatory fit, message engagement, and message effectiveness. As discussed earlier, regulatory fit increases strength of engagement. Indeed, one can think of "feeling right" and increased strength of engagement from regulatory fit as being a mild kind of *flow* experience (see Csikszentmihalyi, 1975; see also Higgins, 2006). Lee and Aaker (2004) found that subjective reports of ease of processing and comprehensibility of the message, accessibility of focus-related words in the message (measured by a perceptual identification task), and number of supportive reasons generated when participants were asked to write down reasons to use the product, were higher in the fit conditions than in the non-fit conditions. Fluency and flow are fit experiences, because when there is fluency or flow, persons' orientation toward what they are doing is being sustained. This is independent of how much effort is expended or experienced (see Higgins, 2006).

A recent study (Semin, Higgins, Gil de Montes, Estourget, & Valencia, 2005) induced fit through a very different kind of persuasive communication manipulation. In this study, predominant promotion and predominant prevention participants received persuasive sports campaign messages that used either abstract or concrete predicates. Similar to the evidence (Förster & Higgins, 2005) of promotion being linked to global processing and prevention being linked to local processing, we (Semin et al., 2005) had found evidence in other studies of promotion being linked to abstract communication and prevention to concrete communication. We found in this study that participants' behavioral intention to engage in sports in the future was greater in the fit conditions (promotion/abstract message, prevention/concrete message) than in the non-fit conditions (promotion/concrete, prevention/abstract). We also found, importantly, that this fit effect was independent of whether the message was framed in terms of positive outcomes (win condition) or negative outcomes (lose condition).

## CONCLUDING COMMENTS

This chapter describes a source of value that has received little prior attention—regulatory fit. When people make decisions or pursue goals, they experience the value of actual or anticipated outcomes that they find attractive or repulsive. But this is not the only way that value is created. Making decisions and pursuing goals are themselves activities, and, as with any activity, people can be more or less engaged in these activities. Although strength of engagement alone does not determine whether something is attractive or repulsive (i.e., valence), it intensifies people's attraction to or repulsion from something. By increasing strength of engagement, then, regulatory fit contributes to value creation. People experience regulatory fit when the manner in which an activity is engaged sustains their current orientation, and this increases the strength of their engagement. The increased strength of engagement produced by fit is experienced as "feeling right" about what they are doing. Fit makes people "feel right" about both their positive and their negative responses to what they are doing. Moreover, it does this not only for the activity that itself produced the fit, but also for later separate activities, as described earlier in the Higgins, Idson, and colleagues (2003) "good-natured dogs" study.

Fit influences the strength of value experiences—how good or how bad people feel about something—independently of the pleasure and pain experiences that are associated with outcomes. Other process properties, such as the efficiency, effectiveness, or hedonic quality of a process, can have value beyond goal outcomes, but fit has been shown to have effects on value that are independent of these other process properties. It is precisely because fit affects value intensity through increasing strength of engagement, rather than through itself determining valence, that its effects are likely to go unnoticed. Failure to recognize its effects can be problematic, however, because fit from one source can be unknowingly transferred to the perceived monetary value of something else.

Even worse, regulatory fit can influence the ethical value of something, as was found in a study (Camacho et al., 2003) where a public policy program that felt "right" because its manner of execution happened to fit the message recipients' orientation (eager execution/promotion recipients, vigilant execution/prevention recipients) was judged to be more morally "right" than when the manner of execution was a non-fit (eager execution/prevention recipients, vigilant execution/promotion recipients). Another Camacho and colleagues (2003) study had participants think back to a time in their lives when they had a conflict with an authority figure (e.g., a parent), and it was that authority figure who determined the manner of conflict resolution. The participants were asked to recall different kinds of resolution. Some participants recalled a resolution where the authority figure encouraged them to succeed (the pleasant/eager condition), whereas other participants remembered a resolution where the authority figure safeguarded them against anything that might go wrong (the pleasant/vigilant condition). Regardless of whether the manner of resolution was itself pleasant or painful, and regardless of their own pleasant or painful mood while making their judgments, participants judged the resolution to be more morally "right" in the fit conditions (promotion participants/eager conflict resolution, prevention participants/vigilant conflict resolution).

Fit has significant implications for improving quality of life. In interpersonal and intergroup conflicts, for example, it is well recognized that the negotiation process needs to be fair, just and equitable. But fit also needs to be considered. When it is ensured that all parties experience fit in how they carry out a negotiation, satisfaction with and commitment to the agreement will increase, independent of outcomes. Of course, when one is a negotiation agent or representative for others, one should also recognize that these others, by not being directly involved in the negotiation, will miss the fit experience, and thus they might not value the agreement as much and might not support it. Finding ways for these others also to experience fit could be critical to the long-term success of the negotiation. It is also important for parents and teachers to allow children their own fit experiences in goal pursuit and decision making, and not simply to provide answers and positive outcomes. More generally, for people to value their lives fully, they need to go beyond pleasant outcomes and "feel right" about what they are doing. When they engage more strongly in their life activities, their experience of life will be enriched.

## REFERENCES


Abelson, R. P., Aronson, E., McGuire, W. J., Newcomb, T. M., Rosenberg, M. J., & Tannenbaum, P. H. (Eds.). (1968). *Theories of cognitive consistency: A sourcebook.* Chicago: Rand McNally.

Abelson, R. P., & Levi, A. (1985). Decision making and decision theory. In G. Lindzey & E. Aronson (Eds.), *The handbook of social psychology* (Vol. 1, pp. 231–309). New York: Random House.

Adler, A. (1964). *Problems of neurosis.* New York: Harper & Row. (Original work published 1929)

Ajzen, I. (1996). The social psychology of decision making. In E. T. Higgins & A. W. Kruglanski (Eds.), *Social psychology: Handbook of basic principles* (pp. 297–325). New York: Guilford Press.

Argyris, C. (1957). Some problems in conceptualizing organizational climate: A case study of a bank. *Administrative Science Quarterly,* 2, 501–520.

Avnet, T., & Higgins, E. T. (2003). Locomotion, assessment, and regulatory fit: Value transfer from "how" to "what." *Journal of Experimental Social Psychology, 39,* 525–530.

Avnet, T., & Higgins, E. T. (2006). How regulatory fit impacts value in consumer choices and opinions. *Journal of Marketing Research, 43,* 1–10.

Bandura, A. (1986). *Social foundations of thought and action: A social cognitive theory.* Englewood Cliffs, NJ: Prentice Hall.

Benjamin, L., & Flynn, F. (in press). Leadership style and regulatory mode: Value from fit? *Organizational Behavior and Human Decision Processes.*

Bianco, A. T., Higgins, E. T., & Klem, A. (2003). How "fun/importance" fit impacts performance: Relating implicit theories to instructions. *Personality and Social Psychology Bulletin, 29,* 1091–1103.

Brendl, C. M., & Higgins, E. T. (1996). Principles of judging valence: What makes events positive or negative? In M. P. Zanna (Ed.), *Advances in experimental social psychology* (Vol. 28, pp. 95–160). San Diego, CA: Academic Press.

Brodscholl, J. C., Kober, H., & Higgins, E. T. (in press). Strategies of self-regulation in goal attainment versus goal maintenance. *European Journal of Social Psychology.*

Cacioppo, J. T., Priester, J. R., & Berntson, G. G. (1993). Rudimentary determinants of attitudes II: Arm flexion and extension have differential effects on attitudes. *Journal of Personality and Social Psychology, 65,* 5–17.

Camacho, C. J., Higgins, E. T., & Luger, L. (2003). Moral value transfer from regulatory fit:"What feels right *is* right" and "what feels wrong *is* wrong." *Journal of Personality and Social Psychology, 84,* 498–510.

Carver, C. S., & Scheier, M. F. (1981). *Attention and self-regulation: A control-theory approach to human behavior.* New York: Springer-Verlag.

Cesario, J., Grant, H., & Higgins, E. T. (2004). Regulatory fit and persuasion: Transfer from "feeling right." *Journal of Personality and Social Psychology, 86,* 388–404.

Clary, E. G., Snyder, M., Ridge, R. D., Miene, P. K., & Haugen, J. A. (1994). Matching messages to motives in persuasion: A functional approach to promoting volunteerism. *Journal of Applied Social Psychology, 24,* 1129–1149.

Crowe, E., & Higgins, E. T. (1997). Regulatory focus and strategic inclinations: Promotion and prevention in decision-making. *Organizational Behavior and Human Decision Processes, 69,* 117–132.

Csikszentmihalyi, M. (1975). *Beyond boredom and anxiety.* San Francisco: Jossey-Bass.

Dawes, R. M. (1998). Behavioral decision making and judgment. In D. T. Gilbert, S. T. Fiske, & G. Lindzey (Eds.), *The handbook of social psychology* (Vol. 1, pp. 497–548). New York: McGraw-Hill.

Deci, E. L., & Ryan, R. M. (1985). *Intrinsic motivation and self-determination in human behavior.* New York: Plenum Press.

DeSteno, D., Petty, R. E., Rucker, D., Wegener, D. T., & Braverman, J. (2004). Discrete emotions and persuasion: The role of emotion-induced expectancies. *Journal of Personality and Social Psychology, 86*, 43–56.

Evans, L. M., & Petty, R. E. (2003). Self-guide framing and persuasion: Responsibly increasing message processing to ideal levels. *Personality and Social Psychology Bulletin, 29*, 313–324.

Fabrigar, L. R., & Petty, R. E. (1999). The role of affective and cognitive bases of attitudes in susceptibility to affectively and cognitively based persuasion. *Personality and Social Psychology Bulletin, 25*, 363–381.

Festinger, L. (1957). *A theory of cognitive dissonance*. Evanston, IL: Row, Peterson.

Fiedler, F. E. (1967). *A theory of leadership effectiveness*. New York: McGraw-Hill.

Förster, J., Grant, H., Idson, L. C., & Higgins, E. T. (2001). Success/failure feedback, expectancies, and approach/avoidance motivation: How regulatory focus moderates classic relations. *Journal of Experimental Social Psychology, 37*, 253–260.

Förster, J., & Higgins, E. T. (2005). How global versus local perception fits regulatory focus. *Psychological Science, 16*(8), 631–636.

Förster, J., Higgins, E. T., & Idson, C. L. (1998). Approach and avoidance strength as a function of regulatory focus: Revisiting the "goal looms larger" effect. *Journal of Personality and Social Psychology, 75*, 1115–1131.

Freitas, A. L., & Higgins, E. T. (2002). Enjoying goal-directed action: The role of regulatory fit. *Psychological Science, 13*, 1–6.

Freitas, A. L., Liberman, N., & Higgins, E. T. (2002). Regulatory fit and resisting temptation during goal pursuit. *Journal of Experimental Social Psychology, 38*, 291–298.

Freud, S. (1961). The ego and the id. In J. Strachey (Ed. & Trans.), *The standard edition of the complete psychological works of Sigmund Freud* (Vol. 19, pp. 3–66). London: Hogarth Press. (Original work published 1923)

Gollwitzer, P. M. (1996). The volitional benefits of planning. In P. M. Gollwitzer & J. A. Bargh (Eds.), *The psychology of action: Linking cognition and motivation to behavior* (pp. 287–312). New York: Guilford Press.

Han, S., & Shavitt, S. (1994). Persuasion and culture: Advertising appeals in individualistic and collectivistic societies. *Journal of Experimental Social Psychology, 30*, 326–350.

Harackiewicz, J. M., & Sansone, C. (1991). Goals and intrinsic motivation: You can get there from here. In M. L. Maehr & P. R. Pintrich (Eds.), *Advances in motivation and achievement* (Vol. 7, pp. 21–49). Greenwich, CT: JAI Press.

Heider, F. (1958). *The psychology of interpersonal relations*. New York: Wiley.

Higgins, E. T. (1987). Self-discrepancy: A theory relating self and affect. *Psychological Review, 94*, 319–340.

Higgins, E. T. (1997). Beyond pleasure and pain. *American Psychologist, 52*, 1280–1300.

Higgins, E. T. (2000). Making a good decision: Value from fit. *American Psychologist, 55*, 1217–1230.

Higgins, E. T. (2002). How self-regulation creates distinct values: The case of promotion and prevention decision making. *Journal of Consumer Psychology, 12*, 177–191.

Higgins, E. T. (2005). Value from regulatory fit. *Current Directions in Psychological Science, 14*, 208–213.

Higgins, E. T. (2006). Value from hedonic experience *and* engagement. *Psychological Review, 113*, 439–460.

Higgins, E. T. (2007). Value. In A. W. Kruglanski & E. T. Higgins (Eds.), *Social psychology: Handbook of basic principles* (2nd ed., pp. 454–472). New York: Guilford Press.

Higgins, E. T., Idson, L. C., Freitas, A. L., Spiegel, S., & Molden, D. C. (2003). Transfer of value from fit. *Journal of Personality and Social Psychology, 84*, 1140–1153.

Higgins, E. T., Kruglanski, A. W., & Pierro, A. (2003). Regulatory mode: Locomotion and assessment as distinct orientations. In M. P. Zanna (Ed.), *Advances in experimental social psychology* (Vol. 35, pp. 293–344). San Diego, CA: Academic Press.

Higgins, E. T., Pittman, T., & Spiegel, S. (2006). *Regulatory fit effects on the attractiveness of redoing an activity.* Unpublished manuscript, Columbia University.

Higgins, E. T., & Silberman, I. (1998). Development of regulatory focus: Promotion and prevention as ways of living. In J. Heckhausen & C. S. Dweck (Eds.), *Motivation and self-regulation across the life span* (pp. 78–113). New York: Cambridge University Press.

Horney, K. (1950). *Neurosis and human growth*. New York: Norton.

Idson, L. C., Liberman, N., & Higgins, E. T. (2004). Imagining how you'd feel: The role of motivational experiences from regulatory fit. *Personality and Social Psychology Bulletin, 30*, 926–937.

Janis, I. L., & Mann, L. (1977). *Decision making: A psychological analysis of conflict, choice, and commitment*. New York: Free Press.

Kahneman, D., Diener, E., & Schwarz, N. (Eds.). (1999). *Well-being: The foundations of hedonic psychology.* New York: Russell Sage Foundation.

Kahneman, D., & Snell, J. (1990). Predicting utility. In R. M. Hogarth (Ed.), *Insights in decision making* (pp. 295–310). Chicago: University of Chicago Press.

Kahneman, D., & Tversky, A. (1979). Prospect theory: An analysis of decision under risk. *Econometrica, 47*, 263–291.

Kruglanski, A. W., Pierro, A., & Higgins, E. T. (in press). Regulatory mode and preferred leadership styles: How fit increases job satisfaction. *Basic and Applied Social Psychology.*

Kruglanski, A. W., Thompson, E. P., Higgins, E. T., Atash, M. N., Pierro, A., Shah, J. Y., et al. (2000). To "do the right thing" or to "just do it": Locomotion and assessment as distinct self-regulatory imperatives. *Journal of Personality and Social Psychology, 79*, 793–815.

Lee, A. Y., & Aaker, J. L. (2004). Bringing the frame into focus: The influence of regulatory fit on processing fluency and persuasion. *Journal of Personality and Social Psychology, 86*, 205–218.

Lewin, K. (1951). *Field theory in social science.* New York: Harper.

Merton, R. K. (1957). *Social theory and social structure.* Glencoe, IL: Free Press.

Millar, M. G., & Tesser, A. (1986). Effects of affective and cognitive focus on the attitude–behavior relation. *Journal of Personality and Social Psychology, 51*, 270–276.

Miller, G. A., Galanter, E., & Pribram, K. H. (1960). *Plans and the structure of behavior.* New York: Holt, Rinehart & Winston.

Navon, D. (1977). Forest before trees: The precedence of global features in visual perception. *Cognitive Psychology, 9*, 353–383.

Ostroff, C. (1993). The effects of climate and personal influences on individual behavior and attitudes in organizations. *Organizational Behavior and Human Decision Processes, 56*, 56–90.

Payne, J. W., Bettman, J. R., & Johnson, E. J. (1993). *The adaptive decision maker.* Cambridge, UK: Cambridge University Press.

Pennington, N., & Hastie, R. (1988). Explanation-based decision making: Effects of memory structure on judgment. *Journal of Experimental Psychology: Learning, Memory, and Cognition, 14*, 521–533.

Petty, R. E., & Wegener, D. T. (1998). Attitude change: Multiple roles for persuasion variables. In D. T. Gilbert, S. T. Fiske, & G. Lindzey (Eds.), *The handbook of social psychology* (4th ed., Vol. 1, pp. 323–390). New York: McGraw-Hill.

Petty, R. E., Wheeler, S. C., & Bizer, G. Y. (2000). Attitude functions and persuasion: An elaboration likelihood approach to matched versus mismatched messages. In G. R. Maio & J. M. Olson (Eds.), *Why we evaluate: Functions of attitudes* (pp. 133–162). Mahwah, NJ: Erlbaum.

Pham, M. T., & Avnet, T. (2004). Ideals and oughts and the reliance on affect versus substance in persuasion. *Journal of Consumer Research, 30*, 503–518.

Pittman, T. S., Cooper, E. E., & Smith, T. W. (1977). Attribution of causality and the overjustification effect. *Personality and Social Psychology Bulletin, 3*, 280–283.

Powers, W. T. (1973). *Behavior: The control of perception.* Chicago: Aldine.

Sansone, C., & Harackiewicz, J. (1996). "I don't feel like it": The function of interest in self-regulation. In L. L. Martin & A. Tesser (Eds.), *Striving and feeling: Interactions among goals, affect, and self-regulation* (pp. 203–228). Mahwah, NJ: Erlbaum.

Schwarz, N. (2000). Emotion, cognition, and decision making. *Cognition and Emotion, 14*, 433–440.

Semin, G. R., Higgins, E. T., Gil de Montes, L., Estourget, Y., & Valencia, J. F. (2005). Linguistic signatures of regulatory focus: How abstraction fits promotion more than prevention. *Journal of Personality and Social Psychology, 89*, 36–45.

Shah, J. Y., Higgins, E. T., & Friedman, R. (1998). Performance incentives and means: How regulatory focus influences goal attainment. *Journal of Personality and Social Psychology, 74*, 285–293.

Shah, J. Y., & Kruglanski, A. W. (2000). Aspects of goal networks: Implications for self-regulation. In M. Boekaerts & P. R. Pintrich (Eds.), *Handbook of self-regulation* (pp. 85–110). San Diego, CA: Academic Press.

Simon, H. A. (1955). A behavioral model of rational choice. *Quarterly Journal of Economics, 69*, 99–118.

Simon, H. A. (1967). Motivational and emotional controls of cognition. *Psychological Review, 74*, 29–39.

Spiegel, S., Grant-Pillow, H., & Higgins, E. T. (2004). How regulatory fit enhances motivational strength during goal pursuit. *European Journal of Social Psychology, 34*, 39–54.

Sullivan, H. S. (1953). *The collected works of Harry Stack Sullivan: Vol. 1. The interpersonal theory of psychiatry* (H. S. Perry & M. L. Gawel, Eds.). New York: Norton.

Tauer, J., & Harackiewicz, J. (1999). Winning isn't everything: Competition, achievement orientation, and intrinsic motivation. *Journal of Experimental Social Psychology, 35*, 209–238.

Taylor, S. E., Pham, L. B., Rivkin, I. D., & Armor, D. A. (1998). Harnessing the imagination: Mental stimulation, self-regulation, and coping. *American Psychologist, 53*, 429–439.

Tetlock, P. E. (1991). An alternative metaphor in the study of judgment and choice: People as politicians. *Theory and Psychology, 1*, 451–475.

Thaler, R. H. (1980). Toward a positive theory of consumer choice. *Journal of Economic Behavior and Organization, 1*, 39–60.

Thaler, R. H. (1999). Mental accounting matters. *Journal of Behavioral Decision Making, 12*, 183–206.

Thibaut, J. W., & Walker, L. (1975). *Procedural justice: A psychological analysis.* Hillsdale, NJ: Erlbaum.

Tversky, A., & Shafir, E. (1992). The disjunction effect in choice under uncertainty. *Psychological Science, 3*, 305–309.

Tyler, T. R., & Lind, E. A. (1992). A relational model of authority in groups. In M. P. Zanna (Ed.), *Advances in experimental social psychology* (Vol. 25, pp. 115–192). San Diego, CA: Academic Press.

*Webster's Ninth New Collegiate Dictionary* (1989). Springfield, MA: Merriam-Webster.

Vallacher, R. R., & Wegner, D. M. (1987). What do people think they are doing?: Action identification and human behavior. *Psychological Review, 94*, 3–15.

Wiener, N. (1948). *Cybernetics: Control and communication in the animal and the machine.* Cambridge, MA: MIT Press.

Chapter 24

# Can Satisfaction Reinforce Wanting?

## A NEW THEORY ABOUT LONG-TERM CHANGES IN STRENGTH OF MOTIVATION

**Kathleen D. Vohs**
**Roy F. Baumeister**

The purpose of this chapter is to provide a preliminary, speculative statement of a new motivational theory. We propose that motivation for a certain outcome can gradually change in strength over time as a function of whether it is satisfied or frustrated. Specifically, we propose that satisfaction will increase the strength of the motivation, whereas nonsatisfaction will gradually weaken it.

This theory runs directly contrary to the standard motivational theories, which have long held that satisfaction will reduce drive (Hull, 1943; Spence, 1956). However, we do not present the new view as a contrary or rival view, but rather a compatible one. The difference lies in the time frames. In the very short run, satisfying a motivation will decrease the drive. In the longer run, however, satisfaction will ensure that when the drive does come back, it will do so with increased strength. Satisfaction reinforces desire, and so when desire emerges again, its strength will be increased. Conversely, to want something without getting it is at best an absence of reinforcement and quite possibly is punishing, and so this experience will gradually diminish and perhaps ultimately extinguish the motivation.

### STATEMENT OF THEORY

From our perspective, the field of motivation theory is hardly full of metatheory or other integrative, overarching theories. The main—and often implicit—integrative model is what we call the *satiation cycle*, which is the presumption that motivation conforms to a standard pattern: A person desires something, pursues satisfaction, and achieves satisfaction, whereupon the motivation diminishes substantially. At some point (and for possibly unexplained reasons), the motivation reemerges, and the cycle of seeking and getting starts again.

We have no quarrel with the satiation cycle. We propose, however, that if one adopts a longer temporal view, there is another pattern that motivation theorists have overlooked. The idealized form of the satiation cycle (wanting, seeking, getting, not wanting, then wanting again) is not a steady state. Rather, when it occurs on a regular basis, the latter wanting may become stronger than the initial wanting, which is what the current theory suggests. Conversely, if the satiation cycle is frustrated, such that wanting and seeking do not meet with satisfaction, the subsequent wanting may be diminished.

Hence our theory proposes two central hypotheses. The first, which we have dubbed *getting begets wanting*, holds that when a motivation leads to satisfaction or some other form of reward and then temporary satiation, the subsequent reemergence of that same desire will be stronger. The subjective feeling of wanting the same outcome will be stronger and possibly longer-lasting as a result of having achieved satisfaction previously. The second hypothesis is that *not getting leads to less wanting*: When a drive repeatedly fails to reach satisfaction, the subsequent desire is likely to be weaker and less frequent. This has also been referred to as "extinction of the wanting response" (A. Baddley, personal communication, July 24, 2004).

Regarding the second hypothesis: If the satiation cycle theory were fully and simply correct, then the experience of not getting (despite wanting) would bring about a state of subjective torture by means of heightened and uncontrollable wanting. Desire would simply increase linearly over time, forever. Clearly, this is not what normally happens. Rather, we propose that a motivation that goes unmet or unsatisfied will be experienced in most cases as only moderately uncomfortable and unlikeable. Furthermore, this state of unsatisfied desire is proposed to grow less uncomfortable with time, in concert with a lessening of desire. In the form of a concrete example, not going jogging for 1 or 2 or 14 days should be experienced by a regular jogger as perhaps unsettling or annoying, but not as a completely horrible state, with the degree of felt annoyance lessening over time and contributing to the weakening of the desire to jog.

Those two central hypotheses require a further assumption: namely, that satisfactions must be somewhat enjoyable in order to strengthen subsequent desire. That is, if the motivation is satisfied in a way that fails to be rewarding—such as if the experience of getting what one has wanted turns out to be either repulsive or simply nonrewarding—then the model would predict that this particular form of getting should not stimulate the wanting response, precisely because the wanting has not been satisfied.

The definition of *reward* ("liking") in the current model is rather broad, because what is rewarding to some people and for some drives may not be the same as what is rewarding to other people pursuing other drives. For the model to be broad enough to cover the range of motivations that seem to be described by the pattern of getting and subsequent wanting, the concept of reward must also be similarly broad. We conceptualize *reward* as being any of the following: a feeling of pleasure from the outcome of a motivated response; satisfaction with an outcome that one deems as the "correct" response in a given situation (e.g., moral or rational decisions that may not feel good but are perceived as the right thing to do); perceptions of progress under novel circumstances or circumstances involving learning; or perhaps a neutral feeling that one is safe, at rest, and out of danger (see Zajonc, 2001, for "all clear" as a reward signal; see also Weiss, 1971).

To reiterate, our theory complements the satiation cycle. Across multiple iterations of the satiation cycle, the strength of the urge will increase or decrease as a function of whether the drive has been met with satisfaction or nonsatisfaction. In this chapter we outline the basic tenets of the getting-begets-wanting model (including contrasting it with the dominant models of satiation and catharsis), discuss possible examples, describe various mechanisms to account for it, and illustrate its utility with some applications.

## THE MECHANICS BEHIND THE MOTIVATION

Why should getting beget wanting? One simple, plausible explanation would invoke reinforcement theory. Wanting something may be regarded as an operant response and, as such, subject to strengthening via positive reinforcement and weakening via negative reinforcement (nonsatisfaction). To be sure, proposing that operant conditioning can modify motivation raises the question of whether such patterns exist throughout the animal world. They may. We think, however, that human beings are plausibly different. The expanded time perspective in humans (the *extended now*; Vohs &

Schmeichel, 2003) should enable rewards and punishments to influence behavior across broader time spans than are possible for other animals. Roberts (2002) has summarized considerable evidence indicating that operant conditioning among most animals requires that the reward or punishment follow the behavior immediately—that is, within a range of 0.5 to 5 seconds. Wanting something therefore cannot be subject to reinforcement or punishment unless the outcome follows immediately. In contrast, the extended now (Vohs & Schmeichel, 2003) of the human psyche should potentially allow responses to be strengthened or weakened as a function of outcomes occurring after substantially greater delays.

Given the extended now, a subjective feeling of desire for an outcome, object, or state that is followed by satisfaction of that desire should result in a subsequent strengthening of that desire. We readily concede that the dynamics of satiation (cf. Carver & Scheier, Chapter 20, this volume) would entail that the immediate effect of getting what one wants will be a reduction in the desire. However, rather soon thereafter the desire may reemerge, and our central hypothesis is that the reemerging desire will be stronger as a function of having recently achieved satisfaction. The gratification of the desire will be deeply rewarding, and this will reinforce the pattern of wanting. The pleasure of satiation will strengthen the desire.

Conversely, if one desires something and fails to get it, the result will be an aversive state (e.g., frustration) that should effectively punish the person for wanting. (At least, it should be a failure to provide the anticipated reward.) The long-term result should be a reduction or extinction of the wanting response. The subjective state of desire without satisfaction should be aversive. In other words, imagine that a woman has a regular habit of jogging four times a week. If she breaks an ankle and is not able to run for, say, 6 weeks, her desire to run will have been unmet during that time and, from the current perspective, will dwindle. After the 6 weeks, her ankle may be fully recovered, but she may not have the same eagerness and enthusiasm to hit the track that she had 2 months ago. Whether such diminishment of drive is pure extinction (in the sense of lack of reward) or counterconditioning (punishment for wanting) is something we do not know, but in either case the desire should be reduced. Most likely both processes are possible: Desire that meets with no satisfaction, with no emotional result, should lead to gradual extinction, whereas acute frustration and other negative states that attend unsatisfied desires should constitute punishment and produce counterconditioning.

Theorists have recently begun to tackle the issue of wanting as separate from liking, although previous attempts to integrate the two concepts date back to Freud's (1915/1957) catharsis theory. We discuss the wrongheadedness of the catharsis theory later, in our review of evidence on catharsis and aggression. A more sophisticated analysis by Berridge (1999) makes the point that liking and wanting are separate concepts, which suggests that an outcome is acted upon with a response that brings about either liking or nonliking. This state of liking or nonliking further paves the way for the theory presented here: namely, that liking or nonliking (generally speaking) not only sates desire for the current moment, but also feeds back and subsequently affects (increase or decrease) the future degree of wanting.

We submit that motivational plasticity is a likely moderating factor. The more hard-wired the motivation is (i.e., the more evolutionarily based it is), the less scope there is for waxing and waning. As a result, culturally constructed motivations (such as money and self-esteem) should show more evidence than innate ones (such as food and sex). In this way, basic motivations, such as the need to belong, sex, and food, may not be affected as much as cultural motivations. In the culturally constructed motivations, wanting may be much more stable, and getting is much more variable—but because of the necessity of stimulating the basic motivations to be strong (probably no one has perished because he or she couldn't satisfy a desire to go running). As an extension, we think of motivational plasticity as an evolutionary adaptation to make people more cultural.

Baumeister (2005) has elaborated a distinction among three levels of motivations. First, there the most basic motivations, such as those for food, shelter, safety, and control, that humans share with almost all animals. Second come the social motivations, such as aggression and belongingness, that are specific to social animals. Third come the cultural motivations, which are more or less unique to humans and possibly a few very close animal relatives. These include the desire for money, fame, a meaningful life, and self-esteem. Baumeister has observed that the cultural motivations typically build on or elaborate some of the more basic, natural motivations, such as how the desire for money is probably based on the motives for control and for social status. In this scheme, the cultural motivations probably have greater plasticity and may therefore be more subject to the pattern of getting begets wanting, though this is not a strong or central prediction of our theory.

One force that is central not only to the current theory, but also to all addictive processes, is the fact that organisms like and strive to feel good. A desire to feel good as an end unto itself is in fact the foundation on which addictive processes are built. If humans were robots, they would not care if an action felt good; they would only make mental notes of whether an action helped to achieve a goal. The clever trick of evolution made the actions that bolstered the odds of securing survival and reproduction feel good. As humans have evolved, feeling good has become a goal itself—and achieving this goal has apparently become paramount, given the myriad behaviors enacted simply because they elicit pleasurable feelings (Baumeister, 2005). As humans have become more oriented toward the conscious experience of pleasure, actions that lead to pleasure have gained in power over the motivation system, thereby setting the stage for getting-begets-wanting effects.

Our theory builds upon and goes beyond an evolutionary explanation of motivation. We differ, first, in that we posit that more than only evolutionarily beneficial behaviors will adhere to the getting–wanting pattern of motivation. We differ, second, in that we posit a specific curve to the forgoing of rewards to which one has been accustomed. On this point, we propose that people slowly but steadily lose motivation for a certain outcome with time since they have last experienced it. The end result is that people will cease to want a certain outcome if they have not been exposed to it in some time. We expand upon these two points throughout the course of this chapter.

## POSSIBLE EVIDENCE

We are proposing a new theory of motivation, and so almost by definition there exist no empirical tests of it. If there were a large mass of relevant findings that we could reinterpret, then our project might succeed as a literature review, but here again the available information falls short of what we might like. Hence in this section we offer a set of observations that could become relevant to testing our theory. This section might also serve as a research agenda.

### Psychoactive Drugs

We do not cover the wide variety of psychoactive drugs that can elicit patterns of addiction (also called *dependence*, as per the American Psychological Association's [APA's] current requirements), but it is important to review the criteria for dependence. According to the APA (2000), substance dependence involves the experience of three of the following criteria within a 12-month period: tolerance; withdrawal symptoms (compensatory reactions that are the opposite of the effects of the drug); increasing doses; unsuccessful efforts to cut down intake of the substance; a considerable amount of time spent obtaining or using the substance; interference with important social, occupational, or recreational activities; and continued use despite recognition of physical or psychological problems. More broad than the APA definition, the World Health Organization's (1977) definition of dependence centers on "a compulsion to take the drug on a continuous or periodic basis."

Addiction is sometimes regarded as a peculiar, highly specific pattern of motivation. Our view is that it is not so atypical after all. In any case, addition seems a relatively straightforward version of the pattern we have hypothesized. The person initially may have no desire to ingest a drug, having never experienced it. The first experiences are rewarding because they bring pleasure, and they cause the person to begin desiring the drug. Repeated and perhaps more frequent experiences cause the craving to intensify, and so the person wants more and takes more. Where initially there was no motivation, now the person has a powerful and frequent desire for the drug.

As the review that follows indicates, many of these criteria can be met by desires for things other than psychoactive drugs. We propose that the behavioral and psychological patterns of people addicted to psychoactive drugs can also be observed in the motivations for aggression, esteem, love, money, and sex, as well as in various other passions.

## Catharsis and Aggression

One of social psychology's early and dramatic contributions to the broader understanding of human behavior was the discrediting of the so-called *catharsis* hypothesis. This hypothesis, which is traced to Freud (1915/1957), regarded aggression as a drive that steadily builds up until it finds satisfaction in any sort of expression, whereupon it should be substantially reduced (until a subsequent buildup). Freud's theories about aggressive displacement also held that almost any outlet should satisfy the drive—a view that still enjoys wide support in the popular (and pop psychology) views, which advise people to vent their anger by hammering nails, hitting walls or pillows, or at most fighting each other with foam bats (Bushman, Baumeister, & Stack, 1999).

The catharsis hypothesis was roundly discredited in many experiments studying the effects of provocation on people who, after they were made angry, were permitted either to watch an aggressive film (Geen & Berkowitz, 1966) or to behave aggressively in another context (Geen & Quanty, 1977). The hypothesized reduction of aggression never materialized, and in general the effect went in the opposite direction. Summarizing the results of multiple studies, Geen and Quanty (1977) said that it was time to regard the catharsis hypothesis as wrong and to discard it. More recent work has continued to discredit this hypothesis, such as by showing that even people who believe in the value of venting anger do not show reduced subsequent aggressiveness (Bushman et al., 1999). On the contrary, they too become more aggressive after venting their anger.

We concur with the conclusion that the catharsis hypothesis is wrong. If it were merely wrong, however, then allowing people an aggressive outlet should simply fail to produce any reduction in subsequent aggression, thereby producing a no-difference finding. However, quite commonly persons who aggress or witness aggression end up being *more* aggressive than others. Why the increase?

A possible answer is that the aggression is pleasant or rewarding in some way, and that this reward serves as a reinforcer for the aggressive impulses. From this perspective, engaging in aggression should elicit a pleasurable response, which then feeds back and produces a desire for more. When people feel angry or upset, they anticipate that aggressing will make them feel better, and so they aggress (Bushman, Baumeister, & Phillips, 2001).

Empirical support comes from research in which some people were induced to kill five bugs, and others were induced to kill only one (Martens, Kosloff, Greenberg, Landau, & Schmader, 2006). A self-paced "extermination" phase followed, which constituted the dependent measure of killing. As would be predicted by the current model, killing increased after participants had earlier killed five bugs, as opposed to one.

## Motivation for Esteem

Although the motivation for aggression may represent a negative interpersonal side of the getting-begets-wanting pattern, there are positive interpersonal reinforcers as well. The first social reinforcer on which we focus is a craving for admiration from others, which leads to a need for more self-esteem; next we turn to love for a specific person as an addictive state.

Although many if not most people desire to be seen positively by others, an addiction-like cycle of wanting ever more social regard is particularly pronounced among narcissists (Baumeister & Vohs, 2001). Although narcissism has several defining features, one key aspect is the need for greater levels of reassurance and admiration over time.

Narcissists love to hear good things about themselves—a characteristic that is a hallmark of both colloquial and clinical descriptions of narcissists. A more nuanced look has shown that narcissists think of themselves not as any more likeable than others, but rather as deserving more respect and admiration (Campbell, Rudich, & Sedikides, 2002; Rhodewalt & Morf, 1995). This difference may help explain why they are insensitive to the reductions in likeability that accompany a constant need for admiration (Campbell et al., 2002).

Narcissists' understanding of themselves as special people allows them to embrace favorable outcomes and positive social feedback (which may or may not be a result of their own abilities, given that they respond similarly to contingent and noncontingent outcomes; see Morf & Rhodewalt, 2001) and derive a boost in self-esteem as a result. Since narcissists care tremendously about being held in high regard, the boost to their self-esteem is great (Rhodewalt, Madrian, & Cheney, 1998) but short-lived. The impact of a self-esteem boost is curtailed among narcissists by two processes, both stemming from the same root: a narcissist's identity as a special person who deserves good outcomes.

Seeing oneself as special and as deserving of good outcomes means first that a narcissist can quickly assimilate the positive information into his or her self-concept, thereby immediately giving it meaning (e.g., "This happened because I am so terrific"). Making meaning of the positive feedback, however, detracts from its peak self-esteem impact and lessens its durability (Wilson, Gilbert, & Centerbar, 2003). That meaning making shortens the durability of the self-esteem boost is crucial from the standpoint of the getting-begets-wanting model, because it suggests that the craving for more self-esteem will begin that much sooner. For a person who is unaccustomed to fluctuations in self-esteem, conversely, a self-esteem boost may be more difficult to incorporate into his or her self-concept ("How did this wonderful thing happen?") and thus will have a longer-lasting, more intense psychological impact (Wilson et al., 2003).

The second process that attenuates the self-esteem boost is that a narcissist readily adjusts to the new level of self-esteem and consequently comes to assume that the new level of adoration is now the baseline. That is, when narcissists encounter positive feedback from others, they soak up the attendant increase in self-esteem (see Rhodewalt et al., 1998), and we suggest they further assume that this state is the new status quo. Adaptation and the assumption of a new status quo, combined with a deep craving for social approval, spur the narcissists to seek new opportunities to accrue social rewards from which to gain another dose of esteem. One instance of this can be seen in narcissists' failure to perform well when the chance for public glory is low (Wallace & Baumeister, 2002). Similar also to people with substance dependence, narcissists are constantly on the lookout for new sources. Research on the romantic style of narcissists show that even in the midst of a current relationship, they are highly attendant to other potential partners in the hope that they can get a better-quality mate (Campbell, 1999).

Regarding the withdrawal aspect of addiction, narcissists hold fast to their positive views of themselves and are generally unwilling to put aside their views or the impression that others adore them. Narcissists are ready to see the world as supporting their uniqueness, but when they perceive that their special selves are not being supported by the social environment, they lash out in hostility and aggression (e.g., Bushman & Baumeister, 1998). We think of these responses as being akin to the aversive reactions of substance-addicted individuals who are denied a much-needed dose.

In sum, the narcissistic pattern of wanting increasingly higher doses of self-esteem is closely aligned with the addictive patterns of reward, tolerance, and withdrawal. Narcissists, like those with other addictions, seem to experience the rewards (a rise in self-esteem with social acclaim) more strongly than do nonnarcissists, who are happy to be seen positively by others but for whom the constant need to feel highly valued is not present. Narcissists work very hard to feed their esteem addiction, seeking more sources and opportunities for social glory. They are distressed when they face hindrances to getting what they want, and are reluctant to give up the idealized views of themselves they possess.

## Motivation for Love (with a Specific Person)

Another positive interpersonal exemplar of the getting-begets-wanting pattern concerns love for another person. In this case, the feelings of love, positivity, and optimism are the reinforcers that follow being in the presence of a loved one. The initial stages of love are strikingly similar to those of addiction: a state of euphoria that conjures up urges to be around the loved one in greater doses. Spending hours on the telephone or an entire weekend by the other's side is not unheard of and only seems to fuel a deeper craving for the other person.

A scholarly treatment of love as addiction was introduced by Peele and Brodsky (1975), who (similar to the current perspective) sought to broaden the use of the term *addiction* to include a variety of interdependences. Peale and Brodsky thought of love as the ideal case to which to apply principles of addiction, given that two people in love show signs of intense dependence. In their view, each person in the couple comes to rely on the presence of the other in order to feel calm, comfort, and security, or experiences distressing symptoms of withdrawal during separation.

Regarding the feeling of being in love, it is our view that being with the person one loves is like a drug that elicits a euphoric high. The high is so pleasurable that the person seeks more time with or attention from the loved one, with the eventual consequence that any time apart renders each lover miserable and experiencing symptoms of withdrawal (cf. the term *lovesick*). There is never enough time with the lover, and even when one is able to spend 24 hours a day with him or her, this still is not enough. Given, however, that one cannot beg, borrow, or steal more time (as an individual with substance dependence can do with money to get the drug), this ceiling effect means that there is no way to achieve more time together than all the time that is available. As a result, the tolerance that comes from becoming accustomed to the love from this person, combined with the fact that no more time is available to increase exposure to the person, renders each dose of the love somewhat less potent with time. Thus the declining rate of passionate love with time can be explained by tolerance and lack of options for increasing the amount of exposure to the loved one.

There are, however, factors that can rejuvenate the sense of love euphoria. Akin to using a drug in a novel environment, which is known to increase the potency of the drug (as well as to increase the risk of overdose; Siegel, Hinson, Krank, & McCully, 1982), people who perform exciting activities together also report increased intimacy and passion (Aron, Norman, Aron, McKenna, & Heyman, 2000). Being apart from one another is like being denied a drug when one is in a craving state, and when one is finally given a dose of the drug, one needs a smaller amount in order to get the standard (or more intense) effect. Similarly, Baumeister and Bratslavsky (1999) showed that interpersonal conflict between romantic lovers spurs feelings of passion. More broadly, Baumeister and Bratslavsky suggested that any upward changes in intimacy bring about similar changes in passion. Thus, from the viewpoint of the current model, sharing exciting activities (akin to taking the drug in a novel environment), as well as being apart or experiencing conflict (as a temporary denial of intimacy), would bring about increased sensitivity to love such that small doses can have a big effect.

### Motivation for Money

Aside from motivations aimed directly at survival or reproduction, the motivation for having money is perhaps the most potent human motivator. What drives people to acquire more money than they could ever possibly need? Aside from considerations such as children's inheritance, retirement years, and general "rainy day" funds to be saved in case of an unfortunate event in the future, we propose that one reason why people seek to attain more money is that the experience of acquiring money has been rewarding in the past. The more money people get, the more they want. Indeed, the fact that Americans are exceptionally materialistic (Kasser & Ryan, 1993), despite being residents of the richest country in the world, attests to the strong pull of the getting-begets-wanting pattern; from most perspectives, Americans should be the most sated when it comes to material goods, since they have the most.

People's happiness or satisfaction is contingent not on absolute level of wealth, but rather on relative changes in wealth levels, either higher or lower. Economists speak of the *hedonic treadmill* to explain these patterns: Increases or decreases in personal wealth make people happier or unhappier; ensuing adaptation processes alter the expected level of wealth or the lifestyle that comes with it; and consequently the new level of wealth is the baseline against which subsequent changes in wealth are experienced. In this way, motivations about money involve processes similar to addiction, with relative adaptation theory echoing drug-related tolerance effects.

Thus, if the current level of wealth sets the baseline for what to expect in terms of forthcoming earnings, then one could examine what happens psychologically when a certain level of expected wealth is not met. Research in consumerism has shown that high materialism is related to lower subjective well-being (e.g., Kasser & Ryan, 1993, 1996; Sirgy, 1998). However, from another position, over three decades of research has pointed to a small but positive link between wealth and happiness (Diener, Suh, Lucas, & Smith, 1999). Why is it that having more money makes most people marginally happier, but a strong desire for having more money makes people less happy and less satisfied with life?

A possible reinterpretation of the data on materialistic values and well-being is suggested by the getting–wanting theory. Work by Sirgy (1998) reported that materialism and well-being are negatively associated—a finding that was interpreted as meaning that a desire to possess many material goods is largely unattainable for most people, and therefore that their preferred standard of living is out of reach. Seen from the viewpoint of the current theory, these persons have probably been given nice products in the past and found them to be highly rewarding, therefore stimulating the desire to have more goods. Not being able to satisfy this want, they are disappointed in their material status, and hence have lower subjective well-being. In other words, negative well-being comes from a lack of positive correlation between getting and wanting.

Related to the want for more money or material goods is an addiction to gambling. There are many aspects of gambling that are unrelated to the monetary payoff, but the reward does matter. Research on schedules of reinforcement demonstrated that the partial reinforcement schedule yielded strong responses that were resistant to extinction (Lewis, 1952). Many of these studies were conducted in a quasi-realistic environment, with slot machines paying out monetary rewards (Lewis & Duncan, 1956, 1957, 1958). Probably, rewards as tickets or points that are not exchangeable for money would still be exciting, but far less so—and very unlikely to develop into an addiction-like pattern.

The APA (2000) classifies pathological gambling as a manifestation of impulse control. Impulse control disorders involve inability to restrain oneself against the temptation of desire, and in this case the desire involves betting and winning money. The emotional states that accompany this disorder include mood swings, depression, anxiety, suicidal thoughts, and worthlessness—all signs of other forms of addiction.

Why does money have these effects? Money is, in some ways, the ultimate cultural reward; among interdependent cultures as well as independent cultures, money still drives much of human behavior. When a person has accomplished something that has worth to the culture, the accomplishment is then rewarded with a token of cultural esteem—namely, money. Thus here money is the reinforcer (like praise to a child from a mother) that signifies accomplishment in the eyes of the culture.

## Motivation for Sex

As will be discussed later, motivations that are likely to be heavily governed by the getting–wanting process are more culturally constructed motivations (e.g., playing video games) rather than need-based motivations (e.g., eating, sleeping). One exception to the rule may be that sex, under some conditions, may conform to the getting–wanting pattern. At other times, conversely, getting and wanting sex may conform to a more consistent pattern of wanting regardless of getting (or perhaps the reverse, of not getting leading to more wanting; we discuss this possibility later).

One distinguishing factor that may predict whether motivation for sex is a function of getting–wanting processes is the strength of the drive. We discuss this in greater depth later in the chapter, but suffice it to say that a stronger *initial* sex drive (i.e., interest in sex prior to recently obtaining sex) should be less susceptible to the reinforcement and extinguishing patterns described in the current model. Instead, people with high initial sex drive should show a weaker getting–wanting relationship, because the wanting should be consistent and not tied as closely to satisfying the desire.

On the topic of types of sex, some ancillary reports suggest that the wilder types of sex (e.g., masochism, bondage) show patterns akin to the getting-begets-wanting model. For instance, the autobiography of pornography star Linda Lovelace (Lovelace with McGrady, 1980) includes a report from an acquaintance of *Playboy* magazine's founder, Hugh Hefner, that although Hefner liked several of Lovelace's movies, he particularly admired a film she made in which she had sex with a dog. He said that he had seen many films of women with animals, but her film was especially good. It appears that Hefner's pornography viewing had escalated to the point that films depicting people-to-people sex were stale and uninteresting; he was looking for more and varied forms of taboo sex, presumably to get him to his standard level of stimulation. This pattern, although reported third-hand, suggests that Hefner was experiencing a getting-begets-wanting cycle of desiring increasingly outrageous sex scenes in order to achieve sexual satisfaction.

## Harmonious and Obsessive Passions

We believe that the types of activities that evoke the getting-begets-wanting pattern can range from the physically and psychologically addicting, such as drugs, to more pedestrian pursuits, such as golf, jogging, cooking, or playing a musical instrument. These latter types of pursuits were the focus of a recent investigation by Vallerand and colleagues (2003), who detailed two different forms of passions. *Passions* are defined as activities that people like, that they deem quite important, and to which they devote energy and time. A *harmonious* passion is characterized by joy, positivity, and a lack of negativity about an activity, whereas an *obsessive* passion is characterized by increased negativity and less positivity about the activity. Furthermore, an obsessive passion is related to negative emotions when one is blocked from engaging in the activity, whereas a harmonious passion does not show such a link. Notably, one particular aspect that seems to divide the two types of passions is the extent to which a passion comes into conflict with other aspects of a person's life; only an obsessive passion shows a strong, positive correlation with the activity as a disruption. For instance, among a community sample of people who continued bicycling outdoors when cold, snowy winter weather arrived in the province of Québec, Canada, there was a significant showing of obsessive passion, as compared to cyclists who cycled in the other three seasons but discontinued cycling during winter weather.

The getting–wanting pattern is prominent in the data on obsessive passions: People who have this type of passion answer affirmatively to items such as "I cannot live without it [the activity]," "I have a tough time controlling my need to do this activity," and "I have difficulty imagining my life without this activity." Vallerand and colleagues (2003) also reported that people with obsessive passions use the activity to regulate their emotions. All of these aspects are concordant with an addiction-like style of first performing an activity and then wanting to do it again and again. We concur with Vallerand and colleagues that much more research is needed in this area, as we believe that there is much convergence between addiction and passions, and that this nexus may be best explained by the getting-begets-wanting model.

Anecdotal observations suggest that many activities can develop from an initial, possibly innate indifference into consuming passions, and it is plausible that these desires are strengthened by satisfaction and extinguished by lack of contact. Being a sports fan seems an excellent model for this, because almost by definition sports contests do not have any material or pragmatic significance. Yet as people watch sports, they can become devoted, passionate followers who keep track of many apparent details (such as sports statistics, survey-based rankings, and betting odds). Conversely, if one stops following a sport on a regular basis, the fascination seems to diminish. Indeed, to some extent the seasonal nature of most sports is dependent on this, or else football fans would become increasingly desperate across the weeks and months after the season ends.

Our impression is that some people follow the news in much the same way. To be sure, factual news may have some impact on individual lives, and so it is arguably rational and self-interested to follow the news. Then again, people who do not follow the news regularly do not seem much worse off because of it, and if one separates the weather forecast from the rest of the news, the benefits of the remainder are even slimmer. Our point is merely that so-called "news junkies" watch and read about news events to an extent that goes far beyond what rational self-interest and pragmatic concerns dictate. In any case, we suspect that following the news for a week will tend to breed increased interest and ultimately an enhanced motivation to follow the news further, whereas ignoring the news for a period of time will allow that interest to dissipate.

Other culturally created pastimes likewise depend on the pattern that getting stimulates wanting. It is hard to argue that people have an innate desire to solve crossword puzzles, watch soap operas, ski, play video games (or billiards or bridge), and so forth, even though some of these might appeal at some level to aspects of basic or innate motivations. (For example, skiing may capitalize on a basic tendency to enjoy motion and speed, and watching soap operas may be based on a basic curiosity, akin to gossip, about people's private affairs.)

## Speculation about the Most Basic Desires

Our theory is essentially one of motivational plasticity, because it allows for people's desires to increase and decrease as a function of how regularly satisfaction is available. If we assume that evolution by means of natural selection helped shape the human psyche to be effective at living in culture (Baumeister, 2005), then it would follow that motivational plasticity would be helpful: It is easier to live in culture if the organism can continue to adjust its cravings according to circumstances than if the basic drives are immune to current, situational pressures. The reason for this is the assumption that a cultural environment is more changeable and more interdependent on other people than a physical environment.

For those reasons, we have emphasized culturally constructed motives as the most likely candidates to confirm the hypothesis that getting stimulates wanting. But what about the unlikeliest candidates—namely, the innate needs that are necessary for survival? A priori, one would suggest that these might be less amenable to environmental influence. In other words, they might remain more constant regardless of satisfaction and nonsatisfaction. Despite this assumption, our impression is that it is at least plausible that the most basic human motives also conform to the pattern that getting begets wanting and nonsatisfaction breeds indifference.

The requirement of food is certainly one of the most basic motivations. It would hardly be surprising if it proved completely impervious to reinforcement and nonsatisfaction in the way our theory proposes. That is, people who are deprived of food should simply become more and more motivated to eat, period. And yet anecdotal reports of starvation suggest that at some point the craving for food does diminish, as if the hunger is extinguished (this effect occurs more strongly among some people than others; see Pinel, Assanand, & Lehman, 2000, for a discussion of the positive incentive value of food). Converging evidence from studies of anorexia nervosa likewise suggests that the desire for food diminishes among people who refrain from eating for a long period of time (Pinel et al., 2000).

Even if the pattern is not true for all food, it may be true for specific foods. Anecdotally, vegetarians report that they lose the desire to eat meat. We have heard this even from reluctant vegetarians, who are pressured by a spouse or by their religion into forgoing meat. Such patterns speak against the explanation that vegetarians do not really like meat to begin with.

In parallel, the late diet mogul Dr. Robert Atkins (1992) proposed that the body's desire for carbohydrates exhibits remarkable plasticity. His views, which are echoed by some devotees (though we do not know of systematic studies of this pattern), suggest that people who live without carbohydrates lose some of the craving for them. Conversely, indulgence in carbohydrates may stimulate increased desire for them. Atkins (1992) and others have noted that pasta-based Italian food was long regarded as fattening, but in the 1970s the anti-fat theories that dominated nutrition research suddenly declared pasta as ideal for losing weight because of its low fat content. As a result, many Americans began consuming more carbohydrates without fat. This shift in national eating patterns was soon followed by an unprecedented rise in the national rate of obesity, which had been stable for decades. Quite possibly, eating more carbohydrates made people crave them more, and so they ate more and gained weight, much to their own discomfiture.

There are reports that the reduction in desire for food (or for a certain food) often reaches a point of either not desiring the food at all or feeling repulsion at the thought of the food. Vegetarians frequently say that they do not miss meat, but their claims are of course also contributed to by the fact that they may not have liked meat initially, which is why (or how) they became vegetarians. Similar reports come from individuals recovering from alcoholism, who no longer drink alcohol and who later report not missing it—or at least not missing it as much as they anticipated they would. These are people who once obviously liked alcohol very much, so they provide somewhat stronger evidence for the not-getting-not-wanting cycle. Stronger evidence comes from people who are put on a specific diet for health reasons, such as people who are allergic to gluten or dairy products. To the extent that substitutes are available (such as soy cheese or gluten-free bread), however, the desire for the food category may not wane, but instead may be satisfied by the substitute food and thus stimulate further demand for the forbidden food. We doubt, however, that craving for water will ever show this pattern, because regular infusions of water are needed for survival, though in some respects fluid consumption can be increased or decreased by culture.

Sleep, however, may be a better bet. Our impression is that some people grow accustomed to lesser amounts of sleep and do not suffer as much as newly deprived individuals. That is, if two people would both naturally like to sleep 8 hours every night, and one regularly does so while the other normally gets only 6, then a particular night of 6 hours of sleep will be much more troubling and tiring to the person who regularly gets 8 hours than to the one who has grown accustomed to getting by with less. The latter has learned to get by with less because the body adjusts its need for sleep.

## Studies Directly Testing the Getting-Begets-Wanting Theory

We conducted two studies to test tenets of the getting-begets-wanting model. In both studies, the goal was to instigate a motivation for an object or state that did not exist prior to the study's commencement. Then, several days later, participants were tested to see which activity they preferred, as a sign of their motivation for the activity.

In one study, we asked participants to take home either a crossword puzzle book filled with puzzles that ranged in difficulty or a handheld electronic game of solitaire (participants were randomly assigned to condition). A third group, a control condition, performed only the pre- and postexperimental tasks to provide a baseline against which we could compare the two motivation conditions. For five days, participants in the solitaire or crossword puzzle conditions played their game for 20 minutes each day and completed questionnaires about their mood (before and after the activity), their success at the activity, and how much they had thought about the activity during the previous 24 hours. Results showed that as the days progressed, participants enjoyed their respective activities more, thought about them more, and felt more successful. They were also significantly more likely to think about their activity than control condition participants. Furthermore, upon completion of the 5-day experiment, participants dropped off their questionnaires, were thanked and given their experimental credit, and then were asked whether they would perform another short experiment that was ongoing in the department. After consent, participants were led into a different room with a different experimenter and given several filler questionnaires, which were intended to allow the concept of the game task to decay. Next, they were given the choice of performing one of several different types of activities; one of these was their activity for the previous 5 days, but the rest of the activities were different games. The results of this part of the study showed that participants were more likely to chose their assigned activity from the previous "experiment" than would have been predicted by chance.

A second study used a different method to test the getting-begets-wanting process. We focused on the desire to take a nap as an activity that entrains the getting–wanting cycle, such that after people start taking naps, they have a subsequent urge to take naps more often and more urgently. In this study, either participants were asked to take a nap for 15 minutes a day for 4 days of 8 possible days, or they were asked to think about taking a nap for a period of 8 minutes on each of 8 subsequent days. We used this method to test whether merely thinking of the activity was sufficient to instigate the getting–wanting cycle, or whether one must actually perform the activity to show the effects. (We grant that this may not have been the strongest test, insofar as we did not train people to engage in visual imagining, which would have been a stronger test of whether a specific, detailed visualization could stimulate getting–wanting patterns. However, we allowed participants to use the visualization processes they would use when naturally imagining an activity.) Much as in the first study, we queried participants in advance of the study as to whether they enjoyed napping, and then asked during the course of the 8-day trial about the degree to which they enjoyed the activity, found it satisfying, and thought about the activity when they were not performing it. We found that participants in the actual-napping conditions thought about the activity more, were more satisfied, and enjoyed the experiment more as the days progressed—as well as relative to participants in the thinking-about-napping condition. Moreover, we asked participants how much they intended to nap after the experiment was over; those in the actual-napping condition reported they were more likely to nap than those in the thinking-about-napping condition. This last comparison is particularly important, given that simply thinking about napping—without being able to engage in it (participants in this condition were instructed not to nap for the duration of the 8-day trial)—may have evoked a desire to nap that went unmet and therefore may have brought about increased likelihood to nap from that day forward. Instead, it did not seem to arouse desire to nap; rather, those participants who engaged in the activity were more likely to say that they would do it in the future.

Results from two experiments directly testing the getting-begets-wanting pattern support the model. We found that getting people to engage in an activity—be it crossword puzzles, a hand-held electronic game, or napping—led them to like the activity more as their practice of the task went on and, more importantly, resulted in choices or reports that they would perform the activity subsequently. Note that a novelty-based explanation would have predicted the opposite: that participants would prefer a new task when given the choice (in Study 1) and would report no increased desire and perhaps less desire to take naps (in Study 2) at the conclusion of the study. We continue to look for new, creative ways to test the getting–wanting model, and we encourage researchers interested in cultivating new methods to contact us for possible collaborative efforts.

## COUNTEREXAMPLES, TYPES OF MOTIVATIONS, AND THEIR RELATION TO THE MODEL

One can imagine outcomes and processes differing from those that have been specified here. For instance, when one considers what happens to an unmet desire, the getting-begets-wanting model anticipates that the desire will wither and decrease drastically, if not fall away altogether. However, one can conjure up instances whereby an unmet desire only serves to strengthen the resolve or desire to achieve a certain outcome. From our understanding, two components are likely to distinguish this from the getting–wanting process: the strength of the initial wanting (before being unmet) and the duration of time in which the desire has gone unrewarded.

Let's take as an example anecdotal evidence suggesting that sex therapists at times attempt to strengthen sexual desire (literally) by making sure that it is not satisfied (a phenomenon similar to marketers' attempts to stimulate demand for a product by reducing its supply). This means that a couple is instructed *not* to have sex for a specified period of time, with the idea that knowing that sex is not available will stimulate urges for sex and then, when sex is allowable again, the couple will experience heightened desire and a better sex life.

First, we submit that one condition that may elicit the pattern of not getting leading to more wanting would be a strong and reliable state of wanting, as is likely to be the case for a motivation as fundamental as sex. This is especially likely to occur for men, whose sex drives are far stronger and more reliable than women's sex drives (Baumeister et al., 2001; but see our earlier discussion for the emergence of getting–wanting patterns among those with low sex drive). To varying extents, motivations to eat, sleep, have positive and stable relationships with others (Baumeister & Leary, 1995), seek meaning in one's life (Heine, Proulx, & Vohs, 2006), and fulfill other basic needs may not die down if unmet and may in fact increase. We would expect this pattern for motivations that guarantee human survival, such as reproduction and the abilities increasing the likelihood that one will be an accepted member of a cultural species (Baumeister, 2005). Hence someone who has gone without water for days upon end would probably not turn down the offer of a glass of water, most likely because the state of dehydration would be so miserable that he or she would want to end it as soon as possible.

On the other hand, there are motivations that are more culturally based, and we would expect these motivations to show the getting–wanting pattern to a much greater degree than more basic motivations. Baumeister's (2005) analysis of humans as a cultural species suggests that culture may have developed the motivational getting-begets-wanting pattern so as to have a mechanism whereby desires outside the few basic motivations could form. Given the wealth and specificity of modern human motivations, it is impossible for nature to have prepared humans with thousands of latent motivations just waiting to be unleashed under the right circumstances. It is more likely that the drive to perform basic behaviors beyond eating, sleeping, having sex, and so on developed on top of the same structure that exists for basic motivations.

Hence, to return to the idea that the strength of the motivation is a crucial component of whether the getting-begets-wanting pattern will arise (particularly after a long period of not getting), cultural motivations are likely to be weaker than basic motivations because they are not, on their own, ultimately necessary for a person's survival and reproduction. The basic motivations may show more consistent wanting patterns, even in conditions when the getting is variable; the cultural motivations may show a stronger link between the getting and subsequent wanting, whereas the association may be weaker among the basic motivations for which nature would have been foolish to link survival-related efforts to a factor as tenuous as whether the behavior has been performed in recent times. Hence a sex therapist may in fact be able to stimulate short-term desire between partners by forbidding them to have sex—an effect that occurs in part because the desire for sex is a strong biological drive that may be less affected by getting–wanting influences.

We now move to the second qualifier of whether and when desire increases in the absence of satisfaction—duration of the not-getting period. Let's consider another example: If the woman jogger in our earlier example was obliged not to jog for a certain period of time, would her motivation to jog increase? Maybe, but only initially. With time we would expect it to decrease, which leads us to our second point that the length of time that the desire has gone unrewarded is crucial to predicting the level of subsequent motivation for the object. As mentioned before, the unique human state of a mental *extended now* (Vohs & Schmeichel, 2003) means that the getting–wanting influences on behavior can take place along a rather broad time span; hence desire for an unobtainable object may rise at first, but then fall and dissipate to a not-wanting state over time.

This may be one explanation for the observation that wanting an unattainable object may initially increase immediately after it is found to be unattainable. This rise would be expected in part, due to a continuation of the getting–wanting cycle: The person was previously getting and wanting and getting and wanting; thus the wanting may continue to rise in the hopes of leading to attainment. A rise in desire may also be due to reactance in response to being denied access to something one wants (Brehm, 1966). However, with the possible exception of basic evolutionary motivations such as food, need to belong, sex, and so on, we predict that desire for other objects after a period of being unobtainable (which may result in a short burst of increased wanting) should drop and eventually dwindle to a lack of drive for the object.

There is also the consideration that people do grow tired of engaging in certain activities or receiving certain pleasures. For instance, a person who goes on a ski trip presumably does not feel an increase each day in desire to ski. The decrease of desire for sex within a stable relationship may be another example. It may be in these cases that when satisfaction is readily and consistently available, the desire (wanting) ceases to build up very far, so there is nothing to reinforce. Although we have no direct evidence, it seems plausible that some level of wanting needs to be present for the reinforcement effects to occur.

## RELATION TO OTHER THEORIES

Our theory bears some resemblance to *adaptation-level theory* (Helson, 1964), which is a more specific theory regarding the experience of positive states. This theory states that people grow accustomed to what they have and consequently will come to crave a more extreme version. Adaptation-level theory says that people's initial pleasure wears off with time, and therefore the same level ceases to have the same positive effect as it did initially. Accordingly, they need more or a stronger version to get pleasure from the object again. (Hence the phrase *hedonic treadmill*, which is often used in conjunction with this theory; Brickman & Campbell, 1971.) Adaptation is a process similar to the getting-begets-wanting process, insofar as it employs concepts akin to *tolerance* and *craving* from addiction theory. However, the current theory differs from adaptation-level theory insofar as the getting-begets-wanting model applies not only to having positive states, but also to the denial of positive states to which one has grown accustomed. We have explicated this point above, in the section addressing seemingly discrepant outcomes.

Our theory differs in some crucial respects from the recent theorizing and data on habits as a form of motivation. One model of habit formation (Wood, Quinn, & Kashy, 2002) posits that the more often someone has engaged in a behavior to meet a goal, the more likely it is that the behavior will become a habit, which is to say that it will occur again in the future. Similarly, our model posits that a motivational drive is strengthened to the extent that it has been met with a satisfactory behavior in the past. However, we posit the presence of a desire and, accordingly, the pairing of a desire and a behavior that over time become linked. The main difference between the desire–behavior link described here and the Wood and colleagues (2002) model of habitual behaviors is that the latter lacks a wanting component, which provides the basis for reinforcement.

Habits are devoid of emotion, drive, or conscious thought, whereas each of these is sufficient to stimulate the getting–wanting model. A second, more speculative difference between this habit formation model and the getting–wanting model is that habits are associated with higher feelings of control (Wood et al., 2002), whereas getting and subsequent wanting, conversely, are characterized by lower feelings of control. Not feeling completely in control of one's wants or of one's ability to obtain relief again mirrors our emphasis on the getting-and-wanting pattern as a process akin to addiction. Thus a habit may be a behavior that is also predicted from earlier enactments of the behavior, but a lack of reinforcement and consequent unemotional process separates habits from getting–wanting processes.

One common and convincing manner of dividing the various human motivations is to think of a drive either to move toward or to recoil away from a target (good or bad, respectively) outcome (Elliot & Thrash, 2002; Higgins, 1997; Shah & Higgins, 2001). For instance, two sisters performing the same behavior of attending their children's school plays may be differentially motivated. One sister is driven by a desire to be a good mother (an approach motivation), whereas the other is drive by a desire not to be a bad mother (an avoidance motivation). Theorists (e.g., Carver, Sutton, & Scheier, 2000) have noted the difficulty of achieving avoidance motivations (e.g., the Nancy Reagan–inspired "Just say no to drugs" is a famous avoidance-motivated slogan that failed miserably). Instead, motivation theorists recommend transforming an avoidance motivation into an approach motivation because it tends to yield better outcomes. One reason, although there are several, for the success of approach-motivated endeavors may be that approach motivations allow for getting–wanting processes. In approach-motivated goals, a person with a drive to satisfy can use getting–wanting processes to his or her advantage. For instance, a woman may want to be in better shape, so she starts jogging. As long as jogging does not cause her severe physical pain or mental anguish, she may jog again—and the more often she jogs, the more she will want to jog, according to the model. Thus her overall goal of getting in shape is being reached. It is less easy to envision how an avoidance motivation can take advantage of the getting–wanting process (see Wegner, Ansfield, & Pilloff, 1998, on the difficulty of avoidance-related control strategies), but there may be some cases that are applicable to the getting–wanting process, such as therapeutic desensitization (discussed next). That said, most of the goals that we detail are approach-motivated, and we are encouraged for now about the ready appeal of the model to approach-motivated outcomes.

The therapeutic tactic of desensitization may be one form of the getting–wanting process that uses avoidance-related goals. This tactic is used in clinical psychology settings among patients who are intensely afraid of an object (e.g., a snake). To treat the phobia, these individuals are exposed to the feared object at different levels of intensity (e.g., first handling a picture of a rubber snake, then touching a rubber snake, then handling a picture of a live snake, and finally being exposed to and later touching a live snake). In a sense, then, the motivation to avoid the object (snake) is not reinforced, so it diminishes.

Two parallel mechanisms by which the getting-begets-wanting pattern may be reinforced are the *valuation* and *devaluation* effects. The valuation effect (Tversky & Kahneman, 1986) pertains to increased worth of an object that is perceived as allowing for the satisfaction of a need, such as the higher prices that people who smoke are willing to pay for cigarettes when they are in a state of nicotine deprivation than when they have recently satisfied their need for nicotine. The devaluation effect (Brendl, Markman, & Messner, 2003), conversely, has been proposed to explain the lower value of objects that are seen as unrelated to satisfying a need. Due to the valuation effect, when a need is satisfied by a particular object at Time 1, then that object will be known to be need-satisfying and therefore will be wanted more (i.e., will have high value) during subsequent occasions when the need is experienced. If the same object ceases to satisfy the need, it will eventually lose its high valuation and become, through the devaluation effect, less important. Eventually, if nothing can or does satisfy the need, the need itself may wither.

## SUMMARY AND CONCLUSION

The statement that someone is highly motivated for success implies a general view that motivations are stable characteristics of a person. The tendency to look for stable dispositions has perhaps led motivation theory to focus inadequately on how a person's level of a particular motivation or drive will change over time. The main such focus is what we have called the *satiation cycle*. When a drive is high, a creature will seek satisfaction, but when satisfaction is achieved the drive diminishes, only to reemerge gradually over time as the satisfaction wears off. When it's been a long time since eating, you feel hungry, which motivates you to seek and obtain food, but after you have eaten you feel less urgency to secure more food.

We have no quarrel with the satiation cycle. It depicts one pattern of within-animal fluctuation in motivation strength, and it seems likely that it is correct. We want to suggest another pattern of systematic fluctuation within the same animal, though possible only creatures with the cognitive flexibility of humans can fully exhibit this pattern.

Specifically, the pattern is what we have called *getting begets wanting* (and *not getting gradually reduces subsequent wanting*). Due possibly to the extended now of human mental processing, people can learn from rewards and punishments that come more than a few seconds after the operant. And we suggest that motivational states operate like operants, such that rewarded ones will become stronger and more frequent, whereas unsatisfied ones will gradually diminish in force and frequency.

The broad implication is that human desires will ebb and flow as a result of whether they find and bring satisfactions. A desire for something that is followed by intense, blissful satisfaction is likely to emerge again soon, and so the person will look again for the satisfaction he or she has found. A desire that leads nowhere except to boredom and frustration may be a bit slower to emerge the next time around, and it may not feel as strong the next time.

To have drive states wax and wane as a function of their apparent consequences should create a broad motivational plasticity. It should allow people to become progressively less troubled by hopeless desires, and conversely it should enable them to zero in on activities and spheres where they can and do find satisfaction. In this way, a person's complement of motivated strivings will shift to feature the motivations that are productive and that therefore ultimately improve survival and reproduction.

Ultimately, this process should to some degree shift the balance of power between person and environment. Essentially, it should allow people to change their hierarchies of motives and strivings toward sets that will be workable in their cultural environments. An organism that can reshuffle its deck of motivations so as to emphasize ones that do bring satisfaction will fit into its environment much better than an organism whose wants and needs stubbornly remain constant, impervious to circumstances and opportunities.

To put it more bluntly: It is better (more useful, more productive, more adaptive) to want what one can get than what one can't get. Thus it would be beneficial for getting to stimulate further wanting, and for chronically unfilled yearnings to diminish over time.

## ACKNOWLEDGMENTS

Preparation of this chapter was supported by National Institutes of Health Grant No. MH12794 (to Kathleen D. Vohs) and Grant No. MH 57039 (to Roy F. Baumeister); funding from the Social Sciences and Humanities Research Council to Kathleen D. Vohs; and support from the Canada Research Chair Council and the McKnight Land-Grant Professorship funds to Kathleen D. Vohs.

## REFERENCES

American Psychiatric Association (APA). (2000). *Diagnostic and statistical manual of mental disorders* (4th ed., text rev.). Washington, DC: Author.

Aron, A., Norman, C. C., Aron, E. N., McKenna, C., & Heyman, R. E. (2000). Couples' shared participation in novel and arousing activities and experienced relationship quality. *Journal of Personality and Social Psychology, 78*, 273–284.

Atkins, R. C. (1992). *Dr. Atkins' new diet revolution.* New York: Avon Books.

Baumeister, R. F. (2005). *The cultural animal: Human nature, meaning, and social life.* New York: Oxford University Press.

Baumeister, R. F., & Bratslavsky, E. (1999). Passion, intimacy, and time: Passionate love as a function of change in intimacy. *Personality and Social Psychology Review, 3*, 49–67.

Baumeister, R. F., & Leary, M. R. (1995). The need to belong: Desire for interpersonal attachments as a fundamental human motivation. *Psychological Bulletin, 117*, 497–529.

Baumeister, R. F., & Vohs, K. D. (2001). Narcissism as addiction to esteem. *Psychological Inquiry, 12*, 206–210.

Berridge, K. C. (1999). Pleasure, pain, desire and dread: Hidden core processes of emotion. In D. Kahneman,

E. Diener, & N. Schwarz (Eds.), *Well-being: The foundations of hedonic psychology* (pp. 525—557). New York: Russell Sage Foundation.

Brehm, J. W. (1966). *A theory of psychological reactance*. New York: Academic Press.

Brendl, C. M., Markman, A. B., & Messner, C. (2003). The devaluation effect: Activating a need devalues unrelated objects. *Journal of Consumer Research, 29*, 463–473.

Brickman, P., & Campbell, D. T. (1971). Hedonic relativism and planning the good society. In M. H. Appley (Ed.), *Adaptation level theory: A symposium* (pp. 287–302). New York: Academic Press.

Bushman, B. J., & Baumeister, R. F. (1998). Threatened egotism, narcissism, self-esteem, and direct and displaced aggression: Does self-love or self-hate lead to violence? *Journal of Personality and Social Psychology, 75*, 219–229.

Bushman, B. J., Baumeister, R. F., & Phillips, C. M. (2001). Do people aggress to improve their mood?: Catharsis beliefs, affect regulation opportunity, and aggressive responding. *Journal of Personality and Social Psychology, 81*, 17–32.

Bushman, B. J., Baumeister, R. F., & Stack, A. D. (1999). Catharsis, aggression, and persuasive influence: Self-fulfilling or self-defeating prophecies? *Journal of Personality and Social Psychology, 76*, 367–376.

Campbell, W. K. (1999). Narcissism and romantic attraction. *Journal of Personality and Social Psychology, 77*, 1254–1270.

Campbell, W. K., Rudich, E. A., & Sedikides, C. (2002). Narcissism, self-esteem, and the positivity of self-views: Two portraits of self-love. *Personality and Social Psychology Bulletin, 28*, 358–368.

Carver, C. S., Sutton, S. K., & Scheier, M. F. (2000). Action, emotion, and personality: Emerging conceptual integration. *Personality and Social Psychology Bulletin, 26*, 741–751.

Diener, E., Suh, E. M., Lucas, R. E., & Smith, H. L. (1999). Subjective well-being: Three decades of progress. *Psychological Bulletin, 125*, 276–302.

Elliot, A. J., & Thrash, T. M. (2002). Approach–avoidance motivation in personality: Approach and avoidance temperaments and goals. *Journal of Personality and Social Psychology, 82*, 804–818.

Freud, S. (1957). Instincts and their vicissitudes. In J. Strachey (Ed. & Trans.), *The standard edition of the complete psychological works of Sigmund Freud* (Vol. 14, pp. 111–142). London: Hogarth Press. (Original work published 1915)

Geen, R. G., & Berkowitz, L. (1966). Name-mediated aggressive cue properties. *Journal of Personality, 34*, 456–465.

Geen, R. G., & Quanty, M. B. (1977). The catharsis of aggression: An evaluation of a hypothesis. In L. Berkowitz (Ed.), *Advances in experimental social psychology* (Vol. 10, pp. 1–37). New York: Academic Press.

Heine, S. J., Proulx, T., & Vohs, K. D. (2006). Meaning maintenance model: On the coherence of social motivations. *Review of Social and Personality Psychology, 10*, 88–110.

Helson, H. (1964). *Adaptation-level theory: An experimental and systematic approach to behavior.* New York: Harper & Row.

Higgins, E. T. (1997). Beyond pleasure and pain. *American Psychologist, 52*, 1280–1300.

Hull, C. L. (1943). *Principles of behavior.* New York: Appleton-Century-Crofts.

Kasser, T., & Ryan, R. M. (1993). A dark side of the American dream: Correlates of financial success as a central life aspiration. *Journal of Personality and Social Psychology, 65*, 410–422.

Kasser, T., & Ryan, R. M. (1996). Further examining the American dream: Differential correlates of intrinsic and extrinsic goals. *Personality and Social Psychology Bulletin, 22*, 280–287.

Lewis, D. J. (1952). Partial reinforcement in a gambling situation. *Journal of Experimental Psychology, 43*, 447–450.

Lewis, D. J., & Duncan, C. P. (1956). Effect of different percentages of money rewards on extinction of a lever-pulling response. *Journal of Experimental Psychology, 52*, 23–27.

Lewis, D. J., & Duncan, C. P. (1957). Expectation and resistence to extinction of a lever-pulling response as functions of percentage of reinforcement and amount of reward. *Journal of Experimental Psychology, 54*, 115–120.

Lewis, D. J., & Duncan, C. P. (1958). Expectation and resistance to extinction of a lever-pulling response as a function of percentage of reinforcement and number of acquisition trials. *Journal of Experimental Psychology, 55*, 121–128.

Lovelace, L., with McGrady, M. (1980). *Ordeal.* Secaucus, NJ: Citadel Press.

Martens, A., Kosloff, S., Greenberg, J., Landau, M., & Schmader, T. (2006, January). *Killing begets killing.* Poster presented at the annual conference of the Society for Personality and Social Psychology, Palm Springs, CA.

Morf, C. C., & Rhodewalt, F. (2001). Unraveling the paradoxes of narcissism: A dynamic self-regulatory processing model. *Psychological Inquiry, 12*, 177–196.

Peele, S., & Brodsky, A. (1975). *Love and addiction.* New York: Taplinger.

Pinel, J. P. J., Assanand, S., & Lehman, D. R. (2000). Hunger, eating, and ill health. *American Psychologist, 55*, 1105–1116

Rhodewalt, F., Madrian, J. C., & Cheney, S. (1998). Narcissism, self-knowledge organization, and emotional reactivity: The effect of daily experiences on self-esteem and affect. *Personality and Social Psychology Bulletin, 24*, 75–87.

Rhodewalt, F., & Morf, C. (1995). Self and interpersonal correlates of the Narcissistic Personality Inventory: A review and new findings. *Journal of Research in Personality, 29*, 1–23.

Roberts, W. A. (2002). Are animals stuck in time? *Psychological Bulletin, 128*, 473–489.

Shah, J., & Higgins, E. T. (2001). Regulatory concerns and appraisal efficiency: The general impact of promotion and prevention. *Journal of Personality and Social Psychology, 80*, 693–705.

Siegel, S., Hinson, R. E., Krank, M. D., & McCully, J. (1982). Heroin "overdose" death: Contribution of drug-associated environmental cues. *Science, 216*, 436–437.

Sirgy, M. J. (1998). Materialism and quality of life. *Social Indicators Research, 43*, 227–260.

Spence, K. W. (1956). *Behavior theory and conditioning.* New Haven, CT: Yale University Press.

Tversky, A., & Kahneman, D. (1986). Judgment under uncertainty: Heuristics and biases. In H. R. Arkes & K. R. Hammond (Eds.), *Judgment and decision making: An interdisciplinary reader* (pp. 38–55). New York: Cambridge University Press.

Vallerand, R. J., Blanchard, C., Mageau, G. A., Koestner, R., Ratelle, C., Léonard, M., et al. (2003). Les passions de l'âme: On obsessive and harmonious passion. *Journal of Personality and Social Psychology, 85*, 756–767.

Vohs, K. D., & Schmeichel, B. J. (2003). Self-regulation and extended now: Controlling the self alters the subjective experience of time. *Journal of Personality and Social Psychology, 85*, 217–230.

Wallace, H. M., & Baumeister, R. F. (2002). The performance of narcissists rises and falls with perceived opportunity for glory. *Journal of Personality and Social Psychology, 82*, 819–834.

Wegner, D. M., Ansfield, M., & Pilloff, D. (1998). The putt and the pendulum: Ironic effects of the mental control of action. *Psychological Science, 9*, 196–199.

Weiss, J. M. (1971). Effects of coping behavior with and without a feedback signal on stress pathology in rats. *Journal of Comparative and Physiological Psychology, 77*, 22–30.

Wilson, T. D., Gilbert, D. T., & Centerbar, D. B. (2003). Making sense: The causes of emotional evanescence. In I. Brocas & J. Carrillo (Eds.), *The psychology of economic decisions: Vol. 1. Rationality and well being* (pp. 209–233). New York: Oxford University Press.

Wood, W., Quinn, J. M., & Kashy, D. A. (2002). Habits in everyday life: Thought, emotion, and action. *Journal of Personality and Social Psychology, 83*, 1281–1297.

World Health Organization. (1977). *Manual of the international statistical classification of diseases, injuries, and causes of death* (Vol. 1). Geneva: Author.

Zajonc, R. B. (2001). Mere exposure: A gateway to the subliminal. *Current Directions in Psychological Science, 10*, 224–228.

# MOTIVATIONAL DIFFERENCES

Chapter 25

# The Role of Goal Investment in Self-Regulation

## BENEFITS AND COSTS

**Eva M. Pomerantz**
**Serena Shim**

Throughout life, individuals are faced with a variety of *goals*—that is, desired ends, such as doing well in school, being well liked by others, taking on an effective leadership role, and raising well-functioning children. A wealth of research indicates that beginning in early childhood and continuing throughout the course of life, individuals differ in how they regulate their progress toward accomplishing their goals (e.g., Dweck & Leggett, 1988; Ziegert, Kistner, Castro, & Robertson, 2001). Because such self-regulation may have implications for individuals' success in meeting their goals, as well as for their emotional functioning, a key issue is that of the characteristics that enhance it. Indeed, much theory and research has been directed toward elucidating this issue (e.g., Crocker & Wolfe, 2001; Dweck & Leggett, 1988; Eccles, 1983; Higgins, 1987).

In this chapter we make the case that when individuals are very invested in their goals, their regulation of their progress toward accomplishing them is intensified, because success and failure in this endeavor are particularly meaningful. We begin with a discussion of what it means to be invested in one's goals, with attention to related phenomena. We then turn to delineating the idea that individuals' heightened goal investment creates an intensified self-regulatory system. Subsequently, we highlight the benefits and costs of the regulatory processes that ensue when individuals are highly invested in their goals. Lastly, we identify potential moderators of the benefits and costs.

### DEFINING GOAL INVESTMENT

The notion of *goal investment* was first raised in psychology by William James (1890) when he proposed that individuals differ in the importance they place on multiple arenas (e.g., academics, social relations, and parenting) of their lives. He argued that the more personally important an arena is, the more likely it is that feelings of competence in the domain contribute to self-esteem. This idea generated much research as investigators in the areas of personality and social psychology sought empirical support for it (e.g., Harter, 1993; Marsh, 1993; Pelham & Swann, 1989). Indeed, since James's writings, constructs similar to that of investment can be found throughout psychology. For example, in theory and research concerned with attitudes (e.g., toward capital punishment, abortion rights, and university tuition increases), the personal importance of the issue appears to play a key role in the strength of the attitude individuals hold (for a review, see Boninger, Krosnick, Berent, & Fabrigar, 1995), with such importance often being tied to individuals' identity (Pomerantz, Chaiken, & Tordesillas, 1995). In the area of organizational psychology, commitment to the organization and its goals has been a topic of central concern, producing a plethora of theory and research focused on understanding job satisfaction and productivity (for a review, see Meyer, 1997).

Notions reflecting investment in one's goals are perhaps most prevalent in the large body of theory and research concerned with motivation. Although the labels, definitions, and methods have varied across research programs, over the last half of the 20th century substantial attention has been directed toward understanding individuals' investment in their goals. Much of the attention has been in the context of work attempting to understand individual differences as they manifest themselves in an alternative unit of analysis to the trait. In this vein, Emmons (1986; Emmons & King, 1988) studied individuals' *personal strivings* (i.e., the goals individuals are attempting to accomplish). One of the characteristics on which he focused was the personal importance individuals assign to their strivings. In a similar endeavor, Little and colleagues (e.g., Little, 1983; Palys & Little, 1983) studied individuals' personal projects (i.e., an interrelated sequence of actions in which individuals engage to achieve their goals). Investment in this work emerged as a central dimension in factor analyses examining multiple aspects of personal projects. For example, McGregor and Little (1998) identified a factor they labeled *integrity*, which included not only the personal importance individuals place on their personal projects and their commitment to them, but also the centrality of individuals' projects to their identity and the congruency of their projects with their values—similar to some extent to Sheldon's (Chapter 30, this volume) idea of *self-concordance*.

Constructs similar to goal investment also characterize other major programs of research related to motivation. First, work using an expectancy–value framework is concerned with goal investment in its focus on *value*, which is commonly defined as the importance individuals place on a particular arena (e.g., Atkinson, 1964; Feather, 1990). Eccles (e.g., Eccles & Wigfield, 2002) distinguished among *attainment value* (i.e., the personal importance of doing well on a task), *utility value* (i.e., the relation of a task to current and future goals), and *intrinsic value* (i.e., the enjoyment individuals get from engaging in goal-related activities or the subjective interest individuals have in the goal-related activities). Although attainment value is most similar to the notion of investment, investment is also likely to be related to utility and intrinsic value. Indeed, Eccles, Wigfield, Harold, and Blumenfeld (1993) combined the three aspects of value because they were strongly associated. Second, Harackiewicz and colleagues (e.g., Elliot et al., 2000; Harackiewicz & Manderlink, 1984) defined *competence valuation* as affective commitment to performing well. According to these investigators, such commitment can be reflected in how much individuals care about doing well at an activity and how personally important it is for them to do so. Third, several investigators have depicted goal investment as reflecting *ego involvement* in goal pursuit (e.g., Robins & Beers, 2001). Perhaps most prominently, in the context of self-completion theory, Wicklund and Gollwitzer (1982) focus on commitment to *self-defining goals*, with the idea that it creates a continual striving to acquire the identity reflected in such goals.

Drawing from these conceptualizations, we define *goal investment* as placing much importance on goal accomplishment and being highly committed to this endeavor. The notion of *commitment* is often a central element in the goal concept, either implicitly or explicitly, so that part of holding a goal is being committed to pursuing the desired end reflected in the goal (Elliot & Fryer, Chapter 15, this volume). We see goal investment as representing commitment beyond that necessary to simply holding a goal. Thus even individuals who are not highly invested in a goal they hold have a minimal amount of commitment to it. Although several lines of evidence indicate that individuals feel that their personal worth is contingent on meeting the goals in which they are highly invested (e.g., McGregor & Little, 1998; Pomerantz, Saxon, & Oishi, 2000), we do not see such feelings as necessarily part of goal investment, unlike some prior conceptualizations (e.g., Robins & Beers, 2001; Wicklund & Gollwitzer, 1982). Individuals' investment may not always be accompanied by the feeling that their worth is contingent on accomplishing their goals (Crocker & Wolfe, 2001). Although the association between investment and contingent self-worth is strong, it does not suggest that the two are completely overlapping (Pomerantz et al., 2000). Indeed, individuals may sometimes be invested in their goals because they see attainment as yielding desirable consequences (e.g., monetary rewards, stimulating opportunities, and increased knowledge) unrelated to their self-worth.

Individuals' investment may manifest itself at multiple levels. James's (1890) general assumption was that most people are invested in attaining competence in at least one arena of their life, with the arena of most importance varying across individuals. In line with this perspective, Pelham (Pelham & Swann, 1989; Pelham, 1995a) highlighted that the relative importance individuals assign to their multiple goals (intrapersonal variability) is essential, regardless of the actual level of importance individuals assign (interpersonal variability). Indeed, most individuals exhibit variability in their investment in their multiple goals (e.g., Pelham & Swann, 1989; Pomerantz et al., 2000), suggesting that they have a hierarchy of investment. However, individuals also differ from one another in how invested they are in their goals overall (see Pomerantz et al., 2000; Shah, Friedman, & Kruglanski, 2002). Hence investment hierarchies are likely to be nested within a general level of investment. Some individuals may generally not be very invested in their goals; thus their differential investment may occur at low levels of investment. In contrast, for others, differential investment may occur at the high end of the investment continuum. Supporting this notion, ratings of personal importance across multiple arenas form one factor, despite the variability in individuals' investment in their multiple goals (Pomerantz et al., 2000). As is the case with other individual differences (see Higgins, 1990), there may be stable differences in investment hierarchies and levels; however, both may be sensitive to situational influences, so that individuals' investment may wax and wane as they encounter a variety of situations. Regardless of whether investment is at an intraindividual or interindividual level, or of whether it is an ongoing individual difference or elicited by the situation, investment is likely to influence individuals' regulation of their progress toward their goals. We now turn to discussing this issue.

## THE ROLE OF GOAL INVESTMENT IN SELF-REGULATION

The term *self-regulation* has been used to refer to various phenomena related to individuals' pursuit of their goals (e.g., Carver & Scheier, 1998; Eccles, Wigfield, & Schiefele, 1998; Higgins, 1996; Ryan & Connell, 1989). Drawing on this prior work, we define *self-regulation* as individuals' management, either conscious or unconscious, of their progress toward their goals. Such management manifests itself in individuals' goal-oriented *behavior* (e.g., the effort children exert to do well in school and the information seeking parents do about their parenting skills). Self-regulation has a *cognitive* component (e.g., children's perceptions of competence to do well in school and parents' worrying over their parenting practices) as well, which may promote or prevent goal pursuit and eventual goal attainment. In addition, *affect* (e.g., children's sadness after failing an exam and parents' happiness when their parenting practices are effective) is a critical aspect of the self-regulatory system, because individuals' affective responses to their success and failure may be instrumental in the goal pursuit process (see Carver & Scheier, Chapter 20, this volume). In this section, we make the case that individuals' regulation of their progress toward the goals in which they are very invested is intensified in terms of their behavior, cognition, and affect. In essence, individuals are highly motivated to promote success and prevent failure in the pursuit of the goals in which they are very invested, because such success and failure are particularly meaningful to them—given the implications either for their self-worth or for realizing desirable consequences (Pomerantz et al., 2000).

### Behavior: Heightened Positive Engagement

As individuals attempt to promote success and prevent failure in the context of meeting the goals in which they are highly invested, they may become exceptionally engaged in goal-related activities. In fact, Brunstein (1993) identified engagement as a key characteristic of investment. In line with the notion that investment heightens engagement, the more both children and adults are invested in their goals, the higher they report their engagement in goal-related activities to be (e.g., Emmons, 1986; Pelham, 1995b; Pomerantz et al., 2000), as well as their intentions for future engagement (Meece, Wigfield, & Eccles, 1990). For example, in a daily diary study with children in elementary and junior high school, we found that on days children felt school was particularly important, they reported being particularly engaged (e.g., paying attention and working hard) in school (Pomerantz & Shim, 2006b). Notably, the effect of investment on engagement extended to the next day, even when children's engagement the prior day was taken into account. Individuals' heightened effort exerted in the mission of meeting the goals in which they are highly invested appears to be particularly pronounced when challenge is encountered (e.g., Parsons, Adler, & Meece, 1984). For example, in a laboratory study with college students (Pomerantz & Shim, 2006b), we manipulated investment by either providing information that a test students were going to take was highly diagnostic of their future success (high investment) or providing no such information (low investment). Students in the high-investment condition spent more time on difficult, but not easy, problems than did students in the low-investment condition.

The engagement fostered by investment is characterized by several positive qualities. Shah and colleagues (2002) showed that the more committed college students are to their goals, the more they are able to suppress alternative goals; this suggests that when individuals are highly engaged in the pursuit of the goals in which they are most invested, they are likely to remain focused even when tempted by other pursuits that may be more enjoyable in the short term. Indeed, Shah and colleagues found that the ability to inhibit alternative goals is associated with heightened persistence. Individuals' engagement in the pursuit of the goals in which they are invested also appears to involve heightened information seeking, which may allow individuals to develop effective strategies for reaching their goals: The more importance college students place on their goals, the more they want information about their competence to meet them (Trope & Pomerantz, 1998). Notably, students report being interested in information about their assets as well as their liabilities; this suggests that their information seeking may be relatively unbiased, allowing them to develop strategies that take into account both there strengths and weaknesses.

### Cognition: Perceiving Oneself as Competent, but Worrying Anyway

As a consequence of their engagement, individuals may perceive themselves as quite capable of meeting the goals in which they are very invested. Moreover, in an effort to protect themselves against the negative implications of failure, individuals may sometimes even construct their reality so that they perceive themselves as capable of meeting their goals when in actuality they are not (see Pelham, 1995b; Pomerantz et al., 2000; Robins & Beers, 2001; Tesser, 1988; Wicklund & Gollwitzer, 1982). Consistent with the idea that individuals view themselves as capable of meeting the goals in which they are very invested, the more invested both children and adults are in meeting their goals, the more they perceive themselves as possessing areas of competence relevant to meeting their goals (e.g., Berndt & Miller, 1990; Eccles & Wigfield, 1995; Emmons, 1986; Pelham, 1995b). In our daily diary research, on the days on which children felt school was particularly important, they perceived themselves as particularly competent in school (Pomerantz & Shim, 2006b). Notably, investment actually appears to foreshadow perceptions of competence. This is true among elementary and middle school children not only from one day to the next (Pomerantz & Shim, 2006b), but also over 6 months (Pomerantz et al., 2000), even when initial perceptions of competence are taken into account. Moreover, when we have manipulated investment in the lab (as described earlier), college students in the high-investment condition expect to do better at the test they are to take than do their counterparts in the low-investment condition (Pomerantz & Shim, 2006b). Although individuals' positive beliefs about their capability to meet the goals in which they are very invested may often be accurate, at times they may be overestimates (Robins & Beers, 2001).

Despite the positive beliefs individuals hold about their capability to meet the goals in which they are highly invested, other aspects of their cognition may not be positive. Individuals may worry over whether or not they will attain the goals in which they are invested, because of the heightened significance of doing so (see Pomerantz et al., 2000). Moreover, their increased engagement in goal-related activities may increase their worrying, as they have more experience with what can go awry. Supportive of the possibility that investment fosters worrying, the more invested individuals are in their goals, the more anxious they are (Kasser & Ryan, 1996).[1] Research from our lab indicates that investment actually foreshadows worrying: Elementary school children who were highly invested in their goals were more prone to worrying a year later, even after we adjusted for their earlier worrying (Pomerantz et al., 2000). We replicated such a foreshadowing effect in the day-to-day analyses of our daily diary study: Children not only worried more about their school progress on days they were very invested in school, but also worried more the next day, even after we adjusted for their prior worrying (Pomerantz & Shim, 2006b).

## Affect: Falling Hard, but Bouncing Back Easily

Given the heightened meaning individuals assign to their success and failure in the pursuit of the goals in which they are invested, they may show heightened affective responses to their success and failure. Indeed, James (1890) speculated that individuals feel particularly positive about themselves when they meet their personally important goals, but feel particularly negative when they fail to do so. In line with James, several investigators have found that children and college students feel more positive about themselves when they perceive themselves as possessing competence in personally important arenas of their lives, but feel more negative about themselves when they perceive themselves as lacking competence in such arenas (e.g., Harter, 1993; Maier & Brunstein, 2001; Pelham, 1995b; Pelham & Swann, 1989). However, several investigators have also failed to find such effects, leading to arguments that they do not exist (e.g., Campbell, 1986; Marsh, 1993, 1995; Pomerantz et al., 2000).

The intensified self-regulatory system generated by heightened goal investment makes it likely that both sets of findings reflect reality. It is just that (contrary to James's original assumption) the negative responses to failure may often only be temporary, because the intensified self-regulatory system ensuing from goal investment involves engagement and perceptions of competence that allow individuals to bounce back easily. Thus, when individuals are invested in their goals, they may fall hard in response to failure as James postulated, but also bounce back from it with ease. Individuals' responses to their failure to meet the goals in which they are highly invested may be an exaggerated version of the affective forecasting effect documented by Gilbert and Wilson (e.g., Gilbert, Pinel, Wilson, Blumberg, & Wheatley, 1998), in which individuals predict that when they fail it will be a long-lasting negative experience from which they will suffer emotionally, but when they actually fail their psychological resources allow them to bounce back relatively quickly.

To directly examine the idea that individuals are highly responsive to their successes and failures in their pursuit of the goals in which they are very invested, we manipulated college students' goal investment (Pomerantz & Shim, 2006a). As in our earlier research, we told students in the high-investment condition that they would be taking a test that is diagnostic of future success; we told students in the low-investment condition that they would be taking a test that was once thought to be diagnostic of future success, but that more recent research has shown is actually not diagnostic. In the context of answering questions on a variety of topics, students indicated how happy they were at the moment. They then took the test. Subsequent to completing the test, half of the students in each condition were given failure feedback, and half were given success feedback. Immediately after receiving this feedback, students again indicated how happy they were at the moment (embedded in a set of filler questions). They were then left alone in the testing room with nothing to do for 8 minutes, allowing them time to contemplate their performance. When the experimenter returned, students again indicated how happy they were at the moment, in the context of a final set of questions.

In the success condition, there was a marginal tendency for students in the high-investment condition to be happier than their counterparts in the low-investment condition immediately after success. However—in line with the idea that individuals often respond more strongly to negative events than to positive ones (Baumeister, Bratslavsky, Finkenauer, & Vohs, 2001)—although all students experienced a dip in their happiness immediately after failure, this was particularly pronounced for students in the high-investment condition, such that they were much less happy than their counterparts in the low-investment condition at this point. Notably, consistent with our proposal that the self-regulatory system produced by investment should prohibit a lasting downward spiral in the face of failure, the high-investment students were no less happy 8 minutes later than the low-investment students. We replicated this affective "falling hard, but bouncing back easily" effect in the face of failure among elementary and junior high school children in our daily diary study. Although children highly invested in school were likely to feel particularly unhappy on days they experienced a failure in school (e.g., did poorly on a test or received a poor grade on a homework assignment), they bounced back in terms of their emotional experience the following day, so that they were no less unhappy than the day before the failure.

Research by Brunstein and Gollwitzer (1996) suggests that one reason why individuals' emotional experience may bounce back so easily after failure at meeting the goals in which they are invested is that they quickly find opportunities to rectify their failure through engagement in other tasks related to such goals (see also Gollwitzer & Wicklund, 1985). These investigators manipulated investment in the laboratory by framing a test on which college students worked as either relevant (high-investment) to success in the profession (e.g., medicine) they were committed to pursuing or irrelevant (low-investment). Participants receiving failure feedback on a relevant test and then given an opportunity to work on another test that was not relevant were particularly likely to do poorly on the subsequent test, due in part to their lack of engagement in the irrelevant test. However, if the subsequent test was relevant to their profession, students were particularly likely to do well, due in part to their engagement in the test. Similarly, in our daily diary study, the engagement in school of children who were very invested in school fell on days they experienced a failure in school; it was actually lower than that of children who were not invested on such days. However, by the next day their engagement increased, so that they were more engaged than their less invested counterparts, as was the case the day before their failure. Thus it appears that individuals can bounce back from their failure in the context of the pursuit of the goals in which they are highly invested when they are given a chance to rectify the situation through enhanced engagement.

Unfortunately, opportunities for engagement may not always be available; even when they are, engagement may not always yield success, particularly in the short term. Under such conditions, individuals may work at cognitively construing the situation so that they are able to view themselves as capable of meeting the goals in which they are invested, thereby allowing themselves to bounce back from failure in terms of their affect (see Robins & Beers, 2001; Tesser, 1988). In one test of such an idea, Wagner, Wicklund, and Shaigan (1990) found that when the success of college students who were committed to becoming psychologists was threatened, such students were more likely than their uncommitted counterparts to further denigrate the competence of a fellow student they already saw as lacking competence. Moreover, they also distanced themselves from the fellow student, reporting that their relationship with the student was not particularly close and that the student was not particularly likeable. Such cognitive constructions may often be a last resort, because although they may lead individuals to feel good and even maintain their motivation, they may mean ignoring important information about how to improve one's ability to attain personally important goals.

## Summary

The self-regulatory system generated by heightened goal investment is one in which goal-related behavior, cognition, and affect are intensified. In terms of behavior, individuals are highly likely to be exceptionally engaged in an often effective manner in the pursuit of the goals in which they are invested. In terms of cognition, a similar intensity is evident: Individuals hold highly positive perceptions of their competence to reach the goals in which they are invested, but also worry over whether they will actually do so. Finally, individuals' self-regulatory affect is heightened: It is highly responsive to their progress, particularly failure, to meet the goals in which they are invested.

## THE BENEFITS AND COSTS OF GOAL INVESTMENT

A key question is that of whether it is worthwhile to promote goal investment in an effort to enhance individuals' psychological functioning, or whether doing so may have some costs that actually interfere with such functioning. In this section we make the case that goal investment and its self-regulatory system have benefits along important dimensions of psychological functioning, but that they also have costs. Hence, although it may be valuable to encourage individuals to become invested in their goals, minimizing the potential costs is essential in this endeavor.

### Benefits

Elevated goal investment and the ensuing self-regulation have several notable benefits. One is that the heightened, often high-quality engagement in goal-related activities may lead to success. In this context, the attention that individuals pay to their failure in the pursuit of the goals in which they are invested may lead them not only to work harder to meet their goals (Brunstein & Gollwitzer, 1996; Pomerantz & Shim, 2006a), but also to develop effective strategies that take into account their past mistakes. Consistent with this, several studies have found that the more invested children and adults are in their goals, the more likely they are to accomplish them (Berndt & Miller, 1990; Meece et al., 1990; Pomerantz & Shim, 2006b; Shah et al., 2002); however, it is not always clear that investment actually foreshadows enhanced performance (Meece et al., 1990; Pomerantz & Shim, 2006b). It is possible that although the worrying individuals do over the goals in which they are invested may spur them to become engaged, it may also disrupt their focus, so that their engagement is less productive than it might otherwise be over time. However, to the extent that individuals are invested in valued goals (e.g., doing well in school and supporting others who are less fortunate), simply being engaged in such activities may be beneficial, in that it gives life meaning (e.g., Csikszentmihalyi, 1997; Dong & Pomerantz, 2006; Hunter & Csikszentmihalyi, 2003) and inhibits engagement in delinquent activities.

The tendency for individuals to fall hard, but bounce back easily, when confronted with failure to meet the goals in which they are invested may have benefits for individuals' regulation of not only the goals at which they have failed, but also the other goals they hold. Carver and Scheier (Chapter 20, this volume) argue that individuals' affect may serve to signal how much effort they should direct toward a task. According to these investigators, negative affect indicates to individuals that they are making less than optimal progress toward their goals; as such, negative affect may serve to boost goal-related efforts. In contrast, positive affect indicates that more than adequate progress has been made. Carver and Scheier argue that such positive affect may place individuals in a coasting mode in which they do not exert effort toward goals triggering such affect, unless there is evidence that something has gone awry. This frees up resources that individuals can devote to pursuing other goals. Thus individuals' heightened affective responsiveness to their progress toward the goals in which they are invested may be beneficial, in that it may create a system in which individuals are able to devote their resources to their multiple goals—some of which may be highly important to them, and some of which may be highly important to significant others.

The intensified self-regulation generated by investment is also likely to have benefits for individuals' emotional functioning. To the extent that engagement involves taking part in meaningful activities, it may produce positive emotional experiences (e.g., Csikszentmihalyi, 1997; Dong & Pomerantz, 2006; Hunter & Csikszentmihalyi, 2003). Individuals' positive perceptions of their competence, as well as their actual success, at meeting the goals in which they are invested has also been identified as important to subsequent emotional functioning (e.g., Cole, Martin, Peeke, Seroczynski, & Fier, 1999; Pomerantz & Rudolph, 2003; Taylor & Brown, 1988). Moreover, individuals' ability to bounce back easily from failure in terms of their affect may allow for the maintenance of positive emotional experiences. In line with these notions, the more invested individuals are in their goals, the more positive their emotional functioning is (e.g., Emmons, 1986; Palys & Little, 1983). Notably, investment appears to produce such experiences. Elementary school children's investment is predictive of decreased depressive symptoms over the course of a year, even after adjustment for their earlier depressive symptoms (Pomerantz et al., 2000). Moreover, elementary and junior high school children's investment in school predicts increased positive, but not negative, emotions from one day to the next as well as over 6 months, even after adjustment for earlier emotions (Dong & Pomerantz, 2006; Pomerantz & Shim, 2006b). A comparable picture emerges when college students are asked to think about either their most important or their least important personal striving: After thinking about their most important one, they report more positive emotional experiences than after thinking about their least important one (Pomerantz & Shim, 2006b).

## Costs

The benefits of goal investment and its self-regulatory system are impressive, in that they cover some of the most important areas of psychological functioning. As such, they may lead to the conclusion that assisting individuals to become very invested in their goals is an efficient aid to enhancing psychological functioning. Such an endeavor has the potential to be very effective indeed. However, caution is warranted about painting too rosy a picture of the intensified self-regulatory system cultivated by investment, because it may have some costs beyond worrying and the anxiety symptoms that may ensue. For one, when individuals are not making adequate progress toward the goals in which they are highly invested, their heightened engagement in pursuing these goals may come at the expense of engagement in the pursuit of other goals (see Carver & Scheier, Chapter 20, this volume; Shah et al., 2002). Over the long term, disregarding the pursuit of the latter goals may have costs if individuals fail to pursue goals that are important to themselves, their significant others, or society more generally. Costs may occur not only because individuals have neglected these other arenas of their lives, but also because in pursuit of the goals in which they are highly invested, individuals may engage in behavior that actually hurts these other arenas. For example, in a study conducted by Tesser and Smith (1980), college students who were told that a task assessed important intellectual skills gave their friends more difficult cues than college students who were told that the task was a game. Thus individuals' efforts to prove to themselves that they are capable of meeting the goals in which they are very invested may come at the expense of being a good friend (see also Gollwitzer & Wicklund, 1985).

Another cost of the self-regulatory system cultivated by investment is the tendency for individuals to overestimate their capability for meeting the goals in which they are invested. Although a number of investigators have argued that such positive illusions may be beneficial (e.g., Taylor & Brown, 1988), the case has also been made that overestimating personal competence can have negative consequences (Colvin & Block, 1994; Paulhus, 1998). Unrealistically positive beliefs may be beneficial, in that they maintain goal pursuit and positive affect in relation to such pursuit. However, such beliefs may not serve such a function indefinitely, because individuals may eventually be forced to realize that they will not be able to accomplish the goals in which they are invested (Robins & Beers, 2001). Such a realization may diminish goal pursuit and positive emotional experiences. In line with this notion, Robins and Beer (2001) demonstrated that perceiving personal capabilities in an overly positive light may have benefits in the short term, but costs in the long term. College students who overestimated their competence in the context of a group task experienced an increase in positive affect right after participating in the task. However, when the longer-term effects of such self-enhancement were examined, a different picture emerged: Students who entered college overestimating their academic competence decreased their investment in doing well in college over their 4 years there. Moreover, although such students entered college with heightened subjective well-being, they experienced a decline in this dimension of functioning during their stay at college.

Costs may also be incurred because opportunities to bounce back from failure, through either enhanced engagement or cognitive distortion, do not always exist. This, in conjunction with the worrying that ensues from investment, may place individuals at risk for negative emotional experiences in certain contexts. As Brunstein and Gollwitzer's (1996) research (described earlier) shows, when individuals encounter failure at meeting the goals in which they are invested and do not have the opportunity to pursue such goals further, they experience costs in terms of their performance on tasks unrelated to the goals in which they are invested. This appears to be due to the tendency to ruminate over failure connected to the goals in which one is highly invested. Similar negative consequences may ensue when individuals do not have the opportunity to construe their reality so that they perceive themselves as capable of meeting the goals in which they are invested. Thus there are times when it may not be easy for individuals to bounce back from their failure, which may create a downward spiral impairing their emotional functioning. In line with this possibility, as noted earlier, there is some evidence (although it is not entirely consistent) that individuals suffer when they view themselves as lacking the competence to fulfill the goals in which they are invested.

### Summary

In all, when individuals are invested in their goals, there are major benefits. These benefits are impressive enough that promoting investment among individuals should be considered a significant endeavor. However, awareness of the costs that can sometimes occur is essential. If investment is to be promoted, it needs to be done so in a context that emphasizes the consequences of ignoring other important arenas of life. In addition, sensitivity to the problems of overestimation of competence and responses to failure need to be considered. Moreover, given the heightened worrying that accompanies investment, preventing worrying from spiraling into heightened anxiety is critical. We now turn to a discussion of the factors that may moderate the benefits and costs of investment and its self-regulatory system. Identifying such factors is key to understanding when investment may be a facilitating force and when it may be a debilitating one.

## MODERATORS OF THE BENEFITS AND COSTS OF GOAL INVESTMENT

Although the benefits-to-costs ratio may be enhanced under some conditions, under others the costs may outweigh the benefits. Individuals are likely to be most vulnerable to the costs of their investment under conditions that heighten their need to avoid failure. When individuals experience an amplified need to do so, their worrying over the goals in which they are invested may intensify, often spiraling into full-blown anxiety. Moreover, when failure in the pursuit of personally important goals does occur, it may be particularly difficult for individuals to recover, given the intensity of their need to avoid failure. The most obvious, and perhaps most proximal, factor influencing individuals' need to avoid failure in the pursuit of the goals in which they are invested is the extent to which individuals have a prevention or avoidance orientation rather than a promotion or approach orientation in relation to such goals (see Elliot, 1999; Molden, Lee, & Higgins, Chapter 11, this volume). However, there may be other factors that intensify individuals' need to avoid failure in their pursuit of the goals in which they are highly invested. We focus in this section on several such factors.

The costs of investment may be heightened when investment develops in a controlled rather than an autonomous context, because individuals may feel a great deal of pressure not to disappoint others (see Deci & Ryan, 2000; Pomerantz & Ruble, 1998). Research by Elliot and Thrash (2004) has demonstrated that a major form of control used by parents—love withdrawal—is associated with fear of failure in college students. Thus it is quite likely that when individuals become highly invested in a controlling rather than an autonomous context, they focus on avoiding failure so as not to disappoint others; this heightens their worrying, and eventually anxiety, about the possibility of failure. To examine the idea that when individuals' investment develops in a controlled rather than an autonomous context there are costs, Cho and Pomerantz (2003) studied how mothers' control versus autonomy support moderates the effects of children's investment on their anxiety symptoms. Elementary school children's goal investment was assessed by having them describe how much they wanted to and felt they should do well in school. Children also reported on their anxiety symptoms. Mothers and their children were then observed interacting on a task that they were told assessed children's cognitive abilities. The task was designed to reflect the homework situation in that mothers and children were told that children would be tested on the task later by themselves. Mothers' control (e.g., telling children how to do the task) and autonomy support (e.g., attending to children as they worked on the task, but not getting involved unless requested) was observed and coded. Children who were highly invested in school experienced more anxiety symptoms than their less invested counterparts when their mothers were controlling, but not when their mothers were autonomy-supportive.

A similar intensification of costs may exist when individuals feel that their personal worth is contingent on meeting the goals in which they are invested; as noted earlier, this may be quite common, albeit not always the case. When individuals are motivated by self-worth concerns to meet the goals in which they are invested, their need to avoid failure may be particularly strong, because failure implies that they are worthless. Crocker and Park (2004) argue that individuals' need to validate their self-worth may lead to a number of costs over the long term, because such a need causes individuals to feel controlled rather than autonomous, which may set off the chain of events described above when individuals are highly invested in their goals. A similar sequence of events may ensue when individuals are focused on performance at the expense of mastery (see Senko, Durik, & Harackiewicz, Chapter 7, this volume; Dweck & Grant, Chapter 26, this volume), given that such a focus is characterized by a concern with validating personal ability (Grant & Dweck, 2003), which is often tied to feelings of self-worth (see Burhans & Dweck, 1995). Notably, individuals focused on performance over mastery disengage when they fail, with their perceptions of competence and affect following suit as they conclude that they will never be able to reach their goals (e.g., Elliott & Dweck, 1988; Grant & Dweck, 2003). This may be intensified when individuals are highly invested in their goals.

## CONCLUSIONS

Beginning with William James's seminal writings, individuals' investment in their goals has been of interest in the areas of personality and social psychology. Drawing on the research and theory that has evolved out of this interest, we proposed in this chapter than individuals' investment in their goals heightens the meaning they attach to their success and failure in the pursuit of their goals. As a consequence, self-regulation may be intensified in terms of goal-related behavior, cognition, and affect. We provided data from our own and others' labs, supporting this idea. In terms of behavior, individuals highly invested in their goals are effectively engaged in goal-related activities. Cognitively, such individuals perceive themselves as possessing the competencies to reach their goals, but also worry extensively about whether or not they will meet their goals. Highly invested individuals are also quite affectively sensitive to their failure to reach their goals. We argued that although there are clear benefits to the self-regulation produced by investment, there are also costs. We presented some preliminary research on possible moderators of the benefits and costs. However, additional research is necessary to determine how to maximize the benefits-to-costs ratio of heightened goal investment.

## ACKNOWLEDGMENT

Preparation of this chapter was supported by a grant from the National Institute of Mental Health (No. R01 MH57505).

## NOTES

1. Meece and colleagues (1990) found that investment in math was negatively associated with anxiety about math. However, their measure may have captured not only anxiety, but also other dimensions of psychological functioning (such as dislike of math and avoidance of math) that may be negatively associated with investment.

## REFERENCES

Atkinson, J. W. (1964). *An introduction to motivation*. Princeton, NJ: Van Nostrand.

Baumeister, R. F., Bratslavsky, E., Finkenauer, C., & Vohs, K. D. (2001). Bad is stronger than good. *Review of General Psychology*, *5*, 323–370.

Berndt, T. J., & Miller, K. E. (1990). Expectancies, values, and achievement in junior high school. *Journal of Educational Psychology*, *82*, 319–326.

Boninger, D. S., Krosnick, J. A., Berent, M. K., & Fabrigar, L. R. (1995). The causes and consequences of attitude importance. In R. E. Petty & J. A. Krosnick (Eds.), *Ohio State University series on attitudes and persuasion: Vol. 4. Attitude strength: Antecedents and consequences* (pp. 159–189). Hillsdale, NJ: Erlbaum.

Brunstein, J. C. (1993). Personal goals and subjective well-being: A longitudinal study. *Journal of Personality and Social Psychology*, *65*, 1065–1070.

Brunstein, J. C., & Gollwitzer, P. M. (1996). Effects of failure on subsequent performance: The importance of self-defining goals. *Journal of Personality and Social Psychology*, *70*, 395–407.

Burhans, K. K., & Dweck, C. S. (1995). Helplessness in early childhood: The role of contingent worth. *Child Development*, *66*, 1719–1738.

Campbell, J. D. (1986). Similarity and uniqueness: The effects of attribute type, relevance, and individual differences in self-esteem and depression. *Journal of Personality and Social Psychology, 50*, 281–294.

Carver, C. S., & Scheier, M. F. (1998). *On the self-regulation of behavior.* New York: Cambridge University Press.

Cho, G., & Pomerantz, E. M. (2003). *The implications of children's goal investment for their anxiety symptoms: The role of maternal control.* Paper presented at the biennial meetings of the Society for Research in Child Development, Tampa, FL.

Cole, D. A., Martin, J. M., Peeke, L. A., Seroczynski, A. D., & Fier, J. (1999). Children's over- and underestimation of academic competence: A longitudinal study of gender differences, depression, and anxiety. *Child Development, 70*, 459–473.

Colvin, C. R., & Block, J. (1994). Do positive illusions foster mental health?: An examination of the Taylor and Brown formulation. *Psychological Bulletin, 116*, 1152–1162.

Crocker, J., & Park, L. E. (2004). The costly pursuit of self-esteem. *Psychological Bulletin, 130*, 392–414.

Crocker, J., & Wolfe, C. T. (2001). Contingencies of self-worth. *Psychological Review, 108*, 593–623.

Csikszentmihalyi, M. (1997). *Finding flow: The psychology of engagement with everyday life.* New York: Basic Books.

Deci, E. L., & Ryan, R. M. (2000). The "what" and "why" of goal pursuits: Human needs and the self-determination of behavior. *Psychological Inquiry, 11*, 227–268.

Dong, W., & Pomerantz, E. M. (2006). *Positive emotional development: The role of children's daily functioning around academics.* Manuscript in preparation.

Dweck, C. S., & Leggett, E. L. (1988). A social-cognitive approach to motivation and personality. *Psychological Review, 95*, 256–273.

Eccles, J. S. (1983). Expectancies, values and academic behaviors. In J. T. Spence (Ed.), *Achievement and achievement motives* (pp. 75–146). San Francisco: Freeman.

Eccles, J. S., & Wigfield, A. (1995). In the mind of the actor: The structure of adolescents' achievement task values and expectancy-related beliefs. *Personality and Social Psychology Bulletin, 21*, 215–225.

Eccles, J. S., & Wigfield, A. (2002). Motivational beliefs, values, and goals. *Annual Review of Psychology, 53*, 109–132.

Eccles, J. S., Wigfield, A., Harold, R. D., & Blumenfeld, P. C. (1993). Age and gender differences in children's self- and task-perceptions during elementary school. *Child Development, 64*, 830–847.

Eccles, J. S., Wigfield, A., & Schiefele, U. (1998). Motivation to succeed. In W. Damon (Series Ed.) & N. Eisenberg (Vol. Ed.), *Handbook of child psychology: Vol. 3. Social, emotional, and personality development* (5th ed., pp. 1017–1095). New York: Wiley.

Elliot, A. J. (1999). Approach and avoidance motivation and achievement goals. *Educational Psychologist, 34*, 169–189.

Elliot, A. J., Faler, J., McGregor, H. A., Campbell, W. K., Sedikides, C., & Harackiewicz, J. M. (2000). Competence valuation as a strategic intrinsic motivation process. *Personality and Social Psychology Bulletin, 26*, 780–794.

Elliot, A. J., & Thrash, T. M. (2004). The intergenerational transmission of fear of failure. *Personality and Social Psychology Bulletin, 30*, 957–971.

Elliott, E. S., & Dweck, C. S. (1988). Goals: An approach to motivation and achievement. *Journal of Personality and Social Psychology, 54*, 5–12.

Emmons, R. A. (1986). Personal strivings: An approach to personality and subjective well-being. *Journal of Personality and Social Psychology, 51*, 1058–1068.

Emmons, R. A., & King, L. A. (1988). Conflict among personal strivings: Immediate and long-term implications for psychological and physical well-being. *Journal of Personality and Social Psychology, 54*, 1040–1048.

Feather, N. T. (1990). Bridging the gap between values and actions: Recent applications of the expectancy value model. In E. T. Higgins & R. M. Sorrentino (Eds.), *Handbook of motivation and cognition: Foundations of social behavior* (Vol. 2, pp. 151–192). New York: Guilford Press.

Gilbert, D. T., Pinel, E. C., Wilson, T. D., Blumberg, S. J., & Wheatley, T. P. (1998). Immune neglect: A source of durability bias in affective forecasting. *Journal of Personality and Social Psychology, 75*, 617–638.

Gollwitzer, P. M., & Wicklund, R. A. (1985). Self-symbolizing and the neglect of others' perspectives. *Journal of Personality and Social Psychology, 48*, 702–715.

Grant, H., & Dweck, C. S. (2003). Clarifying achievement goals and their impact. *Journal of Personality and Social Psychology, 85*, 541–553.

Harackiewicz, J. M., & Manderlink, G. (1984). A process analysis of the effects of performance: Contingent rewards on intrinsic motivation. *Journal of Experimental Social Psychology, 20*, 531–551.

Harter, S. (1993). Causes and consequences of low self-esteem in children and adolescents. In R. F. Baumeister (Ed.), *Self-esteem: The puzzle of low self-regard* (pp. 87–116). New York: Plenum Press.

Higgins, E. T. (1987). Self-discrepancy: A theory relating self and affect. *Psychological Review, 94*, 319–340.

Higgins, E. T. (1990). Personality, social psychology, and person–situation relations: Standards and knowledge activation as a common language. In L. A. Pervin (Ed.), *Handbook of personality: Theory and research* (pp. 301–338). New York: Guilford Press.

Higgins, E. T. (1996). The "self digest": Self-knowledge serving self-regulatory functions. *Journal of Personality and Social Psychology, 72*, 1062–1083.

Hunter, J. P., & Csikszentmihalyi, M. (2003). The positive psychology of interested adolescents. *Journal of Youth and Adolescence, 32*, 27–35.

James, W. (1890). *The principles of psychology* (2 vols.). New York: Holt.

Kasser, T., & Ryan, R. M. (1996). Further examining the American dream: Differential correlates of intrinsic and extrinsic goals. *Journal of Personality and Social Psychology, 65*, 410–422.

Little, B. R. (1983). Personal projects: A rationale and method for investigation. *Environment and Behavior, 15*, 273–309.

Maier, G. W., & Brunstein, J. C. (2001). The role of personal work goals in newcomers' job satisfaction and organizational commitment: A longitudinal analysis. *Journal of Applied Psychology, 86*, 1034–1042.

Marsh, H. W. (1993). Relations between global and specific domains of self: The importance of individual importance, certainty, and ideals. *Journal of Personality and Social Psychology, 65*, 975–992.

Marsh, H. W. (1995). A Jamesian model of self-investment and self-esteem: Comment on Pelham (1995). *Journal of Personality and Social Psychology, 69*, 1151–1160.

McGregor, I., & Little, B. R. (1998). Personal projects, happiness, and meaning: On doing well and being yourself. *Journal of Personality and Social Psychology, 74*, 494–512.

Meece, J. L., Wigfield, A., & Eccles, J. S. (1990). Predictors of math anxiety and its influence on young adolescents' course enrollment intentions and performance in mathematics. *Journal of Educational Psychology, 82*, 60–70.

Meyer, J. P. (1997). Organizational commitment. In C. L. Cooper & I. T. Robertson (Eds.), *International review of industrial and organizational psychology* (Vol. 12, pp. 175–228). New York: Wiley.

Palys, T. S., & Little, B. R. (1983). Perceived life satisfaction and the organization of personal project systems. *Journal of Personality and Social Psychology, 44*, 1221–1230.

Parsons, J. E., Adler, T., & Meece, J. L. (1984). Sex differences in achievement: A test of alternate theories. *Journal of Personality and Social Psychology, 46*, 26–43.

Paulhus, D. L. (1998). Interpersonal and intrapsychic adaptiveness of trait self-enhancement: A mixed blessing. *Journal of Personality and Social Psychology, 74*, 1197–1208.

Pelham, B. W. (1995a). Further evidence for a Jamesian model of self-worth: Reply to Marsh (1995). *Journal of Personality and Social Psychology, 69*, 1161–1165.

Pelham, B. W. (1995b). Self-investment and self-esteem: Evidence for a Jamesian model of self-worth. *Journal of Personality and Social Psychology, 69*, 1141–1150.

Pelham, B. W., & Swann, W. B. (1989). From self-conceptions to self-worth: On the sources and structure of global self-esteem. *Journal of Personality and Social Psychology, 57*, 672–680.

Pomerantz, E. M., Chaiken, S., & Tordesillas, R. (1995). Attitude strength and resistance processes. *Journal of Personality and Social Psychology, 69*, 408–419.

Pomerantz, E. M., & Ruble, D. N. (1998). The role of maternal control in the development of sex differences in child self-evaluative factors. *Child Development, 69*, 458–478.

Pomerantz, E. M., & Rudolph, K. D. (2003). What ensues from emotional distress?: Implications for competence estimates. *Child Development, 74*, 329–346.

Pomerantz, E. M., Saxon, J. L., & Oishi, S. (2000). The psychological tradeoffs of goal investment. *Journal of Personality and Social Psychology, 79*, 617–630.

Pomerantz, E. M., & Shim, S. (2006a). *Falling hard, but bouncing back: The responsivity of goal investment.* Manuscript in preparation.

Pomerantz, E. M., & Shim, S. (2006b). *The role of goal investment in emotional well-being: A process analysis.* Manuscript in preparation.

Robins, R. W., & Beers, J. S. (2001). Positive illusions about the self: Short-term benefits and long-term costs. *Journal of Personality and Social Psychology, 80*, 340–352.

Ryan, R. M., & Connell, J. P. (1989). Perceived locus of causality and internalization: Examining reasons for acting in two domains. *Journal of Personality and Social Psychology, 57*(5), 749–761.

Shah, J. Y., Friedman, R., & Kruglanski, A. W. (2002). Forgetting all else: On the antecedents and consequences of goal shielding. *Journal of Personality and Social Psychology, 83*, 1261–1280.

Taylor, S. E., & Brown, J. D. (1988). Illusion and well-being: A social psychological perspective on mental health. *Psychological Bulletin, 103*, 193–210.

Tesser, A. (1988). Toward a self-evaluation maintenance model of social behavior. In L. Berkowitz (Ed.), *Advances in experimental social psychology: Vol. 21. Social psychological studies of the self: Perspectives and programs* (pp. 181–227). San Diego, CA: Academic Press.

Tesser, A., & Smith, J. (1980). Some effects of task relevance and friendship on helping: You don't always help the one you like. *Journal of Experimental Social Psychology, 16*, 582–590.

Trope, Y., & Pomerantz, E. M. (1998). Resolving conflicts among self-evaluative motives: Positive experiences as a resource for overcoming defensiveness. *Motivation and Emotion, 22*, 53–72.

Wagner, U., Wicklund, R. A., & Shaigan, S. (1990). Open devaluation and rejection of a fellow student: The impact of threat to a self-definition. *Basic and Applied Social Psychology, 11*, 61–76.

Wicklund, R. A., & Gollwitzer, P. M. (1982). *Symbolic self-completion.* Hillsdale, NJ: Erlbaum.

Ziegert, D. I., Kistner, J. A., Castro, R., & Robertson, B. (2001). Longitudinal study of young children's responses to challenging achievement situations. *Child Development, 72*, 609–624.

Chapter 26

# Self-Theories, Goals, and Meaning

**Carol S. Dweck**
**Heidi Grant**

Goals lie at the heart of motivation, and thus of psychology. From Freud, Jung, and Adler, to the learning theorists like Hull and Tolman, to more and more researchers today, motivation has been recognized as the organizing and energizing force behind all actions.

Many chapters in this book deal with the nature and workings of goals, and so, in large part, does this one. But this chapter also deals with the question of what orients people toward certain goals—and *then* what happens once they are so oriented. More specifically, in this chapter we review research on people's self-theories and the goals they give rise to. We then show how the self-theories and goals together create a system of meaning that shapes interpretations of self-relevant stimuli and events, influencing how people understand their own experience, and guiding their affect, cognition, and behavior. In this way, self-theories and their allied goals determine important outcomes in academic, social, business, and sports settings.

## SELF-THEORIES

The self-theories we focus on here are people's beliefs about their personal attributes. Do they believe that their important attributes (such as their intelligence or personality) are fixed traits or malleable qualities—things they can't change or things they can? We measure people's self-theories by asking them to agree or disagree with statements such as "Your intelligence is something basic about you that you can't really change," or "No matter who you are, you can substantially change your level of intelligence." When people predominantly agree with statements like the first, they are said to hold an *entity theory*, or the belief that the quality in question is fixed. However, when they predominantly agree with statements like the second one, they are said to hold an *incremental theory*, or the belief that the quality in question can be increased or cultivated through their efforts.

### Frequency of Endorsement

Both types of theories appear to be equally endorsed in North American society, even though members of our culture have the reputation of being mainly entity theorists. Whether we are measuring children's or adults' self-theories, about 40% of our participants favor an entity theory, another 40% favor an incremental theory, and about 20% are more or less undecided (see Dweck, 1999).

### Stability and Malleability

How stable are people's self-theories? They have been found to be relatively stable individual differences (see, e.g., Robins & Pals, 2002), but at the same time—like many knowledge structures—they can also be taught or experimentally primed. For example, in the laboratory, participants are often taught an entity or an incremental theory by reading persuasive scientific articles that argue the case for one theory or the other (Bergen, 1991; Levy, Stroessner, & Dweck, 1998; Niiya, Crocker, & Bartmess, 2004). The articles present evidence that intelligence or personality is an inborn trait that resists efforts to change it, or, on the other hand, is an attribute that can be developed through effort and experience. After reading these articles, people in these studies respond in a way that mirrors the responses of chronic entity or incremental theorists.

In other studies, people are given instructions that the task they are about to work on either measures an inherent fixed ability or involves skills that can be learned. This has been done for such different abilities as intellectual skills (e.g., Aronson, 1998; Martocchio, 1994), physical skills (e.g., Jourden, Bandura, & Banfield, 1991), and managerial skills (e.g., Wood & Bandura, 1989).

People's self-theories can also be changed in more permanent ways by means of interventions that teach a particular theory and its applicability (Aronson, Fried, & Good, 2002; Blackwell, Trzesniewski, & Dweck, 2007; Good, Aronson, & Inzlicht, 2003). As we will see, these interventions have succeeded in enhancing students' motivation and achievement.

### Generality of Theories

Do people tend to hold the same theory across different attributes? Although there is some correlation of self-theories across attributes, people can hold different theories for different qualities. For example, they can believe that their intelligence is malleable but that their personality is fixed. They can even think that part of their intelligence (say, their verbal ability) is malleable, but that another part (e.g., their mathematical ability) is fixed. The theory they hold for a particular ability or attribute will predict their goals and affect–behavior patterns in that area.

### Accuracy of Theories

Is one theory correct? There are few subjects that have been as hotly debated as the fixity versus malleability of intelligence or human nature. As we're always told, it's never an either–or situation; not genes *or* environment, nature *or* nurture. However, evidence increasingly suggests that key aspects of many abilities can be acquired, thus lending credence to an incremental theory (e.g., Brown, 1997; Nickerson, Perkins, & Smith, 1985; Sternberg, 1985, 2005). It might also surprise people to learn that Alfred Binet, the inventor of the first IQ test, was a strong advocate of an incremental theory of intelligence. He did not invent his test to measure a fixed entity, but to identify children who needed different programs to spur their intellectual growth (Binet, 1909/1973; Siegler, 1992).

Nevertheless, the central point here is that *the self-theory that people adopt* has important consequences for their motivation and achievement.

## THE IMPACT OF SELF-THEORIES ON GOALS, SELF-ESTEEM, AND ACHIEVEMENT

We begin our examination of research with four longitudinal studies that monitored students across challenging educational transitions (Blackwell et al., 2007; Cury, Elliot, Da Fonseca, & Moller, 2006; Robins & Pals, 2002; Trzesniewski & Robins, 2003), since it is in the face of challenge that self-theories matter most. It is when people experience difficulty that it matters what they think they are made of—things they can learn and change or things they can't.

These four studies all measured students' theories of intelligence, their goals, and other motivation-relevant factors, and then tracked their self-esteem and/or their achievement over the next year or more. In every case, students' self-theories significantly predicted changes in their self-esteem or grades (of course, controlling for past self-esteem or grades), and in each case, these changes were significantly mediated by students' goals.

Specifically, students who held an entity theory were often more likely than those with an incremental theory to endorse *performance* goals. Believing that their intelligence was fixed, they were more concerned with documenting their intelligence though their performance. In other words, if they had a fixed amount of intelligence, they believed they had better demonstrate that they had a lot of it. Thus they agreed more with statements that emphasized the goal of getting high grades to validate their ability over the goal of seeking challenges and learning new things.

In contrast, students who held an incremental theory were more likely than those who held an entity theory to endorse *learning* goals. Believing that their intelligence could be cultivated, they were more concerned with gaining skills and knowledge. Thus they agreed more with statements that emphasized the goal of mastering new tasks and acquiring new knowledge (e.g., "The knowledge I gain in school is more important than the grades I receive"; Robins & Pals, 2002).

In the first study, by Robins and Pals (2002), 363 University of California–Berkeley students were followed over their years of college. Self-theories of intelligence (entity vs. incremental theories) significantly predicted the goals students held (learning vs. performance goals) and the changes in their self-esteem (increases vs. decreases). Path models showed that there were significant paths from self-theories through goals to self-esteem change. The more students held an entity theory and the more they endorsed performance goals, the more their self-esteem eroded over their college years. In contrast, the more they held an incremental theory and endorsed learning goals, the more they experienced a growth in self-esteem as they went through college. Moreover, it was the students' self-theories and goals, not differences in their academic success and failure, that accounted for the different trajectories of self-esteem.

With a younger sample, Trzesniewski and Robins (2003) followed students from their last semester of grade school (grade 5) through their first three semesters of middle school. They measured students' theories of intelligence, along with other motivation-relevant variables, and then tracked students' self-esteem and math grades. Path analyses again showed that an incremental (vs. entity) theory, by orienting students toward learning (vs. performance) goals, led to increasing (vs. decreasing) self-esteem and grades (with the change in self-esteem mediating the change in grades). Interestingly, in spite of the fact that the math grades were decreasing for the sample as a whole (as they often do in these transitional years), the students who held an incremental theory showed increasing grades during this time.

In a study by Blackwell and colleagues (2007), students were tracked over their transition to junior high school (seventh grade) until the end of eighth grade. Although both entity and incremental theorists entered junior high with equivalent grades, the two groups diverged in math grades by the end of their first semester and pulled farther and farther apart as time wore on. Again, the grades of the incremental theorists rose every semester. Moreover, path analysis showed that the change in grades was not predicted at all by past grades, but instead by students' self-theories and goals,

Recent research by Cury and colleagues (2006) lends further support to our analysis. Again, following adolescents through a semester of math, Cury and colleagues showed that theories of intelligence predicted students' math grades, and that this effect was mediated through their achievement goals. In a second study, they *manipulated* adolescents' theories of intelligence and showed that this affected their scores on an IQ test. Students who were taught an incremental theory earned higher IQ scores, and this effect was in large part mediated through their achievement goals.

## HOW DOES IT HAPPEN?

How do the self-theories and goals work? That is, what are the processes through which they produce their effects? The studies we have just reviewed, along with other research, shed light on these processes.

### Self-Theories Foster Goals

First, as we have noted, self-theories create a framework in which certain goals become more important than others. A dramatic demonstration of how an entity theory makes validating intelligence more important than learning comes from a study by Hong, Chiu, Dweck, Lin, and Wan (1999). The study was conducted at the University of Hong Kong, perhaps the premier institution of higher learning in Hong Kong, where everything takes place in English—all classes, reading, papers, and exams. In other words, proficiency in English is a necessity for success. Unfortunately, not all the students who enter the university come prepared to conduct their academic lives in English. Thus, for many of them, some language instruction would be highly advantageous.

As entering students registered for their classes, their theories of intelligence were assessed; their English proficiency scores were obtained; and they were asked the following: "If the faculty offered a remedial English class, how likely would you be to take it?" Among students with low proficiency in English, the incremental theorists indicated that they were highly likely to take such a course. However, the entity theorists, in spite of their low proficiency, were not particularly interested. It seems that rather than reveal a deficiency and remedy it, they would prefer to put their academic careers at risk.

## Self-Theories and Goals Foster Helpless versus Mastery-Oriented Reactions

Next, self-theories and goals together set up a framework in which people interpret and respond to setbacks. Within an entity theory and performance goal framework (where people believe in fixed ability and have the goal of validating their ability), setbacks reveal permanent inadequacies. Within an incremental theory and learning goal framework (where people believe in expandable ability and have the goal of augmenting their ability), however, setbacks simply provide information about which strategies work and which do not.

In each of the four longitudinal studies described above, self-theories and goals set up helpless versus mastery-oriented attributions and reactions to difficulty. In all cases, there were significant paths from self-theories though goals to the helpless versus mastery-oriented reactions, although there were typically some direct paths from self-theories to these reactions as well.

The helpless response, which followed from an entity theory and performance goals, included both low-ability attributions for failure (Blackwell et al., 2007; Robins & Pals, 2002; Trzesniewski & Robins, 2003) and ineffective (or no) strategies in the face of setbacks (Blackwell et al., 2007; Cury et al., 2006; Robins & Pals, 2002; Trzesniewski & Robins, 2003). Within this framework, responses to failure or the threat of failure have also been found to include *self-handicapping* (Rhodewalt, 1994), a defensive strategy in which people fail to prepare properly for an upcoming task in an effort to ward off low-ability attributions; the intent to cheat (Blackwell et al., 2007); and the tendency to lie about a poor score (Mueller & Dweck, 1998). Thus, when inadequacies are revealed or are likely to be revealed, this framework provides no good recipe for future success. Instead, it often prompts people to give up or to engage in defensive strategies intended to hide their inadequacies—often at cost to their future learning. La Rochefoucauld, the French master of the epigram, once noted that almost all of our faults are preferable to the methods we devise to hide them.

In contrast, the mastery-oriented reactions (which followed from an incremental theory and learning goals) included effort or strategy attributions for failure (Blackwell et al., 2007; Robins & Pals, 2002; Trzesniewski & Robins, 2003), as well as more vigorous and effective strategies in the face of setbacks (Blackwell et al., 2007; Cury et al., 2006; Robins & Pals, 2002; Trzesniewski & Robins, 2003). Robins and Pals (2002) also measured affective responses to setbacks, and here a helpless response included distress and shame, whereas a mastery-oriented response included feeling determined and enthusiastic.

## Helpless versus Mastery-Oriented Reactions Predict Self-Esteem and Grades

In all of the longitudinal studies discussed above, the helpless versus mastery-oriented reactions were key components of the path models that led from self-theories to changes in self-esteem or grades. These reactions typically constituted the final path to self-esteem or grades. Thus self-theories, both directly and indirectly (i.e., by encouraging certain goals), set up students' reactions to difficulty, which went on to predict the course of their self-esteem and achievement.

A study of ours (Grant & Dweck, 2003) sheds further light on the mastery-oriented reactions that lead to higher grades. In this study, students were followed in their college chemistry course, a highly difficult course that is the gateway to the premedical curriculum. Their goals were assessed at the outset, and periodically throughout the semester, they were asked about the study strategies they used to confront the difficult material. The more students had learning goals, the more they used deeper study strategies (e.g., searching for underlying principles that ran through the material), and this mediated the higher course grades that students with learning goals earned.

In a follow-up study, we (Grant & Dweck, 2004) found that the students with strong learning goals also used other strategies that predicted higher grades. They engaged in active self-regulation of their course-relevant motivation and emotions. For example, they did things to maintain their interest in the material and their motivation to study. They also did things to manage their level of stress. In short, these students took charge of the processes that brought about success in the face of challenge. It is not surprising that they were also the ones who were able to recover from an initially poor exam grade in the course, whereas students with strong performance goals generally did not.

### Implications

These findings have a number of practical and theoretical implications. First, they show that the self-theories (and the allied goals) that students favor as they confront a challenging school environment are important determinants of how they feel about themselves and how well they perform. This raises the question of whether altering students' self-theories might enhance their academic attitudes and performance. We return to this later.

But the findings also show that attributions and coping reactions—as important as they are in this process—*arise* from the self-theories and goals that students hold. Not only has this been shown in the path analyses in the studies described above; it has also been shown in experimental studies in which self-theories have been manipulated (Hong et al., 1999) or goals have been fostered (Mueller & Dweck, 1998). This means that attributions and coping reactions should not be studied in isolation, but rather should be examined as part of the *meaning system* in which they arise. A system that encourages an emphasis on fixed traits and the validation of those traits will lead to different attributions and coping reactions than will one that encourages an emphasis on expandable qualities and the growth of those qualities.

## IMPACT ON INTRINSIC INTEREST

Self-theories can affect performance not only through their impact on helpless versus mastery-oriented reactions to difficulty, but also through their impact on intrinsic interest. Put simply, people working within an entity theory framework do not enjoy learning, if by *learning* we mean working on something they're not (yet) good at. In contrast, those working within an incremental framework do enjoy learning hard things, since this is the way to increase their ability.

In a study by Butler (2000), students worked on a set of problems and were then given results showing that their performance had either decreased or increased over time. Following this feedback, they were asked how interesting they had found the problems to be, how interested they would be in receiving more of these problems to work on, and how interested they would be in working on more problems in their spare time. Those students with an incremental theory indicated higher interest when they believed that their performance had improved rather than declined over time. This is consistent with an emphasis on learning, since an ascending level of performance on the problems would indicate learning over time. In contrast, entity theorists showed a trend toward reporting greater interest when their performance had *decreased* over time. This is consistent with the idea that initially high performance indicates high inherent ability. (This trend was obtained even though decreasing performance could be taken to reflect slackening interest.)

In the Grant and Dweck (2003) study described above, students with learning goals who fared poorly on their initial exams nonetheless maintained their high level of interest in the course. However, students with performance goals who fared poorly initially, showed a marked loss in their interest and enjoyment in the course.

Finally, in a study by Mueller and Dweck (1998), students were given either intelligence-related feedback that induced an entity theory and performance goals, or process-related feedback that induced an incremental theory and learning goals. After a set of hard problems, those in the incremental theory framework retained their zest for the problems, whereas those in the entity theory framework showed a sharp decline. If it isn't easy, it isn't fun.

Dweck, Mangels, and Good (2004; see also Mangels, Butterfield, Lamb, Good, & Dweck, 2006) examined this zest (or lack of zest) for learning at a neural level. Using event-related potentials (ERPs), they tracked people's attentional strategies as they worked on a difficult general information task. College students wore caps outfitted with electrodes as they attempted to answer difficult questions relating to such subjects as history, geography, or popular culture. Shortly after they typed an answer into the computer, they were given information about whether their answer had been right or wrong (ability-related feedback). And shortly after that, they were given information about the correct answer (learning-relevant feedback). Analysis of the ERPs revealed what information the students were most interested in—that is, what kind of information they harnessed their attention for.

Incremental theorists harnessed their attention for both the ability-relevant and learning-relevant feedback, since in fact both types of feedback (in this case, knowing whether they were right or wrong, and determining what the right answer is) are important for learning. In contrast, entity theorists harnessed their attention for the ability-relevant feedback, but once they found out whether they were right or wrong, that was it. They showed little sign of interest in learning the right answer. Not surprisingly, incremental theorists' pattern of attention led to greater learning, as reflected in the number of previously missed questions they got correct on a retest.

It is not simply on intellectual or academic tasks that this effect occurs. A number of researchers have measured or induced self-theories and then tracked people's affect or enjoyment as they learned other kinds of difficult skills. These have included perceptual–motor skills (Jourden et al., 1991), computer skills (Martocchio, 1994), and managerial skills (Tabernero & Wood, 1999).

In the study by Jourden and colleagues (1991), for example, people learned a difficult perceptual–motor skill, but before they did, they were given an entity or incremental orientation toward the task. People in the entity condition were told that performance was determined by inherent aptitude, whereas people in the incremental condition learned that their performance reflected an acquirable skill. As they proceeded on this difficult learning task, entity theorists showed low interest in the activity—and, interestingly, showed no growth in confidence over the learning trials, even though they were getting better. Those in the incremental condition, on the other hand, showed strong interest in the activity, a growth in confidence, and a higher level of skill attainment. For entity theorists, the continued difficulty of the task was a source of distress, whereas for incremental theorists, the progress was a source of growing confidence and of enjoyment.

## INTERVENTIONS

If self-theories underlie important patterns of motivation and behavior, then changing people's self-theories should bring about changes in these patterns. To date, several interventions have demonstrated just this (Aronson et al., 2002; Blackwell et al., 2007; Good et al., 2003). In each case, a relatively modest intervention resulted in appreciable changes in academic motivation and achievement.

In one intervention study, Blackwell and colleagues (2007) designed and administered an eight-session workshop to seventh-grade students. All of the students in the study were given sessions on study skills and learned a host of useful things that could aid them in their schoolwork. However, half of the students were also taught an incremental theory of intelligence and ways to use this concept in their studies. Specifically, students were taught (à la Aronson et al., 2002) that their brains form new connections every time they learn, and that in this sense, learning changes their brains and over time makes them smarter. Thus they were taught that they were in charge of their brains and could choose to make new neural connections if they applied themselves.

Before the intervention, students' math grades had been sharply declining. After the intervention, the math grades of the students in the control group continued to decline, even though they had received study skill training and other potentially useful information. In contrast, the students who had been given the incremental intervention showed a marked recovery in their grades and were now earning significantly higher grades than their peers in the control group. Just as striking was the fact that teachers (who were unaware of students' experimental conditions) singled out significantly more students in the incremental intervention as having shown positive motivational change. The teachers described in detail changes in these students' orientation toward learning and their valuing of improvement—the precise things that one would expect to be fostered by an incremental framework. Interestingly, the gains in achievement were shown mostly for students who entered the intervention holding an entity theory about their intelligence. This underscores the idea that it was a change in self-theory that brought about the beneficial changes, and not some other secret ingredient in the incremental intervention.

Good and colleagues (2003) conducted an impressive intervention, also with junior high school students. In this study, students were taught an incremental self-theory as part of a course on computer skills. The students in the incremental intervention group had college students as mentors, who taught them the incremental theory, helped them design a web page about the incremental theory, and had e-mail exchanges with them on the incremental theme. At the end of the year, statewide achievement tests were administered, and these students were compared to students in the control group, who had engaged in similar activities (having mentors, web page building, e-mailing with mentors) but organized around an anti-drug message. The group that had received the incremental intervention showed substantially and significantly higher achievement test scores in both reading and math.

As noted above, both of these interventions were relatively modest, compared with many lengthy and costly educational interventions. This fact brings home the idea that when one pinpoints a belief that is at the core of a motivational pattern, simply altering that belief (and demonstrating how the new belief can be put into practice) can have a cascade of beneficial effects.

## STEREOTYPE THREAT

Within an entity theory framework, every challenge or difficulty can be a threat to the self. Is this doubly true when an individual is a member of a negatively stereotyped group?

Virtually everyone is now familiar with the phenomenon of *stereotype threat.* Stereotype threat occurs when a member of a negatively stereotyped group feels in danger of confirming the negative stereotype, as when a woman feels in danger of confirming the stereotype of low math ability, or an African American student feels in danger of confirming the stereotype of poor academic ability. This concern has been found to result in seriously impaired performance on difficult tests of ability (Steele & Aronson, 1995).

It is plausible to assume that holding an entity theory of ability may exaggerate the impact of stereotype threat. The entity theory conveys that the ability in question is fixed—"You have it or you don't." And the stereotype is saying, "You don't." Thus entity theorists may be highly concerned about their ability in situations in which stereotypes are evoked. In contrast, an incremental theory conveys the idea that the ability in questions is acquirable or improvable. Thus the stereotype may have less sting. First, an incremental theory makes it less credible that your group has permanently low ability; second, it implies that even if you have less ability now, you can make gains if you apply yourself (i.e., if you pursue learning goals).

Aronson (1998) tested this idea. He gave African American college students a test of intellectual ability that was presented in an entity theory or an incremental theory context. In the entity theory condition, a very strong stereotype threat effect was obtained. However, when an incremental theory of ability was highlighted, the African American students did not fall prey to stereotype threat—even though the negative stereotype was made salient.

Good, Rattan, and Dweck (2004) went on to explore these effects for women and math, in a study of several hundred college women pursuing their first calculus course. In this study, they assessed (1) the degree to which the women in these courses perceived a high degree of negative stereotyping about women and math; and (2) the degree to which the women perceived an entity theory or an incremental theory of math ability in their class environment. They followed these women over the semester, monitoring what happened to their sense of belonging and their intention to take math in the future.

Good and colleagues (2004) found that when women perceived a high degree of stereotyping (stereotype threat) *and* an entity theory environment, their sense of belonging dwindled over the course of the semester. In other words, they felt less and less accepted and comfortable in their math environment as time went on. They also felt decreasing confidence in their math abilities, even though they entered with SAT scores that were at least the equals of those of the other groups. Finally, their lowered sense of belonging led to a decreased intention to take math again in the future—even among women who had performed well. This means that even when stereotype threat does not undermine performance per se, it can still undermine individuals' comfort in an area and their desire to continue in that area. In contrast, when women felt a high degree of stereotype threat but perceived that they were in an incremental math environment, they were able to maintain a strong sense of belonging and retain a commitment to take math in the future. Thus an incremental theory appeared to protect women against the negative effects of the stereotype.

Would an incremental intervention decrease the impact of stereotype threat?

## STEREOTYPE THREAT: AN INCREMENTAL INTERVENTION

Aronson and colleagues (2002) addressed this question in a study of African American (and European American) college students. One-third of students received an incremental intervention, which taught them about the way in which the brain forms new connections each time something new is learned. This lesson was emphasized by having them teach the incremental theory to younger students they were tutoring. There were two control groups: one that received no treatment, and one that learned about *multiple intelligences*—the idea that people have many forms of intelligence (so that a failure in one domain does not mean a lack of intelligence in all domains).

At the end of the semester, the African American students in the three groups did not differ in the degree to which they perceived stereotype threat in their school environment. But they did differ in their ability to enjoy school and perform well in the face of the threat. Compared to the two control groups (which did not differ from each other), the students in the incremental intervention group (1) valued academic work significantly more, (2) enjoyed their academic work significantly more, and (3) earned significantly higher grade point averages for the semester. Once again, a relatively modest self-theory intervention yielded widespread benefits: An incremental theory allowed students to retain pleasure and efficacy in their work, despite stereotypes that might surround them.

## SELF-THEORIES IN OTHER DOMAINS

Self-theories can influence motivation in any domain in which people believe their attributes can be judged or improved. So far we have concentrated on intellectual ability, but self-theories have also been shown to be important to motivation across many other areas, including interpersonal or relationship skills (Beer, 2002; Kammrath & Dweck, 2006; Knee, 1998; Knee, Nanayakkara, Vietor, Neighbors, & Patrick, 2001; Knee, Patrick, Vietor, & Neighbors, 2004; Ruvolo & Rotondo, 1998), sports (Biddle, Wang, Chatzisaray, & Spray, 2003; Ommundsen, 2001, 2003; Sarrazin et al., 1996), and business or managerial skills (Heslin, Vandewalle, & Latham, 2005; Maurer, Wrenn, Pierce, Tross, & Collins, 2003; Tabernero & Wood, 1999; Wood & Bandura, 1989; Wood, Philips, & Tabernero, 2002). In each case, self-theories have been linked to analogous patterns of motivation and behavior.

### Social Relationships

Self-theories influence intimate relationships (Kammrath & Dweck, 2006; Knee, 1998; Knee et al., 2001, 2002; Ruvolo & Rotondo, 1998), as well as peer relationships in both children (Erdley, Cain, Loomis, Dumas-Hines, & Dweck, 1997) and adults (Beer, 2002). Entity and incremental theories predict many of the same patterns of goals, attributions, affective responses, and coping strategies in relationships that have been found in the domain of intelligence. Studies by Beer (2002) nicely illustrate the impact that self-theories have in moderating individuals' reactions to interpersonal threat, as well as their role in determining social competence. Beer measured people's self-theories of shyness, with items such as "My shyness is something about me that I can't change very much" (entity theory) and "I can change aspects of my shyness if I want to" (incremental theory). People also reported on their level of shyness by rating the extent to which they exhibited the physiological (e.g., racing pulse), observable (e.g., reduced eye contact), and cognitive–emotional (feelings of anxiety) components of shyness.

In one study, participants were given a choice: to pursue a learning goal (an opportunity to learn some social skills that might help them overcome their shyness, at the cost of possibly appearing awkward on the videotape), or to pursue a performance goal (an opportunity to be paired with people of lesser social ability, so that the shy participants' social skills would compare favorably to those of the others). As expected, shy incremental theorists were more likely than shy entity theorists to opt for the learning goals. In addition, shy incremental theorists also exhibited more approach tendencies than shy entity theorists (agreeing more that "If the chance comes to meet new people, I often take it") and fewer avoidance tendencies (such as avoiding social situations, avoiding eye contact, or preventing the conversation from focusing on them).

Subsequently, participants engaged in an actual dyadic interaction. During the interaction, they rated themselves over three 5-minute time periods and were also rated by observers. In the first 5-minute period, entity and incremental theorists reported engaging in similar levels of avoidant strategies, and observers rated both groups as exhibiting equally high levels of avoidant behavior. In the second and third periods, however, clear differences emerged. Shy entity theorists reported (and were judged by observers to engage in) significantly higher levels of avoidant behavior than shy incremental theorists. Importantly, whereas all shy people were perceived by observers as shy and nervous throughout the interaction, observers rated shy incremental theorists as having fewer undesirable social consequences of their shyness. Specifically, in the second and third periods they were perceived to be more socially skilled, likeable, and enjoyable to be with than their entity counterparts.

Thus, in this arena as well, people's self-theories are linked to other motivational variables, such as goals (Beer, 2002; Erdley et al., 1997; Knee, 1998), attributions (Erdley et al., 1997), and mastery-oriented versus helpless responses to threat (Beer, 2002; Kammrath & Dweck, 2007; Knee et al., 2002), and lead to more or less favorable outcomes.

## Sports

Entity and incremental theories of athletic ability have been studied by Biddle and his colleagues (Biddle et al., 2003; Sarrazin et al., 1996), who examined the impact of self- theories on young people's motivation for sports and physical activity. To do so, they devised a questionnaire to assess theories of sports ability, containing items such as "You have a certain level of ability in sport and you cannot really do much to change that level" (entity belief), and "How good you are at sport will *always* improve if you work harder at it" (incremental belief). The incremental theory predicted feeling successful when learning goals were achieved ("when I improve and master new things") and overall greater enjoyment of sports. In contrast, the entity theory predicted feeling successful when performance goals were achieved ("when I beat out others") and *amotivation* (the belief that sports are a waste of time).

Complementing these findings, Ommundsen (2001, 2003) showed that an incremental theory predicted better use of self-regulatory strategies in sports (e.g., being willing to ask for help when necessary). Entity beliefs predicted failure to take an analytic stance toward one's learning strategies, not asking for help, and abandoning activities when they became difficult. They also predicted higher anxiety and less enjoyment of physical activity. In addition, entity beliefs predicted use of self-handicapping strategies, as they did in the academic domain.

Thus, in the domain of sports and athleticism, self-theories predict many of the same variables as in the academic domain: learning versus performance goals, mastery-oriented versus helpless learning strategies, and intrinsic motivation versus amotivation or anxiety.

## Organizational Behavior

In the arena of organizational behavior, Wood and his colleagues (Tabernero & Wood, 1999; Wood & Bandura, 1989; Wood et al., 2003) tracked individuals and monitored their development of managerial skills as they worked on a complex task (see also Maurer et al., 2003), both as individuals and in groups. Entity and incremental theories of managerial ability were either measured (in some studies) or experimentally induced (in others). The managerial decision-making task involved matching employees' attributes to the different jobs in the organization, and learning over trials how best to facilitate the attainment of the production quota for each employee. In order to determine the best solutions, participants had to engage in continual hypothesis testing, and had to revise their strategies as a function of the feedback.

In one study (Wood & Bandura, 1989), participants, working as individuals, had self-theories induced by being told either that the required skills were a function of their underlying cognitive capacities (entity induction) or that the skills were developed through practice (incremental induction). Although both groups began the task with confidence, those in the entity group showed a progressive decrease in self-efficacy across trials as they struggled to meet the demanding production quotas of the task. In addition, they set less challenging goals across trials; they became less efficient in their use of strategies; and their performance steadily declined. In contrast, those in the incremental group maintained their sense of efficacy, became more systematic in use of strategies, and sustained a high level of performance.

In another study (Wood et al., 2003, Study 2), people's theories of managerial ability were measured, and work groups were formed; each group was composed of either three incremental theorists or three entity theorists. The groups worked together for several weeks, and were then given the same managerial decision-making task described above. The two groups started out with similar attributions, group efficacy, and group goals, but began to diverge over the course of the task. Whereas the entity groups tended to blame uncontrollable factors (i.e., the task, their ability, luck) for their difficulty, incremental groups chose strategy attributions instead. Compared to the entity groups, the incremental groups also increased in efficacy over trials and set higher goals for themselves on the later trials.

Finally, the processes occurring in the two types of groups differed in important ways. Members of the incremental groups openly stated their opinions and expressed disagreements. They were also, as groups, more focused on the task and more effective in their use of time. This greater focus on the task, the more challenging group goals, and the strategy attributions mediated the effects of people's entity or incremental theories on group performance: Incremental groups' superior performance emerged early and became even more pronounced over time. Entity theorists, more concerned about their fixed managerial ability, appeared to fall prey to a *groupthink* process (Janis, 1972), in which frank discussions were not held and disagreements were not aired.

Kray and Haselhuhn (in press), in new research, looked at the impact of self-theories on success in negotiations. In one study, they manipulated people's entity versus incremental theories about negotiation skills by having them read either an article entitled "Negotiation Ability, like Plaster, Is Pretty Stable over Time," or one entitled "Negotiation Ability Is Changeable and Can Be Developed." Following the manipulation, participants were asked to select goals for the upcoming negotiation task. The performance goal task was described as one in which people could show off their negotiation skills, although they would not learn anything new. In the learning goal task, people were told that they might make mistakes and get confused, but they would learn some useful negotiation skills. Eighty-eight percent of the people who received the incremental theory induction chose the learning goal, whereas only 53% of those in the entity theory condition made this choice. Moreover, the more people adopted an incremental theory, the more likely they were to opt for learning over performance goals. In two subsequent studies, Kray and Haselhuhn went on to demonstrate the causal role of self-theories in negotiation performance. On all measures of negotiation performance, those with an incremental theory outperformed those with an entity theory, due in large part to their mastery-oriented responses to the challenging negotiation tasks.

In summary, many of the same factors that mediate the effects of self-theories on performance in other settings—goals, attributions, and mastery-oriented versus helpless learning strategies—appear to be at play in organizational decision making and negotiation as well.

## CONCLUSION

Psychologists agree that human behavior is largely purposeful, and motivation researchers are documenting the precise ways in which individuals' purposes (or goals) energize and shape their behavior. To this, we bring the ideas (1) that self-theories play an important role in determining the goals that people pursue; and (2) that, together, self-theories and goals create systems of meaning that lend particular significance to events in people's lives, directing their responses to those events. We have presented evidence from a wide variety of domains (the academic, social, business, and sports arenas) to show the influence of people's self-theories and goals on their preferences, actions, feelings, and (ultimately) their success.

## ACKNOWLEDGMENTS

Preparation of this chapter was supported in part by grants from the National Science Foundation (Grant No. BCS-02-17251), the Department of Education (Grant No. R305-H-02-0031) and the William T. Grant Foundation (Grant No. 2379) to Carol S. Dweck.

## REFERENCES

Aronson, J. (1998). *The effects of conceiving ability as fixed or improvable on responses to stereotype threat.* Unpublished manuscript, University of Texas.

Aronson, J., Fried, C., & Good, C. (2002). Reducing the effects of stereotype threat on African American college students by shaping theories of intelligence. *Journal of Experimental Social Psychology, 38,* 113–125.

Beer, J. S. (2002). Implicit self-theories of shyness. *Journal of Personality and Social Psychology, 83,* 1009–1024.

Bergen, R. S. (1991) *Beliefs about intelligence and achievement related behaviors.* Unpublished doctoral dissertation, University of Illinois at Urbana–Champaign.

Biddle, S., Wang, J., Chatzisaray, N., & Spray, C. M. (2003). Motivation for physical activity in young people: Entity and incremental beliefs about athletic ability. *Journal of Sports Sciences, 21,* 973–989.

Binet, A. (1973). *Les idées modernes sur les enfants* [*Modern ideas on children*]. Paris: Flammarion. (Original work published 1909)

Blackwell, L. S., Trzesniewski, K., & Dweck, C. S. (2007). Implicit theories of intelligence predict achievement across an adolescent transition: A longitudinal study and an intervention. *Child Development, 78,* 246–263.

Brown, A. L. (1997). Transforming schools into communities of thinking and learning about serious matters. *American Psychologist, 52,* 399–413.

Butler, R. (2000). Making judgments about ability: The role of implicit theories of ability in moderating inferences from temporal and social comparison information. *Journal of Personality and Social Psychology, 78,* 965–978.

Cury, F., Elliot, A. J., Da Fonseca, D., & Moller, A. C. (2006). The social-cognitive model of achievement motivation and the 2 × 2 achievement goal framework. *Journal of Personality and Social Psychology, 90,* 666–679.

Dweck, C. S. (1999). *Self-theories: Their role in motivation, personality, and development.* Philadelphia: Psychology Press.

Dweck, C. S., Mangels, J. A., & Good, C. (2004). Motivational effects on attention, cognition, and performance. In D. Y. Dai & R. J. Sternberg (Eds.), *Motivation, emotion, and cognition: Integrated perspectives on intellectual functioning and development* (pp. 41–56). Mahwah, NJ: Erlbaum.

Erdley, C., Cain, K., Loomis, C., Dumas-Hines, F., & Dweck, C. S. (1997). The relations among children's social goals, implicit personality theories and response to social failure. *Developmental Psychology, 33,* 263–272.

Good, C., Aronson, J., & Inzlicht, M. (2003). Improving adolescents' standardized test performance: An intervention to reduce the effects of stereotype threat. *Journal of Applied Developmental Psychology, 24,* 645–662.

Good, C., Rattan, A., & Dweck, C. S. (2004). [An incremental theory decreases vulnerability to stereotypes about math ability in college females]. Unpublished raw data, Columbia University.

Grant, H., & Dweck, C. S. (2003). Clarifying achievement goals and their impact. *Journal of Personality and Social Psychology, 85,* 541–553.

Grant, H., & Dweck, C. S. (2004). [Goal orientations influence both knowledge and use of self-regulated learning strategies]. Unpublished raw data, Lehigh University.

Heslin, P. A., Vandewalle, D., & Latham, G. (2005). The effect of implicit person theory on performance appraisals. *Journal of Applied Psychology, 90,* 842–856.

Heslin, P. A., Vandewalle, D., & Latham, G. (2006). Keen to help?: Managers' implicit person theories and their subsequent employee coaching. *Personnel Psychology, 59,* 871–902.

Hong, Y. Y., Chiu, C., Dweck, C. S., Lin, D., & Wan, W. (1999). Implicit theories, attributions, and coping: A meaning system approach. *Journal of Personality and Social Psychology, 77,* 588–599.

Janis, I. L. (1972). *Groupthink: A psychological study of foreign-policy decisions and fiascoes.* Boston: Houghton Mifflin.

Jourden, F. J., Bandura, A., & Banfield, J. T. (1991). The impact of conceptions of ability on self-regulatory factors and motor skill acquisition. *Journal of Sport and Exercise Psychology, 13,* 213–226.

Kammrath, L., & Dweck, C. S. (2006). Voicing conflict: Preferred conflict strategies among incremental and entity theorists. *Personality and Social Psychology Bulletin, 32,* 1497–1508.

Knee, C. R. (1998). Implicit theories of relationships: Assessment and prediction of romantic relationship initiation, coping, and longevity. *Journal of Personality and Social Psychology, 74,* 360–370.

Knee, C. R., Nanayakkara, A., Vietor, N. A., Neighbors, C., & Patrick, H. (2001). Implicit theories of relationships: Who cares if romantic partners are less than ideal? *Personality and Social Psychology Bulletin, 27*, 808–819.

Knee, C. R., Patrick, H., Vietor, N. A., & Neighbors, C. (2004). Implicit theories of relationships: Moderators of the link between conflict and commitment. *Personality and Social Psychology Bulletin, 30*, 617–628.

Kray, L. J., & Haselhuhn, M. (in press). Implicit theories of negotiating ability and performance: Longitudinal and experimental evidence. *Journal of Personality and Social Psychology.*

Levy, S. R., Stroessner, S. J., & Dweck, C. S. (1998). Stereotype formation and endorsement: The role of implicit theories. *Journal of Personality and Social Psychology, 74*(6), 1421–1436.

Mangels, J. A., Butterfield, B., Lamb, J., Good, C. D., & Dweck, C. S. (2006). Why do beliefs about intelligence influence learning success?: A social-cognitive-neuroscience model. *Social, Cognitive, and Affective Neuroscience, 1*, 75–86.

Martocchio, J. J. (1994). Effects of conceptions of ability on anxiety, self-efficacy, and learning in training. *Journal of Applied Psychology, 79*, 819–825.

Maurer, T. J., Wrenn, K. A., Pierce, H. R., Tross, S. A., & Collins, W. C. (2003). Beliefs about improvability of career-relevant skills: Relevance to job/task analysis, competency modeling, and learning orientation. *Journal of Organizational Behavior, 24*, 107–131.

Mueller, C. M., & Dweck, C. S. (1998). Intelligence praise can undermine motivation and performance. *Journal of Personality and Social Psychology, 75*, 33–52.

Nickerson, R. S., Perkins, D. N., & Smith, E. E. (1985). *Teaching thinking*. Hillsdale, NJ: Erlbaum.

Niiya, Y., Crocker, J., & Bartmess, E. N. (2004). From vulnerability to resilience: Learning orientations buffer contingent self-esteem from failure. *Psychological Science, 15*, 801–805.

Ommundsen, Y. (2001). Pupils' affective responses in physical education classes: The association of implicit theories of the nature of ability and achievement goals. *European Physical Education Review, 7*, 219–242.

Ommundsen, Y. (2003). Implicit theories of ability and self-regulation strategies in physical education classes. *Educational Psychology, 23*, 141–157.

Rhodewalt, F. (1994). Conceptions of ability, achievement goals, and individual differences in self-handicapping behavior: On the application of implicit theories. *Journal of Personality, 62*, 67–85.

Robins, R. W., & Pals, J. L. (2002). Implicit self-theories in the academic domain: Implications for goal orientation, attributions, affect, and self-esteem change. *Self and Identity, 1*, 313–336.

Ruvolo, A. P., & Rotondo, J. L. (1998). Diamonds in the rough: Implicit personality theories and views of partner and self. *Personality and Social Psychology Bulletin, 24*, 750–758.

Sarrazin, P., Biddle, S., Famose, J. P., Cury, F., Fox, K., & Durand, M. (1966). Goal orientation and conceptions of the nature of sport ability in children: A social cognitive approach. *British Journal of Social Psychology, 35*, 399–414.

Siegler, R. S. (1992). The other Alfred Binet. *Developmental Psychology, 28*, 179–190.

Steele, C. M., & Aronson, J. (1995). Stereotype threat and the intellectual test performance of African-Americans. *Journal of Personality and Social Psychology, 68*, 797–811.

Sternberg, R. J. (1985). Human intelligence: The model is the message. *Science, 230*, 1111–1118.

Sternberg, R. J. (2005). Intelligence, competency, and expertise. In A. J. Elliot & C. S. Dweck (Eds.), *Handbook of competence and motivation* (pp. 15–30). New York: Guilford Press.

Tabernero, C., & Wood, R. E. (1999). Implicit theories versus the social construal of ability in self-regulation and performance on a complex task. *Organizational Behavior and Human Decision Processes, 78*(2), 104–127.

Trzesniewski, K., & Robins, R. (2003, April). *Integrating Self-Esteem into a Process Model of Academic Achievement.* Paper presented at the biennial meetings of the Society for Research in Child Development, Tampa, FL.

Wood, R., & Bandura, A. (1989). Impact of conceptions of ability on self-regulatory mechanisms and complex decision making. *Journal of Personality and Social Psychology, 56*, 407–415.

Wood, R. E., Phillips, K. W., & Tabernero, C. (2002). *Implicit theories of ability, processing dynamics and performance in decision-making groups.* Unpublished manuscript, University of New South Wales, Sydney, New South Wales, Australia.

Chapter 27

# Culture and Motivation

**Beth Morling**
**Shinobu Kitayama**

Asian American children excel at puzzles that their mothers choose for them; European American children do best when they work on puzzles they choose for themselves. American employees may slack off when they work in a group; Chinese workers appear to work better in a team setting. Japanese students want to work on puzzles they are not good at; American students want to work on puzzles they already do well. These examples demonstrate that some patterns of motivation are not universal. Motivation does not reflect solely the idiosyncratic desires and wants of an individual actor; instead, motivation is enacted via the dominant meanings and recurring settings of the cultural context in which the actor participates.

This chapter argues that many significant human motivations are significantly shaped by the shared, everyday practices and meanings that exist in a particular cultural context. Even motivational patterns that psychologists have long treated as universal (such as the motivation for high self-esteem or the superior performance effects of intrinsic motivation) may be local to European American, middle-class cultures, as we will explain.

In this chapter we review theoretical perspectives and empirical evidence regarding cultural variation in human motivation. We first describe how shared meanings or cultural schemas may have motivational force. Then we explain how human motivations vary. We briefly review cultural variations in the expression of "basic" human drives to sleep, eat, reproduce, and protect the self—motives that humans probably share with many other animals. Then we turn to a more in-depth review of motives that are linked to something more uniquely human: the self. Specifically, we discuss human motives for self-enhancement, control, cognitive consistency, self-determination, attention to work, and prioritization of goals. Because these motives all derive from the self-concept, and because the self-concept is enacted differently in different world cultures, psychologists have documented more significant cultural differences in these motives. Finally, we reflect on some existing taxonomies of human motivation. How might evolution have shaped the universality and plasticity of human motivation?

## MOTIVATION IS CULTURAL

Culture and motivation are inextricably linked. Many cultural differences are fundamentally motivational differences. Common definitions of culture typically emphasize that culture provides humans with access to elaborate and sophisticated information structures (Richerson & Boyd, 2005); "software" for operating their biological "hardware" (Geertz, 1973); or, most simply, shared systems of meaning (Bruner, 1990). More relevant to the current volume, culture's meaning systems have a motivational function: They provide directive goals and intentions. For instance, D'Andrade (1984) defined *culture* as "learned systems of meanings, communicated by means of natural language and other symbol systems, having representational, directive, and affective functions, and capable of creating cultural entities and particular senses of reality" (p. 116). This definition's mention of *directive* function indicates that shared systems of meaning play a role in motivating behavior. In another definition of *culture*, Berlin (1976) specifies that shared "goals, values and pictures of the world" constitute culture. Kroeber and Kluckholn (1952) mention that cultural systems "may, on the one hand, be considered products of action, on the other hand as conditioning elements of further action" (p. 357). According to these prominent anthropological definitions, motivation is one primary aspect of the psyche that is potentially influenced by culture. When researchers document cultural differences in behavior, they are probably documenting motivational differences: People in East Asia, India, North America, and so on all *do* and *want to do* different things.

Admittedly, to say simply that culture influences motivation leaves out the exact mechanisms by which culture motivates an individual. According to D'Andrade (1992), a culture's content consists of *schemas*—organized sets of knowledge about what people do or what things mean (see also Strauss & Quinn, 1997). These schemas can be internalized by individuals, and can take the form of *goals* that have motivational force. For example, Quinn (1992) detailed a culturally specific schema for marriage that can motivate women in a culture to carry out culturally specific actions (often lower-level goals), such as getting one's husband a drink or taking on more of the household labor. In this example, a culturally specific concept of marriage organizes and directs the actions of people in that culture; it directly motivates the actions of people in that culture who have internalized that schema. Importantly, D'Andrade points out that not everyone in a cultural group is motivated by all the culture's schemas, perhaps because not everyone internalizes or uses a culture's schemas. And individuals may idiosyncratically combine several schemas (e.g., wives may internalize and negotiate among conflicting models of marriage; Quinn, 1992). Other schemas motivate only in combination with other goals (e.g., a schema for getting into a line only operates in combination with the goal to pay for one's groceries; D'Andrade, 1992).

We emphasize that culturally specific schemas, whether internalized by individual people or not, are *public* meaning structures. Thus a culturally shared marriage schema will anchor the meaning of people's actions—even those who have not internalized it. Because most other people know about this schema, a wife who does not internalize a "wife as server" aspect of the marriage schema will, for example, have to justify wife role behavior that is counterschematic. Specific public meanings (advertisements about housekeeping) or everyday practices (e.g., school notices tailored to mothers or teachings in school; Quinn, 1992) all contribute to the perpetuation of this schema, and give it power even over individuals who don't internalize it.

Cultural schemas have motivational force because they are associated with moral imperatives such as to be good, to be beautiful, and/or to be right (Shweder, 2003). For example, a newlywed may follow a North American schema for marriage by holding hands with her new husband in public, expressing the joy of the honeymoon period, and perhaps publicly reflecting upon the practical adjustments of living together with him ("If only he'd pick up his socks!"). In acting this way, she enacts what is considered appropriate for a new wife: She expresses her love for her husband and affirms herself as good, right, adequate, and functioning well in the social setting of normal new marriage (Strauss & Quinn, 1997). Shweder (2003) gives the example of the cultural concept of widowhood in one Hindu community, which dictates that widows not eat hot foods. In the eyes of many Americans, Indian widows' avoidance of hot foods seems strange, because this moral imperative appears arbitrary and even oppressive. Nevertheless, upon closer inspection of the culture at issue, one will learn that there is a network of reasons and arguments for moral imperatives such as these. For example, hot foods in Indian culture are considered to stimulate sexual desires. For an Indian widow, then, not to eat hot foods is to affirm her love and dedication to her deceased husband, and to remain a decent member of her extended household and family (Shweder, 2003).

Any given cultural schemas acquire moral force because they are embedded in a larger network of practices and public meanings. This is true whether they are secular and modern, such as the contemporary American work ethic, or more traditional, such as Indian widows' avoidance of hot foods. In other words, moral schemas are powerful, psychologically binding, and motivating because they are reinforced by and grounded in everyday practices and public meanings that provide a convincing rationale for them. Everyday practices—such as what kinds of foods are traditionally offered to a widow or how people may talk to her, or what kinds of questions and advice are offered to American newlyweds by their friends—serve to constitute and reinforce the pertinent moral schemas of avoiding hot foods and adjusting to a romantic partnership, respectively. In sum, daily cultural practices reinforce (indeed, they make up) cultural schemas, and these public meaning structures have motivational consequences.

## CULTURES SHAPE THE EXPRESSION OF "BASIC" HUMAN DRIVES

If culture motivates by providing specific, motivating meanings (via social schemas), then we should be able to document cultural differences in motivated behavior. One category of human motivation contains "basic" drives that humans share with most other animals. These drives probably are evolved, are innate, and have dedicated neural structures across species; they include drives to seek nourishment, to sleep, to procreate, to protect oneself and one's kin, and to form attachment bonds to caregivers. Although our focus in this chapter is on motivations with a uniquely human link to self-awareness (Leary, 2004), psychologists and anthropologists have documented many examples of how cultures provide different norms (via meaning structures) that affect how people fulfill these more "basic" drives. We review a few examples here, in a nonexhaustive review focusing on the work of psychologists (we should note that anthropology has a much larger literature).

### Food

As any traveler knows, people around the world satisfy their need for nourishment with a diverse array of cuisines. Modern cultures vary not only in what types of food they eat, but also in how they eat it and what they cognitively associate with it. For instance, the French eat smaller portions and take longer to eat them than Americans do (Rozin, 1996, 1999; Rozin, Kabnick, Pete, Fischler, & Shields, 2003). Cultures can also shape moral values about food through emotional associations. For instance, a culturally specific emotional response (such as disgust) may signal that it's morally wrong to eat certain foods (Haidt, Rozin, McCauley, & Imada, 1997). In addition, cultures shape people's associations to food. Americans' associations to food show greater concern for health, whereas Belgian and French samples associate food with pleasure, and Japanese samples associate a little of each (Rozin, Fischler, Imada, Sarubin, & Wrzesniewski, 1999).

### Sleep

Cultures set norms for where and with whom people sleep. In the West, cultural norms sanctioned by pediatricians and grandparents, as well as available technologies (such as cribs, bassinets, and baby monitors), encourage parents to sleep in a separate room from their dependent children. However, in many world cultures, parents sleep with their children, either in the same bed or in the same room; infants may not sleep in cribs but in their mothers' arms (Rogoff, 2003). Families follow quantifiable rules about who sleeps with whom, depending on space in the home (Shweder, Balle-Jensen, & Goldstein, 2003). For instance, in a home with three sleeping rooms, almost all Americans in a Chicago sample preferred to have mother and father in one room, sons in a second room, and daughters in a third room. Only half of an Oriya, India sample preferred this arrangement, with many others preferring to have young children sleep with a parent. Middle-class American rules for sleeping prioritize *incest avoidance* (parents should not sleep alone with opposite-sex offspring), followed by a rule dubbed *the sacred couple* (parents should sleep together in a separate space), followed by *autonomy* (children should sleep alone). Oriya rules for sleeping also prioritize incest avoidance, but this is followed by a rule for *protection of the vulnerable* (young children should not sleep alone), *female chastity anxiety* (teenage daughters should not sleep alone or with either a father or opposite-sex siblings), and *respect for hierarchy* (oldest sons should sleep separately) (Shweder et al., 2003).

## Sex

In the realm of sexual behavior, researchers have documented both strong universal tendencies and cultural differences. People universally prefer privacy for their sexual activities (Brown, 1991; Baumeister, 2005). And, universally, men probably have a stronger sex drive than women (Baumeister, Catanese, & Vohs, 2001). Contemporary men and women may also have universally different preferences in sexual partners, with men valuing traits that indicate fertility and women valuing traits that indicate high status (Buss & Kenrick, 1998; cf. Eagly & Wood, 1999). However, at the same time, a global view reveals profound cross-cultural differences in sexual attitudes, morality, and behavior—especially among women, who have greater "erotic plasticity" (Baumeister, 2005). In one notable culture, adolescent boys perform ritualized homosexual acts and yet emerge from adolescence as heterosexual adults—a practice that adds cultural complexity to the question of the nature and nurture of homosexuality (Herdt, 1981). Cultures also differ in how they enhance secondary sex characteristics for physical attractiveness (Morris, 1997); in whether, or how, they enforce female chastity (Baumeister & Twenge, 2003; Shweder et al., 2003); and in the frames they use to justify sexual violence (e.g., Vandello & Cohen, 2003).

## Aggression

Cultures differ in their expressions of aggression, a drive that is probably related to an evolutionarily rewarded drive for self-protection. One now classic example is the *culture of honor* (Cohen & Nisbett, 1996), in which men in the U.S. South have been shown to respond quickly, angrily, aggressively, and biologically (via increases in testosterone) to insults; historically, this pattern is linked to an economy of herding, where a man's entire livelihood could be taken away in a single act of aggression. Southern men are apparently socialized to respond to threats to their honor with immediate hostility, in order to maintain a reputation as a person to be reckoned with. In contrast, Northern men respond to insults with relative amusement and no apparent surge in testosterone (Cohen, Nisbett, Bowdle, & Schwartz, 1996). Cultures also differ greatly at extreme levels of violence, with some endorsing and practicing war, and other cultural communities (such as the Hutterites) promoting nonviolent, communal solutions to conflict (Archer, 2001; Fry, 2001). Similarly, one common emotional precursor to aggression—that is, anger—is expressed and experienced differently across cultures. Particularly in cultural contexts that support highly interdependent concepts of self (see below), anger may be experienced as a selfish or childish emotion, and thus may be expressed, and even felt, rarely (Briggs, 1970).

## Attachment

Like many other social animals, helpless human infants must rely upon adult caregivers for their physical survival, so infant–adult attachment systems provide a context that helps ensure the infants' physical care (Bowlby, 1988). Attachment motives, unlike those we have cited for eating, sleeping, self-protection, and sex, may be innate (and favored by evolution) only among social animals such as humans and apes. By crying, smiling, or approaching, human infants universally must establish emotional attachments with adults, which make it more likely that the adults will care for them. But human cultures vary in how adults respond to infant attachment behaviors (Rothbaum, Weisz, Pott, Miyake, & Morelli, 2000). In

North America, healthy or "secure" attachment is marked by the caregiver's consistent, sensitive responses to an infant's attachment-seeking behaviors. Secure attachment is identified when an infant autonomously explores his or her environment, using the caregiver as a "secure base." Such autonomous exploration (as opposed to clinging to the caregiver or ignoring the caregiver) is the mark of social competence in the North American system.

Japanese caregivers and infants show a very different solution to the problem of infant–caregiver attachment. Rather than responding to their infants' cues, Japanese caregivers ideally develop emotional and physical closeness with their infants, allowing them to anticipate what their infants need. In Japan, the socially competent outcome of healthy attachment is interpersonal dependence, rather than autonomy. Infants in Japan are encouraged to develop empathy, responsiveness to their social world, and adherence to norms (rather than exploration of the environment). Because of this qualitative difference in the attachment system, Japanese infants may actually be misclassified as insecurely attached, if they are evaluated with North American tests of attachment. In North America, attachment is ironically in the service of separation: It gives children the confidence to tackle the world on their own, a skill needed for adult success in North American culture. In Japan, attachment is in the service of future attachment. Japanese attachment serves to develop lifelong skills of dependence that presumably enable Japanese adults to participate in a culture that values empathy and interdependence (Rothbaum et al., 2000). Both attachment systems, however, seem to serve some universal motive to form emotional bonds with a caregiver, in the service of infant survival (Rothbaum et al., 2000). (For a review of adult attachment systems, see Mikulincer & Shaver, Chapter 13, this volume.)

## CULTURES SHAPE THE SELF-CONCEPT

We have suggested above that cultural contexts provide quite different ways of enacting even universal biological drives (to eat, sleep, reproduce, aggress, and form attachments). The fact that we can document cultural differences in such motivations, which probably have evolved, dedicated neural structures, is a testimony to the power of culture to influence human motivation. We now extend our review to motives that may not themselves be universal; these motivations stem from the self-concept. For instance, all humans are motivated to eat, but are all humans motivated to have high self-esteem? Humans seem unique among animal species both in their ability to be self-aware (Leary, 2004) and in their dependence upon cultural meaning systems. Although other animals, such as chimpanzees, have cultures (Whiten et al., 1999), humans are unique in the sophistication of their cultural systems and in the extent of their dependence on culture. Similarly, humans are arguably unique in the extent to which they can self-reflect, take the perspectives of others, and connect their actions to the past and the future (Leary, 2004). In this section we explain how human culture shapes the human self-concept, and in the next we give several examples of what this means for motivation.

Human capabilities for culture and self-concept come together fundamentally, because societies differ in their commitment to particular views of the self. As pointed out by a number of theorists (Markus & Kitayama, 1991, 2004; Shweder & Bourne, 1984; Triandis, 1988), different cultures have their own conceptions about what the self is and what it ought to be. These conceptions are reflected, codified, and embodied in a large number of daily practices and associated lay theories or meanings. Thus this literature suggests that people around the world do not practice "the self" in a universal way. Because these different self-ways provide a matrix by which specific moral imperatives are given meanings and moral tones, this consideration has important implications for motivation.

Many middle-class European Americans practice the self as an autonomous, separable, context-free entity whose behavior reflects internal thoughts, feelings, and motivations. This view of the self is fostered and reinforced by myriad practices (e.g., merit-based pay systems, an emphasis on choice in the marketplace) and public meanings (e.g., advertisements, songs, and news coverage that emphasize autonomy and personal achievement, icons associated with the American dream—Hong, Chiu, Morris, & Benet-Martinez, 2000; Kim & Markus, 1999; Markus, Uchida, Omeregie, Townsend, & Kitayama, 2006; Snibbe & Markus, 2005) that are shared in this cultural group. Because this view is consistent with and constantly bolstered by many public facets of social life, it is often taken for granted and perceived to be "natural" rather than culturally crafted. Indeed, until recently, this "independent" model of the self has been studied as the primary, "normal" model of personhood by mainstream psychology.

Yet abundant evidence from psychology and anthropology has converged to show that the independent practice of self is not a dominant practice in many world cultures (Greenfield, Keller, Fuligni, & Maynard, 2003; Markus & Kitayama, 1991, 2004; Shweder & Bourne, 1984; Triandis, 1988). Many cultures (such as East Asia, South America, or Africa) practice a more interdependent concept of self, in which the self is construed to be inherently connected with others in a relationship. As a consequence, people's thoughts, feelings, and motivations are inextricably linked to this particular social context. Many practices (e.g., gift giving and situation-specific politeness codes) and public meanings (e.g., advertisements and news coverage that highlight relationship; Kim & Markus, 1999; Lee, Hallahan, & Herzog, 1996; Markus et al., 2006) of this cultural group constantly bolster such a view of the self; as a consequence, this view is bound to be taken for granted, perceived to be natural, and thus undoubted most of the time. For people in such cultures, who one is—the self—depends on whom one is with, why, and in what role. Feelings of duty and obligation, social connectedness, and personal flexibility are cognitively salient in such cultures, in contrast to an individualistic focus on personal freedoms, self-reliance, and the stability of personality. Although both independent and interdependent views of self are available in all cultural groups, cultures vary remarkably in terms of the extent to which one or the other view of the self is highlighted, reinforced, and described as "natural."

One important outcome of these culturally sanctioned views of self is that the content and structure of motivation are different. In cultures that foster an independent mode of self-regulation, individual attitudes and cognitions may be more important than social norms as a motivator of one's own behavior. People may be motivated, for example, to act upon their own self-determined choices, or they may be motivated to maintain self-evaluated consistency between their own attitudes and behavior.

In contrast, in cultures whose daily practices support an interdependent mode of self-regulation, the attributes and opinions of social others are highly salient (Kitayama & Uchida, 2003) and provide the most important anchor in self-regulation. Furthermore, the function of social others may be *constitutive* in such cultures; that is, social others play a function in defining the self itself. When it comes to motivation, people's needs may be socially constituted. For example, people may be motivated to fulfill the desires of close others, such as the achievement goals of one's family (Bond, 1986). Or people may be explicitly motivated to perform actions that satisfy socially salient norms for how to be a good group member. In the following section of this chapter, we review several ways in which human motivation is encouraged by, constrained by, or sanctioned by different cultural practices of the self.

## CULTURES SHAPE SELF-RELEVANT MOTIVATIONS

### Motivation for High Self-Esteem

If personal attributes of the self are salient and self-defining, people may be expected to strive to maintain and enhance the perceived worth of these attributes. Consistent with this analysis, one well-established motive in Western populations is the motivation to have high self-esteem (Taylor & Sherman, Chapter 4, this volume). Despite the potential hazards of pursuing self-esteem for self-esteem's sake (Crocker & Park, 2004), many Americans continue to treat self-esteem as a natural striving. However, if the self is constructed as a relational entity, the motivation toward positive self-esteem may not be ubiquitous. In support of this analysis, cultural psychological evidence demonstrates that the goal of enhancing one's self-esteem may be local to European American cultures who practice an independent self (Crocker & Park, 2004; Heine, Lehman, Markus, & Kitayama, 1999). Japanese (and perhaps other East Asians) seem motivated to be accurately self-critical, rather than to self-enhance. In an interdependent cultural context, self-criticism may have two important functions. First, it enables a person to identify his or her shortcomings, so as to improve on and eventually to meet the expectations of significant others. Second, it also enables the person to maintain social harmony by avoiding becoming a "stick that stands out."

Although a lack of self-enhancement might sometimes be due to modesty pressures (Kurman, 2001), evidence is quite unequivocal that Asians do not show self-enhancement, and in fact sometimes show sizable self-criticism even when responses are entirely anonymous (Heine et al., 1999). Recent evidence suggests that whereas Americans feel most happy and satisfied when their personal self is enhanced, Asians feel most happy and satisfied when they are connected, social harmony is achieved, and social strain is minimized (Kitayama, Mesquita, & Karasawa, 2006). Within the latter cultural ethos, little or no motivational push toward self-enhancement may be experienced.

Several studies support this conclusion. Whereas North Americans tend to interpret a wide range of situations (written by people in both cultures) as opportunities to increase their self-esteem, Japanese do not (Kitayama, Markus, Matsumoto, & Norasakkunkit, 1997). Whereas Americans are likely to attribute their successes to their own ability and attribute their failures to external forces, East Asians do this less (Kitayama, Takagi, & Matsumoto, 1995). And whereas North Americans are unrealistically optimistic about their own futures (Heine & Lehman, 1995) and view themselves and their own groups as better than average, East Asians tend to feel that their futures will be ordinary (Ohashi & Yamaguchi, 2004). They may view themselves, their families, and their own groups as average (rather than above average; Heine & Lehman, 1997), and they may show ingroup criticism (Snibbe, Kitayama, Markus, & Suzuki, 2003). However, they tend to hold relatively flattering views of others in relationships, resulting in a relationship-enhancing bias (Endo, Heine, & Lehman, 2000).

Such differences in emphasis on self-enhancement versus self-criticism can be linked to self-concept differences in these populations. Indeed, regardless of culture, measures of independence are correlated with positive self-views (e.g., Heine & Renshaw, 2002). This link makes sense, because when people view themselves as autonomous, they may be better off viewing themselves as talented, competent, and capable (Heine, 2005). Independent selves also emphasize their own internal standards of reference, which, because they are hard to disconfirm, are easier to distort in a positive direction to enhance self-esteem. In contrast, in East Asia, people participate in a cultural context that emphasizes positive "face." To maintain face, people try to obtain the positive attention of other people, something that is attained when people live up to the standards of others. Because such feedback comes from other people, it is less easily manipulated in a self-serving direction (Heine, 2005). In addition, inflated self-views can alienate a person from others—an outcome that may not really bother an individualist, but that might devastate an interdependent person (Paulhus, 1998). In contrast, meeting other people's expectations through criticizing, and subsequently improving, the self is more likely to fulfill the affiliative goals of the interdependent self. To sum up, North Americans may be so motivated to view the self positively (in service to the independent self-concept) that they compromise reality in a self-serving direction. East Asians are motivated to accurately diagnose and to correct the self's shortcomings, in part because they are motivated to meet the goals of an ingroup and thus to achieve social harmony, or at least to avoid any interpersonal strains.

These differences between self-enhancement and self-serving biases on the one hand, and face maintenance via self-criticism and self-improvement on the other hand, have also been documented in the academic learning environment. The social practices in schools serve as a significant set of opportunities to practice and learn the self-ways of a culture. Cultural research has documented two meaningful constellations of motivational, attributional, and behavioral response to academic challenge: one predominant among North Americans, and the other predominant among East Asians. In the North American culture, success in school is more often attributed to ability—an innate, unchanging aspect inside the self (Stevenson & Stigler, 1992). In East Asian culture, success in school is more often attributed to effort—a variable, changeable aspect of the self. Although people can attribute their outcomes to effort or to fixed ability (Dweck & Leggett, 1988), American children and their parents in one study were more likely to make ability attributions (at least after success), and East Asian children and parents to make effort attributions (Stevenson & Stigler, 1992). This basic attributional difference has important classroom repercussions. Teachers in North America tend to pass over a child's errors in the classroom, without explaining why an answer is incorrect. When ability is thought to be innate, a child's error means that the child has less innate ability, and teachers appear reluctant to embarrass a child by correcting him or her. In contrast, East Asian teachers treat errors as opportunities to learn more; they may dwell on a child's error in class, explaining why the answer is incorrect, without a hint of embarrassment for the student. Indeed, the quality of instruction may be higher when teachers helpfully explain errors to students than when they ignore errors (Stevenson & Stigler, 1992).

These schemas about academic performance translate into different motivations for effort at academic tasks. Specifically, North Americans are motivated to work harder on tasks that they know they can already do well. In a lab study, North Americans worked longer at puzzles that they had just learned they were good at; they did not want to work on the puzzles if they knew they were bad at them (Heine et al., 2001). In contrast, East Asians are motivated to work harder on tasks that they do not do well. In the lab study, they worked longer at puzzles when they had just learned they were poor at them. Thus Americans act according to culturally shared schemas that say low ability is intractable (they give up), whereas Japanese act according to a shared schema that low ability can and should be repaired. Interestingly, however, giving "innate ability" feedback to East Asians makes them act more like North Americans, and giving "effort" feedback to North Americans makes them act more like East Asians. Specifically, telling North Americans that performance on the puzzles could be improved by effort (thus overriding the dominant schema content) led the North Americans to work hard at puzzles even if they were bad at them. Telling East Asians that performance on the puzzles was innate, however, led the East Asians to stop working hard on puzzles that they were bad at. The motivational implications of ability and effort attributions for academic success relate to self-esteem. Working hard at tasks they do well, and avoiding tasks they do not do well, help Americans maintain high self-esteem in academic situations. In contrast, for East Asians, working hard at tasks they do not do well may not be conducive to high self-esteem, but it may lead both to future improvement of performance and to humility—a trait that is suited to maintaining group harmony.

## Motivation for Personal Control

Another well-studied, self-relevant motivation is the motivation for *personal control*—the perception that one can intentionally cause outcomes in the environment. Personal control research covers a family of related constructs, including *internal locus of control*, *self-efficacy*, *primary control*, and *perceived control* (Heckhausen & Schultz, 1995; Rotter, 1966; Strickland, 1989). The dominant result from research on North Americans is that people who have a sense of personal, internal control (e.g., people who believe that their own efforts will lead to good grades, that maintaining a healthy diet will keep illness at bay, or that their parenting skills will result in a happy child) tend to be better off. Decades of research on North Americans have found that personal control perceptions motivate social action and are correlated with better mental health, even if perceptions of personal control are illusory (Thompson, Sobolew-Shubin, Galbraith, Schwankovsky, & Cruzen, 1993).

Empirical cultural psychology has revealed two interesting patterns in regard to personal control. First, the concept of agency and personal choice appears to be culturally constructed. European American cultures emphasize *disjoint agency*, in which individual (rather than group) desires are central determinants of behavior; interdependent cultures emphasize *conjoint agency*, in which individual agency is shared with important others, such as coaches and close family members (Hobfoll, 2002; Markus et al., 2006). Even within the United States, middle-class music and working-class music reflect different themes of agency, representing choice and freedom on the one hand, and adjustment and integrity on the other (Snibbe & Markus, 2005). Further evidence for differences in the importance of personal control suggest that among a sample of East Asians, in contrast, lack of personal control is not associated with distress; in fact, the self-sufficiency of personal control violates norms of interdependence in such cultures, so it comes at higher cost (Sastry & Ross, 1998).

Personal control may be contrasted with another motivational tendency to adapt flexibly to situations. So-called *secondary control* occurs when people engage in two simultaneous psychological activities: They adjust themselves, and they accept existing circumstances as they are (Morling & Evered, 2006; Rothbaum, Weisz, & Snyder, 1982). Secondary control is adaptive for people in a large variety of situations, even in North America (Morling & Evered, 2006; Morling, Kitayama, & Miyamoto, 2003). Culturally speaking, however, secondary control has been noted to be relatively more available, valued, and endorsed by people in East Asian cultures (Morling & Evered, 2006; Weisz, Rothbaum, & Blackburn, 1984). For example, in one study, students in Japan reported experiencing secondary control (i.e., adjusting) in various situations more frequently than their American counterparts, and these situations were very effective at promoting perceived relatedness to others. In contrast, Americans reported more frequent instances of influencing their environment via personal control, and American personal control situations were very effective at promoting feelings of efficacy and power (Morling, Kitayama, & Miyamoto, 2002). The Japanese practice of adjusting illustrates well the constitutive role of social others and the salience of social information over individual desires. This view of embeddedness helps people cope: Japanese women who relied more on *social assurance*—that is, the trust that other people would make decisions and influence care for them—coped better with normal pregnancy (Morling et al., 2003).

It is noteworthy that researchers have used the labels *primary control* (attempts to influence the environment) and *secondary control* (attempts to adjust to the environment) to describe these two variations on the motive for control. Given that secondary control is probably more elaborated in interdependent cultural contexts, such ethnocentric labeling has come under fire (Gould, 1999; Morling & Evered, 2006, but see Heckhausen & Schulz, 1999). There have been some attempts to rename the constructs (e.g., calling secondary control *internal self-control* [Gould, 1999] or *harmony control* [Morling & Fiske, 1999]), but the problem lies as much in the noun as in the adjective. There is no indigenous word in Japanese for *control*, for example. And empirically, using the term *control* may be a misnomer, as the process of adjusting oneself and accepting the environment does not seem to result in feelings of efficacy, power, or control (Morling & Evered, 2006). At this time, cultural researchers are increasingly adopting "influence" and "adjustment" as labels (after Morling et al., 2002; e.g., Tsai, Knutson, & Fung, 2006).

In sum, seeing oneself as competent, individually efficacious, and "in control" clearly motivates action among people in middle-class European American cultures (Bandura, 1997). Among people in East Asian cultures, however, people's acts of control may involve conjoint agency rather than disjoint, independent agency. Furthermore, East Asian cultures seem to have elaborated and emphasized the complementary process of flexibly adjusting the self to fit into social networks and other situations.

## Motivation for Internal Consistency

Social psychologist Leon Festinger (1957) originally proposed that people feel *cognitive dissonance* when they become aware of inconsistencies between two or more cognitions. For example, if people are subtly coerced to tell another person that an extremely boring task is actually very interesting, they may feel an uncomfortable dissonance between their own belief about the task and their public statements about it. In response, Festinger argued, people will attempt to change one of the dissonant cognitions; in the example just given, people may change their belief about the task and conclude that it was actually quite interesting. Dissonance reduction efforts are especially likely when dissonance threatens some important aspect of the self. Indeed, research on North Americans shows that people will justify behaviors that have gone against their self-image—a self-image that usually views the self as ethical, decisive, and reasonable. For example, in one paradigm, participants in a media attitudes study are given two options of similarly attractive CDs and asked to choose one for themselves. After choosing one of them, participants typically evaluate the chosen CD more positively than before, and the alternative CD less positively. This *spreading of alternatives* is presumably an attempt to bolster a self-image of being a person who makes reasonable decisions (for a review of other paradigms, see

Harmon-Jones & Harmon-Jones, Chapter 5, this volume).

Extending this general framework, Kitayama, Snibbe, Markus, and Suzuki (2004) have proposed that there are two varieties of cognitive dissonance. One type of dissonance is *personal*, which focuses on a possibility that a behavior might reveal a deficit in one's internal self-attributes, such as ability and moral integrity. Another type of worry or dissonance is *interpersonal*, focusing on the prospect that the behavior might not be fully understood, accepted, or appreciated by social others who are relevant to the self (e.g., ingroup members). Research has supported that European North Americans respond to personal dissonance through spreading of alternatives in response to a personal choice. However, in a cross-cultural replication study, East Asians and Asian Canadians did not justify a personal choice in this way (Heine & Lehman, 1997). Instead, Japanese and East Asian Canadians have been shown to engage in postchoice justifications when they made a choice for a *friend* (Hoshino-Browne et al., 2005). After choosing an object for a friend, these groups enhanced their ratings of the chosen object, as if to justify their choice for the friend.

Other research has suggested particular conditions under which even interdependent selves may justify choices made for themselves. Kitayama and colleagues (2004) have hypothesized that Asians should not show any dissonance effect in a standard free-choice dissonance paradigm, because there is no social cue in that paradigm. So they asked North Americans and Japanese to participate in an altered self-choice dissonance paradigm, in which they asked participants to report what their peers would think. As predicted, under these conditions of other-reference, Japanese did show a reliable dissonance effect. Further analyses suggested that the others in reference need to be important; that is, Japanese showed a reliable dissonance effect in a likeable-other condition, but not in an unlikeable-other condition. It is noteworthy that American participants showed an equal dissonance effect regardless of the presence of the other reference manipulations, indicating that their personal knowledge was so salient that they could easily ignore the manipulations of other-reference. In a follow-up study, Japanese participants even showed a dissonance effect in response to the incidental presence of a poster displaying schematic faces that were gazing at them. This suggests that such a subtle cue of social others is enough to evoke interpersonal worry and dissonance for those with salient knowledge about social others.

## Intrinsic Motivation

Cultural differences in the self-concept also seem to affect the extent to which people are motivated for self-determination. One compelling finding in North American psychology is that when people do an activity of their own choosing, they appear to work more persistently, to enjoy their work more, and to be more creative (Deci & Ryan, 1985). North Americans apparently excel at activities that they do for themselves, because of their own intrinsic interest. The effects of intrinsic motivation may be especially strong for independent selves, however, because daily practices in independent cultural contexts (such as regularly offering an array of options) generally support those who know and express their inner preferences. In cultural contexts that emphasize interdependence, expressing one's inner desires through personal choice is not as important, and fewer everyday practices will encourage personal expression. In contrast, people might be more motivated to do things that important ingroup members want, perhaps in part because such social knowledge is more salient. In a study that tested this idea (Iyengar & Lepper, 1999), European American children performed better at tasks when they got to make their own decisions about certain features of the task, whereas Asian American children performed better at the tasks when they heard that their mothers or classmates (i.e., important ingroup members) had chosen these features for them. The motivation to determine one's own fate is apparently less strong for Asian American children; instead, these children were especially motivated to perform, and in fact performed better, when close other people made choices on their behalf. One view of this outcome states that perhaps the Asian American children wanted not to disappoint their ingroups, and so put forth more effort. It is possible that in an interdependent culture, an ingroup's decisions for an individual may reflect special understanding of that individual and a desire to care for and support him or her. Close others constitute an important—and motivating—source of information about what an individual should do (but see Ryan & Deci, 2002, for a more universalist view on self-determination).

## Relative Priority of Personal and Group Goals

As emphasized by researchers who study individualism and collectivism (Hofstede, 1980; Triandis, 1995), people differ in the extent to which they prioritize ingroup goals over personal goals. These differences have significant motivational consequences. By definition, individualists are motivated to pursue their individual plans, even when they conflict with the outcome of a group (Triandis, Bontempo, Villareal, Asai, & Lucca, 1988). Collectivists are motivated to fulfill their duties to the group (Oyserman, Coon, & Kemmelmeier, 2002). The distinction between individualism and collectivism is closely mapped onto the one between independent and interdependent views of self, discussed earlier.

There are several psychological outcomes of a motivational focus on group duty or a motivational focus on individual autonomy (Oyserman et al., 2002; Triandis, 1995). In some cases these psychological outcomes are directly correlated with measures of individualism and collectivism, but in most cases the pertinent psychological patterns are inferred to be related to individualism and collectivism because they differ in cultural groups that show documented differences in these characteristics (e.g., Americans are usually higher than other groups on individualism and usually lower than other groups on collectivism).

Individualism's motivational focus on personal autonomy is associated with *dispositional reasoning* (attributing the actions of others to their dispositions), whereas collectivism is associated with *situational* reasoning (attributing others' actions to contextual factors) (Choi & Nisbett, 1998; Miller, 1984; Miyamoto & Kitayama, 2002). Moreover, this difference in emphasis on the figural object (person) and its context (situation) can sometimes be observed even with nonsocial, entirely decontextualized stimuli (Kitayama, Duffy, Kawamura, & Larsen, 2003), resulting in culturally divergent patterns of thought and perception called *analytic* versus *holistic* modes (Nisbett, 2003). Though this reasoning style may not be motivated per se, it does reflect the kinds of information that would best serve an individualist's perception goals (Fiske, 1992). Specifically, individualists may tune out contextual information (even when it is potentially important), because according to schemas for the self in their culture, individuals act according to internal preferences and traits. Thus dispositional information may be considered more relevant for individualists. In contrast, collectivists may be better at attending to situational information, because context is highlighted in their cultural models (Markus & Kitayama, 1991; Oyserman et al., 2002). Holistic attention may also be facilitated by cultural differences in human-made physical environments. Actual physical environments are more complex in Japan than in North America, and such environments prime holistic attention to a scene (Miyamoto, Nisbett, & Masuda, 2006).

As for actual social behavior, the data suggest that collectivists' behavior in a group may depend on the group's intimacy and familiarity. For example, Japanese may actually act less cooperatively in economic games with strangers (e.g., Toda, Shinotsuka, McClintock, & Stech, 1978), perhaps because familiar systems of mutually committed relations are absent. In contrast, North Americans may surprisingly act more trusting in novel situations (Yamagishi & Yamagishi, 1994). However, when collectivists work as part of a group, they do not engage in social loafing. For example, one study compared U.S. and Chinese managerial trainees on an in-basket task (Early, 1989). In one condition, participants heard that their group would be evaluated on its shared action, and each *group* was expected to complete 200 items. Other participants heard that they should work their best, and each *individual* was expected to complete 20 items. Another factor in the design manipulated accountability, by having participants write their names on their items or not. Chinese participants worked harder in the shared responsibility conditions than they did in the individual responsibility conditions. This is evidence of the *opposite* of social loafing effects that are often observed in Americans. The American participants, in contrast to the Chinese, worked hard in the shared responsibility task only when their output was made personally accountable. Without accountability, Americans worked less hard in the group setting.

Indeed, the literature on cultural differences in social behavior is extensive; it covers friendship (e.g., Wheeler, Reis, & Bond, 1989), romantic relationships (e.g., Dion & Dion, 1993), and even enemyship (e.g., Adams, 2005). A review of this literature is beyond the limited scope of the present chapter. However, individualism and collectivism can be construed as motivational orientations that are important predictors of a variety of social behaviors (see Triandis, 1995, for one review).

### Summary

In these last several subsections, we have reviewed a variety of evidence for cross-cultural variations in human motivation. In most cases, these motivational patterns can be explained as manifestations of how knowledge about the self versus others is selectively salient. When self-knowledge is salient and others are viewed as instruments by which the self can amplify its qualities, people strive to evaluate the self very positively, to influence the environment, to justify difficult decisions to the self, to put effort into actions that reflect the self's own choices, and to prioritize the self's goals over group goals. When social knowledge is salient and others help to define or constitute the self, people strive to identify and correct their shortcomings, to adjust to social circumstances, to justify difficult choices to others, and to prioritize group goals over the self's goals.

## UNIVERSALITY AND SPECIFICITY OF MOTIVATIONS

In this chapter we have demonstrated cultural differences in a number of social motivations that were once assumed to be universal. This evidence for variability raises a number of interesting questions about the universality and local specificity of human motivation. In this section we review a few theorists' efforts to develop "short lists" of evolved human motives—endeavors that reveal a theoretical tension between cultural psychology and evolutionary psychology, two levels of analysis that are occasionally at odds. Cultural psychologists, who are theoretically disposed to document and explain human variety, are conservative when it comes to identifying universals. In contrast, evolutionary perspectives in psychology strive to explain how selection pressures shaped humans at a universal, biological level. What do these seemingly competing perspectives say about human motivations? At what descriptive level might both cultural and evolutionary psychologists be convinced of universality?

One taxonomy of motivations, provided by Kenrick, Li, and Butner (2003), includes six fundamental human goals, all of which presumably evolved to solve evolutionarily important social problems. The six goals are closely related to the fitness of *individual genes*. The list includes the goals to form and maintain cooperative alliances, to gain or maintain respect from or power over other group members, to protect oneself and one's ingroup, to obtain a mate who will enhance one's fitness, to maintain a mating bond with a desirable partner, and to promote the survival of genetic offspring. Another list of possibly universal human goals (Bugental, 2000) includes five aspects of social development that are important for individual and inclusive fitness: attachment, coalitional group formation, mating, reciprocity, and hierarchical power. The authors of these two lists do argue that cultural content provides specific solutions to these universal "problems" of gene survival. Culturally variable motivations reflect a group's historical solutions to the problems, the ecological pressures provided by the group's physical environment, and even the pressure of idiosyncratic individuals in the group (Kenrick et al., 2003). But overall, these two lists mainly focus on people's ability to survive in a social niche (the setting in which human beings most certainly evolved). Cultural systems of meaning are not explicitly seen as selection pressures in these models.

Another prominent motivational model, by Fiske (2003; see also Fiske, Chapter 1, this volume), includes a set of five ("plus or minus five") human motives. According to Fiske, the overarching human motive is to belong—a motive that, in our ancient past as well as our present, helps individual humans survive. The four other motives on Fiske's list are subordinate to belonging: understanding, controlling, enhancing the self, and trusting. These four motives are subordinate to helping the individual survive in a social niche (e.g., the motive to understand helps people function in groups more effectively). But all five also have culturally specific manifestations. For example, collectivism and individualism can be seen as cultural variations on the belonging motive, and self-enhancement and self-criticism (as described earlier in this chapter) may be regarded as cultural variations on the motive to enhance the self (Fiske, 2003).

Another set of motivational processes are described explicitly with reference to the idea that selection favored people who could function in an existing matrix of cultural meanings. Certainly humans originally evolved to function in groups, but anthropologists and cultural psychologists have argued that beyond this, genes and culture coevolved (Geertz, 1973; Richerson & Boyd, 2005). Culture is not just an add-on to a socially evolved brain. Human brains evolved to take advantage of culture, and primitive cultures created selection pressures—favoring humans who were better adapted to living not just in a social group (like other primates), but in complex cultural settings. For example, humans probably evolved the ability to understand the self as a causal agent, to understand that other people have intentions just like the self, and to imitate accurately the intentional actions of others (Tomasello, 1999). At an early age (9 months, typically), human infants begin to imitate others' goal-directed actions, and this developmental milestone sets up the ability to readily absorb the valuable informational content of his or her cultural world (Tomasello, 1999). This cognitive skill is closely tied to motivation and to understanding of others' motivations. Infants imitate others in order to achieve similar goals (e.g., they may use their head to turn on a light, if they see an adult do so) (Meltzoff, 1988, as cited in Tomasello, 1999), and they selectively imitate actions of others that are intentional, rather than accidental. The early appearance of this species-specific ability suggests that it is an evolved motivation to make the most of culture. Extending this spirit, Baumeister (2005) proposed a set of motives that are tied to surviving in a cultural milieu: language, self-esteem, morality, success, and meaning in life.

Although it has not yet been included in a taxonomy of universals, Heine, Proulx, and Vohs (2006) have recently articulated a human motive for meaning—a need that has strong implications for a culturally evolved animal. In their meaning maintenance model, these authors define a *motive for meaning* as the need to see events in such a way that they fit into a cognitive structure of expected relationships. Heine and colleagues argue that people may be extremely disturbed by disruptions to their meaning systems—such as trusted relationship partners who abandon them, "good" people who die, or even playing cards that are printed in the wrong color. People will revise their meaning structures in response to such events in the world, or revise their perceptions of such events to fit into their meaning structures (e.g., via assimilation or accommodation). But according to Heine and colleagues, the need for meaning can also be met by achieving meaningful frameworks in belonging (Leary & Cox, Chapter 2, this volume), self-esteem (Taylor & Sherman, Chapter 4, this volume), certainty (Harmon-Jones & Harmon-Jones, Chapter 5, this volume), and symbolic immortality (Greenberg, Solomon, & Arndt, Chapter 8, this volume). Furthermore, if a lower-level knowledge structure (such as the need for belonging) is threatened, people can feel better by fluidly compensating their need for meaning at a different domain—perhaps by enhancing their self-esteem or asserting their certainty about moral rules (McGregor, Nail, Marigold, & Kang, 2005). Similarly, if people become uncertain about connections among pieces of knowledge in the world, they can compensate by enhancing their relatedness to others. In the context of this chapter, the most interesting thing about this model is that it presents the need for meaning as an overarching motive for human beings. People seek connections and relationships—between people, between self and the world, between elements in the world (Heine et al., 2006). This flexibly satisfied drive for meaning might in the future be viewed as an evolved "meta"-motivation that makes people exquisitely suited for cultural life (since cultural life is, after all, a network of meaning structures). People who were driven to seek meaning wherever they could were more likely to benefit from the rich opportunities and information afforded by culture, and thereby to survive.

In this section we have briefly presented some taxonomies of universal human motivations. Some taxonomies present universal motives as socially evolved strategies for surviving in groups (where basic motives can be shaped by cultural content). Other taxonomies have added universal motives that may be evolved strategies for surviving in a wider cultural niche of information, tools, and meaning structures.

Before leaving this discussion, we should note that the traditional, evolutionary view certainly suggests that it is valuable to identify *both* universals and cultural differences in human motivation, and some commentators have also argued for the scientific and heuristic value of identifying human universals (e.g., Brown, 1991). But others argue that the search for any universals in motivation may be misguided. For instance, Geertz (1973) argued at length that human nature cannot be described in universal terms; instead, to be human is to be culturally *variable*. Geertz argued that although we can identify universals among all humans (e.g., all human beings have a concept of property, a concept of religion, or a concept of marriage), such universal concepts are "bloodless," doing little to capture the richness of cultural specificity. Therefore, a challenging task for future work is to map out the connections between the two levels of analysis—that is, evolutionary and cultural.

## CONCLUSION

Motivated human action takes place in a particular cultural context. Shared meanings, cultural schematic content, and everyday practices provide very different ways of being, wanting, and acting. Our field is developing some fascinating models of human motivation, invoking constitutive forces that are both cultural and evolutionary. The biological motives that humans share with other animals are hypothetically the least likely to be influenced by culture, but as we review here, even these motives (to eat, to sleep, to reproduce, to aggress, to attach) can be significantly shaped by cultural content. Even more dramatically, because culture significantly shapes the self, motivations that involve the self are significantly filled with specific cultural content. When cultures enable and encourage the practice of an independent self, motivations may be experienced as housed within, and for the benefit of, the self. When cultures enable and encourage the practice of an interdependent self, motivations are experienced as shared with close others, and reflect the needs and standards of those close others.

## REFERENCES


Adams, G. (2005). The cultural grounding of personal relationship: Enemyship in North American and West African worlds. *Journal of Personality and Social Psychology, 88*, 948–968.

Archer, J. (2001). Method and theory in cross-cultural studies of aggression. In J. M. Ramirez & D. S. Richardson (Eds.), *Cross-cultural approaches to research on aggression and reconciliation* (pp. 214–228). Huntington, NY: Nova Science.

Bandura, A. (1997). *Self-efficacy: The exercise of control*. New York: Freeman.

Baumeister, R. F. (2005). *The cultural animal*. Oxford, UK: Oxford University Press.

Baumeister, R. F., Catanese, K. R., & Vohs, K. D. (2001). Is there a gender difference in strength of sex drive?: Theoretical views, conceptual distinctions, and a review of relevant evidence. *Personality and Social Psychology Review, 5*, 242–273.

Baumeister, R. F., & Twenge, J. M. (2003). *The social self*. In T. Millon & M. J. Lerner (Eds.), *Handbook of psychology: Personality and social psychology* (Vol. 5, pp. 327–352). New York: Wiley.

Berlin, I. (1976). *Vico and Herder*. London: Hogarth Press.

Bond, M. H. (1986). *The psychology of the Chinese people*. New York: Oxford University Press.

Bowlby, J. (1988). *A secure base: Parent–child attachment and healthy human development*. New York: Basic Books.

Briggs, J. L. (1970). *Never in anger*. Cambridge, MA: Harvard University Press.

Brown, D. E. (1991). *Human universals*. Philadelphia: Temple University Press.

Bruner, J. (1990). *Acts of meaning: Four lectures on mind and culture*. Cambridge, MA: Harvard University Press.

Bugental, D. B. (2000). Acquisition of the algorithms of social life: A domain-based approach. *Psychological Bulletin, 26*, 187–209.

Buss, D. M., & Kenrick, D. T. (1998). Evolutionary social psychology. In D. T. Gilbert, S. T. Fiske, & G. Lindzey (Eds.), *The handbook of social psychology* (4th ed., Vol. 2, pp. 982–1026). New York: McGraw-Hill.

Choi, I., & Nisbett, R. E. (1998). Situational salience and cultural differences in the correspondence bias and in the actor–observer bias. *Personality and Social Psychology Bulletin, 24*, 949–960.

Cohen, D., & Nisbettt, K. E. (1996). *Culture of honor: The psychology of violence in the South*. Boulder, CO: Westview Press.

Cohen, D., Nisbett, R. E., Bowdle, B. F., & Schwarz, N. (1996). Insult, aggression, and the Southern culture of honor: An "experimental ethnography." *Journal of Personality and Social Psychology, 70*, 945–960.

Crocker, J., & Park, L. E. (2004). The costly pursuit of self-esteem. *Psychological Bulletin, 130*, 392–414.

D'Andrade, R. G. (1984). Cultural meaning systems. In R. A. Shweder & R. A. LeVine (Eds.), *Culture theory: Essays on mind, self, and emotion* (pp. 87–119). Cambridge, UK: Cambridge University Press.

D'Andrade, R. G. (1992). Schemas and motivation. In R. G. D'Andrade & C. Strauss (Eds.), *Human motives and cultural models* (pp. 23–44). Cambridge, UK: Cambridge University Press.

Deci, E. L., & Ryan, R. M. (1985). *Intrinsic motivation and self-determination in human behavior.* New York: Plenum Press.

Dion, K. K., & Dion, K. L. (1993). Individualistic and collectivistic perspectives on gender and the cultural context of love and intimacy. *Journal of Social Issues, 49*, 53–69.

Dweck, C., & Leggett, E. (1988). A social-cognitive approach to motivation and personality. *Psychological Review, 95*, 256–273.

Eagly, A. H., & Wood, W. (1999). The origins of sex differences in human behavior: Evolved dispositions versus social roles. *American Psychologist, 54*, 408–423.

Early, P. C. (1989). Social loafing and collectivism: A comparison of the United States and the People's Republic of China. *Administrative Science Quarterly, 34*, 565–581.

Endo, Y., Heine, S. J., & Lehman, D. R. (2000). Culture and positive illusions in close relationships: How my relationships are better than yours. *Personality and Social Psychology Bulletin, 26*, 1571–1586.

Festinger, L. (1957). *A theory of cognitive dissonance.* Evanston, IL: Row, Peterson.

Fiske, S. T. (1992). Thinking is for doing: Portraits of social cognition from daguerreotype to laserphoto. *Journal of Personality and Social Psychology, 63*, 877–889.

Fiske, S. T. (2003). Five core social motives, plus or minus five. In S. J. Spencer, S. Fein, M. P. Zanna, & J. Oleson (Eds.), *The Ontario Symposium: Vol. 9. Motivated social perception* (pp. 233–246). Mahwah, NJ: Erlbaum.

Fry, D. P. (2001). Is violence getting too much attention? cross-cultural findings on the ways people deal with conflict. In J. M. Ramirez & D. S. Richardson (Eds.), *Cross-cultural approaches to research on aggression and reconciliation* (pp. 123–148). Huntington, NY: Nova Science.

Geertz, C. (1973). *The interpretation of cultures.* New York: Basic Books.

Gould, S. J. (1999). A critique of Heckhausen and Schulz's (1995) life-span theory of control from a cross-cultural perspective. *Psychological Review, 106*, 597–604.

Greenfield, P. M., Keller, H. F., Fuligni, A., & Maynard, A. (2003). Cultural pathways through universal development. *Annual Review of Psychology, 54*, 461–490.

Haidt, J., Rozin, P., McCauley, C., & Imada, S. (1997). Body, psyche, and culture: The relationship between disgust and morality. *Psychology and Developing Societies, 9*, 107–131.

Heckhausen, J., & Schulz, R. (1995). A life-span theory of control. *Psychological Review, 102*, 284–304.

Heckhausen, J., & Schulz, R. (1999). The primacy of primary control is a human universal: A reply to Gould's (1999) critique of the life-span theory of control. *Psychological Review, 106*, 605–609.

Heine, S. J. (2005). Constructing good selves in Japan and North America. In R. M. Sorrentino, D. Cohen, J. M. Olson, & M. P. Zanna (Eds.), *The Ontario Symposium: Vol. 10. Culture and social behavior* (pp. 115–143). Mahwah, NJ: Erlbaum.

Heine, S. J., Kitayama, S., Lehman, D. R., Takata, T., Ide, E., Leung, C., et al. (2001). Divergent consequences of success and failure in Japan and North America: An investigation of self-improving motivations and malleable selves. *Journal of Personality and Social Psychology, 81*, 599–615.

Heine, S. J., & Lehman, D. R. (1995). Cultural variation in unrealistic optimism: Does the West feel more invulnerable than the East? *Journal of Personality and Social Psychology, 68*, 595–607.

Heine, S. J., & Lehman, D. R. (1997). The cultural construction of self-enhancement: An investigation of group-serving biases. *Journal of Personality and Social Psychology, 72*, 1268–1283.

Heine, S. H., Lehman, D. R., Markus, H. R., & Kitayama, S. (1999). Is there a universal need for positive self-regard? *Psychological Review, 106*, 766–794.

Heine, S. J., Proulx, T., & Vohs, K. D. (2006). Meaning maintenance model: On the coherence of social motivations. *Personality and Social Psychology Review, 10*, 88–110.

Heine, S. J., & Renshaw, K. (2002). Interjudge agreement, self-enhancement, and liking: Cross-cultural divergences. *Personality and Social Psychology Bulletin, 28*, 442–451.

Herdt, G. H. (1981). *Guardians of the flute: A study of ritualized homosexual behavior.* New York: McGraw-Hill.

Hobfoll, S. E. (2002). Alone together: Comparing communal versus individualistic resiliency. In E. Frydenberg (Ed.), *Beyond coping: Meeting goals, visions, and challenges* (pp. 63–81). New York: Oxford University Press.

Hofstede, G. (1980). *Culture's consequences: International differences in work-related values.* Beverly Hills, CA: Sage.

Hong, Y., Chiu, C. Y., Morris, M. W., & Benet-Martinez, V. (2000). Multicultural minds: A dynamic constructivist approach to culture and cognition. *American Psychologist, 55*, 709–720.

Hoshino-Browne, E., Zanna, A. S., Spencer, S. J., Zanna, M. P., Kitayama, S., & Lackenbauer, S. (2005). On the cultural guises of cognitive dissonance: The case of Easterners and Westerners. *Journal of Personality and Social Psychology, 89*, 294–310.

Iyengar, S. S., & Lepper, M. R. (1999). Rethinking the value of choice: A cultural perspective on intrinsic motivation. *Journal of Personality and Social Psychology, 76*, 349–366.

Kenrick, D. T., Li, N. P., & Butner, J. (2003). Dynamical evolutionary psychology: Individual decision rules and emergent social norms. *Psychological Review, 110*(1), 3–28.

Kim, H., & Markus, H. R. (1999). Uniqueness or deviance, harmony or conformity: A cultural analysis. *Journal of Personality and Social Psychology, 77*, 785–800.

Kitayama, S., Duffy, S., Kawamura, T., & Larsen, J. (2003). Perceiving an object and its context in different cultures: A cultural look at new look. *Psychological Science, 14*, 201–206.

Kitayama, S., Markus, H., Matsumoto, H., & Norasakkunkit, V. (1997). Individual and collective processes in the construction of the self: Self-enhancement in the United States and self-criticism in Japan. *Journal of Personality and Social Psychology, 72*, 1245–1267.

Kitayama, S., Mesquita, B., & Karasawa, M. (2006). Cultural affordances and emotional experience: Engaging and disengaging emotions in Japan and the United States. *Journal of Personality and Social Psychology, 91*, 890–903.

Kitayama, S., Snibbe, A. C., Markus, H. R., & Suzuki, T. (2004). Is there any "free" choice?: Self and dissonance in two cultures. Psychological Science, *15*, 527–533.

Kitayama, S., Takagi, H., & Matsumoto, H. (1995). Cultural psychology of Japanese self: I. Causal attribution of success and failure. *Japanese Psychological Review, 38*, 247–280.

Kitayama, S., & Uchida, Y. (2003). Explicit self-criticism and implicit self-regard: Evaluating self and friend in two cultures. *Journal of Experimental Social Psychology, 39*, 476–482.

Kroeber, A. L., & Kluckholn, C. (1952). *Culture: A critical review of concepts and definitions*. Cambridge, MA: Harvard University Press.

Kurman, J. (2001). Is self-enhancement related to modesty or to individualism-collectivism? *Asian Journal of Social Psychology, 4*, 225–237.

Leary, M. (2004). *The curse of the self.* Oxford, UK: Oxford University Press.

Lee, F., Hallahan, M., & Herzog, T. (1996). Explaining real life events: How culture and domain shape attributions. *Personality and Social Psychology Bulletin, 22*, 731—747.

Markus, H. R., & Kitayama, S. (1991). Culture and the self: Implications for cognition, emotion, and motivation. *Psychological Review, 98*, 224–253.

Markus, H. R., & Kitayama, S. (2003). Models of agency: Sociocultural diversity in the construction of action. In V. Murphy-Berman & J. J. Berman (Eds.), *Nebraska Symposium on Motivation* (Vol. 49, pp. 18–74). Lincoln: University of Nebraska Press.

Markus, H. R., Uchida, Y., Omoregie, H., Townsend, S. S. M., & Kitayama, S. (2006). Going for the gold: Models of agency in Japanese and American contexts. *Psychological Science, 17*, 103–112.

McGregor, I., Nail, P. R., Marigold, D. C., & Kang, S. (2005). Defensive pride and consensus: Strength in imaginary numbers. *Journal of Personality and Social Psychology, 89*, 978–996.

Miller, J. G. (1984). Culture and the development of everyday social explanation. *Journal of Personality and Social Psychology, 46*, 961–978.

Miyamoto, Y., & Kitayama, S. (2002). Cultural variation in correspondence bias: The critical role of attitude diagnosticity of socially constrained behavior. *Journal of Personality and Social Psychology, 83*, 1239.

Miyamoto, Y., Nisbett, R. E., & Masuda, T. (2006). Culture and the physical environment: Holistic vs. analytic perceptual affordances. *Psychological Science, 17*, 113–119.

Morling, B., & Evered, S. (2006). Secondary control reviewed and redefined. *Psychological Bulletin, 132*, 269–296.

Morling, B., & Fiske, S. T. (1999). Defining and measuring harmony control. *Journal of Research in Personality, 33*, 379–414.

Morling, B., Kitayama, S., & Miyamoto, Y. (2002). Cultural practices emphasize influence in the United States and adjustment in Japan. *Personality and Social Psychology Bulletin, 28*, 311–323.

Morling, B., Kitayama, S., & Miyamoto, Y. (2003). American and Japanese women use different coping strategies during normal pregnancy. *Personality and Social Psychology Bulletin, 29*, 1533–1546.

Morris, D. (1997). *The human sexes.* London: BBC Books.

Nisbett, R. E. (2003). *The geography of thought: Why we think the way we do.* New York: Free Press.

Ohashi, M. M., & Yamaguchi, S. (2004). Superordinary bias in Japanese perception of future expectations. *Asian Journal of Social Psychology, 7*, 169–185.

Oyserman, D., Coon, H., & Kemmelmeier, M. (2002). Rethinking individualism and collectivism: Evaluation of theoretical assumptions and meta-analyses. *Psychological Bulletin, 128*, 3–73.

Paulhus, D.L. (1998). Interpersonal adaptiveness of trait self-enhancement: A mixed blessing? *Journal of Personality and Social Psychology, 74*, 1197–1208.

Quinn, N. (1992). The motivational force of self-understanding: Evidence from wives' inner conflicts. In R. G. D'Andrade & C. Strauss (Eds.), *Human motives and cultural models* (pp. 90–126). Cambridge, UK: Cambridge University Press.

Richerson, P. J., & Boyd, R. (2005). *Not by genes alone.* Chicago: University of Chicago Press.

Rogoff, B. (2003). *The cultural nature of human development.* Oxford, UK: Oxford University Press.

Rothbaum, F., Weisz, J. R., Pott, M., Miyake, K., & Morelli, G. (2000). Attachment and culture: Security in the United States and Japan. *American Psychologist, 55*, 1093–1104.

Rothbaum, F., Weisz, J. R., & Snyder, S. S. (1982). Changing the world and changing the self: A two-process model of perceived control. *Journal of Personality and Social Psychology, 42*, 5–37.

Rotter, J. B. (1966). Generalized expectancies for internal versus external control of reinforcement. *Psychological Monographs, 80*(1, Whole No. 609).

Rozin, P. (1996). Towards a psychology of food and eating: From motivation to module to model to marker, morality, meaning, and metaphor. *Current Directions in Psychological Science, 5*, 18–24.

Rozin, P. (1999). Food is fundamental, fun, frightening, and far-reaching. *Social Research, 66*, 9–30.

Rozin, P., Fischler, C., Imada, S., Sarubin, A., & Wrzesniewski, A. (1999). Attitudes to food and the role of food in life in the U.S.A., Japan, Flemish Belgium and France: Possible implications for the diet–health debate. *Appetite, 33*, 163–180.

Rozin, P., Kabnick, K., Pete, E., Fischler, C., & Shields, C. (2003). The ecology of eating: Smaller portion sizes in France than in the United States help explain the French paradox. *Psychological Science, 14*, 450–454.

Ryan, R. M., & Deci, E. L. (2002). Overview of self-determination theory: An organismic–dialectical perspective. In E. L. Deci & R. M. Ryan (Eds.), *Handbook of self-determination research* (pp. 3–33). Rochester, NY: University of Rochester Press.

Sastry, J., & Ross, C. E. (1998). Asian ethnicity and the sense of personal control. *Social Psychology Quarterly, 61*, 101–120.

Shweder, R. A. (2003). Introduction: Anti-postculturalism (or, the view from manywheres). In R. A. Shweder (Ed.), *Why do men barbecue?* (pp. 1–45). Cambridge, MA: Harvard University Press.

Shweder, R. A., Balle-Jensen, L., & Goldstein, W. (2003). Who sleeps by whom revisited. In R. A. Shweder (Ed.), *Why do men barbecue?* (pp. 46–73). Cambridge, MA: Harvard University Press.

Shweder, R. A., & Bourne, L. (1984). Does the concept of the person vary cross-culturally? In R. A. Shweder & R. A. LeVine (Eds.), *Culture theory: Essays on mind, self, and emotion* (pp. 158–190). Cambridge, UK: Cambridge University Press.

Snibbe, A. C., Kitayama, S., Markus, H. R., & Suzuki, T. (2003). They saw a game: A Japanese and American field study. *Journal of Cross-Cultural Psychology, 34*, 581–595.

Snibbe, A. C., & Markus, H. R. (2005). You can't always get what you want: Educational attainment, agency, and choice. *Journal of Personality and Social Psychology, 88*, 703–720.

Stevenson, H. W., & Stigler, J. W. (1992). *The learning gap: Why our schools are failing and what we can learn from Japanese and Chinese education.* New York: Summit Books.

Strauss, C., & Quinn, N. (1997). *A cognitive theory of cultural meanings.* Cambridge, UK: Cambridge University Press.

Strickland, B. R. (1989). Internal-external control expectancies: From contingency to creativity. *American Psychologist, 44*, 1–12.

Thompson, S. C., Sobolew-Shubin, A., Galbraith, M. E., Schwankovsky, L., & Cruzen, D. (1993). Maintaining perceptions of control: Finding perceived control in low-control circumstances. *Journal of Personality and Social Psychology, 64*, 293–304.

Toda, M., Shinotsuka, H., McClintock, C. G., & Stech, F. J. (1978). Development of competitive behavior as a function of culture, age, and social comparison. *Journal of Personality and Social Psychology, 36*, 825–839.

Tomasello, M. (1999). *The cultural origins of human cognition.* Cambridge, MA: Harvard University Press.

Triandis, H. C. (1988). Collectivism vs. individualism: A reconceptualization of a basic concept in cross-cultural social psychology. In G. K. Verma & C. Bagley (Eds.), *Cross-cultural studies of personality, attitudes and cognition* (pp. 60–95). London: Macmillan.

Triandis, H. C. (1995). *Individualism and collectivism.* Boulder, CO: Westview Press.

Triandis, H. C., Bontempo, R., Villareal, M. J., Asai, M., & Lucca, N. (1988). Individualism and collectivism: Cross-cultural perspectives on self–ingroup relationships. *Journal of Personality and Social Psychology, 54*, 323–338.

Tsai, J. L., Knutson, B., & Fung, H. H. (2006). Cultural variation in affect valuation. *Journal of Personality and Social Psychology, 90*, 288–307.

Vandello, J. A., & Cohen, D. (2003). Male honor and female fidelity: Implicit cultural scripts that perpetuate domestic violence. *Journal of Personality and Social Psychology, 84*, 997–1010.

Weisz, J. R., Rothbaum, F. M., & Blackburn, T. C. (1984). Standing out and standing in: The psychology of control in America and Japan. *American Psychologist, 39*, 955–969.

Wheeler, L., Reis, H. T., & Bond, M. H. (1989). Collectivism–individualism in everyday social life: The Middle Kingdom and the melting pot. *Journal of Personality and Social Psychology, 57*, 79–86.

Whiten, A., Goodall, J., McGrew, W. C., Nishida, T., Reynolds, V., Sugiyama, Y., et al. (1999). Cultures in chimpanzees. *Nature, 399*, 682–685.

Yamagishi, T., & Yamagishi, M. (1994). Trust and commitment in the United States and Japan. *Motivation and Emotion, 18*, 129–166.

Chapter 28

# Of Men, Women, and Motivation

## A ROLE CONGRUITY ACCOUNT

**Amanda B. Diekman**
**Alice H. Eagly**

The questions "What do men want?" and "What do women want?" abound in the popular culture. One prevalent belief is that men and women prioritize different life goals—for example, that women primarily seek close relationships and intimacy, whereas men desire prestige and power. In this chapter, we review the scientific evidence about the similarities and differences in the motivations of men and women. For both sexes, good fit to the opportunities afforded by their society yields rewards in terms of ease of completing important tasks and building satisfying interpersonal relationships. Individuals thus (consciously or not) assess the ways in which they can gain rewards and avoid costs, given the opportunities and constraints of the current role system. To the extent that the sexes typically occupy different social roles, these roles frame opportunities in ways that foster differences in motivations, as well as different methods of fulfilling those motivations. Specific roles afford particular opportunities to pursue goals, and individuals are more likely to seek and attain the goals that are afforded by their roles.

From the *role congruity* perspective, the motivation to achieve role congruity—to align behavior with the demands of roles—is an important force. In the tradition of many attitude–behavior researchers (e.g., Ajzen & Fishbein, 2005; Fishbein & Ajzen, 1975), we assume that behavior is influenced by beliefs about the outcomes of behaviors, as well as beliefs about important others' approval of behaviors (i.e., *subjective norms*). Although role congruity should motivate behavior across different types of roles, we focus here on fit to gender roles (for an account of cultural differences in motivation, see Morling & Kitayama, Chapter 27, this volume). The importance of gender roles stems from their ubiquity across different types of interactions and specific roles, their potential applicability to everyone, and their consensually held content as standards for behavior (see Eagly, Wood, & Diekman, 2000, for a review). The widespread agreement about gender roles lends them particular power: Even individuals who have not internalized societal gender norms are susceptible to their influence, because others bring them to bear on interactions (e.g., Deaux & Major, 1987; Ridgeway & Correll, 2004).

Gender roles follow from the division of labor between the sexes, which reflects the specialization of each sex in activities for which they are physically better suited under the circumstances afforded by their society (Wood & Eagly, 2002). One outcome of this division of labor is that men and women may strive for different goals that are relevant to their sex-differentiated roles. In particular, the roles of men and women diverge in their fostering of *agency* and *communion* motives. Agency motives focus on mastering the environment and promoting oneself, whereas communion motives focus on maintaining interpersonal relationships and benefiting others (Bakan, 1966). From the social role perspective, these agentic and communal orientations stem from the roles typically held by men or women. Men's greater agency orientation results from their occupancy of male-dominated roles, especially higher-status roles and roles yielding authority, whereas women's greater communion results from their occupancy of caretaking roles (Eagly, 1987; Eagly et al., 2000).

Unlike specific roles that only apply in a particular context, gender roles are *diffuse* in their application across a wide range of settings. Gender roles, like other diffuse roles based on demographic characteristics such as age, race, and socioeconomic status, have great scope because they can apply to people who belong to the extremely general social categories of men and women, and thus can apply to all portions of daily life. In contrast, more specific roles based on factors such as family relationships (e.g., father, daughter) and occupation (e.g., kindergarten teacher, police officer) are mainly relevant to behavior in a particular group or organizational context—in the workplace, for example, in the case of occupational roles. This distinction between diffuse and specific roles resembles the distinction in expectation states theory between diffuse status characteristics and specific status characteristics (e.g., Berger, Wagner, & Zelditch, 1985).

Gender roles coexist with specific roles and are relevant to most social interactions, including encounters that are also structured by these specific roles. Consistent with this claim, a meta-analysis of studies of physician behavior revealed that female physicians were more likely than male physicians to enact communal behaviors, including engaging in more positive talk, more medical and psychosocial questions, and more smiling and nodding (Roter, Hall, & Aoki, 2002). Even in the context of the specific occupational role of physician, the impact of the diffuse gender role was reflected in the expression of more communal behaviors by female physicians than by male physicians.

One consequence of sex-differentiated role occupancy is that men and women internalize different goals, which are reflected in self-descriptions of traits or values consistent with these internalized goals. Demonstrating sex differences in goals are the well-documented male–female differences in self-reported communal and agentic traits. For example, a meta-analysis of standardized personality tests (Feingold, 1994) detected greater self-reported assertiveness among men than women ($d = 0.50$) and greater self-reported tender-mindedness among women than men ($d = -0.97$). Such differences have also been shown cross-culturally: In a meta-analysis representing adult samples in 25 different cultures (Costa, Terracciano, & McCrae, 2001), men reported greater assertiveness than did women ($d = 0.27$), and women reported greater warmth ($d = -0.23$) and tender-mindedness ($d = -0.28$) than did men. In addition, sex differences in values reflect relative preferences for agentic or communal goals, as revealed in data integrated across 127 samples (Schwartz & Rubel, 2005). Women, more than men, tended to endorse the values of benevolence ($d = -0.29$) and universalism ($d = -0.21$), whereas men, more than women, endorsed power ($d = 0.32$) and achievement ($d = 0.20$).

In one of the few studies to examine agentic and communal goals directly, Pöhlmann (2001) found that men and women differed in their pursuit of personal goals related to agency and communion. In this study, agentic goals included power, achievement, and seeking new experiences or excitement; communal goals included intimacy, affiliation, and altruism. Although participants of both sexes considered both sets of goals important, the majority of women (60.2%) rated communal goals as more important than agentic goals, whereas a majority of men (61.6%) rated agentic goals as more important. As in other findings of sex differences, a substantial minority of each sex showed a gender-atypical pattern. Although the sexes may differ on average in terms of agentic or communal orientation, individual differences are large within both sexes, and the sex differences are most accurately described as overlapping distributions.

Our role congruity account of sex differences and similarities in motivation focuses on how roles influence the goals and methods of goal pursuit elected by men and women. First, we examine support for the idea that role congruity yields various positive outcomes for individuals. Next, we examine the mechanisms by which placement in different roles might foster differences in motivation. Finally, we examine evidence documenting role-congruous motivational orientations—specifically, agency for men and communion for women.

## CONSEQUENCES OF ROLE CONGRUITY AND INCONGRUITY

The argument that individuals are motivated to maximize role congruity rests upon the assumption that rewards stem from role congruity and punishments from role incongruity. The standards used to evaluate role congruity can be set by others in the social environment, set by oneself, or shared by both. In addition, the consequences of succeeding or failing to meet these standards are both intrapersonal (e.g., negative affect) and interpersonal (e.g., ridicule from others).

As a general principle, individuals experience enhanced well-being when they progress toward specific goals that are congruent with their motivational drives. For example, Brunstein, Schultheiss, and Glassman (1998) found that agency-oriented individuals reported greater emotional well-being with progress toward agency-congruent but not communion-congruent goals. In contrast, communion-oriented individuals reported greater emotional well-being with progress toward communion-congruent but not agency-congruent goals. Consistent with the *self-concordance* model (Sheldon & Elliot, 1999), individuals who pursue goals that are congruent with important aspects of the self are more likely to sustain effort toward the goals, attain the goals, and experience positive changes in well-being with goal attainment.

Behavior that is congruous with gender roles can yield positive outcomes for individuals. For example, an experience-sampling study of the daily lives of high school students found that experiences diverged for boys and girls high in affiliation motivation (Wong & Csikszentmihalyi, 1991). Across situations of being alone or with friends, highly affiliative girls reported more positive affective states than other girls did, whereas highly affiliative boys tended to report less positivity than other boys did. The authors interpreted this finding in terms of the greater congruence of affiliation with the female gender role. In a direct test of the affective consequences of gender role fit, Wood, Christensen, Hebl, and Rothgerber (1997) found that for individuals who internalized gender norms, remembering or witnessing a gender-typical interaction (i.e., communion for women and dominance for men) led to more positive affect. Likewise, a diary study revealed that for individuals who held gender-typed personal standards, behaving in gender-congruent ways led to greater self-esteem and more positive affect (Guerrero Witt & Wood, 2006). In studies of elementary and middle school children, feeling typical of and content with one's gender were positively associated with well-being (Carver, Yunger, & Perry, 2003; Egan & Perry, 2001).

Conversely, role incongruity can lead to negative affective consequences. Illustrative of this principle, one early explanation of women's avoidance of high-status careers proposed that women experience "fear of success," as shown by female participants' inclusion of more fear imagery in essays about a woman in medical school, compared with male participants' essays about a man in medical school (Horner, 1969). Later work revealed that this fear of success was confined to settings that are conventionally gender-inappropriate. When the experimental design was enlarged so that participants wrote about either a male or a female student's success in either a female- or male-dominated field (i.e., nursing or medical school), the results were more complex. Greater fear imagery appeared in both of the gender non-normative conditions—specifically, for the woman in medical school and the man in nursing school (Cherry & Deaux, 1978). Concerns about gender role incongruity thus can be relevant to both sexes.

Another illustration of negative consequences of role incongruity comes from a study examining the physical and mental health outcomes for employees who hold occupations incongruent with their gender roles (Evans & Steptoe, 2002). In this study, women in a male-dominated field (i.e., accounting) and men in a female-dominated field (i.e., nursing), relative to their gender-normative counterparts in the same occupations, experienced more job hassles. In addition, individuals in gender-incongruent occupations also experienced significantly more negative psychological or physical health outcomes (for women, higher anxiety; for men, more sick days).

Individuals who demonstrate their fit to gender roles also tend to benefit because attributes thought to facilitate role success elicit positive evaluation from others. In experimental studies that manipulate the requirements of different occupational roles, individuals or groups who possess characteristics congruent with the occupational demands are valued more than are those who possess role-incongruent characteristics (Diekman, 2007; Glick, 1991; Judd & Oswald, 1997). In addition, participants who envision women in male-dominated roles tend to approve of women adopting agentic characteristics (Diekman & Goodfriend, 2006). From the perspective of perceivers, role congruity leads to positive evaluation.

Although some cases of misfit to one's gender role may be simply ignored, other cases are more severely punished. Children's deviations from gender-normative behavior are negatively evaluated by their peers (Blakemore, 2003; Levy, Taylor, & Gelman, 1995) and by college-age adults (Levy et al., 1995; Martin, 1990). Similarly, women who succeed at male-typical jobs are liked less than their male counterparts or than women in female-typical or gender-neutral jobs (Heilman, Wallen, Fuchs, & Tamkins, 2004). Also, a meta-analysis found that women who displayed a male-stereotypical assertive and directive leadership style were evaluated more negatively than men who displayed the same style (Eagly, Makhijani, & Klonsky, 1992). In addition, men are often penalized for behaving passively and expressing negative emotions such as shame, fear, and embarrassment (e.g., Anderson, John, Keltner, & Kring, 2001; Costrich, Feinstein, Kidder, Maracek, & Pascale, 1975).

In general, role incongruity can be a source of prejudice, because observers devalue individuals with role-incongruent characteristics (Eagly & Diekman, 2005). Rewards are more likely for role-normative than non-normative behavior; thus individuals will generally tend to seek to fulfill basic human needs by gender-normative means. In addition, as we explain in the next section, the placement of men and women in differing social roles can lead to different motivational drives and behavioral expressions.

## HOW DO ROLES ELICIT MOTIVATION?

To examine the processes by which the social roles of men and women lead to different motivations, we explore both external mechanisms, which derive directly from the surrounding role environment, and internalized mechanisms, which emanate from individuals themselves. As we show, the strategies of men and women for pursuing goals are influenced by qualities they internalize and qualities that are externally afforded by their environment (Cantor, 1994).

### External Mechanisms

From the social structural perspective, the division of men and women into different social roles is the root cause of sex differences. Even in childhood, roles are differentiated by sex, and children are generally encouraged to pursue gender-normative activities. Parents use reward and punishment to encourage gender-typed activities and interests, such as chores, toys, games, and sports (Lytton & Romney, 1991). For example, adolescents report that parents tend to assign outdoor chores to boys and indoor chores to girls (Peters, 1994). In this section, we explore how certain role environments afford different types of goal pursuit.

#### *Environmental Affordances*

The different contexts of male- and female-dominated roles allow for the pursuit of distinctive goals. For example, although caretaking roles do not afford many opportunities for self-promotion, they do provide opportunities for understanding others' thoughts and feelings and fostering others' development. To the extent that roles differ in the goal achievements that they afford, individuals should be most attracted to roles that they perceive as affording the pursuit of goals that they personally regard as important. A meta-analysis of sex differences in preference for job attributes (Konrad,

Ritchie, Lieb, & Corrigall, 2000) found that these preferences tended to follow gender-normative patterns: Men more than women valued male-typical attributes such as earnings, promotions, freedom, and power, whereas women more than men valued female-typical attributes such as interpersonal relationships and helping others. Lippa (1998) also demonstrated that the vocational interests of women and men reflected differences in their relative preferences for working with people versus things, with women more than men valuing working with people, and men more than women valuing working with things. Likewise, college students' career interests were predicted by their projected competence in the careers, as well as the extent to which the careers were perceived as involving other people (Morgan, Isaac, & Sansone, 2001). For physical and mathematical science careers, interest was also predicted by the perceived high pay and status of the careers. For all careers, controlling for the perceived goal affordances (i.e., high pay and status, involvement of other people) reduced sex differences in career interest. To the extent that people perceive that occupational roles afford opportunities to pursue their important goals, they are more likely to enter and remain in those occupations.

Some roles afford a range of acceptable female- and male-stereotypical behaviors. For example, leadership roles can be enacted in a variety of more masculine and feminine styles (see Eagly & Johannesen-Schmidt, 2007, for a review). *Transformational leadership*, a style marked by inspiring subordinates and developing their skills and creativity, includes qualities that are consistent with the female gender role, including close mentorship and support of subordinates; women tend more than men to enact this transformational leadership style (Eagly, Johannesen-Schmidt, & van Engen, 2003). Such flexibly enacted roles may be appealing to both men and women, possibly resulting in relatively equal representation of the sexes.

### Social Interaction

Interacting with others who hold gender-stereotypical beliefs can elicit behaviors that confirm these beliefs (Geis, 1993). In this way, gender-normative goals may be sought even among those who have not internalized gender norms. Such processes may underlie the tendency for interaction partners to divide tasks according to gender-stereotypical assumptions. In the classic study by Skrypnek and Snyder (1982), task partners negotiated a more traditional division of labor when they were led to believe that they were interacting with a partner of the other sex, regardless of their partner's actual sex (see also Hollingshead & Fraidin, 2003). Moreover, female physicians' more communal behavior, which has been noted above, may be increased further by patients' tendency to speak more to female than to male physicians, disclose more information, and make more positive comments (see meta-analysis by Hall & Roter, 2002). The pleasant social interactions that result from confirming interaction partners' stereotypical assumptions can increase the likelihood of pursuing those behaviors. The gender-normative expectations of people in interaction thus elicit gender-normative actions and reinforce these expectations (Deaux & Major, 1987). Moreover, specific interactions can lead to widespread, consensually shared beliefs about group differences as people participate in and witness these stereotype-confirming interactions (Ridgeway & Correll, 2004; Ridgeway & Erickson, 2000).

### Automatically Activated Goals

Goals relevant to a role that an individual occupies can be automatically activated by cues inherent to the role or its physical or social environment, without awareness or intention to pursue the goals (see Ferguson, Hassin, & Bargh, Chapter 10, this volume). Specifically, the *auto-motive model* posits that nonconscious goals elicit behavioral goal pursuit (Bargh & Chartrand, 1999; Fitzsimons & Bargh, 2004). Goals can be automatically activated by physical or social environments, both of which are likely to vary with different roles. Individuals primed with nonconscious goals to visit certain environments (e.g., a library) have shown greater accessibility of mental representations of behaviors normative in these environments and greater likelihood of engaging in such behaviors (Aarts & Dijksterhuis, 2003). The social environment also influences the types of goals that are nonconsciously activated. Individuals are more likely to perform goal-consistent behavior (e.g., helping) when primed with a close other who is associated with that goal (e.g., a friend) (Fitzsimons & Bargh, 2003). In addition, when an individual is implicitly primed with a close other who values a goal, that goal is perceived as more attainable, and goal persistence and performance are enhanced (Shah, 2003a, 2003b). The different roles that individuals occupy may automatically activate role-congruent behavior and cognition, thus facilitating individuals' fit with their physical and social environments.

## Internalized Mechanisms

With greater exposure to sex-typed roles, the activities and rewards associated with those roles become chronically associated with the self, so that individuals internalize sex-typical goals (see Bussey & Bandura, 1999, for a review). In this section, we discuss the consequences of these internalized goals.

### *Self-Concept*

A rich history of work has explored the consequences of defining the self in terms of the female or male gender role (e.g., Bem, 1974; Crane & Markus, 1982). In their social cognitive model of gender development, Bussey and Bandura (1999) posit that children learn to identify their gender category and the personal and social evaluative consequences of conforming or deviating from the characteristics associated with this category. Children self-regulate their behavior in order to comply with these personal and social standards. To the extent that gender role is an important aspect of the self-concept, individuals are expected to be especially motivated to pursue gender-normative goals and avoid gender-non-normative goals.

Self-construal also varies by sex, with the general finding that men possess a more collective self-construal that focuses on the self as a member of a group, and women a more relational self-construal that focuses on the self as embedded in dyadic and close relationships (Gabriel & Gardner, 1999; Gardner & Gabriel, 2004). To the extent that women define themselves more relationally than men, close relationships exert a stronger motivating force on them and thus attract their attention to relational opportunities afforded by roles.

Incorporation of gender norms into the self-concept enhances the appeal of gender-typical interactions. In Wood and colleagues' (1997) study of the affective benefits of conformity to sex-typed norms, participants who valued conformity to same-sex ideals reduced the discrepancies between their actual and ideal self-concepts when they remembered or witnessed gender-normative interactions. Similarly, Guerrero Witt and Wood's (2006) diary study found that individuals with gender-typed self-standards reported greater self-esteem and positive affect after engaging in gender-normative social interactions. Thus internalized gender roles may increase the likelihood of an individual engaging in gender-normative interactions by increasing positive self-regard from conforming to personal standards.

### *Self-Efficacy*

If people generally seek to maximize perceived utilities, they should choose to engage in behaviors that they believe they will perform successfully. The resulting self-efficacy beliefs stem in part from actual skill at the behavior, which can be shaped by socialization and experience performing the behavior. Additionally, group stereotypes about task ability shape self-efficacy beliefs (Bussey & Bandura, 1999). The sources and consequences of achievement self-efficacy beliefs have been examined by Eccles and colleagues (Eccles, 1994; see Linnenbrink & Fredricks, Chapter 29, this volume, for a review). In their model, one of the major predictors of achievement choices is expectation of task-related success, which in part stems from beliefs of important others. For example, parents' endorsement of gender stereotypes fostered beliefs that their children had sex-typed abilities in various domains, including mathematics, sports, and social activities (Jacobs, 1991; Jacobs & Eccles, 1992). In turn, parental ability beliefs predicted children's self-perceptions, which predicted their mathematics performance.

Self-efficacy beliefs may play a particularly critical role in career selection. For example, across science, math, education, social services, and medicine, participants' perceived competence strongly predicted career interest (Morgan et al., 2001). Likewise, in Giles and Rea's (1999) study of interest in caring- and action-oriented careers, men intended less than women to pursue caring-oriented careers and reported lower self-efficacy in these careers. In particular, men tended more than women to report that they lacked the patience for the work and feared the responsibility and stress involved in the work. In contrast, men and women showed similar interest and similar self-efficacy in action-oriented careers.

### The Intersection of Internal and External Mechanisms

Interactions between internal and external mechanisms occur in various ways. Individuals who are repeatedly exposed to certain roles internalize role-relevant goals, and those who have internalized such goals are likely to structure their environment to facilitate these motivations. This bidirectional relationship is clearly illustrated in longitudinal studies examining relationships between women's career trajectories and their need for achievement (Jenkins, 1987) and need for power (Jenkins, 1994). Women higher in need for power or achievement tended to select careers that provided opportunities to meet these goals. Moreover, women in occupations that aroused these motives showed the greatest increases in these needs over 14 years. Specifically, women in college teaching or entrepreneurial roles especially increased in need for achievement (Jenkins, 1987), and women in occupations allowing the exercise of interpersonal power with immediate feedback especially increased in need for power (Jenkins, 1994). Motivational strivings thus influence the roles people select, but these roles also continue to shape motivational strivings.

Other data also support the idea that people who internalize goals prefer environments that fulfill those goals. For example, individuals high in affiliation motivation reported more often that they thought about friends and wished to be with friends (Wong & Csikszentmihalyi, 1991), as well as about engaging in other social relational behaviors (see Gable & Strachman, Chapter 37, this volume). The intrapsychic state of holding an affiliative goal attracts people to social interactions, which in turn reinforce affiliative motivation. Likewise, college men with stronger affiliative needs preferred and obtained living situations that allowed more social interaction and less privacy (Switzer & Taylor, 1983). From the perspective of these various internal and external mechanisms by which social roles facilitate some motivations and inhibit others, we now examine sex differences in the important domains of agentic and communal orientations.

## SEX DIFFERENCES IN AGENCY AND COMMUNION

Following from the argument that roles shape motivation is the hypothesis that variation in roles corresponds to variation in motivational orientations. To explore this hypothesis, we examine evidence for sex differences in agentic and communal behavior and personality, with particular attention to change and stability over time. Moreover, we examine the extent to which individuals seek to fulfill motivations in ways that align with their gender roles.

### Agency

As noted earlier, men's greater prominence in roles related to authority or status leads to their greater expression of agency-oriented behaviors relative to women. However, these roles have also undergone substantial change in recent decades. In the late 20th century, women greatly increased their presence in the paid labor force; contrasting with this change is the stability of men's presence in the paid labor force, which has declined only slightly (England, 2003; Fullerton, 1999). This asymmetrical role change leads to the social role theory prediction of increased levels of agency for women but stable levels of agency for men over the latter half of the 20th century. Evidence pertaining to agency-related characteristics largely corresponds to this prediction. A meta-analysis of self-reported personality traits from 1973 to 1993 found that the sex difference in masculine or instrumental characteristics decreased over this time period, predominantly because of women's adoption of these characteristics (Twenge, 1997). Similarly, a meta-analysis of the personality trait of assertiveness (Twenge, 2001) found that women's self-reported assertiveness and dominance rose from 1931 to 1945, dropped from 1946 to 1967, and rose again from 1968 to 1993; men's assertiveness remained stable over this time. Moreover, as shown by relating women's assertiveness to role indicators such as educational attainment, the trends in women's assertiveness mirrored the fluctuations in women's roles and status throughout this period.

Also consistent with increasing agentic motivation among women is evidence from a longitudinal study of sex differences in desire for control (Burger & Solano, 1994). The initial assessment in 1980, when participants were undergraduates, revealed that men reported significantly greater desire for control than women did. In 1990, this difference had disappeared because of women's increase in desire for control and men's stability. The career plans of male and female college students also converged from 1966 to 2001, primarily because of women's increased aspiration for traditionally male-dominated careers, especially law, medicine, and business (Astin, Oseguera, Sax, & Korn, 2002). In fact, a recent study of college students found that women more than men rated personal education as an important goal, consistent with women's higher rate of obtaining university degrees (U.S. Department of Education, 2005). In addition, college-age women ranked being well educated as more important than getting married or having children (Abowitz & Knox, 2003).

With respect to achievement motives, cross-temporal research employing thematic apperception methods revealed that women's achievement imagery rose from 1957 to 1976, whereas men's remained stable (Veroff, Depner, Kulka, & Douvan, 1980). In recent research, men and women have shown similar levels of achievement motivation. For example, a study of gifted high school seniors found no sex differences in reports of desiring to work hard, mastering challenges, or fearing success, although senior boys reported higher levels of competitiveness than senior girls (Mendez & Crawford, 2002). Another study of college students found no sex difference in the importance of economic success (Eskilson & Wiley, 1999), although in earlier studies men valued economic success more than did women (e.g., Kasser & Ryan, 1993).

An extreme form of agency is aggression, in which mastery of one's environment encompasses harming others. Because of its extremity, aggressive behavior in particular may be perceived as more congruous with the male than with the female gender role. Indeed, meta-analyses have typically found an overall tendency for men to be more aggressive than women (Bettencourt & Miller, 1996, $d = 0.23$; Eagly & Steffen, 1986, $d = 0.29$). In Eagly and Steffen's (1986) meta-analysis, men were particularly more likely than women to aggress physically, compared with psychologically (or verbally). In addition, the sex difference was exaggerated to the extent that women believed that aggression would cause harm to the target, cause guilt or anxiety to themselves, or endanger themselves. Meta-analyses have also found that certain contexts reduce the sex difference in aggression—for example, when there is clear provocation to aggress (Bettencourt & Miller, 1996) or when physical aggression occurs in the context of close heterosexual relationships (Archer, 2000).

Also corresponding to role congruity predictions is some evidence that women and girls tend more than men or boys to employ *relational aggression*—that is, they use elements of relationships to harm others, such as ostracism or gossip (Crick & Rose, 2000). Meta-analytic findings (Archer, 2004) suggest considerable variation across different measures of indirect aggression, with the largest effects in the direction of greater female aggression for behavioral observations ($d = -0.74$) and peer ratings ($d = -0.19$). Aggressing in the context of relationships may allow women or girls a mode of aggression that is more gender-normative than physical aggression. Illustrative of the sex-typed norms pertaining to aggression, even children are able to specify what kinds of aggression are more appropriate for girls or boys (Crick, Bigbee, & Howes, 1996). Following these gender norms for aggression also has benefits: Children who aggress in gender-atypical ways have lower levels of social adjustment than those who aggress in gender-typical ways (Crick, 1997).

As women enter male-dominated roles, the sex difference in physical aggression may diminish somewhat, consistent with Hyde's (1984) meta-analytic finding (but see Eagly & Steffen, 1986; Knight, Fabes, & Higgins, 1996). In addition, women and girls have increasingly appeared in the criminal justice system. From 1993 to 2002, the rates of arrest for women rose 14.1%, whereas the rates for men decreased 5.9% (Federal Bureau of Investigation, 2003). Female juveniles' rates of arrests for serious violent crimes steadily increased after 1980, although the arrest rate for male juveniles dropped after 1994 (Lynch, 2002). Although men's self-reported crime and their rates of conviction still far exceed women's, the rate of violent crime has risen among women but fallen among men.

Research relevant to agency reveals that although men tend to behave somewhat more male-stereotypically than women, such sex differences may be decreasing over time. Agentic behaviors by women accompany their entry into male-dominated roles as their behaviors shift to reflect the affordances of these new roles.

## Communion

The roles associated with communal orientations—primarily caretaking roles—have not changed their gender composition over recent decades as much as those associated with agentic orientations have. One reason for this stability is that even when women enter paid work roles, they tend to work in occupations (e.g., teacher, nurse) that emphasize communal characteristics (Cejka & Eagly, 1999) or caring for others (England, Budig, & Folbre, 2002). In addition, the division of labor in family roles has changed little in comparison to changes in paid work roles (England, 2003). Comparisons of time use diaries from 1965 to 2000 to show increases of time spent on child care by both men and women; in the data collected in 2000, women's weekly hours of child care remained nearly double those of men (Bianchi, Robinson, & Milkie, 2006). Also, women, more than men, provide care for their elderly parents (Brewer, 2001; Cancian & Olinker, 2000).

Consistent with this stability in the female dominance of caretaking roles are findings that sex differences in communal orientations have remained relatively unchanged over time. Women's affiliation motivation, as assessed by thematic apperception tests, remained stable from 1957 to 1976, although men's decreased (Veroff et al., 1980). A meta-analysis of self-reported personality characteristics found that feminine or communal characteristics were fairly stable from 1973 to 1993 (Twenge, 1997). Similarly, women's greater tendency to endorse self-reports of caring personality traits has shown stability over time (Feingold, 1994). Other life goals concerning family also retain traditional sex differences: For example, college women, more than men, rated family as an important life goal (Eskilson & Wiley, 1999).

Men and women also differ in their endorsement of communally related attitudes, including compassionate support for disadvantaged groups. Sex differences in communally oriented values (i.e., feelings of responsibility for the welfare of others) persisted from the 1970s to the 1990s (Beutel & Marini, 1995). In analyses of sociopolitical attitudes assessed by the General Social Survey from 1973 to 1998 (Eagly, Diekman, Johannesen-Schmidt, & Koenig, 2004), sex differences in political attitudes remained consistent. In particular, women, relative to men, endorsed attitudes supportive of social compassion (i.e., support for disadvantaged groups), reflecting an orientation to think about others' welfare. In addition, women, relative to men, endorsed attitudes supportive of traditional morality (i.e., disapproval of divorce or extramarital relations, restrictions on drug use or suicide), reflecting an allegiance to conventional norms that uphold communally oriented societal institutions, such as marriage, the family, or the church.

Despite the relative temporal stability of caretaking roles and communal orientation, some specific roles enhance or inhibit communality. For example, the transition to parenthood involves greater emphasis on family goals, especially for women, whose role responsibilities tend to change more after childbirth (Salmela-Aro, Nurmi, Saisto, & Halmesmaeki, 2000). In our study of sex differences in social and political attitudes (Eagly et al., 2004), markers of societal status (e.g., ethnicity) were associated with socially compassionate attitudes, whereas markers of traditional family responsibility (e.g., a child in the home) were associated with traditionally moral attitudes.

The evidence for women's greater communal orientation does not obviate men's needs for affiliation and intimacy. In research using thematic apperception tests, individuals of both sexes who are higher in the need for affiliation place importance on building and maintaining relationships (Stewart & Chester, 1982). In Hill's (1987) delineation of different types of affiliation motivation, women reported affiliating more than men for emotional support and positive stimulation, but the same as men for attracting attention and social comparison. Even so, both sexes regarded positive stimulation as the most important reason for affiliation.

Although needs to affiliate may be similar in the sexes, they may be fulfilled through different means. For example, the need to belong has been posited as a fundamental human motivation occurring throughout various societies and historical periods (Baumeister & Leary, 1995). However, each sex may seek to fulfill this need with gender-normative relationships, such as groups for men and dyadic relationships for women (Baumeister & Sommer, 1997; Gardner & Gabriel, 2004). The friendships of men and women also reflect gender role differences (see

Fehr, 2004, for a review): Men are more likely to engage in behavior or talk related to activities (e.g., sports), whereas women are more likely to engage in self-disclosure about personal topics. However, men and women agree that self-disclosure reveals intimacy and is prototypical of intimacy, as compared to shared activities. Although men and women may define intimacy similarly, women may have greater opportunities in their gender role to pursue such intimacy goals across a range of situations.

Prosocial motivations are also expressed in different ways by men and women (see review by Eagly & Koenig, 2006). The extent to which prosocial behavior involves agentic, risky behaviors or communal, empathic behaviors is associated with the direction of the sex difference. A meta-analysis of helping behavior by Eagly and Crowley (1986) revealed an overall sex difference reflecting men's greater tendency to help ($d = 0.13$). Men tended to offer help more than women, especially in off-campus settings or in situations perceived as less dangerous and more comfortable by men than by women. Also, Becker and Eagly (2004) examined heroism in real-life domains, including highly dangerous situations (emergency rescues resulting in Carnegie Medals and aiding Jews in the Holocaust) and less dangerous contexts (volunteering for Doctors of the World or the Peace Corps and donating a kidney). Although men received Carnegie Medals more often than women, women equally or more often than men participated in the other heroic actions. In situations requiring long-term dedication, women tended to help more often. In contrast, men's heroism appeared especially in situations that required immediate action or physical strength. These patterns suggest that features of the male gender role, especially confidence in physical abilities, contribute to men's greater performance of some types of heroic behaviors.

## CONCLUSIONS AND IMPLICATIONS

In general, fit to important social roles is a critical motivational force. Moreover, the opportunities for goal pursuit afforded by these social roles shape the kinds of goals and methods of goal pursuit elected by individuals. Because gender roles are merely one influence among many, the sex differences in agency and communion reviewed here consist of overlapping distributions, with large individual differences within each sex. Although individuals of both sexes may desire both agency and communion, their methods of pursuit may differ according to gender roles. In addition, agency and communion are much more than simple end-states; instead, these motivational orientations filter incoming stimuli and guide further social interactions. Individuals who vary in their agentic and communal orientations may thus pursue similar goals or experience similar situations quite differently. As Cantor (1994) has described, communal situations may afford the pursuit of agentic goals for some individuals, as in the case of individuals who use social support situations to bolster their academic goals.

Although the motivation to fit with one's social system is certainly functional, this conformity slows social change. One of the most challenging aspects of social change is that individuals who enter nontraditional roles generally meet with resistance (Eagly & Diekman, 2005). Although they may possess the qualities necessary for excellent role performance, they may encounter harsh reactions from others. For example, a study of women in blue-collar occupations found that they experienced sexual harassment (60.0%) and sex discrimination (55.7%) much more than women in female-dominated occupations such as clerical work (Mansfield et al., 1991).

Despite this resistance, the evidence about cross-temporal changes reviewed here demonstrates that behaviors change when underlying roles change. Indeed, the expectation that roles will change may help people prepare for that eventual change. Although people are somewhat constrained by their current-day roles, they also possess a great deal of ability to adapt to changing roles (Eagly & Diekman, 2003). Experiments that manipulate the shape of role change in a novel society showed that observers project role-congruent traits to be especially valued: When people are led to believe that the role system will change in a particular fashion, they predict greater utility and positivity for traits that align with the expected future roles of the group (Diekman & Goodfriend, 2006). Individuals may thus be motivated to seek out roles that align with the anticipated future of their society.

The fact that individuals perceive themselves and others as malleable in the face of changing social roles offers hope for accommodation to a rapidly changing world. This perceived malleability may help to counter the restrictive elements of gender roles: Without doubt, a negative aspect of gender roles is that they constrain people from following individual inclinations that happen to be atypical of their gender. Unhappiness can result from denied or suppressed motives, and thus a humane society, respectful of individual potential, facilitates the ability of people of both sexes to achieve power and mastery, as well as affiliation and intimacy.

## REFERENCES


Aarts, H., & Dijksterhuis, A. (2003). The silence of the library: Environment, situational norm, and social behavior. *Journal of Personality and Social Psychology, 84*, 18–28.

Abowitz, D., & Knox, D. (2003). Goals of college students: Some gender differences. *College Student Journal, 37*, 550–556.

Ajzen, I., & Fishbein, M. (2005). The influence of attitudes on behavior. In D. Albarracin, B. T. Johnson, & M. P. Zanna (Eds.), *Handbook of attitudes and attitude change* (pp. 173–221). Mahwah, NJ: Erlbaum.

Anderson, C., John, O. P., Keltner, D., & Kring, A. M. (2001). Who attains social status? Effects of personality and physical attractiveness in social groups. *Journal of Personality and Social Psychology, 81*, 116–132.

Archer, J. (2000). Sex differences in aggression between heterosexual partners: A meta-analytic review. *Psychological Bulletin, 126*, 651–680.

Archer, J. (2004). Sex differences in aggression in real-world settings: A meta-analytic review. *Review of General Psychology, 8*, 291–322.

Astin, A. W., Oseguera, L., Sax, L. J., & Korn, W. S. (2002). *The American freshman: Thirty-five year trends, 1966–2001*. Los Angeles: Higher Education Research Institute, UCLA.

Bakan, D. (1966). *The duality of human existence: An essay on psychology and religion*. Chicago: Rand McNally.

Bargh, J. A., & Chartrand, T. L. (1999). The unbearable automaticity of being. *American Psychologist, 54*, 462–479.

Baumeister, R. F., & Leary, M. R. (1995). The need to belong: Desire for interpersonal attachments as a fundamental human motivation. *Psychological Bulletin, 117*, 497–529.

Baumeister, R. F., & Sommer, K. L. (1997). What do men want?: Gender differences and two spheres of belongingness. *Psychological Bulletin, 122*, 38–44.

Becker, S. W., & Eagly, A. H. (2004). The heroism of men and women. *American Psychologist, 59*, 163–178.

Bem, S. L. (1974). The measurement of psychological androgyny. *Journal of Consulting and Clinical Psychology, 42*, 155–162.

Berger, J., Wagner, D. G., & Zelditch, M., Jr. (1985). Introduction: Expectation states theory: Review and assessment. In J. Berger & M. Zelditch, Jr. (Eds.), *Status, rewards, and influence* (pp. 1–72). San Francisco: Jossey-Bass.

Bettencourt, B. A., & Miller, N. (1996). Gender differences in aggression as a function of provocation: A meta-analysis. *Psychological Bulletin, 119*, 422–447.

Beutel, A. M., & Marini, M. M. (1995). Gender and values. *American Sociological Review, 60*, 436–448.

Bianchi, S. M., Robinson, J. P., & Milkie, M. A. (2006). *Changing rhythms of American family life*. New York: Sage.

Blakemore, J. E. O. (2003). Children's beliefs about violating gender norms: Boys shouldn't look like girls, and girls shouldn't act like boys. *Sex Roles, 48*, 411–419.

Brewer, L. (2001). Gender socialization and the cultural construction of elder caregivers. *Journal of Aging Studies, 15*, 217–235.

Brunstein, J. C., Schultheiss, O. C., & Grassman, R. (1998). Personal goals and emotional well-being: The moderating role of motive dispositions. *Journal of Personality and Social Psychology, 75*, 494–508.

Burger, J. M., & Solano, C. H. (1994). Changes in desire for control over time: Gender differences in a ten-year longitudinal study. *Sex Roles, 31*, 465–472.

Bussey, K., & Bandura, A. (1999). Social cognitive theory of gender development and differentiation. *Psychological Review, 106*, 676–713.

Cancian, F. M., & Olinker, S. J. (2000). *Caring and gender*. Thousand Oaks, CA: Pine Forge Press.

Cantor, N. (1994). Life task problem solving: Situational affordances and personal needs. *Personality and Social Psychology Bulletin, 20*, 235–243.

Carver, P. R., Yunger, J. L., & Perry, D. G. (2003). Gender identity and adjustment in middle childhood. *Sex Roles, 49*, 95–109.

Cejka, M. A., & Eagly, A. H. (1999). Gender-stereotypic images of occupations correspond to the sex segregation of employment. *Personality and Social Psychology Bulletin, 25*, 413–423.

Cherry, F., & Deaux, K. (1978). Fear of success versus fear of gender-inappropriate behavior. *Sex Roles, 4*, 97–101.

Costa, P. T., Jr., Terracciano, A., & McCrae, R. R. (2001). Gender differences in personality traits across cultures: Robust and surprising findings. *Journal of Personality and Social Psychology, 81*, 322–331.

Costrich, N., Feinstein, J., Kidder, L., Maracek, J., & Pascale, L. (1975). When stereotypes hurt: Three studies of penalties for sex-role reversals. *Journal of Experimental Social Psychology, 11*, 520–530.

Crane, M., & Markus, H. (1982). Gender identity: The benefits of a self-schema approach. *Journal of Personality and Social Psychology, 43*, 1195–1197.

Crick, N. R. (1997). Engagement in gender normative versus nonnormative forms of aggression: Links to social-psychological adjustment. *Developmental Psychology, 33*, 610–617.

Crick, N. R., Bigbee, M. A., & Howes, C. (1996). Gender differences in children's normative beliefs about aggression: How do I hurt thee? Let me count the ways. *Child Development, 67*, 1003–1014.

Crick, N. R., & Rose, A. J. (2000). Toward a gender-balanced approach to the study of social–emotional development: A look at relational aggression. In P. H. Miller & E. K. Scholnick (Eds.), *Toward a feminist developmental psychology* (pp. 153–168). New York: Routledge.

Deaux, K., & Major, B. (1987). Putting gender into context: An interactive model of gender-related behavior. *Psychological Review, 94*, 369–389.

Diekman, A. B. (2007). Negotiating the double bind: A role congruity perspective on evaluations of dominance. *Sex Roles, 22* 551–561.

Diekman, A. B., & Goodfriend, W. (2006). Rolling with the changes: A role congruity perspective on gender norms. *Psychology of Women Quarterly, 30*, 369–383.

Eagly, A. H. (1987). *Sex differences in social behavior: A social-role interpretation.* Hillsdale, NJ: Erlbaum.

Eagly, A. H., & Crowley, M. (1986). Gender and helping behavior: A meta-analytic review of the social psychological literature. *Psychological Bulletin, 100*, 283–308.

Eagly, A. H., & Diekman, A. B. (2003). The malleability of sex differences in response to changing social roles. In L. G. Aspinwall & U. M. Staudinger (Eds.), *A psychology of human strengths* (pp. 103–115). Washington, DC: American Psychological Association.

Eagly, A. H., & Diekman, A. B. (2005). What is the problem? Prejudice as an attitude-in-context. In J. F. Dovidio, P. Glick, & L. A. Rudman (Eds.), *On the nature of prejudice: Fifty years after Allport* (pp. 19–35). Malden, MA: Blackwell.

Eagly, A. H., Diekman, A. B., Johannesen-Schmidt, M. C., & Koenig, A. M. (2004). Gender gaps in sociopolitical attitudes: A social psychological analysis. *Journal of Personality and Social Psychology, 87*, 796–816.

Eagly, A. H., & Johannesen-Schmidt, M. C. (2007). Leadership style matters: The small, but important, style differences between male and female leaders. In D. Bilmoria & S. K. Piderit (Eds.), *Handbook of women in business and management* (pp. 279–303). Northampton, MA: Elgar.

Eagly, A. H., Johannesen-Schmidt, M. C., & van Engen, M. L. (2003). Transformational, transactional, and laissez-faire leadership styles: A meta-analysis comparing women and men. *Psychological Bulletin, 129*, 569–591.

Eagly, A. H., & Koenig, A. M. (2006). Social role theory of sex differences and similarities: Implication for prosocial behavior. In D. J. Canary & K. Dindia (Eds.), *Sex differences and similarities in communication* (2nd ed., pp. 161–194). Mahwah, NJ: Erlbaum.

Eagly, A. H., Makhijani, M. G., & Klonsky, B. G. (1992). Gender and the evaluation of leaders: A meta-analysis. *Psychological Bulletin, 111*, 3–22.

Eagly, A. H., & Steffen, V. J. (1986). Gender and aggressive behavior: A meta-analytic review of the social psychological literature. *Psychological Bulletin, 100*, 309–330.

Eagly, A. H., Wood, W., & Diekman, A. B. (2000). Social role theory of sex differences and similarities: A current appraisal. In T. Eckes & H. M. Trautner (Eds.), *The developmental social psychology of gender* (pp. 123–174). Mahwah, NJ: Erlbaum.

Eccles, J. S. (1994). Understanding women's educational and occupational choices: Applying the Eccles et al. model of achievement-related choices. *Psychology of Women Quarterly, 18*, 585–609.

Egan, S. K., & Perry, D. G. (2001). Gender identity: A multidimensional analysis with implications for psychosocial adjustment. *Developmental Psychology, 37*, 451–463.

England, P. (2003). *Toward gender equality: Progress and bottlenecks.* Working paper. Retrieved from *www.northwestern.edu/ipr/publications/papers/2003/WP-03-13.pdf*

England, P., Budig, M., & Folbre, N. (2002). The wages of virtue: The relative pay of care work. *Social Problems, 49*, 455–473.

Eskilson, A., & Wiley, M. G. (1999). Solving for the *X*: Aspirations and expectations of college students. *Journal of Youth and Adolescence, 28*, 51–70.

Evans, O., & Steptoe, A. (2002). The contribution of gender-role orientation, work factors and home stressors to psychological well-being and sickness absence in male- and female-dominated occupational groups. *Social Science and Medicine, 54*, 481–492.

Federal Bureau of Investigation. (2003). *Crime in the United States, 2002: Uniform crime reports.* Retrieved from *www.fbi.gov/ucr/02cius.htm*

Fehr, B. (2004). Intimacy expectations in same-sex friendships: A prototype interaction-pattern model. *Journal of Personality and Social Psychology, 86*, 265–284.

Feingold, A. (1994). Gender differences in personality: A meta-analysis. *Psychological Bulletin, 116*, 429–456.

Fishbein, M., & Ajzen, I. (1975). *Belief, attitude, intention, and behavior: An introduction to theory and research.* Reading, MA: Addison-Wesley.

Fitzsimons, G. M., & Bargh, J. A. (2003). Thinking of you: Nonconscious pursuit of interpersonal goals associated with relationship partners. *Journal of Personality and Social Psychology, 84*, 148–163.

Fitzsimons, G. M., & Bargh, J. A. (2004). Automatic self-regulation. In R. F. Baumeister & K. D. Vohs (Eds.), *Handbook of self-regulation: Research, theory, and applications* (pp. 151–170). New York: Guilford Press.

Fullerton, H. N., Jr. (1999). Labor force participation: 75 years of change, 1950–98 and 1998–2025. *Monthly Labor Review, 122*, 3–12.

Gabriel, S., & Gardner, W. L. (1999). Are there "his" and "hers" types of interdependence?: The implications of gender differences in collective versus relational interdependence for affect, behavior, and cognition. *Journal of Personality and Social Psychology, 77*, 642–655.

Gardner, W. L., & Gabriel, S. (2004). Gender differences in relational and collective interdependence: Implications for self-views, social behavior, and subjective well-being. In A. H. Eagly, A. E. Beall, & R. J. Sternberg (Eds.), *The psychology of gender* (2nd ed., pp. 169–191). New York: Guilford Press.

Geis, F. L. (1993). Self-fulfilling prophecies: A social psychological view of gender. In A. E. Beall & R. J. Sternberg (Eds.), *The psychology of gender* (pp. 9–54). New York: Guilford Press.

Giles, M., & Rea, A. (1999). Career self-efficacy: An application of the theory of planned behaviour. *Journal of Occupational and Organizational Psychology, 72*, 393–398.

Glick, P. (1991). Trait-based and sex-based discrimination in occupational prestige, occupational salary, and hiring. *Sex Roles, 25*, 351–378.

Guerrero Witt, M., & Wood, W. (2006). *Self-regulation of gendered behavior in everyday life*. Unpublished manuscript, Duke University.

Hall, J. A., & Roter, D. L. (2002). Do patients talk differently to male and female physicians?: A meta-analytic review. *Patient Education and Counseling, 48*, 217–224.

Heilman, M. E., Wallen, A. S., Fuchs, D., & Tamkins, M. M. (2004). Penalties for success: Reactions to women who succeed at male gender-typed tasks. *Journal of Applied Psychology, 89*, 416–427.

Hill, C. A. (1987). Affiliation motivation: People who need people . . . but in different ways. *Journal of Personality and Social Psychology, 52*, 1008–1018.

Hollingshead, A. B., & Fraidin, S. (2003). Gender stereotypes and assumptions about expertise in transactive memory. *Journal of Experimental Social Psychology, 39*, 355–363.

Horner, M. (1969, November). Fail: Bright women. *Psychology Today*, pp. 36–38, 62.

Hyde, J. S. (1984). How large are gender differences in aggression?: A developmental meta-analysis. *Developmental Psychology, 20*, 722–736.

Jacobs, J. E. (1991). Influence of gender stereotypes on parent and child mathematics attitudes. *Journal of Personality and Social Psychology, 83*, 518–527.

Jacobs, J. E., & Eccles, J. S. (1992). The impact of mothers' gender-role stereotypic beliefs on mothers' and children's ability perceptions. *Journal of Personality and Social Psychology, 63*, 932–944.

Jenkins, S. R. (1987). Need for achievement and women's careers over 14 years: Evidence for occupational structure effects. *Journal of Personality and Social Psychology, 53*, 922–932.

Jenkins, S. R. (1994). Need for power and women's careers over 14 years: Structural power, job satisfaction, and motive change. *Journal of Personality and Social Psychology, 66*, 155–165.

Judd, P. C., & Oswald, P. A. (1997). Employment desirability: The interactive effects of gender-typed profile, stimulus sex, and gender-typed occupations. *Sex Roles, 37*, 467–476.

Kasser, T., & Ryan, R. M. (1993). A dark side of the American dream: Correlates of financial success as a central life aspiration. *Journal of Personality and Social Psychology, 65*, 410–422.

Knight, G. P., Fabes, R. A., & Higgins, D. A. (1996). Concerns about drawing causal inferences from meta-analyses: An example in the study of gender differences in aggression. *Psychological Bulletin, 119*, 410–421.

Konrad, A. M., Ritchie, J. E. J., Lieb, P., & Corrigall, E. (2000). Sex differences and similarities in job attribute preferences: A meta-analysis. *Psychological Bulletin, 126*, 593–641.

Levy, G. D., Taylor, M. G., & Gelman, S. A. (1995). Traditional and evaluative aspects of flexibility in gender roles, social conventions, and physical laws. *Child Development, 66*, 515–531.

Lippa, R. (1998). Gender-related individual differences and the structure of vocational interests: The importance of the people–things dimension. *Journal of Personality and Social Psychology, 74*, 996–1009.

Lynch, J. P. (2002, October). Trends in juvenile violent offending: An analysis of victim survey data. *Juvenile Justice Bulletin*. Retrieved from *www.ncjrs.org/pdffiles1/ojjdp/191052.pdf*

Lytton, H., & Romney, D. M. (1991). Parents' differential socialization of boys and girls: A meta-analysis. *Psychological Bulletin, 109*, 267–296.

Mansfield, P. K., Koch, P. B., Henderson, J., Vicary, J. R., Cohn, M., & Young, E. W. (1991). The job climate for women in traditionally male blue-collar occupations. *Sex Roles, 25*, 63–79.

Martin, C. L. (1990). Attitudes and expectations about children with nontraditional and traditional gender roles. *Sex Roles, 22*, 151–165.

Mendez, L. M. R., & Crawford, K. M. (2002). Gender-role stereotyping and career aspirations: A comparison of gifted early adolescent boys and girls. *Journal of Secondary Gifted Education, 13*, 96–107.

Morgan, C., Isaac, J. D., & Sansone, C. (2001). The role of interest in understanding the career choices of female and male college students. *Sex Roles, 44*, 295–320.

Peters, J. F. (1994). Gender socialization of adolescents in the home: Research and discussion. *Adolescence, 29*, 913–929.

Pöhlmann, K. (2001). Agency- and communion-orientation in life goals: Impacts on goal pursuit strategies and psychological well-being. In P. Schmuck & K. M. Sheldon (Eds.), *Life goals and well-being: Towards a positive psychology of human striving* (pp. 68–84). Seattle, WA: Hogrefe & Huber.

Ridgeway, C. L., & Correll, S. J. (2004). Unpacking the gender system: A theoretical perspectives on gender beliefs and social relations. *Gender and Society, 18*, 510–531.

Ridgeway, C. L., & Erickson, K. G. (2000). Creating and spreading status beliefs. *American Journal of Sociology, 106*, 579–615.

Roter, D. L., Hall, J. A., & Aoki, Y. (2002). Physician gender effects in medical communication: A meta-analytic review. *Journal of the American Medical Association, 288*, 756–764.

Salmela-Aro, K., Nurmi, J.-E., Saisto, T., & Halmesmaeki, E. (2000). Women's and men's personal goals during the transition to parenthood *Journal of Family Psychology, 14*, 171–186.

Schwartz, S. H., & Rubel, T. (2005). Sex differences in value priorities: Cross-cultural and multimethod studies. *Journal of Personality and Social Psychology, 89*, 1010–1028.

Shah, J. (2003a). Automatic for the people: How representations of significant others implicitly affect goal pursuit. *Journal of Personality and Social Psychology, 84*, 661–681.

Shah, J. (2003b). The motivational looking glass: How significant others implicitly affect goal appraisals. *Journal of Personality and Social Psychology, 85*, 424–439.

Sheldon, K. M., & Elliot, A. J. (1999). Goal striving, need satisfaction, and longitudinal well-being: The self-concordance model. *Journal of Personality and Social Psychology, 76*, 482–497.

Skrypnek, B. J., & Snyder, M. (1982). On the self-perpetuating nature of stereotypes about women and men. *Journal of Experimental Social Psychology, 18*, 277–291.

Stewart, A. J., & Chester, N. L. (1982). Sex differences in human social motives: Achievement, affiliation, and power. In A. J. Stewart (Ed.), *Motivation and society* (pp. 172–218). San Francisco: Jossey-Bass.

Switzer, R., & Taylor, R. B. (1983). Sociability versus privacy of residential choice: Impacts of personality and local social ties. *Basic and Applied Social Psychology, 4*, 123–136.

Twenge, J. M. (1997). Changes in masculine and feminine traits over time: A meta-analysis. *Sex Roles, 36*, 305–325.

Twenge, J. M. (2001). Changes in women's assertiveness in response to status and roles: A cross-temporal meta-analysis, 1931–1993. *Journal of Personality and Social Psychology, 81*, 133–145.

U.S. Department of Education, National Center for Educational Statistics. (2005). *Digest of educational statistics, 2005* (Table 246). Retrieved from *nces.ed.gov/programs/digest/d05/tables/dt05_256.asp?referrer-list*

Veroff, J., Depner, C., Kulka, R., & Douvan, E. (1980). Comparison of American motives: 1957 versus 1976. *Journal of Personality and Social Psychology, 39*, 1249–1262.

Wong, M. M., & Csikszentmihalyi, M. (1991). Affiliation motivation and daily experience: Some issues on gender differences. *Journal of Personality and Social Psychology, 60*, 154–164.

Wood, W., Christensen, P. N., Hebl, M. R., & Rothgerber, H. (1997). Conformity to sex-typed norms, affect, and the self-concept. *Journal of Personality and Social Psychology, 73*, 523–535.

Wood, W., & Eagly, A. H. (2002). A cross-cultural analysis of the behavior of women and men: Implications for the origins of sex differences. *Psychological Bulletin, 128*, 699–727.

Chapter 29

# Developmental Perspectives on Achievement Motivation

## PERSONAL AND CONTEXTUAL INFLUENCES

**Lisa Linnenbrink-Garcia**
**Jennifer A. Fredricks**

In this chapter we focus on achievement motivation from a developmental perspective, with a specific focus on the basic developmental patterns of competence beliefs, values, and goal orientations, as well as on individual differences in the developmental pathways for motivation (Eccles, Wigfield, & Schiefele, 1998). We can think about developmental pathways as describing children's changing beliefs about whether they can do certain tasks and why they might engage in certain tasks. In the first section of the chapter, we provide an overview of research on competence beliefs, values, and goal orientations, focusing on typical patterns of development during middle childhood and adolescence. These shifting developmental patterns are important, but do not necessarily reflect the complexity of the patterns for individual development. For instance, the examination of mean-level differences does not take into account the changing influences of home and school contexts, nor does it consider that there might be developmental changes in how children and adolescents respond to these varying contexts (e.g., Eccles, 1993; Eccles, Midgley, et al., 1993; Maehr & Midgley, 1991). Accordingly, the second part of this chapter focuses on parental and educational influences on developmental trajectories of achievement motivation, with a specific focus on competence beliefs, values, and goal orientations. In doing so, we consider both the direct influences of home, classroom, and school environments on children's and adolescents' achievement motivation, as well as potential person × environment interactions. Throughout the chapter we seek to highlight the areas of achievement motivation in which there has been the most substantial developmental research, but we do not attempt to provide a thorough review of all areas of research on achievement motivation, which would be well beyond the scope of the chapter.

## PATTERNS OF INDIVIDUAL DEVELOPMENT

### Perceptions of Competence

*Competence* beliefs are a central construct in the motivational literature (see Elliot & Dweck, 2005). Some theorists have defined perceptions of competence in terms of self-concepts of ability and expectations for success in different domains (e.g., Eccles (Parsons), et al., 1983; Harter, 1982; Marsh, 1990). Competence perceptions are also prominent in other motivational models—including self-efficacy theory, or one's perceived capabilities to accomplish a task (Bandura, 1986); and self-worth theory, or one's desire to maintain a positive self-image (Covington, 1992). These two theories illustrate differences in the level of specificity of ability judgments: *Self-efficacy* refers to perceptions of abilities in a specific task situation, and *self-worth* is a more global assessment of one's ability and one's feelings about oneself. Furthermore, self-efficacy includes a belief that one has the skills for performing a task and a willingness to put forth effort in that task. Overall, individuals who perceive that they are competent are more likely to believe that they will succeed, control their outcomes, seek out challenging tasks, and attribute success to their ability and failure to other causes (Eccles et al., 1998). Numerous studies have shown that perceptions of competence are associated with positive affect, task choices, effort, persistence, academic performance, and task engagement (see Elliot & Dweck, 2005, for a review).

Much of the research on the development of children's motivation has focused on changes in children's self-concepts of ability. Researchers have found that even young elementary school children can distinguish their self-perceptions across many different domains, including reading, math, sports, physical appearance, and social interactions (e.g., Eccles, Wigfield, Harold, & Blumenfeld, 1993; Harter, 1982). Using cross-sectional and short-term longitudinal designs, studies have consistently shown a decline in children's perceptions of competence across the elementary and secondary school years in various domains, including mathematics, reading, sports, and music (e.g., Eccles et al., 1998; Stipek & MacIver, 1989; Wigfield et al., 1997). Fredricks and Eccles (2002) extended this work with a 12-year longitudinal study examining the development of children's competence beliefs in math and sports from 1st to 12th grade. Using hierarchical linear modeling techniques, they documented a decline in children's competence beliefs in math and sports over this 12-year period.

These age-related changes in competence beliefs may reflect age-related shifts in the cognitions that underlie competence beliefs. Young children tend to have overly optimistic perceptions of their competence, rely more on wishful thinking, and are less likely to use social comparative standards to judge their ability (Ruble, 1983; Stipek & MacIver, 1989). At about 7–8 years of age, children begin to understand that ability is a potentially stable quality, and they begin to use success and failure feedback in judging their competence in different domains. By 10–12 years of age, children begin to differentiate ability and effort as separate factors (Dweck, 2002). These developmental shifts in competence-related beliefs may also reflect changes in the school environment. Most elementary school teachers use criterion mastery grading, whereas middle school and high school teachers use more normative/social comparative grading that tends to give children information about their ability relative to other children (Eccles, Midgley, et al., 1993). The heightened availability of social comparison information helps children to develop more accurate assessments of their abilities (Dweck, 2002). In fact, perceptions of competence are a stronger predictor of achievement outcomes as children get older and become more accurate in their assessments (Wigfield & Eccles, 1992).

### Values

Other motivational theories have focused on *values*, or the reasons why an individual chooses to engage in a task. For example, values are an important component of the Eccles expectancy–value model, intrinsic motivation theory, and research on personal interest (or individual interest). Although value has been defined somewhat differently across these motivational constructs, these theoretical perspectives share several features. The Eccles expectancy–value model (Eccles (Parsons) et al., 1983) is the most extensive model of task values. Eccles and her colleagues broadly define *task value* as incentives for doing different tasks; individuals will do tasks they positively value and avoid tasks that they negatively value. According to Eccles's model, task value is a function of four distinct components: intrinsic and interest value (enjoyment of the activity), attainment value (importance of doing well on the task for confirming aspects of one's self-schema), utility value/importance (importance of the task for future goals), and cost (negative aspects of engaging in the task). Several studies have shown support for the hypothesized links between task value beliefs and achievement-related choices, including course taking, occupational choices, college majors, and involvement in sports (see Eccles et al., 1998).

*Intrinsic motivation* considers why individuals choose to engage in tasks (Deci & Ryan, 1985; Harter, 1983). Much of the work in this area has focused on the distinction between intrinsic and extrinsic motivation. Deci and Ryan (1985) argued that individuals have a natural need to feel competent and self-determining, or a desire to believe that they are engaging in activities out of their own volition rather than to achieve some external outcome. Individuals who are intrinsically motivated perceive themselves as the cause of their own behavior, whereas individuals who are extrinsically motivated believe they are engaging in an activity because of rewards, punishments, or a desire to please another person (see Ryan & Deci, 2000, for a more detailed discussion of the varying types of extrinsic motivation).

A third construct, *personal* (or *individual*) *interest*, is also important to consider in relation to value. Personal interest refers to an individual's enduring attention to and willingness to engage in a particular activity (or object related to an activity) that develops over time (Hidi & Harackiewicz, 2000; Krapp, Hidi, & Renninger, 1992; Schiefele, 1991). There are varying views regarding the dispositional versus state-like nature of personal interest, and varying views regarding the role of value and knowledge in personal interest (see Hidi, Renninger, & Krapp, 2004, for a discussion). Generally, however, personal interest can be thought of as involving both feeling (affect associated with a particular domain such as liking and enjoyment) and value (importance of a particular domain because it is useful, personally relevant, or central to the self) (Krapp, 2002; Schiefele, 2001).

In comparison to competence beliefs, research on age differences in children's value perceptions is less extensive. Studies generally show age-related declines in children's value beliefs in different academic subjects (see Eccles et al., 1998, for a review). Both contextual and individual factors can explain the decline in task value and interest over time. Declines in task value and interest may reflect increasing public evaluation, competition, and ability grouping. As competition increases, children are more likely to experience a drop in their performance. As a consequence, individuals may lower their perceptions of the task value of an activity to help protect their self-esteem (Wigfield & Eccles, 1992). Furthermore, the increased emphasis on competition and evaluation may provide little support for intrinsic motivation and personal interest, as autonomy support and belonging are likely to decline with these shifting school contexts (Eccles, Midgley, et al., 1993).

It is possible, however, that the declines in value are more of a function of how value is measured and do not reflect true declines in adolescents' personal interest in school. For instance, most studies measure interest and task value at the domain level (e.g., interest in science), rather than assessing specific personal interests (e.g., a personal interest in biology or Newtonian physics) (Krapp, 2002). If adolescents' personal interests become more differentiated into subdomains, but interest is still being measured at the domain level, this pattern of a general decline in domain-level interest may be masking a differentiation of interest into specific subfields (in which interest in some subdisciplines increases while interest in other subdisciplines declines). Thus, if personal interest were to be assessed in relation to specific topics or subspecialties, this same decline in value might not be observed.

Another possibility is that the developmental patterns of task value and personal interest vary based on the underlying components (e.g., the distinction between interest/feeling and importance/value). In their recent study, Fredricks and Eccles (2002) considered developmental changes from 1st to 12th grade in the interest and importance components of task value. They ran four hierarchical linear growth models: math interest, math importance, sport interest, and sport importance. In general, children's perceptions of task value declined over time across these four models, though there were some differences in the developmental patterns. For example, Fredricks and Eccles documented a deceleration in the decline in children's math importance from 1st to 12th grade, with perceptions of math importance slightly increasing at the 10th grade, while children's perceptions of math interest declined from 1st to 12th grade. This differential pattern of change was reversed for sports. Children maintained relatively high interest in sports from childhood through adolescence, despite declining perceptions of its importance. This finding supports Eccles's contention that interest and importance are distinct components of value, and that developmental changes in these constructs will not necessarily follow the same pattern (see Eccles (Parsons) et al., 1983). This finding may have implications for the personal interest research, in that it may be important to assess feeling and value with separate scales.

## Achievement Goal Orientations

A third prominent perspective in research on achievement motivation is that of *achievement goal theory* (Weiner, 1990). According to achievement goal theory, goal orientations provide a framework for interpreting and reacting to events. There are thought to be two primary goals or reasons why students engage in achievement behavior, which in turn differentially predict students' behaviors, thoughts, and affect (Dweck & Leggett, 1988). A *mastery* goal orientation reflects a focus on learning and understanding, while a *performance* goal orientation reflects a focus on demonstrating one's ability or competence, often in relation to others.[1] More recently, a distinction between approach and avoidance orientations has been introduced, such that a student may approach the demonstration of competence (*performance–approach*) or avoid the demonstration of incompetence (*performance–avoidance*) (Elliot, 1999; Middleton & Midgley, 1997).[2] In general, mastery goals are associated with adaptive patterns of socio-emotional and learning outcomes (Dweck & Leggett, 1988; Linnenbrink & Pintrich, 2000), and performance–avoidance goals are linked with negative outcomes (Elliot, 1999). The relation of performance–approach goals to learning-related outcomes is mixed and is not readily explained by considering developmental levels or different patterns based on ability, gender, or ethnicity. In particular, some studies find a positive relation between performance–approach goals and achievement, and other studies report a negative relation; in many studies, performance–approach goals are neither beneficial nor detrimental for socio-emotional outcomes (Harackiewicz, Barron, Pintrich, Elliot, & Thrash, 2002; Linnenbrink, 2005; Midgley, Kaplan, & Middleton, 2001).

Overall, there is less research on the development of achievement goal orientations, and much of the research involves short-term longitudinal studies examining change across 2 years or across school transitions. This research generally suggests that mastery goal orientations are strongly endorsed during the elementary years (for reviews, see Anderman, Austin, & Johnson, 2002; Midgley, Middleton, Gheen, & Kumar, 2002). Although there is some decrease in mastery goal orientations as students make the transition into middle school, the more striking pattern concerns the endorsement of performance–approach goals. In particular, during the transition into middle school and high school, there is an increase in performance–approach goal orientations. Less is known about developmental shifts in performance–avoidance orientations, although there is preliminary evidence that performance–avoidance orientations may develop from performance–approach orientations during the middle school years, especially for students with high perceptions of competence during elementary school (Middleton, Kaplan, & Midgley, 2004).

Two explanations for this shift in performance–approach goal orientations are most prominent. First, Dweck has proposed that beliefs about ability underlie achievement goal orientations (Dweck & Leggett, 1988), and that there are developmental differences in these beliefs about ability (Dweck, 2002). In particular, younger children are more likely to hold *incremental* beliefs about ability, or the belief that ability is malleable. These incremental beliefs are associated with the adoption of learning (or mastery) goal orientations. In contrast, *entity* beliefs about ability, which suggest that ability is fixed, are associated with performance–approach goals; entity beliefs tend to emerge during middle to late childhood, although not all children shift to these entity beliefs. Nicholls (1990) has also proposed that beliefs about ability help to explain developmental patterns in children's goal orientations. In particular, changing conceptions of ability from effort-based to normative ability-based judgments are also important in the shift between mastery and performance orientations during middle childhood and early adolescence. A second approach has focused on changes in the classroom and school environments as critical for developmental shifts in goal orientations (e.g., Midgley et al., 2002). For example, there is a shift in the perceptions of the school and classroom goal structures over time, with students reporting an increase in performance-goal structures at the middle and high school levels (Midgley et al., 2002).

In addition to considering mean-level developmental changes in goal orientations, we can also consider whether the relation of goal orientations to socioemotional and learning outcomes varies as a function of age. Indeed, many researchers have suggested that performance–approach goals may be more beneficial during the college years, because performance orientations are better aligned with the increasing emphasis on competition in educational settings, but detrimental for younger children, whose learning environment still emphasizes mastery and learning (Harackiewicz, Barron, & Elliot, 1998). There is some evidence to support this claim (Pajares, Britner, & Valiante, 2000), at least in terms of the increasing benefits of performance–approach goals across the middle school years. However, across the literature, the consideration of age differences does not clearly explain the mixed findings regarding the benefits and detriments of performance–approach goals, and thus this issue needs to be more closely investigated (Linnenbrink, 2002).

## PARENTAL SOCIALIZATION OF MOTIVATION

An important aspect to consider in the development of achievement motivation is how motivation is socialized via various contextual influences. The family context is critical to consider in this socialization process, as parents convey important messages about schooling to children, and parents may influence children's beliefs about themselves. Eccles and her colleagues have developed the most extensive model of parental socialization of children's motivation, linking parenting practices both to their antecedents and to their socialization consequences (Eccles, 1993; Eccles et al., 1998). According to this model, parents' child-specific beliefs and behaviors are associated with demographic factors (e.g., socioeconomic status, neighborhood resources, and parents' marital status), child characteristics (e.g., gender, aptitude, past performance, and temperament), and parents' general beliefs (e.g., valuing of achievement, childrearing beliefs, values and goals, and gender-typed ideologies). In turn, parents' child-specific beliefs and behaviors are associated with children's competence beliefs, values, goals, and activity choices. Although there is some work linking parenting practices to goal orientations (see Dweck, 2002; Pomerantz, Grolnick, & Price, 2005), the majority of research has focused on parental socialization of competence and values; therefore, we focus our discussion here on these latter two aspects of motivation.

### Parents' Beliefs: Interpreters of Experience

The two primary ways in which parents influence children's motivation are by being interpreters of experience and providers of experience (Eccles, 1993; Eccles et al., 1998). Parents help to interpret their children's experiences by providing messages about the likelihood that their children will attain competence in a particular achievement domain, in combination with messages about the value of participating in that activity. Several studies have shown that parents' perceptions of their children's abilities are associated with children's and adolescents' competence beliefs, even after controlling for performance differences (e.g., Eccles, 1993; Jacobs & Eccles, 1992; Miller, Manhal, & Mee, 1991). In fact, parents' perceptions of their children's abilities are more strongly associated with children's competence beliefs than are teachers' perceptions (Wigfield et al., 1997). There has been less research examining the relation between parents' values and children's motivational constructs. A few studies have shown that when parents perceive that participating in schoolwork and sports is important, elementary school and junior high students have higher academic and sport competence beliefs (Bandura, Barbaranelli, Caprara, & Pastorelli, 1996; Fredricks & Eccles, 2005).

Fredricks and Eccles (2002) extended this work with a longitudinal study that examined the long-term effects of parents' perceptions of children's ability in the elementary school years and changes in children's competence beliefs and value beliefs from 1st to 12th grade. They found that parents' perceptions of children's beliefs in the early elementary school years helped to explain both mean differences in math and sports competence beliefs, and differences in the rate of change in sports competence perceptions and value beliefs over time.

Parents' who had high perceptions of their children's ability in the early elementary school years had children with less dramatic declines in their perceptions of competence, interest, and importance over time, regardless of early ability differences.

### Parents' Behaviors: Provision of Experiences

Parents also can increase children's motivation through their behaviors and provision of specific experiences inside and outside of the home. According to the Eccles model, parents influence motivation through their use of time with their children; teaching of strategies; encouragement of participation in various activities; and provision of toys, equipment, and lessons (Eccles et al., 1998). There have been several studies of the effects of parental involvement on motivation and achievement. Evidence from this work indicates a positive association between parental involvement and children's perceptions of competence (Grolnick, Kurowski, Dunlap, & Hevey, 2000; Grolnick & Ryan, 1989). Other work has explored the effects of parents' autonomy-supportive and controlling behaviors on children's motivation. Parents who support autonomy allow their children to take initiative, work on their own, and take an active role in solving problems. In contrast, controlling parents exert pressure, regulate children's behavior, and inhibit children from solving problems on their own (Grolnick, 2003). In both field and experimental studies, parents' use of autonomy-supportive practices rather than controlling practices has been shown to foster intrinsic motivation (e.g., Deci, Driver, Hotchkiss, Robbins, & Wilson, 1993; Ginsburg & Bronstein, 1993).

## SCHOOL AND CLASSROOM CONTEXTUAL FACTORS

In addition to the family context, school and classroom environments also play an important role in shaping students' motivation. Given the breadth of research on school and classroom environments, we focus our discussion specifically on aspects of the educational environment that are directly related to competence beliefs, values, and goal orientations, rather than providing a comprehensive review of research.

### School Environments

Maehr and Midgley (Maehr & Midgley, 1991, 1996) have suggested that school environments can be thought of as creating a particular culture for learning. Although individual teachers can have a significant impact on students' motivation, the general culture of the school can also have an important influence on student motivation. In support of this view, students' perceptions of school goal structures have been linked to their personal goal orientations (Roeser, Midgley, & Urdan, 1996).

The existence of a schoolwide honor roll is one salient example of how school culture may influence motivation. Schools' use of honor rolls to recognize academic excellence may send the message to students that it is important to demonstrate competence, which may result in higher levels of students' endorsement of performance goal orientations. This practice can also be seen as involving control by others and thus may undermine intrinsic motivation (Ryan & Deci, 2000). As noted previously, honor rolls also place an emphasis on relative ability, which may contribute to decreasing perceptions of competence as children move into the middle grades (Eccles, Midgley, et al., 1993).

More broadly, a variety of changes in school environments may help to explain the declines in competence beliefs and value and the increase in performance goal adoption. For instance, Midgley, Maehr, and their colleagues (e.g., Maehr & Midgley, 1996; Midgley, Anderman, & Hicks, 1995; Midgley et al., 2002) suggest that elementary schools place a greater emphasis on developing competence (mastery), with the use of heterogeneous grouping, support for improvement, and the importance of effort in evaluation practices as just a few of the critical features. In contrast, middle school (and high school) environments place a greater emphasis on demonstrating competence (performance) through the use of tracking and the increased importance placed on academic recognition (e.g., the honor roll). This shifting emphasis on demonstrating competence is also likely to undermine students' perceptions of competence over time.

Greater teacher authority and fewer student choices are also seen as students move from elementary to middle school (Eccles, Midgley, et al., 1993, Maehr & Midgley, 1996). For example, the scheduling requirements of middle school and high schools require that students move through the day according to a strict timetable, whereas more flexibility in scheduling and greater opportunities for students to work on a variety of topics during individual seatwork are seen at the elementary level. This decrease in student autonomy and increase in teacher and administrator authority are likely to undermine task value and intrinsic motivation, as students see fewer opportunities for self-determination and choice.

## Classroom Environments

Research on classroom contexts in relation to the development of achievement motivation has focused on a variety of factors, including the types of tasks that are used, structures of authority and autonomy, and recognition and evaluation systems. Some scholars have argued that motivation and engagement can be increased in classrooms where tasks are authentic, provide opportunities for students to assume ownership, allow students to work collaboratively, and permit diverse forms of talents (Blumenfeld et al., 1991; Newmann, 1991). Unfortunately, the most common instructional approach in most classrooms is the use of tasks that require recall or repetition of procedures rather than active problem solving (Newmann, Wehlage, & Lamborn, 1992).

The use of varied, meaningful, and appropriately challenging tasks is thought to foster mastery goal orientations (Ames, 1992a, 1992b). Challenging tasks may also be important in creating classroom environments that support perceptions of competence, as success on challenging rather than easy tasks is more likely to support higher levels of efficacy and competence beliefs (Pintrich & Schunk, 2002). Tasks that involve fantasy, suspense, novelty, and elements of uncertainty can increase intrinsic motivation (Stipek, 1993). Tasks that stimulate students' attention and help students to see the domain as meaningful and personally relevant may also enhance situational interest, which may in turn lead to the development of personal interest over time (Hidi et al., 2004).

The authority or autonomy structures of the classroom are critical to achievement motivation in terms of both values and goal orientations. With respect to value, Deci and Ryan (1987) suggest that providing students with choice and removing external controls helps to support students' need for self-determination and thus promotes intrinsic motivation. In contrast, perceptions of high control (and low autonomy) in the form of deadlines, surveillance, and extrinsic rewards are much more likely to undermine intrinsic motivation. More specific research on rewards suggests that rewards that are used as an incentive to engage in task (*task-contingent* rewards) have a more deleterious effect on intrinsic motivation than rewards that convey information about mastery (*performance-contingent* rewards) (Deci & Ryan, 1985). The effect of rewards also varies depending on whether the rewards are expected and tangible, with expected and/or tangible rewards leading to lower levels of intrinsic motivation than unexpected and/or intangible rewards (for a more detailed discussion, see Deci, Koestner, & Ryan, 2001).

High levels of autonomy and low levels of authority are also critical to creating a mastery goal structure in the classroom (Ames, 1992a, 1992b; Patrick, Anderman, Ryan, Edelin, & Midgley, 2001). When teachers allow students more control in the classroom, students receive the message that importance and value are placed on engaging in an activity for its own sake, rather than to please their teachers or demonstrate their own competence. Patrick and colleagues (2001) found evidence to support this link between autonomy–authority and mastery goal orientations. They identified four different classrooms where students' perceptions of the classroom goal structure varied across the dimensions of mastery and performance. They found that classrooms were perceived as more mastery-oriented when students participated in rule making, when rules supported autonomy (e.g., students were free to talk as long as the talk was work-related), and when students had more choice in terms of the classroom daily routines (e.g., eating snacks, sharpening pencils). Of course, we must also consider that different forms of autonomy support may be more meaningful than others, with cognitive autonomy support—in which students are given ownership for learning through practices such as the encouragement of multiple strategies for solving a problem or the acceptance of multiple solutions—leading to higher levels of motivation and engagement than autonomy support for classroom organization or procedures (Stefanou, Perencevich, DiCintio, & Turner, 2004).

Finally, evaluation and recognition structures send important messages regarding the emphasis on developing versus demonstrating competence (Ames, 1992a, 1992b; Patrick et al., 2001). In classrooms where evaluation and recognition structures emphasize relative ability and social comparison, students are likely to endorse performance goal orientations (Ames, 1992a, 1992b). In contrast, recognition for improvement and effort sends the message that developing competence is valued, and thus students are more likely to endorse mastery goals. For example, Linnenbrink (2005) altered students' goal orientations by changing the feedback that students received while working on small-group activities during a 5-week mathematics unit. Groups that received feedback about their improvement across a math unit (mastery condition) or their improvement relative to other groups (combined mastery/performance–approach condition) reported higher levels of personal mastery goal orientations at the end of the unit relative to the performance–approach condition. Feedback that was framed in terms of relative ability (based on relative performance or relative improvement) was associated with the endorsement of performance–approach goals at the end of the mathematics unit.

Recognition and evaluation practices can also be framed in terms of supporting or undermining intrinsic motivation, based on the forms of recognition that are used (e.g., tangible, task-contingent, etc.) (Deci et al., 2001), as discussed previously in regard to autonomy support. Finally, evaluation practices may play an important role in students' perceptions of competence (Dweck, 2002; Eccles, Midgley, et al., 1993). When achievement is evaluated in relation to other students, this creates a situation in which some students must fail or do worse than their peers. The experience of failure relative to others is likely to lead to lower perceptions of competence. And when students endorse a view that ability is fixed, this may be especially problematic in creating a downward cycle of decreasing perceptions of competence as they compare themselves to their peers.

## Person × Context Interactions

In addition to considering the relation of the context to students' motivation, a critical feature of many of these theoretical approaches is the potential interplay between what the individual brings to the situation and whether the situation affords support for that individual. One prominent approach for considering person × context interactions is Eccles and Midgley's (Eccles, Midgley, et al., 1993) research on stage–environment fit. They argue that a stage–environment fit model can help to explain declines in motivation during the middle school transition. In particular, the context of most middle schools does not support adolescents' growing need for autonomy, social interactions, self-focus and self-exploration, and capacity for abstract cognitive thought. Instead, middle schools tend to decrease the opportunities for personal choice and responsibility, create lower-quality relationships with teachers, limit social interactions with peers, and create fewer opportunities for challenging work while using higher standards for judging competence. This mismatch between adolescents' developmental needs and the affordances in the environment for meeting those needs may help to explain the decline in self-perceptions of competence and task value during this period.

For instance, early work in this area suggested that students who made the transition from environments with high social support in elementary school to ones with low social support in middle school experienced a decline in task value in mathematics (Midgley, Feldlaufer, & Eccles, 1989). Interestingly, with recent middle school reforms that have focused on reconciling this mismatch between adolescents' developmental needs and school environments during the transition from fifth to sixth grade, these declines in motivation are not as prominent until seventh and eighth grades (Midgley et al., 2002). This suggests that increasing our effort to create school environments that support students' shifting developmental needs across the school years might be one potential pathway to slowing or even eliminating the declines in perceived competence and value across the school years.

A stage–environment fit paradigm has also been applied to research in the family context. Eccles, Midgley, and colleagues (1993) argue that the fit between adolescents' need for autonomy and independence and input in family decision making may also help to explain declines in motivation during the middle school transition. In support of this theory, they find that the opportunity to participate in family decision making during adolescence predicts intrinsic motivation and adjustment to school (Eccles, Midgley, et al., 1993; see also Yee & Flanagan, 1985).

Another example of a motivational theory that focuses on the fit between context and motivation is *self-system theory* (Connell, 1990; Connell & Wellborn, 1991). This theory has been applied to both family and classroom environments. According to this theory, individuals have fundamental psychological needs for relatedness, autonomy, and competence. The degree to which students perceive that either the family or classroom context meets these three needs determines how motivated and engaged they will be. When teachers and parents are involved with children, it is assumed that students will be more likely to feel that their need for relatedness is being met. Students' need for autonomy is more likely to be met in family and classroom contexts where students have choice, opportunities to contribute to decision making, and limited external controls. Finally, it is assumed that individuals' need for competence will be met when expectations are clear and consistent, and when adults respond consistently and contingently. Several studies have documented support for the proposed theoretical links among individuals' perceptions of context, needs, and intrinsic motivation (for reviews, see Connell, 1990; Fredricks, Blumenfeld, & Paris, 2004; Pomerantz et al., 2005). In both school and family contexts where students perceive that their needs for competence, autonomy, and relatedness are met, students report higher intrinsic motivation and engagement.

Although person × environment fit is not explicitly addressed by achievement goal theory, this model can also be used as a guide in considering the potential interplay between personal characteristics and the classroom or school environment. For example, Linnenbrink and Pintrich (2001) have argued that it is essential to consider the interplay between students' personal goal orientations and the goal context by examining the extent to which the classroom environment affords students with the opportunity to pursue their personal goal orientations. They have proposed two distinct patterns that may occur. The first pattern, the matching hypothesis, proposes that students should show more adaptive profiles of motivation and learning when there is a match between their own personal goal orientation and the goal structure of the classroom. In this way, an individual with a performance goal orientation should excel in a performance-focused classroom, whereas an individual with a mastery goal orientation should excel in a mastery-focused classroom. In contrast, the buffering hypothesis suggests that all students benefit from an emphasis on mastery in the classroom. For students with mastery goal orientations, the mastery-oriented classroom goal structure should further support their efforts for learning and understanding. For those with a performance goal orientation, the mastery goal structure should buffer the negative effects of endorsing performance goals.

Barron and Harackiewicz (2001) found initial support for the matching hypothesis for undergraduates, based on the match between students' achievement orientation and the goals students pursued during an experimental mathematics task. Linnenbrink (2005) also addressed this issue in a quasi-experimental design conducted in upper elementary mathematics classrooms. In particular, at the start of the school year, 10 classrooms were assigned to one of three classroom goal conditions (mastery, performance–approach, combined mastery and performance–approach); students' initial personal goal orientations were also assessed during the first week of school. Using a repeated-measures multivariate analysis of covariance, Linnenbrink examined the interaction between initial personal goal orientations and the classroom goal context across 12 indicators of socioemotional well-being, engagement, and learning. Surprisingly, there were no significant personal goal × goal context interactions. There were, however, significant main effects for both the classroom goal structure and personal goal orientations, but the findings yielded different patterns.

In particular, Linnenbrink (2005) found that the combined mastery/performance–approach goal condition was the most beneficial classroom goal context, with students working in this condition engaging in more adaptive forms of help seeking and learning. The mastery goal condition was beneficial for help seeking but detrimental for achievement, while the performance–approach goal condition was beneficial for achievement but detrimental for help seeking. A somewhat different pattern emerged when personal goal orientations were examined. Personal mastery goal orientations were beneficial for 11 of the 12 outcomes, including achievement. Personal performance–approach goal orientations were associated with high positive affect, but also with high test anxiety and low achievement. There were no significant personal mastery × personal performance–approach goal interactions.

Although neither the matching nor the buffering hypothesis was supported in this study, it is interesting that different patterns may emerge when personal goal orientations versus classroom goal contexts are considered. These results suggest the need to consider both personal and contextual factors, but they also suggest that the interaction between these may not be the most important element. However, given the dearth of research in this area, it would be worthwhile for future research to continue to investigate possible personal goal × classroom goal interactions, while also closely considering the possible unique effects of both personal goal orientations and the classroom goal context over time. The consideration of parental beliefs and behaviors—in terms of direct effects on students' goal orientations, as well as the potential interaction with personal goal orientations—would also be worthwhile to consider. Finally, the field in general would benefit if more researchers attended to the interplay between family and school contexts and students' perceived competence, values, and goals, as this research would be likely to provide a more realistic picture of the development of student motivation.

## CONCLUSION AND FUTURE DIRECTIONS

In this chapter we have reviewed research on how different competence beliefs, values, and goal orientations develop during childhood and adolescence. We conclude by first briefly outlining the key findings on developmental changes in these constructs and research on the relation between context and motivation. We then consider the methodological challenges that researchers face in conducting this type of research, and propose some new approaches that may prove fruitful.

### Developmental Changes in Achievement Motivation

In general, indicators of achievement motivation (i.e., competence beliefs, value, and mastery goals) decline across the school grades; the exception is the increase in the endorsement of performance–approach goals in middle school. These developmental differences result from changes in beliefs about ability, increases in the use of social comparative information, and changes in the instructional environment and evaluation practices as students progress through school. Our review also highlights the importance of contextual factors in shaping motivation. Several aspects of the classroom context have been linked to more adaptive forms of motivation, including supportive relationships with teachers, meaningful and varied tasks, opportunities for choice, evaluations that focus on personal improvement, and the use of informational rather than controlling rewards. Other work has linked aspects of the family environment to adaptive patterns of motivation. Parents who have high perceptions of their children's abilities, provide messages that school is valuable, are actively involved in children's lives, and provide learning opportunities in the home have children who report higher perceptions of competence, value, and intrinsic motivation. The relation between context and motivation also appears to vary by developmental level, psychological needs, and goals. These findings suggest that a person–environment model of motivation may fit the empirical data. As such, the key to increasing motivation may be to better appreciate the complex interplay between individual characteristics and the home or school context, so that we can better understand how to create contexts that support adaptive motivational development for most children.

### Future Directions: Challenges and Fruitful New Approaches

Although the field has made great strides in research investigating motivation from a developmental perspective over the past several decades, there are still many challenges in conducting this research and many areas of study that have not been thoroughly investigated. In this section we consider five critical aspects for future research: (1) how to assess patterns of motivation, (2) how to measure individual and contextual factors, (3) how to examine the interplay of the individual with his or her context, (4) how to assess change, and (5) how to study dynamic embedded systems. Within each of these areas, we discuss both challenges and fruitful areas of future inquiry.

### Patterns of Motivation

One methodological challenge that researchers face is how to measure complex patterns of individual development. In general, most studies have tended to use variable-centered techniques, such as regression analyses, to explore the development of achievement motivation and the unique effects of contextual factors on motivational outcomes. Variable-centered techniques assume linear relations among relevant dimensions, after adjusting for all other factors in the model. This may not be the best method to capture rich characteristics of both individuals and environments. Rather, person-centered analysis techniques such as cluster analysis, multidimensional scaling, and cumulative models may be better analytic approaches for assessing synergistic and complex systems. From a developmental perspective, researchers could use person-centered analyses to track personal trajectories over time or to consider whether students' change clusters over time, especially across school transitions.

For example, a pattern-centered approach can be used to consider how contexts shape motivation. In a series of studies, Fredricks and her colleagues (i.e., Fredricks & Eccles, 2005; Fredricks, Simpson, & Eccles, 2005; Simpson, Fredricks, Davis-Kean, & Eccles, 2005) compared a variable-centered model and a pattern-centered analytic model of parental socialization in math, sports, and music. The pattern-centered analyses were modeled on the risk and resiliency research, which has used cutoff points on various risk and promotive factors to examine the impact of cumulative risk and promotive/protective factors on children's functioning (Rutter, 1988; Sameroff, Bartko, Baldwin, Baldwin, & Seifer, 1998). Interestingly, the findings from the two sets of analyses led to different conclusions about the effects of parental socialization. In the regression model, parents' perceptions of their children's ability and value had the strongest unique relations with children's competence beliefs and value in math, sports, and music, both concurrently and over time. In fact, many of the other behavioral aspects of parents' socialization were not associated with children's competence beliefs and value after adjusting for the higher intercorrelation between parents' beliefs (e.g., perceptions of children's ability and value) and children's competence beliefs and value. In contrast, in the pattern-centered model, socialization techniques had an additive positive association with competence and value beliefs over time. One possible explanation for the different findings is that parents' behaviors are closely related to their beliefs, and these constructs operate more synergistically with each other. Another explanation could lie in the fact that pattern-centered approaches do not necessarily assume linear relations between predictors and outcomes. By using a cutoff point method, researchers can identify families who are providing extraordinarily high levels of support on each of the socialization factors.

A person-centered approach can also be taken to consider patterns of motivation, emotional well-being, and engagement in school. For instance, Turner, Thorpe, and Meyer (1998) used cluster analysis to consider how patterns of achievement goals and perceptions of competence combined with emotional well-being and cognitive strategies for early adolescents (see also Braten & Olaussen, 2005, for a cluster analysis linking mastery goals, task value, interest, and efficacy with cognitive strategies and epistemologies). Roeser, Strobel, and Quihuis (2002) also investigated the relation among achievement motivation, emotional well-being, and engagement for adolescents, using median splits to create groups based on two theoretical models. They found that it was especially useful to consider the combination of motivational and emotional variables in understanding students' engagement in school. These studies suggest that it is critical to consider patterns of motivation—something that is not clearly seen in variable-centered approaches. Additional research in which multiple motivational variables and theories are considered in one study would shed further light on how motivational variables might combine to influence learning and motivation.

### Assessing Individual and Contextual Factors

Another methodological question concerns how to measure individual and contextual factors. One measurement issue is the distinction between subjective and objective features of the classroom environment. Ames (1992b) argued that one needs to focus on subjective features, as students' perceptions of the environment are critical for their motivation and engagement. Nevertheless, considerations of more objective features (e.g., the presentation of classroom rules, teachers' evaluation practices, and the features of classrooms tasks) are also important, especially as policy changes for schools and classrooms are proposed and made (Kaplan, Middleton, Urdan, & Midgley, 2002; Linnenbrink, 2004). To date, research has primarily focused on students' perceptions of the goal structure or teachers' self-reported instructional practices, but has not examined the classroom context by experimentally altering the classroom context or by also considering an observer's ratings of the classroom context.

However, several recent studies have attempted to address this issue. For instance, as noted earlier, Linnenbrink (2005) found significant differences in students' personal goal orientations at the end of a 5-week unit that were in line with the quasi-experimental classroom goal conditions; these findings suggest that it is possible to alter students' personal goal orientations by making changes to the classroom goal structure. Classroom observation studies can also be useful in that they often employ a combination of students' self-reports and classroom observations, and are therefore able to examine the classroom from multiple lenses. For instance, Patrick and colleagues (2001) used students' self-reports to categorize classrooms' goal structures as high mastery–low performance, high mastery–high performance, low mastery–high performance, and low mastery–low performance. The authors then examined the way that teachers set up their classrooms and interacted with students to consider how observed goal structures related to students' perceptions of the classroom goal structure. The results of the observed indicators of goal structure were consistent with students' perceptions, suggesting that the studies conducted using student perceptions may have important implications for actual classroom practices. Nevertheless, additional research that addresses both observed and students' perceived features would help to clarify these relations.

An alternative to the use of experimental designs or observations to assess the context is the use of hierarchical linear modeling (HLM) to consider how context-level variables relate to students' motivation or behavior. This also provides a different lens, in that aggregates of students' perceptions of the classroom context, teachers' reports of their classrooms, or observer reports can be used to model classroom-level predictors of individual student behavior. For example, Ryan, Gheen, and Midgley (1998) examined how students' perceptions of the classroom goal structure and teachers' reports of instructional strategies as supporting mastery or performance goal orientations related to students' help-seeking behaviors. They found that there were differences in help seeking between classrooms, and that this difference could be explained, at least in part, by aggregates of students' perceptions of the goal structure at the classroom level. Interestingly, teachers' reported instructional strategies did not predict students' help-seeking behaviors. In another study, Urdan, Midgley, and Anderman (1998) used teacher reports of the goal structure and aggregated students' reports of the classroom goal structure to examine how classroom contexts related to students' use of self-handicapping strategies; they found that both students' perceptions of the classroom as emphasizing performance goal orientations and teachers' reports of using performance-oriented instructional practices were independent and significant predictors of students' reports of self-handicapping. These studies further highlight the need to examine the environment through multiple lenses and the need to move beyond single-level models that do not take into account class- or school-level variables. Furthermore, the HLM, observational, and experimental studies serve to highlight the complexity in capturing contextual elements of the home, school, or classroom, and the need for multiple methodologies to address this complexity more accurately.

### *Person–Environment Models*

As we begin to take into account contextual and personal factors, we also need to think about how best to assess the interplay between the individual and contextual factors. A fruitful area of work is to examine the fit between the person and the family and school context (see work by Connell & Wellborn, 1991, and Eccles & Midgley, 1989, for examples) across samples of children with different individual characteristics. To have a fuller understanding of developmental shifts in motivation, we also need to explore a richer array of person variables. For example, there are probably other individual factors, such as gender, ethnicity, or ability, that should be included in person–environment models. Such research would tell us which aspects of the classroom and family context are most salient, and potentially most important, for increasing adaptive forms of motivation for different types of students.

It is also likely that different contextual changes are more important in increasing motivation at different ages, though few studies have explored differences in the strength of the relations between contextual factors and motivation by age. For example, teacher support may be a more important factor in increasing motivation in elementary schools, because elementary students develop strong relationships with a single teacher throughout a school year, whereas students typically have multiple teachers in a given year during middle school and high school. However, one might also imagine that there is greater variation in perceptions of teacher support and belonging at the middle school and high school levels, so this may be an area where reform efforts could have a stronger influence.

### *Measuring Change*

Another issue for developmental researchers concerns how to best measure change. Much of our understanding of mean-level changes in these motivational constructs has come from cross-sectional and short-term longitudinal studies. With the exception of work by Eccles and her colleagues (e.g., Fredricks & Eccles, 2002), there are few longitudinal studies that have followed individuals over an extended period of time. We also know very little about variations in the developmental trajectories as functions of socioeconomic status and ethnicity. The obstacles faced by minority and low-income students in school have made the study of the development of motivation among these groups a critical area of future inquiry.

When considering change, we also have very little research that considers reciprocal influences between the person and the environment on the change process. We have discussed several studies showing that aspects of family and school context are predictors of motivation. However, socialization is not only a unidirectional process in which parents and teachers shape children. Instead, teachers and parents adjust their beliefs and practices based on children's competence beliefs, values, and goals. For example, there is evidence that teachers prefer students who are academically competent (see Kedar-Voivodas, 1983). This preference is likely to lead teachers to provide different opportunities to students they perceive as higher in competence. There is also evidence that parental socialization is shaped by children's ability level. For example, parents are more likely to spend time with a child on homework when the child is having difficulty (e.g., Chen & Stevenson, 1989). Longitudinal designs that include measures of context and motivation at multiple time points are necessary to test reciprocal links.

### *Dynamic Systems*

A final challenge is how to consider the interplay between the varying contexts in which children live. The reality is that family and school contexts are interrelated and are shaped by the larger social context in which teachers and parents live. For example, conflicting messages between the home and the school may result in different motivational patterns than when home and school environments are matched (Arunkumar, Midgley, & Urdan, 1999). In addition, a teacher's perceptions of parental values regarding schooling may have an impact on the teacher's perceptions of a child's competence and the child's subsequent academic skills (Hauser-Cram, Sirin, & Stipek, 2003). In this way, a dynamic model of the person in multiple environments (Bronfenbrenner, 1986) may be particularly useful in understanding the complexity of motivational development. There is a need for more sophisticated research designs to identify interrelations between different settings and to test the moderating role of social contextual factors in shaping the development of motivation.

## Summary

Scholars have made a great deal of progress in understanding general patterns of development of achievement motivation in terms of mean-level changes. However, we are just starting to understand the complexity of individual trajectories in the development of achievement motivation, and the relation of home and school environments in shaping these patterns. We believe that several broad areas of future research can expand our understanding of these issues in important ways. One area of work is to integrate theoretical models of motivation and employ person-centered analyses to accomplish this integration. A second area of future work is to refine our measures of the individual and context to include multiple types of indicators, rather than relying solely on self-reports. A final area of work is to consider the dynamic interplay between individuals and their multiple environments.

## ACKNOWLEDGMENT

We thank Allison M. Ryan and Steven R. Asher for their helpful feedback and suggestions on this chapter.

## NOTES

1. These goals have also been referred to as *learning* and *performance* goals (Dweck & Leggett, 1988), *task* and *ability* goals (Maehr & Midgley, 1991), and *task-involved* and *ego-involved* goals (Nicholls, 1984, 1990).

2. Pintrich (2000) and Elliot (1999) have proposed the addition of a *mastery–avoidance* orientation; however, this distinction has not yet been fully supported in the literature.

## REFERENCES

Ames, C. (1992a). Achievement goals and the classroom motivational climate. In D. H. Schunk & J. L. Meece (Eds.), *Student perceptions in the classroom* (pp. 327–348). Hillsdale, NJ: Erlbaum.

Ames, C. (1992b). Classrooms: Goals, structures, and student motivation. *Journal of Educational Psychology, 84*, 261–271.

Anderman, E. M., Austin, C. C., & Johnson, D. M. (2002). The development of goal orientation. In A. Wigfield & J. S. Eccles (Eds.), *Development of achievement motivation* (pp. 197–220). San Diego, CA: Academic Press.

Arunkumar, R., Midgley, C., & Urdan, T. (1999). Perceiving high or low home–school dissonance: Longitudinal effects on adolescent emotional and academic well-being. *Journal of Research on Adolescence, 9*, 441–466.

Bandura, A. (1986). *Social foundations of thought and action: A social cognitive theory.* Englewood Cliffs, NJ: Prentice Hall.

Bandura, A., Barbaranelli, C., Caprara, G. V., & Pastorelli, C. (1996). Multi-faceted impact of self-efficacy beliefs on academic functioning. *Child Development, 67*, 1206–1222.

Barron, K. E., & Harackiewicz, J. M. (2001). Achievement goals and optimal motivation: Testing multiple goal models. *Journal of Personality and Social Psychology, 80*, 706–722.

Blumenfeld, P. C., Soloway, E., Marx, R., Krajcik, J. S., Guzdial, M., & Palinscar, A. (1991). Motivating project based learning: Sustaining the doing, supporting the learning. *Educational Psychologist, 26*, 369–398.

Braten, I., & Olaussen, B. S. (2005). Profiling individual differences in student motivation: A longitudinal cluster-analytic study in different academic contexts. *Contemporary Educational Psychology, 30*, 359–396.

Bronfenbrenner, U. (1986). Ecology of the family as a context for human development: Research perspectives. *Developmental Psychology, 22*, 723–742.

Chen, C., & Stevenson, H. W. (1989). Homework: A cross-cultural examination. *Child Development, 60*, 551–561.

Connell, J. P. (1990). Context, self, and action: A motivational analysis of self-system processes across the life-span. In D. Cicchetti (Ed.), *The self in transition: Infancy to childhood* (pp. 61–97). Chicago: University of Chicago Press.

Connell, J. P., & Wellborn, J. G. (1991). Competence, autonomy, and relatedness: A motivational analysis of self-system processes. In M. Gunnar & L. A. Sroufe (Eds.), *Minnesota Symposium on Child Psychology* (Vol. 23, pp. 43–77). Chicago: University of Chicago Press.

Covington, M. V. (1992). *Making the grade: A self-worth perspective on motivation and school reform.* New York: Cambridge University Press.

Deci, E. L., Driver, R. E., Hotchkiss, L., Robbins, R. J., & Wilson, I. M. (1993). The relation of mothers' controlling vocalizations to children's intrinsic motivation. *Journal of Experimental Child Psychology, 55*, 151–162.

Deci, E. L., Koestner, R., & Ryan, R. M. (2001). Extrinsic rewards and intrinsic motivation in education: Reconsidered once again. *Review of Educational Research, 71*, 1–27.

Deci, E. L., & Ryan, R. M. (1985). *Intrinsic motivation and self-determination in human behavior.* New York: Plenum Press.

Deci, E. L., & Ryan, R. M. (1987). The support of autonomy and the control of behavior. *Journal of Personality and Social Psychology, 53*, 1024–1037.

Dweck, C. (2002). The development of ability conceptions. In A. Wigfield & J. S. Eccles (Eds.), *Development of achievement motivation* (pp. 57–88). San Diego, CA: Academic Press.

Dweck, C., & Leggett, E. (1988). A social-cognitive approach to motivation and personality. *Psychological Review, 95*, 256–273.

Eccles, J. S. (1993). School and family effects of the ontogeny of children's interests, self-perceptions, and activity choice. In J. Jacobs (Ed.), *Nebraska Symposium on Motivation: Vol. 40. Developmental perspectives on motivation* (pp. 145–208). Lincoln: University of Nebraska Press.

Eccles (Parsons), J. S., Adler, T. F., Futterman, R., Goff, S .B., Kaczala, C. M., Meece, J. L., et al. (1983). Expectations, values and academic behaviors. In J. T. Spence (Ed.), *Achievement and achievement motivation* (pp. 75–146). San Francisco: Freeman.

Eccles, J. S., & Midgley, C. (1989). Stage–environment fits: Developmentally appropriate classrooms for young adolescents. In C. Ames & R. Ames (Eds.), *Research on motivation in education* (Vol. 3, pp. 139–186). San Diego, CA: Academic Press.

Eccles, J. S., Midgley, C., Wigfield, A., Buchanan, C., Reuman, D., Flanagan, C., et al. (1993). Development during adolescence: The impact of stage–environment fit on young adolescents' experiences in schools and families. *American Psychologist*, *48*, 90–101.

Eccles, J. S., Wigfield, A., Harold, R. D., & Blumenfeld, P. (1993). Ontogeny of children's self-perceptions and subjective task values across activity domains during the early elementary school years. *Child Development*, *64*, 830–847.

Eccles, J. S., Wigfield, A., & Schiefele, U. (1998). Motivation to succeed. In W. Damon (Series Ed.) & N. Eisenberg (Vol. Ed.), *Handbook of child psychology: Vol. 3. Social, emotional, and personality development* (5th ed., pp. 1017–1094). New York: Wiley.

Elliot, A. J. (1999). Approach and avoidance motivation and achievement goals. *Educational Psychologist*, *34*, 169–189.

Elliot, A. J., & Dweck, C. S. (Eds.). (2005). *Handbook of competence and motivation*. New York: Guilford Press.

Fredricks, J. A., Blumenfeld, P. C., & Paris, A. (2004). School engagement: Potential of the concept: State of the evidence. *Review of Educational Research*, *74*, 59–119.

Fredricks, J. A., & Eccles, J. S. (2002). Children's competence and value beliefs from childhood to adolescence: Growth trajectories in two "male-typed" domains. *Developmental Psychology*, *38*, 519–533.

Fredricks, J. A., & Eccles, J. A. (2005). Family socialization, gender, motivation, and competitive sports involvement. *Journal of Sport and Exercise Psychology*, *27*, 3–31.

Fredricks, J., Simpson, S., & Eccles, J. (2005). Family socialization, gender, and participation in sports and instrumental music. In C. R. Cooper, C. Garcia Coll, W. T. Bartko, H. M. Davis, & C. Chatman (Eds.), *Developmental pathways through middle childhood: Rethinking diversity and contexts as resources* (pp. 41–62). Mahwah, NJ: Erlbaum.

Ginsburg, G. S., & Bronstein, P. (1993). Family factors related to children's intrinsic/extrinsic motivational orientation and academic performance. *Child Development*, *64*, 1461–1474.

Grolnick, W. S. (2003). *The psychology of parental control: How well-meant parenting backfires*. Mahwah, NJ: Erlbaum.

Grolnick, W. S., Kurowski, C. O., Dunlap, K. G., & Hevey, C. (2000). Parental resources and the transition to junior high. *Journal of Research on Adolescence*, *10*, 465–488.

Grolnick, W. S., & Ryan, R. M. (1989). Parent styles associated with children's self-regulation and competence in school. *Journal of Educational Psychology*, *81*, 143–154.

Harter, S. (1982). The Perceived Competence Scale for Children. *Child Development*, *53*, 87–97.

Harter, S. (1983). Developmental perspectives on the self-system. In P. H. Mussen (Series Ed.) & E. M. Hetherington (Vol. Ed.), *Handbook of child psychology: Vol. 4. Socialization, personality, and social development* (4th ed., pp. 275–385). New York: Wiley.

Harackiewicz, J. M., Barron, K. E., & Elliot, A. J. (1998). Rethinking achievement goals: When are they adaptive for college students and why? *Educational Psychologist*, *33*, 1–21.

Harackiewicz, J. M., Barron, K. E., Pintrich, P. R., Elliot, A. J., & Thrash, T. M. (2002). Revision of achievement goal theory: Necessary and illuminating. *Journal of Educational Psychology*, *94*, 638–645.

Hauser-Cram, P., Sirin, S. R., & Stipek, D. (2003). When teachers' and parents' values differ: Teachers' ratings of academic competence in children from low-income families. *Journal of Educational Psychology*, *95*, 813–820.

Hidi, S., & Harackiewicz, J. M. (2000). Motivating the academically unmotivated: A critical issue for the 21st century. *Review of Educational Research*, *70*, 151–179.

Hidi, S., Renninger, K. A., & Krapp, A. (2004). Interest, a motivational variable that combines affective and cognitive functioning. In D. Dai & R. Sternberg (Eds.), *Motivation, emotion, and cognition: Perspectives on intellectual development and functioning* (pp. 89–115). Mahwah, NJ: Erlbaum.

Jacobs, J., & Eccles, J. (1992). The impact of mothers' gender stereotypic beliefs on mothers' and children's ability perceptions. *Journal of Personality and Social Psychology*, *63*, 932–944.

Kaplan, A., Middleton, M. J., Urdan, T., & Midgley, C. (2002). Achievement goals and goal structures. In C. Midgley (Ed.), *Goals, goal structures, and patterns of adaptive learning* (pp. 21–53). Mahwah, NJ: Erlbaum.

Kedar-Voivodas, G. (1983). The impact of elementary children's school roles and sex roles on teacher attitudes: An interactional analysis. *Review of Educational Research*, *53*, 415–437.

Krapp, A. (2002). Structural and dynamic aspects of interest development: Theoretical considerations from an ontogenetic perspective. *Learning and Instruction*, *12*, 383–409.

Krapp, A., Hidi, S., & Renninger, K. A. (1992). Interest, learning, and development. In K. A. Renninger, S. Hidi, & A. Krapp (Eds.), *The role of interest in learning and development* (pp. 3–25). Hillsdale, NJ: Erlbaum.

Linnenbrink, E. A. (2002). *The dilemma of performance goals: Promoting students' motivation and learning in cooperative groups*. Unpublished doctoral dissertation, University of Michigan.

Linnenbrink, E. A. (2004). Person and context: Theoretical and practical considerations in achievement goal theory. In P. R. Pintrich & M. L. Maehr (Eds.), *Advances in motivation and achievement: Vol. 31. Motivating students, improving schools: The legacy of Carol Midgley* (pp. 159–184). Greenwich, CT: JAI Press.

Linnenbrink, E. A. (2005). The dilemma of performance–approach goals: The use of multiple goal contexts to promote students' motivation and learning. *Journal of Educational Psychology, 97*, 197–213.

Linnenbrink, E. A., & Pintrich, P. R. (2000). Multiple pathways to learning and achievement: The role of goal orientation in fostering adaptive motivation, affect, and cognition. In C. Sansone & J. M. Harackiewicz (Eds.), *Intrinsic and extrinsic motivation: The search for optimal motivation and performance* (pp. 195–227). San Diego, CA: Academic Press.

Linnenbrink, E. A., & Pintrich, P. R. (2001). Multiple goals, multiple contexts: The dynamic interplay between personal goals and contextual goal stresses. In S. Volet & S. Järvelä (Eds.), *Motivation in learning contexts: Theoretical and methodological implications* (pp. 251–269). New York: Pergamon Press.

Maehr, M. L., & Midgley, C. (1991). Enhancing student motivation: A schoolwide approach. *Educational Psychologist, 26*, 399–427.

Maehr, M. L., & Midgley, C. (1996). *Transforming school cultures*. Boulder, CO: Westview Press.

Marsh, H. W. (1990). A multidimensional, hierarchical self-concept: Theoretical and empirical justification. *Educational Psychology Review, 2*, 77–171.

Middleton, M. J., Kaplan, A., & Midgley, C. (2004). The change in middle school students' achievement goals in mathematics over time. *Social Psychology of Education, 7*, 289–311.

Middleton, M. J., & Midgley, C. (1997). Avoiding the demonstration of lack of ability: An under-explored aspect of goal theory. *Journal of Educational Psychology, 89*, 710–718.

Midgley, C., Anderman, E. M., & Hicks, L. (1995). Differences between elementary and middle school teachers and students: A goal theory approach. *Journal of Early Adolescence, 15*, 195–206.

Midgley, C., Feldlaufer, H., & Eccles, J. S. (1989). Student/teacher relations and attitudes toward mathematics before and after the transition to junior high school. *Child Development, 60*, 981–992.

Midgley, C., Kaplan, A., & Middleton, M. J. (2001). Performance–approach goals: Good for what, for whom, under what circumstances, and at what cost? *Journal of Educational Psychology, 93*, 77–86.

Midgley, C., Middleton, M. J., Gheen, M. H., & Kumar, R. (2002). Stage–environment fit revisited: A goal theory approach to examining school transitions. In C. Midgley (Ed.), *Goals, goal structures, and patterns of adaptive learning* (pp. 109–142). Mahwah, NJ: Erlbaum.

Miller, S. A., Manhal, M., & Mee, L. L. (1991). Parental beliefs, parental accuracy and children's cognitive performance: A search for causal relations. *Developmental Psychology, 27*, 267–276.

Newmann, F. (1991). Student engagement in academic work: Expanding the perspective on secondary school effectiveness. In J. R. Bliss & W. A. Firestone (Eds.), *Rethinking effective schools: Research and practice* (pp. 58–76). Englewood Cliffs, NJ: Prentice Hall.

Newmann, F., Wehlage, G. G., & Lamborn, S. D. (1992). The significance and sources of student engagement. In F. Newmann (Ed.), *Student engagement and achievement in American secondary schools* (pp. 11–39). New York: Teachers College Press.

Nicholls, J. (1990). What is ability and why are we mindful of it?: A developmental perspective. In R. Sternberg & J. Kolligian (Eds.), *Competence considered* (pp. 11–40). New Haven, CT: Yale University Press.

Nicholls, J. G. (1984). Achievement motivation: Conceptions of ability, subjective experience, task choice, and performance. *Psychological Review, 91*, 328–346.

Pajares, F., Britner, S. L., & Valiante, G. (2000). Relation between achievement goals and self-beliefs of middle school students in writing and science. *Contemporary Educational Psychology, 25*, 406–422.

Patrick, H., Anderman, L. H., Ryan, A. M., Edelin, K., & Midgley, C. (2001). Teachers' communication of goal orientations in four fifth-grade classrooms. *Elementary School Journal, 102*, 35–58.

Pintrich, P. R. (2000). The role of goal orientation in self-regulated learning. In M. Boekarts, P. R. Pintrich, & M. Zeidner (Eds.), *Handbook of self-regulation: Theory, research and applications* (pp. 451–502). San Diego, CA: Academic Press.

Pintrich, P. R., & Schunk, D. (2002). *Motivation in education: Theory, research, and applications*. Upper Saddle River, NJ: Merrill.

Pomerantz, E. M., Grolnick, W. S., & Price, C. E. (2005). The role of parents in how children approach achievement. In A. J. Elliot & C. S. Dweck (Eds.), *Handbook of competence and motivation* (pp. 259–278). New York: Guilford Press.

Roeser, R., Strobel, K., & Quihuis, G. (2002). Studying early adolescents' academic motivation, socioemotional functioning, and engagement in learning: Variable- and person-centered approaches. *Anxiety, Stress, and Coping, 15*, 345–368.

Roeser, R. W., Midgley, C., & Urdan, T. C. (1996). Perceptions of the school psychological environment and early adolescents' psychological and behavioral functioning in school: The mediating role of goals and belonging. *Journal of Educational Psychology, 88*, 408–422.

Ryan, A. M., Gheen, M., & Midgley, C. (1998). Why do some students avoid asking for help?: An examination of the interplay among students' academic efficacy, teachers' socio-emotional role, and the classroom goal structure. *Journal of Educational Psychology, 90*, 528–535.

Ruble, D. (1983). The development of social comparison processes and their role in achievement-related self-socialization. In E. T. Higgins, D. N. Ruble, & W. W. Hartup (Eds.), *Social cognition and social development: A sociocultural perspective* (pp. 134–157). New York: Cambridge University Press.

Rutter, M. (Ed.). (1988). *Studies of psychosocial risk: The power of longitudinal data*. New York: Cambridge University Press.

Ryan, R. M., & Deci, E. L. (2000). Self-determination theory and the facilitation of intrinsic motivation, social development, and well-being. *American Psychologist, 55*, 68–78.

Sameroff, A. J., Bartko, W. T., Baldwin, A., Baldwin, C., & Seifer, R. (1998). Family and social influences on the development of child competence. In M. Lewis (Ed.), *Families, risk, and competence* (pp. 161–185). Mahwah, NJ: Erlbaum.

Schiefele, U. (1991). Interest, learning, and motivation. *Educational Psychologist, 26*, 299–323.

Schiefele, U. (2001). The role of interest in motivation and learning. In J. M. Collis & S. Messick (Eds.), *Intelligence and personality: Bridging the gap in theory and measurement* (pp. 163–194). Mahwah, NJ: Erlbaum.

Simpson, S. D., Fredricks, J. A., Davis-Kean, P., & Eccles, J. S. (2005). Healthy minds, healthy habits: The influence of activity involvement in middle childhood. In A. Huston & M. Ripke (Eds.), *Middle childhood: Contexts of development* (pp. 283–302). New York: Cambridge University Press.

Stipek, D. J. (1993). *Motivation to learn: From theory to practice*. Boston: Allyn & Bacon.

Stipek, D. J., & MacIver, D. (1989). Developmental changes in children's assessment of intellectual competence. *Child Development, 60*, 520–538.

Stefanou, C. R., Perencevich, K. C., DiCintio, M., & Turner, J. C. (2004). Supporting autonomy in the classroom: Ways teachers encourage student decision making and ownership. *Educational Psychologist, 39*, 97–110.

Turner, J. C., Thorpe, P. K., & Meyer, D. K. (1998). Students' reports of motivation and negative affect: A theoretical and empirical analysis. *Journal of Educational Psychology, 90*, 758–771.

Urdan, T. C., Midgley, C., & Anderman, E. M. (1998). The role of classroom goal structure in students' use of self-handicapping. *American Educational Research Journal, 35*, 101–122.

Weiner, B. (1990). History of motivational research in education. *Journal of Educational Psychology, 82*, 616–622.

Wigfield, A., & Eccles, J. S. (1992). The development of achievement task values: A theoretical analysis. *Developmental Review, 12*, 265–310.

Wigfield, A., Eccles, J., Yoon, K. S., Harold, R. D., Arbreton, A. J., & Blumenfeld, P. C. (1997). Change in children's competence beliefs and subjective task values across the elementary school years: A three-year study. *Journal of Education Psychology, 89*, 451–469.

Yee, D. K., & Flanagan, C. (1985). Family environment and self-consciousness in early adolescence. *Journal of Early Adolescence, 5*, 59–68.

Chapter 30

# The Interface of Motivation Science and Personology

## SELF-CONCORDANCE, QUALITY MOTIVATION, AND MULTILEVEL PERSONALITY INTEGRATION

**Kennon M. Sheldon**

### MOTIVATION SCIENCE AND THE QUALITY OF MOTIVATION

In this chapter I address an issue that has had an uneasy history within motivation science: namely, the "quality" of a person's motivation. I consider this issue in depth in the next section by explicating the concept of *self-concordance* (Sheldon, 2002; Sheldon & Elliot, 1999), but would first like to begin with some more general remarks. My hope is to place the search for motivational quality in a broader, scientifically valid context.

Notably, most contemporary motivational theories focus on *cognitive* constructs, such as positive expectancies, skill possession, type of priming, type of goal framing, type of implementation intention, type of systemic configuration, and so on (Shah, Kruglanski, & Friedman, 2003). In addition, they could be said to focus primarily upon the "quantity" of motivation, and also upon the quantity of effective performance. However, I would like to consider a more phenomenological issue, in which *a person's relationship to his or her own goal or motive* is of paramount importance. Does the person enjoy and identify with the goal? How does the goal fit with the person's sense of self, with the kind of personality traits he or she has, and with basic human needs more generally? Is the goal or motive the "right" one for the whole person, or might he or she have instead made a mistake in choosing the goal? These qualitative questions invite humanistic and existential analysis—forms of inquiry that cognitively oriented psychologists have long viewed with suspicion. It is notoriously difficult to conceptualize, quantify, and evaluate such complex constructs, and thus there is an ever-present temptation to ignore them or to try to reduce them to simpler, more molecular processes.

However, I contend that motivation science will not be complete until it successfully grapples with these vital personological issues, which transcend "mere cognition." Rather than being dismissable as too vague or too amenable to explanation via more molecular analysis, such questions instead directly address the highest levels of influence upon human behavior—levels that cannot be reduced to lower levels of influence. In other words, in order to understand human motivation fully, we will have to understand what it means to be a motivated person, at a transcognitive level of analysis. I also show in this chapter that it is quite possible to approach these issues by using quantitative methodologies.

## A MULTILEVEL FRAMEWORK FOR VIEWING MOTIVATION AND PERSONALITY

To justify my assertion and to locate my discussion of self-concordance within an appropriate context, I must briefly consider the many levels of influence upon human behavior, and also the relation of the various human sciences to each other. Figure 30.1 attempts to provide such a global context, using a multilevel hierarchical framework. The framework is offered in the spirit of achieving greater consilience within psychology (Wilson, 1998), and between psychology and the other social and natural sciences.

| Level of Analysis: | Science That Studies It: |
|---|---|
| Culture | Sociology, Anthropology |
| ↑↓ | |
| Social Interaction | Social Psychology |
| ↑↓ | |
| Personality | Personality Psychology |
| ↑↓ | |
| Cognition | Cognitive Psychology |
| ↑↓ | |
| Brain/Nervous System | Neuroscience |
| ↑↓ | |
| Organ Tissues | Medicine, Biology |
| ↑↓ | |
| Cells | Microbiology |
| ↑↓ | |
| Molecules | Chemistry |
| ↑↓ | |
| Atoms | Physics |

**FIGURE 30.1.** Potential influences on human behavior. From Sheldon (2004, p. 17). Copyright 2004 by Lawrence Erlbaum. Reprinted by permission.

Space does not permit a full discussion of the figure (see Sheldon, 2004, for such a discussion), but a brief summary is warranted. The assumption is that human behavior is influenced by a nested set of coacting and interacting factors. Lower-level processes tend to supply the "how" of behavior, and also appeal to scientists' desire for parsimony and reductionism. Higher-level processes tend to supply the "why" of behavior, and appeal to scientists' desire for holistic context and broader intelligibility. Lower levels provide the necessary supports and prerequisites for higher-level functioning to emerge, and thus higher levels of organization cannot exist without the lower levels. However, lower levels can never fully account for higher-level effects, precisely because of the characteristic of higher-order emergence. In addition, higher levels can moderate the functioning of lower levels, in ways that also cannot be understood purely in terms of the lower level of analysis. Thus higher levels of analysis have to be considered in their own terms (i.e., in terms of principles or regularities existing at each level of analysis).

As this reasoning suggests, a hierarchical pluralistic perspective is probably necessary for a full understanding of human behavior, in which factors at each level of analysis can have unique main effects upon behavior, and can also evidence cross-level interactions with factors at other levels (Cacioppo, Berntson, & Crites, 1996). Similarly, every type of human science (i.e., at every level of analysis within Figure 30.1) is needed for full understanding: None can be reduced to any other, and each has its own part to play within the "final" model of human behavior. Of course, the relative contribution of factors and sciences at different levels of analysis doubtless depend on the particular behavioral phenomenon being studied (e.g., biologically oriented explanations might best explain a trip to the market, and personality-oriented explanations might best explain a trip to the psychiatrist). Although such variations doubtless exist, the most important point is that no level of analysis is completely reducible to any other level; all of the levels within Figure 30.1 supply explanatory power, at least for some types of behavioral phenomena.

To apply the model, let us take an example. A person is choosing to trust and cooperate with another person, in a situation in which there is some risk of being exploited. This behavior might be explained in terms of neurochemical factors (i.e., elevated dopamine or serotonin levels within the person's brain), cognitive factors (i.e., high expectancies, accessibilities, or calculated utilities within the person's mind), personality factors (i.e., particular values, traits, and self-images within the person's personality), social contextual factors (i.e., particular communication patterns or status relations existing between the two personalities), and cultural factors (i.e., particular norms, traditions, or orientations of the culture in which the two personalities interact). The goal of multilevel empirical analysis would be to determine how best to predict a target behavior (such as cooperation by a given person in a given situation in a given culture), by considering the main and interactive effects of relevant factors at every level (or at least many levels) of analysis. Of course, we do not yet possess the modeling capability to handle multilevel models of this complexity (Hox, 2002), and even if we did, the sheer quantity of data required would be daunting (i.e., samples of thousands of people from around the world upon whom thousands of measurements would be made). Still, thinking in these terms may be a useful exercise.

To restate my earlier claim within the context of Figure 30.1, most contemporary motivational and personality research focuses on the *cognitive* level of analysis, again by focusing on expectancies, framing, action plans, priming and semantic associations, if–then contingencies, and the like. Indeed, there have been some attempts to explain personality completely in terms of cognitive information processing (Cervone, 2004; Shoda & LeeTiernan, 2002). However, I believe it is vital to consider personality processes at their own level, rather than attempting to reduce them to lower levels. What are the unique psychological contingencies and imperatives that operate at this higher level of analysis, and that must be considered on their own terms?

In order to begin to approach this question, it is necessary to further unpack the personality level of analysis in Figure 30.1. One potentially useful framework for doing so is provided in Figure 30.2. The framework builds upon McAdams's proposed "three tiers" of personality and personality theory. McAdams (1996, 1998) has argued that complete personality analysis involves consideration of a person's personality traits (biologically, temperamentally, and historically influenced patterns of thinking and feeling), his or her goals and motives (the conscious objectives, projects, and purposes that he or she pursues), and his or her self and self-concepts (the narratives and self-images in which the person lives). McAdams argues that each of these three levels of analysis supplies independent information about the person, because none of the levels is reducible to other levels.

Self/Life Story
+
Personality = Goals/Intentions
+
Traits/Individual Differences
+
Organismic Foundations

**FIGURE 30.2.** Four "tiers" of personality and personality theory. From Sheldon (2004, p. 47). Copyright 2004 by Lawrence Erlbaum. Reprinted by permission.

Whereas the traits, goals, and selves levels address important domains of individual difference, it also seems important to consider basic personality processes that are common to all individuals, and upon which individual differences rest (Buss, 1995). Thus I have argued (Sheldon, 2004) that there should also be a fourth, "organismic foundations" level appended to the hierarchy (as has been done in Figure 30.2). I have taken an evolutionary perspective in elaborating on this level, specifically by considering innate physical needs and drives, innate social cognitive mechanisms, innate psychological needs and motives, and innate sociocultural universals. In particular, I have focused on basic psychological needs at this level, because of their relevance for optimal functioning and well-being. I have suggested that security, self-esteem, autonomy, competence, and relatedness constitute the universal set of psychological needs that all humans in all cultures need in order to thrive (Sheldon, 2004; Sheldon, Elliot, Kim, & Kasser, 2001).

Notice that the four levels of analysis depicted in Figure 30.2 can be viewed as hierarchically nested, at least to some extent. Personality traits emerge in the interaction between basic human nature and the individual person's unique genetics and developmental history;

goals and motives emerge in the interaction between the person's personality traits and his or her environment and affordances; and selves and self-stories emerge in the interaction between the person's motives, goals, and behaviors and his or her desire to tell a coherent life story. Thus the four tiers described above might be inserted directly into Figure 30.1, as elaborations at the level of personality. Of course, goals are more than emergent products of traits, and selves are more than emergent products of traits and goals. Still, even if the assumption of strong emergence does not hold in the case of the four levels of personality, I still contend that they depict four unique and irreducible forms of personological inquiry, and that together they usefully elaborate upon the personality level of analysis depicted in Figure 30.1.

## THE SELF-CONCORDANCE CONCEPT

Elsewhere (Sheldon, 2002), I have conceptualized *self-concordance* as the extent to which a person's goals correctly represent their deeper personality dispositions, needs, and motives. In terms of Figure 30.2, self-concordance concerns the degree of consistency or fit between the goal level of personality, and the organismic and trait levels of personality. The person has managed to select the "right" goals for him- or herself—the ones that best channel and direct the person's energies in the service of his or her best potentials. This is no small feat, given that self-knowledge and self-access are forever uncertain (Wilson, 2002). Thus people can sometimes select terribly inappropriate goals for themselves, wasting much time and energy in their pursuit.

How can people act against their own best interests? In my view, this is a consequence of the fact that the emergent self has irreducible higher-level influence upon its own behavior. The self creates itself, and in so doing it has the freedom (or the curse) to make poor or incorrect choices with respect to its own deeper nature and lower-level supports. Self-perception is difficult (Wilson, 2002), and people are easily distracted from the subtle internal signals that might indicate the most optimal choices. Of course, the emergent self also has the ability to create excellent solutions to the organism's problems, which is presumably why it evolved (Sedikides & Skowronski, 1997). Still, the constructed nature of the self entails that people can sometimes be "out of touch with themselves," such that there is incongruence between self-concept and underlying organism (Rogers, 1964). In terms of Epstein's (1973) well-known *self-theory* model of the self, people's theories about who they are can be quite inadequate in modeling their actual underlying personalities.

In order to measure the state of self-concordance, I have applied self-determination theory's *perceived locus of causality* (PLOC) concept (Deci & Ryan, 1991, 2000; Ryan & Connell, 1989). This humanistically based concept specifies a continuum of motivational internalization, ranging from *external* (the person acts because the situation or some other person seems to compel it; no internalization) to *introjected* (the person acts because he or she compels him- or herself, to avoid guilt or anxiety; partial internalization) to *identified* (the person acts to express a self-endorsed value or belief, even if the behavior is nonenjoyable or even aversive; full internalization) to *intrinsic* (the person acts because of the interest, stimulation, and pleasure supplied by the behavior itself; inherent internalization). External and introjected motivations represent "controlled" forms of motivation, in which the person does not feel like the cause of his or her behavior. Identified and intrinsic motivations represent self-determined forms of motivation, in which the person feels fully causal with respect to his or her behavior. Deci, Ryan, and colleagues have published a wide variety of studies demonstrating the positive effects of acting for self-determined rather than controlled reasons, within domains as diverse as education, sports, organizations, and medicine (see Deci & Ryan, 2000, for a review).

Because my own work employs the PLOC concept, it might be said to provide simply another way of assessing self-determination. Although this is true, I have argued that the PLOC concept has extended meaning in the case of idiographic personal goals (Sheldon, 2002). Rather than assessing reactive and domain-specific motivation with regard to experimenter-supplied stems, personal goal methodologies instead allow assessment of proactive domain-general motivation, with regard to participant-supplied stems. Such goals and initiatives encompass a wide variety of life contexts, and thus they allow for comprehensive assessment of the motivational aspect of personality (Emmons, 1989). Also, they allow for consideration of important questions about personality development that go beyond domain-specific motivation—questions concerning how people construct and create themselves over time.

Interestingly, personal goal statements are created *ex nihilo*: A participant can identify any goal he or she likes, with no constraints on content. One might expect, then, that people would only write down goals that they truly enjoy and/or believe in. Surprisingly, however, this is not the case: Our data reveal that some people list many goals that they do *not* enjoy and do *not* believe in. I have explained this paradox (Sheldon, 2002) with the above-discussed suggestion that some people do not have the maturity or self-perceptual skills to select the "correct" goals for themselves (i.e., goals that well represent their personalities and that would further their growth and well-being if pursued). The sign of such non-self-concordant goals is that a person does not enjoy them and cannot get behind them.

Notice that my approach to assessing self-concordance does not directly assess the fit of goals (at level 3 of Figure 30.2) with the person's traits and his or her organismic needs (at levels 1 and 2 of Figure 30.2). However, I assume that the latter judgments are difficult to make; they require accurate knowledge of one's own needs and traits, for starters, as well as the ability to estimate the relevance of one's goals for those entities. In contrast, judgments concerning the "humanistic quality" of one's goals (i.e., does one feel pressured and guilty regarding one's goals, or instead interested and identified with them?) are much easier to make, and approach the same basic issues from a phenomenological perspective. Also, many people have ambivalent relationships with their goals, and readily admit to feelings of guilt or pressure with respect to them. Thus the PLOC methodology may provide a valuable shortcut to assessing person–goal fit.

To summarize, self-concordance is conceptualized as the degree to which conscious goals (at level 3 of Figure 30.2) correctly represent the deeper and more stable levels of personality (organismic needs and traits/dispositions, at levels 1 and 2 of Figure 30.2). Selecting self-appropriate goals is viewed as a difficult skill and developmental achievement, upon which individuals vary. Failures to select self-appropriate goals may be indicated when the person endorses relatively controlled, rather than self-determined, reasons for his or her goals. In such cases, the person's choices are perhaps being overly driven by others or by nonintegrated internal pressures, rather than by his or her own underlying needs, traits, and growth impulses.

## EMPIRICAL SUPPORT FOR THE SELF-CONCORDANCE CONSTRUCT

I have begun this chapter by considering the "quality" of motivation, and obviously I see the self-concordance measure as an apt measure of motivational quality. It is, of course, important to back up such a claim with appropriate evidence. One implication of the humanistic perspective outlined above is that self-concordance should be concurrently associated with a wide variety of positive personality characteristics and states. Another implication, given that personal goals are dynamic constructs that energize and regulate the person's behavior over time (Little, 1993), is that self-concordance should be associated with positive *changes* in a person's characteristics and state over time. This section outlines the evidence in support of these two implications.

One study (Sheldon & Kasser, 1995) assessed the self-concordance of participants' 10 most important personal strivings (Emmons, 1989), using the PLOC measure discussed above. Concurrent associations were found between aggregate self-concordance and a wide variety of positive personality and state variables, including self-actualization, vitality, positive affect, openness, empathy, self-esteem, autonomy orientation, life satisfaction, and low negative affect. Another study (Sheldon, 1995) found associations between self-concordance and two different measures of personal creativity. A third study (Sheldon & Elliot, 2000) found that self-concordance for goals within particular life roles was associated with greater satisfaction and better performance of those roles. These findings all support the postulate that self-concordance and many types of positive functioning should be correlated at a given moment in time.

To turn to the second implication, we (Sheldon & Elliot, 1998) evaluated the dynamic effects of self-concordance in a month-long study of personal projects (Little, 1993). In that study, self-concordance predicted greater longitudinal goal attainment—an effect that was mediated by the greater sustained effort that participants gave to more self-concordant goals. We argued that people do not give up as quickly on their self-concordant goals, because such goals accurately represent deeper personality and thus have more stable motivational resources to draw upon. A second study (Sheldon & Elliot, 1999) replicated and extended these findings, supporting an elaborate path model concerning dynamic changes in well-being. In that model, which fit the data well, self-concordance at time 1 predicted greater goal attainment during the semester. Goal attainment in turn predicted greater organismic need satisfaction during the semester (strong experiences of autonomy, competence, and relatedness as assessed at five points during the semester), which in turn predicted rank-order increases in global well-being (positive mood, negative mood, and life satisfaction) from the beginning to the end of the semester.

In the Sheldon and Elliot (1999) study, in addition to influencing goal attainment directly, self-concordance also *interacted* with goal attainment to predict organismic need satisfaction: The more self-concordant the attained goals, the greater the boost in need satisfaction. A similar interaction was obtained in a different longitudinal study (Sheldon & Kasser, 1988): Those with more self-concordant goals derived more well-being benefits from attaining those goals. Note that the finding that self-concordance predicted greater longitudinal need satisfaction supports the assumption, articulated above, that self-concordance as measured by the self-determination theory's PLOC methodology adequately measures the "fit" between the person's goals and his or her deeper personality (which includes organismic needs).

A two-cycle study of personal goal striving over the freshman year (Sheldon & Houser-Marko, 2001) extended this model even further. In that model, which also fit the data well, initial goal self-concordance predicted fall goal attainment, which also predicted increased adjustment over the first semester of college. Fall goal attainment also predicted increased self-concordance for spring semester goals, which predicted greater spring goal attainment compared to fall goal attainment. Finally, spring goal attainment predicted even higher adjustment at the end of the freshman year. Thus it appears that beginning a new period of life with self-concordant goals may lead to an "upward spiral" of positive change.

Notably, in all of the studies discussed above, more conventional and cognitively based constructs were assessed in addition to self-concordance—constructs such as skills, expectancies, plans, commitment, framing (approach vs. avoidance), and implementation intentions. Although these constructs sometimes had their own effects, in all cases self-concordance demonstrated significant independent effects. For example, in the Sheldon and Elliot (1999) study, self-concordance was still a significant predictor of goal attainment even when the significant effects of implementation intentions, approach (vs. avoidance) framing, and life skills were taken account of. This supports the assertion made at the beginning of the chapter that personological or self-level issues cannot be reduced to cognitive-level constructs, but rather need to be given independent voice in any final model of goal striving. Again, I believe that motivation science needs to consider *all* of the levels of analysis listed in Figure 30.1, in order to arrive at a complete picture.

## FURTHER FEATURES OF THE SELF-CONCORDANCE CONSTRUCT

In this section I discuss some of the most recent research concerning the self-concordance construct, to better illustrate the nature of the construct.

### Self-Concordance Effects Are More Than Goal Content Effects

Self-concordance addresses the quality of motivation by asking people "why" they are striving. For what phenomenological reasons are they pursuing a goal? Another important issue for considering the quality of motivation, however, is in terms of the "what" of goals: What are the specific goal contents and targets that people are pursuing? Kasser and Ryan (1993, 1996) proposed a distinction between *intrinsic* (intimacy, community, personal growth) and *extrinsic* (money, fame, beauty) goal contents. Supporting the idea that this measure indexes the "personological health" of motivation, they showed that those who give more importance to intrinsic rather than extrinsic goals also evidence greater well-being and psychological adjustment (see also Kasser, 2002).

Some have argued that "what" and "why" effects upon well-being are essentially the same effect (Carver & Baird, 1998; Srivastava, Locke, & Bartol, 2001), and in particular that content effects are reducible to reason (or motive) effects. However, recent research (Sheldon, Ryan, Deci, & Kasser, & 2004) indicates that the "what" and the "why" factors make independent contributions to predicting well-being and positive outcomes. Because of these additive main effects, those who pursue intrinsic goals for self-concordant reasons are typically best off; those who pursue extrinsic goals for nonconcordant reasons are usually worst off; and those who pursue extrinsic goals for self-concordant reasons, or intrinsic goals for nonconcordant reasons, are generally in the middle.

## Self-Concordance Matters in Collectivist Cultures

Self-determination theory is described as universally applicable—that is, as applying equally to all persons in all cultures (Deci & Ryan, 2000). Because the self-concordance measure is based on self-determination theory's PLOC methodology, this implies that goal self-concordance should predict positive outcomes in any context or culture. This may sound surprising to those familiar with contemporary cross-cultural theory, as cross-culturalists typically view autonomy and self-determination as culturally bound constructs. For example, Markus, Kitayama, and Heiman (1996) and Oishi and Diener (2001) have argued that autonomy and self-determination are primarily important in individualist cultures, whereas in collectivist cultures conformity and group-centeredness are more adaptive and beneficial for the individual. Note that this argument implies that there should be a cross-level interaction between culture (cultural type, at the top level of Figure 30.1) and goal-striving (degree of self-concordance, at the personality level of Figure 30.1), in determining individual well-being. In this view, although self-concordance might predict positive well-being in some cultures, it might predict *negative* well-being in other cultures, in which self-assertion is a cause or sign of social isolation or exclusion.

However, we (Sheldon, Elliot, et al., 2004) found no such interaction. Instead, we showed that self-concordance predicted concurrent psychological well-being to the same extent in each of four different cultural groups: China, Taiwan, South Korea, and the United States. In other words, no matter which subsample the participants came from, they were happier persons if they were more self-concordant persons. This is as would be expected, according to self-determination theory's assumption that all humans need to feel ownership and identification of their own behavior (presumed to be a species-typical and largely invariant characteristic, located at the bottom level of Figure 30.2).

It is worth briefly considering why the data do not seem to support the cross-cultural perspective. Deci and Ryan (2000) have argued that cross-cultural analyses of autonomy often conflate personal autonomy (volition and self-ownership) with social independence (freedom from influence by others). According to self-determination theory, these are very different constructs. One can feel quite proud and independent but still not autonomous and volitional, because one is being driven by implicit fears and self-esteem threats (Crocker & Park, 2004). In contrast, one can feel quite autonomous, even as one is profoundly influenced by another person. From the perspective of self-determination theory, the key question is this: Can one "take possession" of one's behavior in the face of that influence? In short, although the benefits of social independence may vary across cultures, the benefits of autonomy appear to be consistent across cultures, supporting the proposal that autonomy is an inherent human need (see also Chirkov, Ryan, Kim, & Kaplan, 2003).

## Self-Concordance Increases with Age

Self-determination theory is based on an organismic metatheory. Organismic perspectives, in contrast to mechanistic perspectives, assume that living things are fundamentally self-organizing and *autotelic*, or self-moving (Goldstein, 1939; Overton, 1976). Piaget's conception of the exploring child, who actively constructs his or her own mind through self-initiated interactions with the environment, is a good example of an organismic metatheory. Organismic perspectives also tend to make optimistic assumptions about human nature—namely, that humans are inherently growth-oriented, and also have an inherent desire to mesh with and contribute to the broader social environment (Rogers, 1964). These assumptions are based on the essential negentropic nature of life and human life in particular (i.e., humans' drive to move toward greater organization and elaboration over time, both intrapersonally and interpersonally). However, organismic theories also acknowledge that the growth process can be stalled or even regressed, depending on a variety of problematic social contextual and intrapersonal factors. Because of this, Deci and Ryan (2000) stated that the development of greater self-determination is ultimately a dialectical process, in which a person must learn to integrate external influences and internal drives that may initially overwhelm his or her self-regulatory capacity. Again, however, the organismic perspective suggests that if environments are at least reasonably supportive, then positive change should tend to occur over time.

Recent research has provided significant new evidence for these optimistic assumptions, by showing that self-concordance tends to increase with age. For example, a cross-sectional study (Sheldon & Kasser, 2001) showed that chronological age was associated with higher goal self-concordance—an effect that partially mediated the association between chronological age and subjective well-being. Similarly, another study (Sheldon, Houser-Marko, & Kasser, 2006) showed that parents reported higher mean levels of goal self-concordance than their own college-age children did. In a related vein, three studies (Sheldon, Kasser, Houser-Marko, Jones, & Turban, 2005) showed that parents and older participants evidenced greater self-concordance for their social duties and roles. These findings further bolster the evidence base for the self-concordance construct, as they show its consistency with the organismic metatheory from which it springs. They also suggest that people learn to select more self-appropriate goals as they get older, presumably by having paid attention to their own experience. In other words, older persons tend to base their goals less on "what others think," and more on accurate internal information concerning their own needs and personalities. Again, these two sources of information are not necessarily in opposition; those who are better in touch with themselves are typically better able to be in touch with others.

## MORE COMPLEX CONCEPTUAL ISSUES

### The Real Meaning of Self-Concordance

Some readers may have wondered whether the self-concordance construct is misnamed. Conceptually, the construct refers to the fit between conscious goals (at level 3 of Figure 30.2) and the two "deeper" (or lower) levels of personality—that is, needs and traits (at levels 1 and 2 of Figure 30.2). Notice that level 4 of Figure 30.2, the *self* level of personality, is not referred to in this definition. Given this fact, perhaps the construct should be called *need concordance* or *trait concordance*, rather than *self-concordance*. Perhaps the term *self-concordance* should be reserved to refer to a different state, in which one's goals are consistent with one's self-concept and the self-character in which one lives. Is there a difference between the latter and the former forms of concordance? Potentially yes, *if* the self is "out of touch" with itself, such that the lived self does not well reflect the actual personality (i.e., one's deeper traits and needs). One's goals might then match one's sense of self, without matching one's actual personality. In Epstein's (1973) terms, one's self-theory may be a bad theory of its topic (i.e., the personality in which the self is contained).

A related paradox arises when we consider the fact that the self-concordance measure is based on self-report regarding the participant's self-concept. Doesn't this make it a measure of goal–self concordance after all, rather than a measure of goal–needs or goal–trait concordance? Of course, there are also many potential problems with self-report, which prompt us to ask whether participants' self-report ratings should be taken as face-valid indicators of their personality structure. But on the other hand, don't personality psychologists usually take self-reports as valid indicators of people's actual traits and characteristics? Perhaps the latter paradox is not unique to the self-concordance construct, but refers to the more general problems that arise when researchers rely on participants' own models of themselves for information about those participants' personalities.

Obviously, these are sticky issues. I believe that the PLOC-based self-concordance measure really *does* measure goal-to-needs and goal-to-traits fit, given the many documented associations of self-concordance with well-being, need satisfaction, and positive trait expression. In addition, however, the PLOC measure may also measure goal-to-self fit (Sheldon & Emmons, 1995); it seems logical to suppose that if one enjoys, identifies, and does not feel pressured by a goal, then it probably expresses and concords with one's life narratives and sense of self, as well as with one's needs and traits. This conjecture awaits empirical corroboration.

Still, the fact that the PLOC judgments are based on self-report raises further conceptual issues. What if a person appears self-concordant by self-report, but is quite discordant in actuality (i.e., the person manifests "illusory self-concordance")? Doubtless this is sometimes the case. For example, a premedical student might claim to strongly identify with the goal of becoming a doctor, even though he or she hates the sight of blood, is bad at math and science, and seems to have more talent in other domains of life (Sheldon, 2004). Again, Rogers (1964) described such cases in terms of the "incongruence" that can occur between self-concept and underlying organism, such that the self-concept does not accurately represent the actual person and his or her feelings. Incongruence may result when the person is defending an overidealized and inaccurate version of the self due to past ego wounds and threats, or when a person is anxious not to lose the contingent love or approval of a parent or mentor (e.g., in the case of the premedical student, a parent who insists on the medical career). Pinpointing these cases becomes a vital issue, both for reducing measurement error and increasing the predictive power of the self-concordance measure, and also for better understanding the deeper substantive meaning of the construct. How might such "illusory self-concordance" be identified?

## Detecting Implicit Ambivalence or Illusory Self-Concordance

What is needed is a way of measuring implicit ambivalence regarding goals—ambivalence that a person does not, or cannot, admit to. Recently our lab (Sheldon, Houser-Marko, Osbaldiston, & King, 2007) has been exploring various potential measures of implicit ambivalence. The basic goal of the research has been to develop polygraph-like methodologies to uncover potential discrepancies between self-reports and deeper parts of the personality. One series of studies examined the speed and the accuracy with which participants recognized and claimed their own goals (flashed on a computer screen), compared to "decoy" goals. Specifically, we found a predicted response × goal-type interaction, in which "mistake" trials (saying that a decoy goal was one's own, or saying that one's own goal was a decoy) took the most time. Thus one way of identifying implicit ambivalence regarding a goal may be to look for recognition errors regarding that goal, or for hesitation when saying "It is mine." To return to the example, the premedical student might misclassify the doctor goal or recognize it slowly, providing clues to its true character for him or her.

A second study in this research program approached implicit ambivalence in a different way, showing an interaction such that participants took longest when claiming that extrinsic goals (money, fame, beauty) were self-concordant. In a speeded response task, participants were especially slow in responding that identified and intrinsic motivation words went together with extrinsic goals. The fact that the hesitations occurred primarily in conjunction with known problematic goals (Sheldon, Arndt, & Houser-Marko, 2003) suggests that delayed responding may be a reliable indicator of goal problems, even in cases where nothing is known about a goal's content.

We have also begun employing the Implicit Association Test (IAT; Greenwald, Nosek, & Banaji, 2003) as a third means of assessing implicit ambivalence, and also of identifying illusory self-concordance. The IAT asks participants to categorize stimuli into one of two categories, when the categories are associated with either pleasant or unpleasant words. If categorization of a particular type of stimulus is slowed down when that stimulus is associated with pleasant words, and speeded up when it is associated with unpleasant words, then the person is said to have a negative implicit attitude toward the category (relative to the other category). Typically in IAT research, the two contrasting stimulus categories concern social cognitive issues such as participants' occupational stereotypes (doctor vs. nurse), racial biases (blacks vs. whites), or political preferences (Democrat vs. Republican). However, we have applied the methodology to measure relative implicit feelings regarding contrasting types or contents of goals (i.e., intrinsic vs. extrinsic goals, ought goals vs. ideal goals, parent-relevant goals vs. self-relevant goals).

In one study (Sheldon, King, Houser-Marko, Osbaldiston, & Gunz, in press), we contrasted intimacy with power goals; this was deemed an organismically relevant content dichotomy to use, since power has been shown to be negatively related to well-being and intimacy positively related to psychological well-being (Emmons, 1991). Participants generated four goals within each category. The eight goals were entered into an IAT, which participants took during a later laboratory session. Each participant engaged in 140 trials. Each trial had an associated response time, which could be predicted via a 2 (goal type: intimacy or power) × 2 (associated word type: pleasant or unpleasant) analysis. Conceptually replicating the memory and word association interactions discussed above, we found interactions such that participants took longest in categorizing power goals associated with pleasant words and intimacy goals associated with unpleasant words, and were quickest in categorizing intimacy goals associated with pleasant words and power goals associated with unpleasant words. We believe that the slowdown effect was due to interference between the predominantly negative feelings associated with some types of goals, and the participants' attempts to make a positive or affirmative response regarding those goals.

The research discussed above shows promise for revealing people's "deeper" feelings regarding their goals, and perhaps for pinpointing which goals within a person's system are most likely to benefit that person and which goals might better be abandoned. In terms of the premedical student example, these methodologies might help to reveal hidden emotions regarding important personal goals—emotions of which the person is not consciously aware. Such findings have clear and important implications for a variety of issues, including personality assessment, counseling techniques, and the detection of self-deception (Gur & Sackeim, 1979).

## SUMMARY

This chapter has begun with a consideration of the issue of motivational quality: How can we tell if a person is pursuing the "right" goals and motives? Although this kind of question raises concerns regarding value judgments and scientific objectivity, I have argued that it is essential if we want to understand the whole person, not just his or her cognitive systems. To justify this assertion, I have presented a multilevel hierarchical framework for considering and explaining human behavior, arguing that all levels of the framework are necessary for complete exposition. In this point of view, personality and self-level processes cannot be reduced to "mere" cognitive processes; there are transcognitive rules and laws operating at this level. I have also considered a four-level subframework *within* the personality level of analysis, consisting of organismic needs/characteristics, traits/dispositions, goals/intentions, and self/self-narratives. I have contended that each of these spheres of the person operates via unique rules and regularities—processes that cannot be reduced to lower levels of analysis (such as biological, neurological, and cognitive levels of analysis).

Using this model, I have considered the *self-concordance* construct, which is defined as the match or fit between personal goals and the two lower levels of personality (species-typical needs and differences in basic traits). I have reviewed a variety of empirical data to support the contention that self-concordance has both momentary and dynamic influence upon a person's well-being and level of thriving—influence that is independent of the influence of lower-level, more cognitively oriented constructs, and is also independent of the higher-level factor of culture.

I have then considered the potential problems attendant upon the fact that the self-concordance measure is based on self-report. Might some people exhibit "illusory self-concordance," claiming strong interest and identification concerning goals that are in fact inappropriate for them? Our recent studies concerning implicit ambivalence suggest that this can indeed happen, and that it is more likely to happen in the case of goals known to be problematic for well-being, such as extrinsic goals and power goals. The long-term aim of these studies is to produce a technology by which people might get in touch with themselves—that is, access their own implicit knowledge concerning the best or most satisfying goal choices to make.

## REFERENCES

Buss, D. (1995). Evolutionary psychology: A new paradigm for psychological science. *Psychological Inquiry*, *6*, 1–30.

Cacioppo, J., Berntson, G., & Crites, S. (1996). Social neuroscience: Principles of psychophysiological arousal and response. In E. T. Higgins & A. Kruglanski (Eds.), *Social psychology: Handbook of basic principles* (pp. 72–101). New York: Guilford Press.

Carver, C. S., & Baird, E. (1998). The American dream revisited: Is it what you want or why you want it that matters? *Psychological Science*, *9*, 289–292.

Cervone, D. (2004). The architecture of personality. *Psychological Review*, *111*, 183–204.

Chirkov, V. I., Ryan, R. M., Kim, Y., & Kaplan, R. (2003). Differentiating autonomy from individualism and independence: A self-determination theory perspective on internalization of cultural orientations and well-being. *Journal of Personality and Social Psychology*, *84*, 97–109.

Crocker, J., & Park, L. (2004). The costly pursuit of self-esteem. *Psychological Bulletin*, *130*, 392–414.

Deci, E. L., & Ryan, R. M. (1991). A motivational approach to self: Integration in personality. In R. Dienstbier (Ed.), *Nebraska Symposium on Motivation: Vol. 38. Perspectives on motivation* (pp. 237–288). Lincoln: University of Nebraska Press.

Deci, E. L., & Ryan, R. M. (2000). The "what" and "why" of goal pursuits: Human needs and the self-determination of behavior. *Psychological Inquiry*, *11*, 227–268.

Emmons, R. A. (1989). The personal strivings approach to personality. In L. A. Pervin (Ed.), *Goal concepts in personality and social psychology* (pp. 87–126). Hillsdale,NJ: Erlbaum.

Emmons, R. A. (1991). Personal strivings, daily life events, and psychological and physical well-being. *Journal of Personality*, *59*, 453–472.

Epstein, S. (1973). The self-concept revisited: Or a theory of a theory. *American Psychologist*, *28*, 404–416.

Goldstein, K. (1939). *The organism*. New York: American Book.

Greenwald, A. G., Nosek, B. A., & Banaji, M. R. (2003). Understanding and using the Implicit Association Test: I. An improved scoring algorithm. *Journal of Personality and Social Psychology*, *85*, 197–216.

Gur, R. C., & Sackeim, H. (1979). Self-deception: A concept in search of a phenomenon. *Journal of Personality and Social Psychology*, *37*, 147–169.

Hox, J. (2002). *Multilevel analysis: Techniques and applications*. Mahwah, NJ: Erlbaum.

Kasser, T. (2002). *The high price of materialism*. Cambridge, MA: MIT Press.

Kasser, T., & Ryan, R. M. (1993). A dark side of the American dream: Correlates of financial success as a central life aspiration. *Journal of Personality and Social Psychology*, *65*, 410–422.

Kasser, T., & Ryan, R. M. (1996). Further examining the American dream: Differential correlates of intrinsic and extrinsic goals. *Personality and Social Psychology Bulletin*, *22*, 80–87.

Little, B. R. (1993). Personal projects and the distributed self: Aspects of a conative psychology. In J. Suls (Ed.), *Psychological perspectives on the self: Vol. 4. The self in social perspective* (pp. 157–185). Hillsdale, NJ: Erlbaum.

Markus, H., Kitayama, S., & Heiman, R. (1996). Culture and basic psychological principles. In E. T. Higgins & A. W. Kruglanski (Eds.), *Social psychology: Handbook of basic principles* (pp. 857–913). New York: Guilford Press.

McAdams, D. P. (1996). Personality, modernity, and the storied self: A contemporary framework for studying persons. *Psychological Inquiry*, *7*, 295–321.

McAdams, D. P. (1998). Ego, trait, identity. In P. M. Westenberg & A. Blasi (Eds.), *Personality development: Theoretical, empirical, and clinical investigations of Loevinger's conception of ego development* (pp. 27–38). Mahwah, NJ: Erlbaum.

Oishi, S., & Diener, E. (2001). Goals, culture, and subjective well-being. *Personality and Social Psychology Bulletin*, *27*, 1674–1682.

Overton, W. F. (1976). The active organism in structuralism. *Human Development*, *19*, 71–86.

Rogers, C. R. (1964). Toward a modern approach to values: The valuing process in the mature person. *Journal of Abnormal and Social Psychology*, *68*, 160–167.

Ryan, R. M., & Connell, J. P. (1989). Perceived locus of causality and internalization: Examining reasons for acting in two domains. *Journal of Personality and Social Psychology*, *57*, 749–761.

Sedikides, C., & Skowronski, J. J. (1997). The symbolic self in evolutionary content. *Personality and Social Psychology Review*, *1*, 80–102.

Shah, J., Kruglanski, A., & Friedman, R. (2003). Goal systems theory: Integrating the cognitive and motivational aspects of self-regulation. In S. Spence & S. Fein (Eds.), *The Ontario Symposium: Vol. 9. Motivated social perception* (pp. 247–275). Mahwah, NJ: Erlbaum.

Sheldon, K. M. (1995). Creativity and self-determination in personality. *Creativity Research Journal*, *8*, 61–72.

Sheldon, K. M. (2002). The self-concordance model of healthy goal-striving: When personal goals correctly represent the person. In E. L. Deci & R. M. Ryan (Eds.), *Handbook of self-determination research* (pp. 65–86). Rochester, NY: University of Rochester Press.

Sheldon, K. M. (2004). *Optimal human being: An integrated multi-level approach*. Mahwah, NJ: Erlbaum.

Sheldon, K. M., Arndt, J., & Houser-Marko, L. (2003). In search of the organismic valuing process: The human tendency to move towards beneficial goal choices. *Journal of Personality*, *71*, 835–869.

Sheldon, K. M., & Elliot, A. J. (1998). Not all personal goals are personal: Comparing autonomous and controlled reasons as predictors of effort and attainment. *Personality and Social Psychology Bulletin*, *24*, 546–557.

Sheldon, K. M., & Elliot, A. J. (1999). Goal striving, need-satisfaction, and longitudinal well-being: The self-concordance model. *Journal of Personality and Social Psychology*, *76*, 482–497.

Sheldon, K. M., & Elliot, A. J. (2000). Personal goals in social roles: Divergences and convergences across roles and levels of analysis. *Journal of Personality*, *68*, 51–84.

Sheldon, K. M., Elliot, A. J., Kim, Y., & Kasser, T. (2001). What's satisfying about satisfying events?: Comparing ten candidate psychological needs. *Journal of Personality and Social Psychology*, *80*, 325–339.

Sheldon, K. M., Elliot, A. J., Ryan, R. M., Chirkov, V., Kim, Y., Wu, C., et al. (2004). Self-concordance and subjective well-being in four cultures. *Journal of Cross-Cultural Psychology*, *35*, 209–233.

Sheldon, K. M., & Emmons, R. A. (1995). Comparing differentiation and integration within personal goal systems. *Personality and Individual Differences*, *18*, 39–46.

Sheldon, K. M., & Houser-Marko, L. (2001). Self-concordance, goal-attainment, and the pursuit of happiness: Can there be an upward spiral? *Journal of Personality and Social Psychology*, *80*, 152–165.

Sheldon, K. M., Houser-Marko, L., & Kasser, T. (2006). Does autonomy increase with age?: Comparing the motivation and well-being of college students and their parents. *Journal of Research in Personality*, *40*, 168–178.

Sheldon, K. M., Houser-Marko, L., Osbaldiston, R., & King, L. (2007). *Methodologies for assessing implicit ambivalence for personal goals*. Unpublished manuscript.

Sheldon, K. M., & Kasser, T. (1995). Coherence and congruence: Two aspects of personality integration. *Journal of Personality and Social Psychology*, *68*, 531–543.

Sheldon, K. M., & Kasser, T. (1998). Pursuing personal goals: Skills enable progress, but not all progress is beneficial. *Personality and Social Psychology Bulletin*, *24*, 1319–1331.

Sheldon, K. M., & Kasser, T. (2001). Getting older, getting better?: Personal strivings and personality development across the life-course. *Developmental Psychology*, *37*, 491–501.

Sheldon, K. M., Kasser, T., Houser-Marko, L., Jones, T., & Turban, D. (2005). Doing one's duty: Chronological age, felt autonomy, and subjective well-being. *European Journal of Personality*, *19*, 97–115.

Sheldon, K. M., King, L. A., Houser-Marko, L., Osbaldiston, R., & Gunz, A. (in press). Comparing TAT and IAT measures of power versus intimacy motivation. *European Journal of Personality.*

Sheldon, K. M., Ryan, R., Deci, E., & Kasser, T. (2004). The independent effects of goal contents and motives on well-being: It's both what you pursue *and* why you pursue it. *Personality and Social Psychology Bulletin*, *30*, 475–486.

Shoda, Y., & LeeTiernan, S. (2002). What remains invariant?: Finding order within a person's thoughts, feelings, and behaviors across situations. In D. Cervone & W. Mischel (Eds.), *Advances in personality science* (pp. 241–270). New York: Guilford Press.

Srivastava, A., Locke, E. A., & Bartol, K. M. (2001). Money and subjective well-being: It's not the money, it's the motive. *Journal of Personality and Social Psychology*, *80*, 959–971.

Wilson, E. O. (1998). *Consilience: The unity of knowledge*. New York: Knopf.

Wilson, T. D. (2002). *Strangers to ourselves: Discovering the adaptive unconscious*. Cambridge, MA: Belknap Press of Harvard University Press.

# PART IV

# Applications of Motivational Research

# WELL-BEING AND OPTIMAL FUNCTIONING

# Chapter 31

# Challenge, Threat, and Health

**Jim Blascovich**

For several decades, health psychologists and others (e.g., U.S. Surgeons General) have identified behaviors as major factors in the etiologies of chronic diseases—ones with serious and often fatal consequences, such as heart disease, cancer, acquired immune deficiency syndrome (AIDS), and diabetes mellitus (for an early review, see Hamburg, Elliott, & Parron, 1982). Not surprisingly, researchers concerned with promoting healthy lifestyles and ameliorating morbidity and mortality have sought to understand motivational processes in order to create behavioral change interventions to eliminate or diminish unhealthy behaviors.

Prevention and promotion strategies derived from general theoretical models of motivation and behavior change (e.g., fear—Leventhal & Watts, 1966; health beliefs—Becker, 1974; Rosenstock, 1974) can be and have been applied to a plethora of behaviors known or thought to undermine health, such as eating, smoking, alcohol consumption, and sexual behaviors. The promise of such motivation-based interventions rests on the validity of the etiologies linking specific behaviors to diseases (e.g., eating fatty foods to ischemic heart disease, tobacco use to various cancers, and unsafe sexual intercourse to AIDS). Arguably, improvements in public health have resulted from this work.

Over the last few decades, researchers also have begun pursuing another connection between motivation and health—one based on the effects of motivational states themselves. The promise of this type of work rests on the etiologies linking specific motivational states to diseases. The negative health effects of motivational states are believed to be mediated by disruptions in various control systems involving neurological and endocrinological processes, leading in turn to pathophysiological consequences not only in the operative physiology controlled (e.g., the cardiovascular, immune, hepatic, and renal systems), but also in the control systems themselves. Consequently, certain motivational states themselves may be causally related to disease. The work reviewed here supports this premise.

The long history of motivation theory and research reveals a strong tendency among theorists to delineate contrasting bipolar, superordinate motivational states; for example, approach–avoidance, appetition–aversion, promotion–prevention, and challenge–threat. Here, the focus is on the challenge–threat continuum and its associated biopsychosocial (BPS) model (Blascovich & Mendes, 2000; Blascovich, Mendes, Tomaka, Salomon, & Seery, 2003; Blascovich & Tomaka, 1996). The integration of biological, psychological, and social factors within this BPS model has had noted implications for health from the beginning.

## A RETROSPECTIVE REVIEW OF EARLY INSIGHTS AND RESEARCH

### Beginnings: A Brief Autobiographical Account

My reading of a seminal chapter in an early edition of *The Handbook of Social Psychology*, as well as personal experience some 35 years ago, gave birth to our biopsychosocial approach to understanding human motivation and performance. The chapter, "Psychophysiological Approaches in Social Psychology" by David Shapiro and Andrew Crider (1968), detailed the history and underscored the value of combining psychological and social psychological theory with physiological theory and measurement.

My personal experience involved insights gained during several episodes of participant observational research in gambling casinos.[1] An important observational outcome of this research involved visceral perceptions (i.e., interoceptions) during blackjack play. Specifically, with a relatively large bet on the table and the dealer (i.e., the casino) showing a potentially strong hand, I often felt a strong pounding in my thoracic cavity—a sensation that I attributed to my heart. I consciously mentally evaluated or labeled such cardiovascular responses positively during some episodes, and negatively during others. I noticed more winning episodes during those characterized by positive evaluations rather than negative ones. I wondered whether the direction of causality was somewhat counterintuitive—that is, whether winning followed from positively valued interoceptions, rather than the more intuitive notion that positive evaluations of interoceptions followed from winning.

The Shapiro and Crider (1968) chapter, as well as my participant observational experiences, inspired a career-long inquiry into the nature of motivation, performance, and cardiovascular disease, combining social psychological theory and methods with those of autonomic physiology.[2] The first step involved inventing and fabricating a device to simultaneously record ambulatory electrocardiograms (ECGs) of eight poker players during a 4-hour game.[3] Although the recording technology worked well, scoring and analyzing the resultant massive data set proved beyond the capability of existing technology at the time (i.e., 1970); limitations included the use of early mainframe computers, the lack of analog–digital conversion devices, the absence of data-scoring software, and minimal statistical software packages.

### Tightening the Methodology and Broadening the Physiological Perspective

Turning to proven physiological recording technology (i.e., paper polygraph recordings at the time), a traditional laboratory setting, and experimental game procedures, we (Blascovich, Nash, & Ginsburg, 1978) demonstrated experimentally that increased cardiovascular activity was associated with positive performance in a two-person zero-sum experimental game among male participants. The procedural timeline of the experiment was such that 5-minute simultaneous baseline ECG recordings of each player in a same-sex dyad were followed by game instructions and a few practice game trials, a 1-minute simultaneous ECG recording, 25 game trials during which ECG was recorded, another 1-minute resting ECG recording, another 25 trials with ECG, and a final 1-minute resting ECG recording.

On average, eventual male winners and losers evidenced the same heart rate (HR) at baseline, but diverged reliably after instructions and during the game ($p$'s $< .05$), and did not differ after the game (i.e., male winners had higher HRs just before and during the game). Of the 20 male dyads participating in the reported experiments, the winner had the higher HR immediately preceding and during the game in 19 cases. In essence, HR measures following the instructions (but just prior to the game) predicted which of the males in each dyad would have better performance during the experimental game (i.e., would win), confirming our notion that increased cardiac performance preceded performance rather than vice versa, and suggesting the possibility of a causal relationship.

On average, eventual female winners and losers did not differ before, during, or after the game, though they increased from baseline to postinstruction and game-playing periods. Of the 20 female dyads participating, the winner had higher HR immediately preceding and during the game in only half the cases. We speculated that HR increases for females after game instructions were driven by factors not directly related to performance skills per se; these might have included a possible aversive reaction to being placed in a purely competitive situation, and lack of familiarity or comfort with this type of pure competition.[4]

Following this experiment, I became aware of personal shortcomings in my knowledge of physiological theory and measurement techniques. A year-long sabbatical at the laboratory of noted psychophysiologist Edward S. Katkin, then at the State University of New York at Buffalo, ameliorated some of these shortcomings and enabled a long-term collaboration. The collaboration permitted me to return directly to my casino-generated interest in cardiovascular interoception or visceral perception, one of Katkin's fields of expertise.

Several successful experiments demonstrated the validity of a jointly developed signal detection technique for objectively assessing the ability of individuals to perceive heartbeats, as well as discovering sex differences in such abilities (e.g., Katkin, Blascovich, & Goldband, 1981). However, despite several tries, no relationship was found between heartbeat detection ability and task performance (see, e.g., Blascovich et al., 1992)—a finding consistent with the notion that interoceptive ability does not causally interact with cardiovascular responses to produce distinctive motivational states.

## A Turn toward Cardiovascular Reactivity and Cardiovascular Disease

The idea of a positive, benign relationship between increases in cardiac activity and performance was seriously challenged in the late 1970s and early 1980s. At that time, personality and social health psychology researchers and many cardiovascular psychophysiologists became strong proponents of the idea that chronically repeated elevations in HR and other cardiovascular indexes (i.e., cardiovascular reactivity, or CVR) during task performance mediated the relationship between coronary-prone (Type A) personality and cardiovascular disease (e.g., Matthews et al., 1986). Despite the work of a few researchers (most notably "hardiness" researchers Suzanne Kobasa, Salvatore Maddi, and colleagues; Kobasa, 1979; Kobasa, Maddi, & Kahn, 1982) demonstrating that some seemingly coronary-prone individuals were actually thriving and healthy, and because of increasing difficulty in assessing the coronary-prone personality construct via self-report, an interesting shift in focus occurred for many researchers. CVR, originally proposed as the mediator between coronary-prone behavior style and cardiovascular diseases, in some circles became the dispositional construct itself. Individuals were classified as "hot" or "cold" reactors as a function of the intensity of CVR during task performance.[5]

Although this shift in focus did not do much to advance the understanding of the role of personality on cardiovascular disease, it did advance work on the relationship between CVR during task performance and cardiovascular disease. Indeed, some of our own research supported the CVR–disease link. For example, we (Blascovich & Katkin, 1993) reported a study in which patients arriving for inpatient coronary angiograms underwent both a traditional treadmill exercise stress test and an analogous psychological stress test (PST) the day before the angiogram.[6]

The PST consisted of a choice deadline reaction time task in which patients viewed a computer monitor displaying a large plus sign (+). On each trial, either the horizontal or vertical component of the plus sign disappeared. The patients' task was to press a button indicating which component remained before a deadline signal (i.e., a tone). Unknown to the patients, the deadline was based on their own mean reaction time during the previous three trials. Analogously to the elevation in ramp angle for the exercise treadmill test, the PST deadline time became shorter every 2 minutes by a decrease in the multiplier of patients' mean reaction time on the previous three trials. During the first 2 minutes, the multiplier was 1.3; during the second 2 minutes, 1.15; during the third, 1.0; and during the fourth, 0.85. Hence the faster patients responded, the quicker the deadline as the task continued.

The results demonstrated that HR and blood pressure changes during the PST predicted the degree of occlusion in the major coronary arteries, over and above the degree of occlusion predicted by the more traditional cardiological measures (i.e., ST segment depressions, premature ventricular contractions, and reported pain) during the exercise stress test. The percentage of variance of occlusion predicted in this study by the PST cardiovascular reactivity measures was by far the greater of the two (adjusted $R^2$ change for cardiological measures = .08, for PST measures = .48). This work confirmed that CVR is related to ischemic heart disease.[7]

## RESOLVING A PARADOX

The notion that CVR is malignant was suggested by much research on the CVR–disease link. However, doubts about whether all CVR in active coping situations is unhealthy in the long run remained. Although one could argue that propagation of the species is not dependent on the cardiovascular health of aged humans, the idea that all forms of CVR are malignant even in the long run seemed implausible. Indeed, the work of cardiovascular psychophysiologists during the 1980s and 1990s began to tackle this issue.

### Cardiac–Somatic Coupling and Uncoupling

In the classic book *Cardiovascular Psychophysiology*, Paul Obrist (1981) described his theory of cardiac–somatic coupling and uncoupling. Accordingly, in terms of the CVR–disease link, only CVR during active or task-focused coping should be regarded as malignant. For Obrist, cardiac–somatic coupling is benign. During such coupling, increases in cardiovascular activity such as HR are driven by somatic or metabolic demands. It occurs, Obrist maintained, not only during metabolically demanding activities such as aerobic exercise, but also during passive coping situations such as watching a scary movie. In contrast, according to Obrist, cardiac–somatic uncoupling is malignant. It occurs, Obrist maintained, during active coping situations, those concerned with active task performance such as problem solving. Because such increases in cardiovascular activity are not primarily driven by somatic or metabolic demands, they could be regarded as strains on the cardiovascular system.

In light of Obrist's theory and his and others' supporting research, it seemed necessary at the time to think about the health implications of the experimental game findings of the association between increased HR and positive performance for males reported earlier (Blascovich et al., 1978). Specifically, the positive relationship between HR increases and performance for males, though functional for performance in the short term, might prove dysfunctional in terms of cardiovascular health in the long term. For females, the HR increases themselves during the game appeared dysfunctional both for performance in the short term and for health in the long term.

Although Obrist narrowed the domain regarding the CVR–disease relationship to active coping situations, research such as that of Kobasa and Maddi (see above) suggested that even the notion that CVR during active coping is always malignant might not be tenable. Whereas narrowing the domain to active coping situations helped narrow the focus of the malignancy of CVR to certain situations, other work began examining the relationship of reactivity across specific cardiovascular responses.

### Physiological Toughness

In a *Psychological Review* paper, Richard Dienstbier (1989) suggested that certain patterns of increases in CVR during active coping might differ in functionality both in the short term for task performance and in the long term for cardiovascular health. Based primarily on animal work, Dienstbier noted two patterns of cardiovascular responses: one among animals that appeared to thrive during and following active coping, and one among animals that appeared not to fare well (at least in the long run) in the same apparent active coping situations.

According to Dienstbier, both the benign pattern, labeled *physiological toughness*, and the more malignant pattern, labeled *physiological weakness* by default, involve activation of the sympathetic–adrenal medullary (SAM) axis. Accordingly (see Figure 31.1), sympathetic innervation increases left ventricular contractility (VC) and HR. For physiologically tough animals, SAM activation via stimulation of the adrenal medulla also increases the production of epinephrine, further increasing HR and decreasing total systemic vascular resistance (total peripheral resistance, or TPR), and thereby creating relatively large increases in cardiac output (CO). However, for physiologi-

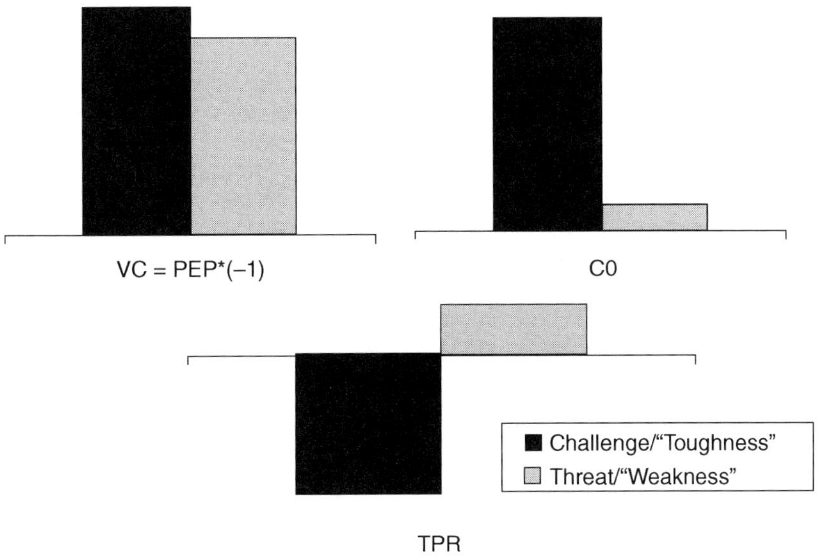


**FIGURE 31.1.** Cardiovascular patterns associated with challenge/physiological toughness and threat/physiological weakness. VC, vascular contractility (i.e., VC = PEP * (–1)); CO, cardiac output; TPR, total peripheral (systemic vascular) resistance.

cally weak animals, near-simultaneous activation of the hypothalamic–pituitary–adrenal (HPA) cortical axis[8] inhibits the SAM effects on HR and TPR via adrenal cortical release of cortisol, thereby attenuating decreases or even causing increases in TPR and attenuating increases in CO.

Hence, by expanding the view of CVR to include measurement of patterns of cardiovascular responses rather than the use of single or multiple unitary responses such as HR or blood pressure, Dienstbier presented a clearer picture of healthy and unhealthy cardiovascular response patterns during active coping situations. Yet questions remained as to whether these response patterns would hold up in humans, and equally, if not more importantly, what the antecedents of physiological toughness and weakness might be for humans.

### Cardiac versus Vascular Reactivity

At the risk of oversimplification, Dienstbier's (1989) cardiovascular patterns of physiological toughness and physiological weakness can be thought of as a cardiac pattern and vascular pattern of CVR, respectively. In the early 1990s, Manuck, Kamarack, Kasprowicz, and Waldstein (1993) reported research pointing to the higher risk of vascular compared to cardiac reactivity for the development of cardiovascular disease. Furthermore, Anderson, McNeilly, and Myers (1993) developed a model of American racial differences in hypertension based on relative differences in vascular reactivity.

## EVOLUTION OF THE BPS MODEL OF CHALLENGE AND THREAT

### Rationale

The major advances in CVR research pioneered by Obrist, Dienstbier, Manuck, their colleagues, and others ameliorated the need to forecast necessarily dire health implications of the CVR–performance link, such as the experimental game scenario we reported (Blascovich et al., 1978). Specifically, it was no longer necessary to assume that the positive relationship between HR increases and performance reported for males might prove dysfunctional for cardiovascular health in the long term. Those HR increases could be ones associated with physiological toughness and cardiac reactivity, rather than physiological weakness and vascular reactivity. However, the psychological antecedents of these patterns, other than a few dispositional ones such as the coronary-prone behavior pattern, remained unspecified by CVR and health researchers.

Fortunately, the work of Richard Lazarus, Susan Folkman, and colleagues (e.g., Lazarus

& Folkman, 1984) on coping with stress suggested that the antecedents of physiological toughness and weakness might involve individuals' cognitive appraisals of goal relevance, coping demands, and coping resources. Similarly but not identically to Lazarus and colleagues' reasoning, we theorized that if an individual perceived[9] sufficient resources to meet the demands of a goal-relevant active coping situation, a positive motivational state would result. We labeled this state *challenge*.[10] On the other hand, we theorized that if an individual perceived insufficient resources to meet the situational demands, a negative motivational state would result. We labeled this motivational state *threat*.

We further theorized that the physiological toughness and weakness patterns specified by Dienstbier (1989) should map onto challenge and threat motivations, respectively. Consequently, we examined these theoretical speculations in correlational, experimental, and (more recently) predictive studies, to ascertain whether Dienstbier's physiological toughness and weakness patterns would map onto challenge and threat motivation.[11] A sample of these studies follows.

## Empirical Studies

Our empirical studies involved the use of laboratory tasks qualifying as active coping tasks,[12] such as serial subtraction (i.e., mental arithmetic) and speech—tasks often used by scientists in the CVR community. The use of ECG, impedance cardiographic, and hemodynamic (i.e., blood pressure) measurement technologies permitted us to assess the cardiovascular responses specified by Dienstbier.[13] In all studies reported below, resting baseline measurements were taken followed by task instructions and task performance. Reactivity scores were calculated by subtracting the last minute of baseline values from corresponding values assessed during the tasks.

### *Correlational Studies*

We conducted a series of correlational experiments to ascertain the relationship between self-reported evaluations of perceived demands and resources prior to active coping performance tasks and patterns of cardiovascular responses during subsequent performance. We hypothesized that an evaluation of resources exceeding demands would result in a motivational state of challenge accompanied by increases in HR, VC, and CO, and a decrease in TPR, and that an evaluation of demands exceeding resources would be accompanied by increases in HR and VC, but little change in CO and little change or even increases in TPR (see Figure 31.1). In three experiments, our hypotheses were confirmed (Tomaka, Blascovich, Kelsey, & Leitten, 1993).

### *Experimental Studies*

In order to strengthen our confidence in the causal relationship between the evaluation of perceived demands and resources, we experimentally manipulated factors likely to create overall challenge and threat evaluations while assessing subsequent CVR patterns. In one experiment (Tomaka, Blascovich, Kibler, & Ernst, 1997), manipulations of the content (e.g., practice vs. criterion) and coupled expression (e.g., friendly vs. hostile vocal tone) of task instructions led to the hypothesized challenge and threat patterns of CVR. In another (Hunter, 2001), participants randomly received instructions that they would be reading or singing the U.S. national anthem while we recorded them. In order to give them some idea of what this experience would be like, participants were instructed to read or sing the first couple of stanzas. Again, the predicted patterns of CVR occurred: Significantly more of the individuals who anticipated singing evidenced the threat pattern than individuals who anticipated reading, and significantly more of the individuals who anticipated reading evidenced the challenge pattern than individuals who anticipated singing.

In order to test the possibility that the patterns or interoceptions of the patterns of cardiovascular responses somehow influence the evaluations of demands and resources, we conducted experiments (Studies 2 and 3 in Tomaka et al., 1997) in which we manipulated cardiovascular patterns mimicking the challenge and threat patterns physically (participants engaged in moderate aerobic exercise, mimicking physiological toughness, vs. no aerobic exercise on a bicycle ergometer in one study; participants experienced a warm pressor, mimicking physiological toughness, vs. a cold pressor, mimicking physiological weakness, in the other) and asked participants to self-report evaluations of demands and resources for an upcoming serial subtraction task during the manipulation. As expected, overall demand–resource evaluations did not differ as a function of the physical manipulations; this suggested that the direction of causality, as indicated by the neo-Jamesian perspective (e.g., Schachter & Singer, 1962), was not from the physiological patterns to the evaluations of demands and resources, but rather vice versa.

### *Predictive Studies*

The studies reported above provided strong evidence to us that Dienstbier's patterns map onto our challenge and threat constructs. Recently, we (Blascovich, Seery, Mugridge, Norris, & Weisbuch, 2004) conducted a study to determine the predictive validity of the challenge–threat patterns of CVR for future performance. We recruited members (position players other than pitchers; i.e., hitters) of the University of California, Santa Barbara varsity baseball and softball teams to serve as participants. Each player gave two 3-minute speeches: a baseball-irrelevant (control) speech ("Why I am a good friend") and a baseball-relevant (target) speech ("How I would approach a critical hitting situation"). We indexed challenge–threat via a unitary physiological index derived from our multiple cardiovascular measures for each task, and we collected offensive (i.e., hitting) statistics during the ensuing varsity league season 6 months later. Our cardiovascular index during the baseball-relevant speech reliably predicted major indexes of offensive baseball performance (the runs-generated index, batting averages, etc.), such that the greater the challenge, the better the performance. Our cardiovascular index during the baseball-irrelevant speech did not predict such performance. Furthermore, because there were no effects of sport (i.e., baseball vs. softball) on these relationships, and because baseball is a men's sport and softball a women's sport, gender was not a factor.

## Brief Summary of the BPS Model

The general components of the BPS model are illustrated in Figure 31.2. The model describes the theoretical processes underlying the generation of challenge–threat states.[14] Accordingly, challenge and threat emerge within the context of motivated performance situations, those perceived as self- and goal-relevant to the individual. Such a situation contains one or more tasks that require active coping (i.e., instrumental behavioral and/or cognitive performance). Evaluations of demands and resources on the part of the individual occur both cognitively and affectively, either of which can occur consciously or unconsciously—and, as Figure 31.2 depicts, the two types of evaluations can interact. As resources begin to equal or outweigh demands, challenge results; when demands begin to outweigh resources, threat results.[15]

Examples of factors or components affecting resources and demands include danger (physical or psychological), uncertainty, required effort, skills and knowledge, and external support. Perceptions of any of these factors can be filtered via dispositional traits and states (coronary-prone behavior style, self-esteem, etc.). Theoretically, these factors can be interactive or synergistic. For example, uncertainty can increase danger and/or required effort.

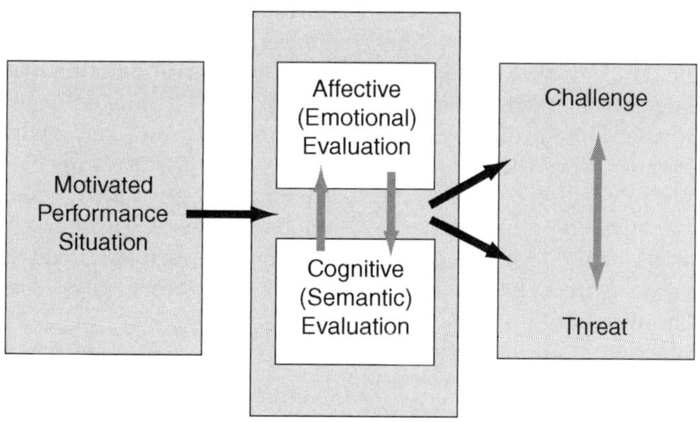


**FIGURE 31.2.** The biopsychosocial model of challenge and threat.

Research supporting and guided by the BPS model of challenge and threat has appeared in the literature (for a recent review, see Blascovich, in press). Work validating the cardiovascular indexes is described above. A substantial body of work using these indexes to test various social psychological theories has also appeared. To the extent that challenge and threat motivational states can be predicted by a social psychological theory, the cardiovascular patterns can be measured to test the theory. For example, attitude theorists have long maintained that attitudes (e.g., attitudes toward food items) are functional in the decision-making domain (e.g., grocery shopping), easing one's way through the myriad decisions faced in everyday life. One would predict that an individual with preexisting attitudes toward decision alternatives would experience challenge during a rapid decision-making task. Such was exactly the case in experimental research (Blascovich et al., 1993).

Additionally, the BPS motivational model and the cardiovascular indexes developed under its aegis have been used successfully to test various hypotheses drawn from various social psychological theories. Such research has focused, for example, on social facilitation (Blascovich, Mendes, Hunter, & Salomon, 1999), social comparison (Mendes, Blascovich, Major, & Seery, 2001), stigma (Blascovich, Mendes, Hunter, Lickel, & Kowai-Bell, 2001), emotional disclosure (Mendes, Reis, Seery, & Blascovich, 2003), self-esteem theory (Seery, Blascovich, Weisbuch, & Vick, 2004), uncertainty (Mendes, Blascovich, Hunter, Lickel, & Jost, 2007), and emotion (Herald & Tomaka, 2002).

It is important to note that the applicability of the BPS model in general and of its CVR-based indexes in particular has limits. Specifically, BPS challenge and threat theorists have not been willing to generalize the theory and indexes beyond the domain of motivated performance situations. Nevertheless, these limitations do not severely limit the value of the BPS model, because motivated performance situations are ubiquitous in modern-day life in nearly every culture on earth. The success of most if not all economies now appears to be based on the production and marketing of goods, services, and/or information and to involve a myriad of ancillary activities, all of which are goal-relevant to workers and require instrumental cognitive and behavioral responses on their part—that is, motivated performance situations (in Lazarian terms, situations requiring *task-focused* coping). Without such responses, a motivated performance situation itself would cease to exist or change its nature (again, in Lazarian terms, perhaps to purely *emotion-focused* coping situations). However, motivated performance situations are not limited to work life. Indeed, they are equally ubiquitous in all manner of interpersonal relationships, "leisure" activities, volunteer activities, and so on. With the increasing intrusion of motivated performance situations into modern-day lives, the possible health consequences of repeated challenge and threat motivational states should not be taken lightly.

## HEALTH IMPLICATIONS OF CHALLENGE AND THREAT STATES

Research strongly suggests both direct and indirect effects of challenge and threat motivational states on health. As stated above challenge can generally be regarded as relatively benign and threat as relatively malignant in terms of physical health, particularly cardiovascular health. Given space limitations, the discussion here focuses on the likely and potential negative health effects of threat, though the positive health effects of challenge should not be underestimated (recall Dienstbier's [1989] physiologically tough animals). Indeed, in motivated performance situations, one can argue that challenge responses contribute to what has become known as *positive psychology* (Seligman, 2002).

### Direct Health Effects of Threat Motivation

Given the demonstration of potentially pathophysiological cardiovascular patterns associated with threat in motivated performance situations, one of the possible direct links between threat motivation and health involves the cardiovascular system. However, the direct health effects of motivational threat are not likely to be limited to the cardiovascular system. For example, motivational threat may well impair immune and other physiological functions directly.

#### *Cardiovascular Disease*

Threat can affect cardiovascular health via at least two direct pathways, one leading to ischemic heart disease and the other to hypertension. Both paths assume repeated episodes of threat, as might occur for individuals who find themselves for whatever reasons (e.g., dispositions, low domain self-efficacy, stereotype threat, war, difficult interpersonal relationships) repeatedly in threatening motivated performance situations.[16]

As described above, the threat pattern of CVR is one in which SAM axis activation is countered by HPA axis activation, putting the heart and vasculature, especially the coronary arteries, in opposition. Arterial constriction in the face of increased VC can lead to acute increases in blood pressure, particularly diastolic blood pressure—thereby creating fluid (i.e., blood) turbulence within the coronary arteries, and consequently causing strain on, and injury (i.e., lesions) to, the endothelial lining of the coronary arteries themselves (Blascovich & Katkin, 1993). Such insults to the coronary arteries lead in turn to scarring of this tissue, the buildup of arterial plaque (i.e., arteriosclerosis) within them, arterial stenosis (i.e., narrowing of the arteries), and thereby ischemia (i.e., lack of oxygen) in the myocardium (i.e., heart muscle); the latter effect can lead to myocardial infarcts (so-called "heart attacks"), which if not fatal often result in necrosis (i.e., death) of the myocardial tissue (i.e., heart muscle) and the accompanying decrease in cardiac efficiency.

Chronic or essential hypertension can result from the repeated transient increases in blood pressure during motivational threat states that over time lead to the failure of hemodynamic regulatory processes (Manuck et al., 1993). Additionally, the accumulation of plaque within the arterial vasculature generally reduces the elasticity of the arteries themselves (so-called "hardening" of the arteries), which also can increase chronic blood pressure levels. Hypertension itself is a risk factor for various cardiac pathologies, including heart attack and stroke.

### *Immune Function*

In the mid-1970s, Ader and Cohen (1975) discovered important connections linking behavior, neural processes, and the immune system. Until that time, the immune system was thought to operate independently of the central nervous system. This seminal discovery led to the establishment of the field of psychoneuroimmunology and later the field of psychoneuroendocrinology. Researchers within these disciplines relatively quickly demonstrated links between stress or threat experiences[17] and immune dysfunction. For example, Glaser and colleagues (1987) reported data linking unhealthy fluctuations in immune responses directly to likely stress or threat fluctuations among medical students; specifically, they compared immune assay data from before and after medical school examination periods. In addition (Kiecolt-Glaser et al., 1987), they reported differences in immune functioning between caregivers of patients with Alzheimer disease and matched controls, such that suppression of immune functioning was more prevalent among the former. In another seminal study, Cohen and colleagues (1998) demonstrated experimentally that repeated stress or threat episodes led to increased susceptibility to rhinoviruses (i.e., common cold viruses), proving the existence of a link among psychological stress states, decreased immune responses, and actual susceptibility to disease. Other psychoneuroimmunological evidence suggests that the evaluation process resulting in challenge (i.e., resources exceeding demands) stimulates anabolic hormone release, which can protect against bacterial infections (Epel, McEwen, & Ickovics, 1998).

## Indirect Health Effects of Threat Motivation

Over the long run, the indirect health effects of threat motivation may contribute to a general weakening of interconnected physiological, psychological, and social systems, increasing many health risks for individuals repeatedly exposed to threatening motivated performance situations.

### *Allostatic Load*

Such a general physiological vulnerability has been described by Bruce McEwen (McEwen with Lasley, 2002) as *allostatic load*. According to McEwen, *allostasis* refers to the physiological changes that help the body maintain or return to homeostasis during episodes of increased activity, such as might be engendered by stress. *Allostatic load* refers to a failure in allostatic systems, resulting from chronically repeated stress or threat episodes, which raises baseline levels of hormonal and autonomically controlled systems (e.g., the cardiovascular system). Thus increasing allostatic load can lead to hypertension, ischemic heart disease, myocardial infarcts, and the like. Hence chronically threatened individuals are more at risk for increased allostatic load on the heart.

### Mental Health

Statistically positive associations exist between repetitive threat or stress episodes and various psychopathologies. That the etiologies of anxiety and depression include constant threat experiences surprises very few. Both anxiety and depression put individuals at increased risk not only for other psychopathologies such as suicide and various addictions, but also for presentations of many "physical" illnesses (headaches, eating disorders, sleep problems, skin diseases, etc.).

### Social Outcomes

Ill health, whether resulting directly from motivational threat experiences, specific pathogens, or interactions between the two, can create a cascade of social problems. For example, to the extent that motivational threat experience results in relatively poor job performance, an individual's socioeconomic outlook may become bleak, leading to job and/or health benefit loss—and thereby increasing that individual's susceptibility to disease, while decreasing the likelihood of his or her receiving appropriate medical care when needed. Furthermore, if a disease actually develops—for example, AIDS—the individual may easily become stigmatized, thereby even further decreasing access to employment opportunities and/or health benefits, as well as causing a loss of social support and increased likelihood of psychopathology. These health outcomes further decrease the individual's resources to cope in motivated performance situations, thereby creating an ever-deepening spiral of health problems.

## Health-Relevant Mediators and Moderators of Threat Motivation

As described above, the balance between an individual's resource and demand evaluations mediates challenge–threat outcomes. Assuming that an individual is motivated to perform in situation in order to reach a self-relevant goal, the BPS model of challenge and threat describes several factors that can moderate the individual's evaluations of demands and resources, and hence can have consequences for health as well.[18] Some of these factors can interact synergistically with each other, and all of them interrelate.

A nonexhaustive set of these factors is described here. One factor involves *danger and safety.* Though potential physical danger is an obvious health-related factor, potential psychological danger, such as loss of self-esteem, negative affective experience, and social sanctions, perhaps plays an even larger role in increasing individuals' demand evaluations in modern society. On the other hand, perceptions of physical and psychological safety decrease demand evaluations. Another factor is *required effort.* The greater the effort required to perform well in a situation, the greater the demand. Again, this effort can be primarily physical or psychological. To the extent that the individual possesses task-relevant *skills, abilities, and knowledge*, the greater the resource evaluation, and the less likely the experience of threat. This factor also probably moderates danger–safety and required effort evaluations in predictable ways.

The *presence of others* can moderate both demand and resource evaluations. Supportive, nonevaluative others are likely to increase resources and perhaps to decrease danger, whereas nonsupportive or evaluative others are likely to increase demands and perhaps to decrease resources; it is assumed, of course, that the individual possesses the resources such as skills, abilities, and knowledge to perform. Indeed, we (Blascovich et al., 1999) have shown that classic social facilitation–inhibition effects are driven by challenge–threat responses, respectively, during motivated situation performance. We (Allen, Blascovich, & Mendes, 2002; Allen, Blascovich, Tomaka, & Kelsey, 1991) have also shown that pets can provide the kind of nonevaluative social support that results in challenge responses. Additionally, we (Mendes, Blascovich, Major, & Seery, 2001) have shown that when the presence of others evokes social comparison processes, challenge or threat can occur as a function of whether the evoked comparison is downward or upward, respectively.

*Individual difference factors* can also moderate demand and resource evaluations in such a way as to cause challenge or threat responses. In numerous experiments, we (Blascovich et al., 2001; Mendes, Blascovich, Lickel, & Hunter, 2002) have demonstrated that motivated performance situations involving interaction, even cooperative interaction, with stigmatized (e.g., by virtue of race, socioeconomic status, physical disfigurement) others evokes threat.

Finally, *dispositions* are very likely to play an important moderating role in demand and resource evaluations. In an early study, we

(Tomaka & Blascovich, 1994) demonstrated that all other things being equal, dispositional beliefs in a just world were probably more related to challenge than to threat motivation. More recently, we (Seery et al., 2004) found predictable relationships among chronic levels of self-esteem, stability of self-esteem, and challenge–threat motivational states. We don't doubt that dispositions related to optimism, confidence, and the like relate to challenge–threat as well. Though we ourselves have never attempted to relate either the Type A or hardiness personality traits to challenge–threat motivational states, the work of others (e.g., Kobasa, 1979; Kobasa et al., 1982) suggests this to be the case.

## FINAL WORD

In this chapter, I have discussed motivation in terms of a challenge and threat model. Although challenge–threat motivation theory can probably be used to develop interventions to motivate individuals to lead healthy lifestyles, the focus here is on the health consequences, direct and indirect, of challenge and threat motivational states themselves. How individuals evaluate their demands and resources affects their motivational states, which in turn lead to differing patterns of physiological responsivity: Motivation in which evaluated individual resources outweigh situational task demands (i.e., challenge) does not appear pathophysiological, and motivation in which evaluated individual resources are outweighed by situational task demands (i.e., threat) does appear pathophysiological.

## NOTES

1. My early research on the risky shift phenomenon used blackjack or 21 as the individual and group laboratory risk-taking task, and bets to index risk taking (e.g., Blascovich, Ginsburg, & Howe, 1974); hence I needed some real-world experience. For those unfamiliar with the game of 21, Thorp (1966) provides an excellent description. The "relatively large bet" referred to in later text typically amounted to $5 or $10 placed before a hand was dealt and played (a not inconsequential proportion of a graduate student's monthly stipend at the time). In terms of today's stipends, this would amount to $50 to $100 on a hand—an important investment in scientific query.

2. A combination of social psychological theory and methods with assessment of endocrine or brain wave activity was nearly inconceivable at the time. Hence, along with a few others, I used the term *social psychophysiology*.

3. The measuring device was a battery-operated, solid-state common-mode rejection amplifier/filter including a then "high-tech" integrated circuit (the forerunner of the computer chip) and the newly invented portable audiotape recorder. Unfortunately, a patent was not sought, and my colleagues and I missed the opportunity that the inventors of ambulatory ECG (i.e., Holter) monitors later seized.

4. In retrospect (see later discussion in the chapter), the male and female HR increases, although obviously confounded with gender, were probably indicative of more variability across the task engagement spectrum for males compared to females, with the latter having both less variability and higher mean HR—hence greater task engagement probably due to greater threat overall.

5. This was a curious case of definitional operationalism (Campbell, 1988).

6. A coronary angiogram involves inserting a cardiac catheter into the aorta (usually via the femoral artery) and guiding it into the major coronary arteries, where radio-opaque dye is injected. During injection, moving radiographic recordings are made, allowing angiographers to measure the extent of ischemia (narrowing) in the coronary arteries. At the time of the reported study, occlusion was quantified by discrete categories labeled as percentages (e.g., 0%, 25%, 50%, 75%, 90%, and 100%).

7. We believe that the relationship between CVR measures taken during PST and coronary ischemia was positive because of the age of the patient participants. Such measures in younger populations (particularly young adults) are not likely to predict coronary ischemia, as the etiology of ischemia is a slow, long-term phenomenon. However, the results are consistent with the notion that CVR during psychological stress eventually leads to heart disease.

8. Dienstbier actually specified the pituitary–adrenal–cortical (PAC) axis. HPA is used here to update the label.

9. The term *perceived* here is used in a general sense to include both conscious and unconscious *perceptions*, *appraisals*, or *evaluations*—the terms we use in more expanded theoretical statements (e.g., Blascovich & Mendes, 2000).

10. It is important to note that we use the term *challenge* in an explicit way to refer to a positive or benign motivational state, in contrast to the way in which cardiological and psychophysiological communities use it to describe a potential stressor to the organism.

11. In addition, these studies served to validate the use of these patterns for indexing challenge and threat motivation online, continuously, and covertly in order to test social psychological theories. However, this use is not the primary focus of this chapter.

12. The active coping tasks must be considered in the whole context or situation in which they take place. For example, the actual mental arithmetic or speech task is

only one element of a situation (in this case, performing in a psychology experiment in a laboratory environment) that influences the perceptions and evaluations of demands and resources. We label these *motivated performance situations*.

13. The ECG provides HR as well as the starting point (depolarization) for left ventricular contraction ($VC_{start}$); the impedance cardiogram (ICG) provides stroke volume (SV) and the ending point (opening of the aortic valve) for left ventricular contraction ($VC_{end}$); and the hemodynamic equipment provides mean arterial pressure (MAP). CO = SV × HR. VC= ($VC_{start} - VC_{end}$) × (–1). TPR = CO × MAP.

14. For a more detailed history and description of the BPS model, see Blascovich and Tomaka (1996), Blascovich and Mendes (2000), Blascovich and colleagues (2002), or Blascovich (in press).

15. Although the two types of motivational states are often described as "challenge *or* threat," we do not intend to connote categorically discrete states. Rather, we view challenge and threat as anchors of a bipolar continuum.

16. Lengthy discussion of the reasons why individuals may constantly subject themselves to threatening motivated performance situations is beyond the scope of this chapter.

17. Proponents of the BPS model of challenge and threat largely avoid the use of the term *stress*, because of its inherent conceptual fuzziness and the myriad ways it has been explicitly and implicitly defined in the literature. In the context of this chapter, *stress* refers to *threat* as defined in the text.

18. Previous theoretical discussions of the BPS model (e.g., Blascovich & Mendes, 2000; Blascovich & Tomaka, 1996) have categorized various antecedents of challenge–threat evaluations as resource or demand components.

## REFERENCES


Ader, R., & Cohen, N. (1975). Behaviorally conditioned immunosuppression. *Psychosomatic Medicine*, *37*, 333–340.

Allen, K. M., Blascovich, J., & Mendes, W. B. (2002). Cardiovascular reactivity and the presence of pets, friends, and spouses: The Truth about cats and dogs. *Psychosomatic Medicine*, *64*, 727–739.

Allen, K. M., Blascovich, J., Tomaka, J., & Kelsey, R. M. (1991). The presence of human friends and pet dogs as moderators of autonomic responses to stress in women. *Journal of Personality and Social Psychology*, *61*, 582–589.

Anderson, N., McNeilly, M., & Myers, H. (1993). A biopsychosocial model of race differences in vascular reactivity. In J. Blascovich & E. S. Katkin (Eds.), *Cardiovascular reactivity to psychological stress and disease* (pp. 83–110). Washington, DC: American Psychological Association.

Becker, M. H. (1974). The health belief model and personal health behavior. *Health Education Monographs*, *2*(4), 1–154.

Blascovich, J. (in press). Challenge and threat. In A. J. Elliot (Ed.), *Handbook of approach and avoidance*. Mahwah, NJ: Erlbaum.

Blascovich, J., Brennan, K., Tomaka, J., Kelsey, R. M., Hughes, P. H., Coad, M. L., et al. (1992). Affect intensity, cardiac arousal, and heartbeat detection. *Journal of Personality and Social Psychology*, *63*, 164–174.

Blascovich, J., Ernst, J. M., Tomaka, J., Kelsey, R. M., Salomon, K. A., & Fazio, R. H. (1993). Attitude as a moderator of autonomic reactivity. *Journal of Personality and Social Psychology*, *64*, 165–176.

Blascovich, J., Ginsburg, G. P., & Howe, R. C. (1974). Risky shifts and gambling: What's at stake? *Personality and Social Psychology Bulletin*, *1*, 246–248.

Blascovich, J., & Katkin, E. S. (1993). Psychological stress testing for coronary heart disease. In J. Blascovich & E. S. Katkin, (Eds.), *Cardiovascular reactivity to psychological stress and disease* (pp. 27–48). Washington, DC: American Psychological Association.

Blascovich, J., & Mendes, W. B. (2000). Challenge and threat appraisals: The role of affective cues. In J. Forgas (Ed.), *Feeling and thinking: The role of affect in social cognition* (pp. 59–82). Cambridge, UK: Cambridge University Press.

Blascovich, J., Mendes, W. B., Hunter, S. B., Lickel, B., & Kowai-Bell, N. (2001). Perceiver threat in social interactions with stigmatized others. *Journal of Personality and Social Psychology*, *80*, 253–267.

Blascovich, J., Mendes, W., Hunter, S., & Salomon, K. (1999). Social facilitation, challenge, and threat. *Journal of Personality and Social Psychology*, *77*, 68–77.

Blascovich, J., Mendes, W. B., Tomaka, J., Salomon, K., & Seery, M. (2003). The robust nature of challenge and threat: A reply to Wright and Kirby. *Personality and Social Psychology Review*, *7*, 234–243.

Blascovich, J., Nash, R. F., & Ginsburg, G. P. (1978). Heart rate and competitive decision making. *Personality and Social Psychology Bulletin*, *4*, 115–118.

Blascovich, J., Seery, M., Mugridge, C., Norris, K., & Weisbuch, M. (2004). Predicting athletic performance from cardiovascular indicators of challenge and threat. *Journal of Experimental Social Psychology*, *40*, 683–688.

Blascovich, J., & Tomaka, J. (1996). The biopsychosocial model of arousal regulation. In M. Zanna (Ed.), *Advances in experimental social psychology* (Vol. 28, pp. 1–51). San Diego, CA: Academic Press.

Campbell, D. T. (1988). Definitional vs multiple operationism. In E. S. Overman (Ed.), *Methodology and epistemology for social science: Selected papers—Donald Campbell* (pp. 31–36). Chicago: University of Chicago Press.

Cohen, S., Frank, E., Doyle, W. J., Skoner, D. P., Rabin, B. S., & Gwaltney, J. M., Jr. (1998). Types of stressors that increase susceptibility to the common cold in adults. *Health Psychology, 17*, 214–223.

Dienstbier, R. A. (1989). Arousal and physiological toughness: Implications for mental and physical health. *Psychological Review, 96*, 84–100.

Epel, E. S., McEwen, B. S., & Ickovics, J. R. (1998). Embodying psychological thriving: Physical thriving in response to stress. *Journal of Social Issues, 54*, 301–322.

Glaser, R., Rice, J., Sheridan, J., Fertel, R., Stout, J., Speicher, C., et al. (1987). Stress-related immune suppression: Health implications. *Brain, Behavior, and Immunity, 1*, 7–20.

Hamburg, D. A., Elliott, G. R., & Parron, D. L. (Eds.). (1982). *Health and behavior: Frontiers of research in the biobehavioral sciences*. Washington, DC: National Academy Press.

Herald, M. M., & Tomaka, J. (2002). Patterns of emotion-specific appraisals, coping and physiological reactivity during an ongoing emotional episode. *Journal of Personality and Social Psychology, 83*, 425–433.

Hunter, S. B. (2001). *Performance under pressure: The impact of challenge and threat states on information processing*. Unpublished doctoral dissertation, University of California, Santa Barbara.

Katkin, E. S., Blascovich, J., & Goldband, S. (1981). Empirical assessment of visceral self-perception: Individual and sex differences in the acquisition of heart beat discrimination. *Journal of Personality and Social Psychology, 40*, 1095–1101.

Kiecolt-Glaser, J. K., Glaser, R., Shuttleworth, E. C., Dyer, C. S., Ogrocki, P., & Speicher, C. E. (1987). Chronic stress and immunity in family caregivers of Alzheimer's disease victims. *Psychosomatic Medicine, 49*, 523–535.

Kobasa, S. C. (1979). Stressful life events, personality, and health: An inquiry into hardiness. *Journal of Personality and Social Psychology, 37*, 1–11.

Kobasa, S. C., Maddi, S. R., & Kahn, S. (1982). Hardiness and health: A prospective study. *Journal of Personality and Social Psychology, 42*, 168–177.

Lazarus, R. S., & Folkman, S. (1984). *Stress, appraisal, and coping*. New York: Springer.

Leventhal, H., & Watts, J. C. (1966). Sources of resistance to fear-arousing communications on smoking and lung cancer. *Journal of Personality, 34*, 155–175.

Manuck, S. B., Kamarack, T. W., Kasprowicz, A. S., & Waldstein, S. R. (1993). Stability and patterning of behaviorally evoked cardiovascular reactivity. In J. Blascovich & E. S. Katkin (Eds.), *Cardiovascular reactivity to psychological stress and disease* (pp. 111–134). Washington, DC: American Psychological Association.

Matthews, K. A., Weiss, S. M., Detre, T., Dembroski, T. M., Faulkner, B., Manuck, S. B., et al. (Eds.). (1986). *Handbook of stress, reactivity, and cardiovascular disease*. New York: Wiley.

McEwen, B., with Lasley, E. N. (2002).*The end of stress as we know it*. Washington, DC: Joseph Henry Press.

Mendes, W. B., Blascovich, J., Hunter, S. B., Lickel, B., & Jost, J. T. (2007). Threatened by the unexpected: Physiological responses during social interactions with expectancy-violating partners. *Journal of Personality and Social Psychology, 92*, 698–716.

Mendes, W. B., Blascovich, J., Lickel, B., & Hunter, S. (2002). Challenge and threat during interactions with white and black men. *Personality and Social Psychology Bulletin, 28*, 939–952.

Mendes, W. B., Blascovich, J., Major, B., & Seery, M. (2001). Effects of social comparisons on challenge and threat reactivity. *European Journal of Social Psychology, 31*, 477–479.

Mendes, W. B., Reis, H. T., Seery, M., & Blascovich, J. (2003). Cardiovascular correlates of emotional disclosure and suppression: Do content and gender context matter? *Journal of Personal and Social Psychology, 84*, 771–792.

Obrist, P. (1981). *Cardiovascular psychophysiology: A perspective*. New York: Plenum Press.

Rosenstock, I. M. (1974). The health belief model and preventive health behavior. *Health Education Monographs, 2*, 354–386.

Schachter, S., & Singer, J. E. (1962). Cognitive, social, and physiological determinants of emotional state. *Psychological Review, 5*, 379–399.

Seery, M., Blascovich, J., Weisbuch, M., & Vick, S. B. (2004). The relationship between self-esteem, self-esteem stability, and cardiovascular reactions to performance feedback. *Journal of Personality and Social Psychology, 87*, 133–145.

Seligman, M. (2002). *Authentic happiness*. New York: Free Press.

Shapiro, D., & Crider, A. (1968). Psychophysiological approaches in social psychology. In G. Lindzey & E. Aronson (Eds.), *The handbook of social psychology* (2nd ed., Vol. 3, pp. 1–49). Reading, MA: Addison-Wesley.

Thorp, E. O. (1966). *Beat the dealer: A winning strategy for the game of Twenty-One* (rev. ed.). New York: Random House.

Tomaka, J., Blascovich, J., Kelsey, R. M., & Leitten, C. L. (1993). Subjective, physiological, and behavioral effects of threat and challenge appraisal. *Journal of Personality and Social Psychology, 65*, 248–260.

Tomaka, J., Blascovich, J., Kibler, J., & Ernst, J. M. (1997). Cognitive and physiological antecedents of threat and challenge appraisal. *Journal of Personality and Social Psychology, 73*, 63–72.

Chapter 32

# Understanding the Determinants of Health Behavior Change

## INTEGRATING THEORY AND PRACTICE

Alexander J. Rothman
Andrew W. Hertel
Austin S. Baldwin
Roger D. Bartels

"This is your brain. This is your brain on drugs." "Be there tomorrow. Stop smoking today." "Do." These appeals provide a small glimpse at the myriad of appeals that are disseminated to persuade people either to avoid an unhealthy pattern of behavior or to adopt a healthy pattern of behavior. The design, and ultimately the effectiveness, of these appeals are predicated on an accurate understanding of the factors that shape the behavioral decisions people make about their health. What motivates people to stop smoking, to avoid binge drinking, to exercise regularly, to eat a healthy diet? Models of behavioral decision making strive to provide investigators with answers to these questions (Conner & Norman, 2005; Rothman & Salovey, 2007; Salovey, Rothman, & Rodin, 1998). In this chapter we examine the factors thought to motivate people's behavior throughout the behavior change process, as well as the implications of this knowledge for the design and implementation of initiatives to promote healthy behavior.[1] In particular, we focus on how people grapple with three distinct phases in the behavior change process: the decision to initiate a new pattern of behavior; the decision to maintain a recently adopted pattern of behavior; and the decision, after a failed effort, to initiate another attempt at behavior change.

### MODELS OF HEALTH BEHAVIOR CHANGE: AN OVERVIEW

Investigators have provided a range of frameworks to account for the factors that shape the decisions people make about their health practices. These include the *health belief model* (Rosenstock, Strecher, & Becker, 1988), *protection motivation theory* (Maddux & Rogers, 1983), *social cognitive theory* (Bandura, 1986), the *theory of planned behavior* (Ajzen, 1991), the *theory of reasoned action* (Ajzen & Fishbein, 1980), and the *transtheoretical model of behavior change* (Prochaska, DiClemente, & Norcross, 1992). The primary application of these models has been either to predict the performance of a given behavior at a specific point in time, or to describe the thoughts and feelings of people who have engaged in a particular pattern of behavior. For example, investigators have worked to specify what predicts whether a woman obtains a mammogram (Aiken, West, Woodward, & Reno, 1994; Rakowski et al., 1992) or why people choose to enroll in a smoking cessation program (Norman, Conner, & Bell, 1999). Although the insights afforded by these investigations are informative, they fail to address the fact that most health practices involve an ongoing series of behavioral decisions. For instance, after age 50 women need to obtain a mammogram every year, and the process of quitting smoking consists of a series of decisions whether or not to smoke.

The working assumption, either implicitly or explicitly, has been that the factors that underlie the decision to initiate a behavior are the same as those that underlie the decision to maintain it (Rothman, 2000; Rothman, Baldwin, & Hertel, 2004). Even stage models (e.g., Prochaska et al., 1992; Weinstein, 1988), which were formulated to describe how the behavior change process unfolds over time, provide little guidance regarding the processes that shape the ongoing performance of behavior. These models do identify behavioral maintenance as a distinct stage, but primarily emphasize how people move from having no interest in a behavior to engaging in the behavior. Thus applications of these models have focused on efforts to motivate people to take action. To the extent that a distinction is made between initial and maintained behavior change, it rests on the length of time a behavior has been performed rather than on stage-specific psychological factors (Prochaska & Velicer, 1997).

Insufficient consideration has been given to modeling the ongoing interplay between people's thoughts and feelings and their behavioral practices, and in particular to determining how people's experiences with a given behavior may affect their interest in sustaining it over time (but see Gerrard, Gibbons, Benthin, & Hessling, 1996; Jeffery et al., 2004). Investigators' ability to develop initiatives that promote sustained healthy behavioral practices will markedly improve if the determinants of ongoing behavioral practices are better specified. To this end, we have proposed that the decision criteria guiding the initiation and maintenance of behavior change are distinct, and that there is value in distinguishing among the following four phases of the behavior change process: *initial response*, *continued response*, *maintenance*, and *habit* (Rothman, 2000; Rothman et al., 2004). These phases capture the behavioral processes that begin once someone attempts to initiate a course of action (e.g., joining a fitness center). Below we provide a general overview of the four phases specified in this model, and then turn to a systematic examination of the psychological factors that are predicted to motivate transitions through the behavior change process.

The *initial response* and *continued response* phases capture the processes that underlie the initiation of a new pattern of behavior. According to our model, initiation is predicated on holding favorable expectations about future outcomes afforded by a new pattern of behavior and about the ability to obtain them.

The first phase of the behavior change process, *initial response*, begins as soon as people embark on an effort to change their behavior and continues until they first manifest a significant change. For example, a person may enroll in a smoking cessation program and subsequently report having been smoke-free for 7 consecutive days. People who fail to perform the desired behavior (e.g., someone who is unable to remain smoke-free for 7 consecutive days) are thought to revert to a consideration of whether they want to begin a new attempt to modify their behavior. In a later section of this chapter, we elaborate on how people may respond to a failed attempt at changing their behavior (at this phase as well as other phases in the behavior change process) and its implications for future behavioral efforts.

Factors that strongly predict successfully completing the initial response phase have been well identified. Specifically, whether people initiate a change in their behavior appears to be mostly a function of both their confidence in their ability to execute the behavior and their belief that engaging in the new pattern of behavior will meaningfully improve their lives (Bandura, 1997; Salovey et al., 1998). Because the onset of this phase of the behavior change process is particularly characterized by a sense of optimism and hope about the future, any factor that undermines a person's ability to generate and sustain this perspective—such as a facet of the individual's personality (e.g., pessimism), an aspect of his or her life situation (e.g., an unsupportive partner), or a lack of investment in the behavior change process (see Pomerantz & Shim, Chapter 25, this volume)—should make it more difficult to pass through this phase.

Once a person has reliably performed the desired behavior, the second phase of the behavioral process, *continued response*, begins. This phase is characterized by a tension between a person's ability and motivation to enact the new pattern of behavior continually, and the challenges and unpleasant experiences that leave him or her vulnerable to lapses and relapses. A key aspect of the continued response phase is that people have to face the reality of engaging in the new pattern of behavior, including the possibility or actuality of slips and lapses. As people begin to accumulate experiences with the new behavior, they must grapple with the challenge of sustaining favorable expectations about change. To the extent that people find the new behavior unpleasant or feel that it demands substantial mental and/or physical energy, their commitment to and confidence in the behavior may weaken, making it difficult for them to complete this phase of the behavior change process (but see Fishbach & Trope, Chapter 18, this volume, for an intriguing observation of how temptation might serve to bolster efforts to change behavior). Moreover, research has shown that the more self-regulatory demands that are overlaid on the behavior change process (e.g., attempting to hide the new behavior from friends or family), the more difficult it will be for people to grapple with the challenges posed by this phase (Baumeister, Heatherton, & Tice, 1994; Schmeichel & Baumeister, 2004). Factors such as the formation of implementation intentions that keep people focused on the specifics of what they need to do—and when and where to do it—may help people grapple with the onslaught of self-regulatory demands (Gollwitzer, 1999; Gollwitzer, Parks-Stamm, Jaudas, & Sheeran, Chapter 21, this volume).

The perceived costs associated with a behavior (e.g., having to get up early to exercise) both emerge and become more salient with direct experience. The heightened salience of these costs may pose a sharp contrast to the optimism and hope that characterized people's initial willingness to commit to the behavior change process.[2] In this case, aspects of a person's personality or life situation that make it difficult for him or her to remain optimistic about the behavior change process are likely to be particularly debilitating. People may find that they can begin to initiate a behavior in the absence of social support or even in the presence of unsupportive others, but that these conditions greatly hinder their ability to sustain their initial efforts over time.

People who are unable to complete the continued response phase are thought to have relapsed and returned to their prior behavioral practices. However, those who successfully complete this phase of the behavior change process have reached a significant milestone in that they have put their prior, unwanted habits behind them; consistently engage in a new, healthy pattern of behavior; and have developed a sense that they are in control of their actions. Up until this point, engaging in the new pattern of behavior has reflected a struggle against pressures to relapse. With the onset of a new phase in the behavior change process, the decision whether to continue the new behavior becomes more volitional. From the perspective of the theory of planned behavior (Ajzen, 1991), by the end of the continued response phase, perceptions of behavioral control should no longer moderate people's ability to translate their intentions into actions.

Whereas decisions regarding behavioral initiation are based on expectations regarding future outcomes, decisions regarding behavioral maintenance are thought to involve a consideration of the behavioral, psychological, and physiological experiences afforded by the new pattern of behavior, and a determination of whether those experiences are sufficiently satisfying to warrant continued action (Rothman, 2000; Rothman et al., 2004). Satisfaction confirms that the initial decision to adopt the behavior was correct and helps to justify continued effort to monitor the behavior. In considering the maintenance of behavior change, we believe it is important to distinguish between two phases. During the *maintenance* phase, the decision regarding what action to take is predicated on a continual assessment of the behavior's value, whereas during the *habit* phase, the behavior is maintained independently of any consideration of a behavioral alternative.

The *maintenance* phase is characterized by the desire to sustain the new, successful pattern of behavior. Having demonstrated that they can successfully perform the behavior over an extended period of time, people shift their attention from questions regarding their ability to engage in the behavior to those regarding the behavior's perceived value. At this point in the behavior change process, people's experiences with the new behavior are likely to be sufficiently informative to allow for an assessment of the relative costs and benefits afforded by the behavior. If they are satisfied with the new behavior, they will choose to sustain it and preserve the gains that have accrued. People can remain in the maintenance phase indefinitely, unlike the prior two phases of the behavior change process.

People continue to monitor the consequences of their behavior during the maintenance phase, and thus are sensitive to changes in both its perceived benefits and costs. For example, people may observe that the effort associated with following a diet or regularly exercising persists, but that over time there has been a decline in the number of compliments they get from friends and family for engaging in those behaviors. If at any point people no longer feel that there is sufficient value in continuing the behavior, they will revert to the earlier, unhealthy pattern of behavior.

The transition to *habit* occurs when people are not actively concerned about either their ability to perform the behavior or their evaluation of the outcomes afforded by the behavior. At this point, people engage in the behavior in the absence of any regular analysis of whether they should or should not continue to take action (Wood, Quinn, & Kashy, 2002). In other words, the behavior sustains itself. For instance, those who consistently wear seat belts—a behavior frequently invoked as a prototypical habit—rarely question their ability to use a seat belt or its value as a safety device. This is not to say that people in this phase do not value the behavior, but rather that they no longer need to verify or test its value. People in this phase should be less sensitive to information about the outcomes afforded by the behavior than are those who remain in the maintenance phase of the behavior change process (e.g., Ferguson & Bibby, 2002). It is assumed that people will continue in the habit phase until an event of sufficient magnitude occurs to cause them to reconsider the value of their behavior. Should this occur, people shift back into the maintenance phase and must determine whether the behavior in question is of sufficient value to maintain.

According to the proposed framework, people's expectations about and perceived satisfaction with their behavior are critical determinants of their ability to initiate and maintain a change in behavior, respectively. Although identifying the predictive value of these constructs is informative, advances in both theory and practice depend on developing a more complete understanding of how people form favorable expectations, what enables them to sustain those expectations, and how they determine they are satisfied with their actions. Too often models of behavioral decision making offer minimal guidance regarding how or even whether critical constructs can be manipulated (Jeffery, 2004; Rothman, 2004). For example, in our own work, the absence of information regarding what can be done to elevate the satisfaction people derive from changes in their behavior makes it difficult for practitioners to design interventions grounded in this theoretical framework.

In the following section, we elaborate on the processes that shape the primary determinants of behavior change. First, we examine how people form and sustain expectations, and then turn to a consideration of what makes behavior change satisfying. Finally, we consider how having failed to change a behavior affects these constructs, and what the implications are for efforts to motivate people to initiate a new attempt at behavior change.

## EXPECTATIONS AND BEHAVIOR INITIATION: A CLOSER LOOK

Successfully initiating behavior change is contingent on holding favorable expectations about that change. Interventions are typically designed to heighten people's belief that a new behavior will provide desirable outcomes and/or that their current behavior will result in a set of undesirable outcomes (King, Rothman, & Jeffery, 2002). As long as they are favorable, are all expectations equally predictive of behavior change? Investigators have developed instruments to assess the concerns or beliefs people say motivate their behavior, but there has been little if any evidence that the specific content of these beliefs affect the likelihood of successful behavior change. For example, researchers have observed that people are motivated to quit smoking for a number of reasons, with the most often cited reason being health concerns, but have been unable to discern a systematic relation between the content of the specific goals people identify and their ability to quit smoking (e.g., Ahluwalia, Resnicow, & Clark, 1998; Eiser, van der Pligt, Raw, & Sutton, 1985; Lichtenstein & Cohen, 1990).

Although the content of people's expectations regarding behavior change may not matter, there is some evidence that how people formulate these expectations does. In the field of education, there is considerable evidence that people who are motivated by goals characterized by the desire to attain a positive state (i.e., an *approach* goal) are more successful than are those who are motivated by goals characterized by the desire to prevent a negative state (i.e., an *avoidance* goal—Elliot & Church, 1997; Elliot & McGregor, 1999, 2001). This finding is predicated on the premise that people find it easier to determine that they are making progress toward a desired state than that they are successfully staying away from an undesired state.

The informative nature of people's goals may be particularly important. In the first study to examine the differential impact of approach and avoidance goals on changing a health behavior (i.e., quitting smoking), Worth, Sullivan, Hertel, Jeffery, and Rothman (2005) found that the more avoidance goals participants generated, the more likely they were to successfully initiate an attempt to quit. At first glance this finding may seem inconsistent with findings obtained in the education domain. However, the observed effect was primarily due to avoidance goals that involved trying to cure a current problem (e.g., getting rid of a hacking cough). Avoidance goals that involved trying to prevent a future unwanted outcome (e.g., not developing cancer) did not predict success. Prior studies had not assessed the potential impact of cure goals (Sullivan & Rothman, 2006). What is intriguing about the observed value of cure goals is that they are informative in a manner similar to that previously ascribed to approach goals. With a cure goal, people have a clear sense of their current undesired state. For example, they know how bad their cough is. As they initiate an attempt to quit smoking, they can monitor changes in their cough and readily detect improvement in their initial undesired state.

Because people's experiences with a new behavior will affect their ability to sustain their expectations about the behavior, the nature and the timing of the consequences afforded by their actions are likely to be critical. People are likely to have greater success initiating a pattern of behavior to the extent that it is motivated by goals affording immediate concrete rewards (e.g., wanting to quit smoking to get rid of the smell of smoke on clothes and belongings) as compared to those affording longer-term benefits (e.g., wanting to quit smoking in order to avoid developing cancer and heart disease). Although this speculation is consistent with current findings, further research is needed to delineate how features of people's expectations affect the thoughts and feelings they have during the behavior change process. For example, investigators need to monitor people's reports of progress toward expected outcomes, their feelings about those changes, and their implications for subsequent behavioral efforts. It would be particularly interesting to examine how having achieved a set of short-term concrete goals (e.g., having clothes that no longer smell of smoke) affects the motivation to sustain the change in behavior.

People are likely to differ in their ability to generate and sustain favorable expectations. For instance, cross-sectional data reveal that favorable expectations are more likely to be generated by those who are dispositionally optimistic (Affleck et al., 2001; Aspinwall & Brunhart, 1996; Cozzarelli, 1993; Gibson & Sanbonmatsu, 2004; Helgeson, 2003) and by those with positive trait self-esteem (Aspinwall & Taylor, 1993; Cozzarelli, 1993; Helgeson, 2003; King & Manaster, 1977).

Those who are more likely to generate favorable expectations initially should also be more likely to maintain favorable expectations throughout the initiation phases of the behavior change process. This may be particularly due to how people respond to difficulties. Laboratory evidence suggests that as long as people experience success in their efforts, a favorable set of expectations should be maintained, regardless of their level of optimism or self-esteem. However, when people experience difficulties or even failure, optimists (Gibson & Sanbonmatsu, 2004) and those with high self-esteem (Campbell & Fairey, 1985) should be more likely than others to maintain their expectations. For optimists, this may be due to their tendency to ignore inconsistencies between their expectations and experiences (Geers & Lassiter, 2002), to evaluate their prior behavioral efforts positively (Gibson & Sanbonmatsu, 2004), and to engage strategically in optimal social comparison processes

(Gibbons, Blanton, Gerrard, Buunk, & Eggleston, 2000). For those with high self-esteem, this may be due to their ability to make external attributions for failures (Campbell & Fairey, 1985).

Thus those with stable personal attributes that are conducive to generating and sustaining favorable expectations should be more likely than others to make the transition through the initiation phases into the maintenance phases of the behavior change process. Those without stable personal attributes that are conducive to generating and maintaining favorable expectations, however, are not necessarily doomed to fail. Prior research has revealed only a moderate correlation between optimism and domain-specific expectations (Peterson, 2000; Scheier et al., 1989), suggesting that it should be possible to encourage even pessimists to generate a favorable set of expectations about change. It is uncertain how stable these expectations would prove to be as these people proceeded through the behavior change process. However, there may be strategies available to buffer the extent to which contradictory experiences undermine initially favorable expectations. For instance, failure experiences may have less of a negative impact on the future expectations of people with low self-esteem, to the extent that they can be encouraged to engage in downward social comparison processes (Aspinwall & Taylor, 1993).

It should be noted that the premise that some people are better able to maintain a set of favorable expectations is predicated on studies that have observed people's reactions to success or failure on laboratory tasks (Campbell & Fairey, 1985; Gibson & Sanbonmatsu, 2004). When possible, investigators should capitalize on opportunities to examine the relation between personality characteristics such as optimism and self-esteem, and the expectations people report as they proceed through the behavior change process. To date, there appear to be no studies that have measured these personality attributes and repeatedly assessed people's expectations about their behavior.

## SATISFACTION AND BEHAVIOR MAINTENANCE: A CLOSER LOOK

It makes intuitive sense that the more satisfied a person is with a behavior, the more likely that person is to continue engaging in the behavior. Yet the effect of such satisfaction on people's health practices has received little empirical scrutiny. Cross-sectional data have supported the predicted impact of satisfaction (see Rothman, 2000), but prospective data regarding the influence of perceived satisfaction on behavioral maintenance have only begun to be collected. Data from two interventions—one designed to promote weight loss (Finch et al., 2005), and a second designed to promote smoking cessation (Hertel et al., in press)—have shown that perceived satisfaction with initial behavior prospectively predicts sustained behavior change. In a more focused set of analyses, Baldwin and colleagues (2006) have shown that whereas perceived self-efficacy predicts whether someone initiates an attempt to quit smoking, perceived satisfaction predicts whether someone maintains an initially successful quit attempt. The pattern of results from these studies is encouraging, but given the limited number of findings, it is difficult to draw any strong conclusions. However, in the consumer domain, the relation between satisfaction and behavior—specifically, repurchase intentions and repurchase behavior—has received considerable scrutiny. The insights afforded by this literature can shed important light on our understanding of how satisfaction affects behavioral maintenance.

### What Shapes Satisfaction?: The Disconfirmation of Expectations

Although it is not difficult to differentiate between the desirable and the undesirable outcomes afforded by changes in people's health practices, in many cases it can be difficult for people to determine how much of a change is sufficient for them to feel satisfied with their efforts. For instance, people may enroll in a weight loss program to improve their social lives or to change the size of the clothes they wear, but have difficulty discerning how many new dates or how much smaller a waist size they need to be satisfied with their efforts. One way people solve this problem is to examine their experiences in light of their expectations (Gollwitzer, 1996; Schwarz & Strack, 1991). How it feels to have had three new dates over a 6-week period will differ, depending on whether one's goal had been to have two or four new dates in that time period. According to the *disconfirmation-of-expectations model*, people are thought to be satisfied when the favorable outcomes they experience meet or surpass their expectations, but are dissatisfied when outcomes fall short of expectations (Szymanski & Henard, 2001).[3]

In response to the observation that the outcomes afforded by changes in health behavior are frequently difficult to evaluate, Rothman (2000; Rothman et al., 2004) has proposed a disconfirmation-of-expectations framework, and moreover has asserted that people's expectations may have a differential effect on the initiation and maintenance of behavior change. To the extent that people's satisfaction with a behavior is predicated on their experiences meeting or exceeding their expectations, the optimistic expectations that initially inspire people to change their behavior may subsequently undermine interest in maintaining the behavior when their experiences fail to meet their expectations. However, to date, two intervention studies have provided no evidence to support the prediction that optimistic expectations undermine feelings of satisfaction (Finch et al., 2005; Hertel et al., in press). These findings are striking, given the empirical evidence in the consumer behavior literature.

There are several reasons why the impact of expectations on satisfaction may have been elusive in studies of health behavior change. Investigators have shown that perceived satisfaction is more likely to depend on people's expectations when people hold their initial expectations with a high degree of confidence (Spreng & Page, 2001), and in situations in which the outcomes afforded by the behavior are difficult to interpret (Anderson & Sullivan, 1993; Yi, 1993). For example, to the extent that people have difficulty assigning meaning to improvements in fitness or in health, their expectations regarding how they would feel may prove critically important. Expectations about the consequences of behaviors studied to date may not have been held with confidence, and the outcomes may have been easy to interpret.

In addition, endeavors such as quitting smoking or losing weight are characterized by factors that make it difficult to discern the impact of people's expectations on satisfaction, such as people holding expectations across a variety of discrete outcomes (Iacobucci, Grayson, & Ostrom, 1994; Spreng, Mackenzie, & Olshavsky, 1996). For example, when evaluating the benefits of quitting smoking, people may have expectations about its impact on their physical fitness, their finances, their social life, and their self-image, to name but four domains. It is not presently clear how best to predict satisfaction when people may be monitoring a number of different comparisons.

It is also possible that the impact expectations have on satisfaction changes over time. At the outset of the behavior change process, when people may have more difficulty ascribing a value to their experiences, the impact should be strong. Over time, people's experiences with the behavior rather than their expectations may prove to be more decisive (Bolton & Drew, 1991; Yi & La, 2004). In this regard, it is worth noting that the preponderance of the evidence for the disconfirmation-of-expectations model in the consumer literature is based on short-term behavioral outcomes.

Finally, investigators must grapple with the fact that people's expectations may shift over time as they accumulate experiences with the new behavior. For example, once people have observed how quitting smoking affects their relations with friends and family, they may update their expectations regarding what will come from successfully changing their behavior. People may also shift their expectations strategically to justify their efforts or increase the likelihood of future satisfaction; some people, such as those who are higher in self-esteem or optimism, may be better able to make these cognitive adjustments (Campbell & Fairey, 1985; Gibson & Sanbonmatsu, 2004). In line with this observation, Zwick, Pieters, and Baumgartner (1995) have proposed that tests of perceived disconfirmation of expectations should be based on comparisons with the expectations people hold after having had some experience with the behavior. One challenge posed by the instability of people's expectations is that it may prove difficult to falsify a disconfirmation-of-expectations framework. Investigators may find themselves unsure as to whether the failure to find an effect of expectations on satisfaction merely indicates that they failed to assess people's expectations correctly. Future work in this area would benefit from a more complete understanding of how and when people's expectations shift in response to behavioral experience.

## Satisfaction and Behavior

Although the available evidence regarding health behavior change suggests that increasing satisfaction increases interest in maintaining behavior, research on consumer behavior has shown the relation between satisfaction and sustained behavior maintenance to be positive, but nonlinear and asymmetrical (Keiningham, Perkins-Munn, & Evans, 2003; Mittal & Kamakura, 2001). As satisfaction increases, so does the repetition of behavior, but the impact of satisfaction on behavior is exaggerated at the extreme ends of the satisfaction continuum. For example, moving from feeling "somewhat satisfied" to feeling "very satisfied" has a disproportionately greater effect on behavior than does an equivalent shift from feeling "neither satisfied nor dissatisfied" to feeling "somewhat satisfied" (Mittal & Kamakura, 2001). Thus the implementation of initiatives to heighten people's sense of satisfaction should be undertaken strategically.

The relation between satisfaction with a behavior and the maintenance of the behavior may depend in part on the behavioral domain. In fact, some behaviors may lead people to be more sensitive to feelings of dissatisfaction, whereas other behaviors may lead them to be more sensitive to feelings of satisfaction (see Yoon & Kim, 2000). People may have relatively modest expectations about some behaviors (e.g., wearing seat belts) and assume from the outset that they will be satisfied. People believe that it makes sense to engage in the behavior and are monitoring primarily for reasons not to continue. In this context, increases in feelings of satisfaction above a given threshold are not likely to affect behavior (e.g., there may be little added benefit in being delighted as opposed to content with how one's seat belt works), but people would be expected to respond quickly if they felt dissatisfied. For behaviors that do not readily invoke feelings of satisfaction, people may need to be persuaded to continue to engage in the behavior. If people are monitoring for favorable outcomes to justify their actions, their behavioral decisions are likely to be very sensitive to variability in satisfaction.

People may also vary in their sensitivity to feelings of dissatisfaction or satisfaction. Higgins (1998, 1999) has proposed that some people primarily focus on hopes and aspirations, and pursue goals that afford them the opportunity to seek out favorable outcomes (i.e., a *promotion* orientation); other people primarily focus on duties and obligations, and pursue goals that afford them the opportunity to avoid unfavorable outcomes (i.e., a *prevention* orientation). The behavioral decisions of people who are promotion-focused may prove to be particularly sensitive to variability in satisfaction, and thus these people would respond favorably to efforts to enhance their satisfaction with their behavior. The behavioral decisions of people who are prevention-focused may prove to be particularly sensitive to signs of dissatisfaction, and thus these people would be responsive to efforts to forestall dissatisfaction but not to efforts to enhance feelings of satisfaction. Future research in this area would benefit from a closer analysis of when and for whom feelings of satisfaction do and do not enhance behavioral performance.

## GETTING STARTED AGAIN: HOW DO PEOPLE RESPOND TO FAILURE?

The dominant focus of most theoretical work regarding health behavior, including our own, has been to delineate the factors that predict successful behavior change. Yet someone who is able to change her or his behavior successfully without having first failed is the exception rather than the rule (Polivy & Herman, 2002; Prochaska et al., 1992). Surveys of people who ultimately succeeded in changing an unwanted behavior reveal that they had to engage in numerous change attempts (e.g., three to four smoking cessation attempts before long-term abstinence [Schachter, 1982]; 5 or more consecutive years of the same New Year's resolution before maintaining the goal for 6 months [Norcross & Vangarelli, 1989]). Thus how people respond to failure is a critical theoretical and practical issue. In particular, we need to understand how the experience of failure affects the motivational factors that underlie the decision to initiate a new attempt at changing the behavior. Does failure always undermine interest in behavior change, and if not, under what conditions might failure facilitate further attempts at behavior change?

When one is considering how people respond to failure, it is important to distinguish between situations in which people have tried and failed to enact a change in their behavior, and those in which people have experienced a slip or a lapse but have not yet relapsed. The decision-making and motivational processes associated with the latter context have received considerable attention (i.e., relapse prevention—Brownell, Marlatt, Lichtenstein,

& Wilson, 1986; Marlatt & Donovan, 2005; Witkiewitz & Marlatt, 2004), and there is ample research tracking people's experiences from slips and lapses to relapses (e.g., Gwaltney et al., 2002; Shiffman et al., 1996, 2000). Considerably less is known about the process by which people move from failure to a new attempt to change their behavior (Norcross & Vangarelli, 1989; Schachter, 1982). Although there is little doubt that failing affects how people think and feel about the behavior in question and about themselves, the time course of these effects is not known; nor is much known about the factors that might exacerbate or ameliorate these effects.

As discussed earlier in this chapter, efforts to initiate a change in behavior are predicated on people's confidence in their ability to enact the change (i.e., their self-efficacy) and their positive expectations about what the change will afford. When people fail in an attempt to change their behavior, they typically experience frustration and self-condemnation (Brownell et al., 1986), which in turn serve to undermine their thoughts about behavior change. However, there may be value in differentiating between different classes of affective reactions to setbacks. According to the framework set forth by Carver and Scheier (Chapter 20, this volume), negative affect signals the need for behavioral adjustment. Specifically, negative affective reactions to failure that involve frustration and anger signify a need to work harder and may lead to increased effort at goal attainment. Thus, in contrast to the perspective set forth by Brownell and colleagues (1986), negative reactions can be beneficial. However, not all negative affective reactions may be beneficial. When a setback elicits feelings of sadness and depression, people may respond with a reduction in effort.

Thus the extent to which people's beliefs and expectations are undermined will determine whether and when they are ready to initiate a new attempt. If, following failure, people are able to sustain their expectations about what the new behavior will afford and their confidence in their ability to change, they should be ready to initiate a new attempt. However, if failing leads people to question the value of changing their behavior and/or their ability to do so, these beliefs will need to be reinstated before a new attempt at behavior change will be initiated.

The observation that people respond to failure by downplaying the benefits afforded by changing their behavior (Chassin, Presson, Sherman, & Kim, 2002) reflects a highly adaptive response to the distress elicited by failure. However, over time the feelings of frustration and the doubts about the merits of the new behavior may fade (see Gibbons, Eggleston, & Benthin, 1997; Hedeker & Mermelstein, 1996). In fact, the rate at which people are able to shake the distress elicited by failure may be a critical determinant of when they will be responsive to a new opportunity to change their behavior. One benefit often attributed to failure is that it can provide people with an opportunity to learn what they need to do (and not to do) in order to be successful (Brownell et al., 1986); this may be particularly true for optimists (Aspinwall, Richter, & Hoffman, 2001). Although these insights may be available immediately after failure, people may not be in a position to recognize and act on any lessons learned until after the distress elicited by failure has receded. Taken together, these observations would suggest that there may be an optimal time following failure at which to implement initiatives to encourage people to initiate another attempt at changing their behavior.

Determining how different psychological factors affect whether people maintain their initial beliefs and expectations following failure, as well as their ability to reinstate these beliefs over time, is critical to determining the most effective ways to motivate people to engage in new behavior change attempts. Below we consider a few factors that we believe may affect how people respond to failure.

## Explanations for Failure

The kinds of attributions that people make for their failure seem to be crucial in determining whether people who have failed will initiate a new change attempt (see Polivy & Herman, 2002). People who respond to failure by attributing it to a lack of effort should be in a good position to maintain or reinstate confidence in their ability to change the behavior, and thus the likelihood of their initiating another attempt at behavior change should be high. However, if people attribute their failure to a lack of ability, their motivation to change will be undermined, and they may need opportunities to regain confidence in their ability before they undertake a new attempt at behavior change. In terms of external attributions, if people believe that their failure was due to things outside of their control (e.g., lack of access to exercise facilities), beliefs about their ability to enact a change will be undermined, and the likelihood of a new attempt will be low until those perceived barriers are addressed. If people attribute their failure to the particular course of action or intervention they chose (e.g., the diet they followed), they may be able to sustain their confidence in their ability to act and in the benefits of action. However, in this case, the likelihood of a new attempt at behavior change will depend on whether a new course of action or intervention strategy is available. As investigators pursue these issues, there may be particular value in assessing both the immediate and delayed impact that people's attributions have on their beliefs regarding behavior change. For instance, variability in the attributions people generate in response to having failed may have a greater effect on the rate at which they recover from the distress elicited by failing than on the magnitude of their initial response to having failed.

### Self-Esteem and Failure

Self-esteem may also play an important role in determining how people respond to failure. In a study of individuals who attempted to quit smoking but failed, Gibbons and colleagues (1997) reported that self-esteem moderated how participants responded to failure. Compared to those with low self-esteem, those with high self-esteem were more likely to change their beliefs about the dangers posed by smoking (i.e., they lowered their estimates of the health risks posed by smoking), and in doing so were able to feel better and to maintain a positive sense of self. However, these changes in beliefs about smoking were accompanied by a reduction in their commitment to a future quit attempt (see also Chassin et al., 2002). Interestingly, over time, high-self-esteem participants' perceptions of the risks posed by smoking and their commitment to a future quit attempt increased. Because this study did not include an assessment of future attempts at cessation, how these changes in beliefs might affect behavior is uncertain. One intriguing possibility is that people low in self-esteem would be responsive to efforts to promote a renewed attempt at behavior change immediately after failure, whereas people high in self-esteem would be better served if there was a delay before those efforts were implemented. Once again, there would appear to be considerable value to documenting the time course of people's responses to failure and to determining how the nature of these trajectories differs for different groups of people.

Given that most people who initiate a change in their behavior fail, there is a need to develop methods to persuade people to initiate a new attempt at behavior change (e.g., Lando, Pirie, Roski, McGovern, & Schmid, 1996). To date, the theoretical insights available to guide the design of these initiatives is quite limited. If a more comprehensive description of how people respond to failure and the time course of those reactions can be developed, it will be likely to spur innovations in efforts to promote repeated efforts at behavior change.

## FUTURE DIRECTIONS: CAPITALIZING ON THE LINKAGES BETWEEN THEORY AND PRACTICE

The proposition that theoretical principles provide invaluable guidance in the design and implementation of interventions is widely endorsed and is thought to justify, at least in part, the pursuit of theoretical innovations. Perhaps the most familiar quote in this regard is Kurt Lewin's statement "that there is nothing so practical as a good theory" (1951, p. 169). Although we heartily agree with Lewin's admonition, we must not fail to recognize that it is critically dependent on the existence of *good* theories (Rothman, 2004). What characterizes a good theory? Although the quality of a theory can be evaluated along numerous dimensions, a critical feature is its ability to accurately specify the relation between constructs; as such, basic behavioral scientists focus their efforts on delineating whether a predicted relationship can be observed (Mook, 1983). From the perspective of an applied behavioral scientist, the accuracy of the relations specified in a theory is an important but not sufficient determinant of its value. Interventionists need theories that specify not only how two constructs are related, but also whether that relation does or does not change across contexts. Because interventionists are typically charged with the task of modifying factors to affect people's behavior, and have to do so within a complex social environment in order for their interventions to be useful, theories regarding the determinants of health behavior need to delineate how those determinants are formed and the contexts in which each determinant is particularly important.

This should not be taken to mean that theories need to be comprehensive and complete when initially proposed. Accurately identifying that a particular set of factors can predict behavior is an important step in the development of a health behavior theory, but it must not be mistaken for the last step. Theories of health behavior need to be treated as dynamic entities that evolve over time. Theory improvement is predicated on a cyclical process that involves the specification of relations between constructs; the testing of those relations; and then, in light of the obtained evidence, the respecification, if needed, of the initial proposition (Weinstein & Rothman, 2005). Although this view of theory development is well known and often advocated, a recent review by Noar and Zimmerman (2005) indicates that research regarding the determinants of health behavior reveals few signs of such a process.

The implementation and evaluation of theory-based interventions afford superb opportunities to spur the refinement and revision of health behavior theories. For example, the effectiveness of initiatives to modify people's expectations regarding the benefits of behavior change can inform our understanding of how people form and sustain these beliefs. Our understanding of relevant theoretical constructs, such as expectations, would also benefit from the comparison of findings across correlational and experimental tests of their impact on behavior. In a recent intervention, we observed that naturally occurring variation in people's expectations about the benefits of weight loss had a more systematic effect on people's weight loss practices than did experimentally induced variation in expectations (Finch et al., 2005). Findings such as these may indicate that even though people can be induced to hold a set of beliefs that are known to lead to a desired outcome (e.g., optimistic expectations regarding behavior change), the strength of these elicited beliefs may not be sufficient to motivate behavior change. Moreover, these findings can then motivate future efforts, both in the laboratory and in the field, to better describe the critical features a given construct must have to motivate behavior. For instance, the confidence with which people hold their expectations about behavior change (cf. Petty, Brinol, & Tormala, 2002) may be a critical determinant of the expectations' influence on people's behavioral practices.

Innovations in our understanding of the determinants of health behavior change are most likely to arise if we capitalize on the opportunities afforded by linking theory and practice. For a theory to evolve, its propositions need to be tested. Of course, the laboratory will continue to be an essential component of this process, but theorists will find that interventions allow for the development of an evidence base that will enable them to see the boundary conditions for their theoretical propositions, and to evaluate the relative contribution of different factors that have been shown previously to predict behavior. The resulting refinements to theory should only enhance its practical utility, which in turn should serve to increase its impact on interventions, creating an even more substantial evidence base on which to evaluate and refine the theory.

## ACKNOWLEDGMENTS

Preparation of this chapter was supported in part by Grant No. NS38441 from the National Institute of Neurological Disorders and Stroke, and a sabbatical supplement grant from the College of Liberal Arts, University of Minnesota.

## NOTES

1. It should be recognized that people's behavior is also shaped by features of the broader environment in which they live, such as public policy decision regarding taxation, access to health care, and the availability of places to exercise (Stokols, 1996; Stokols, Grzywacz, McMahan, & Phillips, 2003). Although they are not the primary focus of this chapter, these structural factors may affect behavior directly by precluding any decision to act, or indirectly by altering people's thoughts and feelings about the behavior.

2. This perspective suggests that the development of a richer description of how the rewards and costs afforded by a behavior unfold over time (e.g., Jeffery et al., 2004) would enable investigators to identify behavioral domains for which this phase in the behavior change process is particularly difficult to negotiate. Again, however, such a description is beyond the scope of this chapter.

3. In those cases in which people anticipate problems with a behavior (e.g., they expect it will be hard to find time to exercise), people will be more satisfied with their actions if their expectations regarding potential problems are not met.

## REFERENCES


Affleck, G., Tennen, H., Zautra, A., Urrows, S., Abeles, M., & Karoly, P. (2001). Women's pursuit of personal goals in daily life with fibromyalgia: A value–expectancy analysis. *Journal of Counseling and Clinical Psychology, 69*, 587–596.

Ahluwalia, J. S., Resnicow, K., & Clark, W. S. (1998). Knowledge about smoking, reasons for smoking, and reasons for wishing to quit in inner-city African Americans. *Ethnicity and Disease, 8*, 385–393.

Aiken, L. S., West, S. G., Woodward, C. K., & Reno, R. R. (1994). Health beliefs and compliance with mammography screening recommendations in asymptomatic women. *Health Psychology, 13*, 122–129.

Ajzen, I. (1991). The theory of planned behavior. *Organizational Behavior and Human Decision Processes, 50*, 179–211.

Ajzen, I., & Fishbein, M. (1980). *Understanding attitudes and predicting social behavior.* Englewood Cliffs, NJ: Prentice Hall.

Anderson, E. W., & Sullivan, M. W. (1993). The antecedents and consequences of customer satisfaction for firms. *Marketing Science, 12*, 125–143.

Aspinwall, L. G., & Brunhart, S. M. (1996). Distinguishing optimism from denial: Optimistic beliefs predict attention to health threats. *Personality and Social Psychology Bulletin, 22*, 993–1003.

Aspinwall, L. G., Richter, L., & Hoffman, R. R., III. (2001). Understanding how optimism works: An examination of optimists' adaptive moderation of belief and behavior. In E. C. Chang (Ed.), *Optimism and pessmism: Implications for theory, research, and practice* (pp. 217–238). Washington, DC: American Psychological Association.

Aspinwall, L. G., & Taylor, S. E. (1993). Effects of social comparison direction, threat, and self-esteem on affect, self-evaluation, and expected success. *Journal of Personality and Social Psychology Bulletin, 64*, 708–722.

Bandura, A. (1986). *Social foundations of thought and action: A social cognitive theory.* Englewood Cliffs, NJ: Prentice Hall.

Bandura, A. (1997). *Self-efficacy: The exercise of control.* New York: Freeman.

Baumeister, R. F., Heatherton, T. F., & Tice, D. M. (1994). *Losing control: How and why people fail at self-regulation.* San Diego, CA: Academic Press.

Baldwin, A. S., Rothman, A. J., Hertel, A. W., Linde, J. A., Jeffery, R. W., Finch, E. A., et al. (2006). Specifying the determinants of the initiation and maintenance of behavior change: An examination of self-efficacy, satisfaction, and smoking cessation. *Health Psychology, 25*(5), 626–634.

Bolton, R. N., & Drew, J. H. (1991). A longitudinal analysis of the impact of service changes on customer attitudes. *Journal of Marketing, 55*, 1–9.

Brownell, K. D., Marlatt, G. A., Lichtenstein, E., & Wilson, G. T. (1986). Understanding and preventing relapse. *American Psychologist, 41*, 765–782.

Campbell, J. D., & Fairey, P. J. (1985). Effects of self-esteem, hypothetical explanations, and verbalization of expectancies on future performance. *Journal of Personality and Social Psychology, 48*, 1097–1111.

Chassin, L., Presson, C. C., Sherman, S. J., & Kim, K. (2002). Long-term psychological sequelae of smoking cessation and relapse. *Health Psychology, 21*, 438–443.

Conner, M., & Norman, P. (2005). *Predicting health behaviour: Research and practice with social cognition models* (2nd ed.). Buckingham, UK: Open University Press.

Cozzarelli, C. (1993). Personality and self-efficacy as predictors of coping with abortion. *Journal of Personality and Social Psychology, 65*, 1224–1236.

Eiser, J. R., van der Pligt, J., Raw, M., & Sutton, S. R. (1985). Trying to stop smoking: Effects of perceived addiction, attributions for failure, and expectancy of success. *Journal of Behavioral Medicine, 8*, 321–341.

Elliot, A. J., & Church, M. A. (1997). A hierarchical model of approach and avoidance achievement motivation. *Journal of Personality and Social Psychology, 72*, 218–232.

Elliot, A. J., & McGregor, H. A. (1999). Test anxiety and the hierarchical model of approach and avoidance achievement motivation. *Journal of Personality and Social Psychology, 76*, 628–644.

Elliot, A. J., & McGregor, H. A. (2001). A 2 × 2 achievement goal framework. *Journal of Personality and Social Psychology, 80*, 501–519.

Ferguson, E., & Bibby, P. A. (2002). Predicting future blood donor returns: Past behavior, intentions, and observer effects. *Health Psychology, 21*, 513–518.

Finch, E. A., Linde, J. A., Jeffery, R. W., Rothman, A. J., King, C. M., & Levy, R. L. (2005). The effects of outcome expectations and satisfaction on weight loss and maintenance: Correlational and experimental analyses. *Health Psychology, 24*, 608–616.

Geers, A. L., & Lassiter, G. D. (2002). Effects of affective expectations on affective experience: The moderating role of optimism–pessimism. *Personality and Social Psychology Bulletin, 28*, 1026–1039.

Gerrard, M., Gibbons, F. X., Benthin, A. C., & Hessling, R. M. (1996). A longitudinal study of the reciprocal nature of risk behaviors and cognitions in adolescents: What you do shapes what you think, and vice versa. *Health Psychology, 16*, 344–354.

Gibbons, F. X., Blanton, H., Gerrard, M., Buunk, B., & Eggleston, T. (2000). Does social comparison make a difference?: Optimism as a moderator of the relation between comparison level and academic performance. *Personality and Social Psychology Bulletin, 26*, 637–648.

Gibbons, F. X., Eggleston, T. J., & Benthin, A. C. (1997). Cognitive reactions to smoking relapse: The reciprocal relation between dissonance and self-esteem. *Journal of Personality and Social Psychology, 72*, 184–195.

Gibson, B., & Sanbonmatsu, D. M. (2004). Optimisim, pessimism, and gambling: The downside of optimism. *Personality and Social Psychology Bulletin*, *30*, 149–160.

Gollwitzer, P. M. (1996). The volitional benefits of planning. In P. M. Gollwitzer & J. A. Bargh (Eds.), *The psychology of action: Linking cognitions and motivation to behavior* (pp. 287–312). New York: Guilford Press.

Gollwitzer, P. M. (1999). Implementation intentions: Strong effects of simple plans. *American Psychologist*, *54*, 493–503.

Gwaltney, C. J., Shiffman, S., Paty, J. A., Liu, K. S., Kassel, J. D., Gnys, M., et al. (2002). Using self-efficacy judgments to predict characteristics of lapses to smoking. *Journal of Consulting and Clinical Psychology*, *70*, 1140–1149.

Hedeker, D., & Mermelstein, R. J. (1996). Application of random-effects regression models in relapse research. *Addiction*, *91*, S211–S229.

Helgeson, V. S. (2003). Cognitive adaptation, psychological adjustment, and disease progression among angioplasty patients: 4 years later. *Health Psychology*, *22*, 30–38.

Hertel, A. W., Finch, E., Kelly, K., King, C., Lando, H., Linde, J., et al. (in press). The impact of outcome expectations and satisfaction on the initiation and maintenance of smoking cessation: An experimental test. *Health Psychology*.

Higgins, E. T. (1998). Promotion and prevention: Regulatory focus as a motivational principle. In M. P. Zanna (Ed.), *Advances in experimental social psychology* (Vol. 30, pp. 1–46). San Diego, CA: Academic Press.

Higgins, E. T. (1999). Promotion and prevention as a motivational duality: Implications for evaluative processes. In S. Chaiken & Y. Trope (Ed.), *Dual-process theories in social psychology* (pp. 503–526). New York: Guilford Press.

Iacobucci, D., Grayson, K. A., & Ostrom, A. L. (1994). The calculus of service quality and customer satisfaction: Theoretical and empirical differentiation and integration. *Advances in Services Marketing and Management*, *3*, 1–67.

Jeffery, R. W. (2004). How can health behavior theory be made more useful for intervention research? *International Journal of Behavioral Nutrition and Physical Activity*, *1*, 10.

Jeffery, R. W., Kelly, K. M., Rothman, A. J., Sherwood, N. E., & Boutelle, K. N. (2004). The weight loss experience: A descriptive analysis. *Annals of Behavioral Medicine*, *27*, 100–106.

Keiningham, T. L., Perkins-Munn, T., & Evans, H. (2003). The impact of customer satisfaction on share-of-wallet in a business-to-business environment. *Journal of Service Research*, *6*, 37–50.

King, C., Rothman, A. J., & Jeffery, R. W. (2002). The challenge study: Theory-based interventions for smoking and weight loss. *Health Education Research*, *17*, 522–530.

King, M. R., & Manaster, G. J. (1977). Body image, self-esteem, expectations, self-assessments, and actual success in a simulated job interview. *Journal of Applied Psychology*, *62*, 589–594.

Lando, H. A., Pirie, P. L., Roski, J., McGovern, P. G., & Schmid, L. A. (1996). Promoting abstinence among relapsed chronic smokers: The effect of telephone support. *American Journal of Public Health*, *86*, 1786–1790.

Lewin, K. (1951). *Field theory in social science: Selected theoretical papers*. New York: Harper & Row.

Lichtenstein, E., & Cohen, S. (1990). Prospective analysis of two modes of unaided smoking cessation. *Health Education Research*, *5*, 63–72.

Maddux, J. E., & Rogers, R. W. (1983). Protection motivation and self-efficacy: A revised theory of fear appeals and attitude change. *Journal of Experimental Social Psychology*, *19*, 469–479.

Marlatt, G. A., & Donovan, D. M. (Eds.). (2005). *Relapse prevention: Maintenance strategies in the treatment of addictive behaviors* (2nd ed.). New York: Guilford Press.

Mittal, V., & Kamakura, W. A. (2001). Satisfaction, repurchase intent, and repurchase behavior: Investigating the moderating effect of customer characteristics. *Journal of Marketing Research*, *38*, 131–142.

Mook, D. G. (1983). In defense of external invalidity. *American Psychologist*, *38*, 379–387.

Noar, S. M., & Zimmerman, R. S. (2005). Health behavior theory and cumulative knowledge regarding health behaviors: Are we moving in the right direction? *Health Education Research*, *20*, 275–290.

Norcross, J. C., & Vangarelli, D. J. (1989). The resolution solution: Longitudinal examination of New Year's change attempts. *Journal of Substance Abuse*, *1*, 127–134.

Norman, P., Conner, M., & Bell, R. (1999). The theory of planned behavior and smoking cessation. *Health Psychology*, *18*, 89–94.

Peterson, C. (2000). The future of optimism. *American Psychologist*, *55*, 44–55.

Petty, R. E., Brinol, P., & Tormala, Z. L. (2002). Thought confidence as a determinant of persuasion: The self-validation hypothesis. *Journal of Personality and Social Psychology*, *82*, 722–741.

Polivy, J., & Herman, C. P. (2002). If at first you don't succeed: False hopes of self-change. *American Psychologist*, *57*, 677–689.

Prochaska, J. O., DiClemente, C. C., & Norcross, J. C. (1992). In search of how people change: Applications to addictive behaviors. *American Psychologist*, *47*, 1102–1114.

Prochaska, J. O., & Velicer, W. F. (1997). The transtheoretical model of health behavior change. *American Journal of Health Promotion*, *12*, 38–48.

Rakowski, W., Dube, C. E., Marcus, B. H., Prochaska, J. O., Velicer, W. F., & Abrams, D. B. (1992). Assessing elements of women's decisions about mammography. *Health Psychology*, *11*, 111–118.

Rosenstock, I. M., Strecher, V. J., & Becker, M. H. (1988). Social learning theory and the health belief model. *Health Education Quarterly*, *15*, 175–183.

Rothman, A. J. (2000) Toward a theory-based analysis of behavioral maintenance. *Health Psychology, 19*, 1–6.

Rothman, A. J. (2004). Is there nothing more practical than a good theory?: Why innovations and advances in health behavior change will arise if interventions are more theory-friendly. *International Journal of Behavioral Nutrition and Physical Activity, 1*, 11.

Rothman, A. J., Baldwin, A. S., & Hertel, A. W. (2004). Self-regulation and behavior change: Disentangling behavioral initiation and behavioral maintenance. In R. F. Baumeister & K. D. Vohs (Eds.), *Handbook of self-regulation: Research, theory, and applications* (pp. 130–148). New York: Guilford Press.

Rothman, A. J., & Salovey, P. (2007). The reciprocal relation between principles and practice: Social psychology and health behavior. In A. W. Kruglanski & E. T. Higgins (Eds.), *Social psychology: Handbook of basic principles* (2nd ed., pp. 826–849). New York: Guilford Press.

Salovey, P., Rothman, A. J., & Rodin, J. (1998). Health behavior. In D. T. Gilbert, S. T. Fiske, & G. Lindzey (Eds.), *The handbook of social psychology* (4th ed., Vol. 2, pp. 633–683). New York: McGraw-Hill.

Schachter, S. (1982). Recidivism and self-cure of smoking and obesity. *American Psychologist, 37*, 436–444.

Scheier, M. F., Matthews, K. A., Owens, J. F., Magovern, G. J., Sr., Lefebvre, R. C., Abbott, R. A., et al. (1989). Dispositional optimism and recovery from coronary artery bypass surgery: The beneficial effects on physical and psychological well-being. *Journal of Personality and Social Psychology, 57*, 1024–1040.

Schmeichel, B. J., & Baumeister, R. (2004). Self-regulatory strength. In R. F. Baumeister & K. D. Vohs (Eds.), *Handbook of self-regulation: Research, theory, and applications* (pp. 84–98). New York: Guilford Press.

Schwarz, N., & Strack, F. (1991). Evaluating one's life: A judgmental model of subjective well-being. In F. Strack, M. Argyle, & N. Schwarz (Eds.), *Subjective well-being: An interdisciplinary perspective* (pp. 27–47). Oxford, UK: Pergamon Press.

Shiffman, S., Balabanis, M. H., Paty, J. A., Engberg, J., Gwaltney, C. J., Liu, K. S., et al. (2000). Dynamic effects of self-efficacy on smoking lapse and relapse. *Health Psychology, 19*, 315–323.

Shiffman, S., Hickcox, M., Paty, J. A., Gnys, M., Kassel, J. D., & Richards, T. J. (1996). Progression from a smoking lapse to relapse: Prediction from abstinence violation effects, nicotine dependence, and lapse characteristics. *Journal of Consulting and Clinical Psychology, 64*, 993–1002.

Spreng, R. A., Mackenzie, S. B., & Olshavsky, R. W. (1996). A reexamination of the determinants of consumer satisfaction. *Journal of Marketing, 60*, 15–32.

Spreng, R. A., & Page, T. J. (2001). The impact of confidence in expectations on consumer satisfaction. *Psychology and Marketing, 18*, 1187–1204.

Stokols, D. (1996). Translating social ecological theory into guidelines for community health promotion. *American Journal of Health Promotion, 10*, 282–298.

Stokols, D., Grzywacz, J. G., McMahan, S., & Phillips, K. (2003). Increasing the health promotive capacity of human environments. *American Journal of Health Promotion, 18*, 4–13.

Sullivan, H., & Rothman, A. J. (2006). *Defining and describing approach and avoidance goals.* Unpublished manuscript, University of Minnesota.

Szymanski, D. M., & Henard, D. H. (2001). Customer satisfaction: A meta-analysis of the empirical evidence. *Journal of the Academy of Marketing Science, 29*, 16–35.

Weinstein, N. D. (1988). The precaution adoption process. *Health Psychology, 7*, 355–386.

Weinstein, N. D., & Rothman, A. J. (2005). Revitalizing research on health behavior theories. *Health Education Research, 20*, 294–297.

Witkiewitz, K., & Marlatt, G. A. (2004). Relapse prevention for alcohol and drug problems: That was Zen, this is Tao. *American Psychologist, 59*, 224–235.

Wood, W., Quinn, J. M., & Kashy, D. A. (2002). Habits in everyday life: Thought, emotion, and action. *Journal of Personality and Social Psychology, 83*, 1281–1297.

Worth, K., Sullivan, H., Hertel, A. W., Jeffery, R. W., & Rothman, A. J. (2005). Are there times when avoidance goals can be beneficial?: A look at smoking cessation. *Basic and Applied Social Psychology, 27*, 107–116.

Yi, Y. (1993). The determinants of consumer satisfaction: The moderating role of ambiguity. In L. McAlister & M. Rothschild (Eds.), *Advances in consumer research series 20* (pp. 502–506). Provo, UT: Advances in Consumer Research.

Yi, Y., & La, S. (2004). What influences the relationship between customer satisfaction and repurchase intention?: Investigating the effects of adjusted expectations and customer loyalty. *Psychology and Marketing, 21*, 351–373.

Yoon, S., & Kim, J. (2000). An empirical validation of a loyalty model based on expectation disconfirmation. *Journal of Consumer Marketing, 17*, 120–136.

Zwick, R., Pieters, R., & Baumgartner, H. (1995). On the practical significance of hindsight bias: The case of the expectancy-disconfirmation model of consumer satisfaction. *Organizational Behavior and Human Decision Processes, 64*, 103–117.

Chapter 33

# Social Exclusion, Motivation, and Self-Defeating Behavior

## WHY BREAKUPS LEAD TO DRUNKENNESS AND ICE CREAM

Jean M. Twenge

Each January, many people make an earnest list of their New Year's resolutions. If you're ambitious, your list might look something like this:

1. Eat better: Eat more fruits and vegetables; take vitamins; avoid unhealthy foods like chips, cookies, candy, and ice cream.
2. Exercise.
3. Lose weight.
4. Stop procrastinating and get important things done.
5. Go to the dentist.
6. Stop watching so much TV, reading so many unenlightening magazines, and playing so many mindless video games.
7. Don't gamble.
8. Don't waste money on clothes, games, and useless things.
9. Drive safely and more slowly.
10. Keep trying at important tasks even when you're frustrated.
11. Stop drinking alcohol.
12. Stop smoking.
13. Lose the number of the drug dealer.

So many good intentions! Yet by February or March, you are right back where you started: You're sitting on the couch, eating handfuls of candy and potato chips, reading *Entertainment Weekly*, and watching TV. You might even be washing down the junk food with a little whiskey or wine (a good merlot goes well with potato chips, you have heard). The night before, you decided to skip aerobics class to go shopping. Because the store was closing in an hour, you drove 80 mph on the freeway to get there. The house hasn't been cleaned in weeks, and you've decided not to work on your novel right now. Depending on your preferences, you might have even bought some cigarettes, scored some weed, and/or called the coke dealer. And the dentist? Too much trouble and pain. "Forget it!" you think. "Let the Cheez Whiz and Pop Rocks rot my teeth! I don't care!"

Why do people make lists of resolutions and not stick to them? In many cases, they make tradeoffs that result in self-defeating behavior (Baumeister & Scher, 1988). These tradeoffs involve choices between two options, one with long-term benefits and the other with short-term benefits. The resolutions listed above have very worthwhile long-term benefits: longer life, better health, saving money for the future, accomplishing important goals, and keeping your teeth. (Not to mention staying out of jail, if your preferences run toward illegal substances.) In other words, why do people fail to keep such resolutions and stupid things? Probably because in the short term, the resolutions either are unpleasant or involve the avoidance of pleasure.

A copious amount of research documents the difficulty people have in postponing pleasure for the sake of long-term gain. Many people drink alcohol, smoke cigarettes, and use illegal drugs due to the pleasant sensations these substances produce (McCollam, Burish, Maisto, & Sobell, 1980). Smoking and drinking alcohol both lead to feelings of relaxation and can provide a pleasant escape from self-awareness (Golding, Burnam, Benjamin, & Wells, 1992; Silverstein, 1982; Wicklund, 1975). Despite the many serious risks to health caused by cigarettes, many people who smoke find it impossible to quit. Even getting a health checkup is difficult for people. Patients fail to appear at more than 25% of medical appointments (Sackett & Snow, 1979). Eating a balanced diet and exercising regularly are also difficult for most people, as the epidemic of obesity in the United States amply demonstrates. Media sources are filled with elusive schemes that promise quick, painless weight loss, and even legitimate medical sources peddle weight loss drugs and gastric bypass surgery. People wish for the quick fix because sticking to a long-term diet regimen is so unpleasant. Overall, people regularly fail at treatment regimens assigned by doctors, particularly if they are time-consuming (Haynes, 1979).

Clearly, it is difficult to sacrifice short-term pleasures for the sake of long-term gains. Doing so requires a large amount of *self-control* or *self-regulation*, commonly defined as the human capacity to alter or override natural responses, including thoughts, emotions, and actions. Several authors have documented the cascade of poor outcomes that occur when the self's reserve of control becomes depleted (e.g., Baumeister, Heatherton, & Tice, 1994; Muraven & Baumeister, 2000; Muraven, Tice, & Baumeister, 1998; Vohs & Heatherton, 2000). Given the speed at which most people abandon their New Year's resolutions, it appears that the self-control system can easily break down, often leading to self-defeating behavior.

Self-control often suffers when control must be exercised over several successive tasks; like a muscle, the system grows tired (Muraven & Baumeister, 2000). For example, it is more difficult to cook and eat a healthy meal when people have been working hard all day and are physically and mentally tired. Dieters find it more difficult to refuse chocolate cake on day 10 of a diet than on day 1. In these circumstances, self-defeating behavior occurs because people have a limited reserve of self-control. However, people sometimes engage in self-defeating behavior even when they have not depleted their self-control on a previous task. For example, people in bad moods are more likely to behave in a self-defeating way. In a series of experiments, people who were angry or sad were more likely to take self-defeating risks (Leith & Baumeister, 1996). Many people also engage in self-defeating behavior after experiencing a romantic breakup or another type of social rejection. Especially for women, typical (or at least stereotypical) postbreakup behavior is to sit on the couch and eat an entire carton of ice cream. For men, the stereotype runs toward getting drunk at a bar, drowning their sorrows in beer and whiskey. Although overeating and getting drunk sound like fairly different reactions, they are both classic self-defeating behaviors. But how true are these images? Do social rejection and exclusion really lead to self-defeating behavior?

## SOCIAL EXCLUSION AND SELF-DEFEATING BEHAVIOR

Beginning in the fall of 1999, my colleagues and I carried out a series of experiments to address this question (Baumeister, DeWall, Ciarocco, & Twenge, 2005; Twenge, Catanese, & Baumeister, 2002). One of these papers focuses specifically on social exclusion and self-defeating behavior (Twenge et al., 2002), and the other addresses social exclusion and self-control/self-regulation (Baumeister et al., 2005). For the purposes of this chapter, however, I interweave the experiments from both papers. Although some self-defeating behaviors do not entail self-control failures (e.g., suicide), most involve tradeoffs between short-term and long-term goals—a process that involves self-control (Baumeister & Scher, 1988). These are the behaviors most relevant to normal variations in self-defeat, and they are also those most linked to self-control. Thus all of the behaviors we studied in these two papers can be seen as self-defeating behaviors, as all reflect the preference for short-term pleasure at the expense of long-term gains.

## Correlational Evidence from the "Real World"

Even before we began to study social exclusion and self-defeating behavior in the laboratory, we found an extraordinary amount of correlational evidence linking the two. Compared to married men, single men are more likely to be arrested for speeding or reckless driving (Harrington & McBride, 1970) and are more likely to be involved in car accidents (Harano, Peck, & McBride, 1975). Single men are especially likely to be involved in alcohol-related crashes (Richman, 1985). Single people are also more likely to abuse alcohol and drugs (Williams, Takeuchi, & Adair, 1992). In addition, married people are often mentally and physically healthier than single, divorced, or widowed individuals (DeLongis, Folkman, & Lazarus, 1988; Goodwin, Hunt, Key, & Samet, 1987; Williams et al., 1992). The health problems experienced by socially isolated individuals may well be linked to self-defeating behaviors and poor self-regulation, because poor regulation of some behaviors (e.g., overeating, smoking, failing to exercise, alcohol and drug addiction) causes harm to health.

In addition, the literature on bereavement links exclusion and self-defeating behavior. Bereaved people are more likely to die from causes related to risky behavior, including accidents and cirrhosis of the liver (usually caused by alcohol abuse). Incredibly, bereaved people are also more likely to be murdered (Stroebe & Stroebe, 1987). Attachment theory suggests that the emotional exclusion produced by the loss of a close relationship should lead to despair and "giving up." This effect goes beyond simple social loneliness, as emotional loneliness from a lack of close relationships leads to the most distress (Stroebe, Stroebe, Abakoumkin, & Schut, 1996).

Although these studies suggest links between social exclusion and self-defeating behavior, they are almost exclusively correlational. Thus we cannot be certain that social exclusion actually causes self-defeating behavior. The converse hypothesis is also plausible: People who engage in self-defeating behaviors may be rejected by others. For example, consider the link between marriage (a common form of social inclusion) and good health. This correlation might mean that marriage leads to good health. On the other hand, it could mean that people in poor health are less likely to marry. Third-variable explanations are also plausible. Perhaps, for example, careless and impulsive people are both less likely to marry and more likely to be in poor health. Another problem with the correlational findings is that most have not measured social exclusion per se. Instead, they examined only current marital status without regard to the quality of the marital relationship or the number and quality of other relationships. Thus these studies do not definitively establish a link between social exclusion and self-defeating behavior.

## Experimental Research

For these reasons, we conducted a series of experimental studies to test the hypothesis that social exclusion causes self-defeating behavior. In these studies, we first manipulated people's perception of social inclusion versus exclusion. We have used two different methods for manipulating social exclusion. The first is a group rejection; it begins when participants meet four to six same-sex peers and talk as a group for 10 minutes. They are then asked to nominate the two people they would like to work with on a subsequent task. By random assignment, half of the participants hear that everyone chose them, and the other half hear that no one chose them. This is similar to getting "voted off the island" or "voted out of the tribe" on the reality TV show *Survivor.* To many people, it evokes the common (and painful) childhood experience of being chosen last for a sports team.

In the other manipulation, participants first complete a personality test. They are given their true score on extroversion, which is used as a segue into a randomly assigned prediction about their future (ostensibly based on their personality profile). In the "Future Alone" condition, participants are told that they are likely to end up alone for much of their adult lives. In the "Future Belonging" condition, participants hear that their future will involve a rich network of personal relationships. A control group, called "Misfortune Control," hears that they will be accident-prone later in life (thus they receive a negative prediction that is unrelated to relationships). We sometimes call this manipulation "No One Will Ever Love You." However, I also favor the suggestion of a colleague (Kent Harber), who suggested I call it "Killer Fortune Cookies."

### Eating Cookies

The first experiment (the first I ever completed on social rejection) used the group manipulation: Participants heard either that no one chose them (rejection) or that everyone chose them (acceptance). I then asked participants to taste-test some cookies; a bowl containing 35 bite-size chocolate chip cookies was placed in front of each person. I told the participants to "eat as much as you need to judge the taste, smell, and texture." They were also given a taste-test form asking them to rate the taste of the cookies. Participants were then left alone with the bowl of cookies and the form for 10 minutes. This presented participants with a clear dilemma: "Should I eat the yummy cookies," they might have thought, "or should I restrain myself from overeating?" A majority of students at Case Western Reserve University, where this study was conducted, rated eating cookies and other fattening snacks as an undesirable, unhealthy behavior that they would prefer to avoid (Tice, Bratslavsky, & Baumeister, 2001). In addition, the need to curtail consumption of fattening foods is widely recognized as a growing, worldwide problem (contributing to the so-called "obesity epidemic") Thus eating a large number of cookies is clearly a self-defeating behavior—not immediately life-threatening, to be sure, but still not a healthy thing to do.

As it turns out, the image of the breakup victim eating a carton of ice cream is fairly accurate: Participants who were rejected by their peers ate twice as many cookies as accepted participants (rejected participants ate an average of 8.94 bite-size cookies, and accepted participants ate 4.40 cookies). This result was unchanged after controlling for time since the participants' last meal and for their rating of how good the cookies tasted. In fact, taste was unrelated to eating for the rejected participants; the correlation between rated taste of cookies and amount eaten failed to reach significance among these participants. In contrast, taste did predict eating among accepted participants. This suggests that accepted participants ate in relative moderation as a response to the good taste, whereas the rejected participants ate in excess regardless of taste. Rejected participants' comments also demonstrated that their eating was not motivated by taste and enjoyment. One said, "I kept eating the cookies and I didn't know why." Another said, "I wasn't hungry, but I ate the cookies anyway." These comments (along with the low correlation between taste and eating) suggest a breakdown of self-regulation and perhaps an absence of meaningful, thought-controlling action. Overall, rejected people were more likely to engage in the self-defeating behavior of overeating an unhealthy snack food.

### Making Other Unhealthy Choices

In another experiment, we tested the effect of social exclusion on healthy versus unhealthy choices. This experiment used the Future Alone manipulation: Some participants heard that they were likely to be alone later in life, whereas others heard that they would have good relationships or that they were likely to be accident-prone later in life. After receiving this feedback, participants were given three choices to make: They could receive a candy bar or a granola bar; read a magazine (such as *People* or *Entertainment Weekly*) or fill out a health questionnaire; and sit or run in place before measuring a pulse. In each case, the second choice was explicitly presented as healthier. Thus the first choice in each pair, despite being more pleasurable, was also less healthy and thus self-defeating in the long run. Consistent with the previous results, socially excluded participants made fewer healthy choices (0.78), compared to 1.94 in the other conditions. Thus excluded participants were more likely to choose the pleasurable yet unhealthy self-defeating behaviors than the less pleasurable but more healthy behaviors. Once again, the image of socially isolated persons is clear: They are sitting on the couch, eating candy, and reading an entertainment magazine.

### Persistence on Unpleasant or Frustrating Tasks

Two additional experiments examined persistence. In the first, participants underwent the Future Alone manipulation and were then presented with a challenge: They would be given a nickel for every ounce of an unpleasant beverage they managed to drink (Muraven, 1998). "Unpleasant" is actually an understatement; the beverage was orange Kool-Aid made with a pint of vinegar. (And yes, the lab did smell like vinegar for weeks afterward.) Participants were told that the drink was healthy, and that there was the small monetary reward involved for drinking it. Twenty small paper cups were arranged in front of each participant, each holding 1 ounce; thus drinking each ounce required a separate act of self-control. Participants were told that the amount they drank was up to them. Participants who had heard they were likely to be alone did not persist at the task as long; they drank a little more than 2 ounces of the vinegar Kool-Aid, compared to 7–8 ounces for those in the control groups. Thus the Future Alone participants drank less of a healthy yet bad-tasting beverage, even when a small monetary reward was involved. Clearly the socially excluded people found it more difficult to force themselves to do something unpleasant, despite the payoff in money and health.

Another experiment examined persistence at unsolvable puzzles. Unsolvable puzzles are frustrating and discouraging, and people may often be inclined to quit trying. However, persistence in the face of failure is admired in our society and is sometimes rewarded with success, so effective self-regulators may override the impulse to quit and instead force themselves to keep trying. Participants underwent the Future Alone manipulation and were then shown how to trace the lines of a puzzle. The sample puzzle was solvable (one could trace the lines completely without picking up the pencil). Participants were then given two additional puzzles; unbeknownst to them, these puzzles were not solvable (the lines could not be traced without picking up the pencil). They were then left alone to work on the puzzles and were told to ring a bell when they were finished or gave up. The amount of time participants chose to work on the puzzles served as a measure of self-regulation (Baumeister, Bratslavsky, Muraven, & Tice, 1998). Consistent with the previous findings, Future Alone participants gave up after 21 minutes, compared to 28 minutes in the control conditions. Given that many difficult tasks in life require persistence, this shows once again that socially excluded people engage in self-defeating behavior.

### Procrastination

If socially excluded people consistently choose short-term pleasures over long-term gains, it seems very likely that they would be tempted to procrastinate rather than do more productive (but possibly boring and unpleasant) things. Recent research has found that procrastinating with frivolous, fun, and distracting activities is a strategy people use to put off their work and feel better immediately (Tice et al., 2001). This strategy is ultimately self-defeating, however. Procrastinators, even those who claim they "work well under pressure," show significant deficits in performance compared to nonprocrastinators (Ferrari & Tice, 2000; Tice & Baumeister, 1997). In addition, procrastinators suffer increased stress and illness (Tice & Baumeister, 1997).

After receiving the Future Alone prediction, participants heard that they would later take a math test that was predictive of overall intelligence. Participants were given 15 minutes to practice for the test, using a series of very boring math problems (such as long division and multiplication of three-digit numbers). Alternatively, they could procrastinate by reading magazines (such as *Maxim* and *Cosmopolitan*) or playing video games; the experimenter mentioned that she sometimes played Tetris on the Game Boy or read the magazines when she was waiting for participants to arrive. The experimenter then left each participant alone, but sat behind a one-way mirror with a view of the participant's room. She then recorded how the participants spent their time during the 15-minute practice period. The results showed that the Future Alone participants spent nearly half of their time procrastinating (7.12 minutes), compared to only 2.98 minutes on average for the participants in the other two conditions. Thus the Future Alone participants were much more likely to procrastinate by doing pleasurable things rather than concentrating on boring math problems that nevertheless might help them do better on an upcoming test. Once again, socially excluded people chose the short-term pleasures of magazines and games over the long-term benefits of superior academic performance. So not only do rejected persons sit on the couch and eat ice cream (or get drunk); they are likely to neglect their work or studies as well.

### *Regulating Attention*

We also examined socially excluded participants' ability to regulate their attention. Similar to the ability to persist and to overcome procrastination, regulating attention is an important skill if one is going to accomplish important goals at work or school. Not concentrating is clearly self-defeating, as it will result in inferior performance at most tasks. In addition, many self-control tasks involve attention regulation. For example, people seeking to control their sexual impulses may avoid exposure to sexual stimuli, and dieters may avoid cues that remind them of tempting, fatty foods.

In this experiment, participants received the Future Alone manipulation and then performed a dichotic listening task. Participants heard a male voice giving a speech on a policy issue in one ear, and a female voice reading a series of words in the other ear. They were told to ignore the speech and listen to the female voice reading the words; they were instructed to write down all of the words that contained a *p* or an *m*. Participants who had heard that they were likely to be alone later in life were not as able to regulate their attention; they wrote down fewer words than participants in the other conditions. This helps explain why socially excluded people find it difficult to get work done or to concentrate on studying. Not only do they feel more like indulging in pleasurable things, but they also find it difficult to concentrate on a task amidst distractions.

### *Taking Risks and Gambling*

Two additional experiments examined the effect of social exclusion on risk taking. As noted previously, single men are more likely to take risks while driving and get into more accidents (Harano et al., 1975). This is a somewhat different image from the rejected couch potato eating ice cream; it suggests that rejected people may make more actively self-defeating choices. Here the image is of a group of unattached young men speeding down the road, planning a risky yet amusing prank (such as hitting mailboxes with baseball bats or spray-painting a highway overpass). It is difficult to imagine a married man with children participating in such an activity, even if he is the same age as the other young men. These acts are clearly self-defeating, as they carry the very real risk of being caught and thrown in jail (or, at the very least, made to work to pay for the damage). The risk may be even more severe in some cases: In the movie *Dazed and Confused*, a group of young men who destroy mailboxes with a baseball bat are chased by a man firing a shotgun.

In our experiments, we were forced to measure more manageable risks. After undergoing the Future Alone manipulation, participants were given a choice between two lotteries. The risky choice offered a small chance of winning a moderate amount of money, whereas the safe choice offered a large chance of winning a small amount of money. In both cases, losing meant hearing a tape of very unpleasant noise. Worked out mathematically, the safe choice was by far the more beneficial, offering the greater payout in the long run and a lesser chance of hearing the unpleasant noise. Thus choosing the risky lottery was a self-defeating choice. In both experiments, socially excluded people were much more likely to choose the risky lottery choice (about 66% of the time), compared to the 15% who chose it in the other conditions. This has an obvious application to gambling, where people often lay out sums of money they are almost certain to lose. Thus socially excluded people are likely to take unnecessary and self-defeating risks.

### *Possible Mediators of the Effect*

Overall, these results show that socially excluded participants are more likely to engage in a full range of self-defeating behaviors, from eating unhealthy food to taking unwise risks. Somewhat to our surprise, none of the effects were mediated by mood. In all of our studies on social exclusion, we have found very few significant differences in mood between socially excluded people and the various control groups. This has been true across four different self-report mood measures, including a one-item measure anchored by "negative" and "positive"; the Positive and Negative Affect Schedule (Watson, Clark, & Tellegen, 1988); the Brief Mood Introspection Scale (Mayer & Gaschke, 1988); and a long list of negative and positive affect words drawn from a number of sources. Apparently social exclusion bypasses negative mood and goes straight to causing self-defeating behavior.

Another possibility for a mediator is a deconstructed state, which includes a loss of future orientation and a failure of rational, meaningful thought (Baumeister, 1990; Twenge et al., 2003). Rather than leading to emotional distress, social exclusion leads to a feeling of dumbstruck numbness that encourages a focus on the present rather than the future. This feeling of numbness may explain why socially excluded people tend to make consistently self-defeating choices. Like a deer mesmerized in a car's headlights, a rejected person freezes and fails to act rationally.

### Escape from Self-Awareness as a Motivation behind Self-Defeating Behavior

The desire to escape from self-awareness may explain why rejection causes self-defeating behavior. Compared to control groups, socially excluded participants were more likely to choose a chair that faced a wall instead of a chair that faced a mirror (Twenge, Catanese, & Baumeister, 2003). Thus excluded participants sought to avoid the heightened self-awareness that comes from facing a mirror. This may explain the link between social exclusion and self-defeating behavior, as many self-defeating behaviors are motivated by the desire to escape self-awareness (for a review, see Baumeister, 1991). For example, alcohol consumption reduces self-attention (Hull, Levenson, Young, & Sher, 1983), as does smoking (Wicklund, 1975). Many of the other self-defeating behaviors we measured also reduce self-awareness (e.g., reading a magazine or playing a game). Even the pleasure of eating sweet, fatty foods probably directs attention away from the self and the rejection. This explanation has intuitive appeal as well; by definition, self-defeating behavior is not rational. However, it makes sense that people who have been rejected might want to forget their troubles for a while. They may want to do anything that will provide a cushion of denial between them and the frightening thought of loneliness or rejection. This explains the common stereotype of the rejected man who promptly gets completely drunk. It may also explain why rejected people sometimes isolate themselves. This seems counterintuitive (rejection should lead to the seeking of new social bonds), but the rejected person finds it easier to be alone than to engage in the self-focus necessary to perform in social situations. Thus the desire to escape from self-awareness may mediate and explain the relationship between social exclusion and self-defeating behavior.

### Applications to Health Issues

As noted previously, correlational research has shown that married people are in better health than single, divorced, or widowed individuals (DeLongis et al., 1988; Goodwin et al., 1987; Williams et al., 1992). The experimental research presented in this chapter provides one reason for these findings: People who feel socially included are less likely to make self-defeating, unhealthy choices. This may occur because socially excluded people enter a state of numbness and tend to favor short-term pleasures over long-term gains. In addition, people with strong social connections may see more value in planning for the future; they may feel they have "something to live for" in a way that unconnected people do not. A recent advertising campaign for Cheerios touted the cholesterol-lowering powers of the cereal and asked, "Who are you eating them for?" In the ads, people talked about eating Cheerios for the sake of their spouses, children, and grandchildren. In other words, the ad campaign assumed that people wouldn't care much about their cholesterol for their own sake, but would want to live a long life in order to be with their loved ones. Similarly, a young man who has a wife and child is less likely to take stupid risks because he has people who are counting on him. An unattached young man, in contrast, may think, "Why not?" Although the underlying mechanisms are still unclear, there is a definite link between social exclusion and self-defeating behavior.

## SOCIAL EXCLUSION AND ANTISOCIAL VERSUS PROSOCIAL BEHAVIOR

Our lab and many others have also examined the link between social exclusion and aggression. We (Twenge, Baumeister, Tice, & Stucke, 2001) randomly assigned participants to experience rejection or acceptance. Rejected participants blasted a higher level of unpleasant white noise, even against an innocent target unconnected to the rejection. Buckley, Winkel, and Leary (2004) randomly assigned participants to be rejected or accepted by an unseen peer; rejected participants assigned the rejecting peer more unpleasant tapes and expressed more hostility. Warburton, Williams, and Cairns (2006) covaried ostracism (vs. inclusion) and level of control in an unpleasant situation. Ostracized participants who had no control were highly aggressive toward a peer who did not like spicy foods, assigning the peer to eat four times as much hot sauce as those in the other conditions. In a quasi-experimental study, Kirkpatrick, Waugh, Valencia, and Webster (2002) found that participants with low social self-esteem (who felt excluded in real life) also allocated more hot sauce to a spice-hating peer. Another set of studies found that socially excluded people were less helpful, cooperative, and prosocial (Twenge, Baumeister, DeWall, Ciarocco, & Bartels, 2007).

In addition, correlational research finds a relationship between social rejection and aggression. A careful study of school shooting incidents during the late 1990s found that almost all of the perpetrators had experienced repeated social rejection (Leary, Kowalski, Smith, & Phillips, 2003). Many other incidents of physical and verbal aggression result from social rejection. The Surgeon General's report on youth violence (Office of the Surgeon General, 2001) found that social rejection (conceptualized as "weak social ties") was the most significant risk factor for adolescent violence—stronger than gang membership, poverty, or drug use. Adults who are socially isolated display similar behavior; single men are more likely to commit crimes than married men, even when age is controlled for (Sampson & Laub, 1990). A review of this research found numerous studies linking the lack of social support to aggressive and antisocial behavior (Leary, Twenge, & Quinlivan, 2006).

Given that aggression is likely to drive people away rather than bring them closer, aggression after social rejection seems counterintuitive and self-defeating. One would expect rejected people to become more prosocial in an attempt to make new friends and compensate for the rejection. In other words, rejected people should be motivated to seek belongingness in the group once again (Baumeister & Leary, 1995). Instead, rejected people are more aggressive and less prosocial. This is clearly another example of self-defeating behavior: Lashing out with aggression will only make more people reject them. Thus the increased aggression and decreased prosocial behavior that follow from social exclusion are additional examples of the self-defeating behavior that often accompanies social isolation.

## CONCLUSIONS

There are many reasons why people engage in self-defeating behaviors. Overall, it is remarkable that people do not act in self-defeating ways more often, as the short-term pleasures often seem so much more real than the long-term payoffs of better health in old age and saving money (Milburn, 1978). Humans are perhaps fortunate that at least some of the pleasurable things in life—such as sex—actually are evolutionarily adaptive. But most other pleasurable things, paradoxically enough, are not particularly adaptive. Perhaps they were at one time (e.g., eating fatty foods), but in the current social environment they have become self-defeating behaviors. Still, it is possible for people to muster the self-control to regulate their behaviors and do the things on their New Year's resolution list; it just isn't very much fun. Thus the process can easily break down. There are many reasons why self-control may fail and people may engage in self-defeating behaviors; social rejection and exclusion appear to be among the proximate causes.

How can this be prevented? In other words, how can you keep from eating the whole carton of ice cream after a breakup? Perhaps knowledge is power in this case: If you know that you're likely to engage in self-defeating behavior after a rejection, maybe you can put the spoon down before it's too late. Realize that there are more effective ways to avoid the painful self-awareness that comes from a social rejection—talk to friends, read a good book, or watch a movie (if you're not supposed to be working or studying, the last two ideas are particularly good ways to escape self-awareness without engaging in self-defeating behavior). In fact, a series of recent experiments found that writing about a valued friend or family member eliminated the usual aggression seen after social exclusion (Twenge, Zhang, et al., 2007).

The work by Pennebaker and his colleagues likewise suggests that writing in a journal may be effective; although it may increase self-awareness in the short term, it tends to cleanse the mind in a way that leads to improved health (e.g., Pennebaker, Kiecolt-Glaser, & Glaser, 1988). It may also be helpful to use the principles of cognitive-behavioral therapy to prevent self-defeating behavior (Giles, 1989). This technique involves stopping negative thoughts about events such as rejection—realizing that the event is not global, not personal, and not permanent. Once the attributions about a rejection are changed, self-defeating behavior may be less tempting. People who are going through a rejection should remember: Things will get better. There is a future for you out there, and you need to take care of yourself to be ready for it. In other words, put that beer back in the fridge, and put down that ice cream scoop right now!

## REFERENCES

Baumeister, R. F. (1990). Suicide as escape from self. *Psychological Review, 97*, 90–113.

Baumeister, R. F. (1991). *Escaping the self: Alcoholism, spirituality, masochism, and other flights from the burden of selfhood.* New York: Basic Books.

Baumeister, R. F., Bratslavsky, E., Muraven, M., & Tice, D. M. (1998). Ego depletion: Is the active self a limited resource? *Journal of Personality and Social Psychology, 74*, 1252–1265.

Baumeister, R. F., DeWall, C. N., Ciarocco, N. J., & Twenge, J. M. (2005). Social exclusion impairs self-regulation. *Journal of Personality and Social Psychology, 88*, 589–604.

Baumeister, R. F., Heatherton, T. F., & Tice, D. M. (1994). *Losing control: How and why people fail at self-regulation.* San Diego, CA: Academic Press.

Baumeister, R. F., & Leary, M. R. (1995). The need to belong: Desire for the interpersonal attachments as a fundamental human motivation. *Psychological Bulletin, 117*, 497–529

Baumeister, R. F., & Scher, S. J. (1988). Self-defeating behavior patters among normal individuals: Review and analysis of common self-destructive tendencies. *Psychological Bulletin, 104*, 3–22.

Buckley, K., Winkel, R., & Leary, M. (2004). Reactions to acceptance and rejection: Effects of level and sequence of relational evaluation. *Journal of Experimental Social Psychology, 40*, 14–28.

DeLongis, A., Folkman, S., & Lazarus, R. S. (1988). The impact of daily stress on health and mood: Psychological and social resources as mediators. *Journal of Personality and Social Psychology, 54*, 486–495.

Ferrari, J. R., & Tice, D. M. (2000). Procrastination as a self-handicap for men and women: A task-avoidance strategy in a laboratory setting. *Journal of Research in Personality, 34*, 73–83.

Giles, C. P. (1989). *Managing stress and controlling self-defeating behavior.* Elmsford, NY: National Publishers.

Golding, J. M., Burnam, M. A., Benjamin, B., & Wells, K. B. (1992). Reasons for drinking, alcohol use, and alcoholism among Mexican Americans and non-Hispanic whites. *Psychology of Addictive Behaviors, 6*, 155–167.

Goodwin, J. S., Hunt, W. C., Key, C. R., & Samet, J. M. (1987). The effect of marital status on stage, treatment, and survival of cancer patients. *Journal of the American Medical Association, 258*, 3125–3130.

Harano, R. M., Peck, R. L., & McBride, R. S. (1975). The prediction of accident liability through biographical data and psychometric tests. *Journal of Safety Research, 7*, 16–52.

Harrington, D. M., & McBride, R. S. (1970). Traffic violations by type, age, sex, and marital status. *Accident Analysis and Prevention, 2*, 67–79.

Haynes, R. B. (1979). Determinants of compliance: The disease and the mechanics of treatment. In R. B. Haynes, D. W. Taylor, & S. L. Sackett (Eds.), *Compliance in health care* (pp. 49–62). Baltimore: Johns Hopkins University Press.

Hull, J. G., Levenson, R. W., Young, R. D., & Sher, K. J. (1983). Self-awareness –reducing effects of alcohol consumption in male social drinkers. *Journal of Personality and Social Psychology, 44*, 461–473.

Kirkpatrick, L. A., Waugh, C. E., Valencia, A., & Webster, G. D. (2002). The functional domain specificity of self-esteem and the differential prediction of aggression. *Journal of Personality and Social Psychology, 82*, 756–767.

Leith, K. P., & Baumeister, R. F. (1996). Why do bad moods increase self-defeating behavior?: Emotion, risk taking, and self-regulation. *Journal of Personality and Social Psychology, 71*, 1250–1267.

Leary, M. R., Kowalski, R. M., Smith, L., & Phillips, S. (2003). Teasing, rejection, and violence: Case studies of the school shootings. *Aggressive Behavior, 29*, 202–214.

Leary, M. R., Twenge, J. M., & Quinlivan, E. (2006). Interpersonal rejection as a determinant of anger and aggression. *Personality and Social Psychology Review, 10*, 111–132.

Mayer, J. D., & Gaschke, Y. N. (1988). The experience and meta-experience of mood. *Journal of Personality and Social Psychology, 55*, 102–111.

McCollum, J. B., Burish, T. G., Maisto, S. A., & Sobell, M. B. (1980). Alcohol's effects on physiological arousal and self-reported affect and sensations. *Journal of Abnormal Psychology, 89*, 224–233.

Milburn, A. (1978). Sources of bias in the prediction of future events. *Organizational Behavior and Human Performance, 21*, 17–26.

Muraven, M. (1998). *Mechanisms of self-control failure: Motivation and limited resources.* Unpublished doctoral dissertation, Case Western Reserve University.

Muraven, M., & Baumeister, R. F. (2000). Self-regulation and depletion of limited resources: Does self-control resemble a muscle? *Psychological Bulletin, 126*, 247–259.

Muraven, M., Tice, D. M., & Baumeister, R. F. (1998). Self-control as limited resource: Regulatory depletion patterns. *Journal of Personality and Social Psychology, 74*, 774–789.

Office of the Surgeon General. (2001). *Youth violence: A report of the Surgeon General.* Retrieved from *www.mentalhealth.org/youthviolence/default.asp*

Pennebaker, J. W., Kiecolt-Glaser, J. K., & Glaser, R. (1988). Disclosure of traumas and immune function: Health implications for psychotherapy. *Journal of Consulting and Clinical Psychology, 56*, 239–245.

Richman, A. (1985). Human risk factors in alcohol-related crashes. *Journal of Studies on Alcohol, 10*, 21–31.

Sackett, D. L., & Snow, J. C. (1979). The magnitude of compliance and noncompliance. In R. B. Haynes, D. W. Taylor, & S. L. Sackett (Eds.), *Compliance in health care* (pp. 11–22). Baltimore: Johns Hopkins University Press.

Sampson, R. J., & Laub, J. H. (1990). Crime and deviance over the life course: The salience of adult social bonds. *American Sociological Review, 55*, 609–627.

Silverstein, B. (1982). Cigarette smoking, nicotine addiction, and relaxation. *Journal of Personality and Social Psychology, 42*, 946–950.

Stroebe, W., & Stroebe, M. S. (1987). *Bereavement and health: The psychological and physical consequences of partner loss.* New York: Cambridge University Press.

Stroebe, W., Stroebe, M. S., Abakoumkin, G., & Schut, H. (1996). The role of loneliness and social support in adjustment to loss: A test of attachment versus stress theory. *Journal of Personality and Social Psychology, 70*, 1241–1249.

Tice, D. M., & Baumeister, R. F. (1997). Longitudinal study of procrastination, performance, stress, and health: The costs and benefits of dawdling. *Psychological Science, 8*, 454–458.

Tice, D. M., Bratslavsky, E., & Baumeister, R. F. (2001). Emotional distress regulation takes precedence over impulse control: If you feel bad, do it! *Journal of Personality and Social Psychology, 80*, 53–67.

Twenge, J. M., Baumeister, R. F., DeWall, C. N., Ciarocco, N. J., & Bartels, J. M. (2007). Social exclusion decreases prosocial behavior. *Journal of Personality and Social Psychology, 92*(1), 56–66.

Twenge, J. M., Baumeister, R. F., Tice, D. M., & Stucke, T. S. (2001). If you can't join them, beat them: Effects of social exclusion on aggressive behavior. *Journal of Personality and Social Psychology, 81*, 1058–1069.

Twenge, J. M., Catanese, K. R., & Baumeister, R. F. (2002). Social exclusion causes self-defeating behavior. *Journal of Personality and Social Psychology, 83*, 606–615.

Twenge, J. M., Catanese, K. R., & Baumeister, R. F. (2003). Social exclusion and the deconstructed state: Time perception, meaninglessness, lethargy, lack of emotion, and self-awareness. *Journal of Personality and Social Psychology, 85*, 409–423.

Twenge, J. M., Zhang, L., Catanese, K. R., Dolan-Pascoe, B., Lyche, L. F., & Baumeister, R. F. (2007). Replenishing connectedness: Reminders of social activity reduce aggression after social exclusion. *British Journal of Social Psychology, 46*, 205–224.

Vohs, K. D., & Heatherton, T. F. (2000). Self-regulatory failure: A resource-depletion approach. *Psychological Science, 11*, 249–254.

Warburton, W. A., Williams, K. D., & Cairns, D. R. (2006). When ostracism leads to aggression: The moderating effects of control deprivation. *Journal of Experimental Social Psychology, 42*, 213–220.

Watson, D., Clark, L. A., & Tellegen, A. (1988). Development and validation of brief measures of positive and negative affect: The PANAS scales. *Journal of Personality and Social Psychology, 54*, 1063–1070.

Wicklund, R. A. (1975). Objective self-awareness. In L. Berkowitz (Ed.), *Advances in experimental social psychology* (Vol. 8, pp. 233–275). New York: Academic Press.

Williams, D. R., Takeuchi, D. T., & Adair, R. K. (1992). Martial status and psychiatric disorders among blacks and whites. *Journal of Health and Social Behavior, 33*, 140–157.

Chapter 34

# Personal Goals and Life Dreams

## POSITIVE PSYCHOLOGY AND MOTIVATION IN DAILY LIFE

Laura A. King

Motivation is the domain in which the basic question of what is essential to and about human beings is identified. Indeed, throughout the history of our field, approaches to motivation have revealed psychologists' views of human nature itself. The Freudian view of human motivation as dominated by unconscious, amoral drives for sex and aggression is the centerpiece of a grand theory of human life. It is worth noting that current (often implicit) psychological views of humanity, as revealed in our approaches to motivation, continue to bear the marks of Freud's influence—a tendency to assume the worst of human nature, and certainly to assume that motivation, lying deep in some secret corner of the human heart, is a dark and potentially vile thing. In contemporary psychology our motives often remain things to be defended against, aspects of our lives about which we'd be better off knowing little. In this chapter I present an alternative conceptualization of motivation, emerging from the positive psychology movement.

### POSITIVE PSYCHOLOGY AND THE SCIENCE OF MOTIVATION

Recently there has been a call for a reexamination of the focus of psychological approaches to human behavior (e.g., Seligman, 2003; Seligman & Csikszentmihalyi, 2000). *Positive psychology* has emerged as a movement emphasizing human strengths and encouraging us to examine what is good and functional in humanity (e.g., Petersen & Seligman, 2004). Many researchers have long been preoccupied with such an "appreciative" view of human nature (see Sheldon & King, 2001). Positive psychology draws our attention to these programs of research, while also pointing out what the "negative bias" in psychology has caused us to ignore. Too often, positive psychologists argue, psychology has focused on what is wrong or ill in human functioning, ignoring the adaptive, functional, or even superior aspects of our lives. Too often, the very "ordinary magic" (Masten, 2001) that characterizes resilience in everyday life has been ignored in favor of the abnormal or dysfunctional. Furthermore, our preference for counterintuitive findings over those that demonstrate the pragmatics of everyday life has led us to denigrate lay notions of functioning (Sheldon & King, 2001). Positive psychology challenges us to open our eyes and our laboratories to the many strengths that humans demonstrate. Importantly, positive psychology is not simply the study of positive thinking (cf. Lazarus, 2004). Rather, it is about recognizing a host of human strengths (Seligman & Peterson, 2004), while acknowledging that even strengths may come at a cost (e.g., King & Burton, 2003). Many of the good things in life must be recognized as having positive and negative characteristics, and it is important to recognize the ambivalence that people may feel about even very good things.

There is no simple positive psychological approach to motivation. Indeed, the views presented in this chapter represent but one positive psychologist's view of what psychological approaches to motivation ought to include. Not all psychologists (positive or otherwise) who study motivation would agree with my assertions here, to be sure. Rather, I hope in this chapter to convey the flavor of one positive psychological approach to motivation. Various approaches to motivation might fit under the rubric of positive psychology; some of these are included in other chapters in this volume (e.g., Sheldon, Chapter 30).

From my perspective, a positive psychological approach to motivation ought to include the following possibilities. First, people should be understood as having the capacity to be motivated toward ends beyond those required for survival. One might recall Maslow's (1970) call to answer the dilemma of human motivation: What does a person do, once his or her belly is chronically full, his or her basic survival needs chronically met? Second, a positive psychological approach to motivation must address the relations of motivation to well-being and functioning. A positive psychological approach to motivation ought to recognize that the capacity for self-regulation implies that human motivation may have an inherent adaptive quality. Negative outcomes of motivation ought to be understood in a context that speaks to the potentially adaptive character of these processes in alternative circumstances. Third, a positive psychological approach to motivation ought at least to address the potential usefulness of conscious experience in motivation. Fourth, a positive psychological approach to motivation might situate motivation in the daily life of normal, garden-variety people. Too often, "everyday folks" have come to believe that psychology has nothing to offer them, is pointedly not *about* them—that psychology is the study of abnormal psychology (e.g., King, 2003). Fifth, positive psychological approaches to motivation ought to look beyond happiness toward various other potentially positive outcomes of the motivational process.

In my view, research on personalized daily goals meets many if not all of these criteria. Thus I briefly review research on personalized goals for this chapter, because I believe that this work exemplifies the mission of positive psychology. First, personalized goals are open to a broad range of human interests beyond the basic needs of survival. Second, research on everyday goals has been focused on the relations of these goal processes to psychological well-being, physical health, and so on. The role of daily goals in negative states has also been examined, particularly as it relates to the reality of everyday life. Personalized goals have not been shown to be a "happiness elixir" that guarantees a pleasant existence. Rather, these constructs have been shown to capture the very ambivalence that is likely to be part and parcel of motivation in human life (see Pomerantz & Shim, Chapter 25, this volume, for a rich treatment of this topic). Third, obviously, research on personalized goals focuses on consciously experienced motivation. Fourth, personalized goals are situated in everyday existence. Research on personalized goals has focused on the person's everyday routine, and as such has brought important empirical attention to bear on everyday life. Fifth, by focusing not only on happiness but on other goods in life (in this case, maturity), research on personalized goals has demonstrated relations between goal processes and human development. Finally, research on daily goals and life goals has been used to draw attention to the "negative bias" in research on expressive writing, and as such demonstrates the potential problems of focusing on only the negative aspects of human life in understanding the breadth of human experience relevant to well-being.

## DAILY GOALS AND LIFE DREAMS: MOTIVATION IN DAILY LIFE

New Year's resolutions, daily to-do lists, and weekly planners: For many of us, these are the ways that motivation is experienced as a part of daily life. Intentions matter to us. We hear about a heinous murder and wonder, "Why?" We receive a bizarre trinket as a birthday gift and remind ourselves, "It's the thought that counts." We feel understood when we can place our behaviors in a motivational context, of not so much *what* we did as *why* we did it. The phenomenology of intentions is an integral part of our intuitive understanding of ourselves and others. Psychologists have long been considered a group of experts on motivation—on what people "really" want, as though motivation itself is essentially unknowable to the uneducated observer. The degree to which people know what they want has certainly been debated (e.g., Brunstein & Maier, 2005; McClelland, Koestner, & Weinberger, 1992). What place, then, do conscious intents have in a science of human motivation?

In the 1980s and 1990s, personality psychology embraced Allport's (1961) radical assertion that if we want to know what someone wants, we'd be best served simply to ask him or her. During this period, various researchers introduced ways to conceptualize personalized everyday goals—the sometimes trivial and sometimes grand pursuits that are experienced by those who embrace them as the motivational forces in their lives. These approaches all assume that goals are available to awareness, and they rely on people's abilities to generate and rate these goals on various dimensions.

What are daily goals? In our research, my colleagues and I often ask people to generate a list of the goals they try to accomplish in their everyday behavior. Responses to this question range from the mundane ("to grow out my bangs," "to cut down on butter") to the magnificent ("to bring God's kingdom to earth," "to fight injustice wherever I see it"). In addition to listing their everyday goals, participants in these studies typically rate their goals on a variety of dimensions, such as importance, value, clarity, difficulty, and conflict (e.g., Emmons, 1989). These goal appraisal dimensions have allowed researchers to transform idiographic goal units into quantifiable nomothetic variables. Everyday, proximal goals (e.g., "to be a friendly person") are thought to exist in a motivational hierarchy, above momentary behavioral plans (e.g., "to have lunch with Jamie today") and below some overarching, more enduring motives or needs (e.g., needs for affiliation, intimacy, or relatedness). Personalized everyday goals can be thought of as midlevel, conscious expressions of a person's desires. As contextualized expressions of motivation, they make most sense within the rich setting that is the person's life. Outside that setting, of course, they may appear rather trivial. Yet research has demonstrated that these everyday goals do demonstrate relations to important variables, such as well-being, thought, mood, and behavior.

## GOALS AND WELL-BEING

The role of goal investment in positive human functioning is well established. Working toward valued goals is an important aspect of psychological (e.g., Brunstein, 1993; Emmons, 1989; King, Richards, & Stemmerich, 1998; Klinger, 1977, 1995, 1999; Omodei & Wearing, 1990; Pervin, 1989), and physical (Emmons & King, 1988) well-being. Research has demonstrated that simply having important, valued goals is related to well-being, as is making progress on those goals. Having daily goals that are in instrumental (rather than conflictful) relations with one another is associated with enhanced physical health.

Furthermore, the level at which individuals construe their everyday goals has been shown to relate to well-being as well. Harkening back to Ach's (1910) classic work on level of aspiration as well as Vallacher and Wegner's (1987/2000) action identification work, Emmons (1992) examined the level of concreteness versus abstraction with which a person approaches his or her daily goals. Low-level goals are those that are quite concrete and that can be easily attained via specific behavior (e.g., "to stop biting my fingernails"). High-level goals are those that are more abstract and more likely to be enduring (e.g., "to fight injustice"). The precise strategies one might use to obtain these goals are not clear, and success at these is likely to be ambiguous. Emmons found that those who pursue high-level, abstract goals tend to be prone to negative affect and distress. Conversely, those who focus their efforts on lower-level goals tend to be happier but prone to physical illness.

## DAILY GOALS AS MOTIVATIONAL CONSTRUCTS

Several types of research have shown that goals are more likely to occur in spontaneous thought if they are important, if a deadline is approaching, or if substantial obstacles are encountered in the pursuit of the goal (e.g., Emmons & King, 1988; Klinger, 1977). Research using daily diary and experience-sampling methods has shown that goal-related events are more likely to be mentioned and more likely to have an impact on mood (e.g., Diener & Fujita, 1995; Emmons, 1989). Singer and his colleagues (e.g., Singer & Blagov, 2004; Singer & Salovey, 1996) have demonstrated that everyday goals relate to important autobiographical memory. For instance, our lingering affective reactions to autobiographical memories can be explained via their relations to our long-term life goals (Singer & Salovey, 1996). Pomerantz, Saxon, and Oishi (2000) found that though investment in and progress toward daily goals was associated with heightened positive feelings, such investment also fostered worry. Indeed, the very goals that were most deeply valued were the most likely to engender concern. The relation of goals to potential worry and preoccupation simply demonstrates their validity as measures of valued ends. Goals may relate to positive or negative emotional experiences, depending on how we are progressing in our goal pursuit. This notion is certainly in accord with models of the role of affect in self-regulation (e.g., Carver & Scheier, Chapter 20, this volume). Goals have been shown to organize daily experience and mediate the relationship between events and daily emotional life (Diener & Fujita, 1995). From this perspective, goal investment is a means by which either positive or negative emotional reactions make sense—suggesting, perhaps, the role of goals in the creation and experience of meaning in daily life.

Motivation has been described as a source of coherence in human behavior. Behaviors make sense to the extent that they are embedded in a motivational context. As such, motivation can be understood as a source of meaning in life. Events have meaning (i.e., matter) to us to the extent that they affect our goals. Daily goal pursuit can be thought of as a way of connecting the past, present, and future, because it meaningfully relates a chain of life events—providing life with beginnings, middles, and ends. Goals may determine which life events are incorporated into memory and eventually become the stuff of the life story. To adopt another metaphor, to the extent that goals direct attention, draw our thoughts to them, and drive the extraction of meaning from life events, they are a kind of psychic "hub" in our mental lives. Thus research supports the ideas that personal goals are indeed motivational units, and that a person's conscious intents reveal important information about his or her well-being, thought, mood, and behavior.

## PERSONALIZED ACCOUNTS OF THE HIERARCHY OF MOTIVATION

As mentioned previously, daily goals are thought to exist in a motivational hierarchy. We might think of the top of the hierarchy as characterized by unconscious needs or motives. Personalized goals may be understood to represent broader motives or needs, but they are not direct reflections of them. The content of personalized goals has been found to relate inconsistently to higher-level social motives (measured via content analyses of imaginative stories; King, 1995). Others have suggested that the degree to which goals map onto a person's motives might itself be a measure of positive functioning. Sheldon's (Chapter 30, this volume) self-concordance model suggests that the extent to which daily goals map onto universal organismic needs relates to and mediates the relation between goal progress and well-being.

In my lab, we have examined the ways that daily goals relate to more abstract life dreams. In these studies, in addition to listing their everyday goals, participants also describe their more distal life dreams, or best possible future selves. *Possible selves* are personalized representations of goals (Markus & Ruvolo, 1989; Niedenthal, Setterlund, & Wherry, 1992). These selves provide a link between the self-concept and motivation. Possible selves and aspects of possible selves have been found to relate to a variety of outcomes (e.g., Hoyle & Sherrill, 2006; Markus & Ruvolo, 1989; Oyserman, Bybee, & Terry, 2006; Quinlan, Jaccard, & Blanton, 2006; Segal, 2006). Previous research has shown that possible selves influence memory (Kato & Markus, 1994) and relate to superior performance (Ruvolo & Markus, 1992)—supporting the notion that these selves are motivational units, comparable to other goal units (Markus & Ruvolo, 1989). Possible selves have been portrayed as psychological resources that motivate the self throughout adult development (Cross & Markus, 1991; Frazier & Hooker, 2006). Possible selves represent the broad range of imaginable futures. One's best possible self is one's most cherished future self, one's best possible outcome. This possible self may be viewed as the fruition of one's more proximal goals.

Our instructions for the generation of possible selves have been the following (e.g., King, 2001a):

> " . . . Imagine that your life has gone as well as it possibly could have. You have worked hard and achieved your goals. Think of this as your 'best possible life' or your 'happily ever after.' In the space below (and on the back of this page, if necessary), write a description of the things you imagined. Be as specific as you can."

After generating goal lists and narrative possible selves, participants (or trained raters) rate the extent to which these daily goals actively lead to participants' best possible futures. We've found that pursuing daily goals that serve as steppingstones to larger future life goals is associated with enhanced well-being (e.g., King et al., 1998). Indeed, progress on goals that are related to life dreams tends to be particularly related to well-being. Thus investing in daily life via everyday goals appears to be a strong correlate of daily well-being. It is not surprising that daily goals have been portrayed as instantiations of the self as agent in daily life (e.g., Harlow & Cantor, 1995; King, 1998).

Note that this approach continues to rely on the phenomenological experience of motivation. Possible selves—though conceptually closer to the self than daily goals, and therefore more likely to represent higher-level motivational constructs—are still conscious, and still carry the person's own sense of the motivational aspects of his or her life. Are these more abstract goals psychologically powerful variables, or simply wishful constructions with few ramifications for the person? One surprising context in which these narrative possible selves have proven useful is the expressive writing paradigm developed by Pennebaker and colleagues.

## BEST POSSIBLE SELVES AND BENEFITS OF WRITING

A large literature has demonstrated that writing about one's most traumatic life events is associated with a variety of health and well-being benefits. Pennebaker and his colleagues have shown that writing about traumatic life experiences has a variety of positive health and well-being benefits (Lepore & Smyth, 2002; Pennebaker & Chun, 2007; Pennebaker, Kiecolt-Glaser, & Glaser, 2004). Several explanatory mechanisms have been suggested to account for these benefits (see King, 2002, for an overview). Importantly, the initial focus of expressive writing studies on traumatic past experience was not dictated by a particular theoretical account of the benefits of writing, but rather by an implicit assumption that negative traumatic events are the rightful focus of psychological attention. There is no question that secret past traumas are inherently interesting, but the early focus on traumatic events led to various conventions in research that were not dictated by theory. This focus certainly colored, and arguably limited, the types of explanatory mechanisms considered for the benefits of writing (King, 2002).

I have proposed (e.g., King, 2002) that we ought to take these writing studies seriously as opportunities to construct narratives about experience. As such, they can be viewed as constructions of meaning, and ultimately as attempts to integrate experience into the self. If writing is a means of integrating experience into the self, we might well ask whether it is valuable to integrate experiences other than traumatic ones from the past into the self as well. I have suggested that our life goals become parts of ourselves via writing—not just things we do, but aspects of our identities.

In order to examine the possibility that integrating goals into the self via writing might have health benefits, we used the construct of possible selves. In a study using the writing paradigm (King, 2001b), participants were asked to write about their most traumatic life experiences, their best possible selves (using the instructions above), or a control topic (their plans for the day). Results demonstrated that the best-possible-self condition led to enhanced positive affect immediately after writing (in contrast to previous studies using only the trauma topic), enhanced psychological well-being weeks after writing, and a lower rate of physical illnesses. Results for physical illness were on par with those found for writing about a traumatic life experience. These results are important because they demonstrate that the focus of earlier writing studies on trauma was not a necessity for gaining benefits. They also suggest that our understanding of the "healing power of writing" might benefit from placing these studies in a motivational context (see also Sheldon & Lyubomirsky, 2006).

Thinking about these writing studies within the context of motivation allows us to explore the potential impact of writing on self-regulation. Perhaps the most influential notion underlying most approaches to motivation is that of self-regulation (see Carver & Scheier, Chapter 20, this volume, for a thorough review of this important construct). *Self-regulation* refers to the organism's capacity to seek desired ends, to track progress toward those ends, and to respond to various environmental contingencies relevant to motivational pursuit. When we write about a life event that is important, we learn about our needs and priorities. The self's story may become increasingly articulated and clear. Such a process may render our own emotional reactions more comprehensible. Our moods may be more clearly goal-relevant. We come to understand what we want in life and what is truly important to us (cf. King, 2001a). In addition, when we write about our life goals, the pursuit of those goals may become less effortful, as these goals become expressions of ourselves rather than tasks that we must complete (cf. Sheldon & Houser-Marko, 2001). Thus individuals who have engaged in writing about some personally meaningful topic can be expected to show signs of enhanced self-regulation, including more efficient goal pursuit, greater contingency between thought and behavior, and greater contingency between mood and goal-relevant events (after Carver & Scheier, Chapter 20, this volume). Thus writing experiences into the self can be expected to influence goal pursuit, rendering goals even more powerful units of agency.

## GOAL LOSS: WHAT HAPPENS WHEN GOALS ARE NO LONGER AVAILABLE?

It is an essential truth of human life that goals, no matter how well chosen or how doggedly pursued, do not always work out. Indeed, setting a goal includes not only the promise of its fulfillment, but the potential for failure, humiliation, and regret. Emotionally investing in one's daily life may mean experiencing disappointment when things don't go well (cf. Kernis, Paradise, Whitaker, Wheatman, & Goldman, 2000; Marsh, 1995; see King & Burton, 2003, for a review). Goal failure is likely to lead to rumination (Brunstein & Gollwitzer, 1996). Not knowing when to disengage from a goal can lead to distress and an inability to engage in new goals (cf. Klinger, 1977, 1995, 1999; Koole & Kuhl, Chapter 19, this volume). The Zeigarnik effect (Zeigarnik, 1938) is a classic example of the tantalizing power of interrupted goals. A true hallmark of successful self-regulation may be the ability to pursue goals *flexibly*—and to disengage from life goals that no longer include the possibility of fulfillment (King, 1996, 1998). What do people do when previously cherished goals are no longer possible? Typically, research indicates that in the face of negative feedback, goal seekers often redouble their efforts. Brunstein and Gollwitzer (1996) found that high involvement in a task was associated with even more involvement after failure. Emmons, Colby, and Kaiser (1998) found that the typical response to life change was not goal change, but rather redoubling of effort on existing goals. These results speak to the power of goals in our lives, but they also point to the problem of neurotic perseverance.

Clearly, sometimes failure is indeed an option, and sometimes quitting is not a bad idea (innumerable movie plots notwithstanding). Klinger (1977) has in fact suggested that failure to disengage from unattainable goals is linked to depressive symptoms. Such distress is considered a normal part of the process of letting go of valued goals, but it can lead to reduced daily goal functioning. Increased psychological distress may result from expending daily thought and emotion on the pursuit of unfulfilled goals. Kuhl and Helle (1986) experimentally demonstrated that individuals who failed to disengage from unattainable goals tended to show depressive symptoms and limited opportunities for new goals. Thus research has typically shown that goal failure is likely to relate, at least in the short term, to distress, neurotic perseverance, and general motivational inertia. Taken at face value, these results might move us to declare that goal investment ought to be avoided to minimize disappointment. Such a conclusion, however, would not only ignore the strong relation between goal progress and well-being, but also require us to forsake the many human accomplishments that have emerged out of the dogged pursuit of difficult goals. Should we surrender our life's passions in favor of a contented existence? Goal investment may ultimately lead to distress, but we needn't pathologize distress per se, or overemphasize the importance of transient fluctuations in self-esteem and mood. It is important to keep in mind that disappointment has a place in human life, and that feeling bad immediately after failure is not a sign of dysfunction. Negative mood has a place in the self-regulation of action.

There may be a better place for lost goals in individuals' lives, particularly in the long term. Goals are representations of motivation that capture people's intuitive sense of why they do the things they do. In this phenomenological context, it is worth considering how individuals understand themselves and their goals. A person may well view a lifetime as a process of writing and revising intentions—of discovering what he or she truly wants and pursuing that ever-changing goal. As such, daily goals, though a strong indicator at any given moment of how a person views him- or herself relative to where he or she wants to be, may also be time-limited and always subject to dismissal. Forsaken goals may eventually be viewed as curiosities in personal history—what the individual thought was important but now realizes is not. Truly understanding the self as agent in everyday life may require a long-term view—one that takes into account the ever-changing motivational landscape of the person's life. Conscious goals may be particularly useful for examining motivation as a dynamic and contextualized phenomenon, because they are themselves highly contextualized and potentially time-limited.

In research on individuals who have experienced major life transitions, my colleagues and I have examined how the goals individuals can no longer pursue relate to other aspects of their lives. Clearly, changes in the self may influence goal pursuit. In the conceptual motivational hierarchy, higher levels are viewed as most definitional of the self. Thus experiences that change the highest levels of the hierarchy should be expected to influence lower-level goals. Focusing on a person's goals as they change over the course of a life transition allows us to track how sources of meaning in life themselves change.

One way to look at the outcome of goal loss or goal change is to focus not on the distress that such an experience might foster, but on such an experience as a potential catalyst for personality development. It is fairly common for individuals who have experienced major life changes to feel that they have grown as a result of the experience (e.g., King, 2002; King & Miner, 2000; King, Scollon, Ramsey, & Williams, 2000; Park & Ai, 2006; Park, Cohen, & Murch, 1996). Loevinger (1976) noted that only when the environment fails to conform to the person's expectations is there potential for growth. Research on difficult life experience has supported this idea (Helson, 1992; Helson & Roberts, 1994; Helson & Wink, 1992). Block (1982) has described the processes by which personality develops, using the Piagetian concepts of *assimilation* and *accommodation*. In assimilation, the individual avoids any meaningful change of orientation and manages simply to interpret and incorporate a new experience into his or her existing framework. When assimilation fails, the person may "construct or invent new schemes that are equilibrating" (Block, 1982, p. 291), or change the self to accommodate the new experience. To some degree, accommodation cannot occur if a person is not invested in his or her preexisting meaning structures. Thus goal investment, though potentially making the person vulnerable to distress in response to failure, may also be seen as predisposing the person toward growth in response to failure. If goal investment is viewed as a source of meaning, then changes in goals may be seen as opportunities for (and manifestations of) accommodative change.

We have examined lost or forsaken goals in groups of individuals who have experienced major life changes. In one study (King & Raspin, 2004), a sample of divorced women, who had been married for an average of 22 years, wrote narrative descriptions of the best possible future selves that they had pursued before divorce (written retrospectively) and the best possible future selves that they were currently pursuing. In addition, they rated the salience of these narratives in their current lives. The *salience* of a possible self refers to its availability in the person's mental life (i.e., the extent to which he or she thinks about this possible self). Salience can be thought of as the mental investment the person makes in a particular possible self—the degree to which the person has actively considered that possible self. In addition to this self-report measure of salience, independent raters coded the narratives for amount of *elaboration*. The elaboration of a narrative possible self refers to the level of rich detail and vividness included in the narration. Although salience and elaboration may be related, they need not be. A very elaborate possible self may be chronically available in a person's mental life (i.e., salient), but it is also possible for someone to describe an elaborate lost possible self that he or she hasn't really thought about in a long time. Below is an example of an elaborate "found" possible self (i.e., the person's current best possible self):

> "In my current or real life, I set goals and experience HARD work as I seek to attain them. I feel fortunate in a back-handed way to have experienced misfortune as a young woman. I feel it taught me humility, to be nonjudgmental, compassion and the ability to regroup. Life is good but not lavish. It's hard work and we have to give each other a hand once in a while. I have changed my goals from material to spiritual. Forgiveness has been key. I have imagined college degrees; a cozy home, educated healthy well-adjusted children, and interesting job; a good marriage."

Not surprisingly, among divorced women, the salience of their lost possible selves (the ones they were seeking prior to the divorce) was negatively related to psychological well-being and positively related to distress, as might be expected from the previous discussion of goal disengagement. In contrast, the salience of their current best possible selves was positively related to well-being and negatively related to distress. Interestingly, the elaboration of the lost selves was associated with personality development, in interaction with time since divorce. That is, over time, women who were able to elaborate with great detail on the goals they had imagined for themselves during their marriages were more likely to develop over time (King & Raspin, 2004).

We also examined these processes in a sample of parents of children with Down syndrome (King & Patterson, 2000). In that study, we examined how lost and found possible selves related to psychological well-being and self-perceived personal growth, using the Stress Related Growth Scale (Park et al., 1996). Parents in that sample wrote narrative descriptions of their life goals prior to and after parenting a child with Down syndrome. An example of a highly elaborate lost possible self follows:

> "When I was pregnant, I used to imagine that I would have the same sort of relationship with my child-to-be that my mother had/has with my youngest sister, who was born late in life at a considerable distance from the first 5 children. Both my mom and dad spent a lot of time with her—she was like an only child. I thought our child would be very bright—his father and I both did well in school and love reading and writing. We love joking around with our nieces and nephews, and I imagined carrying on the same sort of verbal banter with my child. I assumed our child would be healthy, since neither my husband nor I have any health problems. In my wildest dreams, I hoped that we would raise our child in a place of scenic beauty with a strong sense of community and belonging, where he/she would learn compassion for others and respect for the environment. Our child would grow up and become independent and do wonderful things, while my husband and I would retire early and pursue avocations."

An example of a highly elaborate current best possible self follows:

> "At this point, most of my dreams revolve around my son. We're always working on a lot of small goals. Right now, we're working on walking independently, expressive language, and increasing the use of his wrists to do things like turning knobs. He's highly motivated and works hard and cheerfully to do each new thing. When he can't do something, instead of getting frustrated and mad, he simply goes back to the things he can do well. I hope that his attitude and sunny disposition and sociability continue through his life. I'd like for him to be in a regular classroom, where he learns to read and write, and where he can participate in a variety of activities with his classmates. I'd like for him to develop interests and pursue them. For his adulthood, I would hope that he be in good health, that he would be able to live at least semi-independently, that he would be able to make some contribution to the world, and that he have a lot of friends and family. My own future is just a big blur now. I'm working it out a day at a time."

Examining the implications of these lost and found possible selves for well-being, we found that investment in current best possible selves was associated with heightened well-being, as was the case with the divorced women we studied. However, the elaboration of a lost possible self was uniquely related to the perception that one had grown through the experience of parenting a child with Down syndrome.

One potential explanation for this finding is cognitive dissonance. This explanation would hold that individuals who are most aware of the extent to which they have previously invested in lost goals (and who are therefore likely to feel distressed in the face of that loss) ought to be the ones most in need of some rationalization for the depth of their loss. Thus these individuals should conclude that they have grown from the experience. Such a mood management maneuver should make their loss seem worthwhile. However, and importantly, individuals in this study who reported stress-related growth did not necessarily report higher levels of well-being; thus no mood enhancement appeared to be going on (King & Patterson, 2000). A more substantive interpretation of our findings seems appropriate. Individuals who have the capacity to admit to legitimate loss are more likely to report experiencing growth through negative life events. These data provide initial evidence that investment in goals predisposes individuals to growth once those goals are lost.

These studies suggest that investment in current goals has a strong relation to well-being. Furthermore, thinking a great deal about lost goals can indeed be a source of considerable distress and may suggest the wisdom of moving on. Happiness may require that lost goals be relegated to the status of "water under the bridge." However, growth and maturity seem to entail the capacity to elaborate on one's forsaken goals and to be able to focus an unflinching gaze on the goals one is no longer pursuing. This capacity suggests an ability to look back on a less mature, less wise self and to acknowledge one's vulnerability (King, 2000; King & Hicks, 2006). Additionally, these results suggest that the capacity to elaborate on valued goals one is not pursuing may be not only a correlate of maturity, but a predictor of maturity as well.

In the studies of divorced women and parents of children with Down syndrome, we asked individuals to look back in their personal histories and describe retrospectively the goals they once pursued. In another study, we examined whether looking not necessarily back on one's own life, but around at the lives and goals of others, might also relate to well-being and development. In that study (King & Smith, 2004), we asked gay men and lesbians to write narrative descriptions of their straight and gay best possible selves. These participants also rated the salience of these straight and gay possible selves in their current lives. These narratives were again reliably coded for level of elaboration. Straight possible selves might represent lost goals for some in this sample (i.e., if these individuals had assumed themselves to be straight). Even among individuals who had never imagined themselves to be straight, the straight best possible selves might have meaning; it is safe to assume that most gay people are well aware of the heterosexual privileges that are withheld from them and that may be seen as life's precluded possibilities.

Gay individuals' thoughts about their best possible straight selves may be thought of as a specific example of a rather common experience. Anyone whose life circumstances and personal choices have placed them outside "the norm" are likely to consider the benefits of "the road *more* traveled by" (King & Smith, 2004). Yet thinking about unavailable opportunities may serve as a source for envy, regret, and rumination (Niedenthal, Tangney, & Gavanski, 1994; Torges, Stewart, & Miner-Rubino, 2005).

In this sample, the salience of a gay best possible self was related to heightened psychological well-being and lowered distress (concurrently and over 2 years). In addition, participants with highly salient best possible gay selves were more likely to be out of the closet. The more elaborate the gay possible selves were, the less regret individuals felt over their gay identities. As was the case for the lost possible selves among the divorced women, the salience of straight best possible selves was related to increased distress, lowered well-being, and increased closetedness in both gay men and lesbians. Furthermore, the salience of both the gay and the straight best possible selves mediated the relationship between closetedness and well-being, indicating that at least one reason why the closet may be related to lowered well-being is that it hinders goal pursuit.

Examining the narrative descriptions of straight possible selves illustrates the challenge involved in confronting the positives of a life path one cannot pursue. Below is an example of a relatively elaborate straight best possible self:

> "I want to make a life with someone who is my best friend and is understanding of my desire for fulfilling work, whether that would be career or volunteer work. I will be a partner in a relationship that is both giving and forgiving. We will be able to be married if we want to be, as well as having the ability to buy insurance, file taxes, etc., together. We will be able to own homes and cars together. Entertain our families, both biological and chosen families, on special occasions. Our employers will know who our significant others are and what they mean to us. I will be able to spend my free time enjoying that relationship rather than hiding it. My parents and hers will (as well as our other relatives) will be as much and as important a part of our lives as they are now. If we so chose we would be welcomed at each other's high school or college reunions as the 'spouse' of so and so. We would be able to adopt children, given [that] we were deemed suitable parents on an individual basis. We will be [a] financially stable, well traveled, fun loving, optimistic, and hard working couple. We will be able to hold hands in public without fear of being attacked. We won't necessarily have to go to a gay/lesbian-owned store to buy greeting cards, etc., for each other. . . . My lover will be beside me and share my life as I will hers. We'd have a small but spacious home that is warm and welcoming to our friends and family, maybe a dog and my cat."

This example may be contrasted with the relatively less elaborate straight possible self below:

> "I would have more male friends if I were heterosexual. I would have children, which I would love. I would not be affected by cruel gay jokes. Would probably be into sports and cars and using women."

How did elaborating on a straight possible self relate to well-being and personality development? First, elaboration of the best straight possible self was related to experiencing greater levels of regret. Elaboration of the straight possible self, however, also predicted personality development concurrently and prospectively over 2 years (King & Smith, 2004).

These results demonstrate the relation of current goals to well-being, and suggest that happiness is related to the pursuit of identity-consistent goals and the capacity to disengage fully from unattainable goals. Investment in goals that were not consistent with one's identity was associated with lower well-being and hiding one's identity. Yet the capacity to elaborate on such goals, though associated with increasing feelings of regret, predicted personality development over time. Once again, a happy, mature person (King, 2001a) may be one who is able to acknowledge what is regrettable in life without being consumed by it (cf. Torges et al., 2005) and to see the multitude of best possible lives that may be sources of fulfillment (cf. Ryff, 1991). These results speak to the psychological tradeoffs of the "examined life." Individuals who have thought deeply about their possible selves may incur some sense of legitimate regret over missed opportunities or the positives of a road not taken. It is an important lesson for positive psychology, and psychology in general, that the goods of life are sometimes intertwined in unexpected ways. What entails sadness may be the very thing that ultimately provides wisdom. It is interesting to note that while motivation has often been viewed as an area in which psychological defenses are likely to protect the individual from painful self-knowledge, in these studies acknowledgment of such painful truths is an indicator of maturity. We may note that some of the assumptions that psychology has made about humans and human motivation may not apply to the highest-functioning among us.

## THE LIMITATIONS OF FOCUSING ON CONSCIOUS GOALS

Daily goals and consciously generated life dreams are certainly superficial instantiations of motivation. To the extent that we do not know everything about ourselves, personal goals may constitute only the tip of the iceberg of motivation. Furthermore, moments of self-understanding (as may be provided by life-changing experiences) reveal that previously cherished goals may in fact be less important to us than we'd originally imagined. Personal goals are not just expressions of motivation; they are by-products of a larger motivational process. To some extent, goals provide a window into the self-regulatory process. We can fairly easily track goal pursuit via a person's own report of how he or she is doing. Furthermore, the established relations between goal progress and daily mood bear witness to the potential reflection of self regulation in daily goal processes. However, and importantly, conscious goals are also themselves products of the regulatory process. As suggested in Sheldon's (Chapter 30, this volume) examination of motivational quality, goal progress can only be viewed as self-regulatory if the goals themselves are in fact well selected and optimal for a person. Although individuals would ideally select and pursue goals that are optimally adaptive for their talents, skills, and opportunities, clearly this is not always the case. Individuals may "tilt at windmills" for long periods of time, toiling mightily at goals with no promise of fulfillment. Thus, although goals may indicate self-regulation, they may also be products of dysfunction—failure to perceive oneself or one's context accurately. In order for us to fully appreciate the role of goals in self-regulation, they must be placed in a larger motivational and social/environmental context. Surely, in order to evaluate the adaptiveness of a particular set of goals, we must follow a person over time.

Certainly, the research I have described here takes a credulous view of self-reports, perhaps to a fault. Direct measures of defensiveness have not been incorporated in most of the studies I've described. Additionally, I have not engaged in knee-jerk misanthropy that might provoke some to claim that the participants in these studies are either unaware of their motivations or actually lying about their best possible selves. The relations of the variables we've studied to important life outcomes (not all of which are self-reported) lend credence to the notion that these conscious motivations are indeed important to psychological functioning. Whether the underlying processes are in fact fully understandable via the phenomenology of motivation remains for future research.

## THE BREADTH OF POSITIVE PSYCHOLOGY

Positive psychology as a general approach to the science of human behavior calls us to take a broader view of humanity—one that allows for the emergence of human strengths, functionality, and optimal being (Sheldon, 2004). I have described here my own version of a positive psychological approach to motivation, and surely there are many other areas of positive psychology that have relevance to motivation. For instance, from Fredrickson's (1998, 2001) broaden-and-build model of positive emotions, the human drive toward pleasure is transformed from meaningless hedonism to the drive toward the attainment of skills and building of resources. It may be that as a field, we have tended to view what people want from a perspective that is unnecessarily reductionistic: If it feels good, it must be driven by something that's ultimately bad. I suggest that there remains much to be gained by following Allport's (1961) advice just to ask people what we want to know about them—even if our questions pertain to that dark corner of the human heart that propels us to think, to feel, to strive heroically, to fail miserably, and even to grow out our bangs.

## REFERENCES


Ach, N. (1910). *Uber den Willensakt und das Temperament* [Over the will and the temperament]. Leipzig: Quelle & Meyer.

Allport, G. (1961). *Pattern and growth in personality.* New York: Holt, Rinehart, & Winston.

Block, J. (1982). Assimilation, accommodation, and the dynamics of personality development. *Child Development, 53,* 281–295.

Brunstein, J. C. (1993). Personal goals and subjective well-being: A longitudinal study. *Journal of Personality and Social Psychology, 65,* 1061–1070.

Brunstein, J. C., & Gollwitzer, P. M. (1996). Effects of failure on subsequent performance: The importance of self-defining goals. *Journal of Personality and Social Psychology, 70,* 395–407.

Brunstein, J. C., & Maier, G. W. (2005). Implicit and self-attributed motives to achieve: Two separate but interacting needs. *Journal of Personality and Social Psychology, 89,* 205–222.

Cross, S., & Markus, H. (1991). Possible selves across the life span. *Human Development, 34,* 230–255.

Diener, E., & Fujita, F. (1995). Resources, personal strivings, and subjective well-being: A nomothetic and idiographic approach. *Journal of Personality and Social Psychology, 68,* 926–935.

Emmons, R. A. (1989). The personal striving approach to personality. In L. A. Pervin (Ed.), *Goal concepts in personality and social psychology* (pp. 87–126). Hillsdale, NJ: Erlbaum.

Emmons, R. A. (1992). Abstract versus concrete goals: Personal striving level, physical illness, and psychological well-being. *Journal of Personality and Social Psychology, 62,* 292–300.

Emmons, R. A., Colby, P. M., & Kaiser, H. A. (1998). When losses lead to gains: Personal goals and the recovery of meaning. In P. T. P. Wong & P.S. Fry (Eds.), *The human quest for meaning: A handbook of psychological research and clinical applications* (pp. 163–178). Mahwah, NJ: Erlbaum.

Emmons, R. A., & King, L. A. (1988). Conflict among personal strivings: Immediate and long-term implications for psychological and physical well-being. *Jour-*

*nal of Personality and Social Psychology, 53*, 1040–1048.

Frazier, L. D., & Hooker, K. (2006). Possible selves in adult development: Linking theory and research. In C. Dunkel & J. Kerpelman (Eds.), *Possible selves: Theory, research and applications* (pp. 41–59). Hauppauge, NY: Nova Science.

Fredrickson, B. L. (1998). What good are positive emotions? *Review of General Psychology, 2*, 300–319.

Fredrickson, B. L. (2001). The role of positive emotions in positive psychology: The broaden-and-build theory of positive emotions. *American Psychologist, 56*, 218–226.

Harlow, R. E., & Cantor, N. (1995). Overcoming lack of self-assurance in an achievement domain: Creating agency in daily life. In M. H. Kernis (Ed.), *Efficacy, agency, and self-esteem* (pp. 171–191). New York: Plenum Press.

Helson, R. (1992). Women's difficult times and the rewriting of the life story. *Psychology of Women Quarterly, 16*, 331–347.

Helson, R., & Roberts, B. (1994). Ego development and personality change in adulthood. *Journal of Personality and Social Psychology, 66*, 911–920.

Helson, R., & Wink, P. (1992). Two conceptions of maturity examined in findings of a longitudinal study. *Journal of Personality and Social Psychology, 53*, 531–541.

Hoyle, R. H., & Sherrill, M. R. (2006). Future orientation in the self-system: Possible selves, self-regulation, and behavior. *Journal of Personality, 74*, 1673–1696.

Kato, K., & Markus, H. R. (1993). The role of possible selves in memory. *Psychologia: An International Journal of Psychology in the Orient, 36*, 73–83.

Kernis, M. H., Paradise, A. W., Whitaker, D. J., Wheatman, S. R., & Goldman, B. N. (2000). Master of one's psychological domain?: Not likely if one's self-esteem is unstable. *Personality and Social Psychology Bulletin, 26*, 1297–1305.

King, L. A. (1995). Wishes, motives, goals, and personal memories: Relations and correlates of measures of human motivation. *Journal of Personality, 63*, 985–1007.

King, L. A. (1996). Who is regulating what and why?: The motivational context of self-regulation. *Psychological Inquiry, 7*, 57–61.

King, L. A. (1998). Personal goals and personal agency: Linking everyday goals to future images of the self. In M. Kofta, G. Weary, & G. Sedek (Eds.), *Personal control in action: Cognitive and motivational mechanisms* (pp. 109–128). New York: Plenum Press.

King, L. A. (2001a). The hard road to the good life: The happy, mature person. *Journal of Humanistic Psychology, 41*, 51–72.

King, L. A. (2001b). The health benefits of writing about life goals. *Personality and Social Psychology Bulletin, 27*, 798–807.

King, L. A. (2002). Gain without pain: Expressive writing and self regulation. In S. J. Lepore & J. Smythe (Eds.), *The writing cure* (pp. 119–134). Washington, DC: American Psychological Association.

King, L. A. (2003). Some truths behind the trombones? *Psychological Inquiry, 14*, 128–131.

King, L. A., & Burton, C. M. (2003). The hazards of goal pursuit. In E. Chang & L. Sanna (Eds.), *Virtue, vice and personality: The complexity of behavior* (pp. 53–70). Washington, DC: American Psychological Association.

King, L. A., & Hicks, J. A. (2006). Narrating the self in the past and the future: Implications for maturity. *Journal of Research in Human Development, 3*, 121–138.

King, L. A., & Miner, K. N. (2000). Writing about the perceived benefits of traumatic life events: Implications for physical health. *Personality and Social Psychology Bulletin, 26*, 220–230.

King, L. A., & Patterson, C. (2000). Reconstructing life goals after the birth of a child with Down syndrome: Finding happiness and growing. *International Journal of Rehabilitation and Health, 5*, 17–30.

King, L. A., & Raspin, C. (2004). Lost and found possible selves, well-being and ego development in divorced women. *Journal of Personality, 72*, 603–631.

King, L. A., Richards, J. H., & Stemmerich, E. (1998). Daily goals, life goals, and worst fears: Means, ends, and subjective well-being. *Journal of Personality, 66*, 713–744.

King, L. A., Scollon, C. K., Ramsey, C. M., & Williams, T. (2000). Stories of life transition: Happy endings, subjective well-being, and ego development in parents of children with Down syndrome. *Journal of Research in Personality, 34*, 509–536.

King, L. A., & Smith, N. G. (2004). Gay and straight possible selves: Goals, identity, subjective well-being, and personality development. *Journal of Personality, 72*, 967–994.

Klinger, E. (1977). *Meaning and void: Inner experience and the incentives in people's lives.* Minneapolis: University of Minnesota Press.

Klinger, E. (1995). Effects of motivation and emotion on thought flow and cognition: Assessment and findings. In P. E. Shrout & S. Fiske (Eds.), *Personality research, methods, and theory: A festschrift honoring Donald W. Fiske* (pp. 257–270). Hillsdale, NJ: Erlbaum.

Klinger, E. (1999). Thought flow: Properties and mechanisms underlying shifts in content. In J. A. Singer & P. Salovey (Eds.), *At play in the fields of consciousness: Essays in honor of Jerome L. Singer* (pp. 29–50). Mahwah, NJ: Erlbaum.

Kuhl, J., & Helle, P. (1986). Motivational and volitional determinants of depression: The degenerated intention hypothesis. *Journal of Abnormal Psychology, 95*, 247–251.

Lepore, S. J., & Smyth, J. M. (2002). *The writing cure.* Washington, DC: American Psychological Association.

Loevinger, J. (1976). *Ego development: Conceptions and theories.* San Francisco: Jossey-Bass.

Marsh, H. W. (1995). A Jamesian model of self-investment and self-esteem: Comment on Pelham (1995). *Journal of Personality and Social Psychology, 69*, 1151–1160.

Markus, H., & Ruvolo, A. (1989). Possible selves: Personalized representations of goals. In L. A. Pervin (Ed.), *Goal concepts in personality and social psychology* (pp. 211–241). Hillsdale, NJ: Erlbaum.

Maslow, A. (1970). *Motivation and personality* (2nd ed.). New York: Harper & Row.

Masten, A. S. (2001). Ordinary magic: Resilience processes in development. *American Psychologist, 56,* 227–238.

McClelland, D. C., Koestner, R., & Weinberger, J. (1992). How do self-attributed and implicit motives differ? In C. P. Smith (Ed.), *Motivation and personality: Handbook of thematic content analysis* (pp. 49–72). New York: Cambridge University Press.

Niedenthal, P. M., Setterlund, M. B., & Wherry, M. B. (1992). Possible self-complexity and affective reactions to goal-relevant evaluation. *Journal of Personality and Social Psychology, 63,* 5–16.

Niedenthal, P. M., Tangney, J. P., & Gavanski, I. (1994). "If only I weren't" versus "If only I hadn't": Distinguishing shame and guilt in counterfactual thinking. *Journal of Personality and Social Psychology, 67,* 585–595.

Omodei, M. M., & Wearing, A. J. (1990). Need satisfaction and involvement in personal projects: Toward an integrative model of subjective well-being. *Journal of Personality and Social Psychology, 59,* 762–769.

Oyserman, D., Bybee, D., & Terry, K. (2006). Possible selves and academic outcomes: How and when possible selves impel action. *Journal of Personality and Social Psychology, 91,* 188–204.

Park, C. L., & Ai, A. L. (2006). Meaning making and growth: New directions for research on survivors of trauma. *Journal of Loss and Trauma, 11,* 389–407.

Park, C. L., Cohen, L. H., & Murch, R. L. (1996). Assessment and prediction of stress-related growth. *Journal of Personality, 64,* 71–105.

Pennebaker, J. W. (1990). *Opening up: The healing power of confiding in others.* New York: Morrow.

Pennebaker, J. W., & Chung, C. K. (2007). Expressive writing, emotional upheavals, and health. In H. S. Friedman & R. C. Silver (Eds.), *Foundations of health psychology* (pp. 263–284). New York: Oxford University Press.

Pennebaker, J. W., Kiecolt-Glaser, J. K., & Glaser, R. (2004). Disclosure of traumas and immune function: Health implications for psychotherapy. In R. M. Kowalski & M. R. Leary (Eds.), *The interface of social and clinical psychology: Key readings* (pp. 301–312). New York: Psychology Press.

Pervin, L. A. (Ed.). (1989). *Goal concepts in personality and social psychology.* Hillsdale, NJ: Erlbaum.

Peterson, C., & Seligman, M. E. P. (2004). *Character strengths and virtues: A handbook and classification.* Washington, DC: American Psychological Association.

Pomerantz, E. M., Saxon, J. L., & Oishi, S. (2000). The psychological trade-offs of goal investment. *Journal of Personality and Social Psychology, 79,* 617–630.

Quinlan, S. L., Jaccard, J., & Blanton, H. (2006). A decision theoretic and prototype conceptualization of possible selves: Implications for the prediction of risk behavior. *Journal of Personality, 74,* 599–630.

Ruvolo, A. P., & Markus, H. R. (1992). Possible selves and performance: The power of self-relevant imagery. *Social Cognition, 10,* 95–124.

Ryff, C. D. (1991). Possible selves in adulthood and old age: A tale of shifting horizons. *Psychology and Aging, 6,* 286–295.

Segal, H. G. (2006). Possible selves, fantasy distortion, and the anticipated life history: Exploring the role of the imagination in social cognition. In C. Dunkel & J. Kerpelman (Eds.), *Possible selves: Theory, research and applications* (pp. 79–96). Hauppauge, NY: Nova Science.

Seligman, M. E. P. (2003). Positive psychology: Fundamental assumptions. *Psychologist, 16,* 126–127.

Seligman, M. E. P., & Csikszentmihalyi, M. (2000). Positive psychology: An introduction. *American Psychologist, 55,* 5–14.

Sheldon, K. M. (2004). *Optimal human being: An integrated multi-level perspective.* Mahwah, NJ: Erlbaum.

Sheldon, K. M., & Houser-Marko, L. (2001). Self-concordance, goal attainment, and the pursuit of happiness: Can there be an upward spiral? *Journal of Personality and Social Psychology, 80,* 152–165.

Sheldon, K., & King, L. A. (2001). Why positive psychology is necessary. *American Psychologist, 56,* 216–217.

Sheldon, K. M., & Lyubomirsky, S. (2006). How to increase and sustain positive emotion: The effects of expressing gratitude and visualizing best possible selves. *Journal of Positive Psychology, 1,* 73–82.

Singer, J. A., & Blagov, P. (2004). The integrative function of narrative processing: Autobiographical memory, self-defining memories, and the life story of identity. In D. Beike, J. M. Lampinen, & D. A. Behrend (Eds.), *The self and memory* (pp. 117–138). New York: Psychology Press.

Singer, J. A., & Salovey, P. (1996). Motivated memory: Self-defining memories, goals, and affect regulation. In L. Martin & A. Tesser (Eds.), *Striving and feeling: Interactions among goals, affect, and self-regulation* (pp. 229–250). Hillsdale, NJ: Erlbaum.

Torges, C. M., Stewart, A. J., & Miner-Rubino, K. (2005). Personality after the prime of life: Men and women coming to terms with regrets. *Journal of Research in Personality, 39,* 148–165.

Vallacher, R. R., & Wegner, D. M. (2000). What do people think they are doing? In E. T. Higgins & A. Kruglanski (Eds.), *Motivational science: Social and personality perspectives* (pp. 215–228). Philadelphia: Psychology Press. (Original work published 1987)

Ziegarnik, B. (1938). On finished and unfinished tasks. In W. D. Ellis (Ed.), *A sourcebook of gestalt psychology* (pp. 300–314). New York: Harcourt Brace.

# INTERGROUP AND INTERPERSONAL RELATIONS

Chapter 35

# When Self-Protection Hurts

## SATISFYING CONNECTEDNESS MOTIVATIONS IN CLOSE RELATIONSHIPS

Sandra L. Murray

Discerning the quality of another's caring is a preoccupying goal in romantic life. Petals are plucked off daisies, and innocuous events, such as a glance, frown, or smile, are imbued with meaning in the hopes of concluding that another truly cares. Such motivated attentiveness to the evidence is not at all surprising, given the unique interdependence dilemma that romantic relationships pose. Risking thoughts and behaviors that increase closeness necessarily increases both the likelihood and pain of rejection. Imagine that Sally has a bad day at work and comes to Harry for consolation. Her willingness to seek support is critical for establishing satisfying interactions, but in seeking support, she risks Harry's criticism or rebuff. Moreover, the long-term pain of rejection only increases the more Sally comes to depend on Harry for comfort.

Given the potential pain of rejection and relationship loss (Baumeister & Leary, 1995), people should be motivated to think and behave in ways that minimize dependence on their partners, and consequently minimize the likelihood of being hurt (Murray, Holmes, & Collins, 2006). However, people need to risk substantial dependence (Kelley, 1979) to establish the kind of satisfying relationship that can fulfill basic needs for belonging (Baumeister & Leary, 1995). They need to behave in ways that give their partners power over their outcomes, and to think in ways that invest great value and importance in their relationships (see Gagne & Lydon, 2004, and Murray, 1999, for reviews). For instance, people in satisfying relationships excuse their partners' bad behavior (Rusbult, Verette, Whitney, Slovik, & Lipkus, 1991). They also respond to their partners' needs as they arise, and trustingly leave the timing of repayment up to the partners (Clark & Grote, 1998). Taking such risks effectively optimizes the benefits and minimizes the costs afforded by adult relationships (Kelley et al., 2003; Rusbult & Van Lange, 2003).

The coincident need to risk and protect against rejection creates a basic dilemma of interdependence. The thoughts and behaviors that are critical for establishing satisfying close connections with others necessarily increase both the short-term risk of rejection and the long-term pain of rejection. This chapter summarizes a conceptual model of risk regulation developed to explain how people negotiate the resulting conflict between the goal of creating satisfying interpersonal connections and the goal of protecting themselves against rejection (Murray & Derrick, 2005; Murray, Bellavia, Rose, & Griffin, 2003; Murray, Griffin, Rose, & Bellavia, 2003; Murray, Holmes, et al., 2006; Murray, Holmes, & Griffin, 2000; Murray, Holmes, Griffin, Bellavia, & Rose, 2001).[1]

## THE RISK REGULATION SYSTEM IN RELATIONSHIPS

Situations of dependence are fundamental to romantic life. One partner's actions constrain the other's capacity to satisfy important needs and goals. Such dependence is evident from the lowest to the highest level of generality. At the level of specific situations, members of a couple are interdependent in multiple ways, ranging from deciding whose movie preference to favor on a given weekend to deciding what constitutes a fair allocation of household chores. At a broader level, the couple must negotiate different personalities, such as merging one partner's laissez-faire nature with the other's more controlled style (Braiker & Kelley, 1979; Holmes, 2002). At the highest level, the existence of the relationship itself requires both partners' cooperation.

Situations such as these—situations where one partner's responsiveness to the other's needs is in question—routinely activate the threat of rejection in romantic life. Take the mundane example of a couple trying to decide whether to go to the current blockbuster action film or a contemplative arts film. Imagine that Sally confides to Harry that she believes that seeing the action film will help distract her from work worries—concerns that she fears the arts film Harry wants to see will compound. In making this request, Sally is putting her psychological welfare in Harry's hands. As in most situations where sacrifice on Harry's part is required, she risks discovering that Harry is not willing to be responsive to her needs.

Given multiple layers of interdependence, people routinely find themselves in situations where they need to choose how much dependence (and thus how much potential for rejection) they can safely risk (Kelley, 1979). Throughout the course of a relationship, partners need to make iterative and often implicit choices between self-protection (decreasing dependence) and relationship promotion (increasing dependence). Consequently, to risk being in the relationship, the partners need a system in place that functions to keep them feeling reasonably safe in a context of continued vulnerability (Murray, Holmes, et al., 2006).

### Optimizing Assurance: Three If–Then Contingency Rules

The goal of the risk regulation system is to optimize the sense of assurance that is possible given one's relationship circumstances (Murray, Holmes, et al., 2006). This sense of assurance is experienced as a sense of safety in one's level of dependence in the relationship—a feeling of relative invulnerability to hurt. To optimize this sense of assurance, this system functions dynamically, shifting the priority given to the goals of avoiding rejection and seeking closeness so as to accommodate the perceived risks of rejection.

Figure 35.1 illustrates how this system operates. It depicts three if–then contingency rule systems a person needs to gauge the likelihood of a partner's acceptance or rejection and make the *general* situation of being involved in a relationship feel sufficiently safe: (1) an *appraisal* rule system that links situations of dependence to the goal of gauging a partner's acceptance; (2) a *signaling* rule system that links perceptions of a partner's acceptance or rejection to the experience of gratified or hurt feelings and coincident gains or losses in self-esteem; and (3) a *dependence regulation* rule system that links perceptions of a partner's acceptance or rejection to the willingness to risk future dependence. These rule systems operate in concert to prioritize self-protection goals (and the assurance that comes from maintaining psychological distance) when the perceived risks of rejection are high, or relationship promotion goals (and the assurance that comes from feeling connected) when the perceived risks of rejection are low.

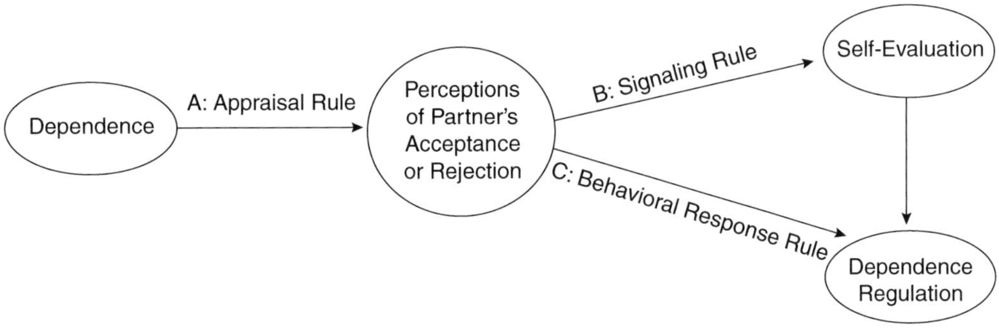


**FIGURE 35.1.** The risk regulation system in relationships.

### *The Appraisal System*

The link between dependence and perceptions of the partner's regard captures the assumption that situations of dependence increase people's need to gauge a partner's regard (Path A in Figure 35.1). This path captures the operation of an appraisal system. This contingency rule takes the form "If dependent, then gauge acceptance or rejection."

To gauge rejection risk accurately, people need to discern whether a chosen partner is willing to meet their needs. If people are to risk connection, the outcome of this appraisal process needs to indicate reason to trust in the partner's responsiveness to needs in situations of dependence (Reis, Holmes, & Clark, 2004; Tooby & Cosmides, 1996). The specific experiences that afford optimistic expectations about responsiveness are likely to vary across relationships, and perhaps across cultures (Berscheid & Regan, 2005). From the perspective of the risk regulation model, the common diagnostic that affords confidence in a partner's responsiveness to needs is the perception that the partner perceives qualities in the self worth valuing—qualities that are not readily available in other partners. In more independent cultures, this sense of confidence requires the inference that a partner perceives valued traits in the self (Murray et al., 2000; Swann, Bosson, & Pelham, 2002). In more interdependent cultures, this sense of confidence requires the further inference that a partner's family also values one's qualities (MacDonald & Jessica, 2006).

### *The Signaling System*

The link between perceived regard and self-evaluations (Path B in Figure 35.1) illustrates the operation of a signaling or emotion system that detects discrepancies between current and desired appraisals of a partner's regard and mobilizes action (Berscheid, 1983). The contingency rule governing the signaling system takes the form "If accepted or rejected, then internalize."

This rule reflects a basic assumption of the *sociometer* model of self-esteem. Leary and his colleagues believe that the need to protect against rejection is so important that people have evolved a system for reacting to rejection threats (Leary & Baumiester, 2000; Leary, Tambor, Terdal, & Downs, 1995; MacDonald & Leary, 2005). They argue that self-esteem is simply a gauge—a *sociometer*—that measures a person's perceived likelihood of being accepted or rejected by others. The sociometer is thought to function such that signs that another's approval is waning diminish self-esteem and motivate compensatory behaviors (Leary et al., 1995). In this sense, the sociometer functions not to preserve self-esteem per se, but to protect people from suffering the serious costs of rejection and not having their needs met.

The need for such a signaling system is amplified in a romantic relationship, because narrowing social connections to focus on one specific partner raises the personal stakes of rejection. In committing himself to Sally, Harry narrows the number of people he can rely on to satisfy his needs, and in so doing makes his welfare all the more dependent on Sally's actions. In his routine interactions, Harry also does not need to seek acceptance from someone he perceives to be rejecting. However, in his relationship with Sally, he is often caught in the position of being hurt by the person whose acceptance he most desires.

Given all that is at stake, the signal that is conveyed by this rule system needs to be sufficiently strong to mobilize action (Berscheid, 1983). Perceiving rejection or drops in a partner's acceptance should hurt and threaten people's general and desired conceptions of themselves as being valuable, efficacious, and worthy of interpersonal connection (Baumeister, 1993; Taylor & Brown, 1988). By making rejection aversive, this signaling system motivates people to avoid situations where relationship partners are likely to be unresponsive and needs for connectedness are likely to be frustrated. In contrast, perceiving acceptance should affirm people's sense of themselves as being good and valuable, mobilizing the desire for greater connection and the likelihood of having their needs met by their partners.

### *The Behavioral Response System*

The link between perceived regard and dependence-regulating behavior captures the assumption that the threat and social pain of rejection in turn shape people's willingness to think and behave in ways that promote dependence and connectedness (Murray et al., 2000). This path illustrates the operation of a behavioral response system—one that proactively minimizes both the likelihood and the pain of *future* rejection experiences by making increased dependence contingent on the perception of acceptance (Paths C and D in Figure 35.1). As the direct and mediated paths illustrate, this system may be triggered directly by the experience of acceptance or rejection (Path C in Figure 35.1), and indirectly through resulting gains or drops in self-esteem (Path D in Figure 35.1). The contingency rule governing this system is "If feeling accepted or rejected, then regulate dependence."

The risk regulation model assumes that the behavioral response system operates to ensure that people only risk as much future dependence as they feel is reasonably safe, given recent experience. Suggesting that felt acceptance is a relatively automatic trigger to safety and the possibility of connection, unconsciously primed words that connote security (e.g., *accepted*) heighten empathy for others (Mikulincer et al., 2001), diminish people's tendency to derogate outgroup members (Mikulincer & Shaver, 2001), and increase people's desire to seek support from others in dealing with a personal crisis (Pierce & Lydon, 1998). In contrast, experiencing rejection elicits a social pain akin to physical pain, so as to trigger automatic responses (e.g., aggression) that increase physical or psychological distance between oneself and the source of the pain (MacDonald & Leary, 2005).

Given the general operation of such a dependence regulation system, and the heightened need to protect against romantic rejection, people should implicitly regulate and structure dependence on a specific partner in ways that allow them to minimize the short-term likelihood and long-term potential pain of rejection (Murray et al., 2000). When a partner's general regard is in question, and rejection seems more likely, people should tread cautiously, reserve judgment, and limit future dependence on the partner.

A first line of defense may involve limiting the situations people are willing to enter within their relationships. Efforts to delimit dependence by choosing such situations carefully may involve conscious decisions to seek support elsewhere, disclose less, or follow exchange norms. These strategies minimize the chance of being in situations where a partner might prove to be unresponsive. A second line of defense might involve shifting the symbolic value attached to the partner and the relationship itself. Such efforts might entail less deliberative shifts in the way people construe their partner's behavior and qualities, such as becoming less willing to excuse specific transgressions (Bradbury & Fincham, 1990), or coming to see the partner's habitual lateness as maddening rather than endearing (Holmes & Rempel, 1989). By diminishing the partner's value as a source of connection, and minimizing the pain of rejection in advance, people can protect a sense of their own worthiness of interpersonal connection against loss.

When confident of a partner's general regard, people can more safely risk increased dependence in the future—entering into situations where the partner has control over immediate outcomes, forgiving transgressions, attaching greater value to the partner's qualities, and risking a stronger sense of commitment to the partner and the relationship.

## Individual Differences: How Perceived Regard Controls Rule Sensitivity

For a relationship risk regulation system to be functional, it needs to adapt itself to suit specific relationship circumstances. If Sally generally perceives Harry to be responsive to her needs, distancing herself from Harry at the first sign of his insensitivity is not likely to be the optimal means of sustaining the needed sense of assurance. If Sally generally perceives Harry to be unresponsive, however, such a response might be Sally's best available means of sustaining some minimal sense of safety from harm. Accordingly, to respond dynamically and adaptively to ongoing events, the regulatory system depicted in Figure 35.1 needs a heuristic means of estimating the level of risk inherent in specific situations.

Figure 35.2 illustrates how this risk calibration occurs. In this individual difference extension of the risk regulation system, people's general or cross-situational sense of confidence in a partner's positive regard and love acts as such an arbiter or barometer—telling people whether it is safe to put self-protection aside and risk thinking and behaving in relationship-promotive ways (Murray, Holmes, et al., 2006). Specifically, feeling more or less positively regarded by a partner interacts with specific event features to control the sensitivity of the appraisal, signaling, and dependence regulation rules people adopt in specific situations.

At the first stage of this process, chronic perceptions of a partner's regard interact with specific event features to control the extent to which people categorize or code specific events as situations of risk. To the extent that Sally is unsure of Harry's regard, even the mundane choice of one movie over another could make concerns about dependence salient. However, to the extent that Sally is more confident of Harry's regard, she might only begin to entertain thoughts about her vulnerability to his actions when they try to negotiate more serious decisions in their relationship, such as deciding whose financial philosophy to follow. Once identified as such, the possibility of rejection inherent in such "dependent" situations activates a situated conflict between self-protection and relationship promotion goals.

The consequent activation of the need for a sense of assurance then triggers the appraisal, signaling, and behavior response systems, respectively (either individually or in concert). A person's habitual means of optimizing feelings of assurance is revealed in the idiosyncratic or signature ways this person tailors these rules to prioritize self-protection or relationship promotion goals in specific situations of dependence.

For people who generally feel less positively regarded by a specific partner, the goal of feeling valued and discerning the partner's caring is likely to be chronically activated (Murray, Bellavia, et al., 2003; Murray, Griffin, et al., 2003). The chronic accessibility of this goal should sensitize people who feel less positively regarded to rejection threats, shaping the if–then contingencies that are activated in ways that put a premium on self-protection.

Why would this be the case? General expectations of rejection, such as those embodied in low self-esteem, make specific rejection experi-

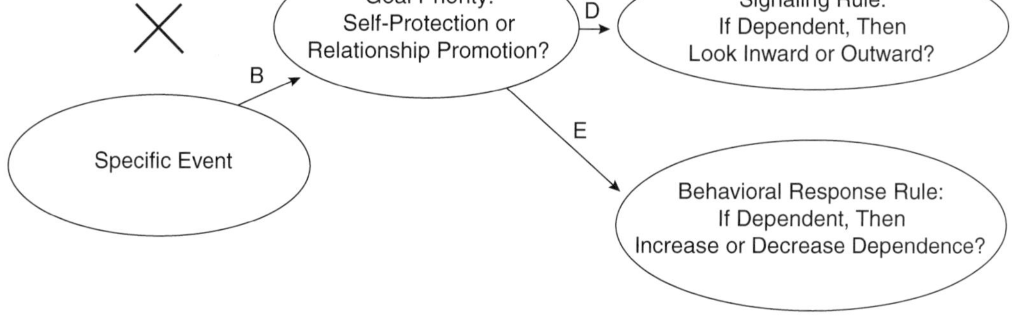


**FIGURE 35.2.** How perceived regard arbitrates the operation of the risk regulation system.

ences all the more painful and all the more motivating (Leary & Baumeister, 2000; Nezlek, Kowalski, Leary, Blevins, & Holgate, 1997; Sommer & Baumeister, 2002). For people who generally feel less positively regarded by a specific partner, situated rejection experiences hurt more because they pose a greater proportional loss to a more precarious, generalized sense of their worthiness of interpersonal connection. Consequently, they are in particular need of a self-protectively weighted or prevention-oriented rule system (Higgins, 1996)—one that quickly detects rejection, strongly signals the possibility of further hurt, and motivates them to take defensive action sooner rather than later (Pietrzak, Downey, & Ayduk, 2005). Thus chronic doubts about Harry's regard require Sally to act as though she believes that minimizing the pain of rejection provides greater assurance or safety from harm than risking closeness.

For people who generally feel more positively regarded by a specific partner, there is little need for such a defensively calibrated rule system. For them, specific rejections pose a smaller proportional loss to a comparably rich resource. Instead, the goal of maintaining the desired level of confidence in the partner's positive regard and caring is likely to prevail (Murray, Bellavia, et al., 2003; Murray, Griffin, et al., 2003). A regulatory system that functions to prioritize relationship promotion goals better affords the person a continued sense of assurance or safety in the relationship. In other words, confidence in Sally's regard allows Harry to act as though he believes that seeking closeness affords the greatest safety from harm.

In appraising the meaning of specific situations of dependence, people who generally feel more positively regarded set a high threshold for detecting rejection. Rather than being primed to see rejection, these people appraise and respond to most situations of dependence in ways that dispel unwanted rejection concerns and uncertainties and protect the desired sense of confidence in their partners' positive regard and caring (Murray & Holmes, 1993). In particular, specific situations of dependence should activate if–then contingencies that link potential threats to motivated cognitive processes that bolster and protect perceptions of their partners' acceptance and caring. Even in situations where they feel rejected, general expectations of partner acceptance should dull the sting of specific hurts, protecting self-esteem from most experiences of rejection. In fact, general expectations of acceptance should give these people reason to believe that seeking greater closeness to their partners will minimize rather than exacerbate the likelihood of future hurts. Consequently, people who generally feel more positively regarded should respond to situated rejections in ways that foster greater dependence.

## THE OPERATION OF THE RISK REGULATION SYSTEM: EMPIRICAL EXAMPLES

The contingencies that govern the thoughts and behavior of people who feel more or less positively regarded should emerge most clearly in situations where the threat of rejection is salient (Holmes, 2002; Mischel & Shoda, 1995). Such differences may be less obvious in more accepting or neutral circumstances. In illustrating the operation of the risk regulation system, I focus on experimental, observational, and daily diary research that best affords this type of comparison. I examine studies that included direct measures of perceived regard (Murray, Bellavia, et al., 2003; Murray, Griffin, et al., 2003), as well as studies that included dispositional proxies for perceived regard, including global self-esteem (Murray et al., 2000), attachment-related anxiety (Murray et al., 2001), and rejection sensitivity (Downey & Feldman, 1996). These dispositional expectations operate similarly to partner-specific expectations of acceptance because people low in self-esteem, high in attachment anxiety, or high in rejection sensitivity report feeling less positively regarded by specific romantic partners.

I highlight the results of a longitudinal daily diary study of married couples conducted in my laboratory. This study utilized a direct measure of expectations of a specific partner's regard and tracked how each couple negotiated a wide variety of dependent situations over 21 days (Murray, Bellavia, et al., 2003; Murray, Griffin, et al., 2003). Participants rated how they believed their partners saw them on positive and negative interpersonal attributes (i.e., perceived regard), such as *warm*, *critical*, and *responsive* (Murray et al., 2000). In each diary, the participant indicated which specific situations of dependence had occurred that day (e.g., "had a minor disagreement," "partner criticized me") and completed state items tapping self-esteem (e.g., felt "good about myself"), feelings of rejection or acceptance by the partner (e.g., felt "rejected or hurt by my partner," "my partner accepts me as I am"), perceptions of the partner's responsiveness (e.g., "my partner is selfish"), and closeness (e.g., "in love with my partner").

## Suiting Appraisal Sensitivity Contingencies to Circumstances

How does the sensitivity of the appraisal rule system shift according to the circumstances afforded by generally feeling more or less valued by a partner in situations that are more or less risky? For people who generally feel less positively regarded by their partners, situations of dependence should readily activate concerns about rejection (i.e., "If dependent situation, then question acceptance"). However, for people who generally feel more positively regarded, the goal of preserving a sense of assurance should activate relationship-promotive contingencies that link situations of dependence to bolstered perceptions of acceptance (i.e., "If dependent situation, then bolster acceptance"). In illustrating these effects, I examine two situations of dependence: self-based situations, in which one person needs support; and relationship-based situations, in which a partner initiates a conflict or behaves negatively.

### *Self-Based Situations*

Imagine that Sally gets criticized at work for failing to complete a project. Such situations activate the attachment system and the need to seek another's literal or symbolic validation (Collins & Feeney, 2000). In fact, priming failure-related thoughts activates thoughts of seeking proximity to others (Mikulincer, Birnbaum, Woddis, & Nachmias, 2000) and increases the accessibility of a romantic partner's name (Mikulincer, Gillath, & Shaver, 2002).

Accordingly, to the extent that Sally feels more confident of Harry's regard, she may readily compensate for her work-related angst by reminding herself how much Harry values her, using him as a resource for self-affirmation. However, if she generally feels uncertain of Harry's ongoing acceptance and positive regard, she may be reluctant to disclose her personal failing for fear that Harry might disparage her. Instead, such a situation may activate if–then contingencies that link her failures to Harry's likely rejection (Baldwin & Sinclair, 1996).

In the diary study, on days after participants felt bad about themselves, people who generally believed that their partners regarded them more positively actually felt more loved and accepted by their partners (Murray, Griffin, et al., 2003). Unfortunately, intimates who generally felt less valued did not find this symbolic source of support or comfort in their partners. Similarly, people who were high in self-esteem, and thus likely to feel more valued by their partners, reacted to threats to self-esteem by becoming even more convinced of their dating partners' acceptance and love (Murray, Holmes, MacDonald, & Ellsworth, 1998). For instance, high-self-esteem participants reacted to failure on a purported test of intelligence by exaggerating their partners' love (relative to high-self-esteem controls). In contrast, dating intimates low in self-esteem reacted to experimentally induced doubts about their intelligence or considerateness by expressing greater concerns about their partners' likely rejection (Murray et al., 1998).

### *Partner-Based Situations of Dependence*

Now imagine that Sally comes home to find Harry in an irritable mood—grumbling about the lack of food in the fridge, and the fact that Sally had promised to replenish the fridge's contents by day's end. If Sally trusts Harry's continuing positive regard, such situations may activate appraisal contingencies that link Harry's irritation to a ready excuse. She may even find some way to see such foibles as signs of Harry's acceptance and love, in a motivated reconstrual of the evidence (e.g., "If Harry grumbles, he's just showing he can be himself around me"). However, if Sally generally feels less valued by Harry, she may have difficulty attributing such negative events to some specific feature of the situation, such as Harry's fatigue. Instead, Sally may attribute such grumbling to an interpersonal disposition—his broader displeasure with her (e.g., "If Harry grumbles, he's upset with me").

In the daily diary study, married intimates who generally felt less positively regarded by their spouses read decidedly more rejection-related meanings into negative situations than intimates who generally felt more positively regarded (Murray, Bellavia, et al., 2003). For instance, people who generally felt less valued by their partners felt more rejected on days after their partners had simply been in a worse than average mood—a mood that had nothing to do with them or their relationships. Such sensitivity to rejection was not at all characteristic of people who generally felt more positively regarded. Instead, they actually recruited more feelings of being loved and accepted by their partners on days after they reported more than their usual amount of conflict or negative partner behavior (and thus had greater actual reason to distrust their partners).

Conceptual parallels of these results are evident in other research. Dating intimates who were low in self-esteem overinterpreted their dating partners' hypothetical negative moods, seeing them as symptomatic of their partners' ill feelings toward them (Bellavia & Murray, 2003). Low-, but not high-, self-esteem participants reacted to experimentally induced signs of their partners' irritation by anticipating rejection (Murray, Rose, Bellavia, Holmes, & Kusche, 2002). Similarly, dating intimates who were high on attachment-related anxiety about acceptance (and were likely to question their specific partners' acceptance) interpreted their partners' hypothetical (Collins, 1996) and actual (Mikulincer, 1998; Simpson, Rholes, & Phillips, 1996) misdeeds in suspicious ways that were likely to exacerbate hurt feelings. People high on attachment-related anxiety even interpreted their partners' ambiguous attempts to be supportive as intentionally hurtful (Collins & Feeney, 2004). They also interpreted daily conflicts as a sign of their partners' waning commitment (Campbell, Simpson, Boldry, & Kashy, 2005). When gauging their dating partners' thoughts about attractive opposite-sex others, intimates high on attachment-related anxiety were more empathically accurate, discerning threatening thoughts that were misunderstood by secure intimates (Simpson, Ickes, & Grich, 1999). People who anticipated interpersonal rejection attributed negative intent to new partners' hypothetical behaviors (Downey & Feldman, 1996). In marriage, people who were less trusting of their partners' responsiveness reacted to reminders of past transgressions by perceiving more hurtful intent in their partners' discussion of a current problem. In contrast, people who were more trusting reacted to past transgressions by seeing their partners' motivations more positively than controls (Holmes & Rempel, 1989).

## Suiting Self-Esteem Sensitivity Contingencies to Circumstances

The signaling system generally operates to detect discrepancies between current and desired appraisals of a partner's regard, thereby mobilizing energy for action. For people who generally feel less valued by their partners, detecting drops in acceptance poses a greater proportional loss to a limited resource. For them, the signal conveyed by this rule needs to be especially strong. Relative to people who feel more positively regarded, people who feel less valued should be hurt more readily, questioning their worth in the face of perceived rejections (i.e., "If feeling acutely rejected, then internalize").

In the diary study, global perceptions of the spouses' regard determined how much daily concerns about the partners' rejection deflated state self-esteem (Murray, Griffin, et al., 2003). People who generally felt less positively regarded by their partners felt worse about themselves on days after they experienced a greater than usual level of anxiety about their partners' acceptance (as compared to low-anxiety days). In contrast, for people who generally felt more positively regarded, one day's anxieties about acceptance did not turn into the next day's self-doubts. In a conceptually parallel experiment, low-, but not high-, self-esteem dating intimates responded to induced fears that their partners perceived important faults in them by questioning their own self-worth (Murray et al., 2002, Experiment 3).

The combination of greater appraisal and self-esteem sensitivity to rejection for people who generally feel less valued by their partners raises an interesting paradox. Namely, why are they so willing to perceive rejection if it is so hurtful? It may be precisely the fact that rejection is more hurtful that makes such people more susceptible to perceiving rejection. In approaching their relationships, people who feel less valued may be attuned for signs of potential rejection so that they might avoid even more hurtful situations in the future (MacDonald & Leary, 2005). Given a minimal level of interdependence, such avoidance attempts are not likely to be wholly successful, however. Prior research on prevention motivations suggests that such ironic effects are quite likely to occur. For instance, people who were highly motivated to avoid negative outcomes (people high on behavioral inhibition) were no more successful in avoiding negative events than people low on such motivation, despite the fact that people high on avoidance motivation reacted more emotionally when such events occurred (Gable, Reis, & Elliot, 2000).

## Suiting Dependence Regulation Contingencies to Circumstances

The behavioral response rule system operates to minimize the likelihood and pain of rejection by only allowing people to risk as much future dependence as feels safe, given recent experience. For people who generally feel less positively regarded, perceiving acute rejections should activate the goal of self-protection and the desire to reduce dependence. For people who feel more positively regarded, perceiving acute rejections should activate the goal of promoting dependence and connectedness.

### *If Rejected, Then Decrease Dependence*

The existing evidence suggests that people who feel less valued by their partners do indeed respond to perceived rejections by reducing dependence (i.e., "If rejected, then decrease dependence"). In the daily diary study (Murray, Bellavia, et al., 2003), people who generally felt less positively regarded responded to feeling acutely rejected by their partners one day by treating their partners in more cold, critical, and negative ways the next day. For these people, feeling rejected activated the behavioral contingency "Distance myself from my partner." These reactions emerged even though the partners of people who felt less valued were not actually upset with them when they felt most rejected. Instead, people who felt less valued responded to an imagined rejection by treating their partners badly.

Conceptual replications of these dynamics are evident in both experimental and field research. People who were likely to doubt their partners' acceptance by virtue of their dispositions reacted to feeling rejected in specific situations in ways that minimized dependence. People with low self-esteem responded to induced anxieties about their partners' possible rejection by depending less on their partners as a source of self-esteem and comfort (Murray et al., 1998). They also evaluated their partners' qualities more negatively (Murray et al., 1998, 2002). The need to downplay the value and importance of the partners (the sources of the hurt) is sufficiently powerful that derogation effects have emerged on the qualities that typically reveal people's positive illusions about their partners (Murray, Holmes, & Griffin, 1996). These devaluing processes have also emerged whether these acute rejection anxieties are imagined in response to a newly discovered fault in the self (Murray et al., 1998) or in response to a partner's behavior (Murray et al., 2002). Such devaluing efforts appear in part to be automatic, as they have also surfaced on implicit measures of partner regard (DeHart, Pelham, & Murray, 2004). For instance, the more difficulties low-self-esteem people currently perceived in their relationships, the less favorably they evaluated their partners' name letters. By diminishing their partners' value, people who feel less valued give their partners less power to hurt them in the future by making the partners less important sources of need satisfaction and less valued informants on their general worthiness of love and connection.

Research in other laboratories further illustrates the model's contention that risky situations activate distancing attempts for people who generally feel less valued by specific partners. Women higher in attachment-related anxiety displayed greater anger toward their partners in a situation in which their partners might not have been as responsive as they hoped (Rholes, Simpson, & Orina, 1999). After discussing a serious relationship problem, more anxiously attached men and women also reported greater anger and hostility (as compared to controls who discussed a minor problem), and they downplayed their feelings of closeness and commitment (Simpson et al., 1996). To the extent that expressions of anger are a means of trying to control a partner's behavior, such sentiments both directly and indirectly reduce dependence.

Intimates high on attachment-related anxiety also reported feeling less close to their partners in a situation where they accurately inferred the (threatening) content of their partners' thoughts about attractive opposite-sex others (Simpson et al., 1999). When dating men in this study were both high on attachment-related anxiety and empathically accurate, their relationships were at the greatest risk of dissolution (Simpson et al., 1999). People high on attachment-related anxiety also reacted to higher levels of daily conflict by minimizing their feelings of closeness to their partners (Campbell et al., 2005). As another example, women chronically high on rejection sensitivity responded to potential partners' disinterest by evaluating those partners more negatively (Ayduk, Downey, Testa, Yen, & Shoda,

1999). Rejection-sensitive women were also more likely to initiate conflicts on days after they felt more rejected by their romantic partners, and simply priming rejection-related words automatically activated hostility-related thoughts for these women (Ayduk et al., 1999).

### *If Rejected, Then Increase Dependence*

For people who generally feel more positively regarded, feeling acutely rejected activates if–then contingencies that link situations of dependence to relationship promotion goals. In the daily diary study, intimates who generally felt more positively regarded actually drew closer to their partners on days after they felt most rejected—a relationship-promotive response (Murray, Bellavia, et al., 2003). Similarly, dating intimates who tended to feel more positively regarded by virtue of higher global self-esteem responded to induced concerns about their dating partners' likely annoyance with them by reporting greater feelings of closeness to those same partners (Murray et al., 2002, Experiment 2). For these people, feeling rejected activated a behavioral contingency "Draw closer." Dating intimates high in global self-esteem also reacted to experimentally induced self-doubts by reporting greater dependence on their partners' reassurance as a source of self-esteem (Murray et al., 1998). Similarly, people low on attachment-related anxiety came to value their partners more after discussing a serious than a minor conflict (Simpson et al., 1996). Such relationship-promotive tendencies even extend to situations where a partner is attracted to another. The closer intimates low on attachment-related anxiety felt to their partners, the more accurate they were in discerning their partners' attraction to opposite-sex others (Simpson et al., 1999).

## THE SELF-DEFEATING EFFECTS OF SELF-PROTECTION

As the experience of slights and hurts at the hands of a romantic partner is inevitable, the challenge in maintaining a satisfying relationship rests in preventing such situated threats from triggering the defensive devaluation of the partner (and the delivery of reciprocal slights). Confident expectations of acceptance seem to dull the self-esteem sting of rejection in ways that allow people to see (occasionally) hurtful partners in the best possible light. However, people who feel less positively regarded are likely to see the slightest offense as a sign of impending rejection, motivating them to self-protect and distance themselves from the sting of any further perceived slights. Such efforts at dependence regulation would be understandable if people who feel less valued actually possessed partners who valued and loved them less, and treated them less well. This does not appear to be the case. Intimates who felt less valued in the diary study still perceived rejection in their partners' behavior, and reacted defensively to feeling hurt, even when the partners' actual behavior and actual regard for them were held constant. Ironically, the desire to protect themselves against hurt seems to lead people who are trying to find acceptance to undermine the resources of admiring partners that they need to preserve.

For instance, women who chronically anticipated rejection behaved more negatively toward their dating partners during conflicts and elicited more rejecting behavior in those specific instances (Downey, Freitas, Michaelis, & Khouri, 1998). Moreover, on days after rejection-sensitive women felt acutely rejected by their dating partners, their partners reported greater dissatisfaction (Downey et al., 1998). In the diary study reported by Murray, Bellavia, and colleagues (2003), the *spouses* of people who felt less positively regarded (correctly) believed they were the target of more hurtful and rejecting behaviors on days after these people had felt most rejected—and it was only then that the spouses finally became annoyed and rejecting. The fact that such perceptions arise suggest that people's self-protective attempts to prospectively blunt the pain of rejection may have the consequence of alienating their partners (Gottman, 1994).

By putting self-protection at a greater premium than relationship promotion, people who feel less positively regarded may create long-term interpersonal realities that defeat their hopes and confirm their fears. Supporting this analysis, a longitudinal daily diary study of married couples suggests that the chronic activation of self-protective appraisal, signaling, and behavioral response rules has a corrosive effect on relationships over time (Murray, Bellavia, et al., 2003; Murray, Griffin, et al., 2003). In this sample, relationship difficulties were more likely to arise when the if–then contingencies underlying people's cognition, affect, and behavior mirrored the if–then contingencies evident among people who felt less valued by their partners.

First, satisfaction declined when people's online systems for appraising rejection threats were calibrated in a more self-protective fashion. In particular, when women linked their own personal self-doubts to their husbands' lessened acceptance, their *husbands* reported relatively greater declines in satisfaction over time (Murray, Griffin, et al., 2003; Murray, Griffin, Rose, & Bellavia, 2006). Conversely, when women compensated for self-doubts by embellishing their husbands' acceptance, their husbands reported relatively greater satisfaction (Murray, Griffin, et al., 2003). Second, satisfaction declined when people's signaling systems were more sensitive to rejection. When people reacted to anxieties about rejection by reporting diminished self-esteem the next day, their *partners* reported significantly greater declines in satisfaction. Third, when women's behavioral response to feeling rejected was to self-protect and behave negatively, their husbands' satisfaction declined over the year (Murray, Griffin, et al., 2003).

Unfortunately, the potential for negative relationship consequences is not likely to be part of the consciousness of a person caught in the immediate experience of trying to blunt the short-term pain of a perceived rejection. People respond to experimentally induced fears of lifelong rejection and social isolation by behaving in self-defeating ways—putting short-term pleasures, such as making risky gambles or unhealthy food choices, ahead of the long-term costs of such endeavors (Twenge, Catanese, & Baumeister, 2002). Induced rejection fears also undermine people's scores on intelligence tests (Baumeister, Twenge, & Nuss, 2002), suggesting that coping with rejection impairs the type of executive functioning necessary for effective self-regulation. Unfortunately, for people low on self-esteem, gauging and then responding to perceived rejections may be sufficiently preoccupying that they exhaust the self-regulatory resources needed to anticipate the costs of self-protection (Finkel & Campbell, 2001).

## AN APPLICATION: UNDERSTANDING WHY LOW SELF-ESTEEM CREATES RELATIONSHIP DIFFICULTIES

Despite people's general needs for belongingness, and the specific goal of establishing a sense of assurance, people troubled by dispositional insecurities such as low self-esteem have difficulty finding evidence of their partners' acceptance in even the most accommodating realities. In both dating and marital relationships, people with low self-esteem underestimate how positively their partners see them on specific traits (Murray et al., 2000) and even underestimate how much their partners love them (Murray et al., 2001). People who are more sensitive to rejection or more preoccupied in attachment style (and thus lower in self-esteem) also underestimate their dating partners' relationship satisfaction and commitment (Downey & Feldman, 1996; Tucker & Anders, 1999). Unfortunately, therefore, the people most in need of relationships may be most vulnerable to the pernicious effects of prioritizing self-protection over connectedness goals. Why would such self-defeating misperceptions arise?

People routinely use their own self-images as heuristics or templates for constructing their perceptions of their partners' beliefs about their specific qualities (e.g., Griffin & Ross, 1991; Kenny, 1994; Shrauger & Schoeneman, 1979). Low-self-esteem people possess less positive, more uncertain, and more conflicted beliefs about themselves than high-self-esteem people (e.g., Baumeister, 1993). Similar self-doubts characterize people troubled by chronic attachment-related anxiety (Collins & Read, 1990) or rejection sensitivity (Downey & Feldman, 1996). Behaving like naive realists, low-self-esteem people in dating and marital relationships then assume that their partners see them in the same relatively negative light as they see themselves (Murray et al., 2000). Compounding this vulnerability, low-self-esteem people also feel inferior to their partners, attributing more desirable interpersonal qualities to their partners than they see in themselves (Murray et al., 2005).

Knowing (at least implicitly) the importance of equivalent social exchange, low-self-esteem people may have trouble explaining why partners who must see so many faults in them, and who seem so superior to them, would really care for them or remain committed. In contrast, the confidently held, positive self-views of high-self-esteem people provide a readily accessible, compelling accounting for their partners' caring and commitment.

Through its focus on partner-specific expectations of acceptance, the risk regulation model helps explain why certain dispositional vulnerabilities, such as low self-esteem (e.g., Murray et al., 1998), chronic rejection sensitivity (Downey et al., 1998), and insecure attachment styles (e.g., Collins & Feeney, 2000; Simpson, Rholes, & Nelligan, 1992), can be so problematic in relationships. More negative models of self go hand in hand with diminished satisfaction, because such self-doubts interfere with people's ability to form representations of specific others that foster a sense of assurance in the partner's positive regard and caring. Consistent with this hypothesis, perceptions of partners' regard mediate the link between self-esteem and satisfaction in both dating and marital relationships (Murray et al., 2000, 2001).

## CONCLUSION

On the brighter side, close romantic relationships offer a unique opportunity for the fulfillment of connectedness needs. On the darker side, the prospect of rejection and relationship loss threatens a profound hurt, which can irrevocably undermine people's sense of self-worth (Baumeister & Leary, 1995). Given such stakes, people only allow themselves to risk seeking connectedness when they trust in their partners' ongoing positive regard and acceptance. People who find this sense of assurance can feel safe in prioritizing connectedness goals—thinking and behaving in ways that ultimately foster stronger relationship bonds. However, people who struggle to find this sense of assurance engage in self-protection—thinking and behaving in ways that provide a sense of safety in the short term, but can ultimately alienate their partners and elicit rejection.

## ACKNOWLEDGMENTS

The preparation of this chapter was supported by grants from the National Science Foundation (No. SBR 9817282) and the National Institute of Mental Health (No. MH 60105-02).

## NOTE

1. The arguments presented in this chapter represent a distilled version of a conceptual model of risk regulation in relationships proposed by Murray, Holmes, and colleagues (2006).

## REFERENCES

Ayduk, O., Downey, G., Testa, A., Yen, Y., & Shoda, Y. (1999). Does rejection elicit hostility in rejection sensitive women? *Social Cognition, 17*, 245–271.

Baldwin, M. W., & Sinclair, L. (1996). Self-esteem and "if . . . then" contingencies of interpersonal acceptance. *Journal of Personality and Social Psychology, 71*, 1130–1141.

Baumeister, R. F. (1993). *Self-esteem: The puzzle of low self-regard*. New York: Plenum Press.

Baumeister, R. F., & Leary, M. R. (1995). The need to belong: Desire for interpersonal attachments as a fundamental human motivation. *Psychological Bulletin, 117*, 497–529.

Baumeister, R. F., Twenge, J. M., & Nuss, C. K. (2002). Effects of social exclusion on cognitive processes: Anticipated aloneness reduces intelligent thought. *Journal of Personality and Social Psychology, 83*, 817–827.

Bellavia, G., & Murray, S. L. (2003). Did I do that?: Self-esteem related differences in reactions to romantic partners' moods. *Personal Relationships, 10*, 77–96.

Berscheid, E. (1983). Emotion. In H. H. Kelley, E. Berscheid, A. Christensen, J. H. Harvey, T. L. Huston, G. Levinger, et al. (Eds.), *Close relationships* (pp. 110–168). New York: Freeman.

Berscheid, E., & Regan, P. (2005). *The psychology of interpersonal relationships*. Upper Saddle River, NJ: Prentice Hall.

Bradbury, T. N., & Fincham, F. D. (1990). Attributions in marriage: Review and critique. *Psychological Bulletin, 107*, 3–23.

Braiker, H. B., & Kelley, H. H. (1979). Conflict in the development of close relationships. In R. L. Burgess & T. L. Huston (Eds.), *Social exchange in developing relationships* (pp. 135–168). New York: Academic Press.

Campbell, L., Simpson, J. A., Boldry, J., & Kashy, D. A. (2005). Perceptions of conflict and support in romantic relationships: The role of attachment anxiety. *Journal of Personality and Social Psychology, 88*, 510–531.

Clark, M. S., & Grote, N. K. (1998). Why aren't indices of relationship costs always negatively related to indices of relationship quality? *Personality and Social Psychology Review, 2*, 2–17.

Collins, N. L. (1996). Working models of attachment: Implications for explanation, emotion and behavior. *Journal of Personality and Social Psychology, 71*, 810–832.

Collins, N. L., & Feeney, B. C. (2000). A safe haven: An attachment theory perspective on support seeking and caregiving in intimate relationships. *Journal of Personality and Social Psychology, 78*, 1053–1073.

Collins, N. L., & Feeney, B. C. (2004). Working models of attachment shape perceptions of social support: Evidence from experimental and observational studies. *Journal of Personality and Social Psychology, 87*, 363–383.

Collins, N. L., & Read, S. J. (1990). Adult attachment, working models, and relationship quality in dating couples. *Journal of Personality and Social Psychology, 58*, 644–663.

DeHart, T., Pelham, B., & Murray, S. L. (2004). Implicit dependency regulation: Self-esteem, relationship closeness, and Implicit evaluations of close others. *Social Cognition, 22*(1), 126–146.

Downey, G., & Feldman, S. I. (1996). Implications of rejection sensitivity for intimate relationships. *Journal of Personality and Social Psychology, 70*, 1327–1343.

Downey, G., Freitas, A. L., Michaelis, B., & Khouri, H. (1998). The self-fulfilling prophecy in close relationships: Rejection sensitivity and rejection by romantic partners. *Journal of Personality and Social Psychology, 75*, 545–560.

Finkel, E. J., & Campbell, W. K. (2001). Self-control and accommodation in close relationships: An interdependence analysis. *Journal of Personality and Social Psychology, 81*, 263–277.

Gable, S. L., Reis, H. T., & Elliot, A. J. (2000). Behavioral activation and inhibition in everyday life. *Journal of Personality and Social Psychology, 78*, 1135–1149.

Gagne, F. M., & Lydon, J. E. (2001). Mind-set and relationship illusions: The moderating effects of domain specificity and relationship commitment. *Personality and Social Psychology Bulletin, 27*, 1144–1155.

Gagne, F. M., & Lydon, J. E. (2004). Bias and accuracy in close relationships: An integrative review. *Personality and Social Psychology Review, 8*, 322–338.

Gottman, J. M. (1994). *What predicts divorce?: The relationship between marital processes and marital outcomes*. Hillsdale, NJ: Erlbaum.

Griffin, D. W., & Ross, L. (1991). Subjective construal, social inference and human misunderstanding. In M. P. Zanna (Ed.), *Advances in experimental social psychology* (Vol. 24, pp. 319–359). San Diego, CA: Academic Press.

Higgins, E. T. (1996). The "self digest": Self-knowledge serving self-regulatory functions. *Journal of Personality and Social Psychology, 71*, 1062–1083.

Holmes, J. G. (2002). Interpersonal expectations as the building blocks of social cognition: An interdependence theory perspective. *Personal Relationships, 9*, 1–26.

Holmes, J. G., & Rempel, J. K. (1989). Trust in close relationships. In C. Hendrick (Ed.), *Review of personality and social psychology: Vol. 10. Close relationships* (pp. 187–219). Newbury Park, CA: Sage.

Kelley, H. H. (1979). *Personal relationships: Their structures and processes*. Hillsdale, NJ: Erlbaum.

Kelley, H. H., Holmes, J. G., Kerr, N., Reis, H., Rusbult, C., & Van Lange, P. A. (2003). *An atlas of interpersonal situations*. Cambridge, UK: Cambridge University Press.

Kenny, D. A. (1994). *Interpersonal perception: A social relations analysis*. New York: Guilford Press.

Leary, M. R., & Baumeister, R. F. (2000). The nature and function of self-esteem: Sociometer theory. In M. P. Zanna (Ed.), *Advances in experimental social psychology* (Vol. 32, pp. 2–51). San Diego, CA: Academic Press.

Leary, M. R., Tambor, E. S., Terdal, S. K., & Downs, D. L. (1995). Self-esteem as an interpersonal monitor: The sociometer hypothesis. *Journal of Personality and Social Psychology, 68*, 518–530.

MacDonald, G., & Jessica, M. (2006). Family approval as a constraint in dependency regulation: Evidence from Australia and Indonesia. *Personal Relationships, 13*, 183–194.

MacDonald, G., & Leary, M. R. (2005). Why does social exclusion hurt?: The relationship between social and physical pain. *Psychological Bulletin, 131*, 202–223.

Mikulincer, M. (1998). Attachment working models and the sense of trust: An exploration of interaction goals and affect regulation. *Journal of Personality and Social Psychology, 74*, 1209–1224.

Mikulincer, M., Birnbaum, G., Woddis, D., & Nachmias, O. (2000). Stress and accessibility of proximity-related thoughts: Exploring the normative and intra-individual components of attachment theory. *Journal of Personality and Social Psychology, 78*, 509–523.

Mikulincer, M., Gillath, O., Halevy, V., Avihou, N., Avidan, S., & Eshkoli, N. (2001). Attachment theory and reactions to others' needs: Evidence that activation of the sense of attachment security promotes empathic responses. *Journal of Personality and Social Psychology, 81*, 1205–1224.

Mikulincer, M., Gillath, O., & Shaver, P. R. (2002). Activation of the attachment system in adulthood: Threat-related primes increase the accessibility of mental representations of attachment figures. *Journal of Personality and Social Psychology, 83*, 881–895.

Mikulincer, M., & Shaver, P. R. (2001). Attachment theory and intergroup bias: Evidence that priming the secure base schema attenuates negative reactions to outgroups. *Journal of Personality and Social Psychology, 81*, 97–115.

Mischel, W., & Shoda, Y. (1995). A cognitive–affective system theory of personality: Reconceptualizing situations, dispositions, dynamics, and invariance in personality structure. *Psychological Review, 102*, 246–268.

Murray, S. L. (1999). The quest for conviction: Motivated cognition in romantic relationships. *Psychological Inquiry, 10*, 23–34.

Murray, S. L., Bellavia, G., Rose, P., & Griffin, D. (2003). Once hurt, twice hurtful: How perceived regard regulates daily marital interaction. *Journal of Personality and Social Psychology, 84*, 126–147.

Murray, S. L., & Derrick, J. (2005). A relationship-specific sense of felt security: How perceived regard regulates relationship-enhancement processes. In M. W. Baldwin (Ed.), *Interpersonal cognition* (pp. 153–179). New York: Guilford Press.

Murray, S. L., Griffin, D. W., Rose, P., & Bellavia, G.

(2003). Calibrating the sociometer: The relational contingencies of self-esteem. *Journal of Personality and Social Psychology, 85*, 63–84.

Murray, S. L., Griffin, D. W., Rose, P., & Bellavia, G. (2006). For better or worse?: Self-esteem and the contingencies of acceptance in marriage. *Personality and Social Psychology Bulletin, 32*, 866–882.

Murray, S. L., & Holmes, J. G. (1993). Seeing virtues in faults: Negativity and the transformation of interpersonal narratives in close relationships. *Journal of Personality and Social Psychology, 65*, 707–722.

Murray, S. L., Holmes, J. G., & Collins, N. L. (2006). Optimizing assurance: The risk regulation system in relationships. *Psychological Bulletin, 132*, 641–666.

Murray, S. L., Holmes, J. G., & Griffin, D. (1996). The benefits of positive illusions: Idealization and the construction of satisfaction in close relationships. *Journal of Personality and Social Psychology, 70*, 79–98.

Murray, S. L., Holmes, J. G., & Griffin, D. W. (2000). Self-esteem and the quest for felt security: How perceived regard regulates attachment processes. *Journal of Personality and Social Psychology, 78*, 478–498.

Murray, S. L., Holmes, J. G., Griffin, D. W., Bellavia, G., & Rose, P. (2001). The mismeasure of love: How self-doubt contaminates relationship beliefs. *Personality and Social Psychology Bulletin, 27*, 423–436.

Murray, S. L., Holmes, J. G., MacDonald, G., & Ellsworth, P. (1998). Through the looking glass darkly?: When self-doubts turn into relationship insecurities. *Journal of Personality and Social Psychology, 75*, 1459–1480.

Murray, S. L., Rose, P., Bellavia, G., Holmes, J., & Kusche, A. (2002). When rejection stings: How self-esteem constrains relationship-enhancement processes. *Journal of Personality and Social Psychology, 83*, 556–573.

Murray, S. L., Rose, P., Holmes, J. G., Derrick, J., Podchaski, E., & Bellavia, G. (2005). Putting the partner within reach: A dyadic perspective on felt security in close relationships. *Journal of Personality and Social Psychology, 88*, 327–347.

Nezlek, J. B., Kowalski, R. M., Leary, M. R., Blevins, T., & Holgate, S. (1997). Personality moderators of reactions to interpersonal rejection: Depression and trait self-esteem. *Personality and Social Psychology Bulletin, 23*, 1235–1244.

Pierce, T., & Lydon, J. (1998). Priming relational schemas: Effects of contextually activated and chronically accessible interpersonal expectations on responses to a stressful event. *Journal of Personality and Social Psychology, 75*, 1441–1448.

Pietrzak, J., Downey, G., & Ayduk, O. (2005). Rejection sensitivity as an interpersonal vulnerability. In M. Baldwin (Ed.), *Interpersonal cognition* (pp. 62–84). New York: Guilford Press.

Reis, H. T., Clark, M. S., & Holmes, J. G. (2004). Perceived partner responsiveness as an organizing construct in the study of intimacy and closeness. In D. Mashek & A. P. Aron (Eds.), *Handbook of closeness and intimacy* (pp. 201–225). Mahwah, NJ: Erlbaum.

Rholes, S. W., Simpson, J. A., & Orina, M. M. (1999). Attachment and anger in an anxiety-provoking situation. *Journal of Personality and Social Psychology, 76*, 940–957.

Rusbult, C. E., & Van Lange, P. A. M. (2003). Interdependence, interaction, and relationships. *Annual Review of Psychology, 54*, 351–375.

Rusbult, C. E., Verette, J., Whitney, G. A., Slovik, L. F., & Lipkus, I. (1991). Accommodation processes in close relationships: Theory and preliminary research evidence. *Journal of Personality and Social Psychology, 60*, 53–78.

Shrauger, J. S., & Schoeneman, T. J. (1979). Symbolic interactionist view of the self-concept: Through the looking glass darkly. *Psychological Bulletin, 86*, 549–573.

Simpson, J. A., Ickes, W., & Grich, J. (1999). When accuracy hurts: Reactions of anxious-ambivalent dating partners to a relationship-threatening situation. *Journal of Personality and Social Psychology, 76*, 754–769.

Simpson, J. A., Rholes, W. S., & Nelligan, J. S. (1992). Support seeking and support giving within couples in an anxiety-provoking situation: The role of attachment styles. *Journal of Personality and Social Psychology, 62*, 434–446.

Simpson, J. A., Rholes, W. S., & Phillips, D. (1996). Conflict in close relationships: An attachment perspective. *Journal of Personality and Social Psychology, 71*, 899–914.

Sommer, K. L., & Baumeister, R. F. (2002). Self-evaluation, persistence, and performance following implicit rejection: The role of trait self-esteem. *Psychological Bulletin, 28*, 926–938.

Swann, W. B., Bosson, J. K., & Pelham, B. W. (2002). Different partners, different selves: Strategic verification of circumscribed identities. *Personality and Social Psychology Bulletin, 28*, 1215–1228.

Taylor, S. E., & Brown, J. D. (1988). Illusion and well-being: A social psychological perspective on mental health. *Psychological Bulletin, 103*, 193–210.

Tooby, J., & Cosmides, L. (1996). Friendship and the banker's paradox: Other pathways to the evolution of adaptations for altruism. *Proceedings of the British Academy, 88*, 119–143.

Tucker, J. S., & Anders, S. L. (1999). Attachment style, interpersonal perception accuracy, and relationship satisfaction in dating couples. *Personality and Social Psychology Bulletin, 25*, 403–412.

Twenge, J. M., Catanese, K. R., & Baumeister, R. F. (2002). Social exclusion causes self-defeating behavior. *Journal of Personality and Social Psychology, 83*, 606–615.

Chapter 36

# Prorelationship Motivation

## AN INTERDEPENDENCE THEORY ANALYSIS OF SITUATIONS WITH CONFLICTING INTERESTS

**Eli J. Finkel**
**Caryl E. Rusbult**

Sometimes involvement in relationships is easy and pleasurable: Communication is effortless, trust is strong, and interaction is suffused with joy and laughter. In such circumstances, partners' preferences are compatible, and neither partner is likely to behave badly. But at other times, relationships are thorny: Conflict emerges, laughter is in short supply, and extra-relationship temptation is fierce. In such circumstances, partners suffer incompatible preferences, and they frequently have to exert themselves to control their less admirable, gut-level impulses (e.g., forgoing the impulse to lash out at the partner or to flirt with a coworker). When gut-level desires conflict with relational well-being, why do people sometimes override their selfish impulses, instead behaving in ways that promote relational interests?

The goal of this chapter is to present an interdependence-based theoretical analysis of self-oriented versus relationship-oriented motivation. The chapter proceeds in four major sections. First, we define *prorelationship motivation* and describe its emergence from interpersonal dynamics. Second, we review the important role of situation structure in understanding this type of motivation. Third, we examine the relevance of temporal processes to understanding prorelationship motivation. And fourth, we consider the potential benefits and dangers of such motivation.

### WHAT IS PRORELATIONSHIP MOTIVATION?

*Prorelationship motivation* describes behavioral preferences that are driven by the desire to benefit one's relationship or partner, despite the fact that enacting such behavior conflicts with one's immediate, gut-level behavioral impulses. For example, if Eleanor wants to watch her alma mater play in the Final Four, but James wants her to accompany him to his cousin's wedding, her prorelationship motivation would be manifested as willingness to skip the game and attend the wedding. Or if Eleanor says something rude, and James is tempted to be equally nasty in return, his prorelationship motivation would be manifested as the inclination to resist retaliating (which would yield escalating conflict), and instead to react in a neutral or considerate manner.

### Forgiveness as an Example of Prorelationship Motivation

Many empirical studies have examined situations in which individuals experience prorelationship motivation despite gut-level impulses to the contrary. As an illustrative example, we review recent findings regarding forgiveness. Forgiveness becomes a relevant interpersonal phenomenon when one partner betrays the other, with *betrayal* defined as "the perceived violation by a partner of an implicit or explicit relationship-relevant norm" (Finkel, Rusbult, Kumashiro, & Hannon, 2002, p. 957). Because the victim frequently experiences such norm violations as moral transgressions, betrayals create an interpersonal debt (Exline & Baumeister, 2000). Perhaps for this reason, immediate impulses in response to betrayal are often retaliatory and vengeful (Finkel et al., 2002; McCullough, Fincham, & Tsang, 2003; Rusbult, Davis, Finkel, Hannon, & Olsen, 2006). Although vengeful impulses may well have some functional value (e.g., reinforcing social norms), it is clear that if a relationship is to flourish in the wake of the betrayal, the victim must find a way to get beyond these impulses.

Moving beyond immediate, retaliatory impulses requires *forgiveness*, defined as "the victim's resumption of prebetrayal behavioral tendencies—as the tendency to forego vengeance and other destructive patterns of interaction, instead behaving toward the perpetrator in a positive and constructive manner" (Finkel et al., 2002, p. 958). Forgiveness rests on prorelationship motivation; individuals are especially likely to forgive a betrayal to the degree that they care about the longevity and well-being of their relationship (Finkel et al., 2002; McCullough et al., 1998). In short, experiencing a betrayal by a close partner illustrates central phenomena relevant to prorelationship motivation: The betrayal frequently leads to retaliatory and vengeful impulses (or *desire* to exact revenge), but prorelationship motivational factors can override these impulses in favor of forgiving responses.

### Sources of Prorelationship Motivation

What "drives" prorelationship motivation? Interdependence theory does not identify a single, overriding source of prorelationship motivation (Kelley & Thibaut, 1978; Thibaut & Kelley, 1959). Rather, the theory suggests that humans possess multiple goals and needs that are likely to vary across situations, partners, and time. The broader considerations that underlie prorelationship motivation may include any or all of the following: motives centering on desire to protect a relationship upon which one is deeply dependent (e.g., strong commitment); motives centering on desire to maximize one's long-term well-being by promoting congenial interaction (e.g., temporally extended positive reciprocity); motives centering on desire to benefit the outcomes of a partner with whom one's well-being is closely linked (e.g., self–other merger, such that promoting a partner's outcomes is tantamount to promoting one's own); or motives centering on desire to "do the right thing," regardless of the consequences to the self (e.g., altruism).

## SITUATION STRUCTURE AND PRORELATIONSHIP MOTIVATION

Our central thesis is that the goals and motives underlying prorelationship motivation can be properly understood only via an analysis of the specific situation in which a given interaction takes place. In this section we examine key structural properties of the situations dyadic partners may confront—emphasizing both the power of situations to influence motivation, and the interplay between personal characteristics and situation structure in predicting prorelationship motivation.

### The Power of the Situation

Although social psychologists frequently pay homage to "the power of the situation" in predicting human behavior, systematic analysis of the meaning of "situation" is rare. More than 70 years ago, Lewin (1936) argued that behavior ($B$) is a function not only of characteristics of the person ($P$), but also of that person's present social environment (*E*). These ideas are summarized in his famous dictum, $B = f(P, E)$. It is readily apparent why we must analyze characteristics of the person (*P*) if we are to apprehend the character of motivation: How could a comprehensive model of human motivation ignore such person-level factors as the drives to survive, to reproduce, to feel safe, to experience close involvement with others, and the like? But examining the person is only part of the story; understanding human motivation also requires a systematic analysis of social situations (see Kelley et al., 2003; Mischel & Shoda, 1995). We adopt a strong form of this argument: Except in extreme cases (e.g., starvation, imminent physical threat), understanding relationship-relevant influences on motivation virtually *requires* an understanding of the social situation in which human behavior transpires.

Recent work in the interdependence tradition proposes an important extension of Lewin's famous dictum. Kelley and Holmes (2006; see also Holmes, 2002) adopt a truly interpersonal analysis of human behavior, suggesting that understanding a given social interaction (*I*) not only requires knowledge of a given actor (*A*), but also knowledge of the interaction partner (*B*) and the specific situation in which their interaction transpires (*S*). These ideas are summarized in an inherently interpersonal dictum regarding behavior, $I = f(S, A, B)$ (also described as the "SABI" model).

The SABI model has important implications for understanding prorelationship motivation. Whereas many perspectives on social motivation focus exclusively on characteristics of the individual who experiences a given motive, interdependence theorists emphasize three classes of variables: the individual (*A*), the partner (*B*), and the situation (*S*). For example, imagine that we want to predict whether Eleanor (*A*) will forgive James (*B*) for talking about their sex life during a dinner party with her family (*S*). If Eleanor feels insecure in her relationship with James (*A*), she may perceive his inconsiderate comments as globally rejecting and therefore virtually unforgivable. If James is relatively indifferent to their relationship (*B*), he may argue that the incident was meaningless and conclude that Eleanor is overreacting. Under circumstances such as these, Eleanor is unlikely to forgive James.

The power of an interdependence theory analysis of social motivation is illustrated by observing that Eleanor's motivation and her interaction with James are likely to differ markedly as a function of changes in any one of the three elements in the SABI model. For example, imagine that James's revelations about their sex life take place during a raucous night on the town with their buddies, rather than at a dinner party with her family (*S*). Or imagine that Eleanor feels completely secure in her relationship with James (*A*). Or imagine that James is strongly committed to maintaining his relationship (*B*), and offers a heartfelt apology and profuse amends. In interactions involving one or more of these modified circumstances, Eleanor may well find her way to complete forgiveness.

### Why Study Situation Structure?

There are two reasons why an analysis of prorelationship motivation requires an understanding of situation structure. First, situations sometimes exert strong effects on individual behavior—effects that are largely independent of the interactants' personal characteristics and motives. For example, most people will forgive another person who bumps into them during a crowded subway ride. This does not mean that most people are dispositionally forgiving; it merely means that forgiveness is a near-universal response to this situation.

A second reason for analyzing situation structure is that particular situations afford specific dyadic problems and opportunities. That is, specific situations (1) render some motives relevant and others irrelevant (e.g., the issue of trust is irrelevant when partners' preferences are in perfect harmony); and (2) allow individuals the opportunity to express or suppress relevant motives (e.g., James cannot demonstrate that he is trustworthy when his outcomes are in perfect harmony with Eleanor's). The term *affordances* describes the possible behaviors, motives, and goals that a particular situation makes possible or may activate in the interactants (Holmes, 2002). For example, if your former friend Bill makes it his sworn mission in life to make you miserable, offering to buy him a beer at the local pub might not be a viable option for resolving the conflict. In contrast, if Bill is angry with you but seems receptive to working things out, offering to buy him a beer might be an effective means of working through problems.

## How Interactants Influence One Another's Outcomes

Thus far, we have characterized situations in a rather informal manner. However, interdependence theory offers a formal, systematic means of analyzing situation structure. In particular, interdependence theorists employ *outcome matrices* to depict both the behavioral options available to each interactant, and the outcomes that will accrue to each individual as a function of both individuals' behavior. For example, Figure 36.1 depicts a variant of the well-known prisoner's dilemma situation (Rusbult & Arriaga, 2000). The house that Eleanor and James share has not been cleaned in several weeks, and both are becoming dissatisfied with its griminess. If they continue to avoid cleaning, both partners will experience poor outcomes (0), as depicted in the lower right cell of Figure 36.1. Given that neither enjoys cleaning, both would prefer that the other clean the house alone (+8); however, each would be irritated by cleaning the house without the other's help (–4). If they clean the house together, both Eleanor and James would enjoy the clean house, and each would experience the cleaning chore as less aversive (+4).

A systematic analysis of prototypical outcome structures allows researchers to explore the implications of a diverse array of interdependence situations (Kelley & Thibaut, 1978). Given that an outcome matrix (such as Figure 36.1) represents a 2 × 2 table of the outcomes that will accrue to each person as a result of both partners' behavioral choices, it is possible to conceptualize the numbers in the matrix by using analysis-of-variance logic. From Eleanor's perspective, a main effect of columns represents her *actor control*, or her ability to exert over control her own outcomes; Eleanor can improve her outcomes by 4 units by not cleaning the house rather than cleaning it, regardless of James's behavior (see Figure 36.1). A main effect of rows represents *partner control* over Eleanor's outcomes, or James's ability to exert control over Eleanor's outcomes; James can improve Eleanor's outcomes by 8 units by cleaning the house rather than not cleaning it, regardless of Eleanor's behavior.

An interaction effect represents *joint control*, or the degree to which Eleanor's outcomes are influenced by the combined behavioral choices of James and herself. In Figure 36.1, James and Eleanor exert no joint control over one another's outcomes. In contrast, Figure 36.2 depicts a new situation in which James and Eleanor experience joint control over one another, but have no actor control or partner control. In this new example, Eleanor and James are deciding at which restaurant they would like to dine on Saturday night. Neither partner has any absolute preference about where they dine (there is no actor control), and neither has any absolute preference about how the partner should behave (there is no partner control). Both have a strong preference, however, to dine together (there is strong joint control). In this

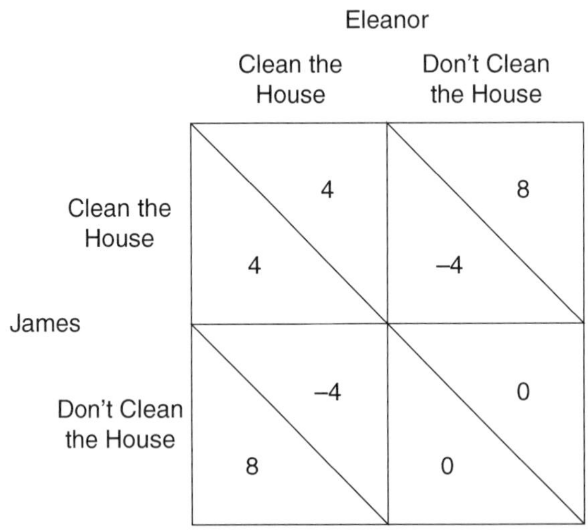


**FIGURE 36.1.** Prisoner's dilemma situation: Cleaning the house.

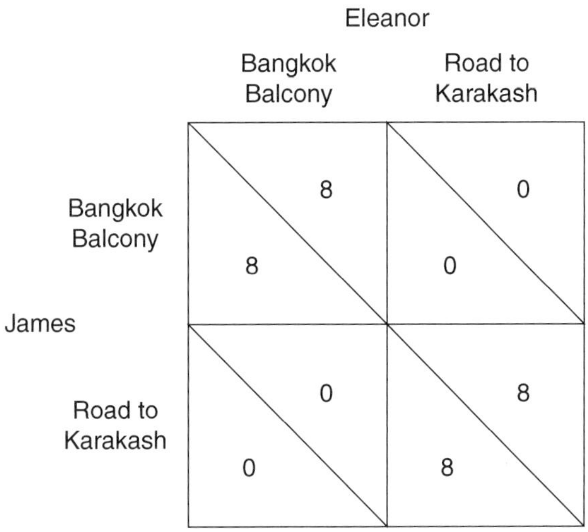


**FIGURE 36.2.** Coordination situation: Where to eat Saturday night?

example, James has joint control over Eleanor, because switching from one restaurant to the other makes it highly desirable for her to change her selection as well. (The interdependence patterns in Figures 36.1 and 36.2 are *symmetrical*, so the analysis would be identical if we were to describe James's outcomes rather than Eleanor's.)

## Four Properties of Situation Structure

In addition to parsing the ways in which interactants can exert control over their own and one another's outcomes, interdependence theorists also define four properties of situation structure (Rusbult & Van Lange, 1996; Thibaut & Kelley, 1959). The first property, *level of dependence*, describes the degree to which an individual's outcomes are influenced by the partner's actions. When Eleanor's outcomes in a given interaction are determined primarily by actor control, she experiences low levels of dependence on James; she can directly control her own outcomes without being influenced by James's behavior. In contrast, when her outcomes are determined primarily by partner control or joint control, she experiences high dependence on James.

The concepts of dependence and power are inextricably linked: Eleanor's level of dependence on James is equivalent to James's power over Eleanor (Huston, 1983). At the same time, power is not always usable. James possesses *usable power* over Eleanor to the extent that (1) when he exercises partner control or joint control over Eleanor's outcomes, his own outcomes are not harmed; and (2) Eleanor cannot obtain better outcomes in an alternative relationship. For example, although James may have the wherewithal to exert power by yelling at Eleanor in a restaurant, he is unlikely to exercise this power because (1) he himself would suffer poor outcomes if he were to engage in such an unseemly public act; and/or (2) if James were to provide her with such terribly poor outcomes, Eleanor might well dump him and opt for an alternative relationship. It is appropriate, therefore, to construe level of dependence in terms of the range of outcomes through which James can *realistically* move Eleanor, with the upper end being defined by the very best outcomes he can cause her to experience, and the lower end being defined by the poorest outcomes he can cause her to experience (without harming himself substantially or causing her to opt out of the relationship).

How does level of dependence influence motivation? Increasing dependence tends to activate increased situation- and person-relevant attention and cognition, in that when Eleanor's outcomes are governed by James's actions, she will dedicate considerable mental resources to discerning what the situation is "about" and to developing expectancies regarding James's future behavior (Arriaga & Rusbult, 1998; Fiske, 1993). Given that dependence constitutes reliance on a partner for fulfilling important needs, increasing dependence tends to promote commitment to relationships (Bui, Peplau, & Hill, 1996; Rusbult, 1983). Also, and as noted earlier, individuals who are highly dependent on a given relationship for good outcomes are likely to experience greater prorelationship motivation than are those who are less dependent. For example, highly dependent individuals are more willing to accommodate when their partners behave badly, and are often willing to make personal sacrifices to benefit their relationships (Rusbult, Verette, Whitney, Slovik, & Lipkus, 1991; Van Lange et al., 1997). Moreover, because dependence sometimes entails vulnerability, it may inspire motivated forms of cognition such as positive illusions and downward social comparison. For example, Eleanor may quell feelings of insecurity by translating James's faults into virtues, or by identifying flaws in other relationships that are not evident in her own (Murray & Holmes, 1993; Rusbult, Van Lange, Wildschut, Yovetich, & Verette, 2000). In short, situations involving high levels of dependence afford cognition, motivation, communication, and interaction centering on issues of comfort (vs. discomfort) with interdependence and independence.

The second property of situation structure, *mutuality of dependence*, describes the degree to which partners experience equal levels of dependence upon one another. When Eleanor is dependent on the relationship for good outcomes but James is not, the relationship is characterized by unilateral dependence; when the partners are similarly dependent, the relationship is characterized by mutual dependence. Again, note that Eleanor's dependence on James is equivalent to James's power over her; if she is unilaterally dependent, then he has power over her, but she has none over him.

How does mutuality of dependence influence prorelationship motivation? When one partner is highly dependent but the other is not, the more dependent partner generally experiences greater prorelationship motivation than the less dependent partner. For example, the less dependent partner tends to exert greater control over decision making and the allocation of resources, whereas the more dependent partner tends to carry the greater burden of interaction costs (forgiveness, accommodation, sacrifice) and is more vulnerable to abandonment (Attridge, Berscheid, & Simpson, 1995; Rusbult, 1983; Witcher, 1999). Therefore, nonmutual dependence tends to magnify the dependent partner's situation- and person-relevant attention and cognition, along with other adaptations geared toward reducing vulnerability. For example, when Eleanor is unilaterally dependent, she is likely to be very attentive to the ways in which her outcomes may be affected by James's actions, to predicting his probable behavior, and to engaging in motivated cognition that may reduce her feelings of vulnerability and anxiety. In contrast, interactions characterized by mutual dependence tend to be more stable and congenial, yielding benefits that accrue from balance of power: more tranquil and positive emotional experience (less anxiety and guilt), reduced use of threat or coercion, and more reciprocal and harmonious interaction (Baumeister, Wotman, & Stillwell, 1993; Drigotas, Rusbult, & Verette, 1999; Fiske, 1993). In short, situations with nonmutual dependence afford the expression of comfort (or discomfort) with vulnerability on the part of the dependent partner, along with comfort (or discomfort) with responsibility on the part of the powerful partner.

A prototypical example of the consequences of unilateral dependence (and of a circumstance where the situation may well overpower personality differences) is the *demand–withdraw pattern* of interaction, involving repeated demands for change by wives and repeated withdrawal behaviors from husbands (Christensen & Heavey, 1993; see Holmes & Murray, 1996). Traditional explanations of this phenomenon might suggest that this pattern of behaviors emerges from fundamental sex differences that cause women to nag and men to withdraw. But a more compelling explanation of the demand–withdraw pattern is that situation structure largely dictates interaction behavior. Because husbands traditionally hold more usable power in many domains, wives are dependent upon their husbands' fairness (e.g., in performing household chores). If a wife perceives that the situation is unfair, her primary recourse is to try to convince her husband to change, which may cause her to complain that the status quo is unfair. In contrast, he may not want to change a status quo that benefits him, so he may try to avoid discussing the topic. In this analysis of the demand–withdraw pattern (Christensen & Heavey, 1993), the situation structure dictates both that the husband has domain-specific power over the wife and that he is more satisfied with his outcomes in this domain (e.g., household chores) than she is with hers. Given this situation structure, the partners' behavior would be easy to predict even without knowing any information about their personality characteristics or motives. The structure of the situation exerts a powerful influence on them; most people facing the same situation, regardless of their gender, may well experience similar motives and exhibit similar behaviors.

The third property of situation structure, *basis of dependence*, describes the way in which partners influence one another's outcomes—whether an individual's dependence emerges from partner control (James's behavior directly controls Eleanor's outcomes, regardless of what she does) or joint control (by changing his behavior, James can make Eleanor want to change hers). Whether dependence on a given relationship is characterized by partner control or joint control leads to important social consequences. For example, when partners face situations characterized by mutual partner control (which renders prorelationship motivation highly relevant), it is frequently adaptive to engage in temporally extended patterns of exchange behaviors ("You scratch my back, I'll scratch yours"), in which James helps Eleanor achieve good outcomes in the present interaction under the assumption that she will help him achieve good outcomes in a future interaction (Axelrod, 1984; Clark & Mills, 1993). In contrast, when partners face situations characterized by mutual joint control, they are less dependent on temporally extended behavioral patterns; rather, they focus their efforts on coordinating their behaviors in such a manner as to maximize efficiency ("You drive, I'll read the map"; see Finkel et al., 2006). In short, basis of dependence affords the expression of motivations relevant to morality and fairness (partner control) versus coordination and assertiveness (joint control).

The first three properties of situation structure (level of dependence, mutuality of dependence, and basis of dependence) pertain to partners' dependence on one another. The fourth property, *covariation of interests*, describes the degree to which *outcomes* from specific behavioral patterns are mutually beneficial rather than unilaterally beneficial. If behavioral patterns that result in good outcomes for Eleanor also generate good outcomes for James, then they experience positive covariation. In contrast, if behavioral patterns that result in good outcomes for her generate poor outcomes for him, they experience negative covariation. If Eleanor's positivity of outcomes is unrelated to James's, they experience zero covariation. Examining the within-cell associations between the two persons' outcomes reveals the degree to which they experience compatible versus incompatible preferences. For example, compare the situations depicted in Figures 36.1 and 36.2. Whereas Figure 36.1 depicts a situation in which Eleanor and James experience moderately negative covariation of interests, Figure 36.2 depicts a situation in which they experience positive covariation of interests. The situation depicted in Figure 36.1 affords the expression of either self-centered goals or relationship-oriented goals, and as a result inspires predictable patterns of cognition (e.g., close monitoring of the partner's behavior) and affect (e.g., fear, greed, gratitude) (Van Lange & Kuhlman, 1994). The situation depicted in Figure 36.2 affords none of these processes; in the bizarre circumstance where the partners fail to coordinate their behaviors to their mutual benefit (i.e., they end up at different restaurants), predictable patterns of cognition (e.g., puzzling over where coordination broke down) and affect (e.g., frustration) differ markedly from those experienced in the former situation.

The association of covariation of outcomes with prorelationship motivation is complex. If partners experience perfectly positive covariation, then the question of prorelationship motivation is irrelevant: What is good for the self is likewise good for the partner, so people do not think about whether they wish to behave well toward one another, and one partner does not worry about whether the other will behave well. At the other extreme, if partners experience perfectly negative covariation, prorelationship motivation becomes irrelevant, because the costs of forgoing self-interest are so high—at least within the context of a particular interaction.[1] In fact, voluntary relationships are likely to dissolve when they are characterized by negative covariation across many situations. Thus, situations with moderate covariation of interests afford the expression of prorelationship versus self-interested motives (e.g., Figure 36.1). In such circumstances, partners' gut-level impulses conflict, but there is plenty of opportunity for them to override these impulses to benefit one another.

Indeed, although situations with moderately negative covariation may be difficult to navigate, they hold an important place in relationship development, because they represent the arena in which partners develop (or fail to develop) trust in one another (Holmes & Rempel, 1989). Eleanor comes to trust James when she observes him engaging in behaviors that are beneficial to her, despite the fact that doing so flies in the face of his immediate preferences (e.g., skipping a Super Bowl party with friends to spend time with her family). Witnessing James make such a sacrifice allows Eleanor to conclude that he cares about her. In short, a partner's prorelationship behavior in situations of moderately negative covariation cause the individual to develop greater trust, thereby enhancing the quality of the relationship (Wieselquist, Rusbult, Foster, & Agnew, 1999).

## TEMPORAL PROCESSES AND PRORELATIONSHIP MOTIVATION

Thus far we have emphasized interactions that take place at a single moment in time (e.g., the examples represented by the outcome matrices in Figures 36.1 and 36.2). We now turn our attention to temporally extended processes relevant to understanding prorelationship motivation.

### Making the Transition from One Situation to the Next

A shortcoming of outcome matrices as theoretical devices is that they only represent snapshots in time, thereby failing to incorporate any of the richness associated with examining relational processes as they develop over time. When researchers are studying prorelationship motivation in close relationships, this is a serious limitation. Interdependence should be conceptualized not only in terms of the immediate outcomes produced by patterns of behavior in a particular situation, but also in terms of the future situations (interdependence structures) that are made available or eliminated as a consequence of present behaviors (Kelley, 1984). For example, in the course of an extended conflict, later behavioral options and outcomes are powerfully influenced by whether, earlier in the conflict, Eleanor has apologized for being inconsiderate rather than insulting James by claiming that he is overly sensitive. In the former case, James may find that hugging Eleanor is a highly available, desirable behavioral option; in the latter, hugging may not be an option for James (or at least not a desirable one).

In understanding prorelationship motivation, there are at least two important implications of the fact that behaviors enacted in the present influence the future situations partners face. First, individuals can enact behaviors in the present that are designed to benefit the relationship or the partner in the future. Second, taking a long-term view of one's relationship allows partners to engage in reciprocity over time. Illustrating the former point, Eleanor may work 80 hours this week to ensure that next week she will not have to bring work with her on a shared vacation. Illustrating the latter, Eleanor and James may decide that they will alternate who gets to select the film for their regular Saturday night date; both Eleanor and James recognize that their relationship is enhanced when both partners' needs are met, and that alternating film choices is an effective means of assuring mutual need fulfillment.

### The Transformation Process

Of course, the temporal processes relevant to understanding prorelationship motivation are not limited to the subsequent situations people create (vs. eliminate) as a consequence of their earlier behavioral choices. Additional temporal processes transpire inside people's heads as they analyze and reinterpret their behavioral options in terms of the broader considerations and values to which they are committed (Kelley & Thibaut, 1978; Rusbult & Van Lange, 1996). That is, temporal processes are relevant to understanding interactions even in the sort of snapshot situations represented by outcome matrices; in both temporally extended interactions and one-shot matrix-like interactions, individuals may subjectively reevaluate situation structure prior to enacting behaviors.

How does this process work? Interdependence theorists distinguish between the given situation and the effective situation (Kelley & Thibaut, 1978). The *given situation* describes the impact on the interactants' outcomes if both were to behave in accord with their own immediate, gut-level behavioral preferences. These outcomes are "given" in that they are not influenced by regard for the partner's preferences, long-term relational concerns, and the like. Individuals sometimes behave in accord with their gut-level, given preferences. Such behavior is especially likely when there are no complex exogenous issues to consider (e.g., "How will this behavior affect my relationship in the long run?"), when an individual lacks the ability to control gut-level behavioral urges (Finkel & Campbell, 2001), or when effortful cognitive processes cause the individual to conclude that gut-level preferences are an exact match with deeply processed preferences.

Behavioral impulses are often altered, however, by broader considerations—by concerns extending beyond the gut-level preferences people experience on the basis of the given situation. Acting on the basis of broader considerations results from a *transformation process*, whereby individuals reconceptualize the given situation so they can be responsive to issues such as strategic concerns, long-term goals, or the desire to influence a partner's outcomes (Kelley & Thibaut, 1978). Outcome values resulting from the transformation process constitute the partners' *effective situation*; their effective preferences guide nonimpulsive behavior.

For example, if Eleanor and James decide that they will enact whatever behaviors yield the best combined outcomes for the two of them (a transformation termed *MaxJoint*), they can reconceptualize the situation depicted in Figure 36.1. This transformation process is depicted in Figure 36.3. The left side of Figure 36.3 reproduces the given situation Eleanor and James confront (from Figure 36.1); the right side portrays their transformed preferences (MaxJoint preferences, wherein each person's effective preferences take into account the sum of both partners' outcomes). After transforming the given situation, both partners experience a clear preference for cleaning the house together, because this option maximizes collective outcomes.

Individuals vary in the degree to which they exhibit different types of transformations, as well as in the likelihood of engaging in any transformation at all. Some people (termed *individualists*) are likely to pursue their simple self-interest, acting on the basis of their given situation preferences. Of course, the theoretical universe of possible transformations is infinite. But realistically, a limited set of relevant transformations is readily available to the interactants for a particular interdependence pattern. Given that the topic at hand is prorelationship motivation, we consider the transformation options available to partners facing situations with conflicting interests, such as the situation illustrated in Figure 36.1. Although some theorists recognize a large number of possible transformation options (e.g., Bornstein et al., 1983), we follow Van Lange's (2000) lead in emphasizing four of them: (1) *MaxJoint*, which maximizes partners' joint outcomes; (2) *MinDiff*, which minimizes differences between partners' outcomes, regardless of the absolute level of these outcomes; (3) *MaxOther*, which maximizes outcomes for the other partner; and (4) *MaxRel*, which maximizes the superiority of the individual's outcomes relative to the other partner's. The first three options are prorelationship transformations; they psychologically alter the given situation to ensure that collective interests are served (MaxJoint), that outcomes are fair (MinDiff), or that the partner is benefited (MaxOther). The fourth option can be construed as a selfish, or antirelationship, transformation; it psychologically alters the given situation to ensure that the indi-

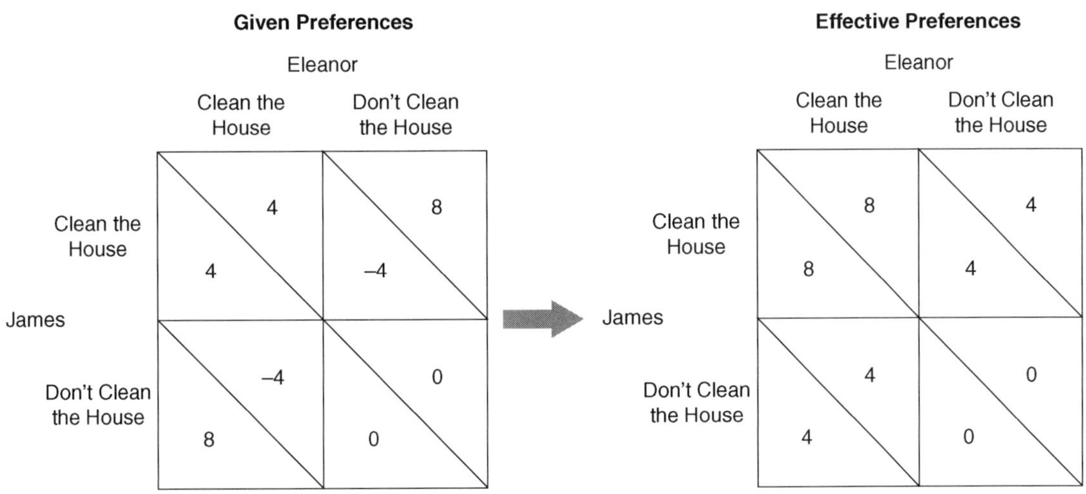


**FIGURE 36.3.** Prorelationship transformation: MaxJoint transformation of motivation.

vidual is advantaged relative to the partner (MaxRel).

One unexplored issue regarding the transformation process concerns the degree to which it can become fully automated over time. For example, is it possible that as a consequence of interacting with James for 30 years, Eleanor undergoes virtually automatic prorelationship transformation if James forgets her birthday? Rather than experiencing an immediate retaliatory impulse, Eleanor may come to experience immediate forgiveness, automatically assuming that James's forgetfulness is attributable to extraneous causes or extenuating circumstances (e.g., James is suffering a bad spell at work).

How might such a process transpire? When they initially confront a new interdependence situation, individuals experience it as a specific opportunity or problem to be addressed. They can either act impulsively (on the basis of their automatic, given situation preferences) or deliberately consider their various options. Repeatedly engaging in cognitively laborious transformations (i.e., consciously and diligently considering their response options, and the implications thereof) is costly and effortful. Early in a relationship, using cognitive resources in this way may well make sense; among other benefits, it allows the individual to determine whether the partner is reliable and cares about the self. However, once a relationship is well established, such laborious mental exertions may be unnecessary. As the partners experience similar given situations over time, they are likely to repeat transformations that previously resulted in good outcomes, and are likely to eschew transformations that previously resulted in poor outcomes. The forgiveness process may well become automated over time to the extent that forgiving each other's minor transgressions has generally been the best course of action.

### Predictors of Prorelationship Transformation of Motivation

In situations involving conflicting interests, three broad categories of variables influence the degree to which individuals are likely to enact prorelationship transformations (Rusbult & Van Lange, 1996). The first category is *dispositions*, including both personal dispositions (e.g., self-control) and interpersonal dispositions (e.g., social value orientation). Personal dispositions are stable characteristics of individuals that are relevant to a broad range of personal and interpersonal tasks. Interpersonal dispositions are actor-specific tendencies to respond to particular interpersonal situations in a specific manner across numerous partners (Kelley, 1983).

An example of a *personal disposition* that reliably facilitates prorelationship transformation is self-control. Individuals with strong self-control are more accommodating and forgiving in response to potentially destructive partner behaviors than are those with weak self-control (Finkel & Campbell, 2001). In particular, people with strong self-control are skilled at inhibiting retaliatory impulses in favor of prorelationship behaviors. An example of an *interpersonal disposition* that is relevant to understanding prorelationship motivation is social value orientation (Van Lange, 2000). Individuals generally fall into one of three social value orientations: *individualists*, *cooperators*, or *competitors*. Individualists are likely to act on the basis of their self-interested, given preferences; cooperators are likely to enact prorelationship transformations; and competitors are likely to enact hostile, antirelationship transformations.

A second category, *relationship-specific motives*, describes tendencies to respond in a consistent manner to particular situations with a specific partner (Holmes, 1981). These motives are especially relevant to situations with conflicting interests. One such motive, relationship commitment, promotes prorelationship motivation across a broad spectrum of situations (Rusbult, Olsen, Davis, & Hannon, 2001), including those in which the individual (1) has been betrayed by the partner (Finkel et al., 2002), (2) must decide whether to make sacrifices to benefit the partner (Van Lange et al., 1997), and (3) is exposed to tempting alternative partners (Miller, 1997). In one study (Finkel et al., 2002, Study 1), participants who were involved in dating relationships were exposed to an experimental manipulation of relationship commitment (i.e., priming of low vs. high commitment) before confronting a series of hypothetical betrayal incidents (e.g., "Your partner becomes sexually intimate with another person"). Participants primed to experience high commitment were more forgiving in response to betrayal incidents than were those primed to experience low commitment. In another study (Van Lange et al., 1997, Study 4), participants with stronger commitment exerted greater physical effort to benefit the partner (stepping up and down a stair to earn money for the partner).

Complementing the effects of commitment, trust is a relationship-specific motive reflecting an individual's confidence that the partner experiences prorelationship motives toward the self (Holmes & Rempel, 1989). As noted earlier, Eleanor develops trust when she perceives that James has behaved in a prorelationship manner in *diagnostic situations* (i.e., situations in which his interests conflict with hers). Such behavior reveals James's willingness to sacrifice for Eleanor, and communicates that her needs are important to him. When Eleanor perceives such behavior, she becomes more willing to commit to their relationship, which in turn increases the likelihood that she will reciprocate James's prorelationship acts (Wieselquist et al., 1999). Thus prorelationship behaviors such as forgiveness and sacrifice produce a pattern of mutual cyclical growth, whereby James's prorelationship motives and behaviors promote Eleanor's confidence in his trustworthiness, which increases her willingness to become dependent, which in turn promotes her own commitment and willingness to exhibit prorelationship motives and behaviors, ultimately yielding patterns of mutual prorelationship motivation and reciprocal prorelationship behavior.

A third category of variables that shapes prorelationship transformation is *social norms*, defined as rule-based, socially transmitted inclinations to respond to specific interdependence situations in a particular manner (Thibaut & Kelley, 1959). Many norms emerge around the goal of promoting prorelationship behavior when immediate impulses might favor selfish motivations. For example, the "golden rule" prescribes that we should treat other people as we ourselves would like to be treated (e.g., with consideration).

A topic worth exploring empirically is the degree to which cultural differences in norms influence prorelationship motivation. For example, it is easy to imagine that people from individualistic cultures such as the United States might experience prorelationship motivation at lower rates (or in fewer circumstances) than those from collectivistic cultures such as Japan (see Markus & Kitayama, 1991). Almost by definition, people who adhere to individualistic norms believe that personal satisfaction is relatively more important—and that relational well-being is relatively less important—than those who adhere to collectivistic norms. Such normative differences are likely to have important and predictable implications for prorelationship motivation.

## BENEFITS AND DANGERS OF PRORELATIONSHIP MOTIVATION

It is difficult—costly and effortful—to sustain a long-term, well-adjusted relationship. A growing literature has examined various relationship maintenance mechanisms (forgiveness, sacrifice, accommodation, etc.), determining that such behaviors are more likely among individuals with greater prorelationship motivation. The question we address in this section is whether and when engaging in relationship maintenance mechanisms is beneficial versus destructive for the self.

### The Benefits of Prorelationship Motivation

Abundant evidence suggests that on average, engaging in prorelationship behavior is associated with positive outcomes for relationships and for individuals. (Less empirical attention has been directed to the obvious prediction that an individual's prorelationship acts are beneficial for the partner.) For example, empirical evidence suggests that prorelationship motivation and behavior are associated with greater couple adjustment and longevity (Carstensen, Gottman, & Levenson, 1995; Van Lange et al., 1997), enhanced mental health (e.g., Coyle & Enright, 1997), and superior physiological functioning (Witvliet, Ludwig, & Vander Laan, 2001). One study demonstrates that prorelationship behavior (accommodation, forgiveness, and conciliatory behavior) is associated with personal well-being (life satisfaction, physical health symptoms, psychological adjustment), and that this effect is driven by the effects of prorelationship behavior on couple well-being (Kumashiro, Finkel, & Rusbult, 2002).

### The Dangers of Prorelationship Motivation

However, the association of prorelationship behavior with positive personal and relational outcomes is not universal. Prorelationship motivation can sometimes result in self-destructive behaviors. For example, extreme levels of commitment may cause individuals to make unhealthy sacrifices for their relationships. One illustration of this point comes from an archival analysis of data from a shelter for battered women: Severely abused women were more likely to return to their abusive partners to the extent that they were highly committed to (and dependent upon) their relationships (Rusbult & Martz, 1995). A plausible interpretation of these results is that because many of these women had exceedingly poor alternatives to their present relationships (e.g., no driver's license, poor work skills, fear of injury or death if they were to leave the partner), they were powerfully motivated to behave in ways that benefited the relationship, even if it meant that they would experience severe physical and psychological abuse as a result.

Less extreme examples corroborate the notion that prorelationship motivation can sometimes be harmful for individuals or relationships. For example, in normal populations, high *unmitigated communion* (i.e., an emphasis on others to the exclusion of the self) is associated with psychological distress (Fritz & Helgeson, 1998). Other research demonstrates that individuals who overprioritize their relationship and thereby neglect their personal needs exhibit poorer subjective well-being, greater psychological distress, and greater physical symptomatology (Kumashiro, Rusbult, & Finkel, 2006). Moreover, an imbalance between partners' commitment levels predicts poorer couple well-being (Drigotas et al., 1999). The conclusion from the corpus of relevant data is that strong prorelationship motivation is beneficial to relationships and to individuals, but that excessive relational motivation—motivation that takes place to the neglect of the self's needs—is self-destructive.

## CONCLUSIONS

Most theories of human motivation look inside the individual, arguing that motivation stems from genetic makeup, biological drives, person-level dispositions, and the like. Although we do not question the importance of these sources of human motivation, they provide an incomplete picture of its character. To understand almost any interpersonal motivation, researchers must take account of the interdependence situations individuals confront. The present analysis of prorelationship motivation recognizes that individuals differ in the strength of their general motivation to benefit the relationship and the partner, but it emphasizes that these differences will be more salient in some situations (e.g., divvying up a limited resource) than in others (e.g., coordinating who will paint which wall of the kitchen). Understanding situation structure provides insight into both (1) the social situations that reliably promote (or inhibit) prorelationship motivation versus the social situations to which prorelationship motivation is irrelevant; and (2) the dispositional, relational, and normative factors that increase the likelihood of prorelationship behavior, even when the situational pull against such behavior is strong.

## NOTE

1. Even in situations with perfectly negative covariation, if partners are forced to interact with one another over an extended period of time, they may sometimes achieve patterns of reciprocal prorelationship behavior. For example, political enemies in the U.S. Senate may find that it is in their long-term interests to support one another's bills, in that such a pattern of reciprocal cooperation enhances the odds that each person will achieve a high rate of successful legislation.

## REFERENCES


Arriaga, X. B., & Rusbult, C. E. (1998). Standing in my partner's shoes: Partner perspective-taking and reactions to accommodative dilemmas. *Personality and Social Psychology Bulletin, 9*, 927–948.

Attridge, M., Berscheid, E., & Simpson, J. A. (1995). Predicting relationship stability from both partners versus one. *Journal of Personality and Social Psychology, 69*, 254–268.

Axelrod, R. (1984). *The evolution of cooperation*. New York: Basic Books.

Baumeister, R. F., Wotman, S. R., & Stillwell, A. M. (1993). Unrequited love: On heartbreak, anger, guilt, scriptlessness, and humiliation. *Journal of Personality and Social Psychology, 64*, 377–394.

Bornstein, G., Crum, L., Wittenbraker, J. Harring, K., Insko, C. A., & Thibaut, J. (1983). On the measurement of social orientations in the minimal group paradigm. *European Journal of Social Psychology, 13*, 321–350.

Bui, K. T., Peplau, L. A., & Hill, C. T. (1996). Testing the Rusbult model of relationship commitment and stability in a 15-year study of heterosexual couples. *Personality and Social Psychology Bulletin, 22*, 1244–1257.

Carstensen, L. L., Gottman, J. M., & Levenson, R. W.

(1995). Emotional behavior in long-term marriage. *Psychology and Aging, 10*, 140–149.

Christensen, A., & Heavey, C. L. (1993). Gender differences in marital conflict: The demand/withdraw interaction pattern. In S. Oskamp & M. Costanzo (Eds.), *Gender issues in contemporary society* (pp. 113–141). Newbury Park, CA: Sage.

Clark, M. S., & Mills, J. (1993). The difference between communal and exchange relationships: What it is and is not. *Personality and Social Psychology Bulletin, 19*, 684–691.

Coyle, C. T., & Enright, R. D. (1997). Forgiveness intervention with postabortion men. *Journal of Consulting and Clinical Psychology, 65*, 1042–1046.

Drigotas, S. M., Rusbult, C. E., & Verette, J. (1999). Level of commitment, mutuality of commitment, and couple well-being. *Personal Relationships, 6*, 389–409.

Exline, J. J., & Baumeister, R. F. (2000). Expressing forgiveness and repentance: Benefits and barriers. In M. E. McCullough, K. I. Pargament, & C. E. Thoresen (Eds.), *Forgiveness: Theory, research, and practice* (pp. 133–155). New York: Guilford Press.

Finkel, E. J., & Campbell, W. K. (2001). Self-control and accommodation in close relationships: An interdependence analysis. *Journal of Personality and Social Psychology, 81*, 263–277.

Finkel, E. J., Campbell, W. K., Brunell, A. B., Dalton, A. N., Scarbeck, S. J., & Chartrand, T. L. (2006). High-maintenance interaction: Inefficient social coordination impairs self-regulation. *Journal of Personality and Social Psychology, 91*, 456–475.

Finkel, E. J., Rusbult, C. E., Kumashiro, M., & Hannon, P. A. (2002). Dealing with betrayal in close relationships: Does commitment promote forgiveness of betrayal? *Journal of Personality and Social Psychology, 82*, 956–974.

Fiske, S. T. (1993). Controlling other people: The impact of power on stereotyping. *American Psychologist, 48*, 621–628.

Fritz, H. L., & Helgeson, V. S. (1998). Distinctions of unmitigated communion from communion: Self-neglect and overinvolvement with others. *Journal of Personality and Social Psychology, 75*, 121–140.

Holmes, J. G. (1981). The exchange process in close relationships: Microbehavior and macromotives. In M. J. Lerner & S. C. Lerner (Eds.), *The justice motive in social behavior* (pp. 261–284). New York: Plenum Press.

Holmes, J. G. (2002). Interpersonal expectations as the building blocks of social cognition: An interdependence theory perspective. *Personal Relationships, 9*, 1–26.

Holmes, J. G., & Murray, S. L. (1996). Conflict in close relationships. In E. T. Higgins & A. Kruglanski (Eds.), *Social psychology: Handbook of basic principles* (pp. 622–654). New York: Guilford Press.

Holmes, J. G., & Rempel, J. K. (1989). Trust in close relationships. *Review of Personality and Social Psychology, 10*, 187–220.

Huston, T. L. (1983). Power. In H. H. Kelley, E. Berscheid, A. Christensen, J. H. Harvey, T. L. Huston, G. Levinger, et al. (Eds.), *Close relationships* (pp. 169–219). New York: Freeman.

Kelley, H. H. (1983). The situational origins of human tendencies: A further reason for the formal analysis of structures. *Personality and Social Psychology Bulletin, 9*, 8–30.

Kelley, H. H. (1984). The theoretical description of interdependence by means of transition lists. *Journal of Personality and Social Psychology, 47*, 956–982.

Kelley, H. H., & Holmes, J. G. (2006). *Interdependence theory: Situations, relationships, and personality.* Unpublished manuscript, University of Waterloo, Waterloo, Ontario, Canada.

Kelley, H. H., Holmes, J. G., Kerr, N. L., Reis, H. T., Rusbult, C. E., & Van Lange, P. A. M. (2003). *An atlas of interpersonal situations.* New York: Cambridge University Press.

Kelley, H. H., & Thibaut, J. W. (1978). *Interpersonal relations: A theory of interdependence.* New York: Wiley.

Kumashiro, M., Finkel, E. J., & Rusbult, C. E. (2002). Self-respect and pro-relationship behavior in marital relationships. *Journal of Personality, 70*, 1009–1049.

Kumashiro, M., Rusbult, C. E., & Finkel, E. J. (2006). *Navigating personal and relational concerns: The quest for equilibrium.* Unpublished manuscript, University of Hamburg, Hamburg, Germany.

Lewin, K. (1936). *Principles of topological psychology.* New York: McGraw-Hill.

Markus, H. R., & Kitayama, S. (1991). Culture and the self: Implications for cognition, emotion, and motivation. *Psychological Review, 98*, 224–253.

McCullough, M. E., Fincham, F. D., & Tsang, J. (2003). Forgiveness, forbearance, and time: The temporal unfolding of transgression-related interpersonal motivations. *Journal of Personality and Social Psychology, 84*, 540–557.

McCullough, M. E., Rachal, K. C., Sandage, S. J., Worthington, E. L., Brown, S. W., & Hight, T. L. (1998). Interpersonal forgiving in close relationships: II. Theoretical elaboration and measurement. *Journal of Personality and Social Psychology, 75*, 1586–1603.

Miller, R. S. (1997). Inattentive and contented: Relationships commitment and attention to alternatives. *Journal of Personality and Social Psychology, 73*, 758–766.

Mischel, W., & Shoda, Y. (1995). A cognitive–affective system theory of personality: Reconceptualizing situations, dispositions, dynamics and invariance in personally structure. *Psychological Review, 102*, 246–268.

Murray, S. L., & Holmes, J. G. (1993). Seeing virtues in faults: Negativity and the transformation of interpersonal narratives in close relationships. *Journal of Personality and Social Psychology, 65*, 707–722.

Rusbult, C. E. (1983). A longitudinal test of the investment model: The development (and deterioration) of satisfaction and commitment in heterosexual involvements. *Journal of Personality and Social Psychology, 45*, 101–117.

Rusbult, C. E., & Arriaga, X. B. (2000). Interdependence in personal relationships. In W. Ickes & S. Duck (Eds.), *The social psychology of personal relationships* (pp. 79–108). New York: Wiley.

Rusbult, C. E., Davis, J. L., Finkel, E. J., Hannon, P. A., & Olsen, N. (2006). *Forgiveness of betrayal in close relationships: A dual process model of the transformation from self-interested impulses to relationship-oriented actions*. Unpublished manuscript, Vrije Universiteit, Amsterdam, The Netherlands.

Rusbult, C. E., & Martz, J. M. (1995). Remaining in an abusive relationship: An investment model analysis of nonvoluntary dependence. *Personality and Social Psychology Bulletin, 21*, 558–571.

Rusbult, C. E., Olsen, N., Davis, J. L., & Hannon, P. A. (2001). Commitment and relationship maintenance mechanisms. In J. H. Harvey & A. Wenzel (Eds.), *Close romantic relationships: Maintenance and enhancement* (pp. 87–113). Mahwah, NJ: Erlbaum.

Rusbult, C. E., & Van Lange, P. A. M. (1996). Interdependence processes. In E. T. Higgins & A. Kruglanski (Eds.), *Social psychology: Handbook of basic principles* (pp. 564–596). New York: Guilford Press.

Rusbult, C. E., Van Lange, P. A. M., Wildschut, T., Yovetich, N. A., & Verette, J. (2000). Perceived superiority in close relationships: Why it exists and persists. *Journal of Personality and Social Psychology, 79*, 521–545.

Rusbult, C. E., Verette, J., Whitney, G. A., Slovik, L. F., & Lipkus, I. (1991). Accommodation processes in close relationships: Theory and preliminary empirical evidence. *Journal of Personality and Social Psychology, 60*, 53–78.

Thibaut, J. W., & Kelley, H. H. (1959). *The social psychology of groups*. New York: Wiley.

Van Lange, P. A. M. (2000). Beyond self-interest: A set of propositions relevant to interpersonal orientations. *European Review of Social Psychology, 11*, 297–330.

Van Lange, P. A. M., & Kuhlman, D. M. (1994). Social value orientations and impressions of a partner's and intelligence: A test of the might versus morality effect. *Journal of Personality and Social Psychology, 67*, 126–141.

Van Lange, P. A. M., Rusbult, C. E., Drigotas, S. M., Arriaga, X. B., Witcher, B. S., & Cox, C. L. (1997). Willingness to sacrifice in close relationships. *Journal of Personality and Social Psychology, 72*, 1373–1395.

Wieselquist, J., Rusbult, C. E., Foster, C. A., & Agnew, C. R. (1999). Commitment, prorelationship behavior, and trust in close relationships. *Journal of Personality and Social Psychology, 77*, 942–966.

Witvliet, C. V., Ludwig, T. E., & Vander Laan, K. L. (2001). Granting forgiveness or harboring grudges: Implications for emotion, physiology, and health. *Psychological Science, 11*, 117–123.

Witcher, B. S. (1999). *The effects of power on relationships and on individuals*. Unpublished doctoral dissertation, University of North Carolina at Chapel Hill.

Chapter 37

# Approaching Social Rewards and Avoiding Social Punishments

## APPETITIVE AND AVERSIVE SOCIAL MOTIVATION

**Shelly L. Gable**
**Amy Strachman**

Close relationships are potent sources of both pleasure and pain. The potential rewards of close relationships, such as companionship, love, and intimacy, are immense. Indeed, social relationships are perhaps the most important sources of life satisfaction and emotional well-being (Berscheid & Reis, 1998). For example, in a recent study by Diener and Seligman (2002), the consistently happiest people (i.e., those scoring in the top 10% of the sample on multiple confirming assessments of happiness) had one thing in common: rewarding social relationships. This finding echoes the Campbell, Converse, and Rodgers (1976) survey of over 2,000 Americans, which found that among the major domains of activity, marriage and family life were the best predictors of overall life satisfaction. The value of rewarding social bonds is recognized by scientists and laypersons alike; the majority of people cite close relationships when asked what gives their lives meaning (Klinger, 1977; Little, 1989), and close friends and family are often at the top of the list when people make retrospective accounts of the sources of happiness in their lives (e.g., Sears, 1977). On the other side of the coin, the potential costs of close relationships present hazards of comparable magnitude (e.g., Burman & Margolin, 1992). Trouble in relationships is the most frequently cited reason for seeking psychotherapy (Pinsker, Nepps, Redfield, & Winston, 1985), and death of a spouse and divorce are among the most stressful of life's events (Holmes & Rahe, 1967). Isolation and rejection from peers in childhood and adolescence predicts myriad psychological and physical problems, both concurrently and in later adulthood (Parker & Asher, 1987). And adults are not immune; for example, conflict and hostility in close relationships are associated with various detriments to well-being and changes in health (Kiecolt-Glaser, 1999). Relationships can also have a direct route to changes in health, as physical violence too often unfolds in the context of close relationships, such as parent–child and spousal partnerships (Straus, 1991). The potential costs and pain of social bonds are commonly known; more than half of the people who were asked to describe the "last bad thing that happened" to them cited disruption, conflict, or loss in a significant relationship (Veroff, Kulka, & Douvan, 1981).

Despite the potential incentives of close bonds, the countless potential threats and costs of social relationships may cause us to wonder why we venture into them at all. However, completely forsaking close relationships is also not a viable option, because failing to form even minimal social connections is linked to mortality risks on a par with those for cigarette smoking (House, Landis, & Umberson, 1988). Without question, despite the precarious balance of incentives and threats in interpersonal relationships, people are tenaciously motivated to form and maintain strong and stable social bonds. For example, when explicitly asked about their life goals, people routinely list successful social relationships as some of their most important strivings (e.g., Emmons, 1999), and many theories of psychological well-being view the fulfillment of relationship needs through forming and maintaining social ties as a central component of health and well-being (e.g., Deci & Ryan, 1985; Ryff, 1995). It should not be a surprise, then, to learn that people who neglect to place social needs in the top tier of life goals have poorer psychological functioning (Kasser & Ryan, 1996).

Reviews of the empirical literature support the idea that human beings across the lifespan have a fundamental *need* for close social bonds (Baumeister & Leary, 1995; Reis, Collins, & Berscheid, 2000). Nonetheless, relatively little work has investigated the processes involved in establishing, maintaining, and dissolving social bonds from a motivational or goal theory perspective. One critical dimension of motivation and the regulation of behavior is the focus of motives and goals. That is, social motives and goals may be focused either on a rewarding or desired end-state (*approach*), or on a punishing, undesired end-state (*avoidance*). Much research on social relationships has been concerned with either the rewarding aspects (e.g., attraction, intimacy) or the punishing aspects (e.g., insecurity, conflict), but rarely has this research examined them in tandem. Given that interpersonal relationships present us with both threats and incentives, research on motives, goals, and the regulation of social behavior needs to address the approach dimension and the avoidance dimension simultaneously. In our view, the approach–avoidance distinction has important implications for attention, cognition, emotions, and behavior in social and relational contexts. Over our human evolutionary history, the social domain presented us with fundamental opportunities (e.g., mating, parenting) and costs (e.g., competition, conflict); therefore, theories of motivation need to address the adaptive strategies arising from relational incentives and threats (Bugental, 2000).

In this chapter we attempt to integrate work from the fields of close relationships and approach and avoidance motivation, in the hopes of enhancing our understanding of interpersonal relationships and motivation more broadly. Understanding the regulation of social incentives and threats is likely to be particularly important, because the majority of life experiences, both meaningful and trivial, take place in the context of close relationships. First we briefly review the prolific literature on the approach–avoidance distinction, including work in general motivation and the achievement motivation domain. Next we summarize previous work on social motivation, including work on affiliation, intimacy, and rejection motives and goals. Finally, we present a model of approach and avoidance social motivation that may be useful for understanding both regulation in the context of specific close relationships and social regulatory processes more broadly, along with preliminary evidence in the support of the model and questions for future research.

## APPROACH AND AVOIDANCE MOTIVES AND GOALS

The approach–avoidance distinction has a lengthy history in psychological theory and research (for reviews, see Elliot, 1999; Higgins, 1998). For instance, Pavlov (1927) detailed two reflexes—one orienting toward the stimulus and the other turning away from the stimulus—and Schneirla (1959) found evidence for this "towardness" and "awayness" distinction across diverse species, suggesting evolutionarily early phylogenic roots. Another salient example lies in Miller's (1959, 1961) classic research on separate approach and withdrawal learning processes, and graphic representations of their interplay in approach and avoidance conflict gradients. In short, although interest in the topic has waxed and waned over the years, work across seemingly diverse areas of psychology has either explicitly or implicitly adopted a view of separate appetitive (i.e., approach) and aversive (i.e., avoidance) systems (for reviews, see Carver, 1996; Gable, Reis, & Elliot, 2003).

Although the majority of theoretical and empirical work on the approach–avoidance distinction has been in the areas of goals and motivation, similar partitions have been made in others areas in psychology, such as in personality, emotion, affect, and coping behavior (e.g., Cacioppo & Gardner, 1999; Gray, 1990; Moos, 1997; Watson, Clark, & Tellegen, 1988). For example, although attitudes have traditionally been assessed on a single dimension, often with a bipolar scale ranging from "agree" to "disagree," Cacioppo and colleagues' research supports the idea that there are separate processes underlying the evaluation of the positive and negative aspects of an attitude object (Cacioppo, Gardner, & Berntson, 1997). In the domain of emotion, there is considerable evidence that activated *positive affect* (PA) is distinct from activated *negative affect* (NA) (Watson et al., 1988; Watson & Tellegen, 1985) (see Russell & Carroll, 1999, for an alternative view of emotion). High PA is characterized by feeling elated, excited, and enthusiastic, and low PA is characterized by feeling dull and sluggish. Feeling distressed, fearful, and hostile describes high NA, whereas feeling calm, placid, and relaxed represents low NA. While PA and NA are not completely orthogonal, they are largely independent, such that low PA does not indicate high NA or vice versa. Recently, and more central to the topic of the current chapter, Watson and his colleagues have argued that PA is the subjective feeling experienced when a biologically based appetitive or approach system is activated, and NA is the subjective feeling experienced when a biologically based aversive or avoidance system is activated (Watson, Wiese, Vaidya, & Tellegen, 1999).

As mentioned, in the domain of motivation and the regulation of behavior, several theories have featured the approach–avoidance distinction, some of which are detailed in this handbook. For example, Carver and Scheier's model of self-regulation (1990; see also Carver & Scheier, Chapter 20, this volume) posits a feedback process such that information from the environment is compared to an internal reference, an output occurs, the environment is reevaluated and compared to the internal reference, and the process continues. Some feedback processes attempt to reduce the discrepancy between the input and the internal reference (*discrepancy-reducing* loops), and some feedback processes attempt to enlarge this discrepancy (*discrepancy-enlarging* loops). Carver (1996) has equated these two systems with approach and avoidance processes, respectively. Elliot (1997) has made the distinction between approach- and avoidance-focused achievement motivation, describing approach motives as those consisting of the need for achievement and avoidance motives as those focused on a fear of failure. Similarly, in his theory of regulatory focus, Higgins (1998) distinguishes between self-regulation of behavior that is focused on positive end-states and self-regulation of behavior that is focused on negative end-states. He refers to the former as a *promotion* focus and the latter as a *prevention* focus. Although promotion and prevention are not theoretically equivalent to approach and avoidance, there are distinct commonalities; for example, promotion foci fulfill needs for growth and prevention foci fulfill needs for security, respectively (see Molden, Lee, & Higgins, Chapter 11, this volume).

Recently, the motivational theory of Jeffrey Gray (1970, 1987, 1994) has attracted considerable attention. Gray posited distinct appetitive and aversive motivational systems, referred to as the *behavioral activation system* (BAS) and the *behavioral inhibition system* (BIS), respectively. Gray's model outlines personality as a function of individual differences in the two systems, which have neuroanatomical and neurophysiological correlates. The appetitive system (BAS) activates behavior in response to signals of reward and nonpunishment, whereas the aversive system (BIS) inhibits behavior in response to signals of punishment, nonreward, and novel stimuli. Gray's (1994) theory also links motivation to emotion: Activation of the BAS is associated with feelings of hope and approach behaviors, whereas activation of the BIS is associated with feelings of anxiety and avoidance behaviors (Gray, 1990).

The approach–avoidance distinction has proved to have important implications for understanding perception, cognition, emotion, behavior, health, and well-being (e.g., Derryberry & Reed, 1994; Elliot & Sheldon, 1998; Higgins, Shah, & Friedman, 1997). For example, Derryberry and Reed (1994) found that individuals with strong approach motivation were biased toward positive cues (i.e., cues indicating gain), and those with strong aversive motivation were biased toward negative cues (i.e., cues indicating loss), during a basic visual target detection task. Higgins and colleagues (1997) have shown that promotion-focused goals (approach) produce cheerfulness–dejection responses and prevention-focused goals (avoidance) produce quiescence–agitation responses. And Elliot and Sheldon (1998) found that higher numbers of avoidance personal goals predicted lower well-being and higher physical symptom reports, both prospectively and retrospectively.

In short, the approach–avoidance distinction has been noted in myriad areas of psychology, most notably in the fields of motivation and emotion. As noted by Carver (1996), "Although these two tendencies [approach and avoidance] are often layered across each other in the topography of behavior, they are conceptually distinct from each other. Being distinct, they may be managed by different structures in the nervous system" (p. 320). Specifically, Gray (1987) has posited that BAS is a function of the limbic circuits and dopaminergic pathways, and that the BIS system is rooted in circuits in the hippocampus, the septum, and related structures.

Recent empirical evidence from neurophysiological investigations provides support for separate structures. For example, Sutton and Davidson (1997) found that Gray's BIS and BAS constructs predicted different components of resting prefrontal asymmetry as measured with electroencephalographic (EEG) technology (see also Harmon-Jones & Allen, 1997). Specifically, subjects with higher BAS showed more relative left prefrontal activation, whereas those with higher BIS scores showed greater relative right prefrontal activation. Similarly, inducing emotions in the laboratory corresponds to neural activity changes as recorded by the EEG: Anticipation of a reward corresponds with left frontal activation, and anticipation of a punishment is associated with right frontal activation (Sobotka, Davidson, & Senulis, 1992). Finally, Reuter and colleagues (2004) found that BAS sensitivity was associated with hippocampus–parahippocampus activity in the left hemisphere in response to erotic stimuli, and that high-BIS subjects showed increased activity in numerous regions of interest in the brain when exposed to fear and disgust images (although it is worth noting that the specific regions activated did not map directly onto Gray's theorized substrates of BIS).

The neurobiological evidence provides a possible reason for the consistent emergence of the approach–avoidance distinction in motivation (as well as in other areas in psychology; Davidson, 1992; Fowles, 1994; Gray, 1987; Schneirla, 1959). Gable and colleagues (2003) conducted a series of confirmatory factor analyses on appetitive and aversive individual difference measures in affect (e.g., PA and NA), personality (e.g., neuroticism and extroversion), motivation (e.g., BAS and BIS), and behavior (e.g., approach and avoidance coping), to test whether a common two-factor solution would be found. They found strong evidence that measures such as PA, BAS, extroversion, and approach-focused coping were tapping a latent appetitive construct, and that measures such as NA, BIS, neuroticism, and avoidance-focused coping were tapping a latent aversive construct. This two-factor model consistently fit the data better than a one-factor model, a domain-based model (i.e., a model with latent variables for personality, affect, motivation, etc.), or a measure-based model (e.g., self-report measures and semiprojective measures). The appetitive and aversive latent variables were negatively correlated (ranging from–.37 to –.60), indicating that the constructs are separate, but not completely independent of one another. Support for a two-factor model (and rejection of a one-factor model) of two relatively independent constructs suggests that appetition is not simply the absence of aversion, and approaching is not equivalent to not avoiding. Rather, the two-factor model implies that these separate physiological systems probably influence many domains of inquiry in psychology, most notably, motivation and emotion.

Moreover, the relative independence of the approach and avoidance systems implies that each may operate through different processes. Gable, Reis, and Elliot (2000) found support for this idea in a study on motivational dispositions and reactions to daily events. In three studies Gable and colleagues operationalized the appetitive dimension in terms of Gray's

BAS, and the aversive dimension in terms of Gray's BIS (see Carver & White, 1994). As predicted, they found that high BIS sensitivity was associated with more daily NA, and that high BAS sensitivity was predictive of increased daily PA. However, the relationship between BAS and PA was explained by a *differential exposure* process, and the relationship between BIS and NA was explained by a *differential sensitivity* hypothesis. People with more sensitive BAS experienced more daily PA because they experienced more frequent and more important positive events (differential exposure). People with more sensitive BIS did not report experiencing more frequent or more important negative events; however, they reacted more strongly to the occurrence of negative events (differential reactivity).

In summary, the approach–avoidance distinction has a long and prolific history; it emerges in several theories of motivation and goal processes; and physiological evidence supports the existence of neuroanatomical correlates for it. The two systems are functionally independent of one another,[1] and thus are correlated with different environmental stimuli and may operate through different processes. As noted in the review above, the large majority of the work on approach and avoidance motivation has not focused specifically on social motivation. However, considerable attention has been paid to the domain of social motivation.

## SOCIAL MOTIVATION: 1950–1975

### Early Thematic Apperception Studies

Murray (1938) postulated several human needs in the social domain (e.g., nurturance, sex); however, the *need for affiliation* has received the most empirical attention. Shipley and Veroff (1952) conducted studies examining how affiliation needs are represented in responses to standard Thematic Apperception Test (TAT) pictures (Morgan & Murray, 1935). In their research, need for affiliation was defined as stemming from insecurity. They compared TAT stories from control groups to those from groups in which need for affiliation was "aroused" by threats of rejection and separation. They then constructed a scoring scheme to measure the strength of the need for affiliation, which was similar to the scoring scheme used by McClelland, Clark, Roby, and Atkinson (1949) to measure the need for achievement with the TAT. In this work, need for affiliation was negatively correlated with popularity.

Subsequently, Atkinson, Heyns, and Veroff (1954) addressed the somewhat narrow definition of need for affiliation used in the previous investigation by expanding this definition to include thoughts concerned with "establishing, maintaining, or restoring a positive affective relationship with another person(s)" (p. 405). Atkinson and colleagues found that need for affiliation was positively correlated with others' ratings of participants' approval-seeking behavior and confidence. These authors interpreted the seemingly mixed results of their study and the previous study by Shipley and Veroff (1952) by suggesting that the arousal conditions differentially activated two types of needs for affiliation: a *hope for affiliation* (approach) and a *fear of rejection* (avoidance). Other studies employing the TAT methodology identified correlates of affiliation motivation (for a review, see Boyatzis, 1973). For example, McKeachie, Lin, Milholland, and Issacson (1966) found that students who scored high on need for affiliation performed better in courses led by instructors who were high in warmth and concern for others than students who were low on need for affiliation did. Lansing and Heyns (1959) found that people with a high need for affiliation made more personal phone calls at work and wrote more letters than those with low affiliative needs. However, in these and other studies that employed the TAT paradigm to study the need for affiliation, no attempt was made to separate hope-for-affiliation needs from fear-of-rejection needs.

DeCharms (1957) attempted to separate approach affiliative motives from avoidance affiliative motives in a study of task performance in groups. He coded TAT imagery concerned with positive relationships and attaining affiliation as *approach affiliation* (+Aff), and TAT imagery concerned with separation and rejection as *avoidance affiliation* (–Aff). He found that people with high –Aff were significantly more productive in competitive groups and less productive in cooperative groups than people with low –Aff. Fishman (1965, as cited in Boyatzis, 1973) also employed deCharms's bivariate coding scheme in a study of small-group interactions. The findings indicated that +Aff (but not–Aff) was associated with observed positive behaviors in the small groups.

These studies were conducted in the context of laboratory-formed groups, however, not with existing or naturally initiated close personal relationships.

### Criticisms and Alternative Conceptualizations

In his review of the existing literature on affiliation motivation, Boyatzis (1973) raised concerns about the existing TAT scoring of approach and avoidance affiliation motivation. His major criticism was that all such scoring procedures (including deCharms's system) were based on variations of the original experiment by Shipley and Veroff (1952), which defined affiliation as a concern with rejection and separation. Moreover, the predominant view of affiliation motivation was based on Murray's (1938) deficit model of needs and Miller's (1959) drive reduction theory of conflict. Boyatzis contended that an approach affiliative need does not conform to such models. That is, the existence of close relationships will not decrease approach affiliative motivation (as predicted by a deficit model); rather, the presence of relationships should stimulate further approach motivation. Boyatzis stated that individuals with high approach motivation will "(a) be relaxed, spontaneous and open in [their] behavior with others; (b) take steps to provide [themselves] with the opportunity to relate to others but not actively pursue others; and (c) be genuinely interested in others" (p. 272).

Boyatzis (1973) went on to speculate that the reason why researchers viewed approach motivation as less influential than avoidance motivation was that the two were evaluated with the same outcome criteria. He reasoned that the distinction between approach and avoidance affiliation motivation is analogous to Maslow's (1968) distinction between *growth* and *deficiency* motivation. Boyatzis suggested that approach concerns should be related to ratings of people's sincerity, sensitivity, and popularity. These criteria differ from those examined in the achievement contexts of earlier studies on affiliation motivation (e.g., productivity in competitive groups).

The theoretical position outlined by Boyatzis is consistent with more contemporary neuroanatomical motivational models, as well as with the model of approach and avoidance social motives and goals presented in this chapter and outlined in detail below. That is, there are two types of affiliative or social motives and goals: Approach motives and goals are focused on positive social outcomes, such as making social contacts and obtaining closeness and intimacy, whereas avoidance motives and goals are focused on negative social outcomes, such as avoiding rejection and preventing conflict in relationships. Moreover, Boyatzis (1973) also outlined a plan for research on affiliation motivation, proposing that future research examine both approach and avoidance affiliative motives. He suggested that the two types of motivation would probably relate to different characteristics of the individual and have different implications for interpersonal relationships. Unfortunately, in over three decades since his ideas were published, little research has separated the approach and avoidance aspects of *social motivation*.

## SOCIAL MOTIVATION: 1975–PRESENT

Although interest in human affiliation motivation has somewhat waned over the past 30-plus years, there are notable exceptions. McAdams (1982) distinguished between affiliation and intimacy motivation; he defined *intimacy motivation* as a "passive, non-controlling, being orientation" (McAdams & Constantian, 1983, p. 852), and he characterized intimate interactions as involving mutual delight, reciprocal dialogue, openness, and harmony. In an experience-sampling study, intimacy motivation was positively related to the frequency of interpersonal thoughts and positive emotions in interpersonal situations, and it was negatively related to desire to be alone during interpersonal interactions. Both affiliation motivation and intimacy motivation predicted time spent in interpersonal communications (oral and written). Only affiliation motivation predicted desire to be interacting with others when alone (McAdams & Constantian, 1983). Intimacy motivation also predicted self-disclosure among friends, listening behavior, and concern for the well-being of friends (McAdams et al., 1984).

The intimacy motive represents an alternative view of affiliative behavior and motivation that seems more appropriate to studying individuals in the context of close personal relationships. However, this approach also does not fully distinguish between appetitive and aversive processes. That is, intimacy motivation by itself cannot distinguish between focus on desired end-states (e.g., hope to obtain intimacy) and undesired end-states (e.g., fear of alienation or conflict).

Mehrabian (1976), however, did distinguish between approach and avoidance affiliation (see also Mehrabian & Ksionzky, 1974; Russell & Mehrabian, 1978), in work largely influenced by expectancy theories. Affiliative characteristics were represented in terms of a two-dimensional scheme based on expectations of positive and negative reinforcements in interpersonal relationships (Mehrabian & Ksionzky, 1974). Mehrabian (1976) developed and validated two measures of affiliative behavior, *affiliative tendency* and *sensitivity to rejection*; he found that people high on affiliative tendency were less anxious, elicited more PA from others, were more self-confident, and saw themselves as similar to others. People high in sensitivity to rejection were less confident, were more anxious, and were judged less positively by others than people low on sensitivity to rejection.[2]

Downey and colleagues have focused on the construct of *rejection sensitivity*, which is defined as the tendency to anxiously expect and intensely react to rejection by significant others. They have found that individual differences in rejection sensitivity predict people's behavior in relationships. For example, high rejection sensitivity was found to be associated with negative behavior and hostility during problem-solving discussions in the lab, and increased negative emotions following conflicts with a romantic partner. For men, high rejection sensitivity has been associated with increased incidents of violence in dating relationship in men (Ayduk et al., 1999; Downey, Feldman, & Ayduk, 2000; Downey, Freitas, Michaelis, & Khouri, 1998). Complementing work focused on rejection in relationships, Sanderson and Cantor (2001) found that individuals with a strong personal focus on intimacy in dating relationships experienced greater relationship satisfaction and were more likely to maintain their relationship over time.

In sum, although social motives have received much less attention than achievement motives, the field has nonetheless seen over 50 years of research on individual differences in affiliation, intimacy, and rejection motivation. However, few theoretical accounts or empirical investigations have emerged that simultaneously addresses social incentive- and threat-based motives and goals. That is, models and investigations of social and relationship motivation have rarely considered both the "towardness" and "awayness" of human beings' fundamental need for social relationships. And precious few have investigated how these goals influence the formation, maintenance, and possible dissolution of actual social bonds. Given the never-ending task of regulating social behavior, and the potential impact of individual differences on these regulatory processes, explicit examination of social motives and goals is long overdue.

## A MODEL OF APPROACH AND AVOIDANCE SOCIAL MOTIVES AND GOALS

### Motives, Goals, and Social Environment Predicting Social Outcomes

Our recent work has focused on the development and validation of a model of approach and avoidance social motives and goals, social processes, and social outcomes (Gable, 2006; Impett, Gable, & Peplau, 2005; Strachman & Gable, 2006). The basic model is shown in Figure 37.1. In the model, the influences of dispositional individual differences (i.e., social motives), environmental factors, and short-term strivings (i.e., social goals) on behaviors and outcomes are simultaneously addressed. Furthermore, dispositional approach social motives and *incentives* in the social environment will predispose people to adopt short-term approach social goals, and dispositional avoidance social motives and *threats* in the social environment will predispose people to adopt avoidance social goals. For example, in a discussion on child care, a husband who has strong appetitive social motives and recently has had pleasant interactions with his wife will be more likely to adopt approach goals, such as "I want for us to have a smooth discussion and for both of us to be happy with the outcome"; a husband who has strong aversive motives and recently has had unpleasant interactions with his wife will be more likely to adopt avoidance goals, such as "I want to avoid a conflict and for neither of us to be unhappy with the outcome." Or, on a first date, a person who has strong approach social motives or who finds him- or herself in an environment rich with dating opportunities will be more likely to adopt approach goals, such as "I want to have

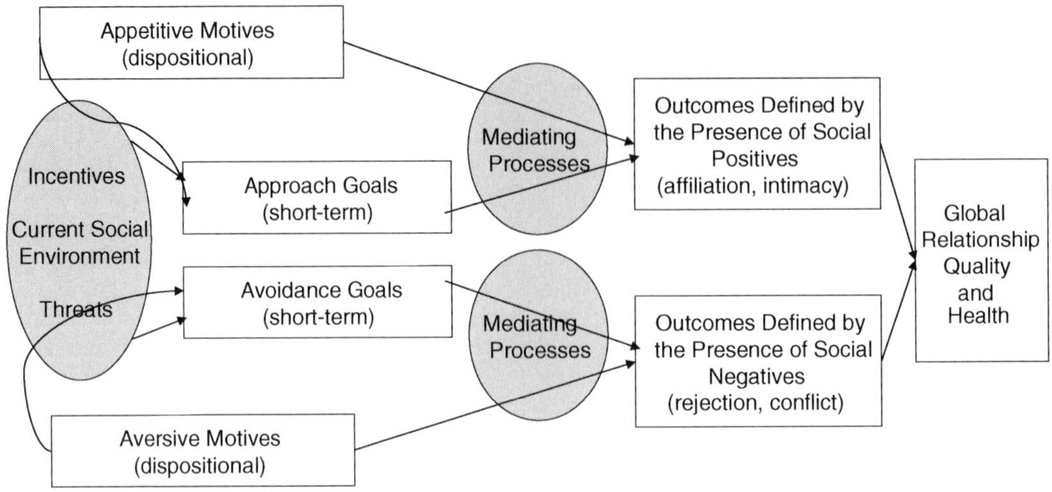


**FIGURE 37.1.** An approach–avoidance model of social motives and goals.

a great time and make a good impression"; someone who has strong aversive motives or finds him- or herself in a hostile and competitive dating environment will be more likely to adopt avoidance goals, such as "I don't want to be bored or make a fool of myself."

Moreover, these two types of goals will be linked to different social outcomes. Approach social goals should be more strongly associated with outcomes defined by the presence or absence of rewarding social bonds, such as affiliation and intimacy. To someone who is mainly approach-oriented (or in an incentive-rich social milieu), successful interactions and relationships are those that provide incentives such as fun, companionship, and understanding; painful relationships are those that fail to provide these rewards. Avoidance social goals should be more strongly associated with outcomes defined by the presence or absence of punishing social bonds, such as rejection, isolation, and conflict. Thus, to someone who is primarily avoidantly motivated (and/or in a high-threat social environment), pleasing interactions and relationships are defined as those that lack uncertainty, disagreements, and anxiety; painful relationships are those that possess these negative qualities. The social outcomes in turn are predicted to combine to form a person's global evaluation of social and relationship quality.

The majority of our empirical work thus far has attempted to establish the links among social motives, goals, and outcomes. For example, three recent studies showed that distal motives predicted more proximal goals: Those with strong approach motives were more likely to adopt short-term approach social goals, and those with strong avoidance motives were more likely to adopt short-term avoidance social goals (Gable, 2006). Sensitivity to social rewards was associated with the adoption of goals focused on obtaining these social rewards (e.g., "To make new friends," "To strengthen my relationships with family"), and sensitivity to punishment was associated with adoption of goals focused on avoiding these social punishments (e.g., "To not be lonely," "To avoid conflicts with my parents"). Moreover, as predicted by the model, approach and avoidance motives and goals were associated with different patterns of social outcomes. Specifically, approach motives and goals were associated with positive social attitudes and more satisfaction with social bonds, whereas avoidance motives and goals were associated with more negative social attitudes and relationship insecurity; both approach and avoidance predicted loneliness, an outcome with both appetitive and aversive features (Gable, 2006). Moreover, hierarchical regression showed that the effects of social goals remained significant even when general sensitivity to reward and punishment (i.e., BIS vs. BAS) was controlled for, and that the regression coefficients for social goals were significantly larger ($p < .05$) than those for general motivation (Gable, 2006, Study 2).

Most recently, we examined approach and avoidance motives and goals in ongoing dyadic relationships (Impett et al., 2005). Romantic couples' motives for everyday relationship sacrifices (enacting a behavior that is not preferred, such as accompanying a partner to a work function, not spending time on a hobby, or having sex when physically tired) were studied in a daily experience study that also included a longitudinal component. We found that on days individuals sacrificed for approach motives (e.g., to promote intimacy), they reported greater PA and relationship satisfaction. But on days when they enacted the same behaviors for avoidance motives (e.g., to avoid conflict), they reported greater NA, lower relationship satisfaction, and more conflict. Sacrificing for avoidance motives was particularly detrimental to the maintenance of relationships over time: The more individuals sacrificed for avoidance motives over the course of the study, the less satisfied they were and the more likely they were to have broken up 6 weeks later, even when initial levels of satisfaction and commitment were controlled for (Impett et al., 2005). Consistent with the Gable (2006) findings, general approach and avoidance motivation did not significantly predict any of the relationship outcomes, and the theoretically predicted results remained significant when general motives were controlled for. These data provide preliminary evidence for the applicability of the model to processes in ongoing relationship maintenance and dissolution.

## Mediating Processes

Our model in Figure 37.1 also predicts that different processes will mediate the relationship between appetitive motivation and social outcomes on the one hand, and between aversive motivation and social outcomes on the other. Preliminary support for this hypothesis was found in our work on general motivation, which has shown that approach motives and goals were associated with increased exposure to positive events. That is, approach motives and goals predicted increased frequency of the occurrence of positive social events (but not frequency of negative social events), which mediated the link between approach motives and outcomes. In contrast, avoidance motives and goals were correlated with increased reactivity to negative social events (and not reactivity to positive events): Avoidance motives did not predict the frequency of experiencing negative social events, but did predict ratings of their impact when they did occur (Gable, 2006, Study 2; see also Gable et al., 2000). Based on this preliminary evidence, our model outlines several mechanisms through which approach and avoidance motives and goals, together with the current social environment, influence social outcomes.

First, individual differences in approach and avoidance motives are likely to influence attention to interpersonal information (incentives and threats, respectively). In order to respond to social stimuli, individuals must first attend to social cues, both incentives and threats. These hypotheses are derived both from work on general motivation and from research on attention in other domains. For example, in two priming experiments, Avila and Parcet (2002) showed that participants higher in BAS (compared to those low in BAS) were more attentive to targets when they were primed with a positive incentive cue than with no cue. In addition, several studies have shown that high trait anxiety (which is closely linked to avoidance motivation; Gable et al., 2003) is associated with increased attention to threatening cues (Mathews & MacLeod, 1994). For example, many studies have employed the emotional Stroop task to study anxiety and attention. In these paradigms participants name the color of a word, and if the word is threatening, people with high anxiety (trait or state) are slower to respond to the threatening word. These delays are thought to reflect enhanced attention to the threatening word (MacLeod & Mathews, 1988). This logic has been extended to study attention to rewards; for example, optimists show more interference (i.e., slower reaction times) on positive words (Segerstrom, 2001). There is also evidence for domain specificity; for example, individuals with spider phobia are slower to respond to spider-related threatening words than those without such phobia, but the two groups do not differ in the response to other threatening words (see Williams, Mathews, & MacLeod, 1996). Thus, although we have not yet directly tested these hypotheses with social motives and attention to social cues, work on general approach and avoidance motivation and on domain-specific attention has shown that individual differences in these motives and environmental cues do predict increased attentional focus toward rewarding and threatening stimuli, respectively.

The second mediating process predicted by our model is concerned with memory. Once social information has been attended to, memory of this information can underlie expectations that are carried into future interactions with the relationship partner or into similar social contexts. Social memory and expectancies are important in ongoing social interaction, because, as Neuberg (1996) has summarized, expectancy confirmation processes can bias future interactions through the way information is gathered from the target, through behavior toward the target, through interpretation of ambiguous signals, and through behavior elicited from the target. We recently collected data showing that the strength of avoidance social goals influenced memory of ambiguous interpersonal events (Strachman & Gable, 2006). Specifically, participants who rated avoidance social goals as more important remembered more negative statements and fewer positive statements from an ambiguous story about a couple than those who rated avoidance social goals as less important. These findings indicate that avoidance motivation heightens memory for socially threatening information. We are currently replicating and expanding these findings and testing how approach goals influence memory.

Equally important to the social information that is retrieved from memory is how this social information is interpreted during the event itself. The third mediating process predicted by our model concerns the interpretation of ambiguous interpersonal information. This is especially relevant in interpersonal relationships, because there is often no clear standard by which to judge another's behavior in an interaction. Many social events are subjective: A spouse's quiet demeanor can be indicative of a bad day at work or a problem with the other spouse; a stranger's smile can be flirtatious or polite. In the study described above (Strachman & Gable, 2006), we also analyzed how accurately participants recalled the original social scenario. The results showed that the more important people rated avoidance goals as being, the more negative a spin they put on the neutral and positive elements of the original story. Thus this work provided initial support for the idea that avoidance motivation negatively biases the interpretation of social events. Our ongoing work focuses on expanding these results and examining how approach goals influence interpretation of social information.

The fourth process that we hypothesize to mediate the links among social goals, environment, and outcomes is the evaluation of progress in terms of goals and subsequent affective experiences. A hallmark of a close relationship is that it persists over time; therefore, goal progress regarding specific relationships is likely to be important. Carver and Scheier's (1982, 1990) control process model predicts that an important element of affective experience is progress on goals. Specifically, their model posits that one's current level of goal attainment is compared to a standard. If progress exceeds the standard, PA is experienced; if progress falls short of the standard, NA is experienced; and if progress is equal to the standard, no affect is experienced. In terms of the focus of goals, the type of PA experienced upon success with avoidance goals (avoiding threat) is relief, and upon success with approach goals (attaining incentive) is joy. The type of NA experienced upon failure with avoidance goals (not avoiding threat) is anxiety, and upon failure with approach goals (not attaining incentive) is disappointment (see Carver, 2004; Carver & Scheier, Chapter 20, this volume; Higgins, 1998). Thus we theorize that the evaluation of goal progress and the subsequent emotional experience play a role in the link between goals and outcomes.

The final mediating process outlined by our approach and avoidance model is the formation of overall relationship quality judgments and subsequent decisions concerning relationship dissolution or escalation.[3] The approach–avoidance model predicts that qualities defined by the presence of positives and the absence of negatives combine to predict overall satisfaction, which then predicts persistence–dissolution decisions in close relationships. In our previous work on general motivation, emotional experience, and life satisfaction, we found that individual differences in approach and avoidance motivations moderated the degree to which people based satisfaction judgments on the presence or absence of positive and negative emotions (Updegraff, Gable, & Taylor, 2004). Specifically, in a lab study and a signal-contingent daily experience study, we found that high-approach participants (those high in BAS) made satisfaction ratings that were more strongly tied to PA than those of low-approach participants were. Although avoidance motivation (BIS) was positively associated with the experience of NA, it did not predict the weighting of negative emotions in life satisfaction judgments. Although we have not yet directly tested these ideas in social relationships, we predict that differences in motivation and goals will influence how different qualities of relationships (e.g., intimacy, trust) are weighted in overall satisfaction and stability. Specifically, we think that approach motives and goals will be positively correlated with appetitive-dimension outcomes, such as passionate love; that avoidance motives and goals will be negatively correlated with aversive-dimension outcomes, such as security; and that those high on approach motives and goals will weigh appetitive outcomes more in overall satisfaction (Gable & Reis, 2001). All three of these processes will predict relationship stability (e.g., escalation, dissolution) over time.

### Correspondence of Current Model with Existing Research

Although work from our own lab is in the initial stages of testing the model of approach and avoidance social motivation presented in Figure 37.1, our predictions are consistent with current findings from other lines of research. For example, researchers have applied an approach and avoidance framework to understanding commitment to romantic relationships. Frank and Brandstätter (2002) found that a previously established tripartite construct of commitment (i.e., personal, moral, and structural) could be reduced to approach commitment and avoidance commitment dimensions. Specifically, approach commitment represents positive incentives for the continuation of the relationship, whereas avoidance commitment represents the negative incentives for the termination of the relationship. By separating commitment into threats and incentives, Frank and Brandstätter were able to predict relationship satisfaction in couples 13 months later, such that approach commitment was associated with increases in satisfaction and avoidance commitment was associated with less satisfaction over time. We draw similar conclusions pertaining to relationship commitment in our own work (see Strachman & Gable, 2006a).

Further support for the role of motivational focus comes from sexual behavior research. Specifically, Cooper, Shapiro, and Power (1998) identified approach motives in sexual relationships as focused on rewarding, desired end-states in the relationship, such as increased intimacy with a partner and physical enhancement. In contrast, avoidance sexual motives are focused on punishing, undesired end-states, such as rejection from the partner and peers, and relief from negative emotions. These sexual motives have been associated with differences in sexual behavior such as age at first sexual encounter, one-night stands, number of lifetime partners, and birth control use (Cooper et al., 1998).

Existing research also provides support for the mediational processes outlined in our model. For example, there is a robust literature regarding the influence of attributions on marital satisfaction (Bradbury & Fincham, 1992; Fincham, 1985; Fincham, Harold, & Gano-Phillips, 2000). This research has shown that attributions accentuating the negative aspects and minimizing the positive aspects of relationship events are associated with lower relationship satisfaction. These maladaptive attributions influence the processing of interpersonal events and create negative interpretations—a process that parallels our data on avoidance goals and interpretation of and memory for social information (see above). In sum, several lines of research have documented the importance of the approach and avoidance distinction and their associated mediational processes in social relationships, in ways that are consistent with the current model.

## IMPLICATIONS AND CONCLUDING COMMENTS

In this chapter we have attempted to apply the approach–avoidance distinction to social and relationship motives and goals. Although the approach and avoidance literature has a distinguished and fruitful history, the framework has not been consistently applied to research on motives and goals in the social domains. One reason for this is that compared to work in the achievement domain, for example, attention to social motives and goals has been small (of course, there are notable exceptions, which we have highlighted in our discussion). We feel that this is a grave oversight, because recent research has shown that the influence of social motivation is not limited to social outcomes; there is also growing evidence that interpersonal goals have a far greater influence on cognition, emotion, and behavior than previously anticipated. That is, recent research shows that close relationship goals affect numerous psychological processes in seemingly unrelated domains, and often without people's explicit knowledge of their power. For example, Shah (2003) recently found that priming goals related to significant others affected goal pursuit for, and performance on, an unrelated achievement task. Moreover, this effect was moderated by degree of closeness to the significant others. Several other studies have found equally compelling evidence for how social goals and internal representations of close relationships influence how people think, feel, and act (e.g., Anderson, Reznik, & Manzella, 1996; Baldwin, Carrell, & Lopez, 1990; Fitzsimons & Bargh, 2003; Mikulincer, 1998). Thus, in conclusion, it is clear that social motives and goals are important constructs for understanding myriad outcomes of interest to psychologists, and we feel that the approach–avoidance distinction is critical in understanding these processes. The future lies in more explicitly understanding how approach and avoidance motives, goals, processes, and outcomes operate in social and close relationships.

## ACKNOWLEDGMENT

Preparation of this chapter was facilitated by Grant No. MH065346 from the National Institutes of Health awarded to Shelly L. Gable.

## NOTES

1. Interactions of the approach and avoidance systems through processes such as coactivation and inhibition are extremely fruitful, and questions about these are likely to constitute the next generation of research issues. Unfortunately, space does not permit full discussion of the possible interactions, but the reader is referred to Cacioppo and colleagues (1997) and Corr, Pickering, and Gray (1997) for examples.

2. Note that this result is consistent with the negative correlation found between need for affiliation and popularity in the early TAT studies (e.g., Atkinson et al., 1954), supporting criticisms that these studies of affiliation were predominantly focused on avoidance or rejection and isolation motives.

3. There are likely to be other processes mediating the links among motives, goals, environment, and outcomes than those focused on here.

## REFERENCES


Anderson, S. M., Reznik, I., & Manzella, L. M. (1996). Eliciting facial affect, motivation, and expectancies in transference: Significant-other representations in social relations. *Journal of Personality and Social Psychology, 71*, 1108–1129.

Atkinson, J. W., Heyns, R. W., & Veroff, J. (1954). The effects of experimental arousal of the affiliation motive on thematic apperception. *Journal of Abnormal and Social Psychology, 49*, 405–410.

Avila, C., & Parcet, M. A. (2002). Individual differences in reward sensitivity and attentional focus. *Personality and Individual Differences, 33*, 979–996.

Ayduk, O., Downey, G., Testa, A., Yen, Y., & Shoda, Y. (1999). Does rejection elicit hostility in rejection sensitive women? *Social Cognition* [Special issue: Social cognition and relationships], *17*(2), 245–271.

Baldwin, M. W., Carrell, S. E., & Lopez, D. F. (1990). Priming relationship schemas: My adviser and the pope are watching me from the back of my mind. *Journal of Experimental Social Psychology, 26*, 435–454.

Baumeister, R. F., & Leary, M. R. (1995). The need to belong: Desire for interpersonal attachments as a fundamental human motivation. *Psychological Bulletin, 117*, 497–529.

Berscheid, E., & Reis, H. T. (1998). Interpersonal attraction and close relationships. In D. T. Gilbert, S. T. Fiske, & G. Lindzey (Eds.), *The handbook of social psychology* (4th ed., Vol. 2, pp. 193–281). New York: McGraw-Hill.

Boyatzis, R. E. (1973). Affiliation motivation. In D. C. McClelland & R. S. Steele (Eds.) *Human motivation: A book of readings* (pp. 252–276). Morristown, NJ: General Learning Press.

Bradbury, T. N., & Fincham, F. D. (1992). Attributions and behavior in marital interaction. *Journal of Personality and Social Psychology, 63*, 613–628.

Bugental, D. B. (2000). Acquisition of the algorithms of social life: A domain-based approach. *Psychological Bulletin, 126*, 187–219.

Burman, B., & Margolin, G. (1992). Analysis of the association between marital relationships and health problems: An interactional perspective. *Psychological Bulletin, 112*, 39–63.

Cacioppo, J. T., & Gardner, W. L. (1999). Emotion. *Annual Review of Psychology, 50*, 191–214.

Cacioppo, J. T., Gardner, W. L., & Berntson, G. G. (1997). Beyond bipolar conceptualizations and measures: The case of attitudes and evaluative space. *Personality and Social Psychology Review, 1*, 3–25.

Campbell, A., Converse, P. E., & Rodgers, W. L. (1976). *The quality of American life*. New York: Russell Sage Foundation.

Carver, C. S. (1996). Emergent integration in contemporary personality psychology. *Journal of Research in Personality, 30*, 319–334.

Carver, C. S. (2004). Negative affects deriving from the behavioral approach system. *Emotion, 4*, 3–22.

Carver, C. S., & Scheier, M. F. (1982). Control theory: A useful conceptual framework for personality-social, clinical, and health psychology. *Psychological Bulletin, 92*, 111–135.

Carver, C. S., & Scheier, M. F. (1990). Origins and functions of positive and negative affect: A control-process view. *Psychological Review, 97*, 19–35.

Carver, C. S., & White, T. L. (1994). Behavioral inhibition, behavioral activation, and affective responses to impending reward and punishment: The BIS/BAS scales. *Journal of Personality and Social Psychology, 67*, 319–333.

Cooper, M. L., Shapiro, C. M., & Powers, A. M. (1998). Motivations for sex and risky sexual behavior among adolescents and young adults: A functional perspective. *Journal of Personality and Social Psychology, 75*, 1528–1558.

Corr, P. J., Pickering, A. D., & Gray, J. A. (1997). Personality, punishment, and procedural learning: A test of J. A. Gray's anxiety theory. *Journal of Personality and Social Psychology, 73*, 337–344.

Davidson, R. J. (1992). Anterior cerebral asymmetry and the nature of emotion. *Brain and Cognition, 20*, 125–151.

DeCharms, R. C. (1957). Affiliation motivation and productivity in small groups. *Journal of Abnormal and Social Psychology, 55*, 222–226.

Deci, E. L., & Ryan, R. M. (1985). *Intrinsic motivation and self-determination in human behavior.* New York: Plenum Press.

Derryberry, D., & Reed, M. A. (1994). Temperament and attention: Orienting toward and away from positive and negative signals. *Journal of Personality and Social Psychology, 66*, 1128–1139.

Diener, E., & Seligman, M. E. P. (2002). Very happy people. *Psychological Science, 13*, 81–84.

Downey, G. Feldman, S., & Ayduk, O. (2000). Rejection sensitivity and male violence in romantic relationships. *Personal Relationships, 7*, 45–61.

Downey, G., Freitas, B. L., Michaelis, B., & Khouri, H. (1998). The self-fulfilling prophecy in close relationships: Rejection sensitivity and rejection by romantic partners. *Journal of Personality and Social Psychology, 75*, 545–560.

Elliot, A. J. (1999). Integrating the "classic" and "contemporary" approaches to achievement motivation: A hierarchical model of approach and avoidance achievement motivation. In M. Maehr & P. Pintrich (Eds.), *Advances in motivation and achievement* (Vol. 10, pp. 243–279). Greenwich, CT: JAI Press.

Elliot, A. J. & Sheldon, K. M. (1998). Avoidance personal goals and the personality–illness relationship. *Journal of Personality and Social Psychology, 75*, 1282–1299.

Emmons, R. A. (1999). *The psychology of ultimate concerns: Motivation and spirituality in personality.* New York: Guilford Press.

Fincham, F. D. (1985). Attribution processes in distressed and nondistressed couples: Responsibility for martial problems. *Journal of Abnormal Psychology, 94*, 183–190.

Fincham, F. D., Harold, G. T., & Gano-Phillips, S. (2000). The longitudinal association between attributions and martial satisfaction: Direction of effects and role of efficacy expectations. *Journal of Family Psychology, 14*, 267–285.

Fishman, D. B. (1965). *Affiliation: Need, expectancy, and small group interaction.* Unpublished doctoral dissertation, Harvard University.

Fitzsimons, G. M., & Bargh, J. A. (2003). Thinking of you: Nonconscious pursuit of interpersonal goals associated with relationship partners. *Journal of Personality and Social Psychology, 84*, 148–164.

Fowles, D. C. (1994). A motivational theory of psychopathology. In W. D. Spaulding (Ed.), *Nebraska Symposium on Motivation: Vol. 41. Integrative views of motivation, cognition, and emotion* (pp. 181–238). Lincoln: University of Nebraska Press.

Frank, E., & Brandstätter, V. (2002). Approach versus avoidance difference types of commitment in intimate relationships. *Journal of Personality and Social Psychology, 82*, 208–221.

Gable, S. L. (2006). Approach and avoidance social motives and goals. *Journal of Personality, 74*, 75–222.

Gable, S. L., & Reis, H. T. (2001). Appetitive and aversive social interaction. In J. H. Harvey & A. E. Wenzel (Eds.), *Close romantic relationship maintenance and enhancement* (pp. 169–194). Mahwah, NJ: Erlbaum.

Gable, S. L., Reis, H. T., & Elliot, A. J. (2000). Behavioral activation and inhibition in everyday life. *Journal of Personality and Social Psychology, 78*, 1135–1149.

Gable, S. L., Reis, H. T., & Elliot, A. J. (2003). Evidence for bivariate systems: An empirical test of appetition and aversion across domains. *Journal of Research in Personality, 37*(5), 349–372.

Gray, J. A. (1970). The psychophysiological basis of introversion–extraversion. *Behaviour Research and Therapy, 8*(3), 249–266.

Gray, J. A. (1987). *The psychology of fear and stress* (2nd ed.). New York: Cambridge University Press.

Gray, J. A. (1990). Brain systems that mediate both emotion and cognition. *Cognition and Emotion, 4*, 269–288.

Gray, J. A. (1994). Three fundamental emotion systems. In P. Ekman & R. J. Davidson (Eds.), *The nature of emotion* (pp. 243–247). New York: Oxford University Press.

Harmon-Jones, E., & Allen, J. J. B. (1997). Behavioral activation sensitivity and resting frontal EEG asymmetry: Covariation of putative indicators related to risk for mood disorders. *Journal of Abnormal Psychology, 106*, 159–163.

Higgins, E. T. (1998). Promotion and prevention: Regulatory focus as a motivational principle. In M. P. Zanna (Ed.), *Advances in experimental social psychology* (Vol. 30, pp. 1–46). San Diego, CA: Academic Press.

Higgins, E. T., Shah, J., & Friedman, R. (1997). Emotional responses to goal attainment: Strength of regulatory focus as moderator. *Journal of Personality and Social Psychology, 72*, 515–525.

Holmes, T. H., & Rahe, R. H. (1967). The Social Readjustment Rating Scale. *Journal of Psychosomatic Research, 11*, 213–218.

House, J. S., Landis, K. R., & Umberson, D. (1988). Social relationships and health. *Science, 241*, 540–545.

Impett, E., Gable, S. L., & Peplau, L. A. (2005). Giving up and giving in: The costs and benefits of daily sacrifice in intimate relationships. *Journal of Personality and Social Psychology, 89*, 327–344.

Kasser, T., & Ryan, R. M. (1996). Further examining the American dream: Differential correlates of intrinsic and extrinsic goals. *Personality and Social Psychology Bulletin, 22*, 280–287.

Kiecolt-Glaser, J. K. (1999). Stress, personal relationships, and immune function: Health implications. *Brain, Behavior, and Immunity, 12*, 61–72.

Klinger, E. (1977). *Meaning and void: Inner experience and the incentives in people's lives*. Minneapolis: University of Minnesota Press.

Lansing, J. B., & Heyns, R. W. (1959). Need for affiliation and four types of communication. *Journal of Abnormal and Social Psychology, 58*, 365–372.

Little, B. R. (1989). Personal projects analysis: Trivial pursuits, magnificent obsessions and the search for coherence. In D. M. Buss & N. Cantor (Eds.), *Personality psychology: Recent trends and emerging directions* (pp. 15–31). New York: Springer-Verlag.

MacLeod, C., & Mathews, A. (1988). Anxiety and the allocation of attention to threat. *Quarterly Journal of Experimental Psychology: Human Experimental Psychology, 40*, 653–670.

Maslow, A. H. (1968). *Toward a psychology of being* (2nd ed.). Princeton, NJ: Van Nostrand.

Mathews, A., & MacLeod, C. (1994). Cognitive approaches to emotion and emotional disorders. *Annual Review of Psychology, 45*, 25–50.

McAdams, D. P. (1982). Intimacy motivation. In A. J. Stewart (Ed.), *Motivation and society* (pp. 133–171). San Francisco: Jossey-Bass.

McAdams, D. P., & Constantian, C. A. (1983). Intimacy and affiliation motives in daily living: An experience sampling analysis. *Journal of Personality and Social Psychology, 45*, 851–861.

McAdams, D. P., Healy, S., & Krause, S. (1984). Social motives and patterns of friendship. *Journal of Personality and Social Psychology, 47*, 828–838.

McClelland, D. C., Clark, R. A., Roby, T. B., & Atkinson, J. W. (1949). The projective expression of needs: IV. The effect of need for achievement on thematic apperception. *Journal of Experimental Psychology, 39*, 242–255.

McKeachie, W. J., Lin, Y., Milholland, J., & Issacson, R. (1966). Student affiliation motives, teacher warmth, and academic achievement. *Journal of Personality and Social Psychology, 4*, 457–461.

Mehrabian A. (1976). Questionnaire measures of affiliative tendency and sensitivity to rejection. *Psychological Reports, 38*, 199–209.

Mehrabian, A., & Ksionzky, S. (1974). *A theory of affiliation*. Lexington, MA: Lexington Books.

Mikulincer, M. (1998). Attachment working models and the sense of trust: An exploration of interaction goals and affect regulation. *Journal of Personality and Social Psychology, 74*, 1209–1224.

Miller, N. (1961). Acquisition of avoidance dispositions by social learning. *Journal of Abnormal and Social Psychology, 63*, 12–19.

Miller, N. E. (1959). Liberalization of basic S-R concepts: Extensions to conflict behavior, motivation, and social learning. In S. Koch (Ed.), *Psychology: A study of a science, Study 1* (pp. 198–292). New York: McGraw-Hill.

Moos, R. H. (1997). Coping Responses Inventory: A measure of approach and avoidance coping skills. In C. P. Zalaquett & R. J. Wood (Eds.), *Evaluating stress: A book of resources* (pp. 51–65). Lanham, MD: Scarecrow Press.

Morgan, C. D., & Murray, H. A. (1935). A method for investigating fantasy: The Thematic Apperception Test. *Archives of Neurology and Psychiatry, 34*, 289–306.

Murray, H. A. (1938). *Explorations in personality*. New York: Oxford University Press.

Neuberg, S. L. (1996). Expectancy influences in social interaction: The moderating role of social goals. In P. M. Gollwitzer & J. A. Bargh (Eds.), *The psychology of action: Linking cognition and motivation to behavior* (pp. 529–552). New York: Guilford Press.

Parker, J. G., & Asher, S. R. (1987). Peer relations and later personal adjustment: Are low-accepted children at risk? *Psychological Bulletin, 102*, 357–389.

Pavlov, I. (1927). *Conditioned reflexes: An investigation into the physiological activity of the cortex* (G. Anrep, Trans.). New York: Dover.

Pinsker, H., Nepps, P., Redfield, J., & Winston, A. (1985). Applicants for short-term dynamic psychotherapy. In A. Winston (Ed.), *Clinical and research issues in short-term dynamic psychotherapy* (pp. 104–116). Washington, DC: American Psychiatric Association.

Reis, H. T., Collins, W. A., & Berscheid, E. (2000). The relationship context of human behavior and development. *Psychological Bulletin, 126*, 844–872.

Reuter, M., Stark, R., Hennig, J., Walter, B., Kirsch, P., Schienle, A., et al. (2004). Personality and emotion: Test of Gray's personality theory by means of an fMRI study. *Behavioral Neuroscience, 118*, 462–469.

Russell, J. A., & Carroll, J. M. (1999). On the bipolarity of positive and negative affect. *Psychological Bulletin, 125*(1), 3–30.

Russell, J. A., & Mehrabian, A. (1978). Approach–avoidance and affiliation as functions of the emotion-eliciting quality of an environment. *Environment and Behavior, 10*, 355–387.

Ryff, C. D. (1995). Psychological well-being in adult life. *Current Directions in Psychological Science, 4*, 99–104.

Sanderson, C. A., & Cantor, N. (2001). The association of intimacy goals and marital satisfaction: A test of four mediational hypotheses. *Personality and Social Psychology Bulletin, 27*, 1567–1577.

Schneirla, T. C. (1959). An evolutionary and developmental theory of biphasic processes underlying approach and withdrawal. In M. R. Jones (Ed.), *Nebraska Symposium on Motivation* (Vol. 7, pp. 1–43). Lincoln: University of Nebraska Press.

Sears, R. R. (1977). Sources of life satisfactions of the Terman gifted men. *American Psychologist, 32*, 119–128.

Segerstrom, S. C. (2001). Optimism and attentional bias for negative and positive stimuli. *Personality and Social Psychology Bulletin, 27*, 1334–1343.

Shah, J. (2003). Automatic for the people: How representations of significant others implicitly affect goal pursuit. *Journal of Personality and Social Psychology, 84*, 661–681.

Shipley, T. E., & Veroff, J. (1952). A projective measure of need for affiliation. *Journal of Experimental Psychology, 43*, 349–356.

Sobotka, S. S., Davidson, R. J., & Senulis, J. A. (1992). Anterior brain electrical asymmetries in response to reward and punishment. *Electroencephalography and Clinical Neurophysiology, 83*, 236–247.

Strachman, A., & Gable, S. L. (2006a). Approach and avoidance relationship commitment. *Motivation and Emotion, 30*, 117–126.

Strachman, A., & Gable, S. L. (2006b). What you want (and don't want) can affect what you see (and don't see): Avoidance social goals and social events. *Personality and Social Psychology Bulletin, 32*, 1446–1458.

Straus, M. A. (1991). Family violence in American families: Incidence rates, causes, and trends. In D. D. Knudsen & J. L. Miller (Eds.), *Abused and battered: Social and legal responses to family violence* (pp. 17–34). New York: Aldine de Gruyter.

Sutton, S. K., & Davidson, R. J. (1997). Prefrontal brain asymmetry: A biological substrate of the behavioral approach and inhibition systems. *Psychological Science, 8*, 204–210.

Updegraff, J. A., Gable, S. L., & Taylor, S. E. (2004). What makes experiences satisfying?: The interaction of approach–avoidance motivations and emotions in well-being. *Journal of Personality and Social Psychology, 86*, 496–504.

Veroff, J., Kulka, R. A., & Douvan, E. (1981). *Mental health in America: Patterns of help-seeking from 1957 to 1976*. New York: Basic Books.

Watson, D., Clark, L. A., & Tellegen, A. (1988). Development and validation of brief measures of positive and negative affect: The PANAS scales. *Journal of Personality and Social Psychology, 54*, 1063–1070.

Watson, D., & Tellegen, A. (1985). Toward a consensual structure of mood. *Psychological Bulletin, 98*, 219–235.

Watson, D., Wiese, D., Vaidya, J., & Tellegen, A. (1999). The two general activation systems of affect: Structural findings, evolutionary considerations, and psychobiological evidence. *Journal of Personality and Social Psychology 76*, 820–838.

Williams, J. M., Mathews, A., & MacLeod, C. (1996). The emotional Stroop task and psychopathology. *Psychological Bulletin, 120*, 3–24.

Chapter 38

# Making Things Better *and* Worse

## MULTIPLE MOTIVES IN STEREOTYPING AND PREJUDICE

**Steven J. Stroessner**
**Abigail A. Scholer**

Of all the topics studied by social psychologists, one might assume that the literatures on stereotyping and prejudice would be replete with motivational concerns.[1] Indeed, much of the early theorizing and empirical research on intergroup perception and behavior had a strong motivational bent, emphasizing in particular intrapsychic bases of stereotyping and prejudice. The frustration–aggression account of prejudice (Dollard, Doob, Miller, Mowrer, & Sears, 1939) sought to identify the roles of projection and displacement in producing aggression toward minority groups as a means for dealing with feelings of frustration, even if those groups were not responsible for the frustrating event. Similarly, work on authoritarianism (Adorno, Frenkel-Brunswik, Levinson, & Sanford, 1950) portrayed prejudice as reflecting an overdeveloped superego produced by a rigid upbringing, resulting in the need to project unconscious desires onto other people or groups. Beyond these neo-Freudian notions, Allport's (1954) classic *The Nature of Prejudice* integrated both cognitive and motivational aspects of stereotyping. Allport emphasized the importance of cognitive factors such as social categorization, but he also emphasized how motives to achieve power, status, and control contribute to disparagement of outgroups.

Despite the strong historical emphasis on motivational factors, the consideration of such factors was largely abandoned for at least several decades from the early 1970s through the mid-1990s. Several reasons led to this neglect of motivational factors. First, theoretical accounts of prejudice through intrapsychic processes proved incomplete, at least in their original formulations. Frustration–aggression theory, for example, could not explain why frustration did not always produce aggression, why certain groups were chosen as agents for displacement, why displacement was sometimes directed at powerful rather than powerless groups, and why displacement tendencies did not vary with prejudice levels. Research on the authoritarian personality also became bogged down by measurement issues. Scales used to identify authoritarianism contained a strong acquiescence demand, tended to produce unreliable and multidimensional responses, and emphasized endorsement of conservative political attitudes. Given these weaknesses, many questioned whether there existed sufficient support for a personality-based account of prejudice. Moreover, and most critically, neither theory produced strong or consistent empirical support (see Duckitt, 2005; Green, Glaser, & Rich, 1998). Neither of these "symptom theories"—accounts that located the genesis of prejudice in motivational consequences of maladaptive psychological development—provided particularly compelling or complete accounts of prejudice.

The waning of the influence of these motivation-based accounts roughly coincided with the rise of social cognition as a theoretical and methodological framework in the early 1970s, and this movement was largely responsible for rejuvenating and sustaining research on stereotyping and prejudice for the subsequent two decades (Fiske, 2004; Schneider, 2004). The social cognition view of stereotyping differed dramatically from previous accounts in several respects. First, stereotyping was viewed as an example of reliance on stored knowledge, judgments, or beliefs about social groups. Although these beliefs might be fraught with error and represent overgeneralizations, stereotypes were thought to function quite similarly to other stored knowledge structures. Thus stereotyping could be compared with and contribute to the understanding of the role of memory structures in general psychological functioning. Second, by emphasizing the normality of prejudgment and reliance on stored beliefs, the social cognition account shifted the focus from *aberrant* individuals who exhibit prejudice as "symptoms" of some underlying disorder to *any* individual. If stereotyping and prejudice result from commonplace cognitive processes, then bias may be exhibited by any person, at least at some times or under some circumstances.

In its first two decades, the social cognitive framework proved incredibly helpful in advancing the understanding of the formation, maintenance, and use of stereotypes (Hamilton, Stroessner, & Driscoll, 1994). Numerous phenomena that had been assumed to be rooted in motivational factors could be explained by deficits in deliberative processing or biases in attention, interpretation, or retrieval of information from memory. Individuals were found to function like "cognitive misers" (Fiske & Taylor, 1984), willing to rely on stereotypes and cognitive heuristics rather than engaging in effortful strategies for avoiding bias. Stereotyping and even prejudice were shown to be quite commonplace, and bias was often found to occur without any intention or awareness by the perpetrator. However, one unfortunate consequence of this success in explaining bias in cognitive terms was the general abandonment of motivational factors in stereotyping, especially at the empirical level (Fiske, 2004). Although motivation was regularly invoked in models of stereotyping and prejudice (e.g., Devine, 1989; Fiske & Neuberg, 1990), little work attempted to measure or to specify the precise nature of relevant motivations.

Fortunately, that has changed over the last decade. A synthesis has emerged recognizing the importance of motivation *and* cognition—and, in fact, their inseparability—as the literature has embraced a view of individuals as "motivated tacticians" (Fiske & Taylor, 1991) who have multiple cognitive strategies available to employ in the service of both fleeting and chronic goals, needs, and values. However, this renewed consideration of motivation is quite different in assumptions and focus from that of the earlier intrapsychic era. It is clear that motivational factors do not invariably produce unified, unidirectional, consistent outcomes. Motivational factors sometimes serve to increase bias (consistent with classic motivational views), but they can also reduce or even eliminate bias in some circumstances. It is also clear that various motives may be activated in different social contexts, and that multiple motives may coexist even within a single context. Understanding the nature of the varied motives that may arise is critical to predicting whether bias is attenuated or exacerbated in any given context. Finally, the new look at motivation has benefited by employing methods and theories that emerged in the era of social cognitive dominance.

Over the last decade, research on motivation and stereotyping has examined topics as diverse as self-esteem, affiliative motives, and social normative factors. As this list implies, motivational factors that influence stereotyping and prejudice are varied in their nature, breadth, and focus. Given the recency of the renewed look at motivation, it is our view that a consideration of only a limited or fundamental set of motivational factors is premature at this point, though it may ultimately prove important to develop a taxonomy of basic motives. For the time being and for the purpose of this chapter, we review lines of work illustrating the breadth and varying foci of the research that has been looking anew at motivation and stereotyping, and we highlight common motivational concerns when possible.

This research demonstrates that whereas some motivational factors tend to ameliorate bias, others exacerbate prejudice. Some motives can do both. In the next section of this chapter, we discuss motivational factors in terms of their demonstrated ability to increase or decrease intergroup bias and discord. Although this framework is somewhat artificial and atheoretical, it reflects the development of research on the impact of motivation on bias. Early studies tended to examine single motives and single outcomes; only recently have the complex roles of motivational factors in bias been reflected in the empirical literature. After reviewing the consequences of various individual motivational states for stereotyping and prejudice, we briefly discuss the importance of considering both motives and means. We conclude by highlighting the importance of studying multiple motives—and of understanding the complex ways in which the same motive can make things better *or* worse for the target *or* the perceiver.

## HOW MOTIVATION MAKES THINGS WORSE

Classic research and theorizing generally assumed that motivational factors affect intergroup perception and behavior negatively. Frustration–aggression and authoritarian personality accounts shared the common assumption that stereotyping and prejudice offer means for dealing with ambiguity and managing deficiencies in self-regulation and ego development, even if doing so has negative consequences for judgments of other individuals and groups.

### The Prejudiced Personality Revisited

More recent research provides evidence that these motivations can increase prejudice, even though contemporary characterizations of these motivational concerns are quite different from those imagined by their original proponents. Altemeyer (e.g., 1981, 1998), for example, has almost single-handedly revived the notion of the authoritarian personality—stripping away its Freudian underpinnings, linking it to perceived threat, and showing how right-wing ideologies are compatible with and supportive of authoritarian orientations. Altemeyer suggests that *right-wing authoritarianism* (RWA) is characterized by a high degree of submissiveness to authorities perceived as legitimate, a general aggressiveness toward people or groups when such actions are believed to be sanctioned by authorities, and a high degree of adherence to established social conventions. Since a core aspect of RWA is an acceptance of existing social hierarchies, it comes as no surprise that RWA scores correlate with acceptance of inequality and generalized prejudice. This work implicates a motivation to justify power and existing social hierarchies, supporting aggression and disparagement of groups seen as deviant or threatening.

The frustration–aggression hypothesis of prejudice has not fared as well. Despite the intuitive appeal and some preliminary evidence supportive of a link between frustration and hate crimes, recent sophisticated reanalyses of these data suggest that there is little evidence supportive of a relationship between economic conditions and outgroup bias (Green et al., 1998), as would be suggested by the theory. Many individuals have also questioned the rationale underlying the link between frustration and prejudice, suggesting that the typical duration of frustration-related emotions (typically lasting seconds to minutes) cannot easily account for patterns of bias that have been consistent from decades to centuries. Recently, however, Glick (2005) has revived the frustration–aggression framework by broadening it to include not just intrapsychic causes, but also external factors involved in the blocking of goal achievement. In addition, he suggests that links among frustration, aggression, and bias should be examined more at the collective level than at the level of individual processes. These reformulations should prove useful in reinvigorating research into the links between frustration and bias.

### The Ubiquitous Need for Self-Regard

Whereas these revised authoritarian and frustration–aggression accounts still suggest that stereotyping and prejudice will tend to be located in a subset of individuals, other recent research has implicated motivational factors that tend to exacerbate bias in people in general. What these factors share in common is that they tend to relate to the fundamental motive to feel good about oneself and, by extension, about the groups to which one belongs. Unlike the earlier theories that focused on dysfunctional personalities, these motivational accounts assume a general and ubiquitous need to acquire and maintain positive self-regard. What this research shows is that engaging in bias against individuals and groups, even subtly and indirectly, provides one way for individuals to maintain a positive view of themselves. The means by which individuals achieve self-enhancement differ, however, among specific motivational accounts.

### Self-Affirmation and Stereotyping

Some findings point to a fairly direct link between self-regard and stereotype endorsement. Fein and Spencer (1997) examined the consequences of self-affirmation manipulations on stereotype use. In one study, participants either received no self-affirmation or were prompted to affirm a value they viewed as important. The former participants derogated the personality of a Jewish (compared with an Italian) woman, whereas the latter did not. In a second study, participants who received negative (but false) feedback regarding their intelligence were more likely to apply stereotypic traits to a gay male than individuals who received no feedback were. Finally, a third study provided evidence that outgroup derogation mediated the relation between self-affirmation threat and self-restoration. Subsequent studies (Spencer, Fein, Wolfe, Fong, & Dunn, 1998) showed that stereotypes tended to be activated following threat even when participants were under cognitive load. These effects are notable both because nonthreatened participants showed no signs of stereotype activation and because previous studies had shown that cognitive load tended to attenuate stereotype accessibility. Being threatened produced accessible stereotypes, which individuals could easily use to restore a positive sense of self. Unfortunately, these data provide support for the notion that individuals often "build themselves up by putting others down."

The specific stereotypes applied to outgroup members are determined at least in part by attempts to maintain a positive view of the self through the process of projection. Freudian notions of projection posited that projecting one's undesired traits onto others serves to deceive and thereby to protect the ego. More contemporary approaches reject this characterization of projection, however, suggesting instead that thought suppression may play a pivotal role (Govorun, Fuegen, & Payne, 2006; Newman, Duff, & Baumeister, 1997). When an individual feels threatened in terms of a particular trait or characteristic, he or she attempts to deal with the threat by suppressing thoughts related to that trait or characteristic. Such attempts often fail, leaving the undesired thought highly accessible and available to color judgments and behavior. Govorun and colleagues (2006) provided evidence consistent with this account. Individuals prompted to think about a time they had failed on a task involving either intelligence or leadership were more likely to derogate sorority members on that specific trait compared with the other trait and compared with conditions in which they had been prompted to think of a success in either domain. Attempts to avoid thinking negatively about a personal failure made those thoughts highly accessible in memory, biasing specific judgments of other individuals and groups.

### Group Affirmation and Stereotyping

Although the work described so far illustrates rather direct links between self-regard and stereotyping, other research clearly shows that there are numerous indirect links as well. Individuals need not explicitly endorse the self to avoid stereotyping or invoke stereotypes to maintain self-esteem. Instead, they can easily obtain benefits indirectly, though affiliation with valued groups. Thus people can acquire and maintain positive self-regard by internalizing strong social identities. These ideas are, of course, at the heart of *social identity theory* (Tajfel & Turner, 1986), which, to its credit, has long recognized the importance of motivation in the era when pure social cognitive analyses were dominant. Social identity theory posits that individuals strive to maintain positive social identities as a means for preserving self-esteem. Positive social identities are derived and maintained through comparison with other groups. To the degree that comparisons favor the ingroup, positive social identities also serve to bolster feelings of individual worth. If, however, intergroup comparisons do not favor the ingroup, various strategies allow maintenance of positive self-regard—including modifying the attribute under consideration, emphasizing dimensions known to favor the ingroup, or seeking to devalue the dimension of comparison. People may also utilize cognitive social mobility, emphasizing certain social identities over others when doing so allows positive ingroup comparisons. Thus social identity theory provides a basis for predicting and understanding ingroup bias, and there is ample research evidence that group memberships, even in relatively meaningless groups, affect intergroup perception and behavior in meaningful ways.

### *Motivated Justification of Inequality*

Two recent theoretical accounts suggest that motivational factors can produce support for social systems that preserve prejudice and discrimination. *Social dominance theory* and *system justification theory* (see Jost & Sidanius, 2004) share the assumption that motivated beliefs about the legitimacy of power relations between groups can serve to justify bias, rationalize prejudice, and ensure superiority over members of oppressed groups. They differ, however, in the specific motivations they invoke to explain these phenomena. Social dominance theory (Sidanius & Pratto, 1999) is rooted in the specific motivation to maintain superiority over groups that activate competitiveness (Duckitt, 2006). Negative attitudes toward competitive groups are justified by invoking various "myths" that explain and legitimize the dominance and privilege of the ingroup. These myths include the belief that dominant groups are necessary for leading and caring for subordinate groups, that both dominant and subordinate groups benefit from status differences, and that status hierarchies reflect divine will. Since dominant groups benefit from preservation of social hierarchies, it should not be surprising that measures of social dominance orientation as an individual difference variable are higher among high-status groups. This orientation has been tied to negative evaluations of women by men, blacks by whites, and working-class by upper-class individuals, and to a general willingness to derogate, punish, or humiliate members of low-status outgroups.

Jost and colleagues' work on system justification theory (Jost & Banaji, 1994; Jost, Banaji, & Nosek, 2004) also suggests that individuals vary in the degree they are motivated to explain systems that preserve inequality between groups. In contrast to social dominance theory, however, system justification theory suggests that rationalizing existing status hierarchies can also meet the motivation to see order in the world and to assume that social systems are fair and just. To preserve a sense of justice and fairness, individuals are motivated to perceive existing differences in social status and power as legitimate, rational, and perhaps inevitable. One critical difference from social dominance theory is that system justification is often exhibited most dramatically by individuals whose group memberships convey low social status. Consequently, a system justification account is able to explain why disadvantaged individuals and groups often justify their lower social status and embrace negative stereotypes of their group. In such cases, the motivation to render the world understandable and predictable can produce endorsement of bias even against the ingroup.

Research on motivational factors that "make things worse" has shifted from a focus on dysfunction within individuals to issues of more widespread motivational concern. A primary motive behind stereotyping and prejudice is the need to see oneself in positive terms, but other motives include a need to preserve privilege and to see order and justice in the world. All these factors tend to produce bias indirectly as consequences of the pursuit of fundamental goals.

## HOW MOTIVATION MAKES THINGS BETTER

So far we have reviewed research that highlights negative roles for motivation in stereotyping and prejudice. Knowledge of the means by which motivation increases bias is, of course, useful in considering interventions for improving intergroup harmony, but more recent research has sought to recognize ways by which motivational factors play a direct and explicit role in improving intergroup relations. In this section we explore the motivations that appear to "make things better" by reducing bias.

In doing so, we distinguish between motives that are explicitly focused on stereotype reduction and motivations that indirectly reduce bias as a side effect of the pursuit of other goals.

Some motives have the effect of reducing reliance on stereotypes, even though that is not the explicit goal, just as we have earlier reviewed that a number of motives can indirectly increase bias. However, there are times that individuals do embrace the explicit goal to be nonprejudiced.

### Motivation to Control Prejudice

We begin by considering several motivations that lead individuals to attempt to control prejudice as an end in itself. The specific motivational theories involved vary in their emphasis: Some highlight differences between external and internal motivations to respond without prejudice (Plant & Devine, 1998); some explore the interplay of controlled attitudes and automatic evaluations (Fazio & Dunton, 1997); some focus on the motivating impact of discrepancies between what one believes one *should* do and what one *would* do (Monteith, 1993); and others emphasize motivations to *avoid* prejudice (Plant & Devine, 1998) versus motivations to *approach* egalitarianism (Moskowitz, Gollwitzer, Wasel, & Schaal, 1999). Despite these differences, these approaches all attempt to explicate the relation between attempts to limit bias and subsequent judgments of and behavior toward groups and their members.

Explicit attempts to avoid bias can fail for several reasons, and one critical factor involves the specific basis of the motivation to be nonprejudiced. Though some attempts to avoid bias are driven by internalized standards of conduct, others reflect a concern with external factors, such as being judged as nonprejudiced by others (Plant & Devine, 1998). Whereas external motivations may inhibit prejudiced responding in public contexts (due to concerns about potential negative reactions from others), internal motivations to avoid prejudice affect behavior in both public and private contexts. Internal motivations to be nonprejudiced also result in different regulatory responses when violated; discrepancies from internalized standards to be nonprejudiced produce negative self-directed affect that motivates subsequent reductions in prejudiced responses (Monteith, 1993; Monteith, Ashburn-Nardo, Voils, & Czopp, 2002).

Plant and Devine (1998) proposed that internal and external motivations to avoid prejudice are independent, and indeed, for individuals who have high internal motivations to avoid prejudice, external motivations to avoid prejudice often make no difference in responding (see also Klonis, Plant, & Devine, 2005). Although the motivations are independent, other studies have shown that individuals who are high in internal motivation and low in external motivation are most effective at regulating prejudice (e.g., Devine, Plant, Amodio, Harmon-Jones, & Vance, 2002). If "high internal, low external" represents a more internalized standard than "high internal, high external," it implies the possibility of conceiving a continuum of motives to avoid prejudice. Recently Legault, Green-Demer, Grant, and Chung (2007) have done just that, building on Deci and Ryan's (1985) self-determination theory. Making finer distinctions along a single continuum, they have decomposed internal motivations into *intrinsic*, *integrated*, and *identified* motivations. All of these motivations predicted lower levels of explicit and implicit prejudice. In contrast, more externalized motivations (introjected and external) to avoid prejudice were unrelated to prejudice expressed on both explicit and implicit measures. This work suggests the value of exploring differing specific motivations and the need to more fully understand the relationships between them.

While much work has shown that internal motivations to avoid being prejudiced affect conscious behaviors and self-reported attitudes, they also appear to interact with and influence automatic processes. Moskowitz and colleagues (1999), for example, found that chronic goals related to egalitarianism toward women can inhibit the automatic activation of the female stereotype. Similarly, individuals with a chronic goal to be egalitarian toward blacks showed no facilitation of stereotype-relevant words after a category prime (i.e., exposure to a black face), but instead showed facilitation for words related to egalitarianism (Moskowitz, Salomon, & Taylor, 2000). Chronically egalitarian individuals were faster to respond to egalitarian words after a category cue (a black face) but not in general, demonstrating that an individual's chronic egalitarian or nonprejudiced goals can change the dominant response that is linked to a particular group or category. Although much of this work has examined chronic motivations to avoid being prejudiced (or to be egalitarian), Lowery, Hardin, and Sinclair (2001) also found that an explicit instruction to try not to be prejudiced can reduce implicit race bias toward blacks for both Asian and white participants.

In addition, the relation between self-reported and automatic evaluations of outgroups depends on an individual's motivation to avoid prejudice. When individuals were not motivated to control prejudice toward blacks, automatic prejudice predicted more negative self-reported evaluations. However, when individuals were motivated to control prejudice, automatic prejudice actually predicted more favorable evaluations of a black student (e.g., Fazio & Dunton, 1997; Towles-Schwen & Fazio, 2003). Dasgupta and Rivera (2006) further found that controlled attitudes (conscious motivation to be egalitarian) influenced even subtle nonverbal and paralinguistic behaviors in actual interactions with gay men. For participants who had low motivation to be egalitarian and who reported low ability to control behavior, automatic prejudice produced biased behavior. However, for individuals who were high in conscious motivation to be egalitarian, there were no differences in positive nonverbal and paralinguistic behavior toward gay men based on automatic attitudes or self-reported ability to control behavior.

## Reduced Bias through Accuracy and Affiliative Motives

Thus far we have reviewed motivational factors that often reduce bias as an end in itself. We now focus on classes of motivational factors that have been linked to reduced stereotyping and prejudice by indirect means—motivations to be accurate (in the service of epistemic concerns or to increase understanding and control) and motivations to form connections and affiliations with others.

### *Motivation for Accuracy*

Accuracy motivation is generally associated with a decreased reliance on stereotypes and increased reliance on individuating information. The motive for accuracy can result from several specific chronic or temporary concerns, including the desire to increase understanding, prediction, and control, and the desire to avoid social costs associated with making mistakes. Chronic goal states, such as need for cognition or fear of invalidity, have been shown to increase accuracy concerns (Cacioppo & Petty, 1982; Freund, Kruglanski, & Shpitzajzen, 1985); accuracy motivation can also arise from situationally activated goal states, such as the need to justify impressions or evaluations to others (e.g., Tetlock, 1992). Moreover, accuracy motivation tends to be high in contexts where one's outcomes are dependent on another. Outcome dependency has been shown to result in processing styles similar to that produced by an explicit accuracy goal, increasing attention to individuating versus categorical information (Neuberg & Fiske, 1987) and to stereotype-inconsistent versus -consistent information (Bogart, Ryan, & Stefanov, 1999; Erber & Fiske, 1984).

However, the structure of the interdependent situation has an impact on accuracy motivation. Within interdependent situations, outcome dependency can be symmetrical or asymmetrical. If one's outcomes are dependent on another, but the reciprocal is not also true, one is in a relatively powerless position. This context can create an even greater motivation for accuracy in the service of prediction and control, and evidence suggests that individuals in relatively powerless roles will form more individuated impressions (Bogart et al., 1999; Depret & Fiske, 1999). Moreover, some interdependent situations are competitive rather than cooperative in nature. Ruscher and Fiske (1990) showed that competitive interdependent situations can also increase attention to inconsistent information and lead to more individualized impressions of opponents. However, when one is faced with the task of sizing up *both* teammates and competitors, there is some evidence that perceivers will allocate more attention to individuating teammates than adversaries (Ruscher, Fiske, Miki, & van Manen, 1991).

The motivation to be accurate has been primarily evaluated via explicit measures of stereotyping, such as attention to and reliance on individuating information. Richeson and Ambady (2001), however, provide evidence that accuracy motivation may also influence measures of *automatic* racial prejudice. In one study, white participants anticipated interacting with a black individual. However, some participants believed they would be interacting in the role of a superior, whereas others believed they would be interacting in a peer or subordinate role. Consistent with earlier findings that employed explicit measures, participants who anticipated being in a subordinate (i.e., relatively powerless) role exhibited the least prejudice on an implicit measure of racial prejudice. In this context, as in the others we've reviewed, it is indeed likely that the motive for predictive accuracy contributed to reducing bias. However, it is probable that affiliative motives, in the service of ingratiation with another who wields power, may also have been operating to reduce bias.

### Motivation for Affiliation

Indeed, the motives to affiliate, to belong to social groups, and to get along with others have been implicated in stereotyping processes. The motivation to have positive and meaningful social interactions with others is posited to be a central human motivation (e.g., Baumeister & Leary, 1995; Fiske, 2003). Desire for connection with others has several potential implications: Individuals may be influenced by social norms regarding attitudes toward stereotypes and prejudice, as well as by relationship concerns with an individual member of a stereotyped outgroup. We return to the issue of social norms in the final section and explore here how the motive to affiliate might lead to decreased stereotyping through relational concerns.

The motive to affiliate can be viewed through the tenets of *shared reality theory* (Hardin & Higgins, 1996). Shared reality theory proposes that social connections are made possible to the extent that social beliefs are shared. Thus a person who is motivated to have a social bond or relationship with another should be motivated to increase shared reality with that individual by, for example, developing shared social beliefs. A motivation to develop shared reality could result either from a strong internal desire to affiliate ("She seems like a wonderful, kind person") or from external situational demands that require social interaction and coordination ("We have to finish this chapter by the deadline").

Lowery and colleagues (2001) tested one implication of shared reality theory in a study of automatic social tuning. If individuals are motivated to shift beliefs and attitudes in line with social contexts to develop relationships, they should shift their attitudes to converge with those of their interaction partners. If the interaction partners are outgroup members, participants should exhibit less prejudice, because they have shifted beliefs and attitudes toward those of the outgroup (whose members are assumed to have less negative attitudes toward their group). Across four studies, Lowery et al. found that participants (white Americans) showed reduced prejudice on an implicit measure in the presence of a black versus a white experimenter.

Sinclair, Lowery, Hardin, and Colangelo (2005) extended this work by separating the social category membership of the interaction partner from his or her ostensible attitudes. If it is a "social tuning" shift in perceiver attitudes that leads to reduced prejudice, presumed attitudes should have a greater impact on bias than social category memberships should. To test this idea, black or white experimenters wore plain or anti-racism t-shirts. When the experimenter was wearing an "anti-racism" t-shirt, participants exhibited reduced stereotype activation regardless of the experimenter's race, though, as would be predicted by shared reality theory, this effect was mediated by liking for the experimenter. A second study in which experimental likeability was directly manipulated again produced the pattern of results that would be predicted by the social tuning hypothesis. When the experimenter was likeable, automatic anti-black prejudice was lower when the experimenter was wearing the anti-racism t-shirt rather than a blank t-shirt. However, when the experimenter was rude (and thus there was no motivation to affiliate), the attitudes of the experimenter did not have an impact on prejudice. These studies provide clear evidence that the motivation to affiliate with another individual can increase the motivation to share beliefs, affecting even measures of automatic attitudes. These studies also extend the work that has been done in interdependent contexts to highlight important moderators of the motivation for belonging. When individuals are unlikeable or when situational demands do not require social coordination, the need for belonging and affiliation may not lead to reduced bias.

As we have reviewed in this section, motives can reduce prejudice both directly (by attempts to avoid bias) and indirectly (by attempts to be accurate and to affiliate). These latter motives are particularly likely to arise in interdependent contexts (Fiske, 2004; Fiske, Lin, & Neuberg, 1999; Fiske & Neuberg, 1990). Under conditions of interdependence, the motivation to avoid bias to increase understanding, prediction, and control becomes paramount (Neuberg & Fiske, 1987). It is also in interdependent situations that the motivation to affiliate and to belong becomes relevant in order to initiate and maintain relationships. Thus it is likely that in many interdependent contexts, motivations for belonging and control contribute jointly to reducing stereotyping. It is important to note, however, that while historically these motivations have been seen to "make things better" in terms of decreased reliance on stereotyping, we are not suggesting that these intentions always produce positive outcomes. Individuals may not have the resources to individuate, even if they are motivated to do so (Biesanz, Neuberg, Smith, Asher, & Judice, 2001; Pendry & Macrae, 1994), or they may rely on individuating information that is itself unreliable.

### The Role of Means in Stereotype Avoidance

No consideration of motivational factors in stereotyping and prejudice would be complete without recognizing the importance of means or strategies for motive fulfillment. Although individuals are often motivated to avoid stereotype use, either directly or because they are pursuing other goals, recent research has shown that different means used to avoid stereotyping produce varying levels of success. In fact, use of improper means can produce the opposite of the effects that were intended, increasing rather than decreasing stereotype activation and use. In particular, given a goal to avoid an undesired end-state (rather than to approach a desired end-state), the means that are utilized can backfire and produce greater stereotyping in some circumstances. Evidence consistent with this contention is provided by studies examining the consequences of thought suppression. In numerous studies (e.g., Macrae, Bodenhausen, Milne, & Jetten, 1994), individuals who are explicitly instructed to try *not* to use stereotypes can produce short-term success, so long as these individuals have both sufficient cognitive capacity and motivation to engage in effortful thought suppression. Unfortunately, attempts to suppress stereotypes tend to increase the accessibility of stereotype-related thoughts, and a lag in ability or effort can allow greater stereotyping than if thought suppression attempts had never been instigated.

Greater success is likely if goals are framed in terms of approaching desired end-states rather than avoiding undesired end-states. When the goal is to become egalitarian, fair, and accurate (rather than *not* prejudiced, unfair, or inaccurate), the means utilized to reach these goals tend to reduce bias without increasing stereotype accessibility. One means that successfully reduces bias is perspective taking. In a series of experiments (see Galinsky, Ku, & Wang, 2005, for a review), manipulations intended to encourage individuals to imagine the point of view of a stereotyped group member produced lower stereotype activation and application, compared with control conditions and conditions in which experimental participants were given stereotype suppression instructions. Imagining life through the eyes of a stereotyped group member seems to increase the overlap in cognitive representations of the self and other, decreasing bias toward outgroups. Unfortunately, the self–other overlap that arises through perspective taking can increase application of the stereotype to the self, suggesting that even this means for stereotype reduction can produce some effects oppositional to an individual's motives.

## SOMETIMES BETTER, SOMETIMES WORSE: THE COMPLEXITY OF MOTIVES IN CONTEXT

We have organized this chapter in terms of motives that have historically been considered to make things worse by increasing stereotyping and prejudice, and motives that have been believed to make things better by decreasing stereotyping and prejudicial responses. During the last decade or so, as researchers became interested anew in issues of motivation with regard to stereotyping and prejudice, the approach has often reflected the framework we have used here: Single motives were typically linked to single outcomes, one at a time. Initial explorations of the role of motivation in stereotyping and prejudice benefited from such an approach, allowing clear explorations of particular motives. Furthermore, it provides a clear, compelling appealing story: Some motives improve and other motives undermine positive intergroup perception and relations, and the goal is to determine which motivation dominates in any interaction. However, we suspect that the story is more complicated. A deeper understanding of the role of motivation in stereotyping and prejudice requires both an exploration of the complexity of even seemingly simple single motives, and a consideration of the existence and interplay of multiple motives.

The need for increased complexity in considering the motivation–bias relationship is illustrated by the fact that the question "What will Motive *X* do?" cannot be addressed successfully without understanding the contextual factors in which the motive is operating—including both external constraints, affordances, and pressures, and internal constraints such as competition from other motives and limited cognitive resources. In this section we highlight two contextual factors that illuminate the complexity of the motivation–bias relationship. First, we present evidence that the impact of a motive on bias will be influenced in part by the other means a situation affords for the motive's fulfillment. Many of the motivational factors we have discussed in this chapter can be served by means both related and unrelated to stereotyping and prejudice. Second, we review how the same motive may produce increased bias in one case and reduced bias in another, depending on the nature of the situation and the content of the stereotypes. In the final section of the chapter, we highlight the need to consider *multiple* motives and goals in accounting for the impact of motivation on bias. Although few studies have explicitly addressed the interaction of multiple motives, it is probably rare that any given situation invokes only a single motivation.

## Opportunities for Motive Fulfillment

We first explore how the impact of any specific motivation on biased responding will be influenced by the opportunities afforded by a situation for motive fulfillment. For instance, the motive to maintain self-esteem can clearly be satisfied in ways other than activating stereotypes or acting in a prejudiced manner. If the motive has been served via different means, it may be less likely to manifest itself in terms of increased bias. Some evidence for this can be found in situations where individuals have had a prior opportunity to self-affirm. Such an opportunity at least temporarily bolsters the sense of self and reduces the need to defend the self by derogating others. Individuals who have recently been self-affirmed by receiving positive feedback, by affirming an important value (Fein & Spencer, 1997), or by receiving reminders of secure attachments to close others (Mikulincer & Shaver, 2001) are less likely to evaluate members of outgroups negatively. Because the motivation has been served through other means, its pursuit is curtailed, and bias is avoided.

Depending on the nature of the motivation, however, prior motive fulfillment may sometimes *increase* stereotyping and prejudice. For example, prior fulfillment of the motive to avoid prejudice may free individuals to engage in behaviors that might otherwise be avoided, for fear of being labeled (by themselves or others) as prejudiced. Monin and Miller (2001) argue, for example, that when individuals have acted in a nonprejudiced manner, they may consequently be more likely to endorse stereotypes because they have established a prior "moral credential." Participants who first selected a female candidate for a job opening were more likely to endorse gender stereotypes in a second hiring decision. Furthermore, individuals did this regardless of chronic internal and external motivations to avoid prejudice (Plant & Devine, 1998), and even when the audience for the second decision (a new experimenter) did not know about their established "credential." This suggests that prior fulfillment of the motive may be as much about proving to oneself that one is nonprejudiced as it is about establishing this for others. Even if individuals have not established a prior "moral credential," they may be more likely to apply stereotypes in ambiguous contexts where other motives could be ascribed (e.g., Gaertner & Dovidio, 1986). Thus simply the possibility of assigning a biased action to a more socially or personally acceptable motive may influence the likelihood of biased responding.

## Same Motive, Different Consequences

Even if we suppose that there are some situations in which the only means available to fulfill a given motive involves stereotyping and prejudice processes, we still cannot predict whether a particular motivation will increase or decrease stereotyping and prejudice without knowing the context in which it is unfolding. For instance, while an accuracy motive often results in decreased stereotyping, sometimes the motive to be accurate leads to increased stereotyping, especially if no other relevant information is available (Kunda, Davies, Adams, & Spencer, 2002; Kunda, Davies, Hoshino-Browne, & Jordan, 2003; Pendry & Macrae, 1994). In these situations, stereotypes may actually be seen as useful categories that can facilitate the motive to comprehend, rather than interfere with it.

Similarly, the motive for positive self-regard may lead to either increased or decreased bias, depending on the particular context. When an individual's self-image is threatened, the motivation to restore a positive sense of self may result in increased stereotyping and prejudice—either because the derogation of others boosts one's self-worth (Fein & Spencer, 1997), or as a way to disparage someone who has provided negative or critical feedback (Sinclair & Kunda, 1999, 2000). However, the motivation to restore a positive sense of self may also decrease stereotyping and prejudice, depending on the nature of the self-image threat, the content of the stereotypes, and whether the target has provided praise or positive feedback.

Spencer, Fein, Strahan, and Zanna (2005) describe a study exploring how different types of self-image threats may either increase or decrease stereotyping. All participants received negative feedback regarding a questionnaire they had completed, but the nature of the feedback differed. In the group that comes closest to replicating the standard self-image threat manipulation, participants were told that they scored high on a "neuroticism" scale and low on a "cognitive complexity" scale. In a different group, participants were told that they scored high on a "contemporary racism" scale and low on a "racial tolerance" scale. Thus, whereas participants in the first group received information that presumably threatened their sense of themselves as intelligent and emotionally stable, participants in the second group received information that threatened their sense of themselves as egalitarian and nonprejudiced. Participants were then primed with black or white faces and completed word stems under cognitive load. Participants who received the "classic" self-image threat showed the typical pattern of results: They exhibited greater stereotype activation under self-image threat. However, when participants were given the racist feedback, they showed inhibition of the stereotype relative to a control group (which had received nonthreatening negative feedback). Both groups received negative self-feedback, and both groups therefore were motivated to restore a positive sense of self. However, stereotyping as a strategy to restore a positive sense of self was ineffective in the racist feedback group. To affirm a positive sense of self, these individuals inhibited stereotype activation.

The content of stereotypes themselves often plays a determining role in whether their activation or inhibition (and/or subsequent application) will serve an underlying motivation (see also Kunda & Spencer, 2003). We can all be categorized as members of multiple groups, and an individual can flexibly and selectively use these multiple identities to protect and enhance the self. In a series of studies, Sinclair and Kunda (1999) showed that participants selectively activated and inhibited negative stereotypes when given negative and positive feedback, respectively, from a black individual (Study 3). In this study, participants received negative or positive feedback from a black doctor. When participants were given positive feedback, they showed increased activation of the positive stereotype, *doctor*, and inhibition of the negative stereotype, *black*. The pattern was reversed for participants who received negative feedback. Thus the impact of the motivation to maintain a positive self-image on stereotyping depends in part on the content of the stereotype (see also Sinclair & Kunda, 2000).

Further evidence of either increased or decreased bias resulting from a single motive is provided by research examining the varied consequences of the affiliative motive in differing contexts. Although we have earlier reviewed research suggesting that the motivate to affiliate with a member of a stereotyped group will often lead to reduced bias, the impact of the motivation to belong more generally depends in large part on the prevailing (and salient) social norms (Crandall, Eshleman, & O'Brien, 2002). If social norms oppose prejudice, then individuals may be less likely to engage in stereotypical or prejudicial responses. If, however, social norms support prejudice, individuals may be more likely to exhibit bias. Sechrist and Stangor (2001) manipulated whether participants believed that there was low or high consensus with their beliefs toward blacks. When highly prejudiced individuals believed that there was low consensus with their beliefs, they sat closer to a black target than when they believed that there was high consensus with their beliefs. Spencer and colleagues (2005) also report evidence that salient social norms influence stereotype activation and application. Participants first watched a video of a panel discussion on gay rights in which the community audience reaction was manipulated to suggest that the audience either favored or opposed gay rights. All participants then received negative feedback on an intelligence test and completed word stems under cognitive load before evaluating a gay or straight target. When the local norms supported gay rights, evaluation of the target were more positive than when local norms opposed gay rights. Interestingly, the relationship between activation and evaluation was also affected by the local norm. When the target was gay, greater activation of the stereotype in the anti-gay-rights condition led to more negative evaluations. In contrast, greater activation of the stereotype in the pro-gay-rights condition led to less negative evaluations of the gay target. It is important to note that in both conditions, participants were presumably motivated to move their own attitudes in alignment with the local norm. However, the nature of the social norm directed the consequences for stereotyping and prejudice.

## CLOSING REMARKS

We hope it is clear from our brief review of the literature that the critical and essential role of motivation in understanding the dynamics of stereotyping and prejudice has been restored over the last decade of research. However, the renewed focus on motivation has emphasized the importance of cognitive factors, exemplifying the synergistic nature of motivation and cognition (Kruglanski et al., 2002). No longer is it a question of motivation *versus* cognition. Both cognitive and motivational factors play integral roles in the formation, maintenance, and regulation of bias, and we suspect that the interplay between motivation and cognition will be a fruitful area of research in the coming years.

We also believe that the interplay among multiple motives, multiple means, and multiple contextual factors will emerge as a critical issue in the further study of motivation and bias. Without a consideration of the complex interrelations linking motives, means, and contexts, it will be nearly impossible to predict the consequence of any given motivational state. For instance, we know that when individuals experience a self-threatening failure, they are more likely to exhibit a biased response, even if they are high in the need to avoid prejudice. However, what may happen if the context affords more than one avenue with which to restore positive self-regard? Such a situation allows exploration of numerous issues. What factors may increase the relative accessibility and dominance of one motive over another? If the motive to restore a positive sense of self dominates, how may the preferred means differ for individuals high and low in the need to avoid prejudice? It seems probable that an individual who is motivated to avoid prejudice will be more likely to choose an alternative means to self-restoration than an individual who is low in the need to avoid prejudice, as such a means will serve both the goal of restoring self-esteem and the goal of avoiding prejudice (the principle of *multifinality*; Kruglanski et al., 2002). Additionally, many situations, like this one, activate numerous (and possibly competing) motivations; when the needs are met for one, resources are freed to address and meet other needs, suggesting that the motivations may wax and wane even within a single context. Thus even a relatively simple example like the one we present here illuminates many significant issues to be explored in understanding the dynamics of motivation in judgment and bias.

While a simple example may illuminate many issues, a simple story cannot adequately capture the role of motivational factors in stereotyping and prejudice. Motivational factors do not always make things worse (as the early research in this field tended to suggest); motivational factors should not be ignored (as the decades of focus on cognitive factors might suggest); and motivational factors do not have unitary consequences. More complex stories, however, often have more interesting plots. We look forward to the unfolding of these intriguing plots in the coming years.

## ACKNOWLEDGMENTS

This chapter was supported by a grant from the Third Millennium Foundation to Steven J. Stroessner, and by a Graduate Research Fellowship from the National Science Foundation to Abigail A. Scholer. We thank Lara Kammrath for her thoughtful comments on an earlier draft of this chapter, and Cara Kantrowitz for her assistance in its preparation.

## NOTE

1. There are important distinctions to be made between stereotyping (generally viewed as the cognitive component of intergroup attitudes) and prejudice (the affective or evaluative component), and the relation between the two can be complex (e.g., Sherman, Stroessner, Conrey, & Azam, 2005). For the purposes of this chapter, however, they are treated in a unitary fashion, and no distinction is made between motivational

factors that have been shown to affect exclusively one or the other.

## REFERENCES


Adorno, T. W., Frenkel-Brunswik, E., Levinson, D. J., & Sanford, R. N. (1950). *The authoritarian personality.* New York: Harper.

Allport, G. W. (1954). *The nature of prejudice.* Cambridge, MA: Addison-Wesley.

Altemeyer, B. (1981). *Right-wing authoritarianism.* Winnipeg: University of Manitoba Press.

Altemeyer, B. (1998). The other "authoritarian personality." In M. P. Zanna (Ed.), *Advances in experimental social psychology* (Vol. 30, pp. 47–92). San Diego, CA: Academic Press.

Baumeister, R. F., & Leary, M. R. (1995). The need to belong: Desire for interpersonal attachments as a fundamental human motivation. *Psychological Bulletin, 117,* 497–529.

Biesanz, J. C., Neuberg, S. L., Smith, D. M., Asher, T., & Judice, T. N. (2001). When accuracy-motivated perceivers fail: Limited attentional resources and the reemerging self-fulfilling prophecy. *Personality and Social Psychology Bulletin, 27,* 621–629.

Bogart, L. M., Ryan, C. S., & Stefanov, M. (1999). Effects of stereotypes and outcome dependency on the processing of information about group members. *Group Processes and Intergroup Relations, 2,* 31–50.

Cacioppo, J. T., & Petty, R. E. (1982). The need for cognition. *Journal of Personality and Social Psychology, 42,* 116–131.

Crandall, C. S., Eshleman, A., & O'Brien, L. (2002). Social norms and the expression and suppression of prejudice: The struggle for internalization. *Journal of Personality and Social Psychology, 82,* 359–378.

Dasgupta, N., & Rivera, L. M. (2006). From automatic antigay prejudice to behavior: The moderating role of conscious beliefs about gender and behavioral control. *Journal of Personality and Social Psychology, 91,* 268–280.

Deci, E. L., & Ryan, R. M. (1985). *Intrinsic motivation and self-determination in human behavior.* New York: Plenum Press.

Depret, E., & Fiske, S. T. (1999). Perceiving the powerful: Intriguing individuals versus threatening groups. *Journal of Experimental Social Psychology, 35,* 461–480.

Devine, P. G. (1989). Stereotypes and prejudice: Their automatic and controlled components. *Journal of Personality and Social Psychology, 56,* 5–18.

Devine, P. G., Plant, E. A., Amodio, D. M., Harmon-Jones, E., & Vance, S. L. (2002). The regulation of explicit and implicit race bias: The role of motivations to respond without prejudice. *Journal of Personality and Social Psychology, 82,* 835–848.

Dollard, J., Doob, L. W., Miller, N. E., Mowrer, O. H., & Sears, R. R. (1939). *Frustration and aggression.* New Haven, CT: Yale University Press.

Duckitt, J. (2005). Personality and prejudice. In J. F. Dovidio, P. Glick, & L. A. Rudman (Eds.), *On the nature of prejudice: Fifty years after Allport* (pp. 395–412). Malden, MA: Blackwell.

Duckitt, J. (2006). Differential effects of right wing authoritarianism and social dominance orientation on outgroup attitudes and their mediation by threat from and competitiveness to outgroups. *Personality and Social Psychology Bulletin, 32,* 684–696.

Erber, R., & Fiske, S. T. (1984). Outcome dependency and attention to inconsistent information. *Journal of Personality and Social Psychology, 47,* 709–726.

Fazio, R. H., & Dunton, B. C. (1997). Categorization by race: The impact of automatic and controlled components of racial prejudice. *Journal of Experimental Social Psychology, 33,* 451–470.

Fein, S., & Spencer, S. J. (1997). Prejudice as self-image maintenance: Affirming the self through derogating others. *Journal of Personality and Social Psychology, 73,* 31–44.

Fiske, S. T. (2003). Five core social motives, plus or minus five. In S. J. Spencer, S. Fein, M. P. Zanna, & J. M. Olson (Eds.), *The Ontario Symposium: Vol. 9. Motivated social perception* (pp. 233–246). Mahwah, NJ: Erlbaum.

Fiske, S. T. (2004). Intent and ordinary bias: Unintended thought and social motivation create casual prejudice. *Social Justice Research, 17,* 117–127.

Fiske, S. T., Lin, M., & Neuberg, S. L. (1999). The continuum model: Ten years later. In S. Chaiken & Y. Trope (Eds.), *Dual-process theories in social psychology* (pp. 231–245). New York: Guilford Press.

Fiske, S. T., & Neuberg, S. L. (1990). A continuum of impression formation, from category-based to individuating processes: Influences of information and motivation on attention and interpretation. In M. P. Zanna (Ed.), *Advances in experimental social psychology* (Vol. 23, pp. 1–74). San Diego, CA: Academic Press.

Fiske, S. T., & Taylor, S. E. (1984). *Social cognition.* Reading, MA: Addison-Wesley.

Fiske, S. T., & Taylor, S. E. (1991). *Social cognition* (2nd ed.). New York: McGraw-Hill.

Freund, T., Kruglanski, A. W., & Shpitzajzen, A. (1985). The freezing and unfreezing of impression primacy: Effects of the need for structure and the fear of invalidity. *Personality and Social Psychology Bulletin, 11,* 479–487.

Gaertner, S. L., & Dovidio, J. F. (1986). The aversive form of racism. In J. F. Dovidio & S. L. Gaertner (Eds.), *Prejudice, discrimination, and racism* (pp. 61–89). Orlando, FL: Academic Press.

Galinsky, A. D., Ku, G., & Wang, C. S. (2005). Perspective-taking and self–other overlap: Fostering social bonds and facilitating social coordination. *Group Processes and Intergroup Relations, 8,* 109–124.

Glick, P. (2005). Choice of scapegoats. In J. F. Dovidio, P. Glick, & L. A. Rudman (Eds.), *On the nature of prejudice: Fifty years after Allport* (pp. 244–261). Malden, MA: Blackwell.

Govorun, O., Fuegen, K., & Payne, B. K. (2006). Stereotypes focus defensive projection. *Personality and Social Psychology Bulletin, 32*, 781–793.

Green, D. P., Glaser, J., & Rich, A. (1998). From lynching to gay bashing: The elusive connection between economic conditions and hate crime. *Journal of Personality and Social Psychology, 75*, 82–92.

Hamilton, D. L., Stroessner, S. J., & Driscoll, D. M. (1994). Social cognition and the study of stereotyping. In P. G. Devine, D. L. Hamilton, & T. M. Ostrom (Eds.), *Social cognition: Impact on social psychology* (pp. 291–321). San Diego, CA: Academic Press.

Hardin, C. D., & Higgins, E. T. (1996). Shared reality: How social verification makes the subjective objective. In R. Sorrentino & E. T. Higgins (Eds.), *Handbook of motivation and cognition: Vol. 3. The interpersonal context* (pp. 28–84). New York: Guilford Press.

Jost, J. T., & Banaji, M. R. (1994). The role of stereotyping in system-justification and the production of false consciousness. *British Journal of Social Psychology, 33*, 1–27.

Jost, J. T., Banaji, M. R., & Nosek, B. A. (2004). A decade of system justification theory: Accumulated evidence of conscious and unconscious bolstering of the status quo. *Political Psychology, 25*, 881–919.

Jost, J. T., & Sidanius, J. (Eds.). (2004). *Political psychology: Key readings*. New York: Psychology Press.

Klonis, S. C., Plant, E. A., & Devine, P. G. (2005). Internal and external motivation to respond without sexism. *Personality and Social Psychology Bulletin, 31*, 1237–1249.

Kruglanski, A. W., Shah, J. Y., Fishbach, A., Friedman, R., Chun, W. Y., & Sleeth-Keppler, D. (2002). A theory of goal systems. In M. P. Zanna (Ed.), *Advances in experimental social psychology* (Vol. 34, pp. 331–378). San Diego, CA: Academic Press.

Kunda, Z., Davies, P. G., Adams, B. D., & Spencer, S. J. (2002). The dynamic time course of stereotype activation: Activation, dissipation, and resurrection. *Journal of Personality and Social Psychology, 82*, 283–299.

Kunda, Z., Davies, P. G., Hoshino-Browne, E., & Jordan, C. (2003). The impact of comprehension goals on the ebb and flow of stereotype activation during interaction. In S. J. Spencer, S. Fein, M. P. Zanna, & J. M. Olson (Eds.), *The Ontario Symposium: Vol. 9. Motivated social perception* (pp. 1–20). Mahwah, NJ: Erlbaum.

Kunda, Z., & Spencer, S. J. (2003). When do stereotypes come to mind and when do they color judgment?: A goal-based theoretical framework for stereotype activation and application. *Psychological Bulletin, 129*, 522–544.

Legault, L., Green-Demers, I., Grant, P., & Chung, C. (2007). On the self-regulation of implicit and explicit prejudice: A self-determination theory perspective. *Personality and Social Psychology Bulletin, 33*, 732–749.

Lowery, B. S., Hardin, C. D., & Sinclair, S. (2001). Social influence effects on automatic racial prejudice. *Journal of Personality and Social Psychology, 81*, 842–855.

Macrae, C. N., Bodenhausen, G. V., Milne, A. B., & Jetten, J. (1994). Out of mind but back in sight: Stereotypes on the rebound. *Journal of Personality and Social Psychology, 67*, 808–817.

Mikulincer, M., & Shaver, P. R. (2001). Attachment theory and intergroup bias: Evidence that priming the secure base schema attenuates negative reactions to out-groups. *Journal of Personality and Social Psychology, 81*, 97–115.

Monin, B., & Miller, D. T. (2001). Moral credentials and the expression of prejudice. *Journal of Personality and Social Psychology, 81*, 5–16.

Monteith, M. J. (1993). Self-regulation of prejudiced responses: Implications for progress in prejudice-reduction effort. *Journal of Personality and Social Psychology, 65*, 469–485.

Monteith, M. J., Ashburn-Nardo, L., Voils, C. I., & Czopp, A. M. (2002). Putting the brakes on prejudice: On the development and operation of cues for control. *Journal of Personality and Social Psychology, 83*, 1029–1050.

Moskowitz, G. B., Gollwitzer, P. M., Wasel, W., & Schaal, B. (1999). Preconscious control of stereotype activation through chronic egalitarian goals. *Journal of Personality and Social Psychology, 77*, 167–184.

Moskowitz, G. B., Salomon, A. R., & Taylor, C. M. (2000). Preconsciously controlling stereotyping: Implicitly activated egalitarian goals prevent the activation of stereotypes. *Social Cognition, 18*, 151–177.

Neuberg, S. L., & Fiske, S. T. (1987). Motivational influences on impression formation: Outcome dependency, accuracy-driven attention, and individuating processes. *Journal of Personality and Social Psychology, 53*, 431–444.

Newman, L. S., Duff, K. J., & Baumeister, R. F. (1997). A new look at defensive projection: Thought suppression, accessibility, and biased person perception. *Journal of Personality and Social Psychology, 72*, 980–1001.

Pendry, L. F., & Macrae, C. N. (1994). Stereotypes and mental life: The case of the motivated but thwarted tactician. *Journal of Experimental Social Psychology, 30*, 303–325.

Plant, E. A., & Devine, P. G. (1998). Internal and external motivation to respond without prejudice. *Journal of Personality and Social Psychology, 75*, 811–832.

Richeson, J. A., & Ambady, N. I. (2001). Who's in charge?: Effects of situational roles on automatic gender bias. *Sex Roles, 44*, 493–512.

Ruscher, J. B., & Fiske, S. T. (1990). Interpersonal competition can cause individuating processes. *Journal of Personality and Social Psychology, 58*, 832–843.

Ruscher, J. B., Fiske, S. T., Miki, H., & van Manen, S. (1991). Individuating processes in competition: Interpersonal versus intergroup. *Personality and Social Psychology Bulletin, 17*, 595–605.

Schneider, D. J. (2004). *The psychology of stereotyping*. New York: Guilford Press.

Sechrist, G. B., & Stangor, C. (2001). Perceived consensus influences intergroup behavior and stereotype accessibility. *Journal of Personality and Social Psychology, 80*, 645–654.

Sherman, J. W., Stroessner, S. J., Conrey, F. R., & Azam, O. A. (2005). Prejudice and stereotype maintenance processes: Attention, attribution, and individuation. *Journal of Personality and Social Psychology, 89*, 607–622.

Sidanius, J., & Pratto, F. (1999). *Social dominance: An intergroup theory of social hierarchy and oppression*. New York: Cambridge University Press.

Sinclair, L., & Kunda, Z. (1999). Reactions to a black professional: Motivated inhibition and activation of conflicting stereotypes. *Journal of Personality and Social Psychology, 77*, 885–904.

Sinclair, L., & Kunda, Z. (2000). Motivated stereotyping of women: She's fine if she praised me but incompetent if she criticized me. *Personality and Social Psychology Bulletin, 26*, 1329–1342.

Sinclair, S., Lowery, B. S., Hardin, C. D., & Colangelo, A. (2005). Social tuning of automatic racial attitudes: The role of affiliative motivation. *Journal of Personality and Social Psychology, 89*, 583–592.

Spencer, S. J., Fein, S., Strahan, E. J., & Zanna, M. P. (2005). The role of motivation in the unconscious: How our motives control the activation of our thoughts and shape our actions. In J. P. Forgas, K. D. Williams, & S. M. Lahan (Eds.), *Social motivation: Conscious and unconscious processes* (pp. 113–129). New York: Cambridge University Press.

Spencer, S. J., Fein, S., Wolfe, C. T., Fong, C., & Dunn, M. A. (1998). Automatic activation of stereotypes: The role of self-image threat. *Personality and Social Psychology Bulletin, 24*, 1139–1152.

Tajfel, H., & Turner, J. C. (1986). The social identity theory of intergroup behavior. In S. Worchel & W. G. Austin (Eds.), *Psychology of intergroup relations* (pp. 7–24). Chicago: Nelson-Hall.

Tetlock, P. E. (1992). The impact of accountability on judgment and choice: Toward a social contingency model. In M. P. Zanna (Ed.), *Advances in experimental social psychology* (Vol. 23, pp. 331–376). San Diego, CA: Academic Press.

Towles-Schwen, T., & Fazio, R. H. (2003). Choosing social situations: The relation between automatically activated racial attitudes and anticipated comfort interacting with African Americans. *Personality and Social Psychology Bulletin, 29*, 170–182.

Chapter 39

# System Justification as Conscious and Nonconscious Goal Pursuit

John T. Jost
Janina Pietrzak
Ido Liviatan
Anesu N. Mandisodza
Jaime L. Napier

The myriad ways in which people, contrary to their own self-interest, "buy into" a social system that objectively harms them constitute the theme of Thomas Frank's (2004) best-selling book *What's the Matter with Kansas?* In seeking to understand the resurgence of blue-collar conservatism and what he calls "The Great Backlash" in middle America, Frank writes:

> The country seems . . . like a panorama of madness and delusion worthy of Hieronymous Bosch: of sturdy blue-collar patriots reciting the Pledge while they strangle their own life chances; of small farmers proudly voting themselves off the land; of devoted family men carefully seeing to it that their children will never be able to afford college or proper health care; of working-class guys in midwestern cities cheering as they deliver up a landslide for a candidate whose policies will end their way of life, will transform their region into a "rust belt," will strike people like them blows from which they will never recover. (p. 10)

The book is full of vivid ethnographic details, but it does relatively little to shed light on the general social psychological mechanisms by which people defend and justify existing social, economic, and political arrangements, often to their own detriment—not just in the midwestern United States in recent years, but around the globe and for as long as anyone can remember (see Jost, Banaji, & Nosek, 2004).

Why is the attraction of the status quo so great? What drives popular ideological support for the existing social system, even among those citizens whose interests it seems not to serve? What inhibits those who are disenfranchised by the status quo from denouncing the system and working toward a better one? What allows those who are privileged by the status quo to suppress guilt and dissonance evoked by the suffering of others? Finally, how does adopting a social psychological perspective on these questions enable us to better understand dynamic processes of change?

In attempting to understand why acquiescence in the face of injustice is so prevalent and why social change is so rare and difficult to accomplish, system justification theory posits that—to varying degrees, depending on both situational and dispositional factors—people are motivated to defend, justify, and rationalize the status quo (e.g., Jost, Banaji, et al., 2004; Jost & Hunyady, 2002, 2005). In this chapter we focus on the motivational basis of system justification, the palliative function it serves, and the implications of the theory for the dynamics of social change. More specifically, we seek to develop the following four theoretical propositions:

1. There is a goal to maintain the status quo. Once a given system or regime is firmly in place, people will be motivated to maintain its existence and stability. Consequently, system-justifying tendencies will display features of goal pursuit.
2. System justification tendencies are moderated by dispositional and situational factors. The extent to which an individual possesses heightened needs to reduce uncertainty and threat will affect his or her system justification tendencies. Similar responses are elicited when the status quo is directly or indirectly threatened.
3. System justification serves a palliative function: It operates as a coping mechanism for members of both advantaged and disadvantaged groups by reducing anxiety and uncertainty when the system's faults are highlighted and promoting positive affect. However, this palliative function inhibits the motivation for social change and therefore may have detrimental long-term consequences for the individual and society.
4. Once change is inevitable, system justification processes should produce rapid conversion to the new status quo.

Before we discuss these four propositions more elaborately, we summarize recent theory and research on system justification processes.

## A BRIEF OVERVIEW OF SYSTEM JUSTIFICATION THEORY

System justification theory provides a sustained, integrated approach to understanding how and why people defend the status quo, even when a different system would better meet their interests (Blasi & Jost, 2006; Jost & Banaji, 1994; Jost & Hunyady, 2002, 2005). We use the term *system justification* to refer to the set of social psychological processes by which the status quo is defended and upheld simply because it exists (Jost & Banaji, 1994; Jost, Pelham, Sheldon, & Sullivan, 2003; Kay, Jimenez, & Jost, 2002; Keller, 2005). To varying degrees, depending on both situational and dispositional factors, people are motivated to accept and perpetuate features of the status quo, even if those features were arrived at accidentally or arbitrarily. System justification efforts are associated with increased ideological support for economic and political systems and arrangements; stereotypic differentiation of social groups; and ingroup favoritism by members of advantaged groups and outgroup favoritism by members of disadvantaged groups (e.g., Jost, Banaji, et al., 2004). These tendencies help to maintain an imperfect but stable status quo.

Typically, system justification efforts are consistent with self-interest for people who are advantaged by the status quo, but harmful to the interests of the disadvantaged. However, research on system justification theory has shown that members of disadvantaged groups engage in system justification processes, even at the expense of their own personal and group interests (Henry & Saul, 2006; Jost, Pelham, et al., 2003). This inherently conservative tendency to maintain the legitimacy of the status quo cannot be explained in terms of theories that emphasize justification on behalf of oneself or one's own group. For members of disadvantaged groups, system justification reactions appear to conflict with ego and group justification goals (Jost & Burgess, 2000; Jost & Thompson, 2000; Kaiser, Dyrenforth, & Hagiwara, 2006; Quinn & Crocker, 1999). For example, stark forms of inequality can create a discrepancy between competing needs to justify the system and to feel good about oneself and one's fellow group members (Glick & Fiske, 2001; Lane, 1962; Sennett & Cobb, 1972).

As a result, members of disadvantaged groups who "buy into" the legitimacy of the status quo (with its attendant degree of inequality) tend to have lower self-esteem and hold more ambivalent attitudes about their own group membership than do those who reject the status quo and strive for social change (Jost & Burgess, 2000; Jost & Thompson, 2000; O'Brien & Major, 2005). Nevertheless, some members of disadvantaged groups even defend and justify the system and its authorities more strongly than do members of advantaged groups, presumably because they have a stronger need to reduce cognitive dissonance by justifying their suffering and their ongoing participation in the status quo (Henry & Saul, 2006; Jost, Pelham, et al., 2003). Under these circumstances, the dissonance that is created by the discrepancy between reality (e.g., widespread disparities in wealth) and one's beliefs about the system ("The economic system is fair") cannot be resolved by rationalizing one's own behavior. Rather, a rationalization of the *system* is necessary to resolve emotional discomfort.

How does system justification theory explain such tendencies? In the remainder of this chapter, we discuss four propositions that may help to explain these findings.

## PROPOSITION 1: THERE IS A GOAL TO MAINTAIN THE STATUS QUO

In previous work, system justification has been operationalized largely in terms of explicit ideologies, such as beliefs and attitudes that are used to justify conservatism about the social system (e.g., Jost & Hunyady, 2002, 2005). Here we consider the notion that system justification operates as a conscious and nonconscious goal: People do not only believe the system is fair and legitimate; they *want* to believe that it is fair and legitimate, and they are prepared to legitimize it despite its evident failings (e.g., Napier, Mandisodza, Andersen, & Jost, 2006). Insofar as system justification can be conceptualized as a psychological striving to maintain the status quo, it should exhibit goal-like properties. When the system's legitimacy is in question, people should persist in system justification efforts until it is restored. Thus the motivational aspects of system justification may provide the key to understanding its effects and consequences.

Theory and research on goals and goal pursuit processes assume that individuals have desired end-states toward which they strive vigorously and purposefully (Gollwitzer & Moskowitz, 1996). Such goal-directed action continues until these end-states are attained (or otherwise altered or abandoned). It is characterized by properties such as persistence (a goal will grow stronger until it is attained or the possibility of attainment is eliminated), substitutability of means (a goal can be reached through a number of different means), flexibility (a goal can be altered upon changes in the individual's needs or in the situational circumstances), and resumption following interruption (a goal will remain activated even if goal pursuit is interrupted, and it will resume when the possibility arises) (Atkinson & Birch, 1970; Bargh, Gollwitzer, Lee-Chai, Barndollar, & Trötschel, 2001; Gollwitzer & Wicklund, 1985; Heckhausen, 1991). Attaining a goal leads to positive affect, whereas failure to attain a goal leads to negative affect (Brendl & Higgins, 1996; Gollwitzer & Bargh, 1996).

Extensive research has shown that goals guide the processing, interpretation, and memory of information (for a review, see Gollwitzer & Moskowitz, 1996). Goals have been found to affect attention to information (e.g., more attention to goal-relevant than goal-irrelevant information), processing of information (e.g., systematic information processing following an accuracy goal), and encoding/recall of information (e.g., organization of information in memory according to the goal), as well as judgment and decision making (e.g., greater reliance on judgmental heuristics upon a goal of reaching closure).

Evidence from decision-making studies similarly indicates that people anchor on the status quo, however arbitrarily it was arrived at, and make insufficient adjustments to it when additional information is provided (Ariely, Loewenstein, & Prelec, 2003). Typically, people compare the status quo to counterfactual alternatives and find the alternatives worse (e.g., Lyubomirsky & Ross, 1999). Indeed, they often disparage alternatives without even attempting to understand them. O'Brien and Crandall (2005) found that people are tempted to dismiss arguments that challenge the status quo as more self-interested than arguments in favor of the status quo. All of these processes can lead to perpetuation of the status quo for reasons that are largely tangential to the real merits of the system (i.e., the benefits it bestows on its citizens). Both those who are advantaged and those who are disadvantaged by the status quo are therefore likely to support it in general (Jost, Banaji, et al., 2004).

### Effects on Information Processing

In a study that examined more directly the effects of system justification tendencies on information processing and memory, Haines and Jost (2000) showed that participants misremembered explanations given for inequality as more legitimate than they actually were, recalling legitimate explanations when no explanation or even an illegitimate explanation was given. Participants were also more likely to judge members of a relatively powerful outgroup as highly intelligent and responsible if they were given an explanation for the power differential than if they were given no explanation at all—regardless of the explanation's legitimacy. Consistent with research on placebic explanations (Langer, Blank, & Chanowitz, 1978), this study suggests that almost *any* justification is a good justification as long as it promotes the attainment of a system justification goal. Haines and Jost suggest that system justification motivates the acceptance of pseudo-explanations that allow people to reconstrue inequality in legitimate terms, and in doing so to satisfy their goal of legitimizing the status quo.

Survey data examining the American public's degree of support for the war in Iraq reveals evidence of rationalization. Public opinion polls suggested that the country was almost evenly split about whether it was a good idea to invade Iraq in early March 2003, but that this changed very rapidly as soon as President George W. Bush announced in mid-March that the U.S. invasion was definitely going to occur. Within a week or so, even before the attack started, public opinion began to shift. In the first poll conducted immediately after the start of the war, popular support rose to approximately 72%. Justification of President Bush's decision was by no means limited to Republicans. Independents and moderate Democrats also showed significant increases in support for the Iraq war as soon as it became the status quo (Pew Research Center, 2003).

Furthermore, there is evidence of reconstructive memory at the collective level. Comparisons of representative national samples just before the start of the war in Iraq (February 2003) and 5 months after the official "end" of the war (August 2003) revealed that by August a substantially larger proportion of respondents than in February believed that at the start of the war the United States had needed to act immediately to invade Iraq, and that they had supported a presidential decision to do so. Mandisodza and Todorov (2007) found that the August respondents overestimated the proportion of Americans who had supported the invasion in February by 20%, and the proportion who had agreed with the presidential decision to invade Iraq by 15%. This suggests that in addition to lending support where it had not previously existed, people tended to overestimate the number of Americans who had supported the war initially—an adjustment in the perception of history to bring it into line with the status quo.

Even when faced with incontrovertible evidence of the system's failings, people tend to support it as the best available option. Enduring support for the status quo is often explained in terms of the power of ideology to explain, justify, and rationalize discrepancies between the ideals of the system and its reality (e.g., Crandall, 2000; Hochschild, 1981; Jost, Glaser, Kruglanski, & Sulloway, 2003; Jost & Hunyady, 2005; Kluegel & Smith, 1986; Lane, 1962; Sidanius & Pratto, 1999; Tyler, 1990). Thus Jost, Blount, Pfeffer, and Hunyady (2003) found that endorsing fair market ideology was associated with the tendency to minimize the seriousness of corporate ethical scandals, such as the Enron Corporation's alleged ethical violations and the Bush–Cheney administration's reluctance to release documents pertaining to meetings with Enron executives.

An additional study by Jost, Blount, and colleagues (2003) investigated ethical inferences concerning real and hypothetical companies based on their profitability. The results showed that people generally believe that companies with profits are more ethical than companies posting losses. For losing companies, people considered a company to be significantly more ethical when an actual company name was used as opposed to a hypothetical name. This research suggests, then, that people are motivated to defend existing or familiar institutions (such as capitalism), and that this system justification goal affects the ways in which people attend to and interpret information about economic actors (see also Mandisodza, Jost, & Unzueta, 2006).

## Properties of Goal Pursuit

In addition to affecting information processing, system justification efforts seem to follow properties of goal-directed behavior as well. One such property is *substitutability of means*. That is, when a system justification goal is activated, there may be a number of substitutable means by which this goal can be attained. Several studies have shown that ideological endorsement, stereotyping, and ingroup (or outgroup) favoritism are all undertaken in response to system threat (Jost, Blount, et al., 2003; Jost & Hunyady, 2002; Jost, Kivetz, Rubini, Guermandi, & Mosso, 2005; Kay, Jost, & Young, 2005; Napier et al., 2006; Ullrich & Cohrs, in press)—suggesting that these are three of the means that can be used, perhaps interchangeably, to justify and rationalize the status quo. That is, the goal of restoring subjective legitimacy and stability to the system should be served just as well by stereotyping or otherwise justifying status differences among groups as by affirming economic or political institutions. Figure 39.1 illustrates the notion that several different means can satisfy the same goal.

The idea that system justification processes are substitutable is analogous to research on the maintenance of self-esteem and substitutability of various mechanisms that can be used to defend the self against ego threat (e.g., Tesser, 2000). However, not every defensive response will serve system justification efforts; the set of substitutable means for satisfying the system justification goal is restricted to those mechanisms that bear directly on the legitimacy or stability of the system. Indirect support for this idea comes from research by Kay and colleagues (2005), who demonstrated that system threat led participants to endorse complementary stereotypes (the means) that justified status differences (the goal). In contrast, personal and collective self-esteem were both unaffected by the experimental manipulation of system threat. In general, we suggest that ego justification means will not necessarily satisfy the goal of system justification.

Research on the *depressed entitlement* effect, another bias that serves to perpetuate and justify social inequalities, supports the idea of system justification as a goal-directed behavior as well. A number of studies have shown that women as well as other individuals in low-paying jobs tend to feel that they deserve lower wages than men or other well-paid individuals (Blanton, George, & Crocker, 2001; Jost, 1997; Major, 1994; Pelham & Hetts, 2001). For example, Jost (1997) documented the depressed entitlement phenomenon with women in an explicitly feminist environment (Yale College in the 1990s). Moreover, Blanton and colleagues (2001) found that women felt they deserved less than men did for past work, but not for future work. This evidence is consistent with the idea that people are motivated to rationalize the current status quo, but not an indeterminate future. Thus, when the circumstances were not applicable to the satisfaction of system justification goals (i.e., the "future work" condition), women were not motivated to justify their low-paid status. However, when the status quo was already established (i.e., "past work" condition) and had to be rationalized, women displayed the system-justifying depressed entitlement tendency.

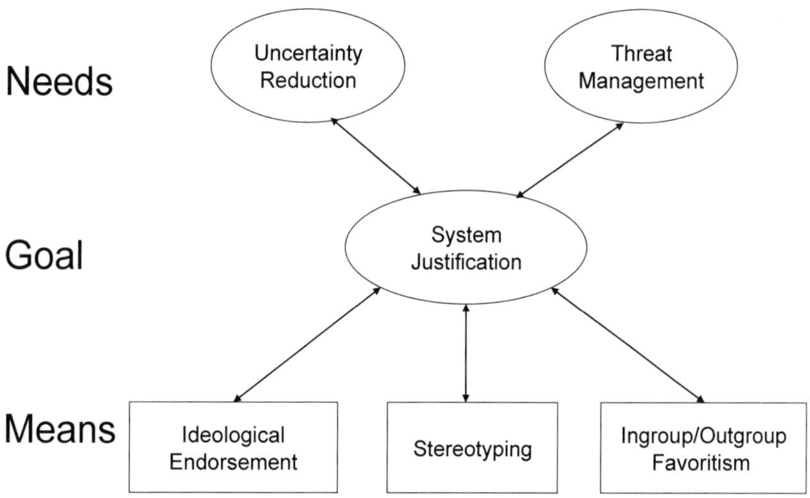


**FIGURE 39.1.** System justification as a goal system.

### System Justification as a Nonconscious Goal

We further postulate that system justification processes can operate nonconsciously, leading people to implicitly accept and defend current social arrangements. Extensive research has demonstrated that goals can be activated outside of awareness, and that subsequent behavior is then guided by these goals to attain the desired end-state (e.g., Bargh et al., 2001; see also Chartrand, Dalton, & Cheng, Chapter 22, and Ferguson, Hassin, & Bargh, Chapter 10, this volume). Hence people may not even be aware of the extent to which they are privileging the status quo and resisting change. Moreover, some forms of system justification efforts are not normatively acceptable, such as stereotyping of and discrimination against low-status groups, and thus may interfere with social desirability concerns at a conscious level (see Jost, Banaji, et al., 2004). Additionally, an explicit acknowledgment of their inferiority may have negative consequences for members of disadvantaged groups. Thus system justification processes may be especially likely to be manifested implicitly rather than explicitly.

Consistent with this assertion, several studies have documented the nonconscious operation of system-justifying biases (e.g., Ashburn-Nardo, Knowles, & Monteith, 2003; Lane, Mitchell, & Banaji, 2005; Rudman, Feinberg, & Fairchild, 2002; Uhlmann, Dasgupta, Elgueta, Greenwald, & Swanson, 2002). For example, Jost, Pelham, and Carvallo (2002) found evidence for outgroup favoritism among members of disadvantaged groups and ingroup favoritism among members of advantaged groups, thereby exhibiting attitudes that legitimize inequality between groups in society. In one study, more than twice as many members of a low-status group (San Jose State University [SJSU] students) exhibited implicit outgroup favoritism on an affective Implicit Association Test (IAT) measure as did members of a high-status group (Stanford University students). Among SJSU students (but not Stanford students), implicit stereotyping of the two groups (Stanford as more academic, SJSU as more involved in "extracurricular" activities) was associated with implicit outgroup favoritism on the affective measure. In a second study, Jost and colleagues showed that European, Hispanic, and Asian American students all preferred to associate with another participant whom they believed to be European American than with a participant whom they believed to be Hispanic or Asian American. Taken together, these studies are consistent with the notion that implicit system justification can serve as a goal.

Similarly, Banaji, Greenwald, and Rosier (1997) have assessed explicit and implicit ingroup and outgroup favoritism among African and European American students, using an explicit "feeling thermometer" measure and the IAT. Their results show that whereas on the explicit measure African Americans expressed significantly more favorable attitudes toward their own group than did European Americans, on the implicit measure African Americans showed less favorable attitudes toward their own group than did European Americans. This pattern of results was replicated with larger and more diverse samples, as well as with other social groups (e.g., young vs. old or heterosexual vs. homosexual samples; see Jost, Banaji, et al., 2004).

In sum, then, system justification goals seem to guide thoughts, feelings, and behaviors through mechanisms that are outside of conscious awareness. As a result, implicit processes seem to conform to the pervasive tendency to justify and rationalize the existing status quo, and to decrease the likelihood that substantive change to existing social arrangements will occur. In general, conceptualizing system justification as a goal-directed tendency is useful for understanding why nearly everyone is motivated (at least to some extent) to explain and justify the status quo in such a way that it is perceived as fair and legitimate (e.g., Jost, Pelham, et al., 2003). A motivated perspective on system justification tendencies is especially well suited to address relatively puzzling cases of conservatism, right-wing allegiance, and outgroup favoritism among members of low-status groups, such as African Americans, Hispanics, women, and members of the working class (e.g., Frank, 2004; Jost, Banaji, et al., 2004; Jost, Glaser, et al., 2003; Lipset, 1960).

## PROPOSITION 2: SYSTEM JUSTIFICATION IS MODERATED BY DISPOSITIONAL AND SITUATIONAL FACTORS

The intensity of goal-directed actions is determined by the individual's motivation, or commitment, to pursue the goal. Thus studies have shown that highly committed individuals are those typically exhibiting the properties commonly attributed to goal pursuit (e.g., studies on self-completion theory, Gollwitzer & Kirchhof, 1998; or studies on goal shielding, Shah, Friedman, & Kruglanski, 2002). In line with this theory and research on the moderating effects of commitment on goal-directed behavior, we propose that system justification tendencies depend on dispositional and situational factors that increase motivation to maintain and defend the status quo and render such goals more accessible.

There are several individual difference variables that gauge the extent to which individuals support versus challenge the status quo (Crandall, 2000; Jost & Hunyady, 2005). Examples of system-justifying ideologies that people endorse to different extents include the Protestant work ethic (Quinn & Crocker, 1999), the belief in a just world (Hafer & Begué, 2005), political conservatism (Jost, Banaji, et al., 2004), opposition to equality (Kluegel & Smith, 1986), and fair market ideology (Jost, Blount, et al., 2003). The degree to which people endorse conservative, system-justifying beliefs is affected by such general dispositional factors as uncertainty avoidance; intolerance of ambiguity; and epistemic needs for order, structure, and closure (Jost, Glaser, et al., 2003; see also Kruglanski & Chun, Chapter 6, this volume). It appears that there is a resonant match between psychological needs to reduce uncertainty and threat and the contents of attitudes that serve to justify the status quo (thereby preserving what is familiar). As illustrated in Figure 39.1, needs for uncertainty reduction and threat management can be satisfied by attaining the system justification goal through various means.

Increased commitment to goals (such as system justification) can be activated by situational as well as dispositional factors (Higgins, 1996; Kruglanski et al., 2002). Much as self-serving biases are accentuated after self-threat and group-serving biases are accentuated after group threat, we find that system justification tendencies increase following system threat. Defensive forms of justification can be triggered by a threat to the legitimacy or stability of the system. Indeed, the need for system justification is greater when a flaw in the system is exposed or the status quo is otherwise threatened. There is reason to think that system-level threats induce negative affect, such as anxiety, cognitive dissonance, and discomfort, and that the endorsement of system-justifying ideologies serves to reduce these negative experiences (Jost & Hunyady, 2002; Kluegel & Smith, 1986; Wakslak, Jost, Tyler, & Chen, 2007).

Anecdotal observation and scientific research both suggest that threats to the status quo—whether direct, as when the system is attacked, or indirect, as when its faults are exposed—provoke negative affect and motivate people to defend the desirability and legitimacy of the social system (e.g., Doty, Peterson, & Winter, 1991; Jost, Glaser, et al., 2003; Napier et al., 2006; Sales, 1973; Ullrich & Cohrs, 2007). That is, threats to the existing system, as long as they are not so severe as to unseat the current regime and establish another, stimulate a defensive motivational response on behalf of the existing system (e.g., Jost & Hunyady, 2002). This defensive response, which can be automatic and unconscious, restores positive affect, but it can have unanticipated consequences.

The responses to the attacks of September 11, 2001 illustrate that support for the regime that is already in place is strengthened following system threat. Support for the U.S. system and its representatives—including President Bush, Congress, the military, and the government in general—increased sharply after the attacks, according to national polling data from the Gallup Poll (2001) organization. Only about half of Americans expressed approval of President Bush from the time he became president until 9/11. Following the attacks, the president's approval rating shot up to almost 90% and remained above 70% for the following year (Gallup Poll, 2005).

Jost, Glaser, and colleagues (2003) found in a meta-analysis that the two strongest situational predictors of conservative, system-justifying responses were system threat and mortality salience. Clearly, the events of 9/11 involved both. Consistent with the Jost, Glaser, and colleagues theoretical analysis, Landau and colleagues (2004) found that people who were experimentally primed to think about the 9/11 attacks 2 years later showed significantly more support for President Bush than did those who were not primed (see also Echebarría & Fernández, 2006; Ullrich & Cohrs, 2007). The control groups included thinking about a negative event or about extreme pain, and these groups did not show increased support for the president, indicating that system threat and mortality salience are especially important motivating factors in determining the degree of system support. Furthermore, Willer (2004) found that between 2001 and 2004, government-issued warnings that resulted in raising the terror alert level had the effect of increasing popular support for President Bush, even on aspects unrelated to terrorism (such as his handling of the economy).

Other research that has manipulated system threat by exposing participants to criticism of the status quo has obtained similar results. For example, in a study conducted in Israel by Jost, Kivetz, Rubini, Guermandi, and Mosso (2005), high (vs. low) system threat was experimentally induced by exposing people to a short passage that was (or was not) highly critical of the system. System threat led to increased complementary stereotypic differentiation between an advantaged group (Ashkenazi Jews) and a disadvantaged group (Sephardic Jews). In a further demonstration, Kay and colleagues (2005) showed that system threat (exposure to a passage ostensibly written by a journalist that was broadly critical of U.S. society) led people to increasingly endorse complementary stereotypes justifying status differences. For example, people in the high-system-threat condition judged overweight people to be lazier but more sociable, and powerful people to be more intelligent but less happy. In this way, strategies of victim blaming on causally relevant traits (e.g., stereotyping obese people as being lazy) and victim enhancement on causally irrelevant traits (e.g., ascribing sociability to obese people) can both serve the goal of system justification (see also Kay et al., 2007, for a comprehensive review).

In sum, then, ample research supports the idea that several dispositional and situational characteristics affect the strength of motivation to justify the system. Under circumstances of system threat, people who endorse system-justifying ideologies may be especially likely to experience negative emotions, such as fear, anxiety, and dissonance. Pursuing system justification efforts reduces these negative emotions as well as promoting positive affect. In the next section of the chapter, we review research that supports this palliative function of system justification processes.

## PROPOSITION 3: SYSTEM JUSTIFICATION SERVES A PALLIATIVE FUNCTION

We have addressed the issues of what people do (i.e., defend, bolster, and justify the status quo), and when they typically do it (i.e., when motivation is increased because of dispositional and/or situational factors). We have only partially dealt with the perplexing question of *why* people support the system so enthusiastically, especially when it clearly does not benefit them. We suggest that justifying the status quo satisfies several social and psychological needs—including epistemic needs for consistency, coherence, and certainty, and existential needs to manage various forms of threat and distress and to find meaning in life (see also Festinger, 1957; Jost, Fitzsimons, & Kay, 2004; Jost & Hunyady, 2005; Lerner, 1980). The status quo has many advantages over counterfactual alternatives: It is familiar, predictable, safe, and (due to system-justifying biases) subjectively experienced as desirable, natural, and just. People often assume that existing arrangements are for the best, and that if alternatives really worked better, then they would have already been adopted. Sticking with the status quo provides a simple and easy way of meeting a variety of psychological needs. Threats to the legitimacy or stability of the system, on the other hand, may elicit feelings of anxiety, uncertainty, and dissonance concerning one's role in the larger system. The fact that attaining the system justification goal satisfies multiple needs and therefore possesses *multifinality* (see Kruglanski et al., 2002) renders it a motivationally powerful factor in human lives (see Figure 39.1).

We propose that in a hierarchical system, both those who are advantaged and those who are disadvantaged by the system are susceptible to experiencing *emotional distress*. The type of emotional distress differs, depending largely on the status of the group, and this in turn influences the system-justifying strategies that advantaged and disadvantaged group members use to manage their emotional distress. The powerful may experience guilt over their relatively advantaged position, particularly when it appears to be undeserved. For example, European Americans experience guilt and dissonance when confronted with evidence of fellow group members' prejudicial or discriminatory actions toward African Americans (Devine, Monteith, Zuwernik, & Elliot, 1991; Swim & Miller, 1999). Similarly, men who are reminded of their gender privilege experience increased guilt and decreased well-being (Branscombe, 1998). To assuage their guilt, ease their consciences, and reduce dissonance arising from inequality in the system, people rationalize their own advantages (Chen & Tyler, 2001) and derogate those who are disadvantaged (Jost, Banaji, et al., 2004; Kay et al., 2005).

The powerless, meanwhile, may feel understandably frustrated and angry about their position in society. They may rail against the system, deriding barriers to individual and social mobility. However, they seldom do. According to system justification theory, the disadvantaged may lower their own aspirations and adapt to the status quo to minimize the anger and resentment evoked by a system with impermeable boundaries. For example, Kluegel and Smith (1986) found that poor people who blamed themselves for their own poverty reported feeling more positive emotion, less guilt, and greater satisfaction than did poor people who made external attributions for their situation. Similarly, Jost, Pelham, and colleagues (2003) found in a national survey that holding the belief that inequality is both legitimate and necessary was associated with increased satisfaction, regardless of a respondent's income level.

Several studies that have examined the relationship between system justification tendencies and affect support the palliative function of system justification. For example, research by Jost, Pelham, and colleagues (2003, Study 5) indicates that ideology is related to satisfaction in terms of one's job, one's financial situation, and life in general. These researchers examined the effects of demographic variables (race and socioeconomic status [SES]) and ideological beliefs concerning meritocracy (e.g., ambition, ability, and hard work are important for "getting ahead in life") and the legitimacy of economic inequality (e.g., "large differences in income are necessary for America's prosperity") on satisfaction. Structural equation modeling revealed that (1) African Americans and people who were lower in SES were *more* likely than others to believe that SES differences were necessary and legitimate, apparently because they had stronger needs to justify the system in order to reduce cognitive dissonance and restore positive affect; and (2) endorsement of meritocratic ideology was positively related to satisfaction for all respondents. That is, the more people believed that hard work, ability, and motivation lead to success, the more they reported being satisfied with their own economic situation, regardless of whether they were rich or poor.

In the United States, stark inequality is a potential indicator of system illegitimacy, and as such it can pose a threat to the system. Placing people in a situation of inequality among peers should therefore activate the system justification goal. Studies conducted by Wakslak and colleagues (2007) explored the dynamic affective consequences of system justification, including effects on discrete negative emotions (e.g., guilt, frustration, anxiety, and uncertainty) associated with advantaged versus disadvantaged positions in hierarchical systems. In a heretofore unpublished study, inequality among peers was artificially created via the "Star Power" exercise, so that a stratified system involving three groups differing in status, power, and privilege was established. Members of all three groups were given the opportunity to endorse meritocratic ideology and consensual stereotypes to justify the system. Results indicated that system justification increased satisfaction in all groups, and that it decreased frustration for members of disadvantaged groups and decreased guilt for members of the advantaged group. The beneficial effects of system-justifying stereotypes and ideologies, then, were evinced by greater self-reported satisfaction and happiness (and less negative affect) on the part of people who were given an opportunity to endorse the legitimacy of the system. For both advantaged and disadvantaged individuals, it appears that system justification processes serve a palliative function.

Endorsing complementary stereotypes of the disadvantaged as lazy but happy can reduce dissonance and guilt for the advantaged, and it can reduce dissonance and frustration for the disadvantaged (see Kay & Jost, 2003). Perhaps this is even more crucial for the disadvantaged, who must come to terms with their complicity in the system (Lane, 1962). Sticking with the status quo provides the added benefits of familiarity, coherence, and security, thereby reducing uncertainty and potential anxiety (e.g., Jost, Glaser, et al., 2003). Thus affirming the system simultaneously restores integrity to the status quo and reduces negative affect.

Although the palliative function of system justification may be adaptive in some ways, it may also have long-term negative consequences, particularly for members of disadvantaged groups. Jost and Banaji (1994) argued that there are three justification motives: ego justification, or the tendency to develop and maintain favorable self-views; group justification, or the tendency to maintain a favorable image of one's social group and defend its actions; and system justification, or the tendency to defend and bolster the social system. For the advantaged group, ego justification, group justification, and system justification goals are concordant. For the disadvantaged group, however, these justification goals are potentially discordant; these conflicts should give rise to attitudinal ambivalence toward ingroup members, and may affect psychological well-being. Indeed, research has shown that conflict among long-term goals is associated with poorer psychological well-being, including lessened life satisfaction and affective problems (Emmons & King, 1988; Riediger & Freund, 2004). Relatedly, Jost and Thompson (2000) found that opposition to equality was positively related to self-esteem and negatively related to depression and neuroticism for members of advantaged groups, but that it was negatively related to self-esteem and positively related to depression and neuroticism for disadvantaged group members (see also O'Brien & Major, 2005). Thus pursuing system justification goals may have positive affective consequences for members of disadvantaged groups in the short term, but it may also have aversive consequences for long-term well-being (Jost & Hunyady, 2002).

In addition to these aversive consequences at the individual level, the palliative effects of system justification may have negative ramifications at the societal level. That is, the positive outcomes of attaining system justification goals may inhibit efforts to improve and change the status quo, thereby producing serious impediments to bringing about substantial change in society's institutions and organizations. Two follow-up studies to the "Star Power" study described above support this notion. These studies indicated that the palliative effect had as its by-product a weakening of support for social policies aimed at eliminating imbalance (Wakslak et al., 2007). In particular, reductions in moral outrage (Montada & Schneider, 1989) mediated the dampening effect of system justification on support for helping the disadvantaged through community service programs. These findings support the notion that system justification tendencies encourage resistance to social change and a reluctance to support policies that would lead to reform and to a more equal redistribution of resources (see also Jost, Glaser, et al., 2003; Jost & Hunyady, 2005). Tendencies to blame individuals rather than systems for poor outcomes, and to minimize the extent of corruption, could also lead to system undercorrection in circumstances in which qualitative change would be beneficial (Jost, Blount, et al., 2003). The palliative function of system justification, therefore, may help to explain many cases of failure to support changes in the system.

## PROPOSITION 4: ONCE CHANGE IS INEVITABLE, SYSTEM JUSTIFICATION PROCESSES PRODUCE RAPID CONVERSION TO THE NEW STATUS QUO

Given system justification tendencies to maintain the status quo and to defend and buttress it in times of trouble, one might expect social change to be virtually impossible. Indeed, collective action and protest are quite rare and occur only when the system is seen as severely unjust (e.g., Gurr, 1970; Moore, 1978; Zinn, 1968). Paradoxically, criticism can make current arrangements seem *more* attractive because of system-justifying processes, as outlined in connection with Proposition 2. If an alternative is considered, system-justifying processes may make its adoption unlikely. Nevertheless, social systems change and evolve in relation to external circumstances, as well as in conjunction with changes to the composition and internal states of the individuals and groups who constitute and control those systems. Economic systems and public policy positions shift, solidify, and shift again. Alternatives to the status quo may be derogated when they are considered improbable, but they become much more attractive as their probability of success increases (Kay et al., 2002; McGuire & McGuire, 1991). According to system justification theory, then, although the idea of change almost always breeds some degree of resistance, innovation is possible because over time people adapt their perceptions of reality—so that what was once seen as untenable eventually becomes accepted and commonplace, and people wonder how and why they could have opposed the change in the first place.

In line with the notion of goal-directed behavior as flexible and adaptive (Gollwitzer & Moskowitz, 1996; see also Ferguson et al., Chapter 10, this volume), we propose that the same processes (e.g., rationalization, stereotyping) that explain inertia also aid social and psychological adaptation to system-level change, provided that change comes quickly and completely (see also Blasi & Jost, 2006). Gradual change can be complicated by resistance to it at each subsequent stage, due to continued justification of the "old" system's remaining elements. Once a new system irrevocably replaces the previous one, however, people should begin to justify its distinctive features (both consciously and nonconsciously) as part of the conversion process. In fact, the rapid change may increase feelings of uncertainty, anxiety, and dissonance, thereby highly activating system justification goals. Thus, when a new status quo is established, people should become motivated to perceive the emerging social arrangements in favorable terms and thus to rationalize the new regime. In contrast, defending the old status quo has no psychological benefits any more, and therefore people will eventually disengage from their previous goal of justifying it.

Such a process was observed in the United States with regard to the relatively rapid shift to a system of racial integration from the earlier norm of racial segregation. Kelman (2001) described a study he conducted in 1954 concerning African American students' attitudes toward maintaining some private all-black colleges in the face of an impending decision by the U.S. Supreme Court regarding racial desegregation in education. After hearing a persuasive message advocating the maintenance of some all-black colleges, students' attitudes were measured just 3 days before the decision and again on the day of the decision. Regardless of the source and degree of the communicator's power, students were significantly more opposed to maintaining all-black colleges after the decision to integrate was made than before. That is, when segregation was the status quo, African Americans professed stronger support for voluntary segregation. When integration became the status quo 3 days later because of the Supreme Court decision, the same group of students became more enthusiastic integrationists.

More direct evidence for our claim that people are motivated to justify an emerging status quo comes from experimental studies by Kay and colleagues (2002). They demonstrated in two studies that system justification processes contribute to anticipatory rationalization for outcomes that have not yet occurred but are likely to occur. In Study 1, a political survey was administered to Democrats, Republicans, and independents/nonpartisans prior to the 2000 presidential election. The survey manipulated the perceived probability of the election's outcome (victory likelihoods: 43/51, 45/49, 47/47, 49/45, or 51/43 in favor of Bush vs. Gore). Participants were asked to indicate how desirable a Bush victory would be for them, and how desirable a Gore victory would be for them. Results showed that for Democrats and Republicans alike, the greater a particular candidate's chances were, the more subjectively desirable his presidency became. For nonpartisans, there was no relationship between likelihood and desirability. When people are motivationally involved in an outcome (as was the case for Democrats and Republicans, but not for nonpartisans), people elevated their evaluation of more likely outcomes (and devalued unlikely outcomes) regardless of their political leanings.

To eliminate potential confounding effects associated with the use of consensus information and impression management concerns, and to generalize beyond the historically unique 2000 presidential election, Kay and colleagues (2002, Study 2) conducted a laboratory study concerning rationalizations of a decision made by university trustees to increase or decrease tuition rates. The researchers again found evidence for rationalization when investment in the decision was high (large tuition changes), so that more probable outcomes were seen as more desirable. This was not true for small changes in tuition. People high in motivational involvement again engaged in rationalization by enhancing the favorability of likely outcomes and derogating unlikely outcomes, regardless of whether they were initially defined as attractive or unattractive.

Gilbert, Pinel, Wilson, Blumberg, and Wheatley (1998) obtained similar results in research on what they termed *immune neglect*. In one of their studies, they contacted citizens who voted in the 1994 Texas gubernatorial election between Ann Richards and George W. Bush, just before the elections and approximately 1 month following them. On the first occasion, voters were asked to predict how happy they would be 1 month after the election if their candidate were to win or lose, as well how they would evaluate Bush or Richards as the winning candidate. One month later, voters were contacted again and were asked about their happiness and about their satisfaction with Bush (who won the election). Gilbert and colleagues found that supporters of Richards were significantly happier than they had expected to be, evaluated Bush more positively after the election than before, and felt better about their new governor than they had expected to feel. The authors explained these results in terms of immune neglect. That is, "people fail to recognize that their negative affect will not merely subside but will be actively antagonized by powerful psychological mechanisms that are specifically dedicated to its amelioration . . . [and therefore] tend to overestimate the longevity of those emotional reactions" (p. 619).

From a system justification perspective, these effects are not merely indicative of people's inability to predict their own internal states, but they also signal a shift in people's motivational concerns. Prior to the Texas election, Richards's voters did not possess the goal of rationalizing a hypothetical victory for Bush, and most likely even had the opposite goal. However, once Bush's authority was firmly in place (i.e., it became the status quo), system justification goals were activated, thereby motivating these people to justify and legitimize Bush's position as governor. Furthermore, research on the effects of goal pursuit on object evaluation has shown that when an object facilitates current goal attainment, it is evaluated more favorably than when the goal is absent (e.g., Shah & Higgins, 2001). Ferguson and Bargh (2004) pointed out that this increased favorability can result from greater accessibility of positive object information, greater inhibition of negative object information, or both. Thus, when Bush's administration became the status quo and people were motivated to justify it, then presumably positive aspects of his tenure became more accessible, negative aspects became less accessible, or both.

In sum, according to our conceptualization of system justification as a motivated process, initial resistance to change should be greater than would be expected on the basis of other theories, and yet adaptation to fully implemented change (i.e., when a new status quo is firmly established) may be easier than expected (Blasi & Jost, 2006). Once change becomes inevitable, support for the former system should dwindle as quickly as support for the emergent system grows, and the old regime should be derogated as much as (or more than) other alternatives to the current status quo. As soon as the new system is completely installed, people begin to rationalize its distinctive features, both consciously and unconsciously. Although there is no way of predicting future events with certainty, it is possible to take advantage of naturally occurring changes to investigate these phenomena. The studies by Kay and colleagues (2002) took advantage of the 2000 presidential election in the United States to demonstrate the increase in support for a new regime as soon as it becomes reality—in this case, support gained by Bush when he was elected. The implication of a system justification analysis for social change is that it will either come not at all or all at once, the way that catastrophic change occurs in dynamic systems and in *tipping point* phenomena (e.g., Gladwell, 2000; Johnson, 1966).

## CONCLUDING REMARKS

In this chapter we have sought to deepen our understanding of the motivational underpinnings of system justification tendencies. Conceptualizing system justification as a goal helps to shed light on why people would defend and justify the status quo, even when it is contrary to their social, economic, and political interests. We propose that there are multiple means (e.g., ideological endorsement, stereotyping, ingroup vs. outgroup favoritism) of satisfying the system justification goal (see also Kay et al., 2005; Napier et al., 2006). In the language of goal systems theory (Kruglanski et al., 2002; Shah et al., 2002), system justification thereby exhibits the property of *equifinality.* More importantly, perhaps, system justification also possesses the property of *multifinality* (see Figure 39.1). That is, it seems to satisfy several epistemic and existential needs, including uncertainty reduction and threat management (Jost, Fitzsimons, et al., 2004; Jost & Hunyady, 2005), and it serves a palliative function in general (Jost & Hunyady, 2002; Wakslak et al., 2007). Ultimately, these psychological benefits may help to explain the prevalence of system-justifying tendencies, the motivational strength that they can acquire, and the extent to which individuals will persist in efforts to justify the status quo.

## ACKNOWLEDGMENTS

The writing of this chapter was based on and supported by National Science Foundation Award No.

BCS-0617558 to John T. Jost. We thank Alison Ledgerwood, Jim Shah, and Hulda Thorisdottir for helpful comments on an earlier draft.

## REFERENCES

Ariely, D., Loewenstein, G., & Prelec, D. (2003). Coherent arbitrariness: Stable demand curves without stable preferences. *Quarterly Journal of Economics, 118*, 73–80.

Ashburn-Nardo, L., Knowles, M. L., & Monteith, M. J. (2003). Black Americans' implicit racial associations and their implications for intergroup judgment. *Social Cognition, 21*, 61–87.

Atkinson, J. W., & Birch, D. (1970). *A dynamic theory of action*. New York: Wiley.

Banaji, M. R., Greenwald, A. G., & Rosier, M. (1997). *Implicit esteem: When collectives shape individuals*. Paper presented at the Preconference on Self, Toronto.

Bargh, J. A., Gollwitzer, P. M., Lee-Chai, A., Barndollar, K., & Trötschel, R. (2001). The automated will: Nonconscious activation and the pursuit of behavioral goals. *Journal of Personality and Social Psychology, 81*, 1014–1027.

Blanton, H., George, G., & Crocker, J. (2001). Contexts of system justification and system evaluation: Exploring the social comparison strategies of the (not yet) contented female worker. *Group Processes and Intergroup Relations, 4*, 127–138.

Blasi, G., & Jost, J. T. (2006). System justification theory and research: Implications for law, legal advocacy, and social justice. *California Law Review, 94*, 1119–1168.

Branscombe, N. R. (1998). Thinking about one's gender groups privileges or disadvantages: Consequences for well-being in women and men. *British Journal of Social Psychology, 37*, 167–184.

Brendl, C. M., & Higgins, E. T. (1996). Principles of judging valence: What makes events positive or negative? In M. P. Zanna (Ed.), *Advances in experimental social psychology* (Vol. 28, pp. 95–160). San Diego, CA: Academic Press.

Chen, E. S., & Tyler, T. R. (2001). Cloaking power: Legitimizing myths and the psychology of the advantaged. In A. Y. Lee-Chai & J. A. Bargh (Eds.), *The use and abuse of power: Multiple perspectives on the causes of corruption* (pp. 241–261). Philadelphia: Psychology Press.

Crandall, C. S. (2000). Ideology and lay theories of stigma: The justification of stigmatization. In T. F. Heatherton, R. E. Kleck, M. R. Hebl, & J. G. Hull (Eds.), *The social psychology of stigma* (pp. 126–150). New York: Guilford Press.

Devine, P. G., Monteith, M. J., Zuwernik, J. R., & Elliot, A. J. (1991). Prejudice with and without compunction. *Journal of Personality and Social Psychology, 60*, 817–830.

Doty, R. M., Peterson, B. E., & Winter, D. G. (1991). Threat and authoritarianism in the United States, 1978–1987. *Journal of Personality and Social Psychology, 61*, 629–640.

Echebarría, A., & Fernández, E. (2006). Effects of terrorism on attitudes and ideological orientation. *European Journal of Social Psychology, 36*, 259–265.

Emmons, R. A., & King, L. A. (1988). Conflict among personal strivings: Immediate and long-term implications for psychological and physical well-being. *Journal of Personality and Social Psychology, 54*, 1040–1048.

Ferguson, M. J., & Bargh, J. A. (2004). How social perception automatically influences behavior. *Trends in Cognitive Sciences, 8*, 33–39.

Festinger, L. (1957). *A theory of cognitive dissonance*. Evanston, IL: Row, Peterson.

Frank, T. (2004). *What's the matter with Kansas?* New York: Metropolitan Books.

Gallup Poll. (2001, September 24). *Confidence in leaders*. Retrieved from *poll.gallup.com/content/default.aspx?ci=4897&pg=1*

Gallup Poll. (2005, December 13). *Presidential ratings—job approval*. Retrieved from *poll.gallup.com/content/default.aspx?ci=1723&pg=1*

Gilbert, D. T., Pinel, E. C., Wilson, T. D., Blumberg, S. J., & Wheatley, T. (1998). Immune neglect: A source of durability bias in affective forecasting. *Journal of Personality and Social Psychology, 75*, 617–638.

Gladwell, M. (2000). *The tipping point: How little things can make a big difference*. Boston: Little, Brown.

Glick, P., & Fiske, S. T. (2001). An ambivalent alliance: Hostile and benevolent sexism as complementary justifications for gender inequality. *American Psychologist, 56*, 109–118.

Gollwitzer, P. M., & Bargh, J. A. (1996). *The psychology of action: Linking cognition and motivation to behavior*. New York: Guilford Press.

Gollwitzer, P. M., & Kirchhof, O. (1998). The willful pursuit of identity. In J. Heckhausen & C. S. Dweck (Eds.), *Life-span perspectives on motivation and control* (pp. 389–423). New York: Cambridge University Press.

Gollwitzer, P. M., & Moskowitz, G. B. (1996). Goal effects on action and cognition. In E. T. Higgins & A. W. Kruglanski (Eds.), *Social psychology: Handbook of basic principles* (pp. 361–399). New York: Guilford Press.

Gollwitzer, P. M., & Wicklund, R. A. (1985). The pursuit of self-defining goals. In J. Kuhl & J. Beckmann (Eds.), *Action control: From cognition to behavior* (pp. 61–85). Berlin: Springer-Verlag.

Gurr, T. R. (1970). *Why men rebel*. Princeton, NJ: Princeton University Press.

Hafer, C. L., & Begué, L. (2005). Experimental research on just-world theory: Problems, developments, and future challenges. *Psychological Bulletin, 131*, 128–167.

Haines, E. L., & Jost, J. T. (2000). Placating the powerless: Effects of legitimate and illegitimate explanation on affect, memory, and stereotyping. *Social Justice Research*, *13*, 219–236.

Heckhausen, H. (1991). *Motivation and action*. Berlin: Springer-Verlag.

Henry, P. J., & Saul, A. (2006). The development of system justification in the developing world. *Social Justice Research*, *19*, 365–378.

Higgins, E. T. (1996). Knowledge activation: Accessibility, applicability, and salience. In E. T. Higgins & A. W. Kruglanski (Eds.), *Social psychology: Handbook of basic principles* (pp. 133–168). New York: Guilford Press.

Hochschild, J. L. (1981). *What's fair?: American beliefs about distributive justice*. Cambridge, MA: Harvard University Press.

Johnson, C. (1966). *Revolutionary change*. Boston: Little, Brown.

Jost, J. T. (1997). An experimental replication of the depressed-entitlement effect among women. *Psychology of Women Quarterly*, *21*, 387–393.

Jost, J. T., & Banaji, M. R. (1994). The role of stereotyping in system-justification and the production of false consciousness. *British Journal of Social Psychology*, *33*, 1–27.

Jost, J. T., Banaji, M. R., & Nosek, B. A. (2004). A decade of system justification theory: Accumulated evidence of conscious and unconscious bolstering of the status quo. *Political Psychology*, *25*, 881–919.

Jost, J. T., Blount, S., Pfeffer, J., & Hunyady, G. (2003). Fair market ideology: Its cognitive-motivational underpinnings. *Research in Organizational Behavior*, *25*, 53–91.

Jost, J. T., & Burgess, D. (2000). Attitudinal ambivalence and the conflict between group and system justification motives in low status groups. *Personality and Social Psychology Bulletin*, *26*, 293–305.

Jost, J. T., Fitzsimons, G., & Kay, A. C. (2004). The ideological animal: A system justification view. In J. Greenberg, S. L. Koole, & T. Pyszczynski (Eds.), *Handbook of experimental existential psychology* (pp. 263–283). New York: Guilford Press.

Jost, J. T., Glaser, J., Kruglanski, A. W., & Sulloway, F. (2003). Political conservatism as motivated social cognition. *Psychological Bulletin*, *129*, 339–375.

Jost, J. T., & Hunyady, O. (2002). The psychology of system justification and the palliative function of ideology. *European Review of Social Psychology*, *13*, 111–153.

Jost, J. T., & Hunyady, O. (2005). Antecedents and consequences of system-justifying ideologies. *Current Directions in Psychological Science*, *14*, 260–265.

Jost, J. T., Kivetz, Y., Rubini, M., Guermandi, G., & Mosso, C. (2005). System-justifying functions of complementary regional and ethnic stereotypes: Cross-national evidence. *Social Justice Research*, *18*, 305–333.

Jost, J. T., Pelham, B. W., & Carvallo, M. (2002). Nonconscious forms of system justification: Cognitive, affective, and behavioral preferences for higher status groups. *Journal of Experimental Social Psychology*, *38*, 586–602.

Jost, J. T., Pelham, B. W., Sheldon, O., & Sullivan, B. N. (2003). Social inequality and the reduction of ideological dissonance on behalf of the system: Evidence of enhanced system justification among the disadvantaged. *European Journal of Social Psychology*, *33*, 13–36.

Jost, J. T., & Thompson, E. P. (2000). Group-based dominance and opposition to equality as independent predictors of self-esteem, ethnocentrism, and social policy attitudes among African Americans and European Americans. *Journal of Experimental Social Psychology*, *36*, 209–232.

Kaiser, C. R., Dyrenforth, P. S., & Hagiwara, N. (2006). Why are attributions to discrimination interpersonally costly?: A test of system- and group-justifying motivations. *Personality and Social Psychology Bulletin*, *32*, 1523–1536.

Kay, A., Jimenez, M. C., & Jost, J. T. (2002). Sour grapes, sweet lemons, and the anticipatory rationalization of the status quo. *Personality and Social Psychology Bulletin*, *28*, 1300–1312.

Kay, A. C., & Jost, J. T. (2003). Complementary justice: Effects of "poor but happy" and "poor but honest" stereotype exemplars on system justification and implicit activation of the justice motive. *Journal of Personality and Social Psychology*, *85*, 823–837.

Kay, A. C., Jost, J. T., Mandisodza, A. N., Sherman, S. J., Petrocelli, J. V., & Johnson, A. L. (2007). Panglossian ideology in the service of system justification: How complementary stereotypes help us to rationalize inequality. In M. P. Zanna (Ed.), *Advances in experimental social psychology* (Vol. 39, pp. 305–358). New York: Elsevier.

Kay, A. C., Jost, J. T., & Young, S. (2005). Victim derogation and victim enhancement as alternate routes to system justification. *Psychological Science*, *16*, 240–246.

Keller, J. (2005). In genes we trust: The biological component of psychological essentialism and its relationship to mechanisms of motivated social cognition. *Journal of Personality and Social Psychology*, *88*, 686–702.

Kelman, H. C. (2001). Reflections on social and psychological processes of legitimization and delegitimization. In J. T. Jost & B. Major (Eds.), *The psychology of legitimacy* (pp. 54–73). New York: Cambridge University Press.

Kluegel, J. R., & Smith, E. R. (1986). *Beliefs about inequality: Americans' view of what is and what ought to be*. New York: Aldine de Gruyter.

Kruglanski, A. W., Shah, J. Y., Fishbach, A., Friedman, R., Chun, W. Y., & Sleeth-Keppler, D. (2002). A theory of goal systems. In M. P. Zanna (Ed.), *Advances in experimental social psychology* (Vol. 34, pp. 331–378). San Diego, CA: Academic Press.

Landau, M. J., Solomon, S., Greenberg, J., Cohen, F., Pyszczynski, T., Arndt, J., et al. (2004). Deliver us from evil: The effects of mortality salience and reminders of 9/11 on support for President George W. Bush. *Personality and Social Psychology Bulletin, 30,* 1136–1150.

Lane, K. A., Mitchell, J. P., & Banaji, M. R. (2005). Me and my group: Cultural status can disrupt cognitive consistency. *Social Cognition, 23,* 353–386.

Lane, R. E. (1962). *Political ideology: Why the American common man believes what he does.* New York: Free Press.

Langer, E. J., Blank, A., & Chanowitz, B. (1978). The mindlessness of ostensibly thoughtful action. *Journal of Personality and Social Psychology, 36,* 635–642.

Lerner, M. J. (1980). *The belief in a just world: A fundamental delusion.* New York: Plenum Press.

Lipset, S. M. (1960). *Political man.* New York: Doubleday.

Lyubomirsky, S., & Ross, L. (1999). Changes in attractiveness of elected, rejected, and precluded alternatives: A comparison of happy and unhappy individuals. *Journal of Personality and Social Psychology, 76,* 988–1007.

Major, B. (1994). From inequality to personal entitlement: The role of social comparisons, legitimacy appraisals, and group memberships. In M. P. Zanna (Ed.), *Advances in experimental social psychology* (Vol. 26, pp. 293–355). San Diego, CA: Academic Press.

Mandisodza, A., Jost, J. T., & Unzueta, M. (2006). "Tall poppies" and "American dreams": Reactions to rich and poor in Australia and the U.S.A. *Journal of Cross-Cultural Psychology, 37,* 659–668.

Mandisodza, A. N., & Todorov, A. (2007). *Differences between prospective and retrospective support for the war with Iraq.* Unpublished manuscript.

McGuire, W. J., & McGuire, C. V. (1991). The content, structure, and operation of thought systems. In R. S. Wyer, Jr. & T. K. Srull (Eds.), *Advances in social cognition* (Vol. 4, pp. 1–78). Hillsdale, NJ: Erlbaum.

Montada, L., & Schneider, A. (1989). Justice and emotional reactions to the disadvantaged. *Social Justice Research, 3,* 313–344.

Moore, B., Jr. (1978). *Injustice: The social bases of obedience and revolt.* White Plains, NY: Sharpe.

Napier, J., Mandisodza, A., Andersen, S. M., & Jost, J. T. (2006). System justification in responding to the poor and displaced in the aftermath of Hurricane Katrina. *Analyses of Social Issues and Public Policy, 6,* 57–73.

O'Brien, L. T., & Crandall, C. S. (2005). Perceiving self-interest: Power, ideology, and maintenance of the status quo. *Social Justice Research, 18,* 1–24.

O'Brien, L. T., & Major, B. (2005). System justifying beliefs and psychological well-being: The roles of group status and identity. *Personality and Social Psychology Bulletin, 31,* 1718–1729.

Pelham, B. W., & Hetts, J. J. (2001). Underworked and overpaid: Elevated entitlement in men's self-pay. *Journal of Experimental Social Psychology, 37,* 93–103.

Pew Research Center. (2003, April 3). *War concerns grow, but support remains steadfast.* Retrieved from *peoplepress.org/reports/display.php3?ReportID=179*

Quinn, D. M., & Crocker, J. (1999). When ideology hurts: Effects of belief in the Protestant ethic and feeling overweight on the psychological well-being of women. *Journal of Personality and Social Psychology, 77,* 402–414.

Riediger, M., & Freund, A. M. (2004). Interference and facilitation among personal goals: Differential association with subjective well-being and persistent goal pursuit. *Personality and Social Psychology Bulletin, 30,* 1511–1523.

Rudman, L. A., Feinberg, J., & Fairchild, K. (2002). Minority members' implicit attitudes: Automatic ingroup bias as a function of group status. *Social Cognition, 20,* 294–320.

Sales, S. M. (1973). Threat as a factor in authoritarianism: An analysis of archival data. *Journal of Personality and Social Psychology, 28,* 44–57.

Sennett, R., & Cobb, J. (1972). *The hidden injuries of class.* New York: Vintage Books.

Shah, J. Y., Friedman, R., & Kruglanski, A. W. (2002). Forgetting all else: On the antecedents and consequences of goal shielding. *Journal of Personality and Social Psychology, 83,* 1261–1280.

Shah, J. Y., & Higgins, E. T. (2001). Regulatory concerns and appraisal efficiency: The general impact of promotion and prevention. *Journal of Personality and Social Psychology, 80,* 693–705.

Sidanius, J., & Pratto, F. (1999). *Social dominance: An intergroup theory of social hierarchy and oppression.* New York: Cambridge University Press.

Swim, J. K., & Miller, D. L. (1999). White guilt: Its antecedents and consequences for attitudes toward affirmative action. *Personality and Social Psychology Bulletin, 25,* 500–514.

Tesser, A. (2000). On the confluence of self-esteem maintenance mechanisms. *Personality and Social Psychology Review, 4,* 290–299.

Tyler, T. R. (1990). *Why people obey the law.* New Haven, CT: Yale University Press.

Uhlmann, E., Dasgupta, N., Elgueta, A., Greenwald, A. G., & Swanson, J. E. (2002). Subgroup prejudice based on skin color among Hispanics in the United States and Latin America. *Social Cognition, 20,* 198–225.

Ullrich, J., & Cohrs, J. C. (2007). Terrorism salience increases system justification: Experimental evidence. *Social Justice Research, 29,* 117–139.

Wakslak, C., Jost, J. T., Tyler, T. R., & Chen, E. (2007). Moral outrage mediates the dampening effect of system justification on support for redistributive social policies. *Psychological Science, 18,* 267–274.

Willer, R. (2004). The effects of government-issued terror warnings on presidential approval ratings. *Current Research in Social Psychology, 10,* 1–12.

Zinn, H. (1968). *Disobedience and democracy.* New York: Random House.

# Author Index

# Subject Index

Page numbers followed by *f* indicate figure; *t* indicate table.